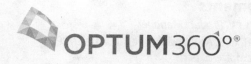

Risk Adjustment Coding and HCC Guide

Simplifying the RA/HCC systems and optimization opportunities

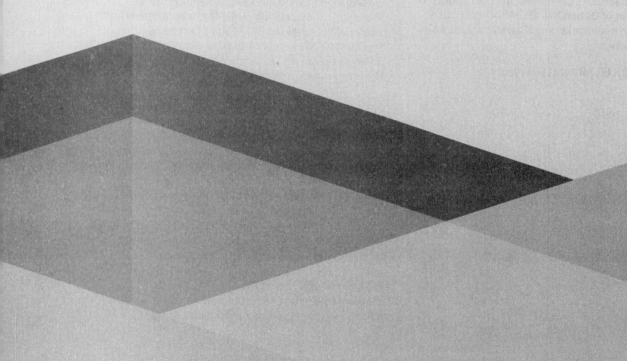

2022   optum360coding.com

Notice

Risk Adjustment Coding and HCC Guide is designed to be an accurate and authoritative source regarding coding and every reasonable effort has been made to ensure accuracy and completeness of the content. However, Optum360 makes no guarantee, warranty, or representation that this publication is accurate, complete, or without errors. It is understood that Optum360 is not rendering any legal or other professional services or advice in this publication and that Optum360 bears no liability for any results or consequences that may arise from the use of this book. Please address all correspondence to:

Optum360
2525 Lake Park Blvd
Salt Lake City, UT 84120

Our Commitment to Accuracy

Optum360 is committed to producing accurate and reliable materials. To report corrections, please email accuracy@optum.com. You can also reach customer service by calling 1.800.464.3649, option 1.

Copyright

Property of Optum360, LLC. Optum360 and the Optum360 logo are trademarks of Optum360, LLC. All other brand or product names are trademarks or registered trademarks of their respective owner.

© 2021 Optum360, LLC. All rights reserved.

Made in the USA
ISBN 978-1-62254-780-7

Acknowledgments

Marianne Randall, CPC, *Product Manager*
Karen Krawzik, RHIT, CCS, AHIMA-approved ICD-10-CM/PCS Trainer, *Subject Matter Expert*
Jacqueline Petersen, BS, RHIA, CHDA, CPC, *Subject Matter Expert*
Stacy Perry, *Manager, Desktop Publishing*
Tracy Betzler, *Senior Desktop Publishing Specialist*
Hope M. Dunn, *Senior Desktop Publishing Specialist*
Katie Russell, *Desktop Publishing Specialist*
Kate Holden, *Editor*

Karen Krawzik, RHIT, CCS, AHIMA, AHIMA-approved ICD-10-CM/PCS Trainer

Ms. Krawzik has expertise in ICD-10-CM, ICD-9-CM, CPT/HCPCS, DRG, and data quality and analytics, with more than 30 years' experience coding in multiple settings, including inpatient, observation, ambulatory surgery, ancillary, and emergency room. She has served as a DRG analyst and auditor of commercial and government payer claims, as a contract administrator, and worked on a team providing enterprise-wide conversion of the ICD-9-CM code set to ICD-10. More recently, she has been developing print and electronic content related to ICD-10-CM and ICD-10-PCS coding systems, MS-DRGs, and HCCs. Ms. Krawzik is credentialed by the American Health Information Management Association (AHIMA) as a Registered Health Information Technician (RHIT) and a Certified Coding Specialist (CCS) and is an AHIMA-approved ICD-10-CM/PCS trainer. She is an active member of AHIMA and the Missouri Health Information Management Association.

Jacqueline Petersen, BS, RHIA, CHDA, CPC

Ms. Petersen has more than 25 years of experience in the health care profession. She has served as Senior Clinical Product Research Analyst with Optum360 developing business requirements for edits to support correct coding and reimbursement for claims processing applications. Her experience includes development of data-driven and system rules for both professional and facility claims and in-depth analysis of claims data inclusive of ICD-10-CM, CPT, HCPCS, and modifiers. Her background also includes consulting work for Optum, serving as a SME, providing coding and reimbursement education to internal and external clients. Ms. Petersen is a member of the American Academy of Professional Coders (AAPC), and the American Health Information Management Association (AHIMA).

Contents

Introduction

The traditional fee-for-service payment model has been widely used since the 1930s when health insurance plans initially gained popularity within the United States. In this payment model, a provider or facility is compensated based on the services provided. This payment model has proven to be very expensive. Closer attention is being paid to healthcare spending versus outcomes and quality of care and this has been compared to the healthcare spending of other nations. This has caused a need to develop a system to evaluate the care being given.

In the 1970s, Medicare began demonstration projects that contracted with health maintenance organizations (HMO) to provide care for Medicare beneficiaries in exchange for prospective payments. In 1985, this project changed from demonstration status to a regular part of the Medicare program, Medicare Part C. The Balanced Budget Act (BBA) of 1997 named Medicare's Part C managed care program Medicare+Choice, and the Medicare Prescription Drug, Improvement and Modernization Act (MMA) of 2003 again renamed it to Medicare Advantage (MA).

Medicare is one of the world's largest health insurance programs, and about one-third of the beneficiaries on Medicare are enrolled in an MA private healthcare plan. Due to the great variance in the health status of Medicare beneficiaries, risk adjustment provides a means of adequately compensating those plans with large numbers of seriously ill patients while not overburdening other plans that have healthier individuals. MA plans have been using the Hierarchical Condition Category (HCC) risk-adjustment model since 2004.

The primary purpose of a risk-adjustment model is to predict (on average) the future healthcare costs for specific consortiums enrolled in MA health plans. The Centers for Medicare and Medicaid Services (CMS) is then able to provide capitation payments to these private health plans. Capitation payments are an incentive for health plans to enroll not only healthier individuals but those with chronic conditions or who are more seriously ill by removing some of the financial burden.

The MA risk-adjustment model uses HCCs to assess the disease burden of its enrollees. HCC diagnostic groupings were created after examining claims data so that enrollees with similar disease processes, and consequently similar healthcare expenditures, could be pooled into a larger data set in which an average expenditure rate could be determined. The medical conditions included in HCC categories are those that were determined to most predictably affect the health status and healthcare costs of any individual.

Section of 1343 of the Affordable Care Act (ACA) of 2010 provides for a risk-adjustment program for non-Medicare Advantage plans that are available in online insurance exchange marketplaces. Beginning in 2014, commercial insurances were able to potentially mitigate increased costs for the insurance plan and increased premiums for higher-risk populations, such as those with chronic illnesses, by using a risk-adjustment model. The risk-adjustment program developed for use by non-Medicare plans is maintained by the Department of Health and Human Services (HHS). This model also uses HCC diagnostic groupings; however, this set of HCCs differs from the CMS-HCCs to reflect the differences in the populations served by each healthcare plan type.

This publication will cover the following:

- History and purpose of risk-adjustment factor (RAF)

- Key terms definitions

- Acceptable provider types

- Payment methodology and timeline

- Coding and documentation

- Tools for risk adjustment

- Coding scenarios

- Guidance for developing internal risk adjustment coding polices

- Audits

- Healthcare Effectiveness Data and Information Set (HEDIS)

- Risk adjustment model tables

Coding is an increasingly complex business. The movement from the fee-for-service payment model to more qualitative models has increased rapidly since 2004. The demand for quality-focused payment models has gained more attention since the ACA introduced a risk-adjustment model to the online insurance exchange marketplace plans in 2017. Coding staff must have knowledge of risk- adjustment practices in this rapidly changing environment. This book provides conceptual and practical knowledge of risk adjustment to coders, coding managers, medical staff, clinical documentation improvement (CDI) professionals, payers, educators, and students. The goal is to develop and enrich the knowledge of the user's understanding of this payment methodology.

This reference is organized by first setting the foundational knowledge of risk adjustment including the history of risk adjustment with key term definitions and the payment timeline. The second section focuses on coding and documentation. This will provide the user with knowledge of the impact of good documentation, common tools used to evaluate documentation for risk-adjustment purposes, and coding scenarios to show real world examples of risk-adjustment coding using the various HCC models. The next section covers audits such as Medicare Risk Adjustment Data Validation (RAD-V). This third section will also cover Health Effectiveness Data and Information Sets (HEDIS) as well as internal quality-improvement audits. Chapter 4 includes the CMS Risk Adjustment Factor (RAF) tables for the various models including the RAF weights.

Risk Adjustment Data Files

To save space in this book and provide more comprehensive references for the user, Optum360 has provided searchable data files for certain features. These data files can be accessed at the following website:

http://www.optum360coding.com/ProductUpdates/

This website is available only to customers who purchase the Risk Adjustment Coding and HCC Guide, using the following password: HCCA21F

Data files available for download:

NOTE: This manual provides the most current information that was available at the time of publication.

CY 2020/2021/2022 CMS-HCC ESRD-HCC V21 Model Tables

This file includes:

CY 2020/2021/2022 CMS ESRD-HCC Model V21 with 2022 Midyear Final ICD-10-CM Mapping, Hierarchies, with Continuing Enrollee Dialysis, Functioning Graft Demographic for Community Population, and Functioning Graft Institutional Population Disease Coefficient Relative Factors

CY 2020/2021/2022 CMS ESRD-HCC Continuing Enrollee Dialysis Demographic Relative Factors

CY 2020/2021/2022 CMS ESRD-HCC Continuing Enrollee Dialysis Disease Interactions Relative Factors

CY 2020/2021/2022 CMS ESRD-HCC Demographic Relative Factors for New Enrollees in Dialysis Status

CY 2020/2021/2022 CMS ESRD-HCC Kidney Transplant Relative Factors for Transplant Beneficiaries

CY 2020/2021/2022 CMS ESRD-HCC Functioning Graft Demographic Relative Factors for Community Population

CY 2020/2021/2022 CMS ESRD-HCC Functioning Graft Disease Interaction Relative Factors for Community Population

CY 2020/2021/2022 CMS ESRD-HCC Functioning Graft Demographic Relative Factors for Institutionalized Population

CY 2020/2021/2022 CMS ESRD-HCC Functioning Graft Disease Interactions Relative Factors for Institutionalized Population

CY 2020/2021/2022 CMS ESRD-HCC Demographic Relative Factors for Functioning Graft New Enrollees Duration Since Transplant of 4-9 Months

CY 2020/2021/2022 CMS ESRD-HCC Demographic Relative Factors for Functioning Graft New Enrollees Duration Since Transplant of 10 Months or More

CMS RxHCC Model Category V05 Tables

This file includes:

CY 2020/2021/2022 RxHCC Model Category V05 with 2022 Midyear Final ICD-10-CM Mapping, Hierarchies, and CY 2022 Disease Coefficients

CY 2022 CMS RxHCC Demographic Relative Factors for Continuing Enrollees

CY 2022 CMS RxHCC Non-Aged Disease Interactions

CY 2022 CMS RxHCC Demographic Relative Factors for New Enrollees, Non-Low Income

CY 2022 CMS RxHCC Demographic Relative Factors for New Enrollees, Low Income

CY 2022 CMS RxHCC Demographic Relative Factors for New Enrollees, Institutional

2021/2022 Benefit Year HHS-HCC Risk Adjustment Model Tables

This file includes:

2021 Benefit Year ICD-10 to V07 HHS-Condition Categories (CC) Crosswalk

2021 Benefit Year Version 07 HHS-Hierarchical Condition Categories (HCC) Hierarchies

Final Coefficients for 2022 Benefit Year Adult Risk Adjustment Models

> Demographic Factors
>
> Diagnosis Factors
>
> Severity Factors
>
> Enrollment Duration Factors
>
> Prescription Drug Category (RXC) Factors
>
> Prescription Drug Interaction Factors

Final Coefficients for 2022 Benefit Year Child Risk Adjustment Models

> Demographic Factors
>
> Diagnosis Factors

2021 Optum360, LLC

Chapter 1. Risk Adjustment Basics

The need to track and report disease and causes of death was recognized in the 18th century. The various popular methodologies were compiled over the course of the First through Fifth International Statistical Institute Conferences in the 20th century; during the Sixth International Conference, the World Health Organization (WHO) was tasked with revising and maintaining the classifications of disease and death. In the 1930s health insurance coverage gained popularity. Many labor groups and companies started offering this type of benefit to their employees. In 1966, the American Medical Association (AMA) published the first edition of the Current Procedural Terminology (CPT®) to standardize the reporting of surgical procedures. This framework created the fee-for-service payment model, which is currently used.

The fee-for-service model, however, does not account for acuity or morbidity of its patients. A medically complex, chronically ill patient's healthcare provider would receive the same reimbursement for the same procedure done on a healthy patient.

In 1997, the Balanced Budget Act mandated that Medicare begin allowing participants to choose between traditional Medicare and managed Medicare plans (now Medicare Advantage), which would incorporate the risk-adjustment payment methodology no later than January 2000. Initially, these managed Medicare plans were paid a fixed dollar amount to care for Medicare members. In 2007, these MA plans were based 100 percent on risk adjustment. This better allocates resources to populations of medically needy patients.

Key Terms

- **Hierarchical condition categories (HCC).** Groupings of clinically similar diagnoses in each risk-adjustment model. Conditions are categorized hierarchically and the highest severity takes precedence over other conditions in a hierarchy. Each HCC is assigned a relative factor that is used to produce risk scores for Medicare beneficiaries, based on the data submitted in the data collection period.

- **Medicare Advantage (MA) plan.** Sometimes called "Part C" or "MA plans," offered by private companies approved by Medicare. If a Medicare Advantage plan is selected by the enrollee, the plan will provide all of Part A (hospital insurance) and Part B (medical insurance) coverage. Medicare Advantage plans may offer extra coverage, such as vision, hearing, dental, and/or health and wellness programs. Most include Medicare prescription drug coverage (Part D).

- **Risk-adjustment factor (RAF).** Risk score assigned to each beneficiary based on his or her disease burden, as well as demographic factors.

- **Sweeps.** Submission deadline for risk adjustment data that occurs three times annually: January, March, and September. Generally, claims continue to be accepted for two weeks after the deadline.

Payment Methodology

Purpose of Risk Adjustment

Risk adjustment allows CMS to pay plans for the risk of the beneficiaries they enroll, instead of an average amount for Medicare beneficiaries. By risk adjusting plan payments, CMS is able to make appropriate and accurate payments for enrollees with differences in expected costs. Risk adjustment is used to adjust bidding and payment based on the health status and demographic characteristics of an enrollee. Risk scores measure individual beneficiaries' relative risk and risk scores are used to adjust payments for each beneficiary's expected expenditures. By risk adjusting plan bids, CMS is able to use standardized bids as base payments to plans.

The primary purpose of a risk-adjustment model is to predict future healthcare costs for specific consortiums enrolled in MA health plans based on current risk factors associated with the covered patient population. CMS is then able to provide capitation payments to these private health plans. Capitation payments that are calculated based on an entire risk pool incentivize health plans to enroll not only healthier individuals but those with chronic conditions or who are more seriously ill by removing some of the financial burden.

The MA risk-adjustment model uses HCCs to assess the disease burden of its enrollees. The HCC diagnostic groupings were created after examining claims data so that enrollees with similar disease processes, and consequently similar healthcare expenditures, could be pooled into a larger data set in which an average expenditure rate could be determined. The medical conditions included in HCC categories are those that were determined to most predictably affect the health status and healthcare costs of any individual.

Hierarchical condition categories (HCC) were first used in 2004 to set capitated payments for private health plans caring for Medicare beneficiaries. The term "risk adjustment" is often used to describe what HCCs do. HCCs predict healthcare resource consumption of individuals. HCC scores are used to "risk adjust" payments to a health plan based on the level of risk the beneficiary presents to the plan. HCCs adjust payments so that there is a higher reimbursement for sicker patients.

The HCC system was developed to improve upon an earlier capitation method that used demographics and inpatient diagnoses to set payments. A major shortcoming of this earlier methodology was that only inpatient diagnoses were used, allowing only patients with an inpatient admission to generate any additional payment to the health plan. Plans that were able to provide adequate ambulatory care received lower payments. Federal law in 2000 required the use of ambulatory diagnoses and specified that the new risk adjustment be phased in beginning in 2004.

Under the current CMS-HCC model, MA organizations collect risk-adjustment data, including beneficiary diagnoses from hospital inpatient facilities, hospital outpatient facilities, and physicians during a data-collection period. MA organizations identify the diagnoses relevant to the CMS model and submit them to CMS. CMS categorizes the diagnoses into groups of clinically related diseases called HCCs and uses the HCCs as well as demographic characteristics to calculate a risk-adjustment factor (RAF) score for each beneficiary. CMS then uses the RAF scores to adjust the monthly capitated payments to MA organizations for the next payment period.

Risk adjustment is a process of adjusting capitation payments to health plans either higher or lower to account for the differences in expected health costs of individuals. Risk adjustment is required for managed care programs that monitor changes in disease progression and population mix, set performance targets to generate outcome data, and identify patients for population health initiatives (disease or case management). RA is used by the government as well as private and commercial insurance entities, and is needed in any value-based purchasing program.

With the transition to ICD-10-CM in 2015, the diagnosis code set was expanded to over 70,000 codes. The conditions that have been determined by CMS or other administering entity, to predict costs are grouped into categories based on similar care costs and body systems affected. In the CMS-HCC model, there are about 86 hierarchical condition categories with about 11,000 ICD-10-CM codes. The HHS-HCC model contains 141 hierarchical condition categories and approximately 10,800 ICD-10-CM codes.

Risk-Adjustment Characteristics

Additive risk-adjustment models are most often compared to the diagnosis related group (DRG) payment methodology. This is partially accurate; multiple conditions may be considered part of the same HCC, such as emphysema and chronic obstructive pulmonary disease (COPD), which belong to HCC 111. Unlike the DRG model, the HCC model is additive. Individual risk scores are calculated by adding the values associated with each beneficiary's disease and demographic factors.

The **multiple diseases** risk-adjustment payment is based on the capture of conditions that map to condition categories. Within the CMS-HCC model, emphasis is on the costs of caring for chronic conditions. Conditions from as many HCCs as necessary to completely report the health status of the patient should be reported. Multiple conditions from the same HCC may also be reported but the value of that HCC is only counted once.

Hierarchical condition categories are placed into hierarchies, which reflect the severity and cost dominance of the conditions. This allows for payments to be based on the most severe conditions, while less severe conditions may co-exist. If multiple conditions from the same HCC are reported for one beneficiary, the most severe will be assigned for that HCC and the other conditions will not be counted. If multiple conditions fall into separate HCCs, trumping logic may apply.

Trumping is the risk adjustment model that recognizes that some conditions can be related to conditions in other categories or that a condition may exist within more than one category. In these instances, CMS and other governing bodies will apply a trumping logic so that the most severe condition is counted in the risk-adjustment factor of the beneficiary. This ensures that related conditions are not double counted. For example, diabetes falls into HCCs 17, 18, and 19. Uncomplicated diabetes (E11.9) falls into HCC 19, but if the patient is found to have a chronic complication (HCC 18) or an acute (HCC 17) complication, the condition from HCC 19 would be trumped by the condition from HCC 17 or 18.

Trumping also occurs within an HCC. The most severe condition in a category will trump the other conditions. For example, a patient is noted to have COPD on one date of service and emphysema on another date of service, both conditions map to HCC 111. The emphysema is considered more specific and, therefore, would trump the COPD.

Disease and disabled interactions allow for an additional weight to be added to the risk score for a beneficiary when certain conditions co-exist or when there is a disability status. This additive factor increases payment accuracy.

Demographic factors are included in most risk-adjustment models: age, sex, disabled status, Medicaid eligibility/low income status, and reason for entitlement (Medicare beneficiaries).

Prospective is included in the CMS-HCC model; Medicare uses diagnostic information from the prior year to predict the costs of covering the beneficiary for the following year.

Unlike other payment models, the CMS-HCC model is **site neutral**; it does not distinguish payment based on a site of care. There are certain sites of services that are not acceptable sources of risk adjustment data for the CMS model including skilled nursing facilities (SNF) and ambulatory surgery centers (ASC). Detailed information on acceptable sites of service and provider types are reviewed on page 19.

Risk Adjustment Beyond Medicare Advantage

Beginning in 2014, individuals and small businesses were able to purchase private health insurance through the online system established by the Affordable Care Act (ACA). Insurers selling policies through these exchanges are not allowed to refuse insurance to anyone or to vary the enrollee premiums based on health status.

Individuals who purchase these plans may also be eligible to premium tax credits that make the insurance more affordable. Without risk adjustment, the plans that enroll a high proportion of high-risk enrollees would normally charge a higher premium across all enrollees to cover risks. For the commercial or Department of Health and Human Services (HHS), the governing body that administers this program, risk adjustment reduces the risk to the plans and levels the playing field so that differences in plan benefits are reflected in premiums and not in the health status of the plan population.

The risk-adjustment model, called the HHS Hierarchical Condition Categories (HHS-HCC) uses an individual's demographic factors and medical diagnoses to determine a risk score. The risk transfer formula created by HHS compensates plans with higher medical risks presented by enrollees as expressed through the HHS-HCCs.

The commercial HCCs were created as a means to transfer risk between health plans participating in the ACA online insurance exchange marketplaces. Outside of this risk-transfer function, plans do not receive risk-adjusted payments. Premiums are paid by the individuals purchasing the insurance. Under the CMS-HCCs, a system that shares the HCC name but uses a somewhat different set of HCC groups, the CMS health plans are paid through a risk-adjusted formula that incorporates the HCC payment system.

The HHS-HCCs were adapted from the MA or CMS model, with three modifications:

- **Prediction year:** The CMS-HCCs use prior year medical and diagnostics to set current year payments. The HHS-HCCs use current year medical status to set current year payments.

- **Population:** The CMS-HCCs were developed based upon data for an aged or disabled population. The HHS-HCCs uses two sets of HCCs: one for children and one for adults.

- **Type of spending:** The HHS-HCCs are configured to include both medical and prescription drug spending. These are separately calculated in the CMS-HCC system, which incorporates a separate RX-HCC drug benefit.

Comparison of Plans

For the majority of this book, the Medicare (CMS-HCC) risk adjustment model is the focus of the discussion. The other main models in use are discussed in the following section. Some of these models predate the CMS risk-adjustment model; however, the overwhelming success and efficacy of the CMS model has brought more attention to these other risk-adjustment models and has inspired plans that traditionally are fully fee for service to consider and implement risk-adjustment models.

Health and Human Services

Section 1343 of the Affordable Care Act provides a risk-adjustment, payment program for the individual and small business markets, which was implemented in 2014. HHS developed a risk-adjustment model, which is based on the CMS model but includes claims information from commercial plans that includes conditions that are expected to be in a non-Medicare, commercial population. The logic governing the hierarchical condition categories is similar to the CMS model but the categories contain different conditions to reflect the population differences. The intent of this model is to eliminate or lessen the influence of risk selection on the plan premiums.

There are two classification systems used in this model. The first classifies beneficiaries into three age groups: adult, child, and infant. The infant age group also has subpopulations used to report additional factors categorized by severity categories. The second classification is by metal level that is used to describe the plan benefits or attributes: gold, silver, bronze, or catastrophic. Payments are adjusted by plan metal category, geographical area, age rating, and induced demand.

Each state operating may use the HHS model or it may propose an alternative model for certification by HHS. If a state does not operate a risk-adjustment model, HHS will operate a risk-adjustment model on the state's behalf.

Aside from the covered population and, therefore, the HCCs used within the model, the main difference between the HHS-HCC and the CMS-HCC models is the type of model being used. The CMS-HCC model is prospective, intended to predict the health costs of the beneficiary for the coming year, whereas the HHS-HCC model is concurrent, focusing on predicting costs during the current year. Unlike Medicare beneficiaries, enrollees in plans offered through healthcare exchanges may move in and out of enrollment in small group and individual markets and change issues. Concurrent models tend to focus and better capture the costs of acute events that include acute exacerbations of chronic conditions.

HHS-HCC	CMS-HCC
Created to transfer risk between health plans paid by premiums from enrolled members in Affordable Care Act marketplace from plans with low-risk enrollees to plans with high-risk enrollees	Created to pay Medicare Advantage plans for enrollees through a risk-adjusted formula
Concurrent - uses current calendar year diagnosis coding to set risk payments in current calendar year	Prospective - uses base calendar year (current calendar year) diagnoses to determine next calendar year rates
For CY 2021 V07 model, 10,816 diagnosis codes map to 141 HCCs	For CY 2021 V24 model, 3,034 diagnosis codes map to 86 HCCs
Developed for patients of all ages	Developed for patients 65 or older and disabled patients of all ages
Includes categories for infants, children and adults, and includes obstetric diagnoses	Pediatric and obstetric diagnosis codes are not assigned risk values
Risk scores represent health status, incorporating age and sex demographics (adult (age 18+), child (age 2-17), and infant (age 0-1), male and female, with "age splits" for certain categories. Classified by the level of plan purchased that determines the percentage of out of pocket healthcare costs a member pays	Risk scores represent a member's heath status and incorporate demographics for age, sex, disabled status, Medicaid eligibility/low income status, and reason for entitlement
Best at capturing acute events such as acute exacerbation of chronic conditions, obstetric cases, severe illness interactions (adult model)	Best at capturing chronic conditions and chronic disease interactions
Includes both medical and prescription drug spending	Incorporates a separate Rx-HCC benefit
Model more recently developed and less well known	Oldest model most widely used

Chronic Illness and Disability Payment Systems

The Chronic Illness and Disability Payment Systems (CDPS) risk-adjustment model has been in use by Medicaid plans since 1996. This model contains significantly more diagnosis codes than other models and includes "personal history" and/or "family history" codes. Conditions within this model are also rated as "high," "medium," or "low" overall risk with ascending trumping. Notable updates to this model include the 2000 addition of Temporary Assistance for Needy Families (TANF). In 2001, a prescription drug risk-adjustment model was created using the CDPS information, known as Medicaid Rx (MRX). In 2008, CDPS and MRX were updated using Medicaid data from 2001 and 2002 from 44 states.

The CDPS and MRX models map diagnosis and pharmaceutical use groups to a group or vector of disease categories. As of 2013, CDPS maps to 16,461 ICD-10-CM codes and to 58 CDPS categories, which lead up to 20 major categories related to major body systems (e.g., cardiovascular) or type of disease (e.g., diabetes). MRX maps to 56, 236 National Drug Codes (NDC) from patient utilization to 45 Medicaid Rx categories.

These mappings lead to "Stage 1 Groups," which help to build the CDPS identification. This groups ICD-10-CM codes, typically at the three-digit level and sometimes at the fourth or fifth digit level when the extra digit describes a more serious condition or version of a diagnosis. Stage 1 Groups are then combined into Major Categories.

The hierarchies in the CDPS model are different from the CMS-HCC model but are based on the same basic principle. The hierarchies are designated using the suffix, which is added to the category names. These include:

- Cardiovascular VH is very high and carries a weight of 2.037.

- Cardiovascular M is medium and carries a weight of 0.805.

- Cardiovascular L is low and carries a weight of 0.368.

- Cardiovascular EL is extra low and carries a weight of 0.130.

The rules that govern acceptable sources of diagnostic data are very similar to the CMS-HCC model. Lab, radiology, or other diagnostic services are not valid sources for diagnostic information. All inpatient and outpatient face-to-face encounters are otherwise acceptable sources. This model also includes the "personal history" and "family history" codes, which often support the suspect logic.

Diagnosis Related Groups

During the 1970's Yale University School of Organizational Management developed the Diagnosis Related Group (DRG) system as part of a contract with CMS to describe all types of patient care in an acute-care hospital. This allowed hospitals to monitor the utilization of resources and quality of service by relating patients' demographics and diagnoses to the costs involved in their care.

The second and all subsequent versions of the DRG definitions have been maintained by 3M Health Information Systems under a contract with CMS . The CMS DRG model is a prospective payment rate model, which was established based on Medicare's hospital reimbursement system. This is a methodology for patient classification that provides a means of relating patient type and treatment (case mix) to the costs incurred by the hospital.

Although DRGs were not initially designed for reimbursement purposes, the state of New Jersey first implemented a DRG-based hospital reimbursement system. In 1982, the Tax Equity and Fiscal Responsibility Act (TEFRA) modified the section 223 Medicare hospital reimbursement limits to include a case-mix adjustment based on the DRG model. Congress incorporated a DRG-based system for Medicare (CMS-DRG) when it created the Inpatient Prospective Payment System (IPPS) in 1983. Draft legislation was quickly appended to the Social Security Amendments of 1983 to include a national DRG-based, hospital prospective payment system for all Medicare beneficiaries.

This case mix includes the following concepts:

- Severity of illness is the relative level of loss of function and mortality that may be experienced by patients with a particular disease.

- Prognosis describes the probable outcome of an illness including the likelihood of improvement or deterioration in the severity of the illness, the likelihood for recurrence and the probable life span.

- Treatment difficulty represents the patient management problems that a particular illness presents to the healthcare provider. Such management problems are associated with illnesses without a clear pattern of symptoms, illnesses requiring sophisticated and technically difficult procedures and illnesses requiring close monitoring and supervision.

- Need for intervention pertains to the consequences in terms of severity of illness that lack of immediate or continuing care would produce.

- Resource intensity relates to the relative volume and types of diagnostic, therapeutic, and bed services used in the management of a particular illness.

The Medicare Severity Diagnosis Related Group (MS-DRG) system was developed to relate case mix to resource utilization. One of the most commonly cited weaknesses of the original DRG system was the absence of levels of severity of illness.

Instead of a two-tiered structure (with and without complication/comorbidity [CC]), MS-DRGs introduced a three-tiered structure: major complication/comorbidity (MCC), complication/comorbidity (CC), and no complication/comorbidity (non-CC).

MCCs are secondary diagnoses of the highest level of severity and CCs are secondary diagnoses of the next lower level of severity.

CMS replaced the old CMS-DRGs with the new MS-DRGs effective with discharges occurring on or after October 1, 2007, with Version 24.0, and the MS-DRGs began with Version 25.0. The most current version, v39.0, was effective October 1, 2021.

The only appropriate site of service for MS-DRG classification and reimbursement is in an inpatient hospital. Unlike most risk-adjustment models, the MS-DRG model is not additive, meaning that a single DRG is reported for each inpatient hospital stay. This single MS-DRG should provide reimbursement for all the services the patient received while in the hospital. MS-DRGs are assigned using the principal diagnosis, which in some cases may also function as a complication/comorbidity (CC) or a major complication/comorbidity (MCC); secondary diagnoses, including CCs and MCCs; surgical or other invasive procedures; sex of the patient; and discharge status. The MS-DRG is affected by comorbid conditions (CC) and/or major comorbid conditions (MCC) by changing the MS-DRG reported instead of being reported in addition as it would with HCC.

HCC Compared to MS-DRG

Feature Payment groups	HCCs (Medicare, non RX) 86 HCCs	MS-DRGs 767 MS-DRGs
ICD-10-CM codes	Just over 10,000 have RAF value.	All ICD-10-CM codes have the potential to affect MS-DRG assignment. Some codes may result in an "ungroupable" MS-DRG.
ICD-10-CM codes are used in one payment group only	An ICD-10-CM code appears in only one HCC, with few exceptions.	Codes may be used in multiple MS-DRGs.
ICD-10-PCS codes	HCCs are not affected by ICD-10-PCS procedure codes.	Thousands of ICD-10-PCS codes, alone or in combination, can affect MS-DRG assignment.
Payment group assignment	An individual may have more than one HCC assigned.	Only one MS-DRG is assigned for each inpatient stay.
Codes used in payment	All HCCs are defined by diagnosis codes, typically chronic conditions.	MS-DRGs may include both procedures and diagnoses, both acute and chronic conditions.
Demographic factors used in payment	Age, sex, institutional status, disability, dual eligibility for Medicare and Medicaid.	Age, sex, discharge status.
Reporting time frame	HCCs are calculated over a calendar year, using scores from all providers that have treated the patient in that time.	MS-DRGs capture one inpatient encounter at a time and for one single provider at a time, based on fiscal year.
Validation	Diagnostic codes reported must follow the coding conventions in the ICD-10-CM classification and the Tabular List and Alphabetic Index and they must adhere to the *ICD-10-CM Official Guidelines for Coding and Reporting*. Chronic diseases treated on an ongoing basis may be coded and reported as many times as the patient receives treatment/care for the condition(s). No sequencing is involved, and codes may be assigned for all properly documented conditions that coexist at the time of the encounter/visit, and require or affect patient care, treatment, or management. Some organizations use mnemonics such as MEAT (Monitor, Evaluate, Assess, Treatment) to assist with identifying reportable conditions.	Diagnostic codes reported must follow the coding conventions in the ICD-10-CM classification and the Tabular List and Alphabetic Index and they must adhere to the *ICD-10-CM Official Guidelines for Coding and Reporting*. Sequencing of Principal and Secondary diagnoses applies, and must meet the Uniform Hospital Discharge Data Set (UHDDS) definitions of Principal and Other Diagnoses.

There is an increasing need for hospital inpatient coders to learn the outpatient coding rules in order to properly capture and report HCC diagnoses, as hospitals frequently acquire physician practices and perform coding and billing functions for these practices. In addition, inpatient coders may not routinely assign codes for chronic conditions that do not qualify as a CC or an MCC for MS-DRG assignment. These chronic conditions are now important elements that can affect the total risk score for the patient.

Programs of All-inclusive Care for the Elderly

The Programs of All-inclusive Care for the Elderly (PACE) program is a Medicare and Medicaid program that aims to assist elderly patients with having their medical needs met within the community instead of in a nursing or other care facility. This program focuses on having a care team that coordinates the services provided in the home community and PACE center.

There are four criteria to determine if a patient qualifies for a PACE program. The patient must:

- Be at least 55 years-old

- Live in the service area of a PACE organization

- Need a nursing home-level of care (meeting state set certification criteria)

- Be able to live safely within the community with assistance from the PACE program

PACE programs are paid a monthly capitation fee by CMS, which is prospective. These payments are calculated using the pre-ACA county rate, which is not adjusted for indirect medical education (IME), multiplied by the beneficiary's total risk score and the organization frailty score. The frailty adjustment is unique to the PACE model of risk adjustment and is added to offset the variations in care expenditures for frail populations. This adjustment accounts for costs that would otherwise be unpredicted by the CMS-HCC model, such as functional impairments. Medicaid-eligible members do not pay a monthly premium. Medicare-eligible members do pay a monthly premium for each the long-term-care portion of the PACE benefit and for the Medicare Part D drugs. There is no copayment or deductible for any drug, service, or care approved by the beneficiary's healthcare team.

Services covered under the PACE model include:

- Adult day primary care

- Dentistry

- Emergency care

- Home care

- Hospital care

- Labs/radiology (such as x-ray)

- Meals

- Medical specialty services

- Nursing home care

- Nutritional counseling

- Occupational therapy

- Physical therapy

- Prescription drugs (the PACE program will cover the Part D benefits)

- Primary care (including doctor & nursing services)

- Recreational therapy

- Social services, such as:

  - respite care

  - support groups

  - training for caregivers

- Social work counseling

- Transportation to the PACE center for activities and medical appointments

End Stage Renal Disease

CMS implemented the End Stage Renal Disease (ESRD) model to improve accuracy for enrollees with end stage renal disease, which includes patients on dialysis, having transplants, and in post-graft status. This model uses the same CMS-HCC model but the coefficients differ to account for costs of caring for a patient who falls into this ESRD category. This model does not vary significantly otherwise from the CMS-HCC model.

RxHCC

In 2006, CMS introduced a second HCC-based risk adjustment model, which covers the Part D (prescription drug) benefit. The Medicare Prescription Drug, Improvement and Modernization Act (MMA) of 2003, created the second major Medicare capitated payment system for the Medicare Part D prescription drug benefit. This model employs a similar structure of the CMS-HCC model wherein conditions are grouped into hierarchical condition categories assigned weights and trumping logic. CMS uses the RxHCC risk adjustment model to adjust the payments for Part D benefits offered by standalone prescription drug plans (PDPs) and MA Part D plans. This model was updated in 2011 based on data from the prescription drug event (PDE) data. This update included more recent cost data and utilization patterns.

For calendar year 2022, CMS will finalize an updated version of the RxHCC risk adjustment model to calculate Part D risk scores, using diagnosis data from 2017 fee for service (FFS) claims and MA encounter data submissions, along with expenditure data from 2018 PDEs. For calendar year 2022, CMS will calculate Part D risk scores using this recalibrated 2017/2018 RxHCC model.

Payment

Unlike the fee-for-service model, risk-adjustment payments from CMS are not paid after services are rendered. The service provider is compensated from the MA plan after the claim is filed but the plan does not receive payment from CMS at that time. The chart below shows the process of a claim within the risk-adjustment model.

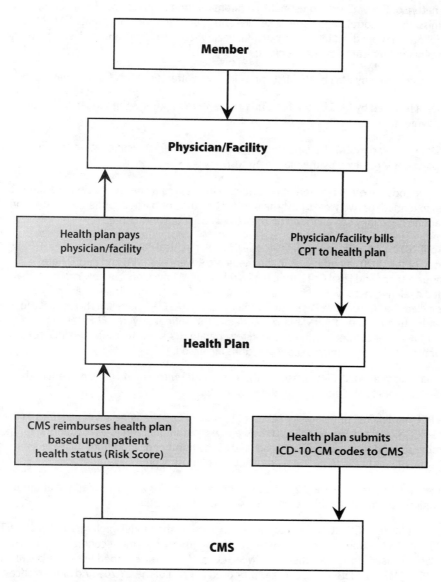

Since risk adjustment is a predictive payment model for CMS, the data from service years must be submitted by deadlines to be included in the disease burden for the payment year. The following table is an example of the deadlines for submission and payment dates associated with those deadlines.

CMS published the payment timelines for risk adjustment in the "2013 National Technical Assistance Risk Adjustment 101 Participant Guide."

Payment Year (PY)	Model Run	Dates of Service Included in Model Run	Payment Date (Following Payment Run)
2013	Final reconciliation	1/1/2012–12/31/2012	7/1/2014*
2014	Initial	7/1/2012–6/30/2013	1/1/2014
2014	Mid-year	1/1/2013–12/31/2013	8/1/2014**
2014	Final reconciliation	1/1/2013–12/31/2013	8/1/2015

* Final risk scores for payment year 2013 will be reflected in the July 2014 payment.

**Mid-year risk scores for payment year 2014 will be reflected in the August 2014 payment.

The nature of the CMS-risk-adjustment-payment method requires specific deadlines for data submission that correlate to dates of service and affect capitation payments. CMS observes the following three deadlines each calendar year when calculating and delivering funding payments to Medicare Advantage plans:

- Data received by CMS by the first Friday in March affects the July funding payment.

- Data received by CMS by the first Friday in September affects the January funding payment.

- Data received by CMS by January 31st is considered a final reconciliation and the payment is received by the plan in August.

These periods are often referred to as "sweeps." In past years, the submission deadline has been extended for two weeks past the original deadline published. Updated information regarding deadlines can be found on the CMS website at www.cms.gov.

In April 2019, CMS released updates to the CMS hierarchical condition categories (HCC) model for the 2020 calendar year in the Medicare Advantage (MA) and Part D Rate Announcement and Final Call Letter. In this release, CMS developed a new category that added a relative factor value based on the number of conditions a beneficiary may have. This was called the "Alternative Payment Condition Count (APCC)" model. In this model the APCC risk-adjustment factor (RAF) value was added to the patient's overall RAF starting when the patient had four conditions that mapped to separate HCCs. The factor added increased up to 10 or more HCCs as the number of conditions increased.

For calendar year 2020, CMS phased in this new model with a blend of 50 percent of the 2017 CMS-HCC model and 50 percent of the new APCC model.

The PCC model CMS proposed for payment year 2020 had the same set of variables as the CMS-HCC model implemented in 2019 except with additional variables accounting for the number of conditions a beneficiary had, and as the number of conditions increased, an adjustment was made to the total predicted cost (or risk score).

As in payment years 2019 and 2020, the model proposed for 2021 included the additional conditions for mental health, substance use disorder, and CKD.

For Calendar Year (CY) 2021, CMS continued to phase in the model implemented in 2020. The 2020 CMS-HCC model (previously known as the alternative payment condition count [APCC] model) was used along with the 2017 CMS-HCC model for the blended risk score calculation. For 2021, CMS calculated risk scores as proposed in Part I of the CY 2021 Advance Notice. Seventy-five percent of the risk score was calculated with the 2020 CMS-HCC model using diagnoses from encounter data, RAPS inpatient records, and FFS, with 25 percent of the risk score using the 2017 CMS-HCC model, using diagnoses from RAPS and FFS.

For CY 2022, CMS will fully phase in the 2020 CMS-HCC model to calculate encounter data-based risk scores for payment to MA organizations and certain demonstrations using only risk-adjustment-eligible diagnoses identified from encounter data submitted by MA organizations and FFS claims. CMS will no longer use the 2017 CMS-HCC model used to calculate risk scores based on data submitted to the Risk Adjustment Processing System (RAPS) for Part C risk adjustment. For CY 2022, CMS will calculate 100 percent of the risk score using the 2020 CMS-HCC model.

This will also complete the transition from the risk adjustment processing system (RAPS) to the encounter data processing system (EDPS). Encounter dates for 2021, for payment year 2022, with a final submission deadline of January 2023, will be submitted under the V24 model entirely via EDPS. Encounter-date submissions prior to this will still use the blended V22 and V24 models using both EDPS and RAPS.

The RAPS system requires dates of service, provider type, diagnosis codes and beneficiary Health Insurance Claim [HIC] numbers and optional date of birth (DOB). Risk adjustment rules are applied by the MA organization and using this filtering logic, diagnoses are assembled into RAPS files and submitted to CMS. CMS reviews these RAPS submissions for duplicates and errors but relies on Risk Adjustment Data Validation (RADV) audits to ensure that the submitted diagnosis codes are valid and supported by the documentation and coding guidelines. EDPS requires all data elements from the HIPAA standard ANSI 837 v5010 claim format and must pass Correct Coding Initiative (CCI) edits used with fee-for-service (FFS) claims.

The following table lists risk adjustment data submission deadlines for calculating risk scores, demonstrating CMS' gradual transition from RAPS to encounter data processing systems (EDPS).

Risk score run	Dates of service	Deadline for submission of risk adjustment data
2019 final run (RAPS and EDPS)	Jan. 1, 2018 – Dec. 31, 2018	Jan. 31, 2020
2020 mid-year run (RAPS and EDPS)	Jan. 1, 2019 – Dec. 31, 2019	March 6, 2020
2021 initial run (RAPS and EDPS)	July 1, 2019 – June 30, 2020	Sept. 4, 2020
2020 interim final run (RAPS and EDPS)	Jan. 1, 2019 – Dec. 31, 2019	Feb. 1, 2021
2021 mid-year run (RAPS and EDPS)	Jan. 1, 2020 – Dec. 31, 2020	March 5, 2021
2020 final run (RAPS and EDPS)	Jan. 1, 2019 – Dec. 31, 2019	Aug. 2, 2021
2022 initial run (EDPS)	July 1, 2020 – June 30, 2021	Sept. 3, 2021
2021 interim final run (RAPS and EDPS)	Jan. 1, 2020 – Dec. 31, 2020	Jan. 31, 2022
2022 mid-year run (EDPS)	Jan. 1, 2020 – Dec. 31, 2021	March 4, 2022
2021 final fun (RAPS and EDPS)	Jan. 1, 2020 – Dec. 31, 2020	Aug. 1, 2022
2023 initial run (EDPS)	July 1, 2021 – June 30, 2022	Sept. 2, 2022
2022 interim final run (EDPS)	Jan. 1, 2020 – Dec. 31, 2021	Jan. 1, 2023
2023 mid-year run (EDPS)	Jan. 1, 2020 – Dec. 31, 2022	March 3, 2023
2022 final run (EDPS)	Jan. 1, 2020 – Dec. 31, 2021	July 31, 2023

Chapter 2. Coding and Documentation

Medical record documentation is one of the cornerstones of the current healthcare system. Whether paper or electronic records are used, these records must be accurate, consistent, and complete to provide the information necessary to ensure clinical quality, substantiate medical necessity, and ensure the most appropriate reimbursement. Health records are the foundation for many decisions that are made, regardless of the setting. Therefore documentation improvement efforts have been on-going for many years and the shift in focus to quality of care further emphasizes the need for quality documentation.

It is not uncommon to find providers who practice medicine in their heads. The provider can review his or her notes for a patient and recall the plan of care he or she had in mind. This can cause issues when the patient needs to coordinate care or transfer care should his or her normal provider be unavailable. Nobody anticipates illness, injury, or even death taking them away from work suddenly, but those situations do happen. Best practice for a provider is to have complete documentation that outlines the status and plan of care for every condition affecting the patient documented at least once a year. The annual wellness visit is an ideal time to take inventory of the patient's overall health. Should any unforeseen event take a provider away from practice, that annual wellness note can serve as an excellent resource for any other providers caring for the patient. In addition to better continuity of care, better documentation can validate and better support insurance claims.

The medical record is an essential component of providing quality care to a patient. It serves as the record of what medical services were provided to a patient and why. The medical record also serves as a communication tool for the care team of a patient, which assists with ensuring continuity of care. It is crucial that medical records meet standards for current, complete, and accurate health information. Ensuring the medical record of the patient meets these standards will assist with ensuring that the patient receives quality and continuous care, precise coding and timely billing are performed, and appropriate reimbursement is made.

According to the 2008 RAPS Participant Guide, the Centers for Medicare and Medicaid Services (CMS) requires the following elements to be considered a valid and complete record:

- The date of service, complete with month, day, and year

- Evidence of a face-to-face encounter with an acceptable provider type and setting

- Acceptable provider signature or authentication

- The provider's credentials

While it is not explicitly required by CMS, it is a standard medical record best practice and either required or recommended by many regulatory agencies and payers that at least two patient identifiers should be used to validate that the medical record matches the patient. Additional identifiers may include the date of birth, Social Security number, or insurance subscriber ID.

In addition, CMS's Contract-Level Risk Adjustment Data Validation Medical Record Reviewer Guidance, In effect as of March 20, 2019, states: "All data fields in Section II contain enrollee data that matches the name on the medical record submitted. The birth date may be used as a secondary identifier for common shortened names if it is present on the medical record." A second identifier, such as a date of birth, is recommended to mitigate Risk Adjustment Data Validation (RAD-V) audit risk.

Medical Record Documentation

Each patient's medical records are the only source of written information about patient encounters and are necessary to assign and substantiate ICD-10-CM, CPT, and/or HCPCS Level II codes. The primary function of the medical record is to provide a record of patient care with emphasis placed on what services were provided to the patient and why. A complete and well-organized medical record will allow any member of the care team to quickly access vital information about the patient's health.

This completeness is even more essential in risk adjustment; provider documentation serves as the main source of risk-adjustment data. While the practice of risk adjustment has expanded to other models such as the Department of Health and Human Services (HHS) model, the original focus of risk adjustment was on Medicare-eligible patients. The Centers for Disease Control and Prevention (CDC) reports that in 2012, half of all adults, about 117 million people, had one or more chronic health conditions and one in four adults had two or more chronic health conditions. Three in four Americans aged 65 and older have at least two chronic conditions that require on-going medical attention and/or limit their activities of daily living.

The increased complexity in treating multiple chronic and comorbid conditions demands clear and complete medical records. It is likely that patients are seeing multiple providers for their care and this healthcare team needs to effectively coordinate care. The Medicare annual wellness visit (AWV) is the perfect opportunity to provide a complete and comprehensive overview of the patient's health. While the AWV is the ideal opportunity to complete the comprehensive review, it is also advisable to address every condition at each face-to-face encounter with the patient since there is no guarantee that the patient will return to the clinic during the rest of the year. Additionally, since most of the CMS-HCC conditions are chronic, they would likely impact the care and/or medical decision making of an encounter, even if the presenting problem is minor, such as suture removal. If a diabetic patient with congestive heart failure (CHF) presented to the clinic for suture removal on his or her foot, the provider should review additional care instructions for this patient as either of those chronic conditions could impact the final healing of the wound that required suturing.

General Standards

Documentation is the recording of pertinent facts and observations about a patient's health history, including past and present illnesses, tests, treatments, and outcomes. The medical record chronologically documents the care of the patient to:

- Enable a physician or other healthcare professional to plan and evaluate the patient's treatment

- Enhance communication and promote continuity of care among physicians and other healthcare professionals involved in the patient's care

- Facilitate claims review and payment

- Assist in utilization review and quality of care evaluations

- Reduce hassles related to medical review

- Provide clinical data for research and education

- Serve as a legal document to verify the care provided (e.g., as defense in the case of a professional liability claim)

- Validate that treatments are appropriate for treating the patient's condition

- Document medical necessity of the diagnosis

Representatives of the American Health Information Management Association (AHIMA), American Health Quality Association (AHQA), American Hospital Association (AHA), American Medical Association (AMA), Blue Cross and Blue Shield Association (BCBSA), and America's Health Insurance Plans (AHIP) have developed several principles of medical record documentation, which expand upon the general standards and include:

- The medical record should be complete and legible.

- The documentation of each patient encounter should include the date; reason for the encounter; appropriate history and physical exam; review of lab, x-ray data, and other ancillary services as appropriate; assessment; and plan for care (including discharge plan, as appropriate).

- Past and present diagnoses should be accessible to the treating or consulting healthcare professional.

- The reasons for, and results of, x-rays, lab tests, and other ancillary services should be documented or included in the medical record.

- Relevant health risk factors should be identified.

- The patient's progress, including response to treatment, change in treatment, change in diagnosis, and patient noncompliance should be documented.

- The written plan for care should include, when appropriate, treatments and medications, specifying frequency and dosage; referrals and consultations; patient and family education; and specific instructions for follow-up.

- The documentation should support the intensity of the patient evaluation and treatment, including thought processes and the complexity of medical decision making.

- All entries to the medical record should be dated and authenticated.

- The codes reported on the health insurance claim form or billing statement should reflect the documentation in the medical record.

Acceptable Sources

CMS requires that Medicare Advantage (MA) organizations use the following sources for risk-adjustment data collection:

- Hospital inpatient facilities

Type of Hospital Inpatient Facility
Short-term (general and specialty) hospitals
Medical assistance facilities/critical access hospitals
Religious nonmedical healthcare institutions
Long-term hospitals
Rehabilitation hospitals
Children's hospitals
Psychiatric hospitals

There is an increasing need for hospital inpatient coders to learn the outpatient coding rules in order to properly capture and report HCC diagnoses. In addition, inpatient coders may not routinely assign codes for chronic conditions that do not qualify as a complication or comorbidity (CC) or a major complication or comorbidity (MCC) for MS-DRG assignment. These chronic conditions are now important elements that can affect the total risk score for the patient. There are also conditions that are only captured in the acute setting, such as stroke and acute exacerbations of chronic illnesses such as chronic obstructive pulmonary disease (COPD) and congestive heart failure (CHF).

- Hospital outpatient facilities

Type of Hospital Outpatient Facility
Short-term (general and specialty) hospitals
Medical assistance facilities/critical access hospitals
Community mental health centers
Federally qualified health centers/religious nonmedical healthcare institutions*[1]
Long-term hospitals
Rehabilitation hospitals
Children's hospitals
Rural health clinics, freestanding and provider-based*[2]
Psychiatric hospitals

* Facilities use a composite bill that covers both the physician and the facility component of the services rendered in these facilities that do not result in an independent physician claim.

1 Community mental health centers (CMHC) provide outpatient services, including specialized outpatient services for children, the elderly, individuals who are chronically ill, and residents of the CMHC's mental health services area who have been discharged from an inpatient treatment facility.

2 Federally qualified health centers (FQHC) are facilities located in a medically underserved area that provide Medicare beneficiaries with preventative primary medical care under the direction of a physician.

- Physicians

Code	Specialty	Code	Specialty	Code	Specialty
1	General Practice	25	Physical Medicine and Rehabilitation	67	Occupational Therapist
2	General Surgery	26	Psychiatry	68	Clinical Psychologist
3	Allergy/Immunology	27	Geriatric Psychiatry	72*	Pain Management
4	Otolaryngology	28	Colorectal Surgery	76*	Peripheral Vascular Disease
5	Anesthesiology	29	Pulmonary Disease	77	Vascular Surgery
6	Cardiology	33*	Thoracic Surgery	78	Cardiac Surgery
7	Dermatology	34	Urology	79	Addiction Medicine
8	Family Practice	35	Chiropractic	80	Licensed Clinical Social Worker
9	Interventional Pain Management (IPM)	36	Nuclear Medicine	81	Critical Care (intensivists)
10	Gastroenterology	37	Pediatric Medicine	82	Hematology
11	Internal Medicine	38	Geriatric Medicine	83	Hematology/Oncology
12	Osteopathic Manipulative Medicine	39	Nephrology	84	Preventive Medicine
13	Neurology	40	Hand Surgery	85	Maxillofacial Surgery
14	Neurosurgery	41	Optometry	86	Neuropsychiatry
15	Speech Language Pathologist	42	Certified Nurse Midwife	89*	Certified Clinical Nurse Specialist
16	Obstetrics/Gynecology	43	Certified Registered Nurse Anesthetist	90	Medical Oncology
17	Hospice And Palliative Care	44	Infectious Disease	91	Surgical Oncology
18	Ophthalmology	46*	Endocrinology	92	Radiation Oncology

* Indicates that a number(s) has been skipped.

Code	Specialty	Code	Specialty	Code	Specialty
19	Oral Surgery	48*	Podiatry	93	Emergency Medicine
20	Orthopedic Surgery	50*	Nurse Practitioner	94	Interventional Radiology
21	Cardiac Electrophysiology	62*	Psychologist	97*	Physician Assistant
22	Pathology	64*	Audiologist	98	Gynecologist/Oncologist
23	Sports Medicine	65	Physical Therapist	99	Unknown Physician Specialty
24	Plastic And Reconstructive Surgery	66	Rheumatology	C0	Sleep Medicine

* Indicates that a number(s) has been skipped.

Signature Issues

CMS provides specific guidance on what is an acceptable and valid signature based on the type of chart being used or submitted—paper or electronic. It is imperative that signatures be compliant and completed within a timely manner.

When using paper charts a handwritten signature or initials is acceptable. If the signature is not legible, it is still acceptable as long as the provider's full name and credentials appear in the note. Signature logs may be used to validate signed paper charts. A signature log contains the provider's name, credentials, and a copy of his or her signed name and initials.

Valid electronic signatures may include:

- Electronically signed by

- Authenticated by

- Approved by

- Closed by

- Finalized by

The provider must include his or her last name, first name or initial. The provider's credential must be found within the note as well.

> It is important, when reviewing paper records, to ensure that a signature stamp is not being used. Stamped signatures are not considered valid by CMS, unless the provider has a physical limitation that prevents him or her from being able to sign the record.

Coding Guidelines

When coding for risk adjustment, it is imperative that the coder pay attention to the entire note for conditions, which are validated by the note and, therefore, appropriate to capture. It is common to have various reasons, such as billing form limitations, clearinghouse limitations, and internal policies that instruct a coder to only code the reason for the encounter or to leave off validated conditions found within other portions of the note. This, however, is not correct based on the ICD-10-CM instructions. In addition, *AHA Coding Clinic*, Fourth Quarter 2017, page 110, indicates that it is not appropriate to develop internal policies to omit codes. Facilities should review documentation to clinically validate diagnoses and develop policies to query the provider to confirm diagnoses that may not meet clinical criteria.

It is also important for coders to have the most up-to-date coding references to assign codes accurately and to the highest level of detail, and to avoid assigning invalid or deleted codes. If diagnosis "cheat sheets" are used, these should be updated in conjunction with the appropriate code set updates.

There is an increasing need for hospital inpatient coders to learn the outpatient coding rules in order to properly capture and report HCC diagnoses, as hospitals frequently acquire physician practices and perform coding and billing functions for these practices.

ICD-10-CM Guidelines

CMS and the National Center for Health Statistics (NCHS) provide the official guidelines for coding and reporting using ICD-10-CM. The guidelines are to be used as a companion to the official version of the ICD-10-CM as published on the NCHS website. In cases where the guidelines conflict with the official classification, the classification takes precedence. Instructions in the ICD-10-CM classification and the guidelines for coding and reporting always take precedence over *AHA Coding Clinic* advice.

The guidelines have been approved by the four organizations that make up the Cooperating Parties for the ICD-10-CM: the AHA, AHIMA, CMS, and NCHS.

The guidelines are organized into sections. Section I includes the structure and conventions of the classification and general guidelines that apply to the entire classification, and chapter-specific guidelines that correspond to the chapters as they are arranged in the classification. Section II includes guidelines for selection of principal diagnosis for non-outpatient settings. Section III includes guidelines for reporting additional diagnoses in non-outpatient settings. Section IV is for outpatient coding and reporting. It is necessary to review all sections of the guidelines to fully understand all of the rules and instructions needed to code properly.

Reporting additional diagnoses guideline section III states: "GENERAL RULES FOR OTHER (ADDITIONAL) DIAGNOSES. For reporting purposes the definition for 'other diagnoses' is interpreted as additional conditions that affect patient care in terms of requiring: clinical evaluation; or therapeutic treatment; or diagnostic procedures; or extended length of hospital stay; or increased nursing care and/or monitoring. The UHDDS item #11-b defines Other Diagnoses as **'all conditions that coexist at the time of admission, that develop subsequently, or that affect the treatment received and/or the length of stay.** Diagnoses that relate to an earlier episode which have no bearing on the current hospital stay are to be excluded.' UHDDS definitions apply to inpatients in acute care, short-term, long term care and psychiatric hospital setting. The UHDDS definitions are used by acute-care-short-term hospitals to report inpatient data elements in a standardized manner. These data elements and their definitions can be found in the July 31, 1985, *Federal Register* (Vol. 50, No. 147), pp. 31038-40.

Since that time the application of the UHDDS definitions has been expanded to include all non-outpatient settings (acute care, short term, long term care and psychiatric hospitals; home health agencies; rehab facilities; nursing homes, etc.). The UHDDS definitions also apply to hospice services (all levels of care)."

Guideline section IV states: "Though the conventions and general guidelines apply to all settings, coding guidelines for outpatient and provider reporting of diagnoses will vary in a number of instances from those for inpatient diagnoses, recognizing that:

The Uniform Hospital Discharge Data Set (UHDDS) definition of principal diagnosis does not apply to hospital-based outpatient services and provider-based office visits.

Coding guidelines for inconclusive diagnoses (probable, suspected, rule out, etc.) were developed for inpatient reporting and do not apply to outpatients."

Diagnostic coding and reporting guidelines for outpatient services guideline section IV states: "Chronic diseases treated on an ongoing basis may be coded and reported as many times as the patient receives treatment and care for the condition(s)."

Example 1

Follow-up visit

S: Patient is seen for follow up on Parkinson's disease. Since last visit, he has noticed an increase in tremors despite maximal medical intervention.

O: Patient is emotional about disease progression. Tremor is pronounced. Wife is assisting with most ADL's. Patient is depressed about loss of independence.

P: Continue current meds. Advised patient he is on maximal therapeutic doses. Started on Paxil for depression.

The Parkinson's disease in example 1 is correct to report as there is on-going care and treatment being dedicated to this condition.

Example 2

Sick Visit

Subjective: Patient is seen today for flu-like symptoms.

Objective: On exam, patient has mild fever and cough on top of emphysema. Patient complains of general malaise with fever and chills.

Assessment: Viral illness in emphysema patient.

Plan: Rest and fluids. Stressed importance of medication adherence for emphysema with the patient. If symptoms do not improve within seven to 10 days, return to clinic or if symptoms get worse or present to the ER for any severe acute symptoms.

In example 2, the emphysema would be correct to capture for risk adjustment as it is mentioned in the exam, assessment, and plan. The provider is clearly demonstrating that the emphysema has impacted the medical decision making, even in an encounter for a minor issue.

Guideline section IV. J states: "Code all documented conditions that coexist."

Code all documented conditions that coexist at the time of the encounter/visit, and require or affect patient care treatment or management. Do not code conditions that were previously treated and no longer exist. However, history codes (categories Z80–Z87) may be used as secondary codes if the historical condition or family history has an impact on current care or influences treatment.

These guidelines instruct coders to capture all conditions that coexist during an encounter. This is a shift in thinking for a large portion of coders, who focus on coding only the reason for the encounter.

Fee for Service vs. Risk-Adjustment Coding

The following example outlines a patient encounter where the patient visited the physician for a specific complaint. During her encounter other patient conditions were addressed.

Example

Date of Service: January 3, 2021

Patient: Juanita Perez

Referral: on file from primary care associates

History of Present Illness

This pleasant 83-year-old female presented to my office with right knee pain. She had a fall on that knee about three years ago and then another fall last year. She has had constant knee pain since the most recent fall and reports occasional giving way or locking up of the knee. Plain standing films showed obliteration of the medial joint spaces, fair preservation of lateral riding patella and mild lateral joint spacing narrowing. An MRI showed a posterior horn medial meniscus tear and obliteration of the articular cartilage at the weight-bearing apex of the femoral condyle. The patient took naproxen for six months without significant relief and four cortisone injections with decreasing efficacy after the second injection.

Past Medical History

Per PCP chart review, the patient has OA, peripheral neuropathy treated with gabapentin, hypertension on lisinopril, a-fib on warfarin, osteoporosis with supplemental vitamin D and calcium, and prediabetes.

Physical Exam

General: well-developed, severely obese female, appears stated age, BMI 51

HEENT: WNL, PERRLA, moist mucous membranes

Heart: normal rate and rhythm

Lungs: clear to auscultation

Abdomen: WNL, no HSM

Extremities: good distal pulses, decreased sensation bilateral feet, marked tenderness on the right knee as expected.

Diagnostic impression: severe degenerative arthritis of the medial compartment of the right knee

Plan: pre-op blood work, Lovenox bridge/stop warfarin, plan for robotic aided MAKOplasty of right knee.

Electronically signed: William C. Jones, MD on Jan. 3, 2021 at 11:42.

Addendum added by William C. Jones, MD on January 5, 2021 at 13:57.

Blood work results: patient's A1C is 9, patient is now diabetic. Schedule diabetic NP teaching and diet plan for tomorrow and PCP will further follow diagnosis. All other blood work WNL. Advised patient of results.

The following table shows the difference between risk-adjustment coding and coding only the reason for the encounter for the example on the previous page. Capturing all coexisting conditions present during the encounter can be impactful to the overall RAF score of the patient.

Outpatient (Non-risk Adjustment) Coding		RAF Value	Risk-Adjustment Coding		RAF Value
M17.11	Unilateral primary osteoarthritis, right knee	0.000	E11.42	Type 2 diabetes mellitus with diabetic polyneuropathy	0.302
Demographics		0.540	E66.01	Morbid (severe) obesity due to excess calories	0.250
			I48.91	Unspecified atrial fibrillation	0.268
			Demographics		0.528
Total:		**0.540**	**Total:**		**1.348**

Linking Diagnoses

The ICD-10-CM guidelines in Section I.A, Conventions for the ICD-10-CM, state:

> **"14. 'And'** The word 'and' should be interpreted to mean either 'and' or 'or' when it appears in a title. For example, cases of 'tuberculosis of bones,' 'tuberculosis of joints' and 'tuberculosis of bones and joints' are classified to subcategory A18.0, Tuberculosis of bones and joints."

Example

> ER CC: leg pain
>
> Exam: left leg is swollen and warm to the touch. Order u/s.
>
> U/S results: DVT seen in left femoral vein
>
> A/P: left leg DVT. start warfarin. Advised patient to wear compression leggings.

In this example, the coder would assign code I82.412 Acute embolism and thrombosis of left femoral vein.

> **"15. 'With'** The word 'with' or 'in' should be interpreted to mean 'associated with' or 'due to' when it appears in a code title, the Alphabetic Index, or an instructional note in the Tabular List. The classification presumes a causal relationship between the two conditions linked by these terms in the Alphabetic Index or Tabular List. These conditions should be coded as related even in the absence of provider documentation explicitly linking them, unless the documentation clearly states the conditions are unrelated or when another guideline exists that specifically requires a documented linkage between two conditions (e.g., sepsis guideline for "acute organ dysfunction that is not clearly associated with the sepsis"). For conditions not specifically linked by these relational terms in the classification or when a guideline requires that a linkage between two conditions be explicitly documented, provider documentation must link the conditions in order to code them as related. The word 'with' in the Alphabetic Index is sequenced immediately following the main term, not in alphabetical order."

With the update in the guidelines regarding the term "with," coding complicated conditions has become less arduous. As long as the linked condition is in the index under the main term, the coder may assume the causal relationship between the two conditions. This concept is imperative. Prior to the change in the guidelines, a provider would need to be queried to provide the linking language. Conditions such as diabetes, chronic kidney disease, or congestive heart failure, have combination codes, which should be reported as appropriate.

Example

A/P: CHF—continue meds and seeing cardiology

Insomnia—practice sleep hygiene and caffeine curfew. Consider Unisom

CKD III—continue lisinopril

RLS—continue gabapentin, poss. increase to BID

OSA—discussed compliance with CPAP

OA—reviewed Rx plan, patient continues to take NSAIDs with CKDHTN—continue to decrease salt intake

DM—A1C is due, patient has missed last three lab appointments, non-fasting today

Incorrect Coding		Correct Coding	
I50.9	Heart failure, unspecified	I50.9	Heart failure, unspecified
N18.30	Chronic kidney disease, stage 3 unspecified (moderate)	N18.30	Chronic kidney disease, stage 3 unspecified (moderate)
I10	Essential (primary) hypertension	**I13.0**	Hypertensive heart and chronic kidney disease with heart failure and stage 1 through stage 4 chronic kidney disease, or unspecified chronic kidney disease
E11.9	Type 2 diabetes mellitus without complications	**E11.22**	Type 2 diabetes mellitus with diabetic chronic kidney disease

When heart failure, chronic kidney disease, and hypertension co-exist, the combination code of I13.0 should be reported. The tabular direction also instructs the coder to use additional codes to identify the type of heart failure and to identify the stage of chronic disease.

Additionally, since chronic kidney disease is listed under the "with" in the index under the main term "Diabetes," the causal relationship can be assumed and E11.22 should be reported.

Care should be taken, however, to avoid assuming a causal relationship in "not elsewhere classified (NEC)" index entries that may cover broad categories of conditions. According to *AHA Coding Clinic*, Fourth Quarter 2017, pages 100 and 101, the "with" guideline does not apply to "not elsewhere classified (NEC)" index entries that cover broad categories of conditions. Specific conditions must be linked by the terms "with," "due to," or "associated with."

CMS Participant Guide Excerpts

In addition to the ICD-10-CM guidelines, which instruct a coder to capture all co-existing conditions, the *CMS Risk Adjustment Processing System (RAPS) Participant Guide* also provides this instruction.

In section 6.4.1 Co-Existing and Related Conditions: "Physicians should code all documented conditions that co-exist at the time of the encounter/visit, and require or affect patient care, treatment, or management. Do not code conditions which were previously treated and no longer exist. However, history codes (V10–V19 not in HCC model) may be used as secondary codes if the historical condition or family history has an impact on the current care or influences treatment."

CMS further clarifies that "co-existing conditions include chronic, ongoing conditions such as diabetes, congestive heart failure, atrial fibrillation, and chronic obstructive pulmonary disease. These conditions are generally managed by ongoing medication and have the potential for acute exacerbations if not treated properly, particularly if the patient is experiencing other acute conditions. It is likely that these diagnoses would be part of a general overview of the patient's health when treating co-existing conditions for all but the most minor of medical encounters. Co-existing conditions also include ongoing conditions such as multiple sclerosis, hemiplegia, rheumatoid arthritis, and Parkinson's disease. Although they may not impact every minor healthcare episode, it is likely that patients having these conditions would have their general health status evaluated within a data reporting period, and these diagnoses would be documented and reportable at that time." Another type of co-existing condition is "symptoms." Symptoms that are integral to an underlying condition should not be coded.

With chronic or ongoing conditions, CMS acknowledges that there is a common error or issue with the use of "history of." The use of "history of" means the patient no longer has the condition and the diagnosis often indexes to an ICD-10-CM "Z" code, which does not map to an HCC category in most models. The documenting provider may designate a current condition as historical or designate a resolved condition as still active. It is important to carefully review all parts of the note for additional information about conditions that may affect care during the encounter. Conditions documented in any portion of the medical record should be evaluated and reported as appropriate. This includes conditions documented in the history of present illness or past history, if the condition is still current; exam, problem lists such as current, on-going, or active; the review of systems; and assessment and plan portions.

On-going Chronic Conditions

Within the *2008 Risk Adjustment Data Technical Assistance for Medicare Advantage Organizations Participant Guide*, CMS acknowledges that there are certain chronic conditions that are not expected to resolve and will continue to require medical management as well as impact future care, even for minor encounters or encounters for an unrelated issue.

While there is no official all-inclusive list, chronic conditions can include:

- Alcohol, drug, or substance abuse/dependence (even in remission)

- Alzheimer's disease and related dementia

- Amputation status

- Asthma

- Atherosclerosis of aorta

- Atherosclerosis of the extremities

- Atrial fibrillation

- Cancer (breast, colorectal, lung, and prostate)

- Chronic kidney disease

- Chronic obstructive pulmonary disease

- Congestive heart failure

- Depression

- Diabetes

- Functional artificial openings

- Hepatitis (chronic viral B & C)

- HIV/AIDS

- Ischemic heart disease

- Multiple sclerosis

- Osteoporosis

- Parkinson's disease

- Rheumatoid arthritis

- Schizophrenia and other psychotic disorders, even single episode (use remission identifier if applicable)

- Stroke sequelae

- Systemic lupus erythematosus (SLE)

- Transplant status for:
  - heart
  - bone marrow
  - stem cell
  - liver
  - lung
  - pancreas
  - kidney

The preceding conditions are recognized as not likely to resolve and to require on-going care; this does not alter the documentation requirements. The supporting documentation should as completely and accurately as possible describe each condition during the face-to-face encounter with the beneficiary. This includes reporting any complications, abnormal findings, or clinical significance during the encounter.

While these conditions are not expected to resolve, that does not mean that there are not exceptions where the condition does resolve. It is important to review the entire record for the encounter for any conflicting or unclear documentation. A few examples of chronic conditions that are considered to be life-long but have resolved, include:

- Diabetes without complications status-post pancreas transplant

- Cirrhosis/end-stage liver disease/hepatitis status-post liver transplant

- COPD/emphysema status-post lung transplant

- CHF/cardiomyopathy status-post heart transplant

Example

Surgical history:
tonsils and adenoids 40 years ago, tah-bso 17 years ago, g-tube three yrs. ago, CV cath placement and removal six months ago.

Exam:
HEENT wnl, PERRLA,

CV: RRR

Resp: normal breath sounds

Abd: no lesions noted, no HSM

Extrem: normal pedal pulses, no clubbing

Skin: no cyanosis

Psych: AO X3

The surgical history documents a gastrostomy being placed but no reversal; however, there is no documentation of a finding of the stoma in the exam and the abdomen is noted to have no lesions. The provider needs to be queried to clarify if the gastrostomy is still functional.

Recapture

On January 1st, each year, the diagnostic information for each beneficiary is reset. This provides a clean slate for the new year of encounter diagnostic data. This practice requires that all chronic and ongoing conditions to be recaptured, otherwise, CMS concludes that the condition has resolved. When a chronic condition is not recaptured, this is referred to as "falling off." Some conditions that are significant to risk adjustment fall off appropriately, such as acute exacerbations of chronic illnesses, acute complications of on-going treatment or management, and acute conditions such as strokes and fractures. In these instances, it is important to capture the chronic condition that is no longer in exacerbation or any sequela from the acute conditions.

Example

Follow-up Visit—Medicare Patient

CC: Fracture Follow-up

HPI: Patient is here for fracture follow-up. Patient has fully recovered from pathological femur fracture, which happened last May. There was no trauma or accident preceding the fracture. Patient has continued to supplement calcium. Follow-up DEXA indicated severe osteoporosis and patient was started on Boniva. PMSH reviewed in EMR, medications reconciled.

Exam: Patient has some tenderness in her back. Strength and reflexes intact in extremities. Patient has bandage from IV site from Boniva therapy two days ago. Affect is wnl.

A/P: s/p pathological fracture. Severe osteoporosis on Boniva and supplemental calcium.

Previous Year		Reported	Current Year		Reported
M84.453A	Pathological fracture, right femur, initial encounter for fracture	Yes	M84.453A	Pathological fracture, right femur, initial encounter for fracture	No

Based on this example, the fracture would have been reported the previous year. But for the current year, this condition would fall off as it has resolved. Osteoporosis without current fracture does not risk adjust within the CMS-HCC model.

Code Set Updates

Annually, on October 1st, the ICD-10-CM updated code set is released. The risk-adjustment model updates typically are released later in the year or early the next year. CMS releases the proposed changes for the coming or current year as early as late December in an Advance Notice. It is more common to see the announcement of the model updates released in February of the current year. These changes are not finalized until the Final Call letter is released in April. The Final Call letter is applicable to the calendar year. Due to timing of the release of the Final Call letter, there may be a need to retroactively review and/or update coding and/or risk-adjustment submissions completed prior to the letter being released.

There are two main parts to the updates released in the Final Call letter. The first is an adjustment to the RAF values assigned to the various categories and models. Typically, most HCCs see a minor decrease in their overall RAF value compared to the prior year. The other change is additions, deletions, or restructuring of HCCs. Examples of this include, removing I25.2 Old myocardial infarction, from the CMS-HCC and making it an Rx-HCC. For example, for the 2019 calendar year, CMS added two more mental health categories (HCC 59 Reactive and Unspecified Psychosis, and HCC 60 Personality Disorders, and the agency split HCC 56 into three separate HCCs. Since these changes were released mid-year, they could impact the data already captured or submitted. Changes in the structure of an HCC category, moving a condition to a different HCC, and removing a condition from an HCC do not take much work on the part of the MA organization or physician/hospital office; these codes will be removed if they are submitted to CMS.

A code or code set being added does take more work. It is best to re-review charts that have been audited or coded to ensure all diagnoses that are risk adjusted have been captured. If organizations have historical data, they may want to target members who have a historical diagnosis on file to see if that condition, which has been added to the conditions list of conditions which risk adjusts, is still present. Additionally, an organization may track diagnoses that have been removed from the HCC model internally; this may assist with capturing the condition if it is added back into the model. For example, chronic kidney disease, stage 3, was added back into the CMS-HCC model for calendar year 2019. Prior to that, it was removed from the model, added to the Rx-HCC model, and subsequently was removed from that model as well. Some healthcare organizations chose to track this condition internally, because they were focused on improving the outcomes for those patients. With this condition being added back into the model, most organizations will want to re-review their charts to ensure that this condition is captured.

The tables included in this reference, which are also available in the online companion, are accurate based on the data and information released in the Final Notice. The information on how to access these tables and data files can be found on page 2 of this book.

Coding Guidelines Discussion

The update to the *ICD-10-CM Official Guidelines for Coding and Reporting*, section 1.A.19 has caused a great deal of controversy. This guideline states: "The assignment of a diagnosis code is based on the provider's diagnostic statement that the condition exists. The provider's statement that the patient has a particular condition is sufficient. Code assignment is not based on clinical criteria used by the provider to establish the diagnosis." It should be noted that the rule has always been that physician documentation of a condition is required in order for it to be coded. This guideline emphasizes that a physician or provider's documentation of a condition is required to code the condition and that it is the responsibility of the physician or provider to ensure that documentation is complete, accurate, and appropriate; not the coder or other staff.

The *AHA Coding Clinic* in the Fourth Quarter 2016 edition indicated that the guideline addresses accurate coding, not clinical validation, which is a separate function from the coding process. The codes assigned by a coder are based on the documentation by the physician, rather than a particular clinical definition or criteria.

In CMS's *MedLearn Matters* Article SE1121, the direction given is "as with all codes, clinical evidence should be present in the medical record to support code assignment."

The ICD-10-CM guidelines also state: "A joint effort between the healthcare provider and the coder is essential to achieve complete and accurate documentation, code assignment, and reporting of diagnoses and procedures. These guidelines have been developed to assist both the healthcare provider and the coder in identifying those diagnoses that are to be reported. The importance of consistent, complete documentation in the medical record cannot be overemphasized. Without such documentation accurate coding cannot be achieved. The entire record should be reviewed to determine the specific reason for the encounter and the conditions treated."

Tools

From a coder's perspective, it may be difficult to determine what conditions co-exist and affect the treatment or management of a patient. Ideally, the provider would document all current conditions with a status and plan of care. Unfortunately, this ideal scenario can take a lot of time and training with the medical staff. There are two common tools specific to risk adjustment that can assist a coder with deciphering if a condition is appropriately documented and, therefore, appropriate to report. Both of these tools are similar and their usage is personal or organizational preference but is not required. They are represented by the mnemonics **MEAT** and **TAMPER**, which are reviewed in more detail on the following page.

- **MEAT**

  - **M**onitor
    Example
    A/P: CKD IV is stable with GFR done today with result of 27. Repeat GFR in six months.

  - **E**valuation
    Example
    Exam: abnormal heart rhythm. EKG ordered.

  - **A**ssessment
    Example
    BMI: 66, patient is morbidly obese.

  - **T**reatment
    Example
    New COPD. Start DuoNeb and Symbicort.

OR

- **TAMPER**

  - **T**reatment
    Example
    Newly diagnosed diabetic patient. Start on sliding scale insulin and metformin

  - **A**ssessment
    Example
    Screening bloodwork shows A1C of 8. Patient is new onset type II diabetic.

  - **M**onitor
    Example
    Patient with uncontrolled DM. A1C today is 9.2, repeat in one month.

  - **P**lan
    Example
    Reminded diabetic patient of importance of regularly testing blood sugar and using sliding scale insulin and carb counting.

  - **E**valuate
    Example
    Diabetic food exam: diminished sensation in bilateral feet with monofilament.

  - **R**eferral
    Example
    Impression: Uncontrolled DM. Refer patient to Endocrinology and Diabetic Educator for further care.

Having knowledge of treatments, medications, therapies, and tests associated with various conditions is imperative when evaluating documentation for risk adjustment purposes. This, however, does not mean that a coder or other allied staff is to be tasked with evaluating the clinical decision making of the documenting provider or the care being provided.

Coders should consider adding an additional element to these tools: **Specificity**. There are several official coding guidelines that mention specificity. For example, ICD-10-CM guideline I.B.2. Level of Detail in Coding, states: "Diagnosis codes are to be used and reported at their highest number of characters available and to the highest level of specificity documented in the medical record." This is similar to guideline IV.F., which states: "Code to the highest level of specificity when supported by the medical record."

Example

> Active problems: COPD followed by pulm, DM getting A1C today, OA continue NSAIDs
>
> A/P: annual exam, encounter for vaccines. RTC in 1 year or PRN

In this example, the COPD and diabetes would both be valid to code for this patient for risk adjustment. While the provider did not document these in the assessment or plan portion of the note, there is a plan for each of these in the active problems list. Documenting that the patient is followed by a pulmonologist for COPD validates that this condition is active and requires treatment. The diabetes mellitus (DM) is validated as an active condition by the provider ordering a lab test to monitor the A1C of the patient.

The supporting documentation to validate a chronic condition does not need to be exhaustive, cumbersome, or an undue burden to the documenting provider, but the more information that is provided, the better the continuity of care for the patient. Using the same note as before, here is how the note could be improved. See page 26 for a list of conditions, which are generally considered chronic and, are therefore, unlikely to be resolved.

Example

> Active problems: COPD followed by pulm, DM getting A1C today, OA continue NSAIDs
>
> *Exam: breath sounds decreased on resp exam, O2 sats 82% RA, pedal pulses intact, normal capillary refill*
>
> A/P: annual exam, encounter for vaccines. *COPD is stable on current Rx, patient sees pulm quarterly; consider supplemental O2 for low room air saturations. DM is stable on metformin, patient to continue regular BS checks, will call with A1C results* RTC in 1 year or PRN.

In the improved documentation, the provider has added additional documentation that further supports that these conditions are active. The physical exam has findings that also support these conditions. The assessment and plan portions of the note give more details into the plan of care discussed with the patient during the encounter.

Clinical Documentation Integrity

The expansion of clinical documentation programs and new technologies such as electronic health record (EHR) "clinical alerts" and Natural Language Understanding (NLU) or Natural Language Processing (NLP) technologies have resulted in the need for prospective clinical documentation health record reviews.

Prospective reviews are performed before the patient is seen by the provider, with the goal of identifying chronic conditions using documentation from previous encounters, medication lists, abnormal laboratory values, etc. These new technologies can be used to prompt providers with "documentation alerts" to be more specific in their documentation, but these alerts still need to be reviewed by a clinical documentation specialist and must be compliant with best practices for clarifying documentation in the legal medical record.

Discussion of the challenges of avoiding leading queries and introducing new information when conducting prospective reviews, as well as examples, are included in the AHIMA Practice Brief, "Prospective Clinical Documentation Integrity (CDI) Reviews and Query/Alert Practice Best Standards." This practice brief stresses the difference between documentation alerts designed to influence a provider's documentation versus a clinical alert for clinical decision-making at the time of entering the clinical information in the health record. It also stresses that the ICD-10-CM Official Guidelines for Coding and Reporting, Uniform Hospital Discharge Data Set (UHDDS) guidelines, and the practice brief "The Guidelines for Achieving a Compliant Query Practice Brief (2019 Update)" should still be followed.

Coding Scenarios with RAF Values

NOTE: RAF scores and calculations provided in this section are estimates using the 2020 Model Relative Factors only. They are provided for example only and are not intended to calculate actual reimbursement or recoupment values.

Coding Scenario 1—CMS-HCC Model

Electronically Signed: Dr. B. Johnson, D.O.

Patient Name: Betty Smith	**Appt. Date/Time:** 4/5/2021
Insurance: Medicare Advantage (HMO)	**Appt. Type:** MCE
Chief Complaint: Follow up hyperlipidemia, HTN, OA, MDD	

Vitals

BP: 134/71 sitting L arm	**BP Cuff Size:** adult	**Pulse:** 61 bpm regular
T: 97.8 F oral	**O2Sat:** 93% RA	**Ht:** 62 in
W: 200lbs	**BMI:** 36.6	

ROS

Patient reports no frequent nosebleeds, no nose problems, and no sinus problems: congestion. She reports dry mouth but reports no sore throat, no bleeding gums, no snoring, no mouth ulcers, and no teeth problems. She reports arthralgia/joint pain (right knee) but reports no muscle aches, no muscle weakness, no back pain, and no swelling in the extremities. She reports frequent or severe headaches but reports no loss of consciousness, no weakness, no numbness, no seizures, no dizziness, and no tremor. She reports fatigue. She reports no fever, no night sweats, no significant weight gain, no significant weight loss, and no exercise intolerance. She reports no dry eyes, no vision change, and no irritation. She reports no difficulty hearing and no ear pain. She reports no chest pain, no arm pain on exertion, no shortness of breath when walking, no shortness of breath when lying down, no palpitations, and no known heart murmur. She reports no cough, no wheezing, no shortness of breath, no coughing up blood. She reports no abdominal pain, no nausea, no vomiting, no constipation, normal appetite, no diarrhea, not vomiting blood, no dyspepsia, and no GERD. She reports no Incontinence, no difficulty urinating, no hematuria, and no increased frequency. She reports no abnormal mole, no jaundice, no rashes, and no laceration. She reports no depression, no sleep disturbances, feeling safe in a relationship, no alcohol abuse, no anxiety, no hallucinations, and no suicidal thoughts. She reports no swollen glands, no bruising, and no excessive bleeding. She reports no runny nose, no sinus pressure, no itching, no hives, and no frequent sneezing.

History—updated 04/05/2021

Breast cancer— stable, sees oncology, on tamoxifen for 2 years

Depressive disorder— major, partially managed on SSRI

OSA— refuses CPAP

Physical Exam

Patient is a 54-year-old female.

Constitutional
General Appearance: well-developed, appears stated age, and obese.

Level of Distress: comfortable.

Psychiatric
Mental Status: alert and normal affect.

Orientation: oriented to time, place, and person. Insight: good judgment.

Cardiovascular
Precordial Exam: no heaves or precordial thrills and non-displaced focal PMI. Rate and rhythm: regular.

Heart Sounds: no rub, gallop, or click and normal S1 and physiologically split S2.

- Systolic Murmur: not heard.
- Diastolic Murmur: not heard

Extremities
No cyanosis, edema, or peripheral signs of emboli

Neurologic
Motor: tremor of neck and face and arms

The provider should also be queried for E66.2 Morbid (severe) obesity with alveolar hypoventilation. The body mass index (BMI) is noted to be 36.6 on the DOS and the patient has comorbidities of hypertension, hyperlipidemia, and obstructive sleep apnea (OSA). Often, providers favor terms to describe obesity that do not validate morbid or severe obesity. It is important that documenting providers use the correct language to describe morbid or severe obesity. Terms such as Class I, II, or III are not terms found in the ICD-10-CM Index.

This note validates that the breast cancer is an active problem, which is being treated. The provider documented that the patient is undergoing treatment with tamoxifen and is seeing an oncology provider. The history portion of this note also shows that it was updated on the date of service (DOS).

Coding Scenario 1—CMS-HCC Model (Continued)

It is necessary to query the provider for additional information about the depression. There is insufficient documentation to code major depressive disorder in remission.

A/P

1. Mixed hyperlipidemia—continue meds
2. Benign essential hypertension—continue meds
3. Insomnia—discussed sleep hygiene/caffeine curfew
4. Anxiety/depression—continue meds/consider seeing psych
5. Obesity—discussed increasing activity and decreasing caloric intake

HCC Category	ICD-10-CM Code Description	RAF Value	Validated by Current Documentation	Improved Documentation
HCC 59	F33.41 Major depressive disorder, recurrent, in partial remission	0.309	No	Yes
HCC 12	C50.919 Malignant neoplasm of unspecified site of unspecified female breast	0.150	Yes	Yes
HCC 22	E66.2 Obesity hypoventilation syndrome (OHS)	0.250	No	Yes
Demographics	54-year-old, female, not Medicaid eligible	0.348	Yes	Yes
Total RAF			0.498	1.057

Condition note: The National Institutes of Health (NIH) uses the following criteria to determine if a patient is morbidly obese. These same criteria are used to validate medical necessity for procedures such as bariatric surgery; therefore, it is advised to ensure all documenting providers are aware of these criteria. According to the NIH, a patient whose BMI is 35 or more with comorbid conditions is at the same risk for developing obesity-related, complicating conditions as a patient whose BMI is 40 or more without comorbid conditions. These comorbid conditions are:

- Coronary heart disease

- History of

  - myocardial infarction

  - angina, stable or unstable

  - coronary artery surgery or procedures such as angioplasty

- Peripheral vascular disease/peripheral artery disease

- Abdominal aortic aneurysm

- Symptomatic carotid artery disease

- Hypertension

- Lipid disorders

- Type II diabetes mellitus

- Sleep apnea

- Gallstones and their complications

- Gynecological abnormalities

2021 Optum360, LLC

- Osteoarthritis

- Urinary stress incontinence

No query is required to report the code for BMI, since the provider documents a diagnosis of obesity. As noted in ICD-10-CM guideline I.C.21.c.3, "BMI codes should only be assigned when there is an associated, reportable diagnosis (such as obesity)." Also, according to ICD-10-CM guideline I.B.14, which states: "Code assignment is based on the documentation by the patient's provider (i.e., physician or other qualified healthcare practitioner legally accountable for establishing the patient's diagnosis). There are a few exceptions when code assignment may be based on medical record documentation from clinicians who are not the patient's provider (i.e., physician or other qualified healthcare practitioner legally accountable for establishing the patient's diagnosis). In this context, 'clinicians' other than the patient's provider refer to healthcare professionals permitted, based on regulatory or ICD-10-CM accreditation requirements or internal hospital policies, to document in a patient's official medical record.

"These exceptions include codes for:

- Body Mass Index (BMI)

- Depth of non-pressure chronic ulcers

- Pressure ulcer stage

- Coma scale

- NIH stroke scale (NIHSS)

- Social determinants of health (SDOH)

- Laterality

- Blood alcohol level

"This information is typically, or may be, documented by other clinicians involved in the care of the patient (e.g., a dietitian often documents the BMI, a nurse often documents the pressure ulcer stages, and an emergency medical technician often documents the coma scale). However, the associated diagnosis (such as overweight, obesity, acute stroke, pressure ulcer, or a condition classifiable to category F10, Alcohol related disorders) must be documented by the patient's provider. If there is conflicting medical record documentation, either from the same clinician or different clinicians, the patient's attending provider should be queried for clarification.

"The BMI, coma scale, NIHSS, blood alcohol level codes and codes for social determinants of health should only be reported as secondary diagnoses."

Coding Scenario 2—CMS-HCC Model

Patient Name: Donald Johnson   **Visit Date/Time:** 9/3/2021

Sex: M   **Age:** 77 years

Chief Complaint
Presents for annual wellness visit

History of Present Illness
Don is an established patient in our office. He is here today for his annual wellness visit. He is doing well on current medication and treatment and there will be no change to current treatment. He is active but has no formal exercise and was encouraged to increase the current level of exercise. Today, his BMI is 35.16 kg/m2, which is down from the most recent BMI of 36.38 kg/m2. The need for continued weight loss was DAL and current diet was assessed. There have been no hospital stays or injuries since the last visit.

Active Problems
Allergic rhinitis, arthritis, chronic kidney disease IV, chronic obstructive pulmonary disease, congestive heart failure, depression, type 2 diabetes, dizziness, hypertension, thrombocytopenia, restless leg syndrome, and vitamin B12 deficiency.

Medication List
Lisinopril, Lantus, Humalog, test strips, Brovana nebulizer, albuterol, CPAP, gabapentin, Wellbutrin SR, Lasix, Singulair, Tofranil, and Ultram

P/F/S history
No changes from AWV on 9/15/2020. Interval history reviewed with patient.

ROS
12-point system reviewed pertinent findings as below.

Resp—SOB, wheezing, DOE

CV—edema increased in legs

Psych—difficulty concentrating, increased tiredness

Neuro—decreased sensation in fingers/toes

Vital Signs

Date	BP	Position	HR	Temp (F)	WT	HT	BMI	BSA
9/3/21	130/69	sitting	106-r	97.6	259	6'0"	35.16	2.44

Exam
Constitutional: well-nourished/well-developed, NAD

HEENT: WNL, PERRL

Respiratory: labored breathing

CV: regular rate and rhythm

GI: WNL, no HSM

GU: deferred, patient refuses

Extremities: abnormal findings with monofilament on both feet, decreased sensation in fingers as well, marked edema in bilateral legs

Psych: PHQ-9 result 4, depressed mood, AOx3

Coding Scenario 2—CMS-HCC Model (Continued)

A/P

Physical Exam V70.0

Severe chronic kidney disease N18.4—sees specialist Dr. Jones

COPD J44.9—stable on current inhalers, considering O2 therapy, uses CPAP as directed

OA left knee M17.12—continues despite replacement surgery in 16, DAL can't take pain meds long term

DM E11.9—monitor BS, take Lantus/Humalog as directed

Edema R60.9—d/t CHF, continue Lasix

CHF I50.9—continue to see cardiology

Major depression F32.5—continue meds

Peripheral neuropathy G62.9—continue meds, DAL blood sugar control to prevent progression

Disposition: home, patient will call or return with any issues

Electronically Signed by: Samantha Fink, NPon 09/05/21

> Per ICD-10-CM coding guidelines, it is appropriate to link the chronic kidney disease and peripheral neuropathy to the diabetes since both of these conditions appear under the "with" directly under the main term "Diabetes" in the index.

> ICD-10-CM guidelines instruct to associate the hypertension, chronic kidney disease, and heart failure.

> It is necessary to query the provider for additional information about the depression. There is insufficient documentation to code major depressive disorder. Additionally, the provider has included the wrong ICD-10-CM code with the code description. The PHQ-9 result in the body of the progress note does not support the depression being resolved.

HCC Category	ICD-10-CM Code Description		RAF Value	Validated by Current Documentation	Improved Documentation
HCC 59	F33.41	Major depressive disorder, recurrent, in partial remission	0.309	No	Yes
HCC 18	E11.22	Type 2 diabetes mellitus with diabetic chronic kidney disease	0.302	Yes	Yes
	Disease Interaction DM + CHF		0.121	Yes	Yes
HCC 22	E66.2	Obesity hypoventilation syndrome (OHS)	0.250	No	Yes
HCC 85	I13.0	Hypertensive heart and chronic kidney disease with heart failure and stage 1 through stage 4 chronic kidney disease, or unspecified chronic kidney disease	0.331	Yes	Yes
HCC 85	I50.9	Heart failure, unspecified	0.000*	Yes	Yes
	Disease Interaction CHF + CKD		0.156	Yes	Yes
HCC 137	N18.4	Chronic kidney disease, stage 4 (severe)	0.289	Yes	Yes
	Disease Interaction CHF + COPD		0.155	Yes	Yes
HCC 111	J44.9	Chronic obstructive pulmonary disease, unspecified	0.335	Yes	Yes
Demographics	77-year-old, male, not Medicaid eligible		0.473	Yes	Yes
D4	4 Payment HCCs		0.006	Yes	Yes
D6	6 Payment HCCs		0.077	No	Yes
Total RAF				2.168	2.798

> *Each HCC category value is only reported/counted once per calendar year; since I13.0 is in the same HCC, the I50.9 would not add to the overall risk-adjustment factor for this patient. The disease interactions between the heart failure with chronic kidney disease, heart failure with COPD, and diabetes with heart failure are also reported.

Coding Scenario 3—CMS-HCC Model

Result type: History and Physical Note

Result date: January 11, 2021

Result status: Auth (Verified)

Result Title/Subject: History and Physical

Performed By/Author: Black MD, Brian on January 11, 2021

Verified By: Black MD, Brian on January 11, 2021

Encounter info: (IPE) Emergency IP, 1/11/2021–1/12/2021

* Final Report *

History and Physical

Patient: Miller, Paul C.   **Age:** 91 years

Sex: Male   **Associated Diagnoses:** None

Author: Black, MD Brian

Chief Complaint
Slurred speech, facial droop, fall

History of Present Illness
91-year-old M PMH significant for A-fib not on anticoagulation, HTN, asthma, colon CA s/p resection 2 years prior who is BIBA for acute onset of slurred speech, left lower facial droop following fall. Patient and wife note around 8:30 p.m. last night, he sustained a slow fall in his home. He is unsure if he lost balance but had difficulty standing back up on his own but was able to be seated into chair by his wife. He then noticed that he had a difficult time speaking and his wife noted he had a left lower facial droop. She suspected he has having a stroke and gave him approximately 250 mg of Aspirin. Wife then called EMS, and patient and wife both note that his symptoms were improving already in the ambulance. Symptoms were essentially resolved by the time he arrived to the ED here, which was approximately 30 mins after onset of symptoms. He had otherwise been feeling well except for a mild cough, which started about 10 days ago and has mostly resolved. He notes he was given a cough suppressant with Bactrim by PCP, which he has since completed. He otherwise denies any fevers, chills, dizziness, shortness of breath, chest pain, palpitations, nausea/vomiting, bowel changes, urinary changes, blood in stool.

Review of Systems
12 point ROS reviewed and negative except as above

Past Medical History
As noted above.

Allergies (1) Active Reaction
quinidine: Affects his liver

Social History
denies tobacco, quit in 1986

denies ETOH or drug use

Family History
Mother—colon CA

Brother—throat CA

Home Medications (6) Active
Atenolol 25 mg oral tablet; see instructions

Finasteride 5 mg oral tablet 5 mg = 1 tab, PO, daily

Loratadine 10 mg, PO, daily

Multivitamin 1 cap, PO, daily

Tamsulosin 0.4 mg oral capsule 0.4 mg = 1 cap, PO, daily

Unlisted Med; see instructions

Coding Scenario 3—CMS-HCC Model (Continued)

Current Vitals (past 48hrs, max 5 results)

Dt/Tm	Temp	BP	MAP	Pulse	RR	SpO2	FiO2	O2 Therapy
01/11/21 00:30	—	122/60	81	88	18	96%	—	Room air
01/11/21 00:11	—	129/58	82	78	18	96%	—	Room air
01/10/21 22:45	36.7	127/75	92	83	18	96%	—	Room air

Tmax 24 Hr: 36.7 DegC (98.1 DegF) 01/10/21 22:45 (Oral)

Tmax 36 Hr: 36.7 DegC (98.1 DegF) 01/10/21 22:45 (Oral)

BMI: 17.44 (01/10/2021 23:10)

> BMI is noted to be less than 19. The provider should be queried for malnutrition or other associated condition such as underweight.

Physical Examination

General: Awake, alert, NAD

HEENT: Normo-cephalic, atraumatic; PERRL. Extraocular muscles are intact, sclera non-icteric

Neck: Trachea midline

Lungs: Clear to auscultation bilaterally

Cardiac: Irregular rate/rhythm, S1 and S2 with no murmurs

Abdomen: Soft, non-tender and non-distended with good bowel sounds

Extremities: No cyanosis or edema

Skin: No rashes or lesion

Neurological: Cranial nerves II through XII grossly intact; motor: 5/5 throughout large muscle groups; sensation-intact throughout; cerebellar: finger to nose wnl; alert and oriented to person, place and time

Psychiatric Evaluation

Normal mood and affect, normal judgment and insight

All Results (36 Hrs):

All labs personally reviewed.

Radiology Results (Past 36 Hours): CT Head w/o Contrast STROKE CO

Performed By/Author: Dr. Moore, MD Sandra M.

Impression: Subtle hyperintensity within an insular branch of the left middle cerebral artery may reflect vessel occlusion or atherosclerotic calcification. Recommend CTA head. No acute intracranial hemorrhage is appreciated. No definite acute parenchymal changes are identified. Probable left basal ganglia infarct. These findings were discussed with Dr. Moore, MD.

XR Hip 2 View Left + Pelvis

Performed By/Author: Dr. Moore, MD Sandra M

Impression: No acute abnormality.

XR Chest 1 View

Performed By/Author: Dr. Moore, MD Sandra M.

Impression: Multifocal airspace opacities suspicious for pneumonia. Recommend follow-up to resolution.

CTA Head/Neck w/ Con STROKE CO

Performed By/Author: Dr. Moore, MD Sandra M.

Impression: Focal complete occlusion of a left middle cerebral artery M2 insular branch. Findings correspond to the dense artery on the non-contrast head CT. 50% right ICA stenosis and 60% left ICA stenosis in the neck. Patchy upper lobe airspace opacities suggestive of multifocal pneumonia. These findings were discussed with Dr. Moore, MD Sandra M.

Coding Scenario 3—CMS-HCC Model (Continued)

Assessment/Plan:

91-year-old M PMH significant for A-fib not on anticoagulation, HTN, asthma, colon CA s/p resection 2 years prior who is BIBA from for acute onset of slurred speech, left lower facial droop following fall.

1. Stroke
   - symptoms resolved
   - CT head with left basal ganglia infarct
   - CTA head/neck w/ focal complete occlusion of left MCA M2 insular branch, 60% left ICA stenosis, 50% right ICA stenosis
   - Neurology consulted in ED—appreciate further recs
   - ASA, statin
   - check MRI brain
   - check 2d echo w/ bubble study
   - PT/OT eval
   - allow for permissive HTN first 24 hrs.

2. Permanent atrial fibrillation—rate controlled
   - not on anticoagulation, dx in late 1980s and has not been on anticoagulation since for > 25 years
   - CHADS2 vasc score of 5 and would likely be candidate for anticoagulation if bleeding risk not significantly elevated
   - will defer timing of anticoagulation to neurology, await MRI results

3. Multifocal PNA—largely asymptomatic
   - incidentally noted on CXR, CTA neck
   - reports recent tx w/ Bactrim
   - possibly remnant of recent PNA; however, given leukocytosis, imaging findings and tx w/ only Bactrim recently, will tx
   - ceftriaxone/doxy
   - f/u sputum cx, pna serologies

4. HTN
   - allow permissive HTN up to SBP 220 first 24 hrs.
   - hold atenolol

5. Chronic asthma
   - no exacerbation > 70 years per patient
   - uses inhalers bid, prn

6. hx colon CA s/p resection 2 years ago
   - pt reports taking vitamins and holistic cures
   - Oncology recs appreciated

FEN/ppx: heart healthy diet, ivsl/SCDS

full code full care: discussed with patient at bedside

> It is necessary to query the provider for additional information about the chronic asthma. There is insufficient documentation to code COPD.

HCC Category	ICD-10-CM Code Description		RAF Value	Validated by Current Documentation	Improved Documentation
HCC 100	I63.9	Cerebral infarction, unspecified	0.380	Yes	Yes
HCC 96	I48.21	Permanent atrial fibrillation	0.384	Yes	Yes
HCC 21	E46	Unspecified protein-calorie malnutrition	0.693	No	Yes
HCC 11	C18.9	Malignant neoplasm of colon, unspecified	0.317	Yes	Yes
HCC 111	J44.9	Chronic obstructive pulmonary disease, unspecified	0.430	No	Yes
Demographics	91-year-old, male, Medicaid eligible		1.142	Yes	Yes
D3	3 Payment HCCs		—	Yes	Yes
D5	5 Payment HCCs		0.042	No	Yes
Total RAF				2.301	3.402

> There is an additional RAF value added for the Medicaid eligibility, which adds to this patient's risk-adjustment factor.

Coding Scenario 4—CMS-HCC Model

Patient: Joe Holmes   **DOS:** 01/23/2021   **Ins:** Medicare

DR: Robert Jacobs, M.D.   **Age:** 78 years

CC:
Annual wellness visit

Subjective
Patient seen for annual wellness visit. He had a colonoscopy in 2016. He refuses the flu vaccine. Patient is compliant with DM management. Patient complains of wound on his leg for 10 days. Med list reviewed in EMR module. No changes to P/F/S hx from last AWV. Patient regularly sees oncology. Today wants to discuss other treatment options. PHQ-9 score is 4. Upset about mets.

Objective
Alert, no acute distress, HEENT:NC, pupils equal, round, sclera white, conj. clear, external nose WNL, on O2 nasal cannula, no lesions, external ear normal, lips/mouth free of lesions, Neuro: no tremor, Neck: trachea midline normal appearance, MS: normal gait and posture, Ext: no edema or clubbing, poss claudication, ulcer noted on distal left calf r/o venous stasis, skin: No rash or lesions, L diminished bs, no wheezing, Hrrr no m/r/c, Abd soft nt +bs.

Assessment
Poss claudication/leg ulcer, bone and lymph mets, prostate ca, DM, IBS, resp insuff syndrome.

Plan
Get ABI—r/o claudication w/ ulcer. DAL patient needs to speak to oncologist about tx for mets and continue "watchful waiting" on prostate ca. Patient is compliant on DM regime, continue. Refer to GI for IBS. Dependent on home O$_2$ increase 5L.

HCC Category	ICD-10-CM Code Description		RAF Value	Validated by Current Documentation	Improved Documentation
HCC 12*	C61	Malignant neoplasm of prostate	0.150	Yes	Yes
HCC 8	C79.51	Secondary malignant neoplasm of bone	2.659	Yes	Yes
HCC 10*	C77.9	Secondary and unspecified malignant neoplasm of lymph node, unspecified	0.675	Yes	Yes
HCC 108	I73.9	Peripheral vascular disease, unspecified	0.288	No	Yes
HCC 18	E11.51	Type 2 diabetes mellitus with diabetic peripheral angiopathy without gangrene	0.302	No	Yes
HCC 59	F32.1	Major depressive disorder, single episode, moderate	0.309	No	Yes
HCC 84	J96.11	Chronic respiratory failure with hypoxia	0.282	No	Yes
Demographics	78-year-old, male, not Medicaid eligible		0.473	Yes	Yes
D1	1 Payment HCC		—	Yes	Yes
D5	5 Payment HCCs		0.042	No	Yes
Total RAF				3.132	4.355

The provider should be queried for major depressive disorder based on the PHQ-9 score 0-4, indicating minimal or no depression.

ICD-10-CM I73.9 is not validated by this note. The provider has indicated that claudication is possible. The provider should be queried for validation of this condition if it exists.

The provider should be queried for chronic respiratory failure and underlying condition. The patient is noted to be dependent on oxygen and the oxygen is being increased. The documentation of "resp insuff syndrome" cannot be indexed in ICD-10-CM, and respiratory insufficiency is a symptom, reported with code R06.89 Other abnormalities of breathing.

*The CMS-HCC trumping logic applies to HCC 12 and HCC 10. Conditions in HCC 8 trump conditions in HCC 10 and HCC 12. Therefore, in this example, the values of HCC 10 and HCC 12 would not be factored into the patient's risk score.

Coding Scenario 5—ESRD-HCC Model

Patient: Diaz, Jenny

Age: 60 years	**Sex:** Female
Associated Diagnoses: None	**Author:** Moore MD, Samuel
DOS: 1/7/2021	**Chief Complaint:** hypotension

History of Present Illness

60-year-old F w/ h/o ESRD on ihd MWF, CAD s/p CABG, a-fib on Eliquis, DM2 , asthma, htn, HL, depression, GERD who p/w hypotension. Her SBP was noted to be in the 80s at the end of dialysis. Her sugar was noted to be in the 40s and her K+ was 2.8. Pt c/o feeling SOB for the past 1 day. C/o mild productive cough. She also notes having several loose stools starting last night. Also c/o generalized body aches and subjective fevers for 2 days. Also w/ R sided frontal headache and neck pain. Denies any recent trauma. Denies recent travel or sick contacts. Denies chills/night sweats/abdominal pain/nausea/vomiting//urinary symptoms/headache/weight loss/visual changes/neck pain.

Review of Systems

12 point ROS reviewed and negative except as stated in HPI

Problem List

Active Problems:

ESRD on ihd MWF, CAD s/p CABG, afib, dm2, asthma, htn, HL, depression, GERD

Past Medical History

See above.

Past Surgical History

CABG

Social History

Denies alcohol use.

Denies tobacco use.

Denies illicit drug use.

Family History

Father w/ HTN

Allergies

NKA

Home Medications (14) Active

Acetaminophen 650 mg, PRN, PO, Q4H

Acyclovir 400 mg oral tablet 800 mg = 2 tab, PO, BID

Aspirin 81 mg, PO, daily

Atorvastatin 10 mg oral tablet 10 mg = 1 tab, PO, daily

Carvedilol 3.125 mg oral tablet 3.125 mg = 1 tab, PO, BIDCC

Crestor 10 mg, PO, daily

Eliquis 2.5 mg, PO, BID

Escitalopram 10 mg oral tablet 10 mg = 1 tab, PO, daily

Gabapentin 100 mg oral capsule 100 mg = 1 cap, PO, TID

Insulin aspart; see scale, SC, AC (before meals)

Metoprolol tartrate 25 mg, PO, BID

Pantoprazole 40 mg, PO, QHS

Senna 8.6 mg oral tablet 17.2 mg = 2 tab, PO, daily

Vancomycin per pharmacy 500 mg = 100 mL, IVPB, Q999H

Vitals

Temp (Oral) 36.9 DegC (98.4 DegF) BP 90/61 mmHg Pulse 96 bpm RR 18 br/min

Coding Scenario 5—ESRD-HCC Model (Continued)

Physical Examination

General: NAD, pleasant, aox3, slightly lethargic but easily arousable

HEENT: PERRL, EOMI, MMM, OP clear

Neck: no thyromegaly, supple, no LAD

CV: RRR, nl s1, s2, no mrg, JVP non-elevated

Pulm: crackles at bases b/l, normal non-labored breathing

ABD: +BS, soft, non-tender, non-distended, no rebound or guarding

Extremities: no cyanosis/clubbing/edema

Neuro: moves all extremities equally, no focal deficits

Labs:

personally reviewed/WNL

Radiology (Past 36 Hours):

XR: Chest 2 Views

Performed By/Author: Johnson MD, Howard M

Impression

Extensive nodular infiltrate throughout the right lung

Fibrotic changes noted in both lungs consistent with pulmonary fibrosis

EKG

None

Assessment/Plan

60-year-old F w/ h/o ESRD on ihd MWF, CAD s/p CABG, Afib not on anticoag b/c fall risk, dm2, asthma, htn, HL, depression, GERD who p/w hypotension, admitted w/ sepsis 2/2 HCAP.

1. Healthcare associated bacterial pneumonia—meets sepsis criteria
    - vancomycin/Zosyn
    - f/u sputum culture
    - f/u blood cultures
    - oxygen protocol
    - urinary strep and legionella ag
    - consult ID
    - influenza screen +
    - trend lactate
2. Hypokalemia
    - replete K+ PRN
3. Diarrhea
    - stool cx
    - c-diff
4. ESRD
    - cont ihd
    - cont home meds
    - consult renal
5. Diabetes mellitus type 2
    - hold home oral hypoglycemics
    - place patient on insulin sliding scale
    - diabetes nurse practitioner consult
6. CAD s/p CABG
7. Afib
    - cont Eliquis
8. anemia
    - check iron levels

> Pulmonary fibrosis belongs to HCC 112. This should not be reported based upon this record because the condition is only noted in the radiology report of the chest x-ray. The attending/treating physician does not address this finding in any other portion of the note. This condition would need further validation to be reported as an HCC for this patient.

> The provider has indicated that she is admitted with sepsis due to healthcare-associated bacterial pneumonia (HCAP), but has also documented that the "patient meets sepsis criteria, and that there is a positive result to the influenza screening." Further clarification would be needed from the physician to validate a condition from HCC 2.

Coding Scenario 5—ESRD-HCC Model (Continued)

Assessment/Plan (Continued)

9. asthma
10. HTN—hold home anti-hypertensives given hypotension
11. Hyperlipidemia—continue statin
12. GERD
    - continue PPI
13. Depression
    - cont home meds

FEN Regular cardiac diabetic renal diet

Prophylaxis—SCDs

Code FCFC

I attest that this patient will require >2 midnight stay due to the nature of the above stated medical conditions.

Result date: January 7, 2021

Result status: Auth (Verified)

Result Title/Subject: History and Physical

Performed By/Author: Moore MD, Samuel on January 7, 2021

Verified By: Moore MD, Samuel on January 7, 2021

HCC Category	ICD-10-CM Code Description		RAF Value	Validated by Current Documentation	Improved Documentation
HCC 58	F32.4	Major depressive disorder, single episode, in partial remission	0.092	No	Yes
HCC 18	E11.22	Type 2 diabetes mellitus with diabetic chronic kidney disease	0.093	Yes	Yes
HCC 136	N18.6	End stage renal disease	0.000*	Yes	Yes
HCC 134	Z99.2	Dependence on renal dialysis	0.000*	Yes	Yes
HCC 136	I12.0	Hypertensive chronic kidney disease with stage 5 chronic kidney disease or end stage renal disease	0.000*	Yes	Yes
HCC 96	I48.91	Unspecified atrial fibrillation	0.094	Yes	Yes
HCC 112	J84.10	Pulmonary fibrosis, unspecified	0.067	No	Yes
HCC 2	A41.9	Sepsis, unspecified organism	0.083	Yes	Yes
Demographics	66-year-old, female, ESRD		0.647	Yes	Yes
Total RAF				0.917	1.076

Sidebar notes:

ICD-10-CM guidelines when hypertension is reported for a patient with chronic kidney disease stage 5 or end stage, use I12.0.

It is necessary to query the provider for additional information about the depression. There is insufficient documentation to code major depressive disorder.

*The ESRD-HCC trumping logic applies to HCC 136. Conditions in HCC 134 trump conditions in HCC 136. So in this example, the RAF value of HCC 136 would not be factored into the patient's risk score.

Clinical Documentation Improvement Education

In today's healthcare environment, it is imperative to ensure that providers recognize that the medical record serves a variety of purposes. These include justification of billed charges, the record of the care or services that have been given to the patient, and also the documentation that affects the codes reported, which become part of statistical data used for quality assurance, research, grants, vital statistics, tumor registry, case management, and utilization management.

Clinical documentation is sometimes seen as a battlefield between clinicians and coding staff. Often, documentation is lacking the necessary details to properly code a claim. There are two main issues that play into this. The fee-for-service model compensated providers based almost solely on procedures performed. The diagnoses assigned were secondary at best and would only be cause for concern if reimbursement policies restricted the approved diagnoses for a particular procedure. The trend of risk-adjustment models has required more emphasis be placed on diagnostic coding and improvement in documentation. In addition to accurately describing the patient's condition, which can validate medical necessity, including any co-existing diagnoses, can validate more complex procedures or services that can result in higher reimbursement. The second issue is that most physicians see the additional work of providing additional clinical detail as having no reward for their extra work. An effective CDI program will give clinicians the requisite tools, which ideally, will cut down on queries and other post-encounter reviews.

Risk-adjustment programs offer additional motivation to improve documentation. As the examples on pages 32–43 demonstrated, more complete documentation can lead to a better description of the health of the beneficiary. About one third of Medicare beneficiaries are currently enrolled in a Medicare Advantage (MA) plan. The payments to these MA plans are capitated, per-member, per-month and the rates are adjusted based on the health status of the patients. A common trend for MA plans, which are allowed to keep a portion of the premiums, not spent on care, is to allow providers to participate in gain sharing. Gain sharing allows participating providers to share in the revenues from the health plan. MA plans recognize that provider documentation is one of the main factors in the revenue of that health plan and often offer tools, trainings, and incentives for improving documentation.

In the table below, assume that the baseline RAF score of 1.0 equates to $700 per-month, per-member.

CMS-HCC Payment Example

No Conditions Coded (Demographics Only)		Some Conditions Coded (Claims Data Only)		All Conditions Coded (Chart Reviewed by Certified Coder)	
76-year-old female	0.451	76-year-old female	0.451	76-year-old female	0.451
Medicaid eligible	0.142	Medicaid eligible	0.142	Medicaid eligible	0.142
DM not coded	0.000	DM coded	0.105	DM w/ hyperglycemia coded	0.302
CHF not coded	0.000	CHF not coded	0.000	CHF coded	0.331
COPD not coded	0.000	Asthma coded	0.000	COPD coded	0.225
Morbid obesity not coded	0.000	Obesity coded	0.000	Morbid obesity coded	0.250
Total RAF	0.613	Total RAF	0.721	Total RAF	2.131
PMPM payment for care	$429	PMPM payment for care	$505	PMPM payment for care	$1,492
Yearly Reserve for Care	$5,149	Yearly Reserve for Care	$6,060	Yearly Reserve for Care	$17,900

The impact of good documentation can be profound within risk adjustment models. The preceding graphic may lead one to assume that the push for good documentation from MA plans is motivated by the desire to make a profit. This is a half-correct assumption; the health plan is reliant on this good documentation to ensure that there is funding from CMS to appropriately provide for the care the plan beneficiaries need. If documentation is lacking, the MA plan will have to cover any deficit from the CMS payments. Additionally, the majority of the profits an insurance company may get through risk adjustment are mandated to go to plan improvement, which could be the addition of other services such as transportation benefits for beneficiaries. It is very common for the portion not spent on plan improvements to be incorporated into a gain sharing arrangement with contracted providers.

As previously mentioned, the completeness of the documentation should not be burdensome to the provider. Typically, a few more words or sentences can vastly improve documentation.

Nonspecific Coding Example

76-year old white female presents today for routine follow up.

During exam, noticed a wound on patient's ankle. Patient states it has been hurting and she has been taking Tylenol to help with the pain. Does appear to have some yellowing tissue at the bottom. Will prescribe Norco to assist in pain management and refer patient to wound specialist.

Patient's diabetes is stable. A1C measured today was at 6.2 percent, patient says she has been trying hard to eat a balanced diet. Continuing Metformin 500 mg at twice per day.

Patient's coronary artery disease is stable. Recommend that she continue regular follow up and medicine regimen as recommended by her cardiologist.

Advised patient to follow up with me in 4 weeks or sooner if wound worsens.

Element	RAF Value
76-year-old female	0.451
Medicaid eligible	0.142
Diabetes w/out complications	0.107
Total	0.700

Specific Coding Example

A 76-year-old white female presents today for routine follow up.

During exam, noticed a *diabetic ulcer* on patient's left ankle. Patient states it has been hurting and she has been taking Tylenol to help with the pain. Does appear to have some yellowing fat tissue exposed at the bottom. Will prescribe Norco to assist in pain management and refer patient to wound specialist. Wound is attributed to patient's existing but otherwise stable *atherosclerosis due to diabetes. Patient has had previous amputation of left great toe due to other diabetic vascular complications*.

Patient's diabetes is stable. A1C measured today was at 6.2 percent, patient says she has been trying hard to eat a balanced diet. Continuing Metformin 500 mg at twice per day.

Patient's *cardiac conditions of cardiomyopathy and CHF are stable*. Recommend that she continue regular follow up and medicine regimen as recommended by her cardiologist.

Advised patient to follow up with me in 4 weeks or sooner if *ulcer* worsens.

Element	RAF Value
76-year-old female	0.451
Medicaid eligible	0.142
Diabetes w/ vascular complications	0.340
Atherosclerosis of extremity w/ ulceration	1.724
Chronic Ulcer of Skin, Except Pressure	0.727
Cardiomyopathy	0.371
Disease interaction (DM+CHF)	0.192
CHF	Same HCC as cardiomyopathy
Amputation of great toe status	0.795
Total	3.742

As the specific coding example shows, the improvement in the documentation would not be taxing to the provider to accomplish. The second example contains pertinent details, which are impactful but did not require a significant effort on the part of the documenting provider.

ICD-10-CM

The transition from ICD-9-CM to ICD-10-CM increased the available diagnosis codes from about 13,000 codes to over 70,000 codes. During this transition from ICD-9-CM to ICD-10-CM, there was a major push for providers to be "more specific" in their documentation. The code set was expanded to include more detail about the conditions such as laterality. This push for the most specific documentation to describe a condition has caused some misunderstandings. In using the most specific language to describe a condition, a provider may provide details, which are very specific, but do not impact the specificity of the code being used to report that condition. It is imperative to any clinical documentation integrity (CDI) training, education, or discussion with providers to review the chapter-specific guidelines. Reviewing the chapter-specific guidelines for ICD-10-CM will give the providers more information about what is needed when they are asked to "be more specific."

Example

Assessment: complex migraine with LUE weakness and tinnitus, hypertension

Plan: No evidence of CVA/TIA on MRI. Referral to neurology given.

In the ICD-10-CM index, under the term "migraine," the term "complex" does not appear, nor does "with LUE weakness" or "tinnitus." A good CDI program will focus on the chapter-specific guidelines for coding to ensure that the specific documentation the provider is giving contains information that will enable the most specific code to be selected. In this example, the provider should have been educated to describe migraines using some of the following terms: with or without refractory migraine, intractable or not intractable, with or without aura, menstrual, etc. In this example, the provider has described a very specific patient experience, which could be his or her understanding of the coding or CDI request for "more specific information."

The ICD-10-CM book includes the chapter-specific guidelines, which should be reviewed and discussed as part of a CDI education or training. The chapter-specific guidelines specify what type of detail is needed for conditions within that chapter. For example, chapter 4, "Endocrine, Nutritional, and Metabolic diseases" indicates that for diabetes, a provider should document:

- Type of diabetes

- Additional codes to assign for the use of insulin, oral hypoglycemics, and injectable non-insulin drugs

- As many codes as necessary to report the associated conditions present

This set of specific criteria is not applicable to conditions found in chapter 5, "Mental, Behavioral, and Neurodevelopmental Disorders." In chapter 5, the specifics necessary to code the most specific condition include:

- Status, including in remission

- Guidance on use, abuse, and dependence reporting

Reviewing these chapter specific-guidelines will ensure that CDI education is more meaningful and impactful to improve documentation.

Queries

The update to the *ICD-10-CM Official Guidelines for Coding and Reporting,* section 1.A.19 has caused a lot of controversy. *AHA Coding Clinic*, Fourth Quarter 2016, p 147 clarified this saying: "This guideline is not a new concept, although it had not been explicitly included in the official coding guidelines until now. *Coding Clinic* and the official coding guidelines have always stated that code assignment should be based on provider documentation. As has been repeatedly stated in *Coding Clinic* over the years, diagnosing a patient's condition is solely the responsibility of the provider. Only the physician, or other qualified healthcare practitioner legally accountable for establishing the patient's diagnosis, can 'diagnose' the patient." This guideline emphasizes that the physician or provider's documentation of a condition is required to code it and that it is the responsibility of the physician or provider to ensure that documentation is complete, accurate, and appropriate; not the coder or other staff. In a recent American Health Information Management Association (AHIMA) brief, the guidance given states:

"When a practitioner documents a diagnosis that does not appear to be supported by the clinical indicators in the health record, it is currently advised that a query be generated to address the conflict or that the conflict be addressed through the facility's escalation policy." Similar advice was also given by the *AHA Coding Clinic* and CMS.

The bottom line is that when the documentation is unclear, incomplete, or conflicting, the provider needs to be queried for more information, if possible.

The following five criteria should be used when reviewing documentation and in determining whether a query is necessary:

- **Legibility:** Poor penmanship, improper use of photocopies, poor document scans, "cut and paste" errors, use of templates, or improperly correcting an error in a medical record can cause problems with legibility, omissions, or additions in text that can result in errors of documentation and code assignment. Does a condition warrant reporting that is a result of "cut and paste" documentation from a previous encounter problem list not addressed on the current encounter?

- **Consistency:** Documentation that is conflicting, inadequate, incomplete, ambiguous, or inconsistent: is the condition exacerbated or is it stable; was the suspected condition ruled out; what is the clinical significance of the abnormal test results; or, does the provider confirm the consultant's diagnosis?

- **Relationships:** Clinical indicators noted without a stated related diagnosis, diagnostic work-up without stated reason, treatment without identified indication or manifestations not linked to an underlying cause: does the notation ↑Na represent a clinically significant diagnosis; what is the reason for the need of continuous O2; what was the indication and final conclusion for the performance of a glucose test; is the ulcer due to a complication of the underlying diabetes?

- **Specificity:** Clinical results, including pathology reports, response to treatment, and/or the patient's clinical condition suggest a more specific diagnosis or level of severity than is documented: based on culture and sensitivity and patient response to treatment, can the condition be further specified as to a causative organism; can the post-op/final diagnosis be further specified due to the pathology report findings; based on the pathology report findings, which additional sites of metastasis are clinically significant?

- **Clinical validation:** There is lack of clinical data or insufficient indicator(s) are met to support a diagnosis or its degree of specificity; the decision to query may require a review by a clinician: does the PACU note stating "post-op respiratory failure" during the routine post-op intubation period without correlating clinical indicators represent a complication due to surgery, other condition, or an expected outcome immediately post-surgery; is the diagnosis of acute exacerbation supported by clinical findings, adjustment of regimen/treatment or clinical manifestation?

After determining that a query is needed, there is additional guidance that should be followed. The main concern is not initiating leading queries. A leading query could cause incorrect code assignment. A leading query is considered to be a query that is not supported by clinical elements within the health record and/or that directs a provider to a specific diagnosis.

A query should not:

- Lead the clinician to a specific diagnosis

- Introduce new information

- Directly or indirectly reference any financial impact of the query response

In risk adjustment, this would include indicating:

- The HCC status of a condition

- The RAF value or HCC category of the HCCs included in the query

Example

Documentation: CXR revealed RLL PNA. Clindamycin ordered.

Dr. Diaz,

Is the patient's pneumonia due to aspiration?

Thanks,

HIM Dept.

This query is an example of a leading query because the coder is directing the provider to a specific diagnosis.

AHIMA provided a practice brief on queries, which was updated in 2019. Within this brief, the use of open-ended queries was indicated as being the preferred format but that multiple choice and/or "yes/no" queries are also acceptable under certain circumstances.

All queries must contain the relevant clinical indicator(s) that demonstrate why a more complete or accurate diagnosis is being requested. The *AHA Coding Clinic* often references clinical indicators associated with particular diagnoses, but it is not an authoritative source for establishing the clinical indicators of a given diagnosis. The clinical indicators used to substantiate a query may include elements from the entire medical record, which may include diagnostic findings or provider impressions and should be from the medical record for the specified encounter.

Of the various acceptable query formats, the open-ended question is the most desirable to use because it requires the responder to use his or her clinical judgment to interpret the clinical indicators without prompting. The multiple choice format is very popular because this format is typically quicker to resolve; the responder reviews the clinical indicator(s) and makes a selection based on his or her clinical knowledge. It is important to note that providing a new diagnosis, which is reasonable based on the included clinical indicators, is not considered to be introducing new information. With the multiple choice format, it is imperative to include choices such as "undetermined," "other" with space to explain, or "not clinically significant," in addition to the reasonable diagnosis options. These additional choices should also be available when using the "yes/no" query format. The caveat to the "yes/no" format is that it is not appropriate when a diagnosis has not been documented and there are only clinical indicators of the condition; new diagnoses cannot be determined from this query format.

Using the same query example as before, here is an example of a compliant, non-leading query.

Example

Documentation: CXR revealed RLL PNA. Clindamycin ordered.

Dr. Diaz,

The chest x-ray indicated that the patient has right lower lobe pneumonia. Speech therapy notes indicated that the patient had a weak swallow reflex and was at risk for aspiration. Using your clinical judgment, please determine the clinical significance of these findings, if any, and update the medical record with an addendum.

Thanks,

HIM Dept.

This query includes more relevant information but does not lead the provider to the aspiration pneumonia. This query uses the open-ended question format. It may be preferable to use the multiple-choice format, with the "other" option including a blank line for the physician to add free text to explain, which would look like this:

Example

Documentation: CXR revealed RLL PNA. Clindamycin ordered.

Dr. Diaz,

The chest x-ray indicated that the patient has right lower lobe pneumonia. Speech therapy notes indicated that the patient had a weak swallow reflex and was at risk for aspiration. Using your clinical judgment, please determine if the patient has:

__ pneumonia, unspecified   __ aspiration pneumonia

__ unable to determine   __ clinically insignificant

__ other, please explain _____

Thanks,

HIM Dept.

Internal Risk Adjustment Policies

The official guidance for risk-adjustment policies should be considered a minimum standard for risk-adjustment coding. Provider practices, facilities, MA plans, etc. may develop internal policies and standards that are more detailed than the official guidelines and that are to be used internally for quality or compliance efforts. Any internal policies created will need to be reviewed to ensure that they are consistent with the official guidelines and do not provide conflicting instructions. If conflicting information is found, the official guidance will take precedence.

An example of a common internal policy, which is stricter than the CMS guidance, is regarding what is considered validated and reportable. The CMS guidance for reporting a diagnosis for risk adjustment is that the condition must be validated by the note. It is common to find that a specific practice or insurance company may require that the physician document a plan of care for the condition to have it be reportable. This type of requirement is more common with insurance-company-employed physicians or within capitation models. Other common examples are requiring patients to be seen at least twice annually for a comprehensive exam or having specific protocols for treatment of specific diseases or conditions. For example, a provider group may require that diabetic patients have an A1C drawn every month instead of the more normal two to four times a year.

The Office of Inspector General (OIG) has developed the *Compliance Program Guidance for Individual and Small Group Physician Practices* to aid in preventing submission of erroneous claims and to combat fraudulent conduct. The agency has also issued compliance program guidance for a variety of other segments of the healthcare industry. These guides were developed to assist healthcare providers with monitoring adherence to applicable statutes, regulations and program requirements. Copies of these compliance program guidances can be found on the OIG website at https://oig.hhs.gov/.

The OIG lists the following six components as part of an effective voluntary compliance program.

- Conducting internal monitoring and auditing

- Implementing compliance and practice standards

- Designating a compliance officer or contact

- Responding appropriately to detected offenses and developing corrective action

- Developing open lines of communication

- Enforcing disciplinary standards through well-publicized

Following these steps can help providers to better protect their practices from potential erroneous or fraudulent conduct. In addition to helping better protect a practice, internal policies like these can assist with reducing billing mistakes, which can optimize the speed of payments. Designating a compliance officer or contact may ensure that the practice or office is up to date on regulatory information without having multiple people looking for the same answers.

Documentation Requirements

There are general principles of medical record documentation that are applicable to all types of medical and surgical services in all settings. The services provided may occur in different settings, physician offices, inpatient hospital, and outpatient ambulatory services within a hospital to name a few. The format of the documentation may vary as well. There are no regulatory standards as to how a record should look (e.g., header templates, location of dates), but there are elements that should be contained within the provider notes that support complete documentation of a face-to-face visit for coding and reporting. The medical record documentation serves as the source for coding. According to *AHA Coding Clinic*, "There are regulatory and accreditation directives that require providers to supply documentation in order to support code assignment. Providers need to have the ability to specifically document the patient's diagnosis, condition and/or problem. It is the provider's responsibility to provide clear and legible documentation of a diagnosis, which is then translated to a code for external reporting purposes" (*AHA Coding Clinic*, Fourth Quarter 2015, page 34 and First Quarter 2012, page 6). The entire encounter note should be reviewed at the time of coding to ensure complete code capture of the conditions documented by the provider in accordance with the official coding guidelines.

Depending on the organization type, documentation standards may be set, which are stricter than the minimum required. Some organizations require a status and plan of care for each condition addressed in the visit. This requirement is typically determined by organization type that determines the influence the requester has on the documenting provider. For example, a provider who is employed by an MA plan is more likely to meet the documentation requirements set by the plan than a contracted physician. CMS conducts Risk Adjustment Data Validation (RAD-V) audits to ensure that the risk-adjustment information being submitted is validated by the medical record. Reviewing the checklists and other referential materials can assist with creating internal documentation requirement policies within the organization. RAD-V audits will be discussed more in the next chapter.

Providers need to be vigilant in documenting patient encounters to support all that is evaluated per patient encounter. Specific details should include the condition and/or test results with the status of the patient's condition regarding any changes using terminology such as "decreased," "increased," "worsening," "improving," or "unchanged," with supporting evidence for tests and future plan of care. The following list provides tips for appropriate documentation:

- Document all cause-and-effect relationships.

- Report the most specific diagnosis code(s) available supported by the medical record.

- Include all diagnoses evaluated during the visit that affect medical decision making.

- Identify diagnoses that are current and/or chronic rather than a past medical history or previous resolved condition.

- Document history of heart attack, status codes, etc., that affect the patient's care as "history of" or "PMH" when they no longer exist or are not current conditions.

- Authenticate all medical record documentation including dated, signed, and credentialed progress notes for each patient encounter.

- Document the thought process used to evaluate each condition.

- Know the high revenue HCCs that are often undiagnosed or under coded.

- Avoid unspecified codes.

- Ensure the codes reported are accurate and supported by detailed documentation.

- Avoid assigning a code in lieu of a documented diagnosis.

Providers should document each clinical diagnosis to the highest degree of specificity per encounter, including all complications and/or manifestations, with clear links to causal conditions. All known conditions, including chronic conditions, that affect the care and treatment of the patient at least once per year should be noted.

Chapter 3. Audits and Quality Improvement

A chart audit is a detailed review of the medical record to determine if the services rendered match the services reported. In risk adjustment, this is ensuring that conditions reported are supported by valid medical records. Most often, audits are performed to ensure accuracy and compliance; however, quality improvement measure audits are increasingly popular.

It is advisable to regularly audit the documentation being used as well as the coding for risk adjustment to ensure compliance.

Step 1

Determine who will perform the audit. An internal audit is typically performed by coding staff within the practice that are proficient in coding and interpreting payer guidelines. Depending upon the size of the practice and the number of services provided annually, a compliance department with full-time auditors may be established. If not, the person performing the audit should not audit claims that he or she coded.

Step 2

Define the scope of the audit. Determine what types of services to include in the review. Use the most recent Office of Inspector General (OIG) Work Plan, recovery audit contractor (RAC) issues, and third-party payer provider bulletins, which will help identify areas that can be targeted for upcoming audits. Review the OIG Work Plan, which is now a web-based work plan updated monthly rather than yearly, to determine if there are issues of concern that apply to the practice. Determine specific coding issues or claim denials that are experienced by the practice. The frequency of coding or claims issues and potential effect on reimbursement or potential risk can help prioritize which areas should be reviewed. Services that are frequently performed or have complex coding and billing issues should also be reviewed, as the potential for mistakes or impact to revenue could be substantial.

Step 3

Determine the type of audit to be performed and the areas to be reviewed. Once the area of review is identified, careful consideration should be given to the type of audit performed. Reviews can be prospective or retrospective. If a service is new to the practice, or if coding and billing guidelines have recently been revised, it may be advisable to create a policy stating that a prospective review is performed on a specified number of claims as part of a compliance plan. The audit should include ensuring the medical record coded meets administrative requirements, such as patient name and date of service are on the record, accuracy of diagnosis codes, compliance of any queries generated, and whether the source document supports code assignment.

Step 4

Assemble reference materials. Reference materials, such as current editions of coding manuals and Centers for Medicare and Medicaid Services (CMS) or other third-party policies pertinent to the services being reviewed, should be collected.

Step 5

Develop customized data capture tools. Use an audit worksheet, see example on page 83. Audit worksheets can aid in the audit process. They help verify that signatures were obtained and that patient identifying information (e.g., complete name, date of birth) is correct.

Step 6

Develop a reporting mechanism for findings. Once the audit is complete, written recommendations should be made. The recommendations can include conducting a more frequent focused audit, implementing improved documentation templates, or conducting targeted education on ICD-10-CM coding. Each practice should have benchmarks set up that all providers must meet. For example, if 10 charts are reviewed, 90 percent must be correct. It is also important to identify claims that may need to be corrected or payments that need to be refunded to the payer.

Step 7

Determine recommendations and corrective actions. The next step is to schedule meetings with the providers to provide feedback, recommendations, and education. Typically it works best to meet with a provider on an individual basis and have his or her audit results and charts available as examples so that they can be reviewed and discussed. The provider should be given the opportunity to explain the rationale behind his or her coding, and perhaps even provide additional information to help the coder further understand a particular clinical term. Allowing the provider to give feedback also helps build a better auditor-provider relationship. This relationship may make the provider feel comfortable enough with the auditor to ask questions about future coding issues, instead of reporting incorrect codes to payers. A word to the wise, when discussing a coding error with a provider, it is a good idea to have a copy of the official source document supporting discussion of the error.

Step 8

Implement quality improvement initiatives. After addressing the identified issues, set up a process to monitor these areas. Formal training programs, one-on-one coaching, and regularly scheduled audits can be beneficial. After an audit process is in place, it may be necessary to update practice policies and procedures that need to be monitored on a regular basis. Lastly, designate an individual who is responsible for each area of compliance and document the follow-through so that providers stay on the right track with billing practices.

Step 9

Determine if corrective actions have resolved issues. Once the corrective actions have been in place for a reasonable time, the practice may wish to perform a second review to determine if the desired results have been achieved. This could be done through a comprehensive audit or a "mini" review. Staff should also be interviewed to determine if additional modifications to the corrective actions are necessary.

Additional considerations for audits would include prevalence data for submitted HCCs compared to normative prevalence. If the practice is frequently reporting uncommon diagnoses or reports a diagnosis more often than other practices regionally and nationally, unless the practice is a specialty group, it would behoove the practice or group to audit those charts to ensure the conditions are correctly reported.

It is fairly common as well to have incorrect or unsubstantiated conditions reported when using electronic medical records, which require the documenting provider to assign diagnosis codes prior to signing an encounter. Very often, this requires the provider to search a key word to find the ICD-10-CM code. The provider then selects a code from the list that populates. This can result in an error in a few ways. The provider may select a code that is not specific to the actual patient condition. For example, reporting E11.9 Type 2 diabetes mellitus without complications, when complications of the diabetes are documented within the note. The provider may also select a diagnosis that is not documented within the note. This type of review can identify those trends, and provider education and/or audits can reduce this error.

The OIG began auditing payments made by CMS in 1996. Billing errors, failure to combine outpatient charges with inpatient stays, and misapplied codes have brought penalties of treble damages, fines, and the threat of criminal prosecution. It has been a visible attempt by the federal government to control fraud and abuse and everyone takes these audits quite seriously. In the 2019 Annual Improper Payments Datasets, published by the federal government, it was estimated that in calendar year (CY) 2019, for Medicare Part C payments of $21.2 billion, approximately $16.7 billion were paid improperly, which is a rate of around 7.87 percent.

The OIG included in its report OEI-03-17-00471, published September 2020, Appendix C, the 10 HCCs that CMS previously identified in November 2017 as having the highest payment error rates for 2014 (the most recent year for which CMS identified high-risk HCCs):

HCC 9	Lung and Other Severe Cancers
HCC 27	End-Stage Liver Disease
HCC 54	Drug/Alcohol Psychosis
HCC 75	Myasthenia Gravis/Myoneural Disorders and Guillain-Barré Syndrome/Inflammatory and Toxic Neuropathy
HCC 87	Unstable Angina and Other Acute Ischemic Heart Disease
HCC 99	Cerebral Hemorrhage
HCC 100	Ischemic or Unspecified Stroke
HCC 106	Atherosclerosis of the Extremities With Ulceration or Gangrene
HCC 114	Aspiration and Specified Bacterial Pneumonias
HCC 136	Chronic Kidney Disease, Stage 5

The conditions listed above, like any submitted for risk adjustment, should be validated by the medical record. It is also necessary to ensure that acute conditions, like stroke, are not being reported incorrectly. It is not uncommon to see providers who are coding their own notes in an electronic medical record incorrectly submit a condition that is not validated by the note. For example, submitting a stroke diagnosis on an outpatient medical record, even when the stroke was many years ago and the patient has no late effects. This type of error can be costly. On-going internal audits should be performed to minimize risk.

Medicare Advantage Risk Adjustment Data Validation

Risk adjustment can be a very lucrative payment methodology for insurance companies and providers. As a result, Medicare Advantage Risk Adjustment Data Validation (RAD-V) audits are the main tool that HHS uses as a corrective action to recoup improper payments. This audit program began with the 2007 payment year, during which two audits were done: Pilot 2007 focused on five Medicare Advantage (MA) contracts and Target 2007 involved 32 MA contracts. CMS auditors reviewed the medical record documentation to substantiate the conditions reported by the MA plans. In this first year of RAD-V audits, CMS recovered $13.7 million in overpayments associated with the sample plans.

CMS published a checklist available to provide guidance on how to ensure that medical records will validate the conditions submitted for risk adjustment by an MA plan. This checklist instructs that records should be reviewed to ensure:

- The record is for the correct patient with sufficient patient identifiers on each page of the medical record.

- The record is legible.

- The service is from a face-to-face visit with a valid provider type.

- The diagnosis is found and supported within the medical record.

- The record contains an acceptable provider signature, which includes the credentials of the provider.

The RAD-V audit process is similar to other OIG/CMS audit procedures. CMS identified all beneficiaries under each MA contract who are "RAD-V eligible," meaning they were continuously enrolled in the same MA contract for the year, did not have end-stage renal disease, were not on hospice, and had at least one risk-adjustment diagnosis during the data collection/payment year. For contract-level audits, CMS may select up to 201 enrollees for audit and this sample size will be adjusted for smaller contracts. The enrollee sampling weights will be used as multipliers to extrapolate the sample payment error findings to the population size. CMS groups the enrollees into three groups: the group with the highest risk-adjustment scores, the group with the lowest risk-adjustment scores, and the rest of the population is assigned to the middle group with mixed risk-adjustment scores. The MA organization is then required to submit medical records to support all CMS-HCCs reported during the payment year. While an MA organization may validate a condition more than once a year using various medical records, for RAD-V purposes, only the "one best" record may be submitted to validate the submission to CMS. Best practice is to address every condition at each visit, as there is no guarantee that a patient will return for an annual wellness visit.

CMS calculates each MA contract's overpayment amount based on the validation results and extrapolates the sample payment error rate using a standard formula based upon the number of enrollees in the plan population and the number of enrollees sampled. For example, if an MA plan has 18,000 RAD-V-eligible enrollees and the sample size is 201 enrollees in three groups of 67, the enrollee sample weight would be 89.552 (18,000 enrollees divided by 201 or 6,000 enrollees in each group of 3 divided by 67). With an average overpayment amount of $200 for each enrollee in the sample, the extrapolated overpayment amount to the MA plan would total $3,600,000 ($200 average overpayment x 89.552 sample weight x 201 total enrollees).

Payment errors at the enrollee level are calculated using the difference between the original payment and the RADV-corrected payment (i.e., per member, per month), and will be either positive (i.e., representing a net overpayment), or negative (i.e., representing a net underpayment). An annual payment error amount will be calculated for each sampled enrollee based on the number of months the person was enrolled in the selected MA contract (and was not in ESRD or hospice status) during the payment year.

Audit Scenarios

NOTE: RAF scores and calculations provided in this section are estimates using the 2020 Model Relative Factors only. They are provided for example only and are not intended to calculate actual reimbursement or recoupment values.

Audit Scenario 1—CMS-HCC Model

Electronically Signed: Dr. B. Johnson, D.O.

Patient Name: Betty Smith   **Appt. Date/Time:** 4/5/2021

Appt. Type: MCE

Insurance: Medicare Advantage (HMO)

Chief Complaint: Follow up hyperlipidemia, HTN, OA, MDD

Vitals

BP: 134/71 sitting L arm	**BP Cuff Size:** adult	**Pulse:** 61 bpm regular
T: 97.8 F oral	**O2Sat:** 93% RA	**Ht:** 5'5"
W: 246 lbs	**BMI:** 41	

ROS

Patient reports no frequent nosebleeds, no nose problems, and no sinus problems: congestion. She reports dry mouth but reports no sore throat, no bleeding gums, no snoring, no mouth ulcers, and no teeth problems. She reports arthralgia/joint pain (right knee) but reports no muscle aches, no muscle weakness, no back pain, and no swelling in the extremities. She reports frequent or severe headaches but reports no loss of consciousness, no weakness, no numbness, no seizures, no dizziness, and no tremor. She reports fatigue and sometimes trouble sleeping, with excessive snoring. She reports no fever, no night sweats, no significant weight gain, no significant weight loss, and no exercise intolerance. She reports no dry eyes, no vision change, and no irritation. She reports no difficulty hearing and no ear pain. She reports no chest pain, no arm pain on exertion, no shortness of breath when walking, no shortness of breath when lying down, no palpitations, and no known heart murmur. She reports no cough, no wheezing, no shortness of breath, no coughing up blood. She reports no abdominal pain, no nausea, no vomiting, no constipation, normal appetite, no diarrhea, not vomiting blood, no dyspepsia, and no GERD. She reports no incontinence, no difficulty urinating, no hematuria, and no increased frequency. She reports no abnormal mole, no jaundice, no rashes, and no laceration. She reports no depression, feels safe in a relationship, no alcohol abuse, no anxiety, no hallucinations, and no suicidal thoughts. She reports no swollen glands, no bruising, and no excessive bleeding. She reports no runny nose, no sinus pressure, no itching, no hives, and no frequent sneezing.

History—updated 04/05/2021—

Hx Breast cancer s/p mastectomy

Depressive disorder— partially managed on SSRI

OSA—refuses CPAP

Physical Exam

Patient is a 65-year-old female.

Constitutional

General Appearance: well-developed, appears stated age, and obese.

Level of Distress: comfortable.

Psychiatric

Mental Status: alert and normal affect.

Orientation: oriented to time, place, and person. Insight: good judgment.

Cardiovascular

Precordial Exam: no heaves or precordial thrills and non-displaced focal PMI. Rate and rhythm: regular.

Heart Sounds: no rub, gallop, or click and normal S1 and physiologically split S2.

- Systolic murmur: not heard.
- Diastolic murmur: not heard

Extremities

No cyanosis, edema, or peripheral signs of emboli

Audit Scenario 1—CMS-HCC Model (Continued)

Neurologic

Motor: tremor of neck and face and arms

A/P

Mixed hyperlipidemia—continue meds

Benign essential hypertension—continue meds

Insomnia—discussed sleep hygiene/caffeine curfew

Anxiety/depression—continue meds/consider seeing psych

Morbid obesity with OSA—discussed increasing activity and decreasing caloric intake. Consider CPAP.

HCC Category Pre-audit	ICD-10-CM Code Submitted		Pre-audit RAF Value	HCC Category Post-audit	ICD-10-CM Validated by Audit		Post-audit RAF Value
HCC 59	F33.41	Major depressive disorder, recurrent, in partial remission	0.309		F41.8	Other specified anxiety disorders	
HCC 12	C50.919	Malignant neoplasm of unspecified site of unspecified female breast	0.150		Z85.3	Personal history of malignant neoplasm of breast	
					Z79.810	Long term (current) use of selective estrogen receptor modulators (SERMs)	
HCC 22	E66.2	Obesity hypoventilation syndrome (OHS)	0.250	HCC 22	E66.2	Obesity hypoventilation syndrome (OHS)	0.250
Demographics	65-year-old, female, not Medicaid eligible		0.323	Demographics	65-year-old, female, not Medicaid eligible		0.323
Total RAF Pre-audit			1.032	Total RAF Post-audit			0.573
RAF x Benchmark $700 Pre-audit (Dollar amount for illustrative purposes only)			$722.00	RAF x Benchmark $700 Post-audit (Dollar amount for illustrative purposes only)			$401.00

Audit Scenario 1 Rationale—CMS-HCC Model

The following codes and corresponding HCCs with associated risk factors have been removed:

| HCC 59 | F33.41 | Major depressive disorder, recurrent, in partial remission | RAF 0.309 |
| HCC 12 | C50.919 | Malignant neoplasm of unspecified site of unspecified female breast | RAF 0.150 |

The ICD-10-CM codes listed above are replaced with the following ICD-10-CM codes with no HCC and no RAF value:

F41.8   Other specified anxiety disorders

Z85.3   Personal history of malignant neoplasm of breast

Z79.810   Long term (current) use of selective estrogen receptor modulators (SERMs)

There is no provider documentation of a major depressive disorder in the record received for review. The provider lists anxiety/depression, which is indexed in ICD-10-CM to code F41.8. Review of the tabular for code F41.8 shows that this code includes "Anxiety depression (mild or not persistent)."

See *ICD-10-CM Official Guidelines for Coding and Reporting*, section I.B.1, which states: "To select a code in the classification that corresponds to a diagnosis or reason for visit documented in a medical record, first locate the term in the Alphabetic Index, and then verify the code in the Tabular List. Read and be guided by instructional notations that appear in both the Alphabetic Index and the Tabular List.

It is essential to use both the Alphabetic Index and Tabular List when locating and assigning a code. The Alphabetic Index does not always provide the full code. Selection of the full code, including laterality and any applicable 7th character can only be done in the Tabular List."

The provider documentation also states that the patient has a history of breast cancer and is status post mastectomy, without documenting breast cancer as an active problem. The provider documented the patient is receiving Tamoxifen to prevent recurrence and is seeing an oncology provider.

See ICD-10-CM guideline section I.C.2.m, which states: "When a primary malignancy has been previously excised or eradicated from its site, there is no further treatment (of the malignancy) directed to that site, and there is no evidence of any existing primary malignancy, a code from category Z85, Personal history of malignant neoplasm, should be used to indicate the former site of the malignancy."

These modifications have resulted in a change from Pre-Audit Total RAF score of 1.032 to Post-Audit Total RAF score of 0.573.

Audit Scenario 2—CMS-HCC Model

Patient Name: Donald Johnson   **Visit Date/Time:** 9/3/2021

Sex: M

Chief Complaint : Presents for annual wellness visit

History of Present Illness

Don is an established patient in our office. He is here today for his annual wellness visit. He is doing well on current medication and treatment and there will be no change to current treatment. He is active but has no formal exercise and was encouraged to increase the current level of exercise. Today, his BMI is 35.16 kg/m2, which is down from the most recent BMI of 36.38 kg/m2. The need for continued weight loss was DAL and current diet was assessed. There have been no hospital stays or injuries since the last visit.

Active Problems

Allergic rhinitis, arthritis, chronic kidney disease IV, chronic obstructive pulmonary disease, heart disease, depression, type 2 diabetes, dizziness, hypertension, thrombocytopenia, restless leg syndrome, and vitamin B12 deficiency.

Medication List

Lisinopril, Lantus, Humalog, test strips, Brovana nebulizer, albuterol, CPAP, gabapentin, Wellbutrin SR, Lasix, Singulair, Tofranil, and Ultram

P/F/S history

No changes from AWV on 9/15/2020. Interval history reviewed with patient.

ROS

12 point system reviewed pertinent findings as below.

Resp—SOB, wheezing, DOE

CV—edema increased in legs

Psych—difficulty concentrating, increased tiredness

Neuro—decreased sensation in fingers/toes

Vital Signs

Date	BP	Position	HR	Temp (F)	WT	HT	BMI	BSA
9/3/21	130/69	sitting	106-r	97.6	259	6'0"	35.16	2.44

Exam

Constitutional: well-nourished/well-developed, NAD

HEENT: WNL, PERRL

Respiratory: labored breathing

CV: regular rate and rhythm

GI: WNL, no HSM

GU: deferred, patient refuses

Extremities: abnormal findings with monofilament on both feet, decreased sensation in fingers as well, marked edema in bilateral legs

Psych: PHQ-9 result 4, depressed mood, AOx3

A/P
Physical Exam

Severe chronic kidney disease due to diabetic nephropathy. Sees specialist Dr. Jones.

COPD—stable on current inhalers, considering O2 therapy, uses CPAP as directed

OA left knee—continues despite replacement surgery in 16, DAL cannot take pain meds long term

Major depression, recurrent, partial remission—continue meds

Peripheral neuropathy—continue meds, DAL blood sugar control to prevent progression

Disposition: home, patient will call or return with any issues

Electronically Signed: Samantha Fink, NP on 09/05/21

HCC Category Pre-audit	ICD-10-CM Code Submitted		Pre-audit RAF Value	HCC Category Post-audit	ICD-10-CM Validated by Audit		Post-audit RAF Value
HCC 59	F33.41-	Major depressive disorder, recurrent, in partial remission	0.309	HCC 59	F33.41-	Major depressive disorder, recurrent, in partial remission	0.309
HCC 18	E11.22	Type 2 diabetes mellitus with diabetic chronic kidney disease	0.302	HCC 18	E11.22	Type 2 diabetes mellitus with diabetic chronic kidney disease	0.302
	Disease Interaction DM + CHF		0.121				
HCC 85	I13.0	Hypertensive heart and chronic kidney disease with heart failure and stage 1 through stage 4 chronic kidney disease, or unspecified chronic kidney disease	0.331		I11.9	Hypertensive heart disease without heart failure	
HCC 85	I50.9	Heart failure, unspecified	0.000		I51.9	Heart disease, unspecified	
	Disease Interaction CHF + CKD		0.156				
HCC 137	N18.4	Chronic kidney disease, stage 4 (severe)	0.289	HCC 137	N18.4	Chronic kidney disease, stage 4 (severe)	0.289
	Disease Interaction CHF + COPD		0.155				
HCC 111	J44.9	Chronic obstructive pulmonary disease, unspecified	0.335	HCC 111	J44.9	Chronic obstructive pulmonary disease, unspecified	0.335
D5	5 Payment HCCs		0.042	D4	4 Payment HCCs		0.006
Demographics	77-year-old, male, not Medicaid eligible		0.473	Demographics	77-year-old, male, not Medicaid eligible		0.473
Total RAF Pre-audit			2.513	Total RAF Post-audit			1.714
RAF x Benchmark $700 Pre-audit (Dollar amount for illustrative purposes only)			$1,759.10	RAF x Benchmark $700 Post-audit (Dollar amount for illustrative purposes only)			$1,199.80

Audit Scenario 2 Rationale—CMS-HCC Model

The following codes and corresponding HCCs with associated risk factors have been removed:

HCC 85	I13.0	Hypertensive heart and chronic kidney disease with heart failure and stage 1 through stage 4 chronic kidney disease, or unspecified chronic kidney disease	RAF 0.331

Is being replaced with

	I11.9	Hypertensive heart disease without heart failure	with no HCC and no RAF

HCC 85	I50.9	Heart failure, unspecified	

Is being replaced with

	I51.9	Heart disease, unspecified	

The physician specifically states the CKD is due to diabetic nephropathy. According to ICD-10-CM coding guidelines, CKD should not be coded as hypertensive if the physician has specifically documented a different cause.

There is also no provider documentation of a diagnosis of heart failure in the record received for review. The physician documents only heart disease. A link between hypertension and heart disease can be presumed according to ICD-10-CM coding guidelines.

These changes drop the HCC Payment count from D5 to D4, changing this RAF from 0.042 to 0.006.

As a result of this coding change, the following disease interactions have also been removed:

Disease Interaction DM + CHF	0.121
Disease Interaction CHF + CKD	0.156
Disease Interaction CHF + COPD	0.155

These modifications have resulted in a change from Pre-Audit Total RAF score of 2.513 to Post-Audit Total RAF score of 1.714.

Audit Scenario 3—CMS-HCC Model

Result type: History and Physical Note

Result date: June 11, 2021

Result status: Auth (Verified)

Result Title/Subject: History and Physical

Performed By/Author: Black MD, Brian on June 11, 2021

Verified By: Black MD, Brian on June 11, 2021

Encounter info: (IPE) Emergency—IP, 6/11/2021–6/12/2021

History and Physical

Patient: Miller, Paul C.

Age: 91 years   **Sex:** Male

Associated Diagnoses: None

Author: Black, MD Brian

Chief Complaint:

slurred speech, facial droop, fall

History of Present Illness:

91-year-old M PMH significant for Afib not on anticoagulation, HTN, COPD, colon CA s/p resection 2 years prior who is BIBA for acute onset of slurred speech, left lower facial droop following fall. Patient and wife note around 8:30 p.m. last night, he sustained a slow fall in his home. He is unsure if he lost balance but had difficulty standing back up on his own but was able to be seated into chair by his wife. He then noticed that he had a difficult time speaking and his wife noted he had a left lower facial droop. She suspected he was having a stroke and gave him approximately 250 mg of Aspirin. Wife then called EMS, and patient and wife both note that his symptoms were improving already in the ambulance. Symptoms were essentially resolved by the time he arrived to the ED here, which was approximately 30 mins after onset of symptoms. He had otherwise been feeling well except for a mild cough, which started about 10 days ago and has mostly resolved. He notes he was given a cough suppressant with Bactrim by PCP, which he has since completed. He otherwise denies any fevers, chills, dizziness, shortness of breath, chest pain, palpitations, nausea/vomiting, bowel changes, urinary changes, blood in stool.

Review of Systems:

12 point ROS reviewed and negative except as above

Past Medical History:

As noted above.

Allergies (1) Active Reaction

Quinidine—Affects his liver

Social History:

Denies tobacco, quit in 1986

Denies ETOH or drug use

Family History:

Mother: colon CA

Brother: throat CA

Home Medications (6) Active

Atenolol 25 mg oral tablet; see Instructions

Finasteride 5 mg oral tablet 5 mg = 1 tab, PO, daily

Loratadine 10 mg, PO, daily

Multivitamin 1 cap, PO, daily

Tamsulosin 0.4 mg oral capsule 0.4 mg = 1 cap, PO, daily

Unlisted Med; see instructions

Current Vitals (past 48 hrs., max 5 results):

Audit Scenario 3—CMS-HCC Model (Continued)

Vital Signs

Dt/Tm	Temp	BP	MAP	Pulse	RR	SpO2	FiO2	O2 Therapy
06/11/21 00:30	—	122/60	81	88	18	96%	—	Room air
06/11/21 00:11	—	129/58	82	78	18	96%	—	Room air
06/10/21 22:45	36.7	127/75	92	83	18	96%	—	Room air

Tmax 24 Hr: 36.7 DegC (98.1 DegF) 01/10/21 22:45 (Oral)

Tmax 36 Hr: 36.7 DegC (98.1 DegF) 01/10/21 22:45 (Oral)

BMI: 17.44 (06/11/2021 23:10)

> BMI is noted to be less than 19. Malnutrition was coded but not documented by the provider.

Physical Examination

General: Awake, alert, NAD

HEENT: Normo-cephalic, atraumatic; PERRL. Extraocular muscles are intact, sclera non-icteric

Neck: Trachea midline

Lungs: Clear to auscultation bilaterally

Cardiac: Irregular rate/rhythm, S1 and S2 with no murmurs

Abdomen: Soft, non-tender and non-distended with good bowel sounds

Extremities: No cyanosis or edema

Skin: No rashes or lesion

Neurological: Cranial nerves II through XII grossly intact, motor- 5/5 throughout large muscle groups, sensation-intact throughout, cerebellar- finger to nose wnl, alert and oriented to person, place and time

Psychiatric Evaluation

Normal mood and affect, normal judgment and insight

All Results (36 Hrs)

All labs personally reviewed.

Radiology results (Past 36 Hours):

CT head w/o contrast STROKE CO

Performed By/Author: Dr. Moore, MD Sandra M.

Impression: Subtle hyper-intensity within an insular branch of the left middle cerebral artery may reflect vessel occlusion or atherosclerotic calcification. Recommend CTA head. No acute intracranial hemorrhage is appreciated. No definite acute parenchymal changes are identified. Probable left basal ganglia infarct. These findings were discussed with Dr. Moore, MD.

XR Hip 2 View Left + Pelvis Performed By/Author: Dr. Moore, MD Sandra M

Impression: No acute abnormality.

XR Chest 1 View

Performed By/Author: Dr. Moore, MD Sandra M

Impression: Multifocal airspace opacities suspicious for pneumonia. Recommend follow-up to resolution.

CTA head/neck w/ Con STROKE CO

Performed By/Author: Dr. Moore, MD Sandra M

Impression: Focal complete occlusion of a left middle cerebral artery M2 insular branch. Findings correspond to the dense artery on the non-contrast head CT. 50% right ICA stenosis and 60% left ICA stenosis in the neck. Patchy upper lobe airspace opacities suggestive of multifocal pneumonia. These findings were discussed with Dr. Moore, MD Sandra M.

Audit Scenario 3—CMS-HCC Model (Continued)

Assessment/Plan

91-year-old M PMH significant for Afib not on anticoagulation, HTN, COPD, colon CA s/p resection 2 years prior who is BIBA from for acute onset of slurred speech, left lower facial droop following fall.

1. Stroke
    - symptoms resolved
    - CT head with left basal ganglia infarct
    - CTA head/neck w/ focal complete occlusion of left MCA M2 insular branch, 60% left ICA stenosis, 50% right ICA stenosis
    - Neurology consulted in ED- confirms infarct due to left MCA occlusion appreciate further recs
    - ASA, statin
    - check MRI brain
    - check 2d echo w/ bubble study
    - PT/OT eval
    - allow for permissive HTN first 24 hrs.

2. Permanent atrial fibrillation–rate controlled
    - not on anticoagulation, dx in late 1980s and has not been on anticoagulation since for > 25 years
    - CHADS2 vasc score of 5 and would likely be candidate for anticoagulation if bleeding risk not significantly elevated
    - will defer timing of anticoagulation to neurology, await MRI results

3. Multifocal PNA– largely asymptomatic
    - incidentally noted on CXR, CTA neck
    - reports recent tx w/ Bactrim
    - possibly remnant of recent PNA, however given leukocytosis, imaging findings and tx w/ only Bactrim recently, will tx
    - ceftriaxone/doxy
    - f/u sputum cx, pna serologies

4. HTN
    - allow permissive HTN up to SBP 220 first 24 hrs.
    - hold atenolol

5. COPD
    - no exacerbation > 70 years per patient
    - uses inhalers bid, prn

6. hx colon CA s/p resection 2 years ago
    - pt reports taking vitamins and holistic cures
    - oncology recs appreciated
    - FEN/ppx: heart healthy diet, ivsl/SCDS
    - full code full care–discussed with patient at bedside

HCC Category Pre-audit	ICD-10-CM Code Submitted		Pre-audit RAF Value	HCC Category Post-audit	ICD-10-CM Validated by Audit		Post-audit RAF Value
HCC 100	I63.9	Cerebral infarction, unspecified	0.230	HCC 100	I63.512	Cerebral infarction due to unspecified occlusion or stenosis of left middle cerebral artery	0.230
HCC 96	I48.21	Permanent atrial fibrillation	0.268	HCC 96	I48.21	Permanent atrial fibrillation	0.268
HCC 21	E46	Unspecified protein-calorie malnutrition	0.455				
HCC 111	J44.9	Chronic obstructive pulmonary disease, unspecified	0.335	HCC 111	J44.9	Chronic obstructive pulmonary disease, unspecified	0.335
D4	4 Payment HCCs		0.006	D3	4 Payment HCCs		–
Demographics	91-year-old, male, non-Medicaid eligible		0.841	Demographics	91-year-old, male, non-Medicaid eligible		0.841
Total RAF Pre-audit			2.135	Total RAF Post-audit			1.674
RAF x Benchmark $700 Pre-audit (Dollar amount for illustrative purposes only)			$1,494.50	RAF x Benchmark $700 Post-audit (Dollar amount for illustrative purposes only)			$1,172.00

Audit Scenario 3 Rationale—CMS-HCC Model
The following codes and corresponding HCCs with associated risk factors have been removed:

| HCC 21 | E46 | Unspecified protein-calorie malnutrition | RAF 0.455 |

There is no provider documentation of a diagnosis of malnutrition. The documentation does indicate a BMI less than 19. The provider should have been queried for a diagnosis of malnutrition.

According to ICD-10-CM guideline I.B.14: "Code assignment is based on the documentation by the patient's provider (i.e., physician or other qualified healthcare practitioner legally accountable for establishing the patient's diagnosis). There are a few exceptions when code assignment may be based on medical record documentation from clinicians who are not the patient's provider (i.e., physician or other qualified healthcare practitioner legally accountable for establishing the patient's diagnosis). In this context, 'clinicians' other than the patient's provider refer to healthcare professionals permitted, based on regulatory or ICD-10-CM accreditation requirements or internal hospital policies, to document in a patient's official medical record.

"These exceptions include codes for:

- Body Mass Index (BMI)

- Depth of non-pressure chronic ulcers

- Pressure ulcer stage

- Coma scale

- NIH stroke scale (NIHSS)

- Social determinants of health (SDOH)

- Laterality

- Blood alcohol level

"This information is typically, or may be, documented by other clinicians involved in the care of the patient (e.g., a dietitian often documents the BMI, a nurse often documents the pressure ulcer stages, and an emergency medical technician often documents the coma scale). However, the associated diagnosis (such as overweight, obesity, acute stroke, pressure ulcer, or a condition classifiable to category F10, Alcohol related disorders) must be documented by the patient's provider. If there is conflicting medical record documentation, either from the same clinician or different clinicians, the patient's attending provider should be queried for clarification.

"The BMI, coma scale, NIHSS, blood alcohol level codes and codes for social determinants of health should only be reported as secondary diagnoses."

In addition, code I63.9 Cerebral infarction, unspecified

Has been changed to:

I63.512   Cerebral infarction due to unspecified occlusion or stenosis of left middle cerebral artery

The documentation in the record confirms cerebral infarction due to left MCA total occlusion. The appropriate code assignment is I63.512 Cerebral infarction due to unspecified occlusion or stenosis of left middle cerebral artery.

This change results in the same HCC and same RAF score and is for accurate code assignment only.

These changes drop the HCC Payment count from D4 to D3, changing this RAF from 0.006 to 0.

These modifications have resulted in a change from Pre-audit Total RAF score of 2.135 to Post-audit Total RAF score of 1.674.

Audit Scenario 4—CMS-HCC Model

Patient: Joe Holmes   **DOS:** 01/23/2021   **Ins:** Managed Care Medicare

DR: Robert Jacobs, M.D.

CC:

annual wellness visit

S

Patient seen for annual wellness visit. He had a colonoscopy in 2016. He refuses the flu vaccine. Patient is compliant with DM management. Patient complains of wound on his leg for 10 days. Med list reviewed in EMR module. No changes to P/F/S hx from last AWV. Patient regularly sees oncology. Today wants to discuss other treatment options. PHQ-9 score is 4. Upset about mets.

O

Alert, no acute distress, HEENT:NC, pupils equal, round, sclera white, conj. clear, external nose WNL, on O2 nasal cannula, no lesions, external ear normal, lips/mouth free of lesions, Neuro: no tremor, Neck: trachea midline normal appearance, MS: normal gait and posture, Ext: no edema or clubbing, poss claudication, ulcer noted on distal left calf with r/o venous stasis, skin: no rash or lesions, L diminished bs, no wheezing, HRRR no m/r/c, Abd soft nt +bs.

A

Poss claudication/leg skin ulcer, bone and lymph mets, prostate ca, DM, IBS, resp insuff syndrome.

P

Get ABI – r/o claudication w/ ulcer with breakdown of skin. DAL patient needs to speak to oncologist about tx for mets and continue "watchful waiting" on prostate ca. Patient is compliant on DM regime, continue. Dependent on home O2 increase 5L.

ICD-10-CM I73.9 is not validated by this note. The provider has indicated that claudication is possible. The provider should be queried for validation of this condition if it exists.

HCC Category Pre-audit	ICD-10-CM Code Submitted		Pre-audit RAF Value	HCC Category Post-audit	ICD-10-CM Validated by Audit		Post-audit RAF Value
HCC 12*	C61	Malignant neoplasm of prostate	0.150	HCC 12*	C61	Malignant neoplasm of prostate	0.150
HCC 8	C79.51	Secondary malignant neoplasm of bone	2.659	HCC 8	C79.51	Secondary malignant neoplasm of bone	2.659
HCC 10*	C77.9	Secondary and unspecified malignant neoplasm of lymph node, unspecified	0.675	HCC 10*	C77.9	Secondary and unspecified malignant neoplasm of lymph node, unspecified	0.675
HCC 108	I73.9	Peripheral vascular disease, unspecified	0.288	HCC 161	L97.221	Non-pressure chronic ulcer of left calf limited to breakdown of skin	0.515
HCC 18	E11.51	Type 2 diabetes mellitus with diabetic peripheral angiopathy without gangrene	0.302	HCC 18	E11.622	Type 2 diabetes mellitus with other skin ulcer	0.302
HCC 108	E11.51	Type 2 diabetes mellitus with diabetic peripheral angiopathy without gangrene	0.288	HCC 161	E11.622	Type 2 diabetes mellitus with other skin ulcer	0.515
HCC 59	F32.1	Major depressive disorder, single episode, moderate	0.309				
HCC 84	J96.11	Chronic respiratory failure with hypoxia	0.282				
D5	5 Payment HCCs		0.042	D3	3 Payment HCCs		–
Demographics	78-year-old, female		0.451	Demographics	78-year-old, male		0.473
Total RAF Pre-audit			4.333	Total RAF Post-audit			3.949
RAF x Benchmark $700 Pre-audit (Dollar amount for illustrative purposes only)			$3,033.10	RAF x Benchmark $700 Post-audit (Dollar amount for illustrative purposes only)			$2,764.30

The CMS-HCC trumping logic applies to HCC 12 and HCC 10. Conditions in HCC 8 trump conditions in HCC 10 and HCC 12. So in this example, the values of HCC 10 and HCC 12 would not be factored into the patient's risk score.

Audit Scenario 4 Rationale—CMS-HCC Model

The following codes and corresponding HCCs with associated risk factors have been removed:

HCC 108	I73.9	Peripheral vascular disease, unspecified	RAF 0.288
HCC 58	F32.1	Major depressive disorder, single episode, moderate	RAF 0.309
HCC 84	J96.11	Chronic respiratory failure with hypoxia	RAF 0.282

There is no provider documentation of diabetic peripheral vascular disease, major depressive disorder, single episode, moderate, or chronic respiratory failure with hypoxia in records received for review.

The provider has documented "Poss claudication," "r/o claudication," and "r/o venous stasis, skin."

According to the *ICD-10-CM Guidelines for Coding and Reporting*, section IV. Diagnostic Coding and Reporting Guidelines for Outpatient Services, "Coding guidelines for inconclusive diagnoses (probable, suspected, rule out, etc.) were developed for inpatient reporting and do not apply to outpatients."

When the documentation in the medical record is clear and consistent, coders may assign and report codes. If there is evidence of a diagnosis within the medical record, and the coder is uncertain whether it is a valid diagnosis because the documentation is incomplete, vague, or contradictory, it is the coder's responsibility to query the provider to determine if this diagnosis should be included.

The following codes and corresponding HCCs with associated risk factors have been changed or added:

Change

HCC 18	E11.51	Type 2 diabetes mellitus with diabetic peripheral angiopathy without gangrene	RAF 0.302
HCC 18	E11.622	Type 2 diabetes mellitus with other skin ulcer	RAF 0.302

Add

HCC 161	L97.221	Non-pressure chronic ulcer of left calf limited to breakdown of skin	RAF 0.515

The provider documentation states that the patient has an ulcer of the left calf with skin breakdown. Skin ulcer is listed under the subterm "with" in the index under the main term Diabetes; therefore, a causal relationship can be assumed and E11.622, with an additional code to report the ulcer site and severity, should be reported.

See ICD-10-CM guideline I.A.15, which states: "The word 'with' or 'in' should be interpreted to mean 'associated with' or 'due to' when it appears in a code title, the Alphabetic Index, or an instructional note in the Tabular List. The classification presumes a causal relationship between the two conditions linked by these terms in the Alphabetic Index or Tabular List. These conditions should be coded as related even in the absence of provider documentation explicitly linking them, unless the documentation clearly states the conditions are unrelated or when another guideline exists that specifically requires a documented linkage between two conditions (e.g., sepsis guideline for 'acute organ dysfunction that is not clearly associated with the sepsis'). For conditions not specifically linked by these relational terms in the classification or when a guideline requires that a linkage between two conditions be explicitly documented, provider documentation must link the conditions in order to code them as related. The word 'with' in the Alphabetic Index is sequenced immediately following the main term, not in alphabetical order."

In addition, there has been a change in the RAF for demographics. This 78-year old male patient was incorrectly identified as a 78-year-old female. Original RAF of 0.452 has been changed to 0.472. The HCC Payment count changed from D4 to D3, changing this RAF from 0.006 to 0. These modifications have resulted in a change from Pre-audit Total RAF score of 4.333 to 3.949.

Audit Scenario 5—ESRD-HCC Model

Patient: Diaz, Jenny   **Age:** 66 years   **Sex:** Female

Associated Diagnoses: None

Author: Moore MD, Samuel   **DOS:** 1/7/2021

Chief Complaint: hypotension

History of Present Illness

66-year-old F w/ h/o ESRD on ihd MWF, CAD s/p CABG, Afib on Eliquis, DM2, asthma, htn, HL, depression, GERD who p/w hypotension. Her SBP was noted to be in the 80s at the end of dialysis. Her sugar was noted to be in the 40s and her K+ was 2.8. Pt c/o feeling SOB for the past 1 day. C/o mild productive cough. She also notes having several loose stools starting last night. Also c/o generalized body aches and subjective fevers for 2 days. Also w/ R sided frontal headache and neck pain. Denies any recent trauma. Denies recent travel or sick contacts. Denies chills/night sweats/abdominal pain/nausea/vomiting/urinary symptoms/headache/weight loss/visual changes/neck pain.

Review of Systems

12 point ROS reviewed and negative except as stated in HPI

Problem List

Active Problems:

ESRD on ihd MWF, CAD s/p CABG, afib, dm2, asthma, htn, HL, depression, GERD

Past Medical History

See above.

Past Surgical History

CABG

Social History

Denies alcohol use

Denies tobacco use

Denies illicit drug use

Family History

Father w/ HTN

Allergies

NKA

Home Medications (14) Active

Acetaminophen 650 mg, PRN, PO, Q4H

Acyclovir 400 mg oral tablet 800 mg = 2 tab, PO, BID

Aspirin 81 mg, PO, daily

Atorvastatin 10 mg oral tablet 10 mg = 1 tab, PO, daily

Carvedilol 3.125 mg oral tablet 3.125 mg = 1 tab, PO, BIDCC

Crestor 10 mg, PO, daily

Eliquis 2.5 mg, PO, BID

Escitalopram 10 mg oral tablet 10 mg = 1 tab, PO, daily

Gabapentin 100 mg oral capsule 100 mg = 1 cap, PO, TID

Insulin aspart See scale, SC, AC (before meals)

Metoprolol tartrate 25 mg, PO, BID

Pantoprazole 40 mg, PO, QHS

Senna 8.6 mg oral tablet 17.2 mg = 2 tab, PO, daily

Vancomycin per pharmacy 500 mg = 100 mL, IVPB, Q999H

Vitals

Temp (Oral) 36.9 DegC (98.4 DegF) BP 90/61 mmHg Pulse 96 bpm RR 18 br/min

Audit Scenario 5—ESRD-HCC Model (Continued)

Physical Examination

General: NAD, pleasant, aox3, slightly lethargic but easily arousable

HEENT: PERRL, EOMI, MMM, OP clear

Neck: no thyromegaly, supple, no LAD

CV: RRR, nl s1, s2, no mrg, JVP non-elevated

Pulm: crackles at bases b/l, normal non-labored breathing

ABD: +BS, soft, non-tender, non-distended, no rebound or guarding

Extremities: no cyanosis/clubbing/edema

Neuro: moves all extremities equally, no focal deficits

Labs

personally reviewed/WNL

Radiology (Past 36 Hours)

XR Chest 2 Views

Performed By/Author: Johnson MD, Howard M

Impression

1. Extensive nodular infiltrate throughout the right lung.
2. Fibrotic changes noted in both lungs consistent with Pulmonary Fibrosis

EKG: None

Assessment Plan

66 yo F w/ h/o ESRD on ihd MWF, CAD s/p CABG, afib not on anticoag b/c fall risk, dm2, asthma, htn, HL, depression, GERD who p/w hypotension, admitted w/HCAP.

1. Influenza B with healthcare associated bacterial pneumonia–meets sepsis criteria
   - vancomycin/Zosyn
   - f/u sputum culture
   - f/u blood cultures
   - oxygen protocol
   - urinary strep and legionella ag
   - consult ID
   - influenza screen +
   - trend lactate
2. Hypokalemia
   - replete K+ PRN
3. Diarrhea
   - stool cx
   - c-diff
4. ESRD
   - cont ihd
   - cont home meds
   - consult renal
5. Diabetes mellitus type 2
   - hold home oral hypoglycemics
   - place patient on insulin sliding scale
   - diabetes nurse practitioner consult
6. CAD s/p CABG
7. Afib
   - cont Eliquis
8. Anemia
   - check iron levels
9. Asthma

Audit Scenario 5—ESRD-HCC Model (Continued)

Assessment Plan (Continued)

10. HTN-hold home anti-hypertensives given hypotension

11. Hyperlipidemia-continue statin

12. GERD

   - continue PPI

13. Depression

   - cont home meds

14. FEN-regular cardiac diabetic renal diet

15. Prophylaxis-SCDs

16. Code-FCFC

I attest that this patient will require >2 midnight stay due to the nature of the above stated medical conditions.

Result date: January 7, 2021

Result status: Auth (Verified)

Result Title/Subject: History and physical

Performed By/Author: Moore MD, Samuel on January 7, 2021

Verified By: Moore MD, Samuel on January 7, 2021

HCC Category Pre-audit	ICD-10-CM Code Submitted		Pre-audit RAF Value	HCC Category Post-audit	ICD-10-CM Validated by Audit		Post-audit RAF Value
HCC 58	F32.4	Major depressive disorder, single episode, in partial remission	0.092		F32.9	Major depressive disorder, single episode, unspecified	
HCC 18	E11.22	Type 2 diabetes mellitus with diabetic chronic kidney disease	0.093	HCC 18	E11.22	Type 2 diabetes mellitus with diabetic chronic kidney disease	0.093
HCC 136	N18.6	End stage renal disease	0.000*	HCC 136	N18.6	End stage renal disease	0.000*
HCC 134	Z99.2	Dependence on renal dialysis	0.000*	HCC 134	Z99.2	Dependence on renal dialysis	0.000*
HCC 136	I12.0	Hypertensive chronic kidney disease with stage 5 chronic kidney disease or end stage renal disease	0.000*	HCC 136	I12.0	Hypertensive chronic kidney disease with stage 5 chronic kidney disease or end stage renal disease	0.000*
HCC 96	I48.91	Unspecified atrial fibrillation	0.094	HCC 96	I48.91	Unspecified atrial fibrillation	0.094
HCC 112	J84.10	Pulmonary fibrosis, unspecified	0.067		J15.9	Unspecified bacterial pneumonia	
					J10.08	Influenza due to other identified influenza virus with other specified pneumonia	
HCC 2	A41.9	Sepsis, unspecified organism	0.083				
Demo-graphics	66-year-old, female		0.647	Demo-graphics	66-year-old, female		0.647
Total RAF Pre-audit			1.076	Total RAF Post-audit			0.834
RAF x Benchmark $700 Pre-audit (Dollar amount for illustrative purposes only)			$753.00	RAF x Benchmark $700 Post-audit (Dollar amount for illustrative purposes only)			$584.00

* This patient is on the ESRD model. Within this model, the end stage renal disease and dialysis are not assigned a value.

Audit Scenario 5 Rationale—ESRD-HCC Model

The following codes and corresponding HCCs with associated risk factors have been removed:

HCC 58	F32.4	Major depressive disorder, single episode, in partial remission	RAF 0.092
HCC 112	J84.10	Pulmonary fibrosis, unspecified	RAF 0.067
HCC 2	A41.9	Sepsis, unspecified organism	RAF 0.083

The ICD-10-CM codes listed below have been added, with no corresponding HCC and no RAF value:

F32.9   Major depressive disorder, single episode, unspecified

J15.9   Unspecified bacterial pneumonia

J10.08   Influenza due to other identified influenza virus with other specified pneumonia

There is insufficient documentation to code major depressive disorder, single episode, in partial remission. Provider documentation in records reviewed indicates depression without further specificity. This is indexed in ICD-10-CM to code F32.9 Major depressive disorder, single episode, unspecified.

See *ICD-10-CM Official Guidelines for Coding and Reporting*, section I.B.1, which states: "To select a code in the classification that corresponds to a diagnosis or reason for visit documented in a medical record, first locate the term in the Alphabetic Index, and then verify the code in the Tabular List. Read and be guided by instructional notations that appear in both the Alphabetic Index and the Tabular List.

It is essential to use both the Alphabetic Index and Tabular List when locating and assigning a code. The Alphabetic Index does not always provide the full code. Selection of the full code, including laterality and any applicable 7th character can only be done in the Tabular List."

The code for pulmonary fibrosis in HCC 112 should not be reported, as this is noted only on the radiology report of the chest x-ray. There is no attending physician documentation of the clinical significance, if any, of this abnormal finding.

See *ICD-10-CM Official Guidelines for Coding and Reporting*, section III.B, which states: "Abnormal findings (laboratory, x-ray, pathologic, and other diagnostic results) are not coded and reported unless the provider indicates their clinical significance. If the findings are outside the normal range and the attending provider has ordered other tests to evaluate the condition or prescribed treatment, it is appropriate to ask the provider whether the abnormal finding should be added.

Please note: This differs from the coding practices in the outpatient setting for coding encounters for diagnostic tests that have been interpreted by a provider."

There is no attending physician documentation of a diagnosis of sepsis in the records reviewed. The physician documents that the patient meets sepsis criteria, and a blood culture was ordered. The physician should have been queried prior to assigning a diagnosis of sepsis.

When the documentation in the medical record is clear and consistent, coders may assign and report codes. If there is evidence of a diagnosis within the medical record, and the coder is uncertain whether it is a valid diagnosis because the documentation is incomplete, vague, or contradictory, it is the coder's responsibility to query the provider to determine if this diagnosis should be included.

Codes J15.9 Unspecified bacterial pneumonia, and J10.08 Influenza due to other identified influenza virus with other specified pneumonia, have been added. The provider documents the patient was admitted with influenza B with healthcare associated bacterial pneumonia (HCAP). Both of these codes are required to capture the diagnostic statement.

These modifications have resulted in a change from Pre-Audit Total RAF score of 1.076 to Post-Audit Total RAF score of 0.834.

RAD-V Audit Steps

As part of an audit, the MA organization will notify the service-rendering providers and request records for the identified beneficiaries from the providers who rendered services for the time frame indicated by the audit scope. The MA organization will prioritize sources to find the "one best" record that most completely and accurately reflects the condition being reported. Typically, these record requests are sent via mail but an MA organization may provide close follow up with emails and phone calls to ensure these requests are completed in an expeditor's manner. After receiving the requested records, the records are compiled into a database and reviewed. If the records received are not complete or additional documentation is required a second or third round of record requests may be initiated by the MA organization.

While electronic medical records are increasingly common, both paper and electronic medical records pose specific challenges to the MA organization requesting the records. The work of retrieving paper records may be a hindrance to provider offices complying with a request. It may be necessary to incentivize providers to return the requested medical records or to use the services of a medical record retrieval company to go on-site to obtain copies of the requested medical records. Paper medical records require additional work such as scanning an indexing. It is also imperative to ensure that the image quality is good and that the scanned image is legible. Electronic medical records also pose challenges. Most electronic medical records have various formats that may be viewed, printed, etc. It is imperative that the correct record format be submitted to the MA plan to ensure that all required administrative elements are present. A common error is sending the incorrect version of a note that may show as a draft or pending encounter note that is still awaiting signature and validation from the performing physician. Sending the finalized version will ensure that the MA plan will not have to request the signed version or perform a signature chase.

It is best practice to have multiple reviewers independently review the records to ensure that the documentation is objectively valid. Once the records have been reviewed within the MA organization, the one best record is selected for each condition in question and is submitted to CMS with the CMS form(s) required.

If the HCC is not validated by the available documentation, the MA organization may reach out to the beneficiary to see if he or she was treated by acceptable provider types. The MA organization should also review to see if other conditions within that HCC are validated by the record. New HCCs discovered during an audit should be submitted to CMS. This can include HCCs that have not been reported for the patient or a different diagnosis being submitted to validate an HCC in question.

Some common issues found during an audit are:

- Invalid medical records

- Unacceptable data sources or dates

- Missing provider signatures or invalid authentication

- Missing medical records

  - missing portions of the medical records

  - missing dates of service

- Insufficient or incomplete documentation

- No medical record to validate the reported HCC

- Coding discrepancies that change the HCC

After the medical records are received by CMS and the audit has been completed, the MA organization will receive an audit report, which includes the following results:

- Detailed enrollee-level information relating to confirmed enrollee HCC discrepancies

- The contract-level RAD-V payment error estimate in dollars

- The contract-level payment adjustment amount to be made in dollars

- The approximate time frame for the payment adjustment

- The appeal rights of the MA organization for the audit findings

After the findings of a RAD-V audit are released, MA plans have a three-step appeals process available to address any findings. This process only applies to error determinations from the review of the one best medical record submitted by the MA organization audited by the RAD-V contractor. The request for reconsideration must be received within 30 days of the date of issuance of the RAD-V audit report.

- Level 1: request for reconsideration

  The MA organization may, in writing, request reconsideration and in that request specify the determinations with which the MA organization disagrees and the reason(s) for the appeal. In this review process, the MA organization is not able to submit new documentation to the reviewer except for RAD-V generated attestation, which can remedy signature issues.

- Level 2: request for CMS hearing official review

  If the MA organization, disagrees with the findings of the reconsideration, the organization may request an official hearing, which must be submitted within 60 days of receiving the determination of the reconsideration request. The CMS hearing officer reviews the medical record documentation submitted to the initial auditor without additional evidence or testimony. The hearing officer will provide written notice of the determination made.

- Level 3: request for CMS administrator review

  The MA organization may request that the CMS administrator review the decision made by the hearing officer within 60 days of receiving the decision from the hearing officer. In this level of review, new evidence may be introduced but is limited to the hearing record, written arguments submitted by CMS or the MA organization, and any materials used by the hearing official to reach his or her determination. The CMS administrator may also decline to hear the case.

Any request that does not strictly adhere to the procedures and requirements specified by the RAD-V audit process, will render the request, from the MA organization for appeal, invalid.

Medicare Advantage Risk Adjustment Data Validation—Recovery Audit Contractors

Under the Affordable Care Act (ACA) enacted in March 2010, CMS was required to expand the Recovery Audit program to the MA RAD-V audit program. However, this has not yet occurred. On December 22, 2015, CMS released a request for information (RFI) and a proposed statement of work (SOW) seeking industry feedback on the expansion of the Recovery Audit Contractor (RAC) program into CMS's RAD-V audit process. The agency's proposal would use the RACs to select MA plan enrollees for review, identify underpayments and overpayments associated with diagnosis data submitted to CMS, and calculate the final overpayment/underpayment amounts. CMS intends "to have all MA contracts subject to either a comprehensive or condition-specific RAD-V audit for each payment year."

CMS currently contracts with RACs to identify and correct overpayments and underpayments in Medicare Parts A and B, but there is no definitive timeline for when the new Medicare Part C program will go into effect. The Medicare Part C RAC program, like the others, also proposes to use a contingency fee payment structure, under which the RACs receive a percentage of the amount of the improper payment. Under the new program, in addition to general comprehensive RAD-V audits, RACs will conduct condition-specific RAD-V audits, which focus on specific diagnostic codes or conditions such as diabetes and malnutrition that have high payment error rates. It is also possible that RACs will include the highest weighted diagnoses in their condition-specific audits. These are HIV, sepsis, opportunistic infections, and current cancers. The RACs identify issues based upon their past audit experience, but CMS must approve these issues, and the RACs must publish them.

CMS also is proposing that each payment error identified by the RACs must be reviewed and verified by a secondary review RAD-V contractor. This contractor is tasked with re-reviewing the documentation to validate the initial findings and to confirm the overpayment.

Health and Human Services Risk Adjustment Data Validation

Risk adjustment validation audits are required for commercial risk-adjusted health plans as part of the Affordable Care Act. The Department of Health and Human Services (HHS) Risk Adjustment Data Validation (HHS-RAD-V) review is performed in two steps: (1) an initial validation audit (IVA) performed by an independent auditor selected by the health plan, and (2) a secondary validation audit (SVA) performed by a secondary auditor retained by CMS. The ACA HHS-RAD-V program reviews claims on a post-payment basis, limited to claims submitted in the previous federal fiscal year. The HHS-RAD-V process verifies that the diagnosis codes submitted for payment by the health plan are supported by the medical records.

Under the ACA HHS-RAD-V, IVA, and SVA auditors review a stratified random sample of 200 ACA plan members selected by CMS. The health plan provides enrollment and claims data and the medical records for the 200 members to their IVA auditor. The audit process includes six stages:

- Sample selection

- Initial validation audit

- Secondary validation audit

- Error rate estimation

- Appeals

- Payment adjustments

If both the IVA and SVA identify overpayments, CMS uses the error rate to determine a payment adjustment to calculate the recoupment amount. CMS gives health plans the option of appealing the audit results or the application of the payment adjustment through the RAD-V administrative appeals process.

Health Effectiveness Data and Information Set

The Health Effectiveness Data and Information Set (HEDIS) is a tool that was developed and is maintained by the National Committee for Quality Assurance (NCQA). More than 90 percent of health plans in the U.S. use HEDIS to evaluate the performance of important portions of care and service. HEDIS measures tie into risk adjustment as they impact the reimbursement an MA plan receives from CMS.

Risk adjustment is validation of the overall health status of a population being cared for by a provider or group. Some HEDIS measures are incorporated into the CMS STAR Ratings system and evaluate the efficacy of the healthcare that population has received.

Currently, there are 81 measures within the six domains of care. The specificity of the data used for each measure makes HEDIS a very effective tool to compare health plans. These measures address a broad range of health issues such as:

- Antidepressant medication management

- Comprehensive diabetes care

  - A1C testing

  - diabetic eye exams

- Controlling high blood pressure

- Screenings for cancers such as colorectal and breast

When HEDIS measures are discussed or studied, the "open gaps" are the focus. Gaps are beneficiaries who fall into the age group for the specific measure but have not completed a specific activity or are not compliant with an aspect of their care plan. These beneficiaries can be excluded from the measure based on measure-specific criteria. For example, a patient is excluded from the breast cancer screening measure if there is documentation of a bilateral mastectomy or two unilateral mastectomies in the patient's medical record. Refusal to complete a screening or study does not exclude a patient. The more "closed gaps," the higher the HEDIS score.

It is not common for coding staff to be working on HEDIS-related activities. Typically, this type of activity is completed by nurses with specialized training for HEDIS review and audits. HEDIS audits require in-depth clinical knowledge that is beyond the scope of coding staff. While audit type activities are not commonly completed by coding staff, some HEDIS measures can use coding data. Within the comprehensive diabetes care measure, there is a submeasure that addresses diabetic eye exams. A coder can assist with capturing this information by reporting CPT Category I, II, and/or III codes, such as 2022F, 2024F, 2026F, and 3072F.

This HEDIS information can be used by health plans to identify areas where improvement is needed and to develop strategies for improvement.

Medicare STAR Ratings

The Medicare STAR rating is a pay for performance program for MA and prescription drug plans. CMS uses HEDIS as part of the criteria for the STAR rating system. This program rates MA and prescription drug plans on a scale of one to five with five being the highest, on various performance categories and measures. The STAR ratings are calculated using the following:

- Claim and medical record chart data (Data source: Healthcare Effectiveness Data and Information Set from the National Committee on Quality Assurance)

- Member survey focusing on service experience and access to care (Data source: Consumer Assessment of Healthcare Providers and Systems)

- Member survey focusing on members' perception of health status (Data source: Health Outcomes Survey)

- Pharmacy measures (Data source: Prescription Drug Event)

- Members' complaints, and appeals and grievances (Data source: Health Plan Operations)

The information taken from the above-listed measures is then calculated in the following categories. Each measure and category has a different weight, which impacts the overall STAR rating. These weights may change year over year depending on a variety of factors, such as past performance or other trending indicators.

The STAR categories are:

- Staying healthy; screenings, tests and vaccines: Includes whether members got various screening tests, a yearly flu shot, and other check-ups that help them stay healthy.

- Managing chronic, long-term conditions: Includes how often members with different conditions got certain tests and treatments that help them manage their condition.

- Member experience: Includes ratings of member satisfaction with the plan.

- Member complaints, problems getting services and improvement in the plan's performance: Includes how often Medicare found problems with the plan and how often members filed complaints against the plan and then chose to leave the plan. Includes how much the plan's performance has improved (if at all) over the last two years.

- Customer service: Includes how well the plan handles calls from members, makes decisions about member appeals for health coverage, and handles new enrollment request in a timely way.

Starting in 2014, plans have to have a 4-STAR rating or higher to receive a quality bonus payment from CMS. Prior to that, plans could receive a bonus for a STAR rating of 3, which was about 91 percent of plans in 2012.

The STAR ratings are displayed for beneficiaries to view on Medicare.gov and are intended to assist members in making a decision about their Medicare benefits.

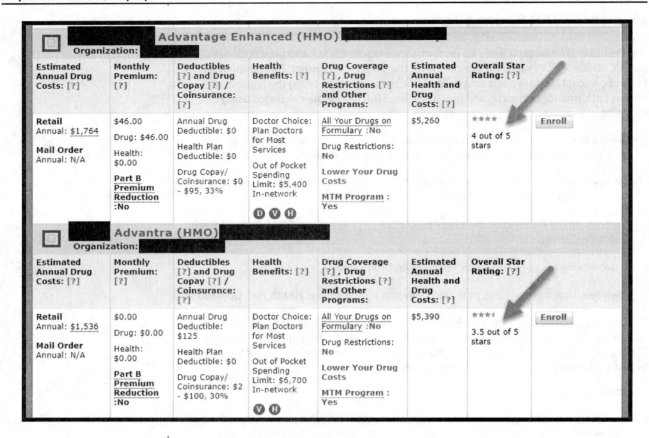

Internal Care and Quality Improvement Audits

Performing chart audits requires careful planning.

Each practice should implement an internal auditing program. Auditing provider charges and billing practices is a large task to undertake, but the results typically lead to improved claims management processes, cash flow, and compliance with payer rules and regulations. Chart audits can serve many purposes, from compliance to research to administrative to clinical. A practice can conduct a chart audit on virtually any aspect of care that is documented in the medical record. Auditing charts allows practices to identify specific coding issues that may occur in claims submissions. There may be a high number of similar types of claim errors that can be identified and, in this case, pre-submission monitoring and review of these may safeguard against repeated errors that result in a claim denial and decreased revenue.

Strategies for risk-adjustment auditing can include an abstract audit of a sample of patients or focusing on a specific condition. It is advisable to incorporate the HHS targeted conditions as well as OIG work plans into internal audits. These work plans and lists are based on widespread trending issues. An internal audit allows the provider and staff to identify incorrect billing patterns before claims are denied or payer audits arise and penalties are assessed.

An audit can be conducted on virtually any aspect of the chart, including diagnostic coding and reporting. The data should be complete, accurate, and must be available in the chart. A chart audit also involves reviewing data that may be deemed confidential; therefore, it is necessary that the internal privacy guidelines be consulted prior to reviewing charts. While most frequently performed to determine compliance with coding and billing requirements, chart audits may also be performed for clinical care quality improvement. A chart audit for quality improvement measures how often and how well something is being done (or not done). For example, a chart audit may involve reviewing a senior citizen care practice's charts to see how often the pneumonia vaccine is offered, administered, or declined. If the audit determines that the vaccine is not being offered or administered as recommended, then there is room for improvement. The HEDIS measures that are appropriate to the practice's population are an excellent source of actionable areas for improvement. Additionally, a practice or institution may develop internal improvement items, such as increasing correct practice for taking a patient's blood pressure.

There are a few steps that can be taken by clinical staff to help avoid mistakes, including:

- Developing written policies and procedures and distributing them to the clinical and administrative staff.

- Creating a written compliance plan and educate all employees on its content.

- Ensuring adherence with internal compliance policies and procedures by all clinical and administrative staff.

- Providing coding and billing education to clinical staff on a regular basis (i.e., annual code and guideline changes).

- Providing access to current coding books and regulation manuals as references.

- Conducting periodic internal audits and documenting the results.

It is imperative to ensure the most accurate coding and billing that staff receive on-going education and training to stay up to date on the annual code updates and changes as well as any updates to guidelines. A thorough understanding of the code sets, medical terminology, and proper use of coding books and other resources is essential to not only reducing claim denials but also to limiting liability from erroneous or fraudulent claims processing practices. It is not only detrimental to the revenue cycle process and the practice's bottom line to code improperly but it can also increase risk and liability while exposing the practice to audits and ongoing reviews of claims. Most coding errors found are easily remedied with focused education and training.

Best practices are to establish a formal audit process. Develop policies and procedures identifying a designated audit coordinator to manage all audit activity and outlining the audit process. Designate the roles and responsibilities of all applicable staff at each step of the process, including record requests and appropriate time frames, audit result tracking, and appeals. Provide education to staff on the types of validation audits and the need for clear and concise documentation.

CMS Requirements

Item	Yes	No
Patient Name/Identifiers Present		
Date of Service		
Face-to-Face Encounter		
Provider Credential Present		
Provider Validation/Signature in Valid Format		

HCC Coding

ICD-10-CM Code	Validated	Comments

Findings/Notes:

Mock Audit Protocol

It may be helpful to test internal audits or audit preparedness with a mock official audit.

The first step in this is to ensure that the members of the team who respond to audits are aware that these duties are part of their role. These team members may include a medical director, project manager(s), auditing staff, and other team members. If a mock audit is being conducted as part of an MA organization, a process should be in place that outlines protocol for reaching out to the various clinics and providers to request medical records. Part of this outreach will include matching the patients listed on the audit with the providers they saw during the indicated time frame.

Next, practices will want to start collecting the records. A clinic or provider's office should review the process for collecting records either paper or electronic. They should identify who will be pulling those records. For an electronic medical record, ensure that whomever is tasked with the record retrieval is aware of which format is the most correct to pull/send. An MA organization will want to have a designated team to follow up on medical record request letters, such as a provider advocate or medical director.

After the needed medical records are collected, the next step is to review the records. If possible, the auditor should not be the person who coded the record initially. The auditor should have advanced knowledge about what is being audited. The records should be reviewed to ensure all required administrative elements are present in the medical record; this type of issue is "low hanging fruit" for official audits such as RAD-V. It is important to track results. Once the audit has been completed, the practice should review any trends found and provide education to remedy these issues.

Once the mock audit is completed, the final step is to evaluate the efficacy of the audit. A practice should identify what went well and what needs to be improved and develop an action plan to address the needed improvements. Some common issues identified are needing vendor help for record collection, improvement in internal reporting to assist with trending issues, additional guidance needed for internal staff on policies or procedures, and the need for additional resources to ensure audits run smoothly, such as a specific dedicated staff member to serve as the main point of contact.

Chapter 4. CMS-HCC Model Category V24

2020/2021/2022 CMS-HCC V24 Model Disease Coefficient Relative Factors and Hierarchies for Continuing Enrollees Community and Institutional Beneficiaries with 2022 Midyear Final ICD-10-CM Mappings

According to the Announcement of Calendar Year (CY) 2022 Medicare Advantage (MA) Capitation Rates and Part C and Part D Payment Policies, published on January 15, 2021, as noted in Part I of the CY 2022 Advance Notice, published on September 14, 2020, and Part II of the CY 2022 Advance Notice, published on October 30, 2020, CMS will continue to use the 2020 risk adjustment model for 2022, completely phasing in the 2020 CMS-HCC model (previously known as the alternative payment condition count [APCC] model) with no blending for the risk score calculation.

ICD-10-CM Code	ICD-10-CM Code Description	V24 CMS-HCC	V24 CMS-HCC Disease Group	V24 CMS-HCC Hierarchies	Community, NonDual, Aged	Community, NonDual, Disabled	Community, FBDual, Aged	Community, FBDual, Disabled	Community, PBDual, Aged	Community, PBDual, Disabled	Institutional
A01.03	Typhoid pneumonia	115	Pneumococcal Pneumonia, Empyema, Lung Abscess		0.130	—	0.258	—	0.093	0.082	0.156
A01.04	Typhoid arthritis	39	Bone/Joint/Muscle Infections/Necrosis		0.401	0.378	0.558	0.682	0.443	0.435	0.401
A01.05	Typhoid osteomyelitis	39	Bone/Joint/Muscle Infections/Necrosis		0.401	0.378	0.558	0.682	0.443	0.435	0.401
A02.1	Salmonella sepsis	2	Septicemia, Sepsis, Systemic Inflammatory Response Syndrome/Shock		0.352	0.414	0.453	0.530	0.316	0.297	0.324
A02.22	Salmonella pneumonia	115	Pneumococcal Pneumonia, Empyema, Lung Abscess		0.130	—	0.258	—	0.093	0.082	0.156
A02.23	Salmonella arthritis	39	Bone/Joint/Muscle Infections/Necrosis		0.401	0.378	0.558	0.682	0.443	0.435	0.401
A02.24	Salmonella osteomyelitis	39	Bone/Joint/Muscle Infections/Necrosis		0.401	0.378	0.558	0.682	0.443	0.435	0.401
A06.5	Amebic lung abscess	115	Pneumococcal Pneumonia, Empyema, Lung Abscess		0.130	—	0.258	—	0.093	0.082	0.156
A07.2	Cryptosporidiosis	6	Opportunistic Infections		0.424	0.740	0.572	0.803	0.318	0.658	0.534
A20.2	Pneumonic plague	115	Pneumococcal Pneumonia, Empyema, Lung Abscess		0.130	—	0.258	—	0.093	0.082	0.156
A20.7	Septicemic plague	2	Septicemia, Sepsis, Systemic Inflammatory Response Syndrome/Shock		0.352	0.414	0.453	0.530	0.316	0.297	0.324
A21.2	Pulmonary tularemia	115	Pneumococcal Pneumonia, Empyema, Lung Abscess		0.130	—	0.258	—	0.093	0.082	0.156
A22.1	Pulmonary anthrax	115	Pneumococcal Pneumonia, Empyema, Lung Abscess		0.130	—	0.258	—	0.093	0.082	0.156
A22.7	Anthrax sepsis	2	Septicemia, Sepsis, Systemic Inflammatory Response Syndrome/Shock		0.352	0.414	0.453	0.530	0.316	0.297	0.324
A26.7	Erysipelothrix sepsis	2	Septicemia, Sepsis, Systemic Inflammatory Response Syndrome/Shock		0.352	0.414	0.453	0.530	0.316	0.297	0.324
A31.0	Pulmonary mycobacterial infection	6	Opportunistic Infections		0.424	0.740	0.572	0.803	0.318	0.658	0.534
A31.2	Disseminated mycobacterium avium-intracellulare complex (DMAC)	6	Opportunistic Infections		0.424	0.740	0.572	0.803	0.318	0.658	0.534
A32.7	Listerial sepsis	2	Septicemia, Sepsis, Systemic Inflammatory Response Syndrome/Shock		0.352	0.414	0.453	0.530	0.316	0.297	0.324
A36.81	Diphtheritic cardiomyopathy	85	Congestive Heart Failure		0.331	0.447	0.371	0.486	0.336	0.422	0.203
A39.1	Waterhouse-Friderichsen syndrome	23	Other Significant Endocrine and Metabolic Disorders		0.194	0.378	0.211	0.299	0.174	0.319	0.379
A39.2	Acute meningococcemia	2	Septicemia, Sepsis, Systemic Inflammatory Response Syndrome/Shock		0.352	0.414	0.453	0.530	0.316	0.297	0.324
A39.3	Chronic meningococcemia	2	Septicemia, Sepsis, Systemic Inflammatory Response Syndrome/Shock		0.352	0.414	0.453	0.530	0.316	0.297	0.324
A39.4	Meningococcemia, unspecified	2	Septicemia, Sepsis, Systemic Inflammatory Response Syndrome/Shock		0.352	0.414	0.453	0.530	0.316	0.297	0.324
A39.83	Meningococcal arthritis	39	Bone/Joint/Muscle Infections/Necrosis		0.401	0.378	0.558	0.682	0.443	0.435	0.401
A39.84	Postmeningococcal arthritis	39	Bone/Joint/Muscle Infections/Necrosis		0.401	0.378	0.558	0.682	0.443	0.435	0.401

ICD-10-CM Code	ICD-10-CM Code Description	V24 CMS-HCC	V24 CMS-HCC Disease Group	V24 CMS-HCC Hierarchies	Community, NonDual, Aged	Community, NonDual, Disabled	Community, FBDual, Aged	Community, FBDual, Disabled	Community, PBDual, Aged	Community, PBDual, Disabled	Institutional
A40.0	Sepsis due to streptococcus, group A	2	Septicemia, Sepsis, Systemic Inflammatory Response Syndrome/Shock		0.352	0.414	0.453	0.530	0.316	0.297	0.324
A40.1	Sepsis due to streptococcus, group B	2	Septicemia, Sepsis, Systemic Inflammatory Response Syndrome/Shock		0.352	0.414	0.453	0.530	0.316	0.297	0.324
A40.3	Sepsis due to Streptococcus pneumoniae	2	Septicemia, Sepsis, Systemic Inflammatory Response Syndrome/Shock		0.352	0.414	0.453	0.530	0.316	0.297	0.324
A40.8	Other streptococcal sepsis	2	Septicemia, Sepsis, Systemic Inflammatory Response Syndrome/Shock		0.352	0.414	0.453	0.530	0.316	0.297	0.324
A40.9	Streptococcal sepsis, unspecified	2	Septicemia, Sepsis, Systemic Inflammatory Response Syndrome/Shock		0.352	0.414	0.453	0.530	0.316	0.297	0.324
A41.01	Sepsis due to Methicillin susceptible Staphylococcus aureus	2	Septicemia, Sepsis, Systemic Inflammatory Response Syndrome/Shock		0.352	0.414	0.453	0.530	0.316	0.297	0.324
A41.02	Sepsis due to Methicillin resistant Staphylococcus aureus	2	Septicemia, Sepsis, Systemic Inflammatory Response Syndrome/Shock		0.352	0.414	0.453	0.530	0.316	0.297	0.324
A41.1	Sepsis due to other specified staphylococcus	2	Septicemia, Sepsis, Systemic Inflammatory Response Syndrome/Shock		0.352	0.414	0.453	0.530	0.316	0.297	0.324
A41.2	Sepsis due to unspecified staphylococcus	2	Septicemia, Sepsis, Systemic Inflammatory Response Syndrome/Shock		0.352	0.414	0.453	0.530	0.316	0.297	0.324
A41.3	Sepsis due to Hemophilus influenzae	2	Septicemia, Sepsis, Systemic Inflammatory Response Syndrome/Shock		0.352	0.414	0.453	0.530	0.316	0.297	0.324
A41.4	Sepsis due to anaerobes	2	Septicemia, Sepsis, Systemic Inflammatory Response Syndrome/Shock		0.352	0.414	0.453	0.530	0.316	0.297	0.324
A41.50	Gram-negative sepsis, unspecified	2	Septicemia, Sepsis, Systemic Inflammatory Response Syndrome/Shock		0.352	0.414	0.453	0.530	0.316	0.297	0.324
A41.51	Sepsis due to Escherichia coli [E. coli]	2	Septicemia, Sepsis, Systemic Inflammatory Response Syndrome/Shock		0.352	0.414	0.453	0.530	0.316	0.297	0.324
A41.52	Sepsis due to Pseudomonas	2	Septicemia, Sepsis, Systemic Inflammatory Response Syndrome/Shock		0.352	0.414	0.453	0.530	0.316	0.297	0.324
A41.53	Sepsis due to Serratia	2	Septicemia, Sepsis, Systemic Inflammatory Response Syndrome/Shock		0.352	0.414	0.453	0.530	0.316	0.297	0.324
A41.59	Other Gram-negative sepsis	2	Septicemia, Sepsis, Systemic Inflammatory Response Syndrome/Shock		0.352	0.414	0.453	0.530	0.316	0.297	0.324
A41.81	Sepsis due to Enterococcus	2	Septicemia, Sepsis, Systemic Inflammatory Response Syndrome/Shock		0.352	0.414	0.453	0.530	0.316	0.297	0.324
A41.89	Other specified sepsis	2	Septicemia, Sepsis, Systemic Inflammatory Response Syndrome/Shock		0.352	0.414	0.453	0.530	0.316	0.297	0.324
A41.9	Sepsis, unspecified organism	2	Septicemia, Sepsis, Systemic Inflammatory Response Syndrome/Shock		0.352	0.414	0.453	0.530	0.316	0.297	0.324
A42.0	Pulmonary actinomycosis	115	Pneumococcal Pneumonia, Empyema, Lung Abscess		0.130	—	0.258	—	0.093	0.082	0.156

ICD-10-CM Code	ICD-10-CM Code Description	V24 CMS-HCC	V24 CMS-HCC Disease Group	V24 CMS-HCC Hierarchies	Community, NonDual, Aged	Community, NonDual, Disabled	Community, FBDual, Aged	Community, FBDual, Disabled	Community, PBDual, Aged	Community, PBDual, Disabled	Institutional
A42.7	Actinomycotic sepsis	2	Septicemia, Sepsis, Systemic Inflammatory Response Syndrome/ Shock		0.352	0.414	0.453	0.530	0.316	0.297	0.324
A43.0	Pulmonary nocardiosis	115	Pneumococcal Pneumonia, Empyema, Lung Abscess		0.130	—	0.258	—	0.093	0.082	0.156
A48.0	Gas gangrene	106	Atherosclerosis of the Extremities with Ulceration or Gangrene	107,108, 161,189	1.488	1.521	1.724	1.748	1.504	1.525	0.867
A48.1	Legionnaires' disease	114	Aspiration and Specified Bacterial Pneumonias	115	0.517	0.236	0.641	0.375	0.514	0.198	0.156
A48.3	Toxic shock syndrome	2	Septicemia, Sepsis, Systemic Inflammatory Response Syndrome/ Shock		0.352	0.414	0.453	0.530	0.316	0.297	0.324
A50.55	Late congenital syphilitic arthropathy	39	Bone/Joint/Muscle Infections/Necrosis		0.401	0.378	0.558	0.682	0.443	0.435	0.401
A54.40	Gonococcal infection of musculoskeletal system, unspecified	39	Bone/Joint/Muscle Infections/Necrosis		0.401	0.378	0.558	0.682	0.443	0.435	0.401
A54.41	Gonococcal spondylopathy	39	Bone/Joint/Muscle Infections/Necrosis		0.401	0.378	0.558	0.682	0.443	0.435	0.401
A54.42	Gonococcal arthritis	39	Bone/Joint/Muscle Infections/Necrosis		0.401	0.378	0.558	0.682	0.443	0.435	0.401
A54.43	Gonococcal osteomyelitis	39	Bone/Joint/Muscle Infections/Necrosis		0.401	0.378	0.558	0.682	0.443	0.435	0.401
A54.49	Gonococcal infection of other musculoskeletal tissue	39	Bone/Joint/Muscle Infections/Necrosis		0.401	0.378	0.558	0.682	0.443	0.435	0.401
A54.84	Gonococcal pneumonia	115	Pneumococcal Pneumonia, Empyema, Lung Abscess		0.130	—	0.258	—	0.093	0.082	0.156
A54.85	Gonococcal peritonitis	33	Intestinal Obstruction/Perforation		0.219	0.503	0.258	0.538	0.232	0.552	0.352
A54.86	Gonococcal sepsis	2	Septicemia, Sepsis, Systemic Inflammatory Response Syndrome/ Shock		0.352	0.414	0.453	0.530	0.316	0.297	0.324
A66.6	Bone and joint lesions of yaws	39	Bone/Joint/Muscle Infections/Necrosis		0.401	0.378	0.558	0.682	0.443	0.435	0.401
A69.23	Arthritis due to Lyme disease	39	Bone/Joint/Muscle Infections/Necrosis		0.401	0.378	0.558	0.682	0.443	0.435	0.401
A81.00	Creutzfeldt-Jakob disease, unspecified	52	Dementia Without Complication		0.346	0.224	0.453	0.256	0.420	0.257	—
A81.01	Variant Creutzfeldt-Jakob disease	52	Dementia Without Complication		0.346	0.224	0.453	0.256	0.420	0.257	—
A81.09	Other Creutzfeldt-Jakob disease	52	Dementia Without Complication		0.346	0.224	0.453	0.256	0.420	0.257	—
A81.1	Subacute sclerosing panencephalitis	52	Dementia Without Complication		0.346	0.224	0.453	0.256	0.420	0.257	—
A81.2	Progressive multifocal leukoencephalopathy	52	Dementia Without Complication		0.346	0.224	0.453	0.256	0.420	0.257	—
A81.81	Kuru	52	Dementia Without Complication		0.346	0.224	0.453	0.256	0.420	0.257	—
A81.82	Gerstmann-Straussler-Scheinker syndrome	52	Dementia Without Complication		0.346	0.224	0.453	0.256	0.420	0.257	—
A81.83	Fatal familial insomnia	52	Dementia Without Complication		0.346	0.224	0.453	0.256	0.420	0.257	—
A81.89	Other atypical virus infections of central nervous system	52	Dementia Without Complication		0.346	0.224	0.453	0.256	0.420	0.257	—
A81.9	Atypical virus infection of central nervous system, unspecified	52	Dementia Without Complication		0.346	0.224	0.453	0.256	0.420	0.257	—
B00.7	Disseminated herpesviral disease	2	Septicemia, Sepsis, Systemic Inflammatory Response Syndrome/ Shock		0.352	0.414	0.453	0.530	0.316	0.297	0.324
B00.82	Herpes simplex myelitis	72	Spinal Cord Disorders/Injuries	169	0.481	0.369	0.532	0.377	0.512	0.336	0.289
B01.12	Varicella myelitis	72	Spinal Cord Disorders/Injuries	169	0.481	0.369	0.532	0.377	0.512	0.336	0.289
B02.24	Postherpetic myelitis	72	Spinal Cord Disorders/Injuries	169	0.481	0.369	0.532	0.377	0.512	0.336	0.289
B06.82	Rubella arthritis	39	Bone/Joint/Muscle Infections/Necrosis		0.401	0.378	0.558	0.682	0.443	0.435	0.401
B18.0	Chronic viral hepatitis B with delta-agent	29	Chronic Hepatitis		0.147	0.314	0.042	0.292	0.181	0.238	0.485
B18.1	Chronic viral hepatitis B without delta-agent	29	Chronic Hepatitis		0.147	0.314	0.042	0.292	0.181	0.238	0.485
B18.2	Chronic viral hepatitis C	29	Chronic Hepatitis		0.147	0.314	0.042	0.292	0.181	0.238	0.485
B18.8	Other chronic viral hepatitis	29	Chronic Hepatitis		0.147	0.314	0.042	0.292	0.181	0.238	0.485

ICD-10-CM Code	ICD-10-CM Code Description	V24 CMS-HCC	V24 CMS-HCC Disease Group	V24 CMS-HCC Hierarchies	Community, NonDual, Aged	Community, NonDual, Disabled	Community, FBDual, Aged	Community, FBDual, Disabled	Community, PBDual, Aged	Community, PBDual, Disabled	Institutional
B18.9	Chronic viral hepatitis, unspecified	29	Chronic Hepatitis		0.147	0.314	0.042	0.292	0.181	0.238	0.485
B20	Human immunodeficiency virus [HIV] disease	1	HIV/AIDS		0.335	0.287	0.595	0.396	0.482	0.200	1.722
B25.0	Cytomegaloviral pneumonitis	6	Opportunistic Infections		0.424	0.740	0.572	0.803	0.318	0.658	0.534
B25.1	Cytomegaloviral hepatitis	6	Opportunistic Infections		0.424	0.740	0.572	0.803	0.318	0.658	0.534
B25.2	Cytomegaloviral pancreatitis	6	Opportunistic Infections		0.424	0.740	0.572	0.803	0.318	0.658	0.534
B25.8	Other cytomegaloviral diseases	6	Opportunistic Infections		0.424	0.740	0.572	0.803	0.318	0.658	0.534
B25.9	Cytomegaloviral disease, unspecified	6	Opportunistic Infections		0.424	0.740	0.572	0.803	0.318	0.658	0.534
B26.85	Mumps arthritis	39	Bone/Joint/Muscle Infections/Necrosis		0.401	0.378	0.558	0.682	0.443	0.435	0.401
B33.24	Viral cardiomyopathy	85	Congestive Heart Failure		0.331	0.447	0.371	0.486	0.336	0.422	0.203
B37.1	Pulmonary candidiasis	6	Opportunistic Infections		0.424	0.740	0.572	0.803	0.318	0.658	0.534
B37.7	Candidal sepsis	2	Septicemia, Sepsis, Systemic Inflammatory Response Syndrome/Shock		0.352	0.414	0.453	0.530	0.316	0.297	0.324
B37.7	Candidal sepsis	6	Opportunistic Infections		0.424	0.740	0.572	0.803	0.318	0.658	0.534
B37.81	Candidal esophagitis	6	Opportunistic Infections		0.424	0.740	0.572	0.803	0.318	0.658	0.534
B38.0	Acute pulmonary coccidioidomycosis	115	Pneumococcal Pneumonia, Empyema, Lung Abscess		0.130	—	0.258	—	0.093	0.082	0.156
B38.1	Chronic pulmonary coccidioidomycosis	115	Pneumococcal Pneumonia, Empyema, Lung Abscess		0.130	—	0.258	—	0.093	0.082	0.156
B38.2	Pulmonary coccidioidomycosis, unspecified	115	Pneumococcal Pneumonia, Empyema, Lung Abscess		0.130	—	0.258	—	0.093	0.082	0.156
B39.0	Acute pulmonary histoplasmosis capsulati	115	Pneumococcal Pneumonia, Empyema, Lung Abscess		0.130	—	0.258	—	0.093	0.082	0.156
B39.1	Chronic pulmonary histoplasmosis capsulati	115	Pneumococcal Pneumonia, Empyema, Lung Abscess		0.130	—	0.258	—	0.093	0.082	0.156
B39.2	Pulmonary histoplasmosis capsulati, unspecified	115	Pneumococcal Pneumonia, Empyema, Lung Abscess		0.130	—	0.258	—	0.093	0.082	0.156
B40.0	Acute pulmonary blastomycosis	115	Pneumococcal Pneumonia, Empyema, Lung Abscess		0.130	—	0.258	—	0.093	0.082	0.156
B40.1	Chronic pulmonary blastomycosis	115	Pneumococcal Pneumonia, Empyema, Lung Abscess		0.130	—	0.258	—	0.093	0.082	0.156
B40.2	Pulmonary blastomycosis, unspecified	115	Pneumococcal Pneumonia, Empyema, Lung Abscess		0.130	—	0.258	—	0.093	0.082	0.156
B41.0	Pulmonary paracoccidioidomycosis	115	Pneumococcal Pneumonia, Empyema, Lung Abscess		0.130	—	0.258	—	0.093	0.082	0.156
B42.82	Sporotrichosis arthritis	39	Bone/Joint/Muscle Infections/Necrosis		0.401	0.378	0.558	0.682	0.443	0.435	0.401
B44.0	Invasive pulmonary aspergillosis	6	Opportunistic Infections		0.424	0.740	0.572	0.803	0.318	0.658	0.534
B44.1	Other pulmonary aspergillosis	6	Opportunistic Infections		0.424	0.740	0.572	0.803	0.318	0.658	0.534
B44.2	Tonsillar aspergillosis	6	Opportunistic Infections		0.424	0.740	0.572	0.803	0.318	0.658	0.534
B44.7	Disseminated aspergillosis	6	Opportunistic Infections		0.424	0.740	0.572	0.803	0.318	0.658	0.534
B44.81	Allergic bronchopulmonary aspergillosis	112	Fibrosis of Lung and Other Chronic Lung Disorders		0.219	0.237	0.161	0.275	0.200	0.229	0.110
B44.89	Other forms of aspergillosis	6	Opportunistic Infections		0.424	0.740	0.572	0.803	0.318	0.658	0.534
B44.9	Aspergillosis, unspecified	6	Opportunistic Infections		0.424	0.740	0.572	0.803	0.318	0.658	0.534
B45.0	Pulmonary cryptococcosis	6	Opportunistic Infections		0.424	0.740	0.572	0.803	0.318	0.658	0.534
B45.1	Cerebral cryptococcosis	6	Opportunistic Infections		0.424	0.740	0.572	0.803	0.318	0.658	0.534
B45.2	Cutaneous cryptococcosis	6	Opportunistic Infections		0.424	0.740	0.572	0.803	0.318	0.658	0.534
B45.3	Osseous cryptococcosis	6	Opportunistic Infections		0.424	0.740	0.572	0.803	0.318	0.658	0.534
B45.7	Disseminated cryptococcosis	6	Opportunistic Infections		0.424	0.740	0.572	0.803	0.318	0.658	0.534
B45.8	Other forms of cryptococcosis	6	Opportunistic Infections		0.424	0.740	0.572	0.803	0.318	0.658	0.534
B45.9	Cryptococcosis, unspecified	6	Opportunistic Infections		0.424	0.740	0.572	0.803	0.318	0.658	0.534
B46.0	Pulmonary mucormycosis	6	Opportunistic Infections		0.424	0.740	0.572	0.803	0.318	0.658	0.534
B46.1	Rhinocerebral mucormycosis	6	Opportunistic Infections		0.424	0.740	0.572	0.803	0.318	0.658	0.534
B46.2	Gastrointestinal mucormycosis	6	Opportunistic Infections		0.424	0.740	0.572	0.803	0.318	0.658	0.534

ICD-10-CM Code	ICD-10-CM Code Description	V24 CMS-HCC	V24 CMS-HCC Disease Group	V24 CMS-HCC Hierarchies	Community, NonDual, Aged	Community, NonDual, Disabled	Community, FBDual, Aged	Community, FBDual, Disabled	Community, PBDual, Aged	Community, PBDual, Disabled	Institutional
B46.3	Cutaneous mucormycosis	6	Opportunistic Infections		0.424	0.740	0.572	0.803	0.318	0.658	0.534
B46.4	Disseminated mucormycosis	6	Opportunistic Infections		0.424	0.740	0.572	0.803	0.318	0.658	0.534
B46.5	Mucormycosis, unspecified	6	Opportunistic Infections		0.424	0.740	0.572	0.803	0.318	0.658	0.534
B46.8	Other zygomycoses	6	Opportunistic Infections		0.424	0.740	0.572	0.803	0.318	0.658	0.534
B46.9	Zygomycosis, unspecified	6	Opportunistic Infections		0.424	0.740	0.572	0.803	0.318	0.658	0.534
B48.4	Penicillosis	6	Opportunistic Infections		0.424	0.740	0.572	0.803	0.318	0.658	0.534
B48.8	Other specified mycoses	6	Opportunistic Infections		0.424	0.740	0.572	0.803	0.318	0.658	0.534
B58.2	Toxoplasma meningoencephalitis	6	Opportunistic Infections		0.424	0.740	0.572	0.803	0.318	0.658	0.534
B58.3	Pulmonary toxoplasmosis	6	Opportunistic Infections		0.424	0.740	0.572	0.803	0.318	0.658	0.534
B59	Pneumocystosis	6	Opportunistic Infections		0.424	0.740	0.572	0.803	0.318	0.658	0.534
B66.4	Paragonimiasis	115	Pneumococcal Pneumonia, Empyema, Lung Abscess		0.130	—	0.258	—	0.093	0.082	0.156
B67.1	Echinococcus granulosus infection of lung	115	Pneumococcal Pneumonia, Empyema, Lung Abscess		0.130	—	0.258	—	0.093	0.082	0.156
B97.35	Human immunodeficiency virus, type 2 [HIV 2] as the cause of diseases classified elsewhere	1	HIV/AIDS		0.335	0.287	0.595	0.396	0.482	0.200	1.722
C01	Malignant neoplasm of base of tongue	11	Colorectal, Bladder, and Other Cancers	12	0.307	0.345	0.317	0.355	0.330	0.351	0.294
C02.0	Malignant neoplasm of dorsal surface of tongue	11	Colorectal, Bladder, and Other Cancers	12	0.307	0.345	0.317	0.355	0.330	0.351	0.294
C02.1	Malignant neoplasm of border of tongue	11	Colorectal, Bladder, and Other Cancers	12	0.307	0.345	0.317	0.355	0.330	0.351	0.294
C02.2	Malignant neoplasm of ventral surface of tongue	11	Colorectal, Bladder, and Other Cancers	12	0.307	0.345	0.317	0.355	0.330	0.351	0.294
C02.3	Malignant neoplasm of anterior two-thirds of tongue, part unspecified	11	Colorectal, Bladder, and Other Cancers	12	0.307	0.345	0.317	0.355	0.330	0.351	0.294
C02.4	Malignant neoplasm of lingual tonsil	11	Colorectal, Bladder, and Other Cancers	12	0.307	0.345	0.317	0.355	0.330	0.351	0.294
C02.8	Malignant neoplasm of overlapping sites of tongue	11	Colorectal, Bladder, and Other Cancers	12	0.307	0.345	0.317	0.355	0.330	0.351	0.294
C02.9	Malignant neoplasm of tongue, unspecified	11	Colorectal, Bladder, and Other Cancers	12	0.307	0.345	0.317	0.355	0.330	0.351	0.294
C03.0	Malignant neoplasm of upper gum	11	Colorectal, Bladder, and Other Cancers	12	0.307	0.345	0.317	0.355	0.330	0.351	0.294
C03.1	Malignant neoplasm of lower gum	11	Colorectal, Bladder, and Other Cancers	12	0.307	0.345	0.317	0.355	0.330	0.351	0.294
C03.9	Malignant neoplasm of gum, unspecified	11	Colorectal, Bladder, and Other Cancers	12	0.307	0.345	0.317	0.355	0.330	0.351	0.294
C04.0	Malignant neoplasm of anterior floor of mouth	11	Colorectal, Bladder, and Other Cancers	12	0.307	0.345	0.317	0.355	0.330	0.351	0.294
C04.1	Malignant neoplasm of lateral floor of mouth	11	Colorectal, Bladder, and Other Cancers	12	0.307	0.345	0.317	0.355	0.330	0.351	0.294
C04.8	Malignant neoplasm of overlapping sites of floor of mouth	11	Colorectal, Bladder, and Other Cancers	12	0.307	0.345	0.317	0.355	0.330	0.351	0.294
C04.9	Malignant neoplasm of floor of mouth, unspecified	11	Colorectal, Bladder, and Other Cancers	12	0.307	0.345	0.317	0.355	0.330	0.351	0.294
C05.0	Malignant neoplasm of hard palate	11	Colorectal, Bladder, and Other Cancers	12	0.307	0.345	0.317	0.355	0.330	0.351	0.294
C05.1	Malignant neoplasm of soft palate	11	Colorectal, Bladder, and Other Cancers	12	0.307	0.345	0.317	0.355	0.330	0.351	0.294
C05.2	Malignant neoplasm of uvula	11	Colorectal, Bladder, and Other Cancers	12	0.307	0.345	0.317	0.355	0.330	0.351	0.294
C05.8	Malignant neoplasm of overlapping sites of palate	11	Colorectal, Bladder, and Other Cancers	12	0.307	0.345	0.317	0.355	0.330	0.351	0.294
C05.9	Malignant neoplasm of palate, unspecified	11	Colorectal, Bladder, and Other Cancers	12	0.307	0.345	0.317	0.355	0.330	0.351	0.294
C06.0	Malignant neoplasm of cheek mucosa	11	Colorectal, Bladder, and Other Cancers	12	0.307	0.345	0.317	0.355	0.330	0.351	0.294
C06.1	Malignant neoplasm of vestibule of mouth	11	Colorectal, Bladder, and Other Cancers	12	0.307	0.345	0.317	0.355	0.330	0.351	0.294

ICD-10-CM Code	ICD-10-CM Code Description	V24 CMS-HCC	V24 CMS-HCC Disease Group	V24 CMS-HCC Hierarchies	Community, NonDual, Aged	Community, NonDual, Disabled	Community, FBDual, Aged	Community, FBDual, Disabled	Community, PBDual, Aged	Community, PBDual, Disabled	Institutional
C06.2	Malignant neoplasm of retromolar area	11	Colorectal, Bladder, and Other Cancers	12	0.307	0.345	0.317	0.355	0.330	0.351	0.294
C06.80	Malignant neoplasm of overlapping sites of unspecified parts of mouth	11	Colorectal, Bladder, and Other Cancers	12	0.307	0.345	0.317	0.355	0.330	0.351	0.294
C06.89	Malignant neoplasm of overlapping sites of other parts of mouth	11	Colorectal, Bladder, and Other Cancers	12	0.307	0.345	0.317	0.355	0.330	0.351	0.294
C06.9	Malignant neoplasm of mouth, unspecified	11	Colorectal, Bladder, and Other Cancers	12	0.307	0.345	0.317	0.355	0.330	0.351	0.294
C07	Malignant neoplasm of parotid gland	11	Colorectal, Bladder, and Other Cancers	12	0.307	0.345	0.317	0.355	0.330	0.351	0.294
C08.0	Malignant neoplasm of submandibular gland	11	Colorectal, Bladder, and Other Cancers	12	0.307	0.345	0.317	0.355	0.330	0.351	0.294
C08.1	Malignant neoplasm of sublingual gland	11	Colorectal, Bladder, and Other Cancers	12	0.307	0.345	0.317	0.355	0.330	0.351	0.294
C08.9	Malignant neoplasm of major salivary gland, unspecified	11	Colorectal, Bladder, and Other Cancers	12	0.307	0.345	0.317	0.355	0.330	0.351	0.294
C09.0	Malignant neoplasm of tonsillar fossa	11	Colorectal, Bladder, and Other Cancers	12	0.307	0.345	0.317	0.355	0.330	0.351	0.294
C09.1	Malignant neoplasm of tonsillar pillar (anterior) (posterior)	11	Colorectal, Bladder, and Other Cancers	12	0.307	0.345	0.317	0.355	0.330	0.351	0.294
C09.8	Malignant neoplasm of overlapping sites of tonsil	11	Colorectal, Bladder, and Other Cancers	12	0.307	0.345	0.317	0.355	0.330	0.351	0.294
C09.9	Malignant neoplasm of tonsil, unspecified	11	Colorectal, Bladder, and Other Cancers	12	0.307	0.345	0.317	0.355	0.330	0.351	0.294
C10.0	Malignant neoplasm of vallecula	11	Colorectal, Bladder, and Other Cancers	12	0.307	0.345	0.317	0.355	0.330	0.351	0.294
C10.1	Malignant neoplasm of anterior surface of epiglottis	11	Colorectal, Bladder, and Other Cancers	12	0.307	0.345	0.317	0.355	0.330	0.351	0.294
C10.2	Malignant neoplasm of lateral wall of oropharynx	11	Colorectal, Bladder, and Other Cancers	12	0.307	0.345	0.317	0.355	0.330	0.351	0.294
C10.3	Malignant neoplasm of posterior wall of oropharynx	11	Colorectal, Bladder, and Other Cancers	12	0.307	0.345	0.317	0.355	0.330	0.351	0.294
C10.4	Malignant neoplasm of branchial cleft	11	Colorectal, Bladder, and Other Cancers	12	0.307	0.345	0.317	0.355	0.330	0.351	0.294
C10.8	Malignant neoplasm of overlapping sites of oropharynx	11	Colorectal, Bladder, and Other Cancers	12	0.307	0.345	0.317	0.355	0.330	0.351	0.294
C10.9	Malignant neoplasm of oropharynx, unspecified	11	Colorectal, Bladder, and Other Cancers	12	0.307	0.345	0.317	0.355	0.330	0.351	0.294
C11.0	Malignant neoplasm of superior wall of nasopharynx	11	Colorectal, Bladder, and Other Cancers	12	0.307	0.345	0.317	0.355	0.330	0.351	0.294
C11.1	Malignant neoplasm of posterior wall of nasopharynx	11	Colorectal, Bladder, and Other Cancers	12	0.307	0.345	0.317	0.355	0.330	0.351	0.294
C11.2	Malignant neoplasm of lateral wall of nasopharynx	11	Colorectal, Bladder, and Other Cancers	12	0.307	0.345	0.317	0.355	0.330	0.351	0.294
C11.3	Malignant neoplasm of anterior wall of nasopharynx	11	Colorectal, Bladder, and Other Cancers	12	0.307	0.345	0.317	0.355	0.330	0.351	0.294
C11.8	Malignant neoplasm of overlapping sites of nasopharynx	11	Colorectal, Bladder, and Other Cancers	12	0.307	0.345	0.317	0.355	0.330	0.351	0.294
C11.9	Malignant neoplasm of nasopharynx, unspecified	11	Colorectal, Bladder, and Other Cancers	12	0.307	0.345	0.317	0.355	0.330	0.351	0.294
C12	Malignant neoplasm of pyriform sinus	11	Colorectal, Bladder, and Other Cancers	12	0.307	0.345	0.317	0.355	0.330	0.351	0.294
C13.0	Malignant neoplasm of postcricoid region	11	Colorectal, Bladder, and Other Cancers	12	0.307	0.345	0.317	0.355	0.330	0.351	0.294
C13.1	Malignant neoplasm of aryepiglottic fold, hypopharyngeal aspect	11	Colorectal, Bladder, and Other Cancers	12	0.307	0.345	0.317	0.355	0.330	0.351	0.294
C13.2	Malignant neoplasm of posterior wall of hypopharynx	11	Colorectal, Bladder, and Other Cancers	12	0.307	0.345	0.317	0.355	0.330	0.351	0.294
C13.8	Malignant neoplasm of overlapping sites of hypopharynx	11	Colorectal, Bladder, and Other Cancers	12	0.307	0.345	0.317	0.355	0.330	0.351	0.294

ICD-10-CM Code	ICD-10-CM Code Description	V24 CMS-HCC	V24 CMS-HCC Disease Group	V24 CMS-HCC Hierarchies	Community, NonDual, Aged	Community, NonDual, Disabled	Community, FBDual, Aged	Community, FBDual, Disabled	Community, PBDual, Aged	Community, PBDual, Disabled	Institutional
C13.9	Malignant neoplasm of hypopharynx, unspecified	11	Colorectal, Bladder, and Other Cancers	12	0.307	0.345	0.317	0.355	0.330	0.351	0.294
C14.0	Malignant neoplasm of pharynx, unspecified	11	Colorectal, Bladder, and Other Cancers	12	0.307	0.345	0.317	0.355	0.330	0.351	0.294
C14.2	Malignant neoplasm of Waldeyer's ring	11	Colorectal, Bladder, and Other Cancers	12	0.307	0.345	0.317	0.355	0.330	0.351	0.294
C14.8	Malignant neoplasm of overlapping sites of lip, oral cavity and pharynx	11	Colorectal, Bladder, and Other Cancers	12	0.307	0.345	0.317	0.355	0.330	0.351	0.294
C15.3	Malignant neoplasm of upper third of esophagus	9	Lung and Other Severe Cancers	10,11,12	1.024	0.910	1.010	1.001	1.001	0.880	0.623
C15.4	Malignant neoplasm of middle third of esophagus	9	Lung and Other Severe Cancers	10,11,12	1.024	0.910	1.010	1.001	1.001	0.880	0.623
C15.5	Malignant neoplasm of lower third of esophagus	9	Lung and Other Severe Cancers	10,11,12	1.024	0.910	1.010	1.001	1.001	0.880	0.623
C15.8	Malignant neoplasm of overlapping sites of esophagus	9	Lung and Other Severe Cancers	10,11,12	1.024	0.910	1.010	1.001	1.001	0.880	0.623
C15.9	Malignant neoplasm of esophagus, unspecified	9	Lung and Other Severe Cancers	10,11,12	1.024	0.910	1.010	1.001	1.001	0.880	0.623
C16.0	Malignant neoplasm of cardia	9	Lung and Other Severe Cancers	10,11,12	1.024	0.910	1.010	1.001	1.001	0.880	0.623
C16.1	Malignant neoplasm of fundus of stomach	9	Lung and Other Severe Cancers	10,11,12	1.024	0.910	1.010	1.001	1.001	0.880	0.623
C16.2	Malignant neoplasm of body of stomach	9	Lung and Other Severe Cancers	10,11,12	1.024	0.910	1.010	1.001	1.001	0.880	0.623
C16.3	Malignant neoplasm of pyloric antrum	9	Lung and Other Severe Cancers	10,11,12	1.024	0.910	1.010	1.001	1.001	0.880	0.623
C16.4	Malignant neoplasm of pylorus	9	Lung and Other Severe Cancers	10,11,12	1.024	0.910	1.010	1.001	1.001	0.880	0.623
C16.5	Malignant neoplasm of lesser curvature of stomach, unspecified	9	Lung and Other Severe Cancers	10,11,12	1.024	0.910	1.010	1.001	1.001	0.880	0.623
C16.6	Malignant neoplasm of greater curvature of stomach, unspecified	9	Lung and Other Severe Cancers	10,11,12	1.024	0.910	1.010	1.001	1.001	0.880	0.623
C16.8	Malignant neoplasm of overlapping sites of stomach	9	Lung and Other Severe Cancers	10,11,12	1.024	0.910	1.010	1.001	1.001	0.880	0.623
C16.9	Malignant neoplasm of stomach, unspecified	9	Lung and Other Severe Cancers	10,11,12	1.024	0.910	1.010	1.001	1.001	0.880	0.623
C17.0	Malignant neoplasm of duodenum	9	Lung and Other Severe Cancers	10,11,12	1.024	0.910	1.010	1.001	1.001	0.880	0.623
C17.1	Malignant neoplasm of jejunum	9	Lung and Other Severe Cancers	10,11,12	1.024	0.910	1.010	1.001	1.001	0.880	0.623
C17.2	Malignant neoplasm of ileum	9	Lung and Other Severe Cancers	10,11,12	1.024	0.910	1.010	1.001	1.001	0.880	0.623
C17.3	Meckel's diverticulum, malignant	9	Lung and Other Severe Cancers	10,11,12	1.024	0.910	1.010	1.001	1.001	0.880	0.623
C17.8	Malignant neoplasm of overlapping sites of small intestine	9	Lung and Other Severe Cancers	10,11,12	1.024	0.910	1.010	1.001	1.001	0.880	0.623
C17.9	Malignant neoplasm of small intestine, unspecified	9	Lung and Other Severe Cancers	10,11,12	1.024	0.910	1.010	1.001	1.001	0.880	0.623
C18.0	Malignant neoplasm of cecum	11	Colorectal, Bladder, and Other Cancers	12	0.307	0.345	0.317	0.355	0.330	0.351	0.294
C18.1	Malignant neoplasm of appendix	11	Colorectal, Bladder, and Other Cancers	12	0.307	0.345	0.317	0.355	0.330	0.351	0.294
C18.2	Malignant neoplasm of ascending colon	11	Colorectal, Bladder, and Other Cancers	12	0.307	0.345	0.317	0.355	0.330	0.351	0.294
C18.3	Malignant neoplasm of hepatic flexure	11	Colorectal, Bladder, and Other Cancers	12	0.307	0.345	0.317	0.355	0.330	0.351	0.294
C18.4	Malignant neoplasm of transverse colon	11	Colorectal, Bladder, and Other Cancers	12	0.307	0.345	0.317	0.355	0.330	0.351	0.294
C18.5	Malignant neoplasm of splenic flexure	11	Colorectal, Bladder, and Other Cancers	12	0.307	0.345	0.317	0.355	0.330	0.351	0.294
C18.6	Malignant neoplasm of descending colon	11	Colorectal, Bladder, and Other Cancers	12	0.307	0.345	0.317	0.355	0.330	0.351	0.294
C18.7	Malignant neoplasm of sigmoid colon	11	Colorectal, Bladder, and Other Cancers	12	0.307	0.345	0.317	0.355	0.330	0.351	0.294
C18.8	Malignant neoplasm of overlapping sites of colon	11	Colorectal, Bladder, and Other Cancers	12	0.307	0.345	0.317	0.355	0.330	0.351	0.294

ICD-10-CM Code	ICD-10-CM Code Description	V24 CMS-HCC	V24 CMS-HCC Disease Group	V24 CMS-HCC Hierarchies	Community, NonDual, Aged	Community, NonDual, Disabled	Community, FBDual, Aged	Community, FBDual, Disabled	Community, PBDual, Aged	Community, PBDual, Disabled	Institutional
C18.9	Malignant neoplasm of colon, unspecified	11	Colorectal, Bladder, and Other Cancers	12	0.307	0.345	0.317	0.355	0.330	0.351	0.294
C19	Malignant neoplasm of rectosigmoid junction	11	Colorectal, Bladder, and Other Cancers	12	0.307	0.345	0.317	0.355	0.330	0.351	0.294
C20	Malignant neoplasm of rectum	11	Colorectal, Bladder, and Other Cancers	12	0.307	0.345	0.317	0.355	0.330	0.351	0.294
C21.0	Malignant neoplasm of anus, unspecified	11	Colorectal, Bladder, and Other Cancers	12	0.307	0.345	0.317	0.355	0.330	0.351	0.294
C21.1	Malignant neoplasm of anal canal	11	Colorectal, Bladder, and Other Cancers	12	0.307	0.345	0.317	0.355	0.330	0.351	0.294
C21.2	Malignant neoplasm of cloacogenic zone	11	Colorectal, Bladder, and Other Cancers	12	0.307	0.345	0.317	0.355	0.330	0.351	0.294
C21.8	Malignant neoplasm of overlapping sites of rectum, anus and anal canal	11	Colorectal, Bladder, and Other Cancers	12	0.307	0.345	0.317	0.355	0.330	0.351	0.294
C22.0	Liver cell carcinoma	9	Lung and Other Severe Cancers	10,11,12	1.024	0.910	1.010	1.001	1.001	0.880	0.623
C22.1	Intrahepatic bile duct carcinoma	9	Lung and Other Severe Cancers	10,11,12	1.024	0.910	1.010	1.001	1.001	0.880	0.623
C22.2	Hepatoblastoma	9	Lung and Other Severe Cancers	10,11,12	1.024	0.910	1.010	1.001	1.001	0.880	0.623
C22.3	Angiosarcoma of liver	9	Lung and Other Severe Cancers	10,11,12	1.024	0.910	1.010	1.001	1.001	0.880	0.623
C22.4	Other sarcomas of liver	9	Lung and Other Severe Cancers	10,11,12	1.024	0.910	1.010	1.001	1.001	0.880	0.623
C22.7	Other specified carcinomas of liver	9	Lung and Other Severe Cancers	10,11,12	1.024	0.910	1.010	1.001	1.001	0.880	0.623
C22.8	Malignant neoplasm of liver, primary, unspecified as to type	9	Lung and Other Severe Cancers	10,11,12	1.024	0.910	1.010	1.001	1.001	0.880	0.623
C22.9	Malignant neoplasm of liver, not specified as primary or secondary	9	Lung and Other Severe Cancers	10,11,12	1.024	0.910	1.010	1.001	1.001	0.880	0.623
C23	Malignant neoplasm of gallbladder	9	Lung and Other Severe Cancers	10,11,12	1.024	0.910	1.010	1.001	1.001	0.880	0.623
C24.0	Malignant neoplasm of extrahepatic bile duct	9	Lung and Other Severe Cancers	10,11,12	1.024	0.910	1.010	1.001	1.001	0.880	0.623
C24.1	Malignant neoplasm of ampulla of Vater	9	Lung and Other Severe Cancers	10,11,12	1.024	0.910	1.010	1.001	1.001	0.880	0.623
C24.8	Malignant neoplasm of overlapping sites of biliary tract	9	Lung and Other Severe Cancers	10,11,12	1.024	0.910	1.010	1.001	1.001	0.880	0.623
C24.9	Malignant neoplasm of biliary tract, unspecified	9	Lung and Other Severe Cancers	10,11,12	1.024	0.910	1.010	1.001	1.001	0.880	0.623
C25.0	Malignant neoplasm of head of pancreas	9	Lung and Other Severe Cancers	10,11,12	1.024	0.910	1.010	1.001	1.001	0.880	0.623
C25.1	Malignant neoplasm of body of pancreas	9	Lung and Other Severe Cancers	10,11,12	1.024	0.910	1.010	1.001	1.001	0.880	0.623
C25.2	Malignant neoplasm of tail of pancreas	9	Lung and Other Severe Cancers	10,11,12	1.024	0.910	1.010	1.001	1.001	0.880	0.623
C25.3	Malignant neoplasm of pancreatic duct	9	Lung and Other Severe Cancers	10,11,12	1.024	0.910	1.010	1.001	1.001	0.880	0.623
C25.4	Malignant neoplasm of endocrine pancreas	9	Lung and Other Severe Cancers	10,11,12	1.024	0.910	1.010	1.001	1.001	0.880	0.623
C25.7	Malignant neoplasm of other parts of pancreas	9	Lung and Other Severe Cancers	10,11,12	1.024	0.910	1.010	1.001	1.001	0.880	0.623
C25.8	Malignant neoplasm of overlapping sites of pancreas	9	Lung and Other Severe Cancers	10,11,12	1.024	0.910	1.010	1.001	1.001	0.880	0.623
C25.9	Malignant neoplasm of pancreas, unspecified	9	Lung and Other Severe Cancers	10,11,12	1.024	0.910	1.010	1.001	1.001	0.880	0.623
C26.0	Malignant neoplasm of intestinal tract, part unspecified	11	Colorectal, Bladder, and Other Cancers	12	0.307	0.345	0.317	0.355	0.330	0.351	0.294
C26.1	Malignant neoplasm of spleen	11	Colorectal, Bladder, and Other Cancers	12	0.307	0.345	0.317	0.355	0.330	0.351	0.294
C26.9	Malignant neoplasm of ill-defined sites within the digestive system	11	Colorectal, Bladder, and Other Cancers	12	0.307	0.345	0.317	0.355	0.330	0.351	0.294
C30.0	Malignant neoplasm of nasal cavity	11	Colorectal, Bladder, and Other Cancers	12	0.307	0.345	0.317	0.355	0.330	0.351	0.294
C30.1	Malignant neoplasm of middle ear	11	Colorectal, Bladder, and Other Cancers	12	0.307	0.345	0.317	0.355	0.330	0.351	0.294
C31.0	Malignant neoplasm of maxillary sinus	11	Colorectal, Bladder, and Other Cancers	12	0.307	0.345	0.317	0.355	0.330	0.351	0.294

ICD-10-CM Code	ICD-10-CM Code Description	V24 CMS-HCC	V24 CMS-HCC Disease Group	V24 CMS-HCC Hierarchies	Community, NonDual, Aged	Community, NonDual, Disabled	Community, FBDual, Aged	Community, FBDual, Disabled	Community, PBDual, Aged	Community, PBDual, Disabled	Institutional
C31.1	Malignant neoplasm of ethmoidal sinus	11	Colorectal, Bladder, and Other Cancers	12	0.307	0.345	0.317	0.355	0.330	0.351	0.294
C31.2	Malignant neoplasm of frontal sinus	11	Colorectal, Bladder, and Other Cancers	12	0.307	0.345	0.317	0.355	0.330	0.351	0.294
C31.3	Malignant neoplasm of sphenoid sinus	11	Colorectal, Bladder, and Other Cancers	12	0.307	0.345	0.317	0.355	0.330	0.351	0.294
C31.8	Malignant neoplasm of overlapping sites of accessory sinuses	11	Colorectal, Bladder, and Other Cancers	12	0.307	0.345	0.317	0.355	0.330	0.351	0.294
C31.9	Malignant neoplasm of accessory sinus, unspecified	11	Colorectal, Bladder, and Other Cancers	12	0.307	0.345	0.317	0.355	0.330	0.351	0.294
C32.0	Malignant neoplasm of glottis	11	Colorectal, Bladder, and Other Cancers	12	0.307	0.345	0.317	0.355	0.330	0.351	0.294
C32.1	Malignant neoplasm of supraglottis	11	Colorectal, Bladder, and Other Cancers	12	0.307	0.345	0.317	0.355	0.330	0.351	0.294
C32.2	Malignant neoplasm of subglottis	11	Colorectal, Bladder, and Other Cancers	12	0.307	0.345	0.317	0.355	0.330	0.351	0.294
C32.3	Malignant neoplasm of laryngeal cartilage	11	Colorectal, Bladder, and Other Cancers	12	0.307	0.345	0.317	0.355	0.330	0.351	0.294
C32.8	Malignant neoplasm of overlapping sites of larynx	11	Colorectal, Bladder, and Other Cancers	12	0.307	0.345	0.317	0.355	0.330	0.351	0.294
C32.9	Malignant neoplasm of larynx, unspecified	11	Colorectal, Bladder, and Other Cancers	12	0.307	0.345	0.317	0.355	0.330	0.351	0.294
C33	Malignant neoplasm of trachea	9	Lung and Other Severe Cancers	10,11,12	1.024	0.910	1.010	1.001	1.001	0.880	0.623
C34.00	Malignant neoplasm of unspecified main bronchus	9	Lung and Other Severe Cancers	10,11,12	1.024	0.910	1.010	1.001	1.001	0.880	0.623
C34.01	Malignant neoplasm of right main bronchus	9	Lung and Other Severe Cancers	10,11,12	1.024	0.910	1.010	1.001	1.001	0.880	0.623
C34.02	Malignant neoplasm of left main bronchus	9	Lung and Other Severe Cancers	10,11,12	1.024	0.910	1.010	1.001	1.001	0.880	0.623
C34.10	Malignant neoplasm of upper lobe, unspecified bronchus or lung	9	Lung and Other Severe Cancers	10,11,12	1.024	0.910	1.010	1.001	1.001	0.880	0.623
C34.11	Malignant neoplasm of upper lobe, right bronchus or lung	9	Lung and Other Severe Cancers	10,11,12	1.024	0.910	1.010	1.001	1.001	0.880	0.623
C34.12	Malignant neoplasm of upper lobe, left bronchus or lung	9	Lung and Other Severe Cancers	10,11,12	1.024	0.910	1.010	1.001	1.001	0.880	0.623
C34.2	Malignant neoplasm of middle lobe, bronchus or lung	9	Lung and Other Severe Cancers	10,11,12	1.024	0.910	1.010	1.001	1.001	0.880	0.623
C34.30	Malignant neoplasm of lower lobe, unspecified bronchus or lung	9	Lung and Other Severe Cancers	10,11,12	1.024	0.910	1.010	1.001	1.001	0.880	0.623
C34.31	Malignant neoplasm of lower lobe, right bronchus or lung	9	Lung and Other Severe Cancers	10,11,12	1.024	0.910	1.010	1.001	1.001	0.880	0.623
C34.32	Malignant neoplasm of lower lobe, left bronchus or lung	9	Lung and Other Severe Cancers	10,11,12	1.024	0.910	1.010	1.001	1.001	0.880	0.623
C34.80	Malignant neoplasm of overlapping sites of unspecified bronchus and lung	9	Lung and Other Severe Cancers	10,11,12	1.024	0.910	1.010	1.001	1.001	0.880	0.623
C34.81	Malignant neoplasm of overlapping sites of right bronchus and lung	9	Lung and Other Severe Cancers	10,11,12	1.024	0.910	1.010	1.001	1.001	0.880	0.623
C34.82	Malignant neoplasm of overlapping sites of left bronchus and lung	9	Lung and Other Severe Cancers	10,11,12	1.024	0.910	1.010	1.001	1.001	0.880	0.623
C34.90	Malignant neoplasm of unspecified part of unspecified bronchus or lung	9	Lung and Other Severe Cancers	10,11,12	1.024	0.910	1.010	1.001	1.001	0.880	0.623
C34.91	Malignant neoplasm of unspecified part of right bronchus or lung	9	Lung and Other Severe Cancers	10,11,12	1.024	0.910	1.010	1.001	1.001	0.880	0.623
C34.92	Malignant neoplasm of unspecified part of left bronchus or lung	9	Lung and Other Severe Cancers	10,11,12	1.024	0.910	1.010	1.001	1.001	0.880	0.623
C37	Malignant neoplasm of thymus	11	Colorectal, Bladder, and Other Cancers	12	0.307	0.345	0.317	0.355	0.330	0.351	0.294
C38.0	Malignant neoplasm of heart	11	Colorectal, Bladder, and Other Cancers	12	0.307	0.345	0.317	0.355	0.330	0.351	0.294
C38.1	Malignant neoplasm of anterior mediastinum	11	Colorectal, Bladder, and Other Cancers	12	0.307	0.345	0.317	0.355	0.330	0.351	0.294
C38.2	Malignant neoplasm of posterior mediastinum	11	Colorectal, Bladder, and Other Cancers	12	0.307	0.345	0.317	0.355	0.330	0.351	0.294

ICD-10-CM Code	ICD-10-CM Code Description	V24 CMS-HCC	V24 CMS-HCC Disease Group	V24 CMS-HCC Hierarchies	Community, NonDual, Aged	Community, NonDual, Disabled	Community, FBDual, Aged	Community, FBDual, Disabled	Community, PBDual, Aged	Community, PBDual, Disabled	Institutional
C38.3	Malignant neoplasm of mediastinum, part unspecified	11	Colorectal, Bladder, and Other Cancers	12	0.307	0.345	0.317	0.355	0.330	0.351	0.294
C38.4	Malignant neoplasm of pleura	9	Lung and Other Severe Cancers	10,11,12	1.024	0.910	1.010	1.001	1.001	0.880	0.623
C38.8	Malignant neoplasm of overlapping sites of heart, mediastinum and pleura	11	Colorectal, Bladder, and Other Cancers	12	0.307	0.345	0.317	0.355	0.330	0.351	0.294
C39.0	Malignant neoplasm of upper respiratory tract, part unspecified	11	Colorectal, Bladder, and Other Cancers	12	0.307	0.345	0.317	0.355	0.330	0.351	0.294
C39.9	Malignant neoplasm of lower respiratory tract, part unspecified	11	Colorectal, Bladder, and Other Cancers	12	0.307	0.345	0.317	0.355	0.330	0.351	0.294
C40.00	Malignant neoplasm of scapula and long bones of unspecified upper limb	10	Lymphoma and Other Cancers	11,12	0.675	0.663	0.717	0.756	0.648	0.667	0.461
C40.01	Malignant neoplasm of scapula and long bones of right upper limb	10	Lymphoma and Other Cancers	11,12	0.675	0.663	0.717	0.756	0.648	0.667	0.461
C40.02	Malignant neoplasm of scapula and long bones of left upper limb	10	Lymphoma and Other Cancers	11,12	0.675	0.663	0.717	0.756	0.648	0.667	0.461
C40.10	Malignant neoplasm of short bones of unspecified upper limb	10	Lymphoma and Other Cancers	11,12	0.675	0.663	0.717	0.756	0.648	0.667	0.461
C40.11	Malignant neoplasm of short bones of right upper limb	10	Lymphoma and Other Cancers	11,12	0.675	0.663	0.717	0.756	0.648	0.667	0.461
C40.12	Malignant neoplasm of short bones of left upper limb	10	Lymphoma and Other Cancers	11,12	0.675	0.663	0.717	0.756	0.648	0.667	0.461
C40.20	Malignant neoplasm of long bones of unspecified lower limb	10	Lymphoma and Other Cancers	11,12	0.675	0.663	0.717	0.756	0.648	0.667	0.461
C40.21	Malignant neoplasm of long bones of right lower limb	10	Lymphoma and Other Cancers	11,12	0.675	0.663	0.717	0.756	0.648	0.667	0.461
C40.22	Malignant neoplasm of long bones of left lower limb	10	Lymphoma and Other Cancers	11,12	0.675	0.663	0.717	0.756	0.648	0.667	0.461
C40.30	Malignant neoplasm of short bones of unspecified lower limb	10	Lymphoma and Other Cancers	11,12	0.675	0.663	0.717	0.756	0.648	0.667	0.461
C40.31	Malignant neoplasm of short bones of right lower limb	10	Lymphoma and Other Cancers	11,12	0.675	0.663	0.717	0.756	0.648	0.667	0.461
C40.32	Malignant neoplasm of short bones of left lower limb	10	Lymphoma and Other Cancers	11,12	0.675	0.663	0.717	0.756	0.648	0.667	0.461
C40.80	Malignant neoplasm of overlapping sites of bone and articular cartilage of unspecified limb	10	Lymphoma and Other Cancers	11,12	0.675	0.663	0.717	0.756	0.648	0.667	0.461
C40.81	Malignant neoplasm of overlapping sites of bone and articular cartilage of right limb	10	Lymphoma and Other Cancers	11,12	0.675	0.663	0.717	0.756	0.648	0.667	0.461
C40.82	Malignant neoplasm of overlapping sites of bone and articular cartilage of left limb	10	Lymphoma and Other Cancers	11,12	0.675	0.663	0.717	0.756	0.648	0.667	0.461
C40.90	Malignant neoplasm of unspecified bones and articular cartilage of unspecified limb	10	Lymphoma and Other Cancers	11,12	0.675	0.663	0.717	0.756	0.648	0.667	0.461
C40.91	Malignant neoplasm of unspecified bones and articular cartilage of right limb	10	Lymphoma and Other Cancers	11,12	0.675	0.663	0.717	0.756	0.648	0.667	0.461
C40.92	Malignant neoplasm of unspecified bones and articular cartilage of left limb	10	Lymphoma and Other Cancers	11,12	0.675	0.663	0.717	0.756	0.648	0.667	0.461
C41.0	Malignant neoplasm of bones of skull and face	10	Lymphoma and Other Cancers	11,12	0.675	0.663	0.717	0.756	0.648	0.667	0.461
C41.1	Malignant neoplasm of mandible	10	Lymphoma and Other Cancers	11,12	0.675	0.663	0.717	0.756	0.648	0.667	0.461
C41.2	Malignant neoplasm of vertebral column	10	Lymphoma and Other Cancers	11,12	0.675	0.663	0.717	0.756	0.648	0.667	0.461
C41.3	Malignant neoplasm of ribs, sternum and clavicle	10	Lymphoma and Other Cancers	11,12	0.675	0.663	0.717	0.756	0.648	0.667	0.461

2021 Optum360, LLC

ICD-10-CM Code	ICD-10-CM Code Description	V24 CMS-HCC	V24 CMS-HCC Disease Group	V24 CMS-HCC Hierarchies	Community, NonDual, Aged	Community, NonDual, Disabled	Community, FBDual, Aged	Community, FBDual, Disabled	Community, PBDual, Aged	Community, PBDual, Disabled	Institutional
C41.4	Malignant neoplasm of pelvic bones, sacrum and coccyx	10	Lymphoma and Other Cancers	11,12	0.675	0.663	0.717	0.756	0.648	0.667	0.461
C41.9	Malignant neoplasm of bone and articular cartilage, unspecified	10	Lymphoma and Other Cancers	11,12	0.675	0.663	0.717	0.756	0.648	0.667	0.461
C43.0	Malignant melanoma of lip	12	Breast, Prostate, and Other Cancers and Tumors		0.150	0.212	0.158	0.212	0.154	0.181	0.210
C43.10	Malignant melanoma of unspecified eyelid, including canthus	12	Breast, Prostate, and Other Cancers and Tumors		0.150	0.212	0.158	0.212	0.154	0.181	0.210
C43.111	Malignant melanoma of right upper eyelid, including canthus	12	Breast, Prostate, and Other Cancers and Tumors		0.150	0.212	0.158	0.212	0.154	0.181	0.210
C43.112	Malignant melanoma of right lower eyelid, including canthus	12	Breast, Prostate, and Other Cancers and Tumors		0.150	0.212	0.158	0.212	0.154	0.181	0.210
C43.121	Malignant melanoma of left upper eyelid, including canthus	12	Breast, Prostate, and Other Cancers and Tumors		0.150	0.212	0.158	0.212	0.154	0.181	0.210
C43.122	Malignant melanoma of left lower eyelid, including canthus	12	Breast, Prostate, and Other Cancers and Tumors		0.150	0.212	0.158	0.212	0.154	0.181	0.210
C43.20	Malignant melanoma of unspecified ear and external auricular canal	12	Breast, Prostate, and Other Cancers and Tumors		0.150	0.212	0.158	0.212	0.154	0.181	0.210
C43.21	Malignant melanoma of right ear and external auricular canal	12	Breast, Prostate, and Other Cancers and Tumors		0.150	0.212	0.158	0.212	0.154	0.181	0.210
C43.22	Malignant melanoma of left ear and external auricular canal	12	Breast, Prostate, and Other Cancers and Tumors		0.150	0.212	0.158	0.212	0.154	0.181	0.210
C43.30	Malignant melanoma of unspecified part of face	12	Breast, Prostate, and Other Cancers and Tumors		0.150	0.212	0.158	0.212	0.154	0.181	0.210
C43.31	Malignant melanoma of nose	12	Breast, Prostate, and Other Cancers and Tumors		0.150	0.212	0.158	0.212	0.154	0.181	0.210
C43.39	Malignant melanoma of other parts of face	12	Breast, Prostate, and Other Cancers and Tumors		0.150	0.212	0.158	0.212	0.154	0.181	0.210
C43.4	Malignant melanoma of scalp and neck	12	Breast, Prostate, and Other Cancers and Tumors		0.150	0.212	0.158	0.212	0.154	0.181	0.210
C43.51	Malignant melanoma of anal skin	12	Breast, Prostate, and Other Cancers and Tumors		0.150	0.212	0.158	0.212	0.154	0.181	0.210
C43.52	Malignant melanoma of skin of breast	12	Breast, Prostate, and Other Cancers and Tumors		0.150	0.212	0.158	0.212	0.154	0.181	0.210
C43.59	Malignant melanoma of other part of trunk	12	Breast, Prostate, and Other Cancers and Tumors		0.150	0.212	0.158	0.212	0.154	0.181	0.210
C43.60	Malignant melanoma of unspecified upper limb, including shoulder	12	Breast, Prostate, and Other Cancers and Tumors		0.150	0.212	0.158	0.212	0.154	0.181	0.210
C43.61	Malignant melanoma of right upper limb, including shoulder	12	Breast, Prostate, and Other Cancers and Tumors		0.150	0.212	0.158	0.212	0.154	0.181	0.210
C43.62	Malignant melanoma of left upper limb, including shoulder	12	Breast, Prostate, and Other Cancers and Tumors		0.150	0.212	0.158	0.212	0.154	0.181	0.210
C43.70	Malignant melanoma of unspecified lower limb, including hip	12	Breast, Prostate, and Other Cancers and Tumors		0.150	0.212	0.158	0.212	0.154	0.181	0.210
C43.71	Malignant melanoma of right lower limb, including hip	12	Breast, Prostate, and Other Cancers and Tumors		0.150	0.212	0.158	0.212	0.154	0.181	0.210
C43.72	Malignant melanoma of left lower limb, including hip	12	Breast, Prostate, and Other Cancers and Tumors		0.150	0.212	0.158	0.212	0.154	0.181	0.210
C43.8	Malignant melanoma of overlapping sites of skin	12	Breast, Prostate, and Other Cancers and Tumors		0.150	0.212	0.158	0.212	0.154	0.181	0.210
C43.9	Malignant melanoma of skin, unspecified	12	Breast, Prostate, and Other Cancers and Tumors		0.150	0.212	0.158	0.212	0.154	0.181	0.210
C45.0	Mesothelioma of pleura	9	Lung and Other Severe Cancers	10,11,12	1.024	0.910	1.010	1.001	1.001	0.880	0.623
C45.1	Mesothelioma of peritoneum	9	Lung and Other Severe Cancers	10,11,12	1.024	0.910	1.010	1.001	1.001	0.880	0.623
C45.2	Mesothelioma of pericardium	9	Lung and Other Severe Cancers	10,11,12	1.024	0.910	1.010	1.001	1.001	0.880	0.623
C45.7	Mesothelioma of other sites	9	Lung and Other Severe Cancers	10,11,12	1.024	0.910	1.010	1.001	1.001	0.880	0.623
C45.9	Mesothelioma, unspecified	9	Lung and Other Severe Cancers	10,11,12	1.024	0.910	1.010	1.001	1.001	0.880	0.623
C46.0	Kaposi's sarcoma of skin	10	Lymphoma and Other Cancers	11,12	0.675	0.663	0.717	0.756	0.648	0.667	0.461

ICD-10-CM Code	ICD-10-CM Code Description	V24 CMS-HCC	V24 CMS-HCC Disease Group	V24 CMS-HCC Hierarchies	Community, NonDual, Aged	Community, NonDual, Disabled	Community, FBDual, Aged	Community, FBDual, Disabled	Community, PBDual, Aged	Community, PBDual, Disabled	Institutional
C79.31	Secondary malignant neoplasm of brain	8	Metastatic Cancer and Acute Leukemia	9,10,11,12	2.659	2.714	2.566	2.801	2.455	2.659	1.303
C79.32	Secondary malignant neoplasm of cerebral meninges	8	Metastatic Cancer and Acute Leukemia	9,10,11,12	2.659	2.714	2.566	2.801	2.455	2.659	1.303
C79.40	Secondary malignant neoplasm of unspecified part of nervous system	8	Metastatic Cancer and Acute Leukemia	9,10,11,12	2.659	2.714	2.566	2.801	2.455	2.659	1.303
C79.49	Secondary malignant neoplasm of other parts of nervous system	8	Metastatic Cancer and Acute Leukemia	9,10,11,12	2.659	2.714	2.566	2.801	2.455	2.659	1.303
C79.51	Secondary malignant neoplasm of bone	8	Metastatic Cancer and Acute Leukemia	9,10,11,12	2.659	2.714	2.566	2.801	2.455	2.659	1.303
C79.52	Secondary malignant neoplasm of bone marrow	8	Metastatic Cancer and Acute Leukemia	9,10,11,12	2.659	2.714	2.566	2.801	2.455	2.659	1.303
C79.60	Secondary malignant neoplasm of unspecified ovary	8	Metastatic Cancer and Acute Leukemia	9,10,11,12	2.659	2.714	2.566	2.801	2.455	2.659	1.303
C79.61	Secondary malignant neoplasm of right ovary	8	Metastatic Cancer and Acute Leukemia	9,10,11,12	2.659	2.714	2.566	2.801	2.455	2.659	1.303
C79.62	Secondary malignant neoplasm of left ovary	8	Metastatic Cancer and Acute Leukemia	9,10,11,12	2.659	2.714	2.566	2.801	2.455	2.659	1.303
C79.63	Secondary malignant neoplasm of bilateral ovaries	8	Metastatic Cancer and Acute Leukemia	9,10,11,12	2.659	2.714	2.566	2.801	2.455	2.659	1.303
C79.70	Secondary malignant neoplasm of unspecified adrenal gland	8	Metastatic Cancer and Acute Leukemia	9,10,11,12	2.659	2.714	2.566	2.801	2.455	2.659	1.303
C79.71	Secondary malignant neoplasm of right adrenal gland	8	Metastatic Cancer and Acute Leukemia	9,10,11,12	2.659	2.714	2.566	2.801	2.455	2.659	1.303
C79.72	Secondary malignant neoplasm of left adrenal gland	8	Metastatic Cancer and Acute Leukemia	9,10,11,12	2.659	2.714	2.566	2.801	2.455	2.659	1.303
C79.81	Secondary malignant neoplasm of breast	10	Lymphoma and Other Cancers	11,12	0.675	0.663	0.717	0.756	0.648	0.667	0.461
C79.82	Secondary malignant neoplasm of genital organs	10	Lymphoma and Other Cancers	11,12	0.675	0.663	0.717	0.756	0.648	0.667	0.461
C79.89	Secondary malignant neoplasm of other specified sites	8	Metastatic Cancer and Acute Leukemia	9,10,11,12	2.659	2.714	2.566	2.801	2.455	2.659	1.303
C79.9	Secondary malignant neoplasm of unspecified site	8	Metastatic Cancer and Acute Leukemia	9,10,11,12	2.659	2.714	2.566	2.801	2.455	2.659	1.303
C7A.00	Malignant carcinoid tumor of unspecified site	12	Breast, Prostate, and Other Cancers and Tumors		0.150	0.212	0.158	0.212	0.154	0.181	0.210
C7A.010	Malignant carcinoid tumor of the duodenum	12	Breast, Prostate, and Other Cancers and Tumors		0.150	0.212	0.158	0.212	0.154	0.181	0.210
C7A.011	Malignant carcinoid tumor of the jejunum	12	Breast, Prostate, and Other Cancers and Tumors		0.150	0.212	0.158	0.212	0.154	0.181	0.210
C7A.012	Malignant carcinoid tumor of the ileum	12	Breast, Prostate, and Other Cancers and Tumors		0.150	0.212	0.158	0.212	0.154	0.181	0.210
C7A.019	Malignant carcinoid tumor of the small intestine, unspecified portion	12	Breast, Prostate, and Other Cancers and Tumors		0.150	0.212	0.158	0.212	0.154	0.181	0.210
C7A.020	Malignant carcinoid tumor of the appendix	12	Breast, Prostate, and Other Cancers and Tumors		0.150	0.212	0.158	0.212	0.154	0.181	0.210
C7A.021	Malignant carcinoid tumor of the cecum	12	Breast, Prostate, and Other Cancers and Tumors		0.150	0.212	0.158	0.212	0.154	0.181	0.210
C7A.022	Malignant carcinoid tumor of the ascending colon	12	Breast, Prostate, and Other Cancers and Tumors		0.150	0.212	0.158	0.212	0.154	0.181	0.210
C7A.023	Malignant carcinoid tumor of the transverse colon	12	Breast, Prostate, and Other Cancers and Tumors		0.150	0.212	0.158	0.212	0.154	0.181	0.210
C7A.024	Malignant carcinoid tumor of the descending colon	12	Breast, Prostate, and Other Cancers and Tumors		0.150	0.212	0.158	0.212	0.154	0.181	0.210
C7A.025	Malignant carcinoid tumor of the sigmoid colon	12	Breast, Prostate, and Other Cancers and Tumors		0.150	0.212	0.158	0.212	0.154	0.181	0.210
C7A.026	Malignant carcinoid tumor of the rectum	12	Breast, Prostate, and Other Cancers and Tumors		0.150	0.212	0.158	0.212	0.154	0.181	0.210

ICD-10-CM Code	ICD-10-CM Code Description	V24 CMS-HCC	V24 CMS-HCC Disease Group	V24 CMS-HCC Hierarchies	Community, NonDual, Aged	Community, NonDual, Disabled	Community, FBDual, Aged	Community, FBDual, Disabled	Community, PBDual, Aged	Community, PBDual, Disabled	Institutional
C7A.Ø29	Malignant carcinoid tumor of the large intestine, unspecified portion	12	Breast, Prostate, and Other Cancers and Tumors		0.150	0.212	0.158	0.212	0.154	0.181	0.210
C7A.Ø9Ø	Malignant carcinoid tumor of the bronchus and lung	12	Breast, Prostate, and Other Cancers and Tumors		0.150	0.212	0.158	0.212	0.154	0.181	0.210
C7A.Ø91	Malignant carcinoid tumor of the thymus	12	Breast, Prostate, and Other Cancers and Tumors		0.150	0.212	0.158	0.212	0.154	0.181	0.210
C7A.Ø92	Malignant carcinoid tumor of the stomach	12	Breast, Prostate, and Other Cancers and Tumors		0.150	0.212	0.158	0.212	0.154	0.181	0.210
C7A.Ø93	Malignant carcinoid tumor of the kidney	12	Breast, Prostate, and Other Cancers and Tumors		0.150	0.212	0.158	0.212	0.154	0.181	0.210
C7A.Ø94	Malignant carcinoid tumor of the foregut, unspecified	12	Breast, Prostate, and Other Cancers and Tumors		0.150	0.212	0.158	0.212	0.154	0.181	0.210
C7A.Ø95	Malignant carcinoid tumor of the midgut, unspecified	12	Breast, Prostate, and Other Cancers and Tumors		0.150	0.212	0.158	0.212	0.154	0.181	0.210
C7A.Ø96	Malignant carcinoid tumor of the hindgut, unspecified	12	Breast, Prostate, and Other Cancers and Tumors		0.150	0.212	0.158	0.212	0.154	0.181	0.210
C7A.Ø98	Malignant carcinoid tumors of other sites	12	Breast, Prostate, and Other Cancers and Tumors		0.150	0.212	0.158	0.212	0.154	0.181	0.210
C7A.1	Malignant poorly differentiated neuroendocrine tumors	12	Breast, Prostate, and Other Cancers and Tumors		0.150	0.212	0.158	0.212	0.154	0.181	0.210
C7A.8	Other malignant neuroendocrine tumors	12	Breast, Prostate, and Other Cancers and Tumors		0.150	0.212	0.158	0.212	0.154	0.181	0.210
C7B.ØØ	Secondary carcinoid tumors, unspecified site	8	Metastatic Cancer and Acute Leukemia	9,10,11, 12	2.659	2.714	2.566	2.801	2.455	2.659	1.303
C7B.Ø1	Secondary carcinoid tumors of distant lymph nodes	8	Metastatic Cancer and Acute Leukemia	9,10,11, 12	2.659	2.714	2.566	2.801	2.455	2.659	1.303
C7B.Ø2	Secondary carcinoid tumors of liver	8	Metastatic Cancer and Acute Leukemia	9,10,11, 12	2.659	2.714	2.566	2.801	2.455	2.659	1.303
C7B.Ø3	Secondary carcinoid tumors of bone	8	Metastatic Cancer and Acute Leukemia	9,10,11, 12	2.659	2.714	2.566	2.801	2.455	2.659	1.303
C7B.Ø4	Secondary carcinoid tumors of peritoneum	8	Metastatic Cancer and Acute Leukemia	9,10,11, 12	2.659	2.714	2.566	2.801	2.455	2.659	1.303
C7B.Ø9	Secondary carcinoid tumors of other sites	8	Metastatic Cancer and Acute Leukemia	9,10,11, 12	2.659	2.714	2.566	2.801	2.455	2.659	1.303
C7B.1	Secondary Merkel cell carcinoma	8	Metastatic Cancer and Acute Leukemia	9,10,11, 12	2.659	2.714	2.566	2.801	2.455	2.659	1.303
C7B.8	Other secondary neuroendocrine tumors	8	Metastatic Cancer and Acute Leukemia	9,10,11, 12	2.659	2.714	2.566	2.801	2.455	2.659	1.303
C8Ø.Ø	Disseminated malignant neoplasm, unspecified	8	Metastatic Cancer and Acute Leukemia	9,10,11, 12	2.659	2.714	2.566	2.801	2.455	2.659	1.303
C8Ø.1	Malignant (primary) neoplasm, unspecified	12	Breast, Prostate, and Other Cancers and Tumors		0.150	0.212	0.158	0.212	0.154	0.181	0.210
C8Ø.2	Malignant neoplasm associated with transplanted organ	12	Breast, Prostate, and Other Cancers and Tumors		0.150	0.212	0.158	0.212	0.154	0.181	0.210
C81.ØØ	Nodular lymphocyte predominant Hodgkin lymphoma, unspecified site	10	Lymphoma and Other Cancers	11,12	0.675	0.663	0.717	0.756	0.648	0.667	0.461
C81.Ø1	Nodular lymphocyte predominant Hodgkin lymphoma, lymph nodes of head, face, and neck	10	Lymphoma and Other Cancers	11,12	0.675	0.663	0.717	0.756	0.648	0.667	0.461
C81.Ø2	Nodular lymphocyte predominant Hodgkin lymphoma, intrathoracic lymph nodes	10	Lymphoma and Other Cancers	11,12	0.675	0.663	0.717	0.756	0.648	0.667	0.461
C81.Ø3	Nodular lymphocyte predominant Hodgkin lymphoma, intra-abdominal lymph nodes	10	Lymphoma and Other Cancers	11,12	0.675	0.663	0.717	0.756	0.648	0.667	0.461
C81.Ø4	Nodular lymphocyte predominant Hodgkin lymphoma, lymph nodes of axilla and upper limb	10	Lymphoma and Other Cancers	11,12	0.675	0.663	0.717	0.756	0.648	0.667	0.461

ICD-10-CM Code	ICD-10-CM Code Description	V24 CMS-HCC	V24 CMS-HCC Disease Group	V24 CMS-HCC Hierarchies	Community, NonDual, Aged	Community, NonDual, Disabled	Community, FBDual, Aged	Community, FBDual, Disabled	Community, PBDual, Aged	Community, PBDual, Disabled	Institutional
C81.05	Nodular lymphocyte predominant Hodgkin lymphoma, lymph nodes of inguinal region and lower limb	10	Lymphoma and Other Cancers	11,12	0.675	0.663	0.717	0.756	0.648	0.667	0.461
C81.06	Nodular lymphocyte predominant Hodgkin lymphoma, intrapelvic lymph nodes	10	Lymphoma and Other Cancers	11,12	0.675	0.663	0.717	0.756	0.648	0.667	0.461
C81.07	Nodular lymphocyte predominant Hodgkin lymphoma, spleen	10	Lymphoma and Other Cancers	11,12	0.675	0.663	0.717	0.756	0.648	0.667	0.461
C81.08	Nodular lymphocyte predominant Hodgkin lymphoma, lymph nodes of multiple sites	10	Lymphoma and Other Cancers	11,12	0.675	0.663	0.717	0.756	0.648	0.667	0.461
C81.09	Nodular lymphocyte predominant Hodgkin lymphoma, extranodal and solid organ sites	10	Lymphoma and Other Cancers	11,12	0.675	0.663	0.717	0.756	0.648	0.667	0.461
C81.10	Nodular sclerosis Hodgkin lymphoma, unspecified site	10	Lymphoma and Other Cancers	11,12	0.675	0.663	0.717	0.756	0.648	0.667	0.461
C81.11	Nodular sclerosis Hodgkin lymphoma, lymph nodes of head, face, and neck	10	Lymphoma and Other Cancers	11,12	0.675	0.663	0.717	0.756	0.648	0.667	0.461
C81.12	Nodular sclerosis Hodgkin lymphoma, intrathoracic lymph nodes	10	Lymphoma and Other Cancers	11,12	0.675	0.663	0.717	0.756	0.648	0.667	0.461
C81.13	Nodular sclerosis Hodgkin lymphoma, intra-abdominal lymph nodes	10	Lymphoma and Other Cancers	11,12	0.675	0.663	0.717	0.756	0.648	0.667	0.461
C81.14	Nodular sclerosis Hodgkin lymphoma, lymph nodes of axilla and upper limb	10	Lymphoma and Other Cancers	11,12	0.675	0.663	0.717	0.756	0.648	0.667	0.461
C81.15	Nodular sclerosis Hodgkin lymphoma, lymph nodes of inguinal region and lower limb	10	Lymphoma and Other Cancers	11,12	0.675	0.663	0.717	0.756	0.648	0.667	0.461
C81.16	Nodular sclerosis Hodgkin lymphoma, intrapelvic lymph nodes	10	Lymphoma and Other Cancers	11,12	0.675	0.663	0.717	0.756	0.648	0.667	0.461
C81.17	Nodular sclerosis Hodgkin lymphoma, spleen	10	Lymphoma and Other Cancers	11,12	0.675	0.663	0.717	0.756	0.648	0.667	0.461
C81.18	Nodular sclerosis Hodgkin lymphoma, lymph nodes of multiple sites	10	Lymphoma and Other Cancers	11,12	0.675	0.663	0.717	0.756	0.648	0.667	0.461
C81.19	Nodular sclerosis Hodgkin lymphoma, extranodal and solid organ sites	10	Lymphoma and Other Cancers	11,12	0.675	0.663	0.717	0.756	0.648	0.667	0.461
C81.20	Mixed cellularity Hodgkin lymphoma, unspecified site	10	Lymphoma and Other Cancers	11,12	0.675	0.663	0.717	0.756	0.648	0.667	0.461
C81.21	Mixed cellularity Hodgkin lymphoma, lymph nodes of head, face, and neck	10	Lymphoma and Other Cancers	11,12	0.675	0.663	0.717	0.756	0.648	0.667	0.461
C81.22	Mixed cellularity Hodgkin lymphoma, intrathoracic lymph nodes	10	Lymphoma and Other Cancers	11,12	0.675	0.663	0.717	0.756	0.648	0.667	0.461
C81.23	Mixed cellularity Hodgkin lymphoma, intra-abdominal lymph nodes	10	Lymphoma and Other Cancers	11,12	0.675	0.663	0.717	0.756	0.648	0.667	0.461
C81.24	Mixed cellularity Hodgkin lymphoma, lymph nodes of axilla and upper limb	10	Lymphoma and Other Cancers	11,12	0.675	0.663	0.717	0.756	0.648	0.667	0.461
C81.25	Mixed cellularity Hodgkin lymphoma, lymph nodes of inguinal region and lower limb	10	Lymphoma and Other Cancers	11,12	0.675	0.663	0.717	0.756	0.648	0.667	0.461
C81.26	Mixed cellularity Hodgkin lymphoma, intrapelvic lymph nodes	10	Lymphoma and Other Cancers	11,12	0.675	0.663	0.717	0.756	0.648	0.667	0.461
C81.27	Mixed cellularity Hodgkin lymphoma, spleen	10	Lymphoma and Other Cancers	11,12	0.675	0.663	0.717	0.756	0.648	0.667	0.461
C81.28	Mixed cellularity Hodgkin lymphoma, lymph nodes of multiple sites	10	Lymphoma and Other Cancers	11,12	0.675	0.663	0.717	0.756	0.648	0.667	0.461

ICD-10-CM Code	ICD-10-CM Code Description	V24 CMS-HCC	V24 CMS-HCC Disease Group	V24 CMS-HCC Hierarchies	Community, NonDual, Aged	Community, NonDual, Disabled	Community, FBDual, Aged	Community, FBDual, Disabled	Community, PBDual, Aged	Community, PBDual, Disabled	Institutional
C81.29	Mixed cellularity Hodgkin lymphoma, extranodal and solid organ sites	10	Lymphoma and Other Cancers	11,12	0.675	0.663	0.717	0.756	0.648	0.667	0.461
C81.30	Lymphocyte depleted Hodgkin lymphoma, unspecified site	10	Lymphoma and Other Cancers	11,12	0.675	0.663	0.717	0.756	0.648	0.667	0.461
C81.31	Lymphocyte depleted Hodgkin lymphoma, lymph nodes of head, face, and neck	10	Lymphoma and Other Cancers	11,12	0.675	0.663	0.717	0.756	0.648	0.667	0.461
C81.32	Lymphocyte depleted Hodgkin lymphoma, intrathoracic lymph nodes	10	Lymphoma and Other Cancers	11,12	0.675	0.663	0.717	0.756	0.648	0.667	0.461
C81.33	Lymphocyte depleted Hodgkin lymphoma, intra-abdominal lymph nodes	10	Lymphoma and Other Cancers	11,12	0.675	0.663	0.717	0.756	0.648	0.667	0.461
C81.34	Lymphocyte depleted Hodgkin lymphoma, lymph nodes of axilla and upper limb	10	Lymphoma and Other Cancers	11,12	0.675	0.663	0.717	0.756	0.648	0.667	0.461
C81.35	Lymphocyte depleted Hodgkin lymphoma, lymph nodes of inguinal region and lower limb	10	Lymphoma and Other Cancers	11,12	0.675	0.663	0.717	0.756	0.648	0.667	0.461
C81.36	Lymphocyte depleted Hodgkin lymphoma, intrapelvic lymph nodes	10	Lymphoma and Other Cancers	11,12	0.675	0.663	0.717	0.756	0.648	0.667	0.461
C81.37	Lymphocyte depleted Hodgkin lymphoma, spleen	10	Lymphoma and Other Cancers	11,12	0.675	0.663	0.717	0.756	0.648	0.667	0.461
C81.38	Lymphocyte depleted Hodgkin lymphoma, lymph nodes of multiple sites	10	Lymphoma and Other Cancers	11,12	0.675	0.663	0.717	0.756	0.648	0.667	0.461
C81.39	Lymphocyte depleted Hodgkin lymphoma, extranodal and solid organ sites	10	Lymphoma and Other Cancers	11,12	0.675	0.663	0.717	0.756	0.648	0.667	0.461
C81.40	Lymphocyte-rich Hodgkin lymphoma, unspecified site	10	Lymphoma and Other Cancers	11,12	0.675	0.663	0.717	0.756	0.648	0.667	0.461
C81.41	Lymphocyte-rich Hodgkin lymphoma, lymph nodes of head, face, and neck	10	Lymphoma and Other Cancers	11,12	0.675	0.663	0.717	0.756	0.648	0.667	0.461
C81.42	Lymphocyte-rich Hodgkin lymphoma, intrathoracic lymph nodes	10	Lymphoma and Other Cancers	11,12	0.675	0.663	0.717	0.756	0.648	0.667	0.461
C81.43	Lymphocyte-rich Hodgkin lymphoma, intra-abdominal lymph nodes	10	Lymphoma and Other Cancers	11,12	0.675	0.663	0.717	0.756	0.648	0.667	0.461
C81.44	Lymphocyte-rich Hodgkin lymphoma, lymph nodes of axilla and upper limb	10	Lymphoma and Other Cancers	11,12	0.675	0.663	0.717	0.756	0.648	0.667	0.461
C81.45	Lymphocyte-rich Hodgkin lymphoma, lymph nodes of inguinal region and lower limb	10	Lymphoma and Other Cancers	11,12	0.675	0.663	0.717	0.756	0.648	0.667	0.461
C81.46	Lymphocyte-rich Hodgkin lymphoma, intrapelvic lymph nodes	10	Lymphoma and Other Cancers	11,12	0.675	0.663	0.717	0.756	0.648	0.667	0.461
C81.47	Lymphocyte-rich Hodgkin lymphoma, spleen	10	Lymphoma and Other Cancers	11,12	0.675	0.663	0.717	0.756	0.648	0.667	0.461
C81.48	Lymphocyte-rich Hodgkin lymphoma, lymph nodes of multiple sites	10	Lymphoma and Other Cancers	11,12	0.675	0.663	0.717	0.756	0.648	0.667	0.461
C81.49	Lymphocyte-rich Hodgkin lymphoma, extranodal and solid organ sites	10	Lymphoma and Other Cancers	11,12	0.675	0.663	0.717	0.756	0.648	0.667	0.461
C81.70	Other Hodgkin lymphoma, unspecified site	10	Lymphoma and Other Cancers	11,12	0.675	0.663	0.717	0.756	0.648	0.667	0.461
C81.71	Other Hodgkin lymphoma, lymph nodes of head, face, and neck	10	Lymphoma and Other Cancers	11,12	0.675	0.663	0.717	0.756	0.648	0.667	0.461

ICD-10-CM Code	ICD-10-CM Code Description	V24 CMS-HCC	V24 CMS-HCC Disease Group	V24 CMS-HCC Hierarchies	Community, NonDual, Aged	Community, NonDual, Disabled	Community, FBDual, Aged	Community, FBDual, Disabled	Community, PBDual, Aged	Community, PBDual, Disabled	Institutional
C81.72	Other Hodgkin lymphoma, intrathoracic lymph nodes	10	Lymphoma and Other Cancers	11,12	0.675	0.663	0.717	0.756	0.648	0.667	0.461
C81.73	Other Hodgkin lymphoma, intra-abdominal lymph nodes	10	Lymphoma and Other Cancers	11,12	0.675	0.663	0.717	0.756	0.648	0.667	0.461
C81.74	Other Hodgkin lymphoma, lymph nodes of axilla and upper limb	10	Lymphoma and Other Cancers	11,12	0.675	0.663	0.717	0.756	0.648	0.667	0.461
C81.75	Other Hodgkin lymphoma, lymph nodes of inguinal region and lower limb	10	Lymphoma and Other Cancers	11,12	0.675	0.663	0.717	0.756	0.648	0.667	0.461
C81.76	Other Hodgkin lymphoma, intrapelvic lymph nodes	10	Lymphoma and Other Cancers	11,12	0.675	0.663	0.717	0.756	0.648	0.667	0.461
C81.77	Other Hodgkin lymphoma, spleen	10	Lymphoma and Other Cancers	11,12	0.675	0.663	0.717	0.756	0.648	0.667	0.461
C81.78	Other Hodgkin lymphoma, lymph nodes of multiple sites	10	Lymphoma and Other Cancers	11,12	0.675	0.663	0.717	0.756	0.648	0.667	0.461
C81.79	Other Hodgkin lymphoma, extranodal and solid organ sites	10	Lymphoma and Other Cancers	11,12	0.675	0.663	0.717	0.756	0.648	0.667	0.461
C81.90	Hodgkin lymphoma, unspecified, unspecified site	10	Lymphoma and Other Cancers	11,12	0.675	0.663	0.717	0.756	0.648	0.667	0.461
C81.91	Hodgkin lymphoma, unspecified, lymph nodes of head, face, and neck	10	Lymphoma and Other Cancers	11,12	0.675	0.663	0.717	0.756	0.648	0.667	0.461
C81.92	Hodgkin lymphoma, unspecified, intrathoracic lymph nodes	10	Lymphoma and Other Cancers	11,12	0.675	0.663	0.717	0.756	0.648	0.667	0.461
C81.93	Hodgkin lymphoma, unspecified, intra-abdominal lymph nodes	10	Lymphoma and Other Cancers	11,12	0.675	0.663	0.717	0.756	0.648	0.667	0.461
C81.94	Hodgkin lymphoma, unspecified, lymph nodes of axilla and upper limb	10	Lymphoma and Other Cancers	11,12	0.675	0.663	0.717	0.756	0.648	0.667	0.461
C81.95	Hodgkin lymphoma, unspecified, lymph nodes of inguinal region and lower limb	10	Lymphoma and Other Cancers	11,12	0.675	0.663	0.717	0.756	0.648	0.667	0.461
C81.96	Hodgkin lymphoma, unspecified, intrapelvic lymph nodes	10	Lymphoma and Other Cancers	11,12	0.675	0.663	0.717	0.756	0.648	0.667	0.461
C81.97	Hodgkin lymphoma, unspecified, spleen	10	Lymphoma and Other Cancers	11,12	0.675	0.663	0.717	0.756	0.648	0.667	0.461
C81.98	Hodgkin lymphoma, unspecified, lymph nodes of multiple sites	10	Lymphoma and Other Cancers	11,12	0.675	0.663	0.717	0.756	0.648	0.667	0.461
C81.99	Hodgkin lymphoma, unspecified, extranodal and solid organ sites	10	Lymphoma and Other Cancers	11,12	0.675	0.663	0.717	0.756	0.648	0.667	0.461
C82.00	Follicular lymphoma grade I, unspecified site	10	Lymphoma and Other Cancers	11,12	0.675	0.663	0.717	0.756	0.648	0.667	0.461
C82.01	Follicular lymphoma grade I, lymph nodes of head, face, and neck	10	Lymphoma and Other Cancers	11,12	0.675	0.663	0.717	0.756	0.648	0.667	0.461
C82.02	Follicular lymphoma grade I, intrathoracic lymph nodes	10	Lymphoma and Other Cancers	11,12	0.675	0.663	0.717	0.756	0.648	0.667	0.461
C82.03	Follicular lymphoma grade I, intra-abdominal lymph nodes	10	Lymphoma and Other Cancers	11,12	0.675	0.663	0.717	0.756	0.648	0.667	0.461
C82.04	Follicular lymphoma grade I, lymph nodes of axilla and upper limb	10	Lymphoma and Other Cancers	11,12	0.675	0.663	0.717	0.756	0.648	0.667	0.461
C82.05	Follicular lymphoma grade I, lymph nodes of inguinal region and lower limb	10	Lymphoma and Other Cancers	11,12	0.675	0.663	0.717	0.756	0.648	0.667	0.461
C82.06	Follicular lymphoma grade I, intrapelvic lymph nodes	10	Lymphoma and Other Cancers	11,12	0.675	0.663	0.717	0.756	0.648	0.667	0.461
C82.07	Follicular lymphoma grade I, spleen	10	Lymphoma and Other Cancers	11,12	0.675	0.663	0.717	0.756	0.648	0.667	0.461
C82.08	Follicular lymphoma grade I, lymph nodes of multiple sites	10	Lymphoma and Other Cancers	11,12	0.675	0.663	0.717	0.756	0.648	0.667	0.461
C82.09	Follicular lymphoma grade I, extranodal and solid organ sites	10	Lymphoma and Other Cancers	11,12	0.675	0.663	0.717	0.756	0.648	0.667	0.461
C82.10	Follicular lymphoma grade II, unspecified site	10	Lymphoma and Other Cancers	11,12	0.675	0.663	0.717	0.756	0.648	0.667	0.461

ICD-10-CM Code	ICD-10-CM Code Description	V24 CMS-HCC	V24 CMS-HCC Disease Group	V24 CMS-HCC Hierarchies	Community, NonDual, Aged	Community, NonDual, Disabled	Community, FBDual, Aged	Community, FBDual, Disabled	Community, PBDual, Aged	Community, PBDual, Disabled	Institutional
C82.11	Follicular lymphoma grade II, lymph nodes of head, face, and neck	10	Lymphoma and Other Cancers	11,12	0.675	0.663	0.717	0.756	0.648	0.667	0.461
C82.12	Follicular lymphoma grade II, intrathoracic lymph nodes	10	Lymphoma and Other Cancers	11,12	0.675	0.663	0.717	0.756	0.648	0.667	0.461
C82.13	Follicular lymphoma grade II, intra-abdominal lymph nodes	10	Lymphoma and Other Cancers	11,12	0.675	0.663	0.717	0.756	0.648	0.667	0.461
C82.14	Follicular lymphoma grade II, lymph nodes of axilla and upper limb	10	Lymphoma and Other Cancers	11,12	0.675	0.663	0.717	0.756	0.648	0.667	0.461
C82.15	Follicular lymphoma grade II, lymph nodes of inguinal region and lower limb	10	Lymphoma and Other Cancers	11,12	0.675	0.663	0.717	0.756	0.648	0.667	0.461
C82.16	Follicular lymphoma grade II, intrapelvic lymph nodes	10	Lymphoma and Other Cancers	11,12	0.675	0.663	0.717	0.756	0.648	0.667	0.461
C82.17	Follicular lymphoma grade II, spleen	10	Lymphoma and Other Cancers	11,12	0.675	0.663	0.717	0.756	0.648	0.667	0.461
C82.18	Follicular lymphoma grade II, lymph nodes of multiple sites	10	Lymphoma and Other Cancers	11,12	0.675	0.663	0.717	0.756	0.648	0.667	0.461
C82.19	Follicular lymphoma grade II, extranodal and solid organ sites	10	Lymphoma and Other Cancers	11,12	0.675	0.663	0.717	0.756	0.648	0.667	0.461
C82.20	Follicular lymphoma grade III, unspecified, unspecified site	10	Lymphoma and Other Cancers	11,12	0.675	0.663	0.717	0.756	0.648	0.667	0.461
C82.21	Follicular lymphoma grade III, unspecified, lymph nodes of head, face, and neck	10	Lymphoma and Other Cancers	11,12	0.675	0.663	0.717	0.756	0.648	0.667	0.461
C82.22	Follicular lymphoma grade III, unspecified, intrathoracic lymph nodes	10	Lymphoma and Other Cancers	11,12	0.675	0.663	0.717	0.756	0.648	0.667	0.461
C82.23	Follicular lymphoma grade III, unspecified, intra-abdominal lymph nodes	10	Lymphoma and Other Cancers	11,12	0.675	0.663	0.717	0.756	0.648	0.667	0.461
C82.24	Follicular lymphoma grade III, unspecified, lymph nodes of axilla and upper limb	10	Lymphoma and Other Cancers	11,12	0.675	0.663	0.717	0.756	0.648	0.667	0.461
C82.25	Follicular lymphoma grade III, unspecified, lymph nodes of inguinal region and lower limb	10	Lymphoma and Other Cancers	11,12	0.675	0.663	0.717	0.756	0.648	0.667	0.461
C82.26	Follicular lymphoma grade III, unspecified, intrapelvic lymph nodes	10	Lymphoma and Other Cancers	11,12	0.675	0.663	0.717	0.756	0.648	0.667	0.461
C82.27	Follicular lymphoma grade III, unspecified, spleen	10	Lymphoma and Other Cancers	11,12	0.675	0.663	0.717	0.756	0.648	0.667	0.461
C82.28	Follicular lymphoma grade III, unspecified, lymph nodes of multiple sites	10	Lymphoma and Other Cancers	11,12	0.675	0.663	0.717	0.756	0.648	0.667	0.461
C82.29	Follicular lymphoma grade III, unspecified, extranodal and solid organ sites	10	Lymphoma and Other Cancers	11,12	0.675	0.663	0.717	0.756	0.648	0.667	0.461
C82.30	Follicular lymphoma grade IIIa, unspecified site	10	Lymphoma and Other Cancers	11,12	0.675	0.663	0.717	0.756	0.648	0.667	0.461
C82.31	Follicular lymphoma grade IIIa, lymph nodes of head, face, and neck	10	Lymphoma and Other Cancers	11,12	0.675	0.663	0.717	0.756	0.648	0.667	0.461
C82.32	Follicular lymphoma grade IIIa, intrathoracic lymph nodes	10	Lymphoma and Other Cancers	11,12	0.675	0.663	0.717	0.756	0.648	0.667	0.461
C82.33	Follicular lymphoma grade IIIa, intra-abdominal lymph nodes	10	Lymphoma and Other Cancers	11,12	0.675	0.663	0.717	0.756	0.648	0.667	0.461
C82.34	Follicular lymphoma grade IIIa, lymph nodes of axilla and upper limb	10	Lymphoma and Other Cancers	11,12	0.675	0.663	0.717	0.756	0.648	0.667	0.461
C82.35	Follicular lymphoma grade IIIa, lymph nodes of inguinal region and lower limb	10	Lymphoma and Other Cancers	11,12	0.675	0.663	0.717	0.756	0.648	0.667	0.461
C82.36	Follicular lymphoma grade IIIa, intrapelvic lymph nodes	10	Lymphoma and Other Cancers	11,12	0.675	0.663	0.717	0.756	0.648	0.667	0.461

ICD-10-CM Code	ICD-10-CM Code Description	V24 CMS-HCC	V24 CMS-HCC Disease Group	V24 CMS-HCC Hierarchies	Community, NonDual, Aged	Community, NonDual, Disabled	Community, FBDual, Aged	Community, FBDual, Disabled	Community, PBDual, Aged	Community, PBDual, Disabled	Institutional
C82.37	Follicular lymphoma grade IIIa, spleen	10	Lymphoma and Other Cancers	11,12	0.675	0.663	0.717	0.756	0.648	0.667	0.461
C82.38	Follicular lymphoma grade IIIa, lymph nodes of multiple sites	10	Lymphoma and Other Cancers	11,12	0.675	0.663	0.717	0.756	0.648	0.667	0.461
C82.39	Follicular lymphoma grade IIIa, extranodal and solid organ sites	10	Lymphoma and Other Cancers	11,12	0.675	0.663	0.717	0.756	0.648	0.667	0.461
C82.40	Follicular lymphoma grade IIIb, unspecified site	10	Lymphoma and Other Cancers	11,12	0.675	0.663	0.717	0.756	0.648	0.667	0.461
C82.41	Follicular lymphoma grade IIIb, lymph nodes of head, face, and neck	10	Lymphoma and Other Cancers	11,12	0.675	0.663	0.717	0.756	0.648	0.667	0.461
C82.42	Follicular lymphoma grade IIIb, intrathoracic lymph nodes	10	Lymphoma and Other Cancers	11,12	0.675	0.663	0.717	0.756	0.648	0.667	0.461
C82.43	Follicular lymphoma grade IIIb, intra-abdominal lymph nodes	10	Lymphoma and Other Cancers	11,12	0.675	0.663	0.717	0.756	0.648	0.667	0.461
C82.44	Follicular lymphoma grade IIIb, lymph nodes of axilla and upper limb	10	Lymphoma and Other Cancers	11,12	0.675	0.663	0.717	0.756	0.648	0.667	0.461
C82.45	Follicular lymphoma grade IIIb, lymph nodes of inguinal region and lower limb	10	Lymphoma and Other Cancers	11,12	0.675	0.663	0.717	0.756	0.648	0.667	0.461
C82.46	Follicular lymphoma grade IIIb, intrapelvic lymph nodes	10	Lymphoma and Other Cancers	11,12	0.675	0.663	0.717	0.756	0.648	0.667	0.461
C82.47	Follicular lymphoma grade IIIb, spleen	10	Lymphoma and Other Cancers	11,12	0.675	0.663	0.717	0.756	0.648	0.667	0.461
C82.48	Follicular lymphoma grade IIIb, lymph nodes of multiple sites	10	Lymphoma and Other Cancers	11,12	0.675	0.663	0.717	0.756	0.648	0.667	0.461
C82.49	Follicular lymphoma grade IIIb, extranodal and solid organ sites	10	Lymphoma and Other Cancers	11,12	0.675	0.663	0.717	0.756	0.648	0.667	0.461
C82.50	Diffuse follicle center lymphoma, unspecified site	10	Lymphoma and Other Cancers	11,12	0.675	0.663	0.717	0.756	0.648	0.667	0.461
C82.51	Diffuse follicle center lymphoma, lymph nodes of head, face, and neck	10	Lymphoma and Other Cancers	11,12	0.675	0.663	0.717	0.756	0.648	0.667	0.461
C82.52	Diffuse follicle center lymphoma, intrathoracic lymph nodes	10	Lymphoma and Other Cancers	11,12	0.675	0.663	0.717	0.756	0.648	0.667	0.461
C82.53	Diffuse follicle center lymphoma, intra-abdominal lymph nodes	10	Lymphoma and Other Cancers	11,12	0.675	0.663	0.717	0.756	0.648	0.667	0.461
C82.54	Diffuse follicle center lymphoma, lymph nodes of axilla and upper limb	10	Lymphoma and Other Cancers	11,12	0.675	0.663	0.717	0.756	0.648	0.667	0.461
C82.55	Diffuse follicle center lymphoma, lymph nodes of inguinal region and lower limb	10	Lymphoma and Other Cancers	11,12	0.675	0.663	0.717	0.756	0.648	0.667	0.461
C82.56	Diffuse follicle center lymphoma, intrapelvic lymph nodes	10	Lymphoma and Other Cancers	11,12	0.675	0.663	0.717	0.756	0.648	0.667	0.461
C82.57	Diffuse follicle center lymphoma, spleen	10	Lymphoma and Other Cancers	11,12	0.675	0.663	0.717	0.756	0.648	0.667	0.461
C82.58	Diffuse follicle center lymphoma, lymph nodes of multiple sites	10	Lymphoma and Other Cancers	11,12	0.675	0.663	0.717	0.756	0.648	0.667	0.461
C82.59	Diffuse follicle center lymphoma, extranodal and solid organ sites	10	Lymphoma and Other Cancers	11,12	0.675	0.663	0.717	0.756	0.648	0.667	0.461
C82.60	Cutaneous follicle center lymphoma, unspecified site	10	Lymphoma and Other Cancers	11,12	0.675	0.663	0.717	0.756	0.648	0.667	0.461
C82.61	Cutaneous follicle center lymphoma, lymph nodes of head, face, and neck	10	Lymphoma and Other Cancers	11,12	0.675	0.663	0.717	0.756	0.648	0.667	0.461
C82.62	Cutaneous follicle center lymphoma, intrathoracic lymph nodes	10	Lymphoma and Other Cancers	11,12	0.675	0.663	0.717	0.756	0.648	0.667	0.461
C82.63	Cutaneous follicle center lymphoma, intra-abdominal lymph nodes	10	Lymphoma and Other Cancers	11,12	0.675	0.663	0.717	0.756	0.648	0.667	0.461
C82.64	Cutaneous follicle center lymphoma, lymph nodes of axilla and upper limb	10	Lymphoma and Other Cancers	11,12	0.675	0.663	0.717	0.756	0.648	0.667	0.461

ICD-10-CM Code	ICD-10-CM Code Description	V24 CMS-HCC	V24 CMS-HCC Disease Group	V24 CMS-HCC Hierarchies	Community, NonDual, Aged	Community, NonDual, Disabled	Community, FBDual, Aged	Community, FBDual, Disabled	Community, PBDual, Aged	Community, PBDual, Disabled	Institutional
C82.65	Cutaneous follicle center lymphoma, lymph nodes of inguinal region and lower limb	10	Lymphoma and Other Cancers	11,12	0.675	0.663	0.717	0.756	0.648	0.667	0.461
C82.66	Cutaneous follicle center lymphoma, intrapelvic lymph nodes	10	Lymphoma and Other Cancers	11,12	0.675	0.663	0.717	0.756	0.648	0.667	0.461
C82.67	Cutaneous follicle center lymphoma, spleen	10	Lymphoma and Other Cancers	11,12	0.675	0.663	0.717	0.756	0.648	0.667	0.461
C82.68	Cutaneous follicle center lymphoma, lymph nodes of multiple sites	10	Lymphoma and Other Cancers	11,12	0.675	0.663	0.717	0.756	0.648	0.667	0.461
C82.69	Cutaneous follicle center lymphoma, extranodal and solid organ sites	10	Lymphoma and Other Cancers	11,12	0.675	0.663	0.717	0.756	0.648	0.667	0.461
C82.80	Other types of follicular lymphoma, unspecified site	10	Lymphoma and Other Cancers	11,12	0.675	0.663	0.717	0.756	0.648	0.667	0.461
C82.81	Other types of follicular lymphoma, lymph nodes of head, face, and neck	10	Lymphoma and Other Cancers	11,12	0.675	0.663	0.717	0.756	0.648	0.667	0.461
C82.82	Other types of follicular lymphoma, intrathoracic lymph nodes	10	Lymphoma and Other Cancers	11,12	0.675	0.663	0.717	0.756	0.648	0.667	0.461
C82.83	Other types of follicular lymphoma, intra-abdominal lymph nodes	10	Lymphoma and Other Cancers	11,12	0.675	0.663	0.717	0.756	0.648	0.667	0.461
C82.84	Other types of follicular lymphoma, lymph nodes of axilla and upper limb	10	Lymphoma and Other Cancers	11,12	0.675	0.663	0.717	0.756	0.648	0.667	0.461
C82.85	Other types of follicular lymphoma, lymph nodes of inguinal region and lower limb	10	Lymphoma and Other Cancers	11,12	0.675	0.663	0.717	0.756	0.648	0.667	0.461
C82.86	Other types of follicular lymphoma, intrapelvic lymph nodes	10	Lymphoma and Other Cancers	11,12	0.675	0.663	0.717	0.756	0.648	0.667	0.461
C82.87	Other types of follicular lymphoma, spleen	10	Lymphoma and Other Cancers	11,12	0.675	0.663	0.717	0.756	0.648	0.667	0.461
C82.88	Other types of follicular lymphoma, lymph nodes of multiple sites	10	Lymphoma and Other Cancers	11,12	0.675	0.663	0.717	0.756	0.648	0.667	0.461
C82.89	Other types of follicular lymphoma, extranodal and solid organ sites	10	Lymphoma and Other Cancers	11,12	0.675	0.663	0.717	0.756	0.648	0.667	0.461
C82.90	Follicular lymphoma, unspecified, unspecified site	10	Lymphoma and Other Cancers	11,12	0.675	0.663	0.717	0.756	0.648	0.667	0.461
C82.91	Follicular lymphoma, unspecified, lymph nodes of head, face, and neck	10	Lymphoma and Other Cancers	11,12	0.675	0.663	0.717	0.756	0.648	0.667	0.461
C82.92	Follicular lymphoma, unspecified, intrathoracic lymph nodes	10	Lymphoma and Other Cancers	11,12	0.675	0.663	0.717	0.756	0.648	0.667	0.461
C82.93	Follicular lymphoma, unspecified, intra-abdominal lymph nodes	10	Lymphoma and Other Cancers	11,12	0.675	0.663	0.717	0.756	0.648	0.667	0.461
C82.94	Follicular lymphoma, unspecified, lymph nodes of axilla and upper limb	10	Lymphoma and Other Cancers	11,12	0.675	0.663	0.717	0.756	0.648	0.667	0.461
C82.95	Follicular lymphoma, unspecified, lymph nodes of inguinal region and lower limb	10	Lymphoma and Other Cancers	11,12	0.675	0.663	0.717	0.756	0.648	0.667	0.461
C82.96	Follicular lymphoma, unspecified, intrapelvic lymph nodes	10	Lymphoma and Other Cancers	11,12	0.675	0.663	0.717	0.756	0.648	0.667	0.461
C82.97	Follicular lymphoma, unspecified, spleen	10	Lymphoma and Other Cancers	11,12	0.675	0.663	0.717	0.756	0.648	0.667	0.461
C82.98	Follicular lymphoma, unspecified, lymph nodes of multiple sites	10	Lymphoma and Other Cancers	11,12	0.675	0.663	0.717	0.756	0.648	0.667	0.461
C82.99	Follicular lymphoma, unspecified, extranodal and solid organ sites	10	Lymphoma and Other Cancers	11,12	0.675	0.663	0.717	0.756	0.648	0.667	0.461
C83.00	Small cell B-cell lymphoma, unspecified site	10	Lymphoma and Other Cancers	11,12	0.675	0.663	0.717	0.756	0.648	0.667	0.461
C83.01	Small cell B-cell lymphoma, lymph nodes of head, face, and neck	10	Lymphoma and Other Cancers	11,12	0.675	0.663	0.717	0.756	0.648	0.667	0.461
C83.02	Small cell B-cell lymphoma, intrathoracic lymph nodes	10	Lymphoma and Other Cancers	11,12	0.675	0.663	0.717	0.756	0.648	0.667	0.461

ICD-10-CM Code	ICD-10-CM Code Description	V24 CMS-HCC	V24 CMS-HCC Disease Group	V24 CMS-HCC Hierarchies	Community, NonDual, Aged	Community, NonDual, Disabled	Community, FBDual, Aged	Community, FBDual, Disabled	Community, PBDual, Aged	Community, PBDual, Disabled	Institutional
C83.Ø3	Small cell B-cell lymphoma, intra-abdominal lymph nodes	10	Lymphoma and Other Cancers	11,12	0.675	0.663	0.717	0.756	0.648	0.667	0.461
C83.Ø4	Small cell B-cell lymphoma, lymph nodes of axilla and upper limb	10	Lymphoma and Other Cancers	11,12	0.675	0.663	0.717	0.756	0.648	0.667	0.461
C83.Ø5	Small cell B-cell lymphoma, lymph nodes of inguinal region and lower limb	10	Lymphoma and Other Cancers	11,12	0.675	0.663	0.717	0.756	0.648	0.667	0.461
C83.Ø6	Small cell B-cell lymphoma, intrapelvic lymph nodes	10	Lymphoma and Other Cancers	11,12	0.675	0.663	0.717	0.756	0.648	0.667	0.461
C83.Ø7	Small cell B-cell lymphoma, spleen	10	Lymphoma and Other Cancers	11,12	0.675	0.663	0.717	0.756	0.648	0.667	0.461
C83.Ø8	Small cell B-cell lymphoma, lymph nodes of multiple sites	10	Lymphoma and Other Cancers	11,12	0.675	0.663	0.717	0.756	0.648	0.667	0.461
C83.Ø9	Small cell B-cell lymphoma, extranodal and solid organ sites	10	Lymphoma and Other Cancers	11,12	0.675	0.663	0.717	0.756	0.648	0.667	0.461
C83.1Ø	Mantle cell lymphoma, unspecified site	10	Lymphoma and Other Cancers	11,12	0.675	0.663	0.717	0.756	0.648	0.667	0.461
C83.11	Mantle cell lymphoma, lymph nodes of head, face, and neck	10	Lymphoma and Other Cancers	11,12	0.675	0.663	0.717	0.756	0.648	0.667	0.461
C83.12	Mantle cell lymphoma, intrathoracic lymph nodes	10	Lymphoma and Other Cancers	11,12	0.675	0.663	0.717	0.756	0.648	0.667	0.461
C83.13	Mantle cell lymphoma, intra-abdominal lymph nodes	10	Lymphoma and Other Cancers	11,12	0.675	0.663	0.717	0.756	0.648	0.667	0.461
C83.14	Mantle cell lymphoma, lymph nodes of axilla and upper limb	10	Lymphoma and Other Cancers	11,12	0.675	0.663	0.717	0.756	0.648	0.667	0.461
C83.15	Mantle cell lymphoma, lymph nodes of inguinal region and lower limb	10	Lymphoma and Other Cancers	11,12	0.675	0.663	0.717	0.756	0.648	0.667	0.461
C83.16	Mantle cell lymphoma, intrapelvic lymph nodes	10	Lymphoma and Other Cancers	11,12	0.675	0.663	0.717	0.756	0.648	0.667	0.461
C83.17	Mantle cell lymphoma, spleen	10	Lymphoma and Other Cancers	11,12	0.675	0.663	0.717	0.756	0.648	0.667	0.461
C83.18	Mantle cell lymphoma, lymph nodes of multiple sites	10	Lymphoma and Other Cancers	11,12	0.675	0.663	0.717	0.756	0.648	0.667	0.461
C83.19	Mantle cell lymphoma, extranodal and solid organ sites	10	Lymphoma and Other Cancers	11,12	0.675	0.663	0.717	0.756	0.648	0.667	0.461
C83.3Ø	Diffuse large B-cell lymphoma, unspecified site	10	Lymphoma and Other Cancers	11,12	0.675	0.663	0.717	0.756	0.648	0.667	0.461
C83.31	Diffuse large B-cell lymphoma, lymph nodes of head, face, and neck	10	Lymphoma and Other Cancers	11,12	0.675	0.663	0.717	0.756	0.648	0.667	0.461
C83.32	Diffuse large B-cell lymphoma, intrathoracic lymph nodes	10	Lymphoma and Other Cancers	11,12	0.675	0.663	0.717	0.756	0.648	0.667	0.461
C83.33	Diffuse large B-cell lymphoma, intra-abdominal lymph nodes	10	Lymphoma and Other Cancers	11,12	0.675	0.663	0.717	0.756	0.648	0.667	0.461
C83.34	Diffuse large B-cell lymphoma, lymph nodes of axilla and upper limb	10	Lymphoma and Other Cancers	11,12	0.675	0.663	0.717	0.756	0.648	0.667	0.461
C83.35	Diffuse large B-cell lymphoma, lymph nodes of inguinal region and lower limb	10	Lymphoma and Other Cancers	11,12	0.675	0.663	0.717	0.756	0.648	0.667	0.461
C83.36	Diffuse large B-cell lymphoma, intrapelvic lymph nodes	10	Lymphoma and Other Cancers	11,12	0.675	0.663	0.717	0.756	0.648	0.667	0.461
C83.37	Diffuse large B-cell lymphoma, spleen	10	Lymphoma and Other Cancers	11,12	0.675	0.663	0.717	0.756	0.648	0.667	0.461
C83.38	Diffuse large B-cell lymphoma, lymph nodes of multiple sites	10	Lymphoma and Other Cancers	11,12	0.675	0.663	0.717	0.756	0.648	0.667	0.461
C83.39	Diffuse large B-cell lymphoma, extranodal and solid organ sites	10	Lymphoma and Other Cancers	11,12	0.675	0.663	0.717	0.756	0.648	0.667	0.461
C83.5Ø	Lymphoblastic (diffuse) lymphoma, unspecified site	10	Lymphoma and Other Cancers	11,12	0.675	0.663	0.717	0.756	0.648	0.667	0.461
C83.51	Lymphoblastic (diffuse) lymphoma, lymph nodes of head, face, and neck	10	Lymphoma and Other Cancers	11,12	0.675	0.663	0.717	0.756	0.648	0.667	0.461

ICD-10-CM Code	ICD-10-CM Code Description	V24 CMS-HCC	V24 CMS-HCC Disease Group	V24 CMS-HCC Hierarchies	Community, NonDual, Aged	Community, NonDual, Disabled	Community, FBDual, Aged	Community, FBDual, Disabled	Community, PBDual, Aged	Community, PBDual, Disabled	Institutional
C83.52	Lymphoblastic (diffuse) lymphoma, intrathoracic lymph nodes	10	Lymphoma and Other Cancers	11,12	0.675	0.663	0.717	0.756	0.648	0.667	0.461
C83.53	Lymphoblastic (diffuse) lymphoma, intra-abdominal lymph nodes	10	Lymphoma and Other Cancers	11,12	0.675	0.663	0.717	0.756	0.648	0.667	0.461
C83.54	Lymphoblastic (diffuse) lymphoma, lymph nodes of axilla and upper limb	10	Lymphoma and Other Cancers	11,12	0.675	0.663	0.717	0.756	0.648	0.667	0.461
C83.55	Lymphoblastic (diffuse) lymphoma, lymph nodes of inguinal region and lower limb	10	Lymphoma and Other Cancers	11,12	0.675	0.663	0.717	0.756	0.648	0.667	0.461
C83.56	Lymphoblastic (diffuse) lymphoma, intrapelvic lymph nodes	10	Lymphoma and Other Cancers	11,12	0.675	0.663	0.717	0.756	0.648	0.667	0.461
C83.57	Lymphoblastic (diffuse) lymphoma, spleen	10	Lymphoma and Other Cancers	11,12	0.675	0.663	0.717	0.756	0.648	0.667	0.461
C83.58	Lymphoblastic (diffuse) lymphoma, lymph nodes of multiple sites	10	Lymphoma and Other Cancers	11,12	0.675	0.663	0.717	0.756	0.648	0.667	0.461
C83.59	Lymphoblastic (diffuse) lymphoma, extranodal and solid organ sites	10	Lymphoma and Other Cancers	11,12	0.675	0.663	0.717	0.756	0.648	0.667	0.461
C83.70	Burkitt lymphoma, unspecified site	10	Lymphoma and Other Cancers	11,12	0.675	0.663	0.717	0.756	0.648	0.667	0.461
C83.71	Burkitt lymphoma, lymph nodes of head, face, and neck	10	Lymphoma and Other Cancers	11,12	0.675	0.663	0.717	0.756	0.648	0.667	0.461
C83.72	Burkitt lymphoma, intrathoracic lymph nodes	10	Lymphoma and Other Cancers	11,12	0.675	0.663	0.717	0.756	0.648	0.667	0.461
C83.73	Burkitt lymphoma, intra-abdominal lymph nodes	10	Lymphoma and Other Cancers	11,12	0.675	0.663	0.717	0.756	0.648	0.667	0.461
C83.74	Burkitt lymphoma, lymph nodes of axilla and upper limb	10	Lymphoma and Other Cancers	11,12	0.675	0.663	0.717	0.756	0.648	0.667	0.461
C83.75	Burkitt lymphoma, lymph nodes of inguinal region and lower limb	10	Lymphoma and Other Cancers	11,12	0.675	0.663	0.717	0.756	0.648	0.667	0.461
C83.76	Burkitt lymphoma, intrapelvic lymph nodes	10	Lymphoma and Other Cancers	11,12	0.675	0.663	0.717	0.756	0.648	0.667	0.461
C83.77	Burkitt lymphoma, spleen	10	Lymphoma and Other Cancers	11,12	0.675	0.663	0.717	0.756	0.648	0.667	0.461
C83.78	Burkitt lymphoma, lymph nodes of multiple sites	10	Lymphoma and Other Cancers	11,12	0.675	0.663	0.717	0.756	0.648	0.667	0.461
C83.79	Burkitt lymphoma, extranodal and solid organ sites	10	Lymphoma and Other Cancers	11,12	0.675	0.663	0.717	0.756	0.648	0.667	0.461
C83.80	Other non-follicular lymphoma, unspecified site	10	Lymphoma and Other Cancers	11,12	0.675	0.663	0.717	0.756	0.648	0.667	0.461
C83.81	Other non-follicular lymphoma, lymph nodes of head, face, and neck	10	Lymphoma and Other Cancers	11,12	0.675	0.663	0.717	0.756	0.648	0.667	0.461
C83.82	Other non-follicular lymphoma, intrathoracic lymph nodes	10	Lymphoma and Other Cancers	11,12	0.675	0.663	0.717	0.756	0.648	0.667	0.461
C83.83	Other non-follicular lymphoma, intra-abdominal lymph nodes	10	Lymphoma and Other Cancers	11,12	0.675	0.663	0.717	0.756	0.648	0.667	0.461
C83.84	Other non-follicular lymphoma, lymph nodes of axilla and upper limb	10	Lymphoma and Other Cancers	11,12	0.675	0.663	0.717	0.756	0.648	0.667	0.461
C83.85	Other non-follicular lymphoma, lymph nodes of inguinal region and lower limb	10	Lymphoma and Other Cancers	11,12	0.675	0.663	0.717	0.756	0.648	0.667	0.461
C83.86	Other non-follicular lymphoma, intrapelvic lymph nodes	10	Lymphoma and Other Cancers	11,12	0.675	0.663	0.717	0.756	0.648	0.667	0.461
C83.87	Other non-follicular lymphoma, spleen	10	Lymphoma and Other Cancers	11,12	0.675	0.663	0.717	0.756	0.648	0.667	0.461
C83.88	Other non-follicular lymphoma, lymph nodes of multiple sites	10	Lymphoma and Other Cancers	11,12	0.675	0.663	0.717	0.756	0.648	0.667	0.461
C83.89	Other non-follicular lymphoma, extranodal and solid organ sites	10	Lymphoma and Other Cancers	11,12	0.675	0.663	0.717	0.756	0.648	0.667	0.461
C83.90	Non-follicular (diffuse) lymphoma, unspecified, unspecified site	10	Lymphoma and Other Cancers	11,12	0.675	0.663	0.717	0.756	0.648	0.667	0.461

2021 Optum360, LLC

ICD-10-CM Code	ICD-10-CM Code Description	V24 CMS-HCC	V24 CMS-HCC Disease Group	V24 CMS-HCC Hierarchies	Community, NonDual, Aged	Community, NonDual, Disabled	Community, FBDual, Aged	Community, FBDual, Disabled	Community, PBDual, Aged	Community, PBDual, Disabled	Institutional
C83.91	Non-follicular (diffuse) lymphoma, unspecified, lymph nodes of head, face, and neck	10	Lymphoma and Other Cancers	11,12	0.675	0.663	0.717	0.756	0.648	0.667	0.461
C83.92	Non-follicular (diffuse) lymphoma, unspecified, intrathoracic lymph nodes	10	Lymphoma and Other Cancers	11,12	0.675	0.663	0.717	0.756	0.648	0.667	0.461
C83.93	Non-follicular (diffuse) lymphoma, unspecified, intra-abdominal lymph nodes	10	Lymphoma and Other Cancers	11,12	0.675	0.663	0.717	0.756	0.648	0.667	0.461
C83.94	Non-follicular (diffuse) lymphoma, unspecified, lymph nodes of axilla and upper limb	10	Lymphoma and Other Cancers	11,12	0.675	0.663	0.717	0.756	0.648	0.667	0.461
C83.95	Non-follicular (diffuse) lymphoma, unspecified, lymph nodes of inguinal region and lower limb	10	Lymphoma and Other Cancers	11,12	0.675	0.663	0.717	0.756	0.648	0.667	0.461
C83.96	Non-follicular (diffuse) lymphoma, unspecified, intrapelvic lymph nodes	10	Lymphoma and Other Cancers	11,12	0.675	0.663	0.717	0.756	0.648	0.667	0.461
C83.97	Non-follicular (diffuse) lymphoma, unspecified, spleen	10	Lymphoma and Other Cancers	11,12	0.675	0.663	0.717	0.756	0.648	0.667	0.461
C83.98	Non-follicular (diffuse) lymphoma, unspecified, lymph nodes of multiple sites	10	Lymphoma and Other Cancers	11,12	0.675	0.663	0.717	0.756	0.648	0.667	0.461
C83.99	Non-follicular (diffuse) lymphoma, unspecified, extranodal and solid organ sites	10	Lymphoma and Other Cancers	11,12	0.675	0.663	0.717	0.756	0.648	0.667	0.461
C84.00	Mycosis fungoides, unspecified site	10	Lymphoma and Other Cancers	11,12	0.675	0.663	0.717	0.756	0.648	0.667	0.461
C84.01	Mycosis fungoides, lymph nodes of head, face, and neck	10	Lymphoma and Other Cancers	11,12	0.675	0.663	0.717	0.756	0.648	0.667	0.461
C84.02	Mycosis fungoides, intrathoracic lymph nodes	10	Lymphoma and Other Cancers	11,12	0.675	0.663	0.717	0.756	0.648	0.667	0.461
C84.03	Mycosis fungoides, intra-abdominal lymph nodes	10	Lymphoma and Other Cancers	11,12	0.675	0.663	0.717	0.756	0.648	0.667	0.461
C84.04	Mycosis fungoides, lymph nodes of axilla and upper limb	10	Lymphoma and Other Cancers	11,12	0.675	0.663	0.717	0.756	0.648	0.667	0.461
C84.05	Mycosis fungoides, lymph nodes of inguinal region and lower limb	10	Lymphoma and Other Cancers	11,12	0.675	0.663	0.717	0.756	0.648	0.667	0.461
C84.06	Mycosis fungoides, intrapelvic lymph nodes	10	Lymphoma and Other Cancers	11,12	0.675	0.663	0.717	0.756	0.648	0.667	0.461
C84.07	Mycosis fungoides, spleen	10	Lymphoma and Other Cancers	11,12	0.675	0.663	0.717	0.756	0.648	0.667	0.461
C84.08	Mycosis fungoides, lymph nodes of multiple sites	10	Lymphoma and Other Cancers	11,12	0.675	0.663	0.717	0.756	0.648	0.667	0.461
C84.09	Mycosis fungoides, extranodal and solid organ sites	10	Lymphoma and Other Cancers	11,12	0.675	0.663	0.717	0.756	0.648	0.667	0.461
C84.10	Sezary disease, unspecified site	10	Lymphoma and Other Cancers	11,12	0.675	0.663	0.717	0.756	0.648	0.667	0.461
C84.11	Sezary disease, lymph nodes of head, face, and neck	10	Lymphoma and Other Cancers	11,12	0.675	0.663	0.717	0.756	0.648	0.667	0.461
C84.12	Sezary disease, intrathoracic lymph nodes	10	Lymphoma and Other Cancers	11,12	0.675	0.663	0.717	0.756	0.648	0.667	0.461
C84.13	Sezary disease, intra-abdominal lymph nodes	10	Lymphoma and Other Cancers	11,12	0.675	0.663	0.717	0.756	0.648	0.667	0.461
C84.14	Sezary disease, lymph nodes of axilla and upper limb	10	Lymphoma and Other Cancers	11,12	0.675	0.663	0.717	0.756	0.648	0.667	0.461
C84.15	Sezary disease, lymph nodes of inguinal region and lower limb	10	Lymphoma and Other Cancers	11,12	0.675	0.663	0.717	0.756	0.648	0.667	0.461
C84.16	Sezary disease, intrapelvic lymph nodes	10	Lymphoma and Other Cancers	11,12	0.675	0.663	0.717	0.756	0.648	0.667	0.461
C84.17	Sezary disease, spleen	10	Lymphoma and Other Cancers	11,12	0.675	0.663	0.717	0.756	0.648	0.667	0.461
C84.18	Sezary disease, lymph nodes of multiple sites	10	Lymphoma and Other Cancers	11,12	0.675	0.663	0.717	0.756	0.648	0.667	0.461

ICD-10-CM Code	ICD-10-CM Code Description	V24 CMS-HCC	V24 CMS-HCC Disease Group	V24 CMS-HCC Hierarchies	Community, NonDual, Aged	Community, NonDual, Disabled	Community, FBDual, Aged	Community, FBDual, Disabled	Community, PBDual, Aged	Community, PBDual, Disabled	Institutional
C84.19	Sezary disease, extranodal and solid organ sites	10	Lymphoma and Other Cancers	11,12	0.675	0.663	0.717	0.756	0.648	0.667	0.461
C84.40	Peripheral T-cell lymphoma, not classified, unspecified site	10	Lymphoma and Other Cancers	11,12	0.675	0.663	0.717	0.756	0.648	0.667	0.461
C84.41	Peripheral T-cell lymphoma, not classified, lymph nodes of head, face, and neck	10	Lymphoma and Other Cancers	11,12	0.675	0.663	0.717	0.756	0.648	0.667	0.461
C84.42	Peripheral T-cell lymphoma, not classified, intrathoracic lymph nodes	10	Lymphoma and Other Cancers	11,12	0.675	0.663	0.717	0.756	0.648	0.667	0.461
C84.43	Peripheral T-cell lymphoma, not classified, intra-abdominal lymph nodes	10	Lymphoma and Other Cancers	11,12	0.675	0.663	0.717	0.756	0.648	0.667	0.461
C84.44	Peripheral T-cell lymphoma, not classified, lymph nodes of axilla and upper limb	10	Lymphoma and Other Cancers	11,12	0.675	0.663	0.717	0.756	0.648	0.667	0.461
C84.45	Peripheral T-cell lymphoma, not classified, lymph nodes of inguinal region and lower limb	10	Lymphoma and Other Cancers	11,12	0.675	0.663	0.717	0.756	0.648	0.667	0.461
C84.46	Peripheral T-cell lymphoma, not classified, intrapelvic lymph nodes	10	Lymphoma and Other Cancers	11,12	0.675	0.663	0.717	0.756	0.648	0.667	0.461
C84.47	Peripheral T-cell lymphoma, not classified, spleen	10	Lymphoma and Other Cancers	11,12	0.675	0.663	0.717	0.756	0.648	0.667	0.461
C84.48	Peripheral T-cell lymphoma, not classified, lymph nodes of multiple sites	10	Lymphoma and Other Cancers	11,12	0.675	0.663	0.717	0.756	0.648	0.667	0.461
C84.49	Peripheral T-cell lymphoma, not classified, extranodal and solid organ sites	10	Lymphoma and Other Cancers	11,12	0.675	0.663	0.717	0.756	0.648	0.667	0.461
C84.60	Anaplastic large cell lymphoma, ALK-positive, unspecified site	10	Lymphoma and Other Cancers	11,12	0.675	0.663	0.717	0.756	0.648	0.667	0.461
C84.61	Anaplastic large cell lymphoma, ALK-positive, lymph nodes of head, face, and neck	10	Lymphoma and Other Cancers	11,12	0.675	0.663	0.717	0.756	0.648	0.667	0.461
C84.62	Anaplastic large cell lymphoma, ALK-positive, intrathoracic lymph nodes	10	Lymphoma and Other Cancers	11,12	0.675	0.663	0.717	0.756	0.648	0.667	0.461
C84.63	Anaplastic large cell lymphoma, ALK-positive, intra-abdominal lymph nodes	10	Lymphoma and Other Cancers	11,12	0.675	0.663	0.717	0.756	0.648	0.667	0.461
C84.64	Anaplastic large cell lymphoma, ALK-positive, lymph nodes of axilla and upper limb	10	Lymphoma and Other Cancers	11,12	0.675	0.663	0.717	0.756	0.648	0.667	0.461
C84.65	Anaplastic large cell lymphoma, ALK-positive, lymph nodes of inguinal region and lower limb	10	Lymphoma and Other Cancers	11,12	0.675	0.663	0.717	0.756	0.648	0.667	0.461
C84.66	Anaplastic large cell lymphoma, ALK-positive, intrapelvic lymph nodes	10	Lymphoma and Other Cancers	11,12	0.675	0.663	0.717	0.756	0.648	0.667	0.461
C84.67	Anaplastic large cell lymphoma, ALK-positive, spleen	10	Lymphoma and Other Cancers	11,12	0.675	0.663	0.717	0.756	0.648	0.667	0.461
C84.68	Anaplastic large cell lymphoma, ALK-positive, lymph nodes of multiple sites	10	Lymphoma and Other Cancers	11,12	0.675	0.663	0.717	0.756	0.648	0.667	0.461
C84.69	Anaplastic large cell lymphoma, ALK-positive, extranodal and solid organ sites	10	Lymphoma and Other Cancers	11,12	0.675	0.663	0.717	0.756	0.648	0.667	0.461
C84.70	Anaplastic large cell lymphoma, ALK-negative, unspecified site	10	Lymphoma and Other Cancers	11,12	0.675	0.663	0.717	0.756	0.648	0.667	0.461
C84.71	Anaplastic large cell lymphoma, ALK-negative, lymph nodes of head, face, and neck	10	Lymphoma and Other Cancers	11,12	0.675	0.663	0.717	0.756	0.648	0.667	0.461

ICD-10-CM Code	ICD-10-CM Code Description	V24 CMS-HCC	V24 CMS-HCC Disease Group	V24 CMS-HCC Hierarchies	Community, NonDual, Aged	Community, NonDual, Disabled	Community, FBDual, Aged	Community, FBDual, Disabled	Community, PBDual, Aged	Community, PBDual, Disabled	Institutional
C84.72	Anaplastic large cell lymphoma, ALK-negative, intrathoracic lymph nodes	10	Lymphoma and Other Cancers	11,12	0.675	0.663	0.717	0.756	0.648	0.667	0.461
C84.73	Anaplastic large cell lymphoma, ALK-negative, intra-abdominal lymph nodes	10	Lymphoma and Other Cancers	11,12	0.675	0.663	0.717	0.756	0.648	0.667	0.461
C84.74	Anaplastic large cell lymphoma, ALK-negative, lymph nodes of axilla and upper limb	10	Lymphoma and Other Cancers	11,12	0.675	0.663	0.717	0.756	0.648	0.667	0.461
C84.75	Anaplastic large cell lymphoma, ALK-negative, lymph nodes of inguinal region and lower limb	10	Lymphoma and Other Cancers	11,12	0.675	0.663	0.717	0.756	0.648	0.667	0.461
C84.76	Anaplastic large cell lymphoma, ALK-negative, intrapelvic lymph nodes	10	Lymphoma and Other Cancers	11,12	0.675	0.663	0.717	0.756	0.648	0.667	0.461
C84.77	Anaplastic large cell lymphoma, ALK-negative, spleen	10	Lymphoma and Other Cancers	11,12	0.675	0.663	0.717	0.756	0.648	0.667	0.461
C84.78	Anaplastic large cell lymphoma, ALK-negative, lymph nodes of multiple sites	10	Lymphoma and Other Cancers	11,12	0.675	0.663	0.717	0.756	0.648	0.667	0.461
C84.79	Anaplastic large cell lymphoma, ALK-negative, extranodal and solid organ sites	10	Lymphoma and Other Cancers	11,12	0.675	0.663	0.717	0.756	0.648	0.667	0.461
C84.7A	Anaplastic large cell lymphoma, ALK-negative, breast	10	Lymphoma and Other Cancers	11,12	0.675	0.663	0.717	0.756	0.648	0.667	0.461
C84.9Ø	Mature T/NK-cell lymphomas, unspecified, unspecified site	10	Lymphoma and Other Cancers	11,12	0.675	0.663	0.717	0.756	0.648	0.667	0.461
C84.91	Mature T/NK-cell lymphomas, unspecified, lymph nodes of head, face, and neck	10	Lymphoma and Other Cancers	11,12	0.675	0.663	0.717	0.756	0.648	0.667	0.461
C84.92	Mature T/NK-cell lymphomas, unspecified, intrathoracic lymph nodes	10	Lymphoma and Other Cancers	11,12	0.675	0.663	0.717	0.756	0.648	0.667	0.461
C84.93	Mature T/NK-cell lymphomas, unspecified, intra-abdominal lymph nodes	10	Lymphoma and Other Cancers	11,12	0.675	0.663	0.717	0.756	0.648	0.667	0.461
C84.94	Mature T/NK-cell lymphomas, unspecified, lymph nodes of axilla and upper limb	10	Lymphoma and Other Cancers	11,12	0.675	0.663	0.717	0.756	0.648	0.667	0.461
C84.95	Mature T/NK-cell lymphomas, unspecified, lymph nodes of inguinal region and lower limb	10	Lymphoma and Other Cancers	11,12	0.675	0.663	0.717	0.756	0.648	0.667	0.461
C84.96	Mature T/NK-cell lymphomas, unspecified, intrapelvic lymph nodes	10	Lymphoma and Other Cancers	11,12	0.675	0.663	0.717	0.756	0.648	0.667	0.461
C84.97	Mature T/NK-cell lymphomas, unspecified, spleen	10	Lymphoma and Other Cancers	11,12	0.675	0.663	0.717	0.756	0.648	0.667	0.461
C84.98	Mature T/NK-cell lymphomas, unspecified, lymph nodes of multiple sites	10	Lymphoma and Other Cancers	11,12	0.675	0.663	0.717	0.756	0.648	0.667	0.461
C84.99	Mature T/NK-cell lymphomas, unspecified, extranodal and solid organ sites	10	Lymphoma and Other Cancers	11,12	0.675	0.663	0.717	0.756	0.648	0.667	0.461
C84.AØ	Cutaneous T-cell lymphoma, unspecified, unspecified site	10	Lymphoma and Other Cancers	11,12	0.675	0.663	0.717	0.756	0.648	0.667	0.461
C84.A1	Cutaneous T-cell lymphoma, unspecified lymph nodes of head, face, and neck	10	Lymphoma and Other Cancers	11,12	0.675	0.663	0.717	0.756	0.648	0.667	0.461
C84.A2	Cutaneous T-cell lymphoma, unspecified, intrathoracic lymph nodes	10	Lymphoma and Other Cancers	11,12	0.675	0.663	0.717	0.756	0.648	0.667	0.461

ICD-10-CM Code	ICD-10-CM Code Description	V24 CMS-HCC	V24 CMS-HCC Disease Group	V24 CMS-HCC Hierarchies	Community, NonDual, Aged	Community, NonDual, Disabled	Community, FBDual, Aged	Community, FBDual, Disabled	Community, PBDual, Aged	Community, PBDual, Disabled	Institutional
C84.A3	Cutaneous T-cell lymphoma, unspecified, intra-abdominal lymph nodes	10	Lymphoma and Other Cancers	11,12	0.675	0.663	0.717	0.756	0.648	0.667	0.461
C84.A4	Cutaneous T-cell lymphoma, unspecified, lymph nodes of axilla and upper limb	10	Lymphoma and Other Cancers	11,12	0.675	0.663	0.717	0.756	0.648	0.667	0.461
C84.A5	Cutaneous T-cell lymphoma, unspecified, lymph nodes of inguinal region and lower limb	10	Lymphoma and Other Cancers	11,12	0.675	0.663	0.717	0.756	0.648	0.667	0.461
C84.A6	Cutaneous T-cell lymphoma, unspecified, intrapelvic lymph nodes	10	Lymphoma and Other Cancers	11,12	0.675	0.663	0.717	0.756	0.648	0.667	0.461
C84.A7	Cutaneous T-cell lymphoma, unspecified, spleen	10	Lymphoma and Other Cancers	11,12	0.675	0.663	0.717	0.756	0.648	0.667	0.461
C84.A8	Cutaneous T-cell lymphoma, unspecified, lymph nodes of multiple sites	10	Lymphoma and Other Cancers	11,12	0.675	0.663	0.717	0.756	0.648	0.667	0.461
C84.A9	Cutaneous T-cell lymphoma, unspecified, extranodal and solid organ sites	10	Lymphoma and Other Cancers	11,12	0.675	0.663	0.717	0.756	0.648	0.667	0.461
C84.Z0	Other mature T/NK-cell lymphomas, unspecified site	10	Lymphoma and Other Cancers	11,12	0.675	0.663	0.717	0.756	0.648	0.667	0.461
C84.Z1	Other mature T/NK-cell lymphomas, lymph nodes of head, face, and neck	10	Lymphoma and Other Cancers	11,12	0.675	0.663	0.717	0.756	0.648	0.667	0.461
C84.Z2	Other mature T/NK-cell lymphomas, intrathoracic lymph nodes	10	Lymphoma and Other Cancers	11,12	0.675	0.663	0.717	0.756	0.648	0.667	0.461
C84.Z3	Other mature T/NK-cell lymphomas, intra-abdominal lymph nodes	10	Lymphoma and Other Cancers	11,12	0.675	0.663	0.717	0.756	0.648	0.667	0.461
C84.Z4	Other mature T/NK-cell lymphomas, lymph nodes of axilla and upper limb	10	Lymphoma and Other Cancers	11,12	0.675	0.663	0.717	0.756	0.648	0.667	0.461
C84.Z5	Other mature T/NK-cell lymphomas, lymph nodes of inguinal region and lower limb	10	Lymphoma and Other Cancers	11,12	0.675	0.663	0.717	0.756	0.648	0.667	0.461
C84.Z6	Other mature T/NK-cell lymphomas, intrapelvic lymph nodes	10	Lymphoma and Other Cancers	11,12	0.675	0.663	0.717	0.756	0.648	0.667	0.461
C84.Z7	Other mature T/NK-cell lymphomas, spleen	10	Lymphoma and Other Cancers	11,12	0.675	0.663	0.717	0.756	0.648	0.667	0.461
C84.Z8	Other mature T/NK-cell lymphomas, lymph nodes of multiple sites	10	Lymphoma and Other Cancers	11,12	0.675	0.663	0.717	0.756	0.648	0.667	0.461
C84.Z9	Other mature T/NK-cell lymphomas, extranodal and solid organ sites	10	Lymphoma and Other Cancers	11,12	0.675	0.663	0.717	0.756	0.648	0.667	0.461
C85.10	Unspecified B-cell lymphoma, unspecified site	10	Lymphoma and Other Cancers	11,12	0.675	0.663	0.717	0.756	0.648	0.667	0.461
C85.11	Unspecified B-cell lymphoma, lymph nodes of head, face, and neck	10	Lymphoma and Other Cancers	11,12	0.675	0.663	0.717	0.756	0.648	0.667	0.461
C85.12	Unspecified B-cell lymphoma, intrathoracic lymph nodes	10	Lymphoma and Other Cancers	11,12	0.675	0.663	0.717	0.756	0.648	0.667	0.461
C85.13	Unspecified B-cell lymphoma, intra-abdominal lymph nodes	10	Lymphoma and Other Cancers	11,12	0.675	0.663	0.717	0.756	0.648	0.667	0.461
C85.14	Unspecified B-cell lymphoma, lymph nodes of axilla and upper limb	10	Lymphoma and Other Cancers	11,12	0.675	0.663	0.717	0.756	0.648	0.667	0.461
C85.15	Unspecified B-cell lymphoma, lymph nodes of inguinal region and lower limb	10	Lymphoma and Other Cancers	11,12	0.675	0.663	0.717	0.756	0.648	0.667	0.461
C85.16	Unspecified B-cell lymphoma, intrapelvic lymph nodes	10	Lymphoma and Other Cancers	11,12	0.675	0.663	0.717	0.756	0.648	0.667	0.461
C85.17	Unspecified B-cell lymphoma, spleen	10	Lymphoma and Other Cancers	11,12	0.675	0.663	0.717	0.756	0.648	0.667	0.461
C85.18	Unspecified B-cell lymphoma, lymph nodes of multiple sites	10	Lymphoma and Other Cancers	11,12	0.675	0.663	0.717	0.756	0.648	0.667	0.461

ICD-10-CM Code	ICD-10-CM Code Description	V24 CMS-HCC	V24 CMS-HCC Disease Group	V24 CMS-HCC Hierarchies	Community, NonDual, Aged	Community, NonDual, Disabled	Community, FBDual, Aged	Community, FBDual, Disabled	Community, PBDual, Aged	Community, PBDual, Disabled	Institutional
C85.19	Unspecified B-cell lymphoma, extranodal and solid organ sites	10	Lymphoma and Other Cancers	11,12	0.675	0.663	0.717	0.756	0.648	0.667	0.461
C85.20	Mediastinal (thymic) large B-cell lymphoma, unspecified site	10	Lymphoma and Other Cancers	11,12	0.675	0.663	0.717	0.756	0.648	0.667	0.461
C85.21	Mediastinal (thymic) large B-cell lymphoma, lymph nodes of head, face, and neck	10	Lymphoma and Other Cancers	11,12	0.675	0.663	0.717	0.756	0.648	0.667	0.461
C85.22	Mediastinal (thymic) large B-cell lymphoma, intrathoracic lymph nodes	10	Lymphoma and Other Cancers	11,12	0.675	0.663	0.717	0.756	0.648	0.667	0.461
C85.23	Mediastinal (thymic) large B-cell lymphoma, intra-abdominal lymph nodes	10	Lymphoma and Other Cancers	11,12	0.675	0.663	0.717	0.756	0.648	0.667	0.461
C85.24	Mediastinal (thymic) large B-cell lymphoma, lymph nodes of axilla and upper limb	10	Lymphoma and Other Cancers	11,12	0.675	0.663	0.717	0.756	0.648	0.667	0.461
C85.25	Mediastinal (thymic) large B-cell lymphoma, lymph nodes of inguinal region and lower limb	10	Lymphoma and Other Cancers	11,12	0.675	0.663	0.717	0.756	0.648	0.667	0.461
C85.26	Mediastinal (thymic) large B-cell lymphoma, intrapelvic lymph nodes	10	Lymphoma and Other Cancers	11,12	0.675	0.663	0.717	0.756	0.648	0.667	0.461
C85.27	Mediastinal (thymic) large B-cell lymphoma, spleen	10	Lymphoma and Other Cancers	11,12	0.675	0.663	0.717	0.756	0.648	0.667	0.461
C85.28	Mediastinal (thymic) large B-cell lymphoma, lymph nodes of multiple sites	10	Lymphoma and Other Cancers	11,12	0.675	0.663	0.717	0.756	0.648	0.667	0.461
C85.29	Mediastinal (thymic) large B-cell lymphoma, extranodal and solid organ sites	10	Lymphoma and Other Cancers	11,12	0.675	0.663	0.717	0.756	0.648	0.667	0.461
C85.80	Other specified types of non-Hodgkin lymphoma, unspecified site	10	Lymphoma and Other Cancers	11,12	0.675	0.663	0.717	0.756	0.648	0.667	0.461
C85.81	Other specified types of non-Hodgkin lymphoma, lymph nodes of head, face, and neck	10	Lymphoma and Other Cancers	11,12	0.675	0.663	0.717	0.756	0.648	0.667	0.461
C85.82	Other specified types of non-Hodgkin lymphoma, intrathoracic lymph nodes	10	Lymphoma and Other Cancers	11,12	0.675	0.663	0.717	0.756	0.648	0.667	0.461
C85.83	Other specified types of non-Hodgkin lymphoma, intra-abdominal lymph nodes	10	Lymphoma and Other Cancers	11,12	0.675	0.663	0.717	0.756	0.648	0.667	0.461
C85.84	Other specified types of non-Hodgkin lymphoma, lymph nodes of axilla and upper limb	10	Lymphoma and Other Cancers	11,12	0.675	0.663	0.717	0.756	0.648	0.667	0.461
C85.85	Other specified types of non-Hodgkin lymphoma, lymph nodes of inguinal region and lower limb	10	Lymphoma and Other Cancers	11,12	0.675	0.663	0.717	0.756	0.648	0.667	0.461
C85.86	Other specified types of non-Hodgkin lymphoma, intrapelvic lymph nodes	10	Lymphoma and Other Cancers	11,12	0.675	0.663	0.717	0.756	0.648	0.667	0.461
C85.87	Other specified types of non-Hodgkin lymphoma, spleen	10	Lymphoma and Other Cancers	11,12	0.675	0.663	0.717	0.756	0.648	0.667	0.461
C85.88	Other specified types of non-Hodgkin lymphoma, lymph nodes of multiple sites	10	Lymphoma and Other Cancers	11,12	0.675	0.663	0.717	0.756	0.648	0.667	0.461
C85.89	Other specified types of non-Hodgkin lymphoma, extranodal and solid organ sites	10	Lymphoma and Other Cancers	11,12	0.675	0.663	0.717	0.756	0.648	0.667	0.461
C85.90	Non-Hodgkin lymphoma, unspecified, unspecified site	10	Lymphoma and Other Cancers	11,12	0.675	0.663	0.717	0.756	0.648	0.667	0.461
C85.91	Non-Hodgkin lymphoma, unspecified, lymph nodes of head, face, and neck	10	Lymphoma and Other Cancers	11,12	0.675	0.663	0.717	0.756	0.648	0.667	0.461

ICD-10-CM Code	ICD-10-CM Code Description	V24 CMS-HCC	V24 CMS-HCC Disease Group	V24 CMS-HCC Hierarchies	Community, NonDual, Aged	Community, NonDual, Disabled	Community, FBDual, Aged	Community, FBDual, Disabled	Community, PBDual, Aged	Community, PBDual, Disabled	Institutional
C85.92	Non-Hodgkin lymphoma, unspecified, intrathoracic lymph nodes	10	Lymphoma and Other Cancers	11,12	0.675	0.663	0.717	0.756	0.648	0.667	0.461
C85.93	Non-Hodgkin lymphoma, unspecified, intra-abdominal lymph nodes	10	Lymphoma and Other Cancers	11,12	0.675	0.663	0.717	0.756	0.648	0.667	0.461
C85.94	Non-Hodgkin lymphoma, unspecified, lymph nodes of axilla and upper limb	10	Lymphoma and Other Cancers	11,12	0.675	0.663	0.717	0.756	0.648	0.667	0.461
C85.95	Non-Hodgkin lymphoma, unspecified, lymph nodes of inguinal region and lower limb	10	Lymphoma and Other Cancers	11,12	0.675	0.663	0.717	0.756	0.648	0.667	0.461
C85.96	Non-Hodgkin lymphoma, unspecified, intrapelvic lymph nodes	10	Lymphoma and Other Cancers	11,12	0.675	0.663	0.717	0.756	0.648	0.667	0.461
C85.97	Non-Hodgkin lymphoma, unspecified, spleen	10	Lymphoma and Other Cancers	11,12	0.675	0.663	0.717	0.756	0.648	0.667	0.461
C85.98	Non-Hodgkin lymphoma, unspecified, lymph nodes of multiple sites	10	Lymphoma and Other Cancers	11,12	0.675	0.663	0.717	0.756	0.648	0.667	0.461
C85.99	Non-Hodgkin lymphoma, unspecified, extranodal and solid organ sites	10	Lymphoma and Other Cancers	11,12	0.675	0.663	0.717	0.756	0.648	0.667	0.461
C86.0	Extranodal NK/T-cell lymphoma, nasal type	10	Lymphoma and Other Cancers	11,12	0.675	0.663	0.717	0.756	0.648	0.667	0.461
C86.1	Hepatosplenic T-cell lymphoma	10	Lymphoma and Other Cancers	11,12	0.675	0.663	0.717	0.756	0.648	0.667	0.461
C86.2	Enteropathy-type (intestinal) T-cell lymphoma	10	Lymphoma and Other Cancers	11,12	0.675	0.663	0.717	0.756	0.648	0.667	0.461
C86.3	Subcutaneous panniculitis-like T-cell lymphoma	10	Lymphoma and Other Cancers	11,12	0.675	0.663	0.717	0.756	0.648	0.667	0.461
C86.4	Blastic NK-cell lymphoma	10	Lymphoma and Other Cancers	11,12	0.675	0.663	0.717	0.756	0.648	0.667	0.461
C86.5	Angioimmunoblastic T-cell lymphoma	10	Lymphoma and Other Cancers	11,12	0.675	0.663	0.717	0.756	0.648	0.667	0.461
C86.6	Primary cutaneous CD30-positive T-cell proliferations	10	Lymphoma and Other Cancers	11,12	0.675	0.663	0.717	0.756	0.648	0.667	0.461
C88.0	Waldenstrom macroglobulinemia	23	Other Significant Endocrine and Metabolic Disorders		0.194	0.378	0.211	0.299	0.174	0.319	0.379
C88.2	Heavy chain disease	10	Lymphoma and Other Cancers	11,12	0.675	0.663	0.717	0.756	0.648	0.667	0.461
C88.3	Immunoproliferative small intestinal disease	10	Lymphoma and Other Cancers	11,12	0.675	0.663	0.717	0.756	0.648	0.667	0.461
C88.4	Extranodal marginal zone B-cell lymphoma of mucosa-associated lymphoid tissue [MALT-lymphoma]	10	Lymphoma and Other Cancers	11,12	0.675	0.663	0.717	0.756	0.648	0.667	0.461
C88.8	Other malignant immunoproliferative diseases	10	Lymphoma and Other Cancers	11,12	0.675	0.663	0.717	0.756	0.648	0.667	0.461
C88.9	Malignant immunoproliferative disease, unspecified	10	Lymphoma and Other Cancers	11,12	0.675	0.663	0.717	0.756	0.648	0.667	0.461
C90.00	Multiple myeloma not having achieved remission	9	Lung and Other Severe Cancers	10,11,12	1.024	0.910	1.010	1.001	1.001	0.880	0.623
C90.01	Multiple myeloma in remission	9	Lung and Other Severe Cancers	10,11,12	1.024	0.910	1.010	1.001	1.001	0.880	0.623
C90.02	Multiple myeloma in relapse	9	Lung and Other Severe Cancers	10,11,12	1.024	0.910	1.010	1.001	1.001	0.880	0.623
C90.10	Plasma cell leukemia not having achieved remission	9	Lung and Other Severe Cancers	10,11,12	1.024	0.910	1.010	1.001	1.001	0.880	0.623
C90.11	Plasma cell leukemia in remission	9	Lung and Other Severe Cancers	10,11,12	1.024	0.910	1.010	1.001	1.001	0.880	0.623
C90.12	Plasma cell leukemia in relapse	9	Lung and Other Severe Cancers	10,11,12	1.024	0.910	1.010	1.001	1.001	0.880	0.623
C90.20	Extramedullary plasmacytoma not having achieved remission	9	Lung and Other Severe Cancers	10,11,12	1.024	0.910	1.010	1.001	1.001	0.880	0.623
C90.21	Extramedullary plasmacytoma in remission	9	Lung and Other Severe Cancers	10,11,12	1.024	0.910	1.010	1.001	1.001	0.880	0.623

ICD-10-CM Code	ICD-10-CM Code Description	V24 CMS-HCC	V24 CMS-HCC Disease Group	V24 CMS-HCC Hierarchies	Community, NonDual, Aged	Community, NonDual, Disabled	Community, FBDual, Aged	Community, FBDual, Disabled	Community, PBDual, Aged	Community, PBDual, Disabled	Institutional
C90.22	Extramedullary plasmacytoma in relapse	9	Lung and Other Severe Cancers	10,11,12	1.024	0.910	1.010	1.001	1.001	0.880	0.623
C90.30	Solitary plasmacytoma not having achieved remission	10	Lymphoma and Other Cancers	11,12	0.675	0.663	0.717	0.756	0.648	0.667	0.461
C90.31	Solitary plasmacytoma in remission	10	Lymphoma and Other Cancers	11,12	0.675	0.663	0.717	0.756	0.648	0.667	0.461
C90.32	Solitary plasmacytoma in relapse	10	Lymphoma and Other Cancers	11,12	0.675	0.663	0.717	0.756	0.648	0.667	0.461
C91.00	Acute lymphoblastic leukemia not having achieved remission	8	Metastatic Cancer and Acute Leukemia	9,10,11,12	2.659	2.714	2.566	2.801	2.455	2.659	1.303
C91.01	Acute lymphoblastic leukemia, in remission	8	Metastatic Cancer and Acute Leukemia	9,10,11,12	2.659	2.714	2.566	2.801	2.455	2.659	1.303
C91.02	Acute lymphoblastic leukemia, in relapse	8	Metastatic Cancer and Acute Leukemia	9,10,11,12	2.659	2.714	2.566	2.801	2.455	2.659	1.303
C91.10	Chronic lymphocytic leukemia of B-cell type not having achieved remission	10	Lymphoma and Other Cancers	11,12	0.675	0.663	0.717	0.756	0.648	0.667	0.461
C91.11	Chronic lymphocytic leukemia of B-cell type in remission	10	Lymphoma and Other Cancers	11,12	0.675	0.663	0.717	0.756	0.648	0.667	0.461
C91.12	Chronic lymphocytic leukemia of B-cell type in relapse	10	Lymphoma and Other Cancers	11,12	0.675	0.663	0.717	0.756	0.648	0.667	0.461
C91.30	Prolymphocytic leukemia of B-cell type not having achieved remission	10	Lymphoma and Other Cancers	11,12	0.675	0.663	0.717	0.756	0.648	0.667	0.461
C91.31	Prolymphocytic leukemia of B-cell type, in remission	10	Lymphoma and Other Cancers	11,12	0.675	0.663	0.717	0.756	0.648	0.667	0.461
C91.32	Prolymphocytic leukemia of B-cell type, in relapse	10	Lymphoma and Other Cancers	11,12	0.675	0.663	0.717	0.756	0.648	0.667	0.461
C91.40	Hairy cell leukemia not having achieved remission	10	Lymphoma and Other Cancers	11,12	0.675	0.663	0.717	0.756	0.648	0.667	0.461
C91.41	Hairy cell leukemia, in remission	10	Lymphoma and Other Cancers	11,12	0.675	0.663	0.717	0.756	0.648	0.667	0.461
C91.42	Hairy cell leukemia, in relapse	10	Lymphoma and Other Cancers	11,12	0.675	0.663	0.717	0.756	0.648	0.667	0.461
C91.50	Adult T-cell lymphoma/leukemia (HTLV-1-associated) not having achieved remission	10	Lymphoma and Other Cancers	11,12	0.675	0.663	0.717	0.756	0.648	0.667	0.461
C91.51	Adult T-cell lymphoma/leukemia (HTLV-1-associated), in remission	10	Lymphoma and Other Cancers	11,12	0.675	0.663	0.717	0.756	0.648	0.667	0.461
C91.52	Adult T-cell lymphoma/leukemia (HTLV-1-associated), in relapse	10	Lymphoma and Other Cancers	11,12	0.675	0.663	0.717	0.756	0.648	0.667	0.461
C91.60	Prolymphocytic leukemia of T-cell type not having achieved remission	10	Lymphoma and Other Cancers	11,12	0.675	0.663	0.717	0.756	0.648	0.667	0.461
C91.61	Prolymphocytic leukemia of T-cell type, in remission	10	Lymphoma and Other Cancers	11,12	0.675	0.663	0.717	0.756	0.648	0.667	0.461
C91.62	Prolymphocytic leukemia of T-cell type, in relapse	10	Lymphoma and Other Cancers	11,12	0.675	0.663	0.717	0.756	0.648	0.667	0.461
C91.90	Lymphoid leukemia, unspecified not having achieved remission	10	Lymphoma and Other Cancers	11,12	0.675	0.663	0.717	0.756	0.648	0.667	0.461
C91.91	Lymphoid leukemia, unspecified, in remission	10	Lymphoma and Other Cancers	11,12	0.675	0.663	0.717	0.756	0.648	0.667	0.461
C91.92	Lymphoid leukemia, unspecified, in relapse	10	Lymphoma and Other Cancers	11,12	0.675	0.663	0.717	0.756	0.648	0.667	0.461
C91.A0	Mature B-cell leukemia Burkitt-type not having achieved remission	10	Lymphoma and Other Cancers	11,12	0.675	0.663	0.717	0.756	0.648	0.667	0.461
C91.A1	Mature B-cell leukemia Burkitt-type, in remission	10	Lymphoma and Other Cancers	11,12	0.675	0.663	0.717	0.756	0.648	0.667	0.461
C91.A2	Mature B-cell leukemia Burkitt-type, in relapse	10	Lymphoma and Other Cancers	11,12	0.675	0.663	0.717	0.756	0.648	0.667	0.461
C91.Z0	Other lymphoid leukemia not having achieved remission	10	Lymphoma and Other Cancers	11,12	0.675	0.663	0.717	0.756	0.648	0.667	0.461
C91.Z1	Other lymphoid leukemia, in remission	10	Lymphoma and Other Cancers	11,12	0.675	0.663	0.717	0.756	0.648	0.667	0.461

ICD-10-CM Code	ICD-10-CM Code Description	V24 CMS-HCC	V24 CMS-HCC Disease Group	V24 CMS-HCC Hierarchies	Community, NonDual, Aged	Community, NonDual, Disabled	Community, FBDual, Aged	Community, FBDual, Disabled	Community, PBDual, Aged	Community, PBDual, Disabled	Institutional
C91.Z2	Other lymphoid leukemia, in relapse	10	Lymphoma and Other Cancers	11,12	0.675	0.663	0.717	0.756	0.648	0.667	0.461
C92.00	Acute myeloblastic leukemia, not having achieved remission	8	Metastatic Cancer and Acute Leukemia	9,10,11,12	2.659	2.714	2.566	2.801	2.455	2.659	1.303
C92.01	Acute myeloblastic leukemia, in remission	8	Metastatic Cancer and Acute Leukemia	9,10,11,12	2.659	2.714	2.566	2.801	2.455	2.659	1.303
C92.02	Acute myeloblastic leukemia, in relapse	8	Metastatic Cancer and Acute Leukemia	9,10,11,12	2.659	2.714	2.566	2.801	2.455	2.659	1.303
C92.10	Chronic myeloid leukemia, BCR/ABL-positive, not having achieved remission	9	Lung and Other Severe Cancers	10,11,12	1.024	0.910	1.010	1.001	1.001	0.880	0.623
C92.11	Chronic myeloid leukemia, BCR/ABL-positive, in remission	9	Lung and Other Severe Cancers	10,11,12	1.024	0.910	1.010	1.001	1.001	0.880	0.623
C92.12	Chronic myeloid leukemia, BCR/ABL-positive, in relapse	9	Lung and Other Severe Cancers	10,11,12	1.024	0.910	1.010	1.001	1.001	0.880	0.623
C92.20	Atypical chronic myeloid leukemia, BCR/ABL-negative, not having achieved remission	9	Lung and Other Severe Cancers	10,11,12	1.024	0.910	1.010	1.001	1.001	0.880	0.623
C92.21	Atypical chronic myeloid leukemia, BCR/ABL-negative, in remission	9	Lung and Other Severe Cancers	10,11,12	1.024	0.910	1.010	1.001	1.001	0.880	0.623
C92.22	Atypical chronic myeloid leukemia, BCR/ABL-negative, in relapse	9	Lung and Other Severe Cancers	10,11,12	1.024	0.910	1.010	1.001	1.001	0.880	0.623
C92.30	Myeloid sarcoma, not having achieved remission	9	Lung and Other Severe Cancers	10,11,12	1.024	0.910	1.010	1.001	1.001	0.880	0.623
C92.31	Myeloid sarcoma, in remission	9	Lung and Other Severe Cancers	10,11,12	1.024	0.910	1.010	1.001	1.001	0.880	0.623
C92.32	Myeloid sarcoma, in relapse	9	Lung and Other Severe Cancers	10,11,12	1.024	0.910	1.010	1.001	1.001	0.880	0.623
C92.40	Acute promyelocytic leukemia, not having achieved remission	8	Metastatic Cancer and Acute Leukemia	9,10,11,12	2.659	2.714	2.566	2.801	2.455	2.659	1.303
C92.41	Acute promyelocytic leukemia, in remission	8	Metastatic Cancer and Acute Leukemia	9,10,11,12	2.659	2.714	2.566	2.801	2.455	2.659	1.303
C92.42	Acute promyelocytic leukemia, in relapse	8	Metastatic Cancer and Acute Leukemia	9,10,11,12	2.659	2.714	2.566	2.801	2.455	2.659	1.303
C92.50	Acute myelomonocytic leukemia, not having achieved remission	8	Metastatic Cancer and Acute Leukemia	9,10,11,12	2.659	2.714	2.566	2.801	2.455	2.659	1.303
C92.51	Acute myelomonocytic leukemia, in remission	8	Metastatic Cancer and Acute Leukemia	9,10,11,12	2.659	2.714	2.566	2.801	2.455	2.659	1.303
C92.52	Acute myelomonocytic leukemia, in relapse	8	Metastatic Cancer and Acute Leukemia	9,10,11,12	2.659	2.714	2.566	2.801	2.455	2.659	1.303
C92.60	Acute myeloid leukemia with 11q23-abnormality not having achieved remission	8	Metastatic Cancer and Acute Leukemia	9,10,11,12	2.659	2.714	2.566	2.801	2.455	2.659	1.303
C92.61	Acute myeloid leukemia with 11q23-abnormality in remission	8	Metastatic Cancer and Acute Leukemia	9,10,11,12	2.659	2.714	2.566	2.801	2.455	2.659	1.303
C92.62	Acute myeloid leukemia with 11q23-abnormality in relapse	8	Metastatic Cancer and Acute Leukemia	9,10,11,12	2.659	2.714	2.566	2.801	2.455	2.659	1.303
C92.90	Myeloid leukemia, unspecified, not having achieved remission	9	Lung and Other Severe Cancers	10,11,12	1.024	0.910	1.010	1.001	1.001	0.880	0.623
C92.91	Myeloid leukemia, unspecified in remission	9	Lung and Other Severe Cancers	10,11,12	1.024	0.910	1.010	1.001	1.001	0.880	0.623
C92.92	Myeloid leukemia, unspecified in relapse	9	Lung and Other Severe Cancers	10,11,12	1.024	0.910	1.010	1.001	1.001	0.880	0.623
C92.A0	Acute myeloid leukemia with multilineage dysplasia, not having achieved remission	8	Metastatic Cancer and Acute Leukemia	9,10,11,12	2.659	2.714	2.566	2.801	2.455	2.659	1.303
C92.A1	Acute myeloid leukemia with multilineage dysplasia, in remission	8	Metastatic Cancer and Acute Leukemia	9,10,11,12	2.659	2.714	2.566	2.801	2.455	2.659	1.303
C92.A2	Acute myeloid leukemia with multilineage dysplasia, in relapse	8	Metastatic Cancer and Acute Leukemia	9,10,11,12	2.659	2.714	2.566	2.801	2.455	2.659	1.303
C92.Z0	Other myeloid leukemia not having achieved remission	9	Lung and Other Severe Cancers	10,11,12	1.024	0.910	1.010	1.001	1.001	0.880	0.623

ICD-10-CM Code	ICD-10-CM Code Description	V24 CMS-HCC	V24 CMS-HCC Disease Group	V24 CMS-HCC Hierarchies	Community, NonDual, Aged	Community, NonDual, Disabled	Community, FBDual, Aged	Community, FBDual, Disabled	Community, PBDual, Aged	Community, PBDual, Disabled	Institutional
C92.Z1	Other myeloid leukemia, in remission	9	Lung and Other Severe Cancers	10,11,12	1.024	0.910	1.010	1.001	1.001	0.880	0.623
C92.Z2	Other myeloid leukemia, in relapse	9	Lung and Other Severe Cancers	10,11,12	1.024	0.910	1.010	1.001	1.001	0.880	0.623
C93.00	Acute monoblastic/monocytic leukemia, not having achieved remission	8	Metastatic Cancer and Acute Leukemia	9,10,11,12	2.659	2.714	2.566	2.801	2.455	2.659	1.303
C93.01	Acute monoblastic/monocytic leukemia, in remission	8	Metastatic Cancer and Acute Leukemia	9,10,11,12	2.659	2.714	2.566	2.801	2.455	2.659	1.303
C93.02	Acute monoblastic/monocytic leukemia, in relapse	8	Metastatic Cancer and Acute Leukemia	9,10,11,12	2.659	2.714	2.566	2.801	2.455	2.659	1.303
C93.10	Chronic myelomonocytic leukemia not having achieved remission	9	Lung and Other Severe Cancers	10,11,12	1.024	0.910	1.010	1.001	1.001	0.880	0.623
C93.11	Chronic myelomonocytic leukemia, in remission	9	Lung and Other Severe Cancers	10,11,12	1.024	0.910	1.010	1.001	1.001	0.880	0.623
C93.12	Chronic myelomonocytic leukemia, in relapse	9	Lung and Other Severe Cancers	10,11,12	1.024	0.910	1.010	1.001	1.001	0.880	0.623
C93.30	Juvenile myelomonocytic leukemia, not having achieved remission	9	Lung and Other Severe Cancers	10,11,12	1.024	0.910	1.010	1.001	1.001	0.880	0.623
C93.31	Juvenile myelomonocytic leukemia, in remission	9	Lung and Other Severe Cancers	10,11,12	1.024	0.910	1.010	1.001	1.001	0.880	0.623
C93.32	Juvenile myelomonocytic leukemia, in relapse	9	Lung and Other Severe Cancers	10,11,12	1.024	0.910	1.010	1.001	1.001	0.880	0.623
C93.90	Monocytic leukemia, unspecified, not having achieved remission	9	Lung and Other Severe Cancers	10,11,12	1.024	0.910	1.010	1.001	1.001	0.880	0.623
C93.91	Monocytic leukemia, unspecified in remission	9	Lung and Other Severe Cancers	10,11,12	1.024	0.910	1.010	1.001	1.001	0.880	0.623
C93.92	Monocytic leukemia, unspecified in relapse	9	Lung and Other Severe Cancers	10,11,12	1.024	0.910	1.010	1.001	1.001	0.880	0.623
C93.Z0	Other monocytic leukemia, not having achieved remission	9	Lung and Other Severe Cancers	10,11,12	1.024	0.910	1.010	1.001	1.001	0.880	0.623
C93.Z1	Other monocytic leukemia, in remission	9	Lung and Other Severe Cancers	10,11,12	1.024	0.910	1.010	1.001	1.001	0.880	0.623
C93.Z2	Other monocytic leukemia, in relapse	9	Lung and Other Severe Cancers	10,11,12	1.024	0.910	1.010	1.001	1.001	0.880	0.623
C94.00	Acute erythroid leukemia, not having achieved remission	8	Metastatic Cancer and Acute Leukemia	9,10,11,12	2.659	2.714	2.566	2.801	2.455	2.659	1.303
C94.01	Acute erythroid leukemia, in remission	8	Metastatic Cancer and Acute Leukemia	9,10,11,12	2.659	2.714	2.566	2.801	2.455	2.659	1.303
C94.02	Acute erythroid leukemia, in relapse	8	Metastatic Cancer and Acute Leukemia	9,10,11,12	2.659	2.714	2.566	2.801	2.455	2.659	1.303
C94.20	Acute megakaryoblastic leukemia not having achieved remission	8	Metastatic Cancer and Acute Leukemia	9,10,11,12	2.659	2.714	2.566	2.801	2.455	2.659	1.303
C94.21	Acute megakaryoblastic leukemia, in remission	8	Metastatic Cancer and Acute Leukemia	9,10,11,12	2.659	2.714	2.566	2.801	2.455	2.659	1.303
C94.22	Acute megakaryoblastic leukemia, in relapse	8	Metastatic Cancer and Acute Leukemia	9,10,11,12	2.659	2.714	2.566	2.801	2.455	2.659	1.303
C94.30	Mast cell leukemia not having achieved remission	9	Lung and Other Severe Cancers	10,11,12	1.024	0.910	1.010	1.001	1.001	0.880	0.623
C94.31	Mast cell leukemia, in remission	9	Lung and Other Severe Cancers	10,11,12	1.024	0.910	1.010	1.001	1.001	0.880	0.623
C94.32	Mast cell leukemia, in relapse	9	Lung and Other Severe Cancers	10,11,12	1.024	0.910	1.010	1.001	1.001	0.880	0.623
C94.40	Acute panmyelosis with myelofibrosis not having achieved remission	8	Metastatic Cancer and Acute Leukemia	9,10,11,12	2.659	2.714	2.566	2.801	2.455	2.659	1.303
C94.41	Acute panmyelosis with myelofibrosis, in remission	8	Metastatic Cancer and Acute Leukemia	9,10,11,12	2.659	2.714	2.566	2.801	2.455	2.659	1.303
C94.42	Acute panmyelosis with myelofibrosis, in relapse	8	Metastatic Cancer and Acute Leukemia	9,10,11,12	2.659	2.714	2.566	2.801	2.455	2.659	1.303
C94.6	Myelodysplastic disease, not classified	48	Coagulation Defects and Other Specified Hematological Disorders		0.192	0.312	0.221	0.298	0.186	0.330	0.190

ICD-10-CM Code	ICD-10-CM Code Description	V24 CMS-HCC	V24 CMS-HCC Disease Group	V24 CMS-HCC Hierarchies	Community, NonDual, Aged	Community, NonDual, Disabled	Community, FBDual, Aged	Community, FBDual, Disabled	Community, PBDual, Aged	Community, PBDual, Disabled	Institutional
D89.3	Immune reconstitution syndrome	47	Disorders of Immunity		0.665	0.860	0.452	0.691	0.674	0.594	0.576
D89.40	Mast cell activation, unspecified	47	Disorders of Immunity		0.665	0.860	0.452	0.691	0.674	0.594	0.576
D89.41	Monoclonal mast cell activation syndrome	47	Disorders of Immunity		0.665	0.860	0.452	0.691	0.674	0.594	0.576
D89.42	Idiopathic mast cell activation syndrome	47	Disorders of Immunity		0.665	0.860	0.452	0.691	0.674	0.594	0.576
D89.43	Secondary mast cell activation	47	Disorders of Immunity		0.665	0.860	0.452	0.691	0.674	0.594	0.576
D89.44	Hereditary alpha tryptasemia	47	Disorders of Immunity		0.665	0.860	0.452	0.691	0.674	0.594	0.576
D89.49	Other mast cell activation disorder	47	Disorders of Immunity		0.665	0.860	0.452	0.691	0.674	0.594	0.576
D89.810	Acute graft-versus-host disease	47	Disorders of Immunity		0.665	0.860	0.452	0.691	0.674	0.594	0.576
D89.811	Chronic graft-versus-host disease	47	Disorders of Immunity		0.665	0.860	0.452	0.691	0.674	0.594	0.576
D89.812	Acute on chronic graft-versus-host disease	47	Disorders of Immunity		0.665	0.860	0.452	0.691	0.674	0.594	0.576
D89.813	Graft-versus-host disease, unspecified	47	Disorders of Immunity		0.665	0.860	0.452	0.691	0.674	0.594	0.576
D89.82	Autoimmune lymphoproliferative syndrome [ALPS]	47	Disorders of Immunity		0.665	0.860	0.452	0.691	0.674	0.594	0.576
D89.89	Other specified disorders involving the immune mechanism, not elsewhere classified	47	Disorders of Immunity		0.665	0.860	0.452	0.691	0.674	0.594	0.576
D89.9	Disorder involving the immune mechanism, unspecified	47	Disorders of Immunity		0.665	0.860	0.452	0.691	0.674	0.594	0.576
E03.5	Myxedema coma	23	Other Significant Endocrine and Metabolic Disorders		0.194	0.378	0.211	0.299	0.174	0.319	0.379
E08.00	Diabetes mellitus due to underlying condition with hyperosmolarity without nonketotic hyperglycemic-hyperosmolar coma (NKHHC)	17	Diabetes with Acute Complications	18,19	0.302	0.351	0.340	0.423	0.326	0.373	0.440
E08.01	Diabetes mellitus due to underlying condition with hyperosmolarity with coma	17	Diabetes with Acute Complications	18,19	0.302	0.351	0.340	0.423	0.326	0.373	0.440
E08.10	Diabetes mellitus due to underlying condition with ketoacidosis without coma	17	Diabetes with Acute Complications	18,19	0.302	0.351	0.340	0.423	0.326	0.373	0.440
E08.11	Diabetes mellitus due to underlying condition with ketoacidosis with coma	17	Diabetes with Acute Complications	18,19	0.302	0.351	0.340	0.423	0.326	0.373	0.440
E08.21	Diabetes mellitus due to underlying condition with diabetic nephropathy	18	Diabetes with Chronic Complications	19	0.302	0.351	0.340	0.423	0.326	0.373	0.440
E08.22	Diabetes mellitus due to underlying condition with diabetic chronic kidney disease	18	Diabetes with Chronic Complications	19	0.302	0.351	0.340	0.423	0.326	0.373	0.440
E08.29	Diabetes mellitus due to underlying condition with other diabetic kidney complication	18	Diabetes with Chronic Complications	19	0.302	0.351	0.340	0.423	0.326	0.373	0.440
E08.311	Diabetes mellitus due to underlying condition with unspecified diabetic retinopathy with macular edema	18	Diabetes with Chronic Complications	19	0.302	0.351	0.340	0.423	0.326	0.373	0.440
E08.319	Diabetes mellitus due to underlying condition with unspecified diabetic retinopathy without macular edema	18	Diabetes with Chronic Complications	19	0.302	0.351	0.340	0.423	0.326	0.373	0.440
E08.3211	Diabetes mellitus due to underlying condition with mild nonproliferative diabetic retinopathy with macular edema, right eye	18	Diabetes with Chronic Complications	19	0.302	0.351	0.340	0.423	0.326	0.373	0.440
E08.3212	Diabetes mellitus due to underlying condition with mild nonproliferative diabetic retinopathy with macular edema, left eye	18	Diabetes with Chronic Complications	19	0.302	0.351	0.340	0.423	0.326	0.373	0.440

ICD-10-CM Code	ICD-10-CM Code Description	V24 CMS-HCC	V24 CMS-HCC Disease Group	V24 CMS-HCC Hierarchies	Community, NonDual, Aged	Community, NonDual, Disabled	Community, FBDual, Aged	Community, FBDual, Disabled	Community, PBDual, Aged	Community, PBDual, Disabled	Institutional
E08.3213	Diabetes mellitus due to underlying condition with mild nonproliferative diabetic retinopathy with macular edema, bilateral	18	Diabetes with Chronic Complications	19	0.302	0.351	0.340	0.423	0.326	0.373	0.440
E08.3219	Diabetes mellitus due to underlying condition with mild nonproliferative diabetic retinopathy with macular edema, unspecified eye	18	Diabetes with Chronic Complications	19	0.302	0.351	0.340	0.423	0.326	0.373	0.440
E08.3291	Diabetes mellitus due to underlying condition with mild nonproliferative diabetic retinopathy without macular edema, right eye	18	Diabetes with Chronic Complications	19	0.302	0.351	0.340	0.423	0.326	0.373	0.440
E08.3292	Diabetes mellitus due to underlying condition with mild nonproliferative diabetic retinopathy without macular edema, left eye	18	Diabetes with Chronic Complications	19	0.302	0.351	0.340	0.423	0.326	0.373	0.440
E08.3293	Diabetes mellitus due to underlying condition with mild nonproliferative diabetic retinopathy without macular edema, bilateral	18	Diabetes with Chronic Complications	19	0.302	0.351	0.340	0.423	0.326	0.373	0.440
E08.3299	Diabetes mellitus due to underlying condition with mild nonproliferative diabetic retinopathy without macular edema, unspecified eye	18	Diabetes with Chronic Complications	19	0.302	0.351	0.340	0.423	0.326	0.373	0.440
E08.3311	Diabetes mellitus due to underlying condition with moderate nonproliferative diabetic retinopathy with macular edema, right eye	18	Diabetes with Chronic Complications	19	0.302	0.351	0.340	0.423	0.326	0.373	0.440
E08.3312	Diabetes mellitus due to underlying condition with moderate nonproliferative diabetic retinopathy with macular edema, left eye	18	Diabetes with Chronic Complications	19	0.302	0.351	0.340	0.423	0.326	0.373	0.440
E08.3313	Diabetes mellitus due to underlying condition with moderate nonproliferative diabetic retinopathy with macular edema, bilateral	18	Diabetes with Chronic Complications	19	0.302	0.351	0.340	0.423	0.326	0.373	0.440
E08.3319	Diabetes mellitus due to underlying condition with moderate nonproliferative diabetic retinopathy with macular edema, unspecified eye	18	Diabetes with Chronic Complications	19	0.302	0.351	0.340	0.423	0.326	0.373	0.440
E08.3391	Diabetes mellitus due to underlying condition with moderate nonproliferative diabetic retinopathy without macular edema, right eye	18	Diabetes with Chronic Complications	19	0.302	0.351	0.340	0.423	0.326	0.373	0.440
E08.3392	Diabetes mellitus due to underlying condition with moderate nonproliferative diabetic retinopathy without macular edema, left eye	18	Diabetes with Chronic Complications	19	0.302	0.351	0.340	0.423	0.326	0.373	0.440
E08.3393	Diabetes mellitus due to underlying condition with moderate nonproliferative diabetic retinopathy without macular edema, bilateral	18	Diabetes with Chronic Complications	19	0.302	0.351	0.340	0.423	0.326	0.373	0.440
E08.3399	Diabetes mellitus due to underlying condition with moderate nonproliferative diabetic retinopathy without macular edema, unspecified eye	18	Diabetes with Chronic Complications	19	0.302	0.351	0.340	0.423	0.326	0.373	0.440
E08.3411	Diabetes mellitus due to underlying condition with severe nonproliferative diabetic retinopathy with macular edema, right eye	18	Diabetes with Chronic Complications	19	0.302	0.351	0.340	0.423	0.326	0.373	0.440

ICD-10-CM Code	ICD-10-CM Code Description	V24 CMS-HCC	V24 CMS-HCC Disease Group	V24 CMS-HCC Hierarchies	Community, NonDual, Aged	Community, NonDual, Disabled	Community, FBDual, Aged	Community, FBDual, Disabled	Community, PBDual, Aged	Community, PBDual, Disabled	Institutional
E08.3412	Diabetes mellitus due to underlying condition with severe nonproliferative diabetic retinopathy with macular edema, left eye	18	Diabetes with Chronic Complications	19	0.302	0.351	0.340	0.423	0.326	0.373	0.440
E08.3413	Diabetes mellitus due to underlying condition with severe nonproliferative diabetic retinopathy with macular edema, bilateral	18	Diabetes with Chronic Complications	19	0.302	0.351	0.340	0.423	0.326	0.373	0.440
E08.3419	Diabetes mellitus due to underlying condition with severe nonproliferative diabetic retinopathy with macular edema, unspecified eye	18	Diabetes with Chronic Complications	19	0.302	0.351	0.340	0.423	0.326	0.373	0.440
E08.3491	Diabetes mellitus due to underlying condition with severe nonproliferative diabetic retinopathy without macular edema, right eye	18	Diabetes with Chronic Complications	19	0.302	0.351	0.340	0.423	0.326	0.373	0.440
E08.3492	Diabetes mellitus due to underlying condition with severe nonproliferative diabetic retinopathy without macular edema, left eye	18	Diabetes with Chronic Complications	19	0.302	0.351	0.340	0.423	0.326	0.373	0.440
E08.3493	Diabetes mellitus due to underlying condition with severe nonproliferative diabetic retinopathy without macular edema, bilateral	18	Diabetes with Chronic Complications	19	0.302	0.351	0.340	0.423	0.326	0.373	0.440
E08.3499	Diabetes mellitus due to underlying condition with severe nonproliferative diabetic retinopathy without macular edema, unspecified eye	18	Diabetes with Chronic Complications	19	0.302	0.351	0.340	0.423	0.326	0.373	0.440
E08.3511	Diabetes mellitus due to underlying condition with proliferative diabetic retinopathy with macular edema, right eye	18	Diabetes with Chronic Complications	19	0.302	0.351	0.340	0.423	0.326	0.373	0.440
E08.3511	Diabetes mellitus due to underlying condition with proliferative diabetic retinopathy with macular edema, right eye	122	Proliferative Diabetic Retinopathy and Vitreous Hemorrhage		0.222	0.231	0.271	0.269	0.182	0.201	0.394
E08.3512	Diabetes mellitus due to underlying condition with proliferative diabetic retinopathy with macular edema, left eye	18	Diabetes with Chronic Complications	19	0.302	0.351	0.340	0.423	0.326	0.373	0.440
E08.3512	Diabetes mellitus due to underlying condition with proliferative diabetic retinopathy with macular edema, left eye	122	Proliferative Diabetic Retinopathy and Vitreous Hemorrhage		0.222	0.231	0.271	0.269	0.182	0.201	0.394
E08.3513	Diabetes mellitus due to underlying condition with proliferative diabetic retinopathy with macular edema, bilateral	18	Diabetes with Chronic Complications	19	0.302	0.351	0.340	0.423	0.326	0.373	0.440
E08.3513	Diabetes mellitus due to underlying condition with proliferative diabetic retinopathy with macular edema, bilateral	122	Proliferative Diabetic Retinopathy and Vitreous Hemorrhage		0.222	0.231	0.271	0.269	0.182	0.201	0.394
E08.3519	Diabetes mellitus due to underlying condition with proliferative diabetic retinopathy with macular edema, unspecified eye	18	Diabetes with Chronic Complications	19	0.302	0.351	0.340	0.423	0.326	0.373	0.440
E08.3519	Diabetes mellitus due to underlying condition with proliferative diabetic retinopathy with macular edema, unspecified eye	122	Proliferative Diabetic Retinopathy and Vitreous Hemorrhage		0.222	0.231	0.271	0.269	0.182	0.201	0.394

ICD-10-CM Code	ICD-10-CM Code Description	V24 CMS-HCC	V24 CMS-HCC Disease Group	V24 CMS-HCC Hierarchies	Community, NonDual, Aged	Community, NonDual, Disabled	Community, FBDual, Aged	Community, FBDual, Disabled	Community, PBDual, Aged	Community, PBDual, Disabled	Institutional
E08.3521	Diabetes mellitus due to underlying condition with proliferative diabetic retinopathy with traction retinal detachment involving the macula, right eye	18	Diabetes with Chronic Complications	19	0.302	0.351	0.340	0.423	0.326	0.373	0.440
E08.3521	Diabetes mellitus due to underlying condition with proliferative diabetic retinopathy with traction retinal detachment involving the macula, right eye	122	Proliferative Diabetic Retinopathy and Vitreous Hemorrhage		0.222	0.231	0.271	0.269	0.182	0.201	0.394
E08.3522	Diabetes mellitus due to underlying condition with proliferative diabetic retinopathy with traction retinal detachment involving the macula, left eye	18	Diabetes with Chronic Complications	19	0.302	0.351	0.340	0.423	0.326	0.373	0.440
E08.3522	Diabetes mellitus due to underlying condition with proliferative diabetic retinopathy with traction retinal detachment involving the macula, left eye	122	Proliferative Diabetic Retinopathy and Vitreous Hemorrhage		0.222	0.231	0.271	0.269	0.182	0.201	0.394
E08.3523	Diabetes mellitus due to underlying condition with proliferative diabetic retinopathy with traction retinal detachment involving the macula, bilateral	18	Diabetes with Chronic Complications	19	0.302	0.351	0.340	0.423	0.326	0.373	0.440
E08.3523	Diabetes mellitus due to underlying condition with proliferative diabetic retinopathy with traction retinal detachment involving the macula, bilateral	122	Proliferative Diabetic Retinopathy and Vitreous Hemorrhage		0.222	0.231	0.271	0.269	0.182	0.201	0.394
E08.3529	Diabetes mellitus due to underlying condition with proliferative diabetic retinopathy with traction retinal detachment involving the macula, unspecified eye	18	Diabetes with Chronic Complications	19	0.302	0.351	0.340	0.423	0.326	0.373	0.440
E08.3529	Diabetes mellitus due to underlying condition with proliferative diabetic retinopathy with traction retinal detachment involving the macula, unspecified eye	122	Proliferative Diabetic Retinopathy and Vitreous Hemorrhage		0.222	0.231	0.271	0.269	0.182	0.201	0.394
E08.3531	Diabetes mellitus due to underlying condition with proliferative diabetic retinopathy with traction retinal detachment not involving the macula, right eye	18	Diabetes with Chronic Complications	19	0.302	0.351	0.340	0.423	0.326	0.373	0.440
E08.3531	Diabetes mellitus due to underlying condition with proliferative diabetic retinopathy with traction retinal detachment not involving the macula, right eye	122	Proliferative Diabetic Retinopathy and Vitreous Hemorrhage		0.222	0.231	0.271	0.269	0.182	0.201	0.394
E08.3532	Diabetes mellitus due to underlying condition with proliferative diabetic retinopathy with traction retinal detachment not involving the macula, left eye	18	Diabetes with Chronic Complications	19	0.302	0.351	0.340	0.423	0.326	0.373	0.440
E08.3532	Diabetes mellitus due to underlying condition with proliferative diabetic retinopathy with traction retinal detachment not involving the macula, left eye	122	Proliferative Diabetic Retinopathy and Vitreous Hemorrhage		0.222	0.231	0.271	0.269	0.182	0.201	0.394

ICD-10-CM Code	ICD-10-CM Code Description	V24 CMS-HCC	V24 CMS-HCC Disease Group	V24 CMS-HCC Hierarchies	Community, NonDual, Aged	Community, NonDual, Disabled	Community, FBDual, Aged	Community, FBDual, Disabled	Community, PBDual, Aged	Community, PBDual, Disabled	Institutional
E08.3533	Diabetes mellitus due to underlying condition with proliferative diabetic retinopathy with traction retinal detachment not involving the macula, bilateral	18	Diabetes with Chronic Complications	19	0.302	0.351	0.340	0.423	0.326	0.373	0.440
E08.3533	Diabetes mellitus due to underlying condition with proliferative diabetic retinopathy with traction retinal detachment not involving the macula, bilateral	122	Proliferative Diabetic Retinopathy and Vitreous Hemorrhage		0.222	0.231	0.271	0.269	0.182	0.201	0.394
E08.3539	Diabetes mellitus due to underlying condition with proliferative diabetic retinopathy with traction retinal detachment not involving the macula, unspecified eye	18	Diabetes with Chronic Complications	19	0.302	0.351	0.340	0.423	0.326	0.373	0.440
E08.3539	Diabetes mellitus due to underlying condition with proliferative diabetic retinopathy with traction retinal detachment not involving the macula, unspecified eye	122	Proliferative Diabetic Retinopathy and Vitreous Hemorrhage		0.222	0.231	0.271	0.269	0.182	0.201	0.394
E08.3541	Diabetes mellitus due to underlying condition with proliferative diabetic retinopathy with combined traction retinal detachment and rhegmatogenous retinal detachment, right eye	18	Diabetes with Chronic Complications	19	0.302	0.351	0.340	0.423	0.326	0.373	0.440
E08.3541	Diabetes mellitus due to underlying condition with proliferative diabetic retinopathy with combined traction retinal detachment and rhegmatogenous retinal detachment, right eye	122	Proliferative Diabetic Retinopathy and Vitreous Hemorrhage		0.222	0.231	0.271	0.269	0.182	0.201	0.394
E08.3542	Diabetes mellitus due to underlying condition with proliferative diabetic retinopathy with combined traction retinal detachment and rhegmatogenous retinal detachment, left eye	18	Diabetes with Chronic Complications	19	0.302	0.351	0.340	0.423	0.326	0.373	0.440
E08.3542	Diabetes mellitus due to underlying condition with proliferative diabetic retinopathy with combined traction retinal detachment and rhegmatogenous retinal detachment, left eye	122	Proliferative Diabetic Retinopathy and Vitreous Hemorrhage		0.222	0.231	0.271	0.269	0.182	0.201	0.394
E08.3543	Diabetes mellitus due to underlying condition with proliferative diabetic retinopathy with combined traction retinal detachment and rhegmatogenous retinal detachment, bilateral	18	Diabetes with Chronic Complications	19	0.302	0.351	0.340	0.423	0.326	0.373	0.440
E08.3543	Diabetes mellitus due to underlying condition with proliferative diabetic retinopathy with combined traction retinal detachment and rhegmatogenous retinal detachment, bilateral	122	Proliferative Diabetic Retinopathy and Vitreous Hemorrhage		0.222	0.231	0.271	0.269	0.182	0.201	0.394
E08.3549	Diabetes mellitus due to underlying condition with proliferative diabetic retinopathy with combined traction retinal detachment and rhegmatogenous retinal detachment, unspecified eye	18	Diabetes with Chronic Complications	19	0.302	0.351	0.340	0.423	0.326	0.373	0.440

ICD-10-CM Code	ICD-10-CM Code Description	V24 CMS-HCC	V24 CMS-HCC Disease Group	V24 CMS-HCC Hierarchies	Community, NonDual, Aged	Community, NonDual, Disabled	Community, FBDual, Aged	Community, FBDual, Disabled	Community, PBDual, Aged	Community, PBDual, Disabled	Institutional
E08.3549	Diabetes mellitus due to underlying condition with proliferative diabetic retinopathy with combined traction retinal detachment and rhegmatogenous retinal detachment, unspecified eye	122	Proliferative Diabetic Retinopathy and Vitreous Hemorrhage		0.222	0.231	0.271	0.269	0.182	0.201	0.394
E08.3551	Diabetes mellitus due to underlying condition with stable proliferative diabetic retinopathy, right eye	18	Diabetes with Chronic Complications	19	0.302	0.351	0.340	0.423	0.326	0.373	0.440
E08.3551	Diabetes mellitus due to underlying condition with stable proliferative diabetic retinopathy, right eye	122	Proliferative Diabetic Retinopathy and Vitreous Hemorrhage		0.222	0.231	0.271	0.269	0.182	0.201	0.394
E08.3552	Diabetes mellitus due to underlying condition with stable proliferative diabetic retinopathy, left eye	18	Diabetes with Chronic Complications	19	0.302	0.351	0.340	0.423	0.326	0.373	0.440
E08.3552	Diabetes mellitus due to underlying condition with stable proliferative diabetic retinopathy, left eye	122	Proliferative Diabetic Retinopathy and Vitreous Hemorrhage		0.222	0.231	0.271	0.269	0.182	0.201	0.394
E08.3553	Diabetes mellitus due to underlying condition with stable proliferative diabetic retinopathy, bilateral	18	Diabetes with Chronic Complications	19	0.302	0.351	0.340	0.423	0.326	0.373	0.440
E08.3553	Diabetes mellitus due to underlying condition with stable proliferative diabetic retinopathy, bilateral	122	Proliferative Diabetic Retinopathy and Vitreous Hemorrhage		0.222	0.231	0.271	0.269	0.182	0.201	0.394
E08.3559	Diabetes mellitus due to underlying condition with stable proliferative diabetic retinopathy, unspecified eye	18	Diabetes with Chronic Complications	19	0.302	0.351	0.340	0.423	0.326	0.373	0.440
E08.3559	Diabetes mellitus due to underlying condition with stable proliferative diabetic retinopathy, unspecified eye	122	Proliferative Diabetic Retinopathy and Vitreous Hemorrhage		0.222	0.231	0.271	0.269	0.182	0.201	0.394
E08.3591	Diabetes mellitus due to underlying condition with proliferative diabetic retinopathy without macular edema, right eye	18	Diabetes with Chronic Complications	19	0.302	0.351	0.340	0.423	0.326	0.373	0.440
E08.3591	Diabetes mellitus due to underlying condition with proliferative diabetic retinopathy without macular edema, right eye	122	Proliferative Diabetic Retinopathy and Vitreous Hemorrhage		0.222	0.231	0.271	0.269	0.182	0.201	0.394
E08.3592	Diabetes mellitus due to underlying condition with proliferative diabetic retinopathy without macular edema, left eye	18	Diabetes with Chronic Complications	19	0.302	0.351	0.340	0.423	0.326	0.373	0.440
E08.3592	Diabetes mellitus due to underlying condition with proliferative diabetic retinopathy without macular edema, left eye	122	Proliferative Diabetic Retinopathy and Vitreous Hemorrhage		0.222	0.231	0.271	0.269	0.182	0.201	0.394
E08.3593	Diabetes mellitus due to underlying condition with proliferative diabetic retinopathy without macular edema, bilateral	18	Diabetes with Chronic Complications	19	0.302	0.351	0.340	0.423	0.326	0.373	0.440
E08.3593	Diabetes mellitus due to underlying condition with proliferative diabetic retinopathy without macular edema, bilateral	122	Proliferative Diabetic Retinopathy and Vitreous Hemorrhage		0.222	0.231	0.271	0.269	0.182	0.201	0.394
E08.3599	Diabetes mellitus due to underlying condition with proliferative diabetic retinopathy without macular edema, unspecified eye	18	Diabetes with Chronic Complications	19	0.302	0.351	0.340	0.423	0.326	0.373	0.440
E08.3599	Diabetes mellitus due to underlying condition with proliferative diabetic retinopathy without macular edema, unspecified eye	122	Proliferative Diabetic Retinopathy and Vitreous Hemorrhage		0.222	0.231	0.271	0.269	0.182	0.201	0.394

ICD-10-CM Code	ICD-10-CM Code Description	V24 CMS-HCC	V24 CMS-HCC Disease Group	V24 CMS-HCC Hierarchies	Community, NonDual, Aged	Community, NonDual, Disabled	Community, FBDual, Aged	Community, FBDual, Disabled	Community, PBDual, Aged	Community, PBDual, Disabled	Institutional
E08.36	Diabetes mellitus due to underlying condition with diabetic cataract	18	Diabetes with Chronic Complications	19	0.302	0.351	0.340	0.423	0.326	0.373	0.440
E08.37X1	Diabetes mellitus due to underlying condition with diabetic macular edema, resolved following treatment, right eye	18	Diabetes with Chronic Complications	19	0.302	0.351	0.340	0.423	0.326	0.373	0.440
E08.37X2	Diabetes mellitus due to underlying condition with diabetic macular edema, resolved following treatment, left eye	18	Diabetes with Chronic Complications	19	0.302	0.351	0.340	0.423	0.326	0.373	0.440
E08.37X3	Diabetes mellitus due to underlying condition with diabetic macular edema, resolved following treatment, bilateral	18	Diabetes with Chronic Complications	19	0.302	0.351	0.340	0.423	0.326	0.373	0.440
E08.37X9	Diabetes mellitus due to underlying condition with diabetic macular edema, resolved following treatment, unspecified eye	18	Diabetes with Chronic Complications	19	0.302	0.351	0.340	0.423	0.326	0.373	0.440
E08.39	Diabetes mellitus due to underlying condition with other diabetic ophthalmic complication	18	Diabetes with Chronic Complications	19	0.302	0.351	0.340	0.423	0.326	0.373	0.440
E08.40	Diabetes mellitus due to underlying condition with diabetic neuropathy, unspecified	18	Diabetes with Chronic Complications	19	0.302	0.351	0.340	0.423	0.326	0.373	0.440
E08.41	Diabetes mellitus due to underlying condition with diabetic mononeuropathy	18	Diabetes with Chronic Complications	19	0.302	0.351	0.340	0.423	0.326	0.373	0.440
E08.42	Diabetes mellitus due to underlying condition with diabetic polyneuropathy	18	Diabetes with Chronic Complications	19	0.302	0.351	0.340	0.423	0.326	0.373	0.440
E08.43	Diabetes mellitus due to underlying condition with diabetic autonomic (poly)neuropathy	18	Diabetes with Chronic Complications	19	0.302	0.351	0.340	0.423	0.326	0.373	0.440
E08.44	Diabetes mellitus due to underlying condition with diabetic amyotrophy	18	Diabetes with Chronic Complications	19	0.302	0.351	0.340	0.423	0.326	0.373	0.440
E08.49	Diabetes mellitus due to underlying condition with other diabetic neurological complication	18	Diabetes with Chronic Complications	19	0.302	0.351	0.340	0.423	0.326	0.373	0.440
E08.51	Diabetes mellitus due to underlying condition with diabetic peripheral angiopathy without gangrene	18	Diabetes with Chronic Complications	19	0.302	0.351	0.340	0.423	0.326	0.373	0.440
E08.51	Diabetes mellitus due to underlying condition with diabetic peripheral angiopathy without gangrene	108	Vascular Disease		0.288	0.301	0.294	0.267	0.297	0.314	0.093
E08.52	Diabetes mellitus due to underlying condition with diabetic peripheral angiopathy with gangrene	18	Diabetes with Chronic Complications	19	0.302	0.351	0.340	0.423	0.326	0.373	0.440
E08.52	Diabetes mellitus due to underlying condition with diabetic peripheral angiopathy with gangrene	106	Atherosclerosis of the Extremities with Ulceration or Gangrene	107,108, 161,189	1.488	1.521	1.724	1.748	1.504	1.525	0.867
E08.59	Diabetes mellitus due to underlying condition with other circulatory complications	18	Diabetes with Chronic Complications	19	0.302	0.351	0.340	0.423	0.326	0.373	0.440
E08.610	Diabetes mellitus due to underlying condition with diabetic neuropathic arthropathy	18	Diabetes with Chronic Complications	19	0.302	0.351	0.340	0.423	0.326	0.373	0.440
E08.618	Diabetes mellitus due to underlying condition with other diabetic arthropathy	18	Diabetes with Chronic Complications	19	0.302	0.351	0.340	0.423	0.326	0.373	0.440
E08.620	Diabetes mellitus due to underlying condition with diabetic dermatitis	18	Diabetes with Chronic Complications	19	0.302	0.351	0.340	0.423	0.326	0.373	0.440

ICD-10-CM Code	ICD-10-CM Code Description	V24 CMS-HCC	V24 CMS-HCC Disease Group	V24 CMS-HCC Hierarchies	Community, NonDual, Aged	Community, NonDual, Disabled	Community, FBDual, Aged	Community, FBDual, Disabled	Community, PBDual, Aged	Community, PBDual, Disabled	Institutional
E08.621	Diabetes mellitus due to underlying condition with foot ulcer	18	Diabetes with Chronic Complications	19	0.302	0.351	0.340	0.423	0.326	0.373	0.440
E08.621	Diabetes mellitus due to underlying condition with foot ulcer	161	Chronic Ulcer of Skin, Except Pressure		0.515	0.592	0.727	0.583	0.541	0.542	0.294
E08.622	Diabetes mellitus due to underlying condition with other skin ulcer	18	Diabetes with Chronic Complications	19	0.302	0.351	0.340	0.423	0.326	0.373	0.440
E08.622	Diabetes mellitus due to underlying condition with other skin ulcer	161	Chronic Ulcer of Skin, Except Pressure		0.515	0.592	0.727	0.583	0.541	0.542	0.294
E08.628	Diabetes mellitus due to underlying condition with other skin complications	18	Diabetes with Chronic Complications	19	0.302	0.351	0.340	0.423	0.326	0.373	0.440
E08.630	Diabetes mellitus due to underlying condition with periodontal disease	18	Diabetes with Chronic Complications	19	0.302	0.351	0.340	0.423	0.326	0.373	0.440
E08.638	Diabetes mellitus due to underlying condition with other oral complications	18	Diabetes with Chronic Complications	19	0.302	0.351	0.340	0.423	0.326	0.373	0.440
E08.641	Diabetes mellitus due to underlying condition with hypoglycemia with coma	17	Diabetes with Acute Complications	18,19	0.302	0.351	0.340	0.423	0.326	0.373	0.440
E08.649	Diabetes mellitus due to underlying condition with hypoglycemia without coma	18	Diabetes with Chronic Complications	19	0.302	0.351	0.340	0.423	0.326	0.373	0.440
E08.65	Diabetes mellitus due to underlying condition with hyperglycemia	18	Diabetes with Chronic Complications	19	0.302	0.351	0.340	0.423	0.326	0.373	0.440
E08.69	Diabetes mellitus due to underlying condition with other specified complication	18	Diabetes with Chronic Complications	19	0.302	0.351	0.340	0.423	0.326	0.373	0.440
E08.8	Diabetes mellitus due to underlying condition with unspecified complications	18	Diabetes with Chronic Complications	19	0.302	0.351	0.340	0.423	0.326	0.373	0.440
E08.9	Diabetes mellitus due to underlying condition without complications	19	Diabetes without Complication		0.105	0.124	0.107	0.145	0.087	0.122	0.178
E09.00	Drug or chemical induced diabetes mellitus with hyperosmolarity without nonketotic hyperglycemic-hyperosmolar coma (NKHHC)	17	Diabetes with Acute Complications	18,19	0.302	0.351	0.340	0.423	0.326	0.373	0.440
E09.01	Drug or chemical induced diabetes mellitus with hyperosmolarity with coma	17	Diabetes with Acute Complications	18,19	0.302	0.351	0.340	0.423	0.326	0.373	0.440
E09.10	Drug or chemical induced diabetes mellitus with ketoacidosis without coma	17	Diabetes with Acute Complications	18,19	0.302	0.351	0.340	0.423	0.326	0.373	0.440
E09.11	Drug or chemical induced diabetes mellitus with ketoacidosis with coma	17	Diabetes with Acute Complications	18,19	0.302	0.351	0.340	0.423	0.326	0.373	0.440
E09.21	Drug or chemical induced diabetes mellitus with diabetic nephropathy	18	Diabetes with Chronic Complications	19	0.302	0.351	0.340	0.423	0.326	0.373	0.440
E09.22	Drug or chemical induced diabetes mellitus with diabetic chronic kidney disease	18	Diabetes with Chronic Complications	19	0.302	0.351	0.340	0.423	0.326	0.373	0.440
E09.29	Drug or chemical induced diabetes mellitus with other diabetic kidney complication	18	Diabetes with Chronic Complications	19	0.302	0.351	0.340	0.423	0.326	0.373	0.440
E09.311	Drug or chemical induced diabetes mellitus with unspecified diabetic retinopathy with macular edema	18	Diabetes with Chronic Complications	19	0.302	0.351	0.340	0.423	0.326	0.373	0.440
E09.319	Drug or chemical induced diabetes mellitus with unspecified diabetic retinopathy without macular edema	18	Diabetes with Chronic Complications	19	0.302	0.351	0.340	0.423	0.326	0.373	0.440

ICD-10-CM Code	ICD-10-CM Code Description	V24 CMS-HCC	V24 CMS-HCC Disease Group	V24 CMS-HCC Hierarchies	Community, NonDual, Aged	Community, NonDual, Disabled	Community, FBDual, Aged	Community, FBDual, Disabled	Community, PBDual, Aged	Community, PBDual, Disabled	Institutional
E09.3211	Drug or chemical induced diabetes mellitus with mild nonproliferative diabetic retinopathy with macular edema, right eye	18	Diabetes with Chronic Complications	19	0.302	0.351	0.340	0.423	0.326	0.373	0.440
E09.3212	Drug or chemical induced diabetes mellitus with mild nonproliferative diabetic retinopathy with macular edema, left eye	18	Diabetes with Chronic Complications	19	0.302	0.351	0.340	0.423	0.326	0.373	0.440
E09.3213	Drug or chemical induced diabetes mellitus with mild nonproliferative diabetic retinopathy with macular edema, bilateral	18	Diabetes with Chronic Complications	19	0.302	0.351	0.340	0.423	0.326	0.373	0.440
E09.3219	Drug or chemical induced diabetes mellitus with mild nonproliferative diabetic retinopathy with macular edema, unspecified eye	18	Diabetes with Chronic Complications	19	0.302	0.351	0.340	0.423	0.326	0.373	0.440
E09.3291	Drug or chemical induced diabetes mellitus with mild nonproliferative diabetic retinopathy without macular edema, right eye	18	Diabetes with Chronic Complications	19	0.302	0.351	0.340	0.423	0.326	0.373	0.440
E09.3292	Drug or chemical induced diabetes mellitus with mild nonproliferative diabetic retinopathy without macular edema, left eye	18	Diabetes with Chronic Complications	19	0.302	0.351	0.340	0.423	0.326	0.373	0.440
E09.3293	Drug or chemical induced diabetes mellitus with mild nonproliferative diabetic retinopathy without macular edema, bilateral	18	Diabetes with Chronic Complications	19	0.302	0.351	0.340	0.423	0.326	0.373	0.440
E09.3299	Drug or chemical induced diabetes mellitus with mild nonproliferative diabetic retinopathy without macular edema, unspecified eye	18	Diabetes with Chronic Complications	19	0.302	0.351	0.340	0.423	0.326	0.373	0.440
E09.3311	Drug or chemical induced diabetes mellitus with moderate nonproliferative diabetic retinopathy with macular edema, right eye	18	Diabetes with Chronic Complications	19	0.302	0.351	0.340	0.423	0.326	0.373	0.440
E09.3312	Drug or chemical induced diabetes mellitus with moderate nonproliferative diabetic retinopathy with macular edema, left eye	18	Diabetes with Chronic Complications	19	0.302	0.351	0.340	0.423	0.326	0.373	0.440
E09.3313	Drug or chemical induced diabetes mellitus with moderate nonproliferative diabetic retinopathy with macular edema, bilateral	18	Diabetes with Chronic Complications	19	0.302	0.351	0.340	0.423	0.326	0.373	0.440
E09.3319	Drug or chemical induced diabetes mellitus with moderate nonproliferative diabetic retinopathy with macular edema, unspecified eye	18	Diabetes with Chronic Complications	19	0.302	0.351	0.340	0.423	0.326	0.373	0.440
E09.3391	Drug or chemical induced diabetes mellitus with moderate nonproliferative diabetic retinopathy without macular edema, right eye	18	Diabetes with Chronic Complications	19	0.302	0.351	0.340	0.423	0.326	0.373	0.440
E09.3392	Drug or chemical induced diabetes mellitus with moderate nonproliferative diabetic retinopathy without macular edema, left eye	18	Diabetes with Chronic Complications	19	0.302	0.351	0.340	0.423	0.326	0.373	0.440
E09.3393	Drug or chemical induced diabetes mellitus with moderate nonproliferative diabetic retinopathy without macular edema, bilateral	18	Diabetes with Chronic Complications	19	0.302	0.351	0.340	0.423	0.326	0.373	0.440

ICD-10-CM Code	ICD-10-CM Code Description	V24 CMS-HCC	V24 CMS-HCC Disease Group	V24 CMS-HCC Hierarchies	Community, NonDual, Aged	Community, NonDual, Disabled	Community, FBDual, Aged	Community, FBDual, Disabled	Community, PBDual, Aged	Community, PBDual, Disabled	Institutional
E09.3399	Drug or chemical induced diabetes mellitus with moderate nonproliferative diabetic retinopathy without macular edema, unspecified eye	18	Diabetes with Chronic Complications	19	0.302	0.351	0.340	0.423	0.326	0.373	0.440
E09.3411	Drug or chemical induced diabetes mellitus with severe nonproliferative diabetic retinopathy with macular edema, right eye	18	Diabetes with Chronic Complications	19	0.302	0.351	0.340	0.423	0.326	0.373	0.440
E09.3412	Drug or chemical induced diabetes mellitus with severe nonproliferative diabetic retinopathy with macular edema, left eye	18	Diabetes with Chronic Complications	19	0.302	0.351	0.340	0.423	0.326	0.373	0.440
E09.3413	Drug or chemical induced diabetes mellitus with severe nonproliferative diabetic retinopathy with macular edema, bilateral	18	Diabetes with Chronic Complications	19	0.302	0.351	0.340	0.423	0.326	0.373	0.440
E09.3419	Drug or chemical induced diabetes mellitus with severe nonproliferative diabetic retinopathy with macular edema, unspecified eye	18	Diabetes with Chronic Complications	19	0.302	0.351	0.340	0.423	0.326	0.373	0.440
E09.3491	Drug or chemical induced diabetes mellitus with severe nonproliferative diabetic retinopathy without macular edema, right eye	18	Diabetes with Chronic Complications	19	0.302	0.351	0.340	0.423	0.326	0.373	0.440
E09.3492	Drug or chemical induced diabetes mellitus with severe nonproliferative diabetic retinopathy without macular edema, left eye	18	Diabetes with Chronic Complications	19	0.302	0.351	0.340	0.423	0.326	0.373	0.440
E09.3493	Drug or chemical induced diabetes mellitus with severe nonproliferative diabetic retinopathy without macular edema, bilateral	18	Diabetes with Chronic Complications	19	0.302	0.351	0.340	0.423	0.326	0.373	0.440
E09.3499	Drug or chemical induced diabetes mellitus with severe nonproliferative diabetic retinopathy without macular edema, unspecified eye	18	Diabetes with Chronic Complications	19	0.302	0.351	0.340	0.423	0.326	0.373	0.440
E09.3511	Drug or chemical induced diabetes mellitus with proliferative diabetic retinopathy with macular edema, right eye	18	Diabetes with Chronic Complications	19	0.302	0.351	0.340	0.423	0.326	0.373	0.440
E09.3511	Drug or chemical induced diabetes mellitus with proliferative diabetic retinopathy with macular edema, right eye	122	Proliferative Diabetic Retinopathy and Vitreous Hemorrhage		0.222	0.231	0.271	0.269	0.182	0.201	0.394
E09.3512	Drug or chemical induced diabetes mellitus with proliferative diabetic retinopathy with macular edema, left eye	18	Diabetes with Chronic Complications	19	0.302	0.351	0.340	0.423	0.326	0.373	0.440
E09.3512	Drug or chemical induced diabetes mellitus with proliferative diabetic retinopathy with macular edema, left eye	122	Proliferative Diabetic Retinopathy and Vitreous Hemorrhage		0.222	0.231	0.271	0.269	0.182	0.201	0.394
E09.3513	Drug or chemical induced diabetes mellitus with proliferative diabetic retinopathy with macular edema, bilateral	18	Diabetes with Chronic Complications	19	0.302	0.351	0.340	0.423	0.326	0.373	0.440
E09.3513	Drug or chemical induced diabetes mellitus with proliferative diabetic retinopathy with macular edema, bilateral	122	Proliferative Diabetic Retinopathy and Vitreous Hemorrhage		0.222	0.231	0.271	0.269	0.182	0.201	0.394

ICD-10-CM Code	ICD-10-CM Code Description	V24 CMS-HCC	V24 CMS-HCC Disease Group	V24 CMS-HCC Hierarchies	Community, NonDual, Aged	Community, NonDual, Disabled	Community, FBDual, Aged	Community, FBDual, Disabled	Community, PBDual, Aged	Community, PBDual, Disabled	Institutional
E09.3519	Drug or chemical induced diabetes mellitus with proliferative diabetic retinopathy with macular edema, unspecified eye	18	Diabetes with Chronic Complications	19	0.302	0.351	0.340	0.423	0.326	0.373	0.440
E09.3519	Drug or chemical induced diabetes mellitus with proliferative diabetic retinopathy with macular edema, unspecified eye	122	Proliferative Diabetic Retinopathy and Vitreous Hemorrhage		0.222	0.231	0.271	0.269	0.182	0.201	0.394
E09.3521	Drug or chemical induced diabetes mellitus with proliferative diabetic retinopathy with traction retinal detachment involving the macula, right eye	18	Diabetes with Chronic Complications	19	0.302	0.351	0.340	0.423	0.326	0.373	0.440
E09.3521	Drug or chemical induced diabetes mellitus with proliferative diabetic retinopathy with traction retinal detachment involving the macula, right eye	122	Proliferative Diabetic Retinopathy and Vitreous Hemorrhage		0.222	0.231	0.271	0.269	0.182	0.201	0.394
E09.3522	Drug or chemical induced diabetes mellitus with proliferative diabetic retinopathy with traction retinal detachment involving the macula, left eye	18	Diabetes with Chronic Complications	19	0.302	0.351	0.340	0.423	0.326	0.373	0.440
E09.3522	Drug or chemical induced diabetes mellitus with proliferative diabetic retinopathy with traction retinal detachment involving the macula, left eye	122	Proliferative Diabetic Retinopathy and Vitreous Hemorrhage		0.222	0.231	0.271	0.269	0.182	0.201	0.394
E09.3523	Drug or chemical induced diabetes mellitus with proliferative diabetic retinopathy with traction retinal detachment involving the macula, bilateral	18	Diabetes with Chronic Complications	19	0.302	0.351	0.340	0.423	0.326	0.373	0.440
E09.3523	Drug or chemical induced diabetes mellitus with proliferative diabetic retinopathy with traction retinal detachment involving the macula, bilateral	122	Proliferative Diabetic Retinopathy and Vitreous Hemorrhage		0.222	0.231	0.271	0.269	0.182	0.201	0.394
E09.3529	Drug or chemical induced diabetes mellitus with proliferative diabetic retinopathy with traction retinal detachment involving the macula, unspecified eye	18	Diabetes with Chronic Complications	19	0.302	0.351	0.340	0.423	0.326	0.373	0.440
E09.3529	Drug or chemical induced diabetes mellitus with proliferative diabetic retinopathy with traction retinal detachment involving the macula, unspecified eye	122	Proliferative Diabetic Retinopathy and Vitreous Hemorrhage		0.222	0.231	0.271	0.269	0.182	0.201	0.394
E09.3531	Drug or chemical induced diabetes mellitus with proliferative diabetic retinopathy with traction retinal detachment not involving the macula, right eye	18	Diabetes with Chronic Complications	19	0.302	0.351	0.340	0.423	0.326	0.373	0.440
E09.3531	Drug or chemical induced diabetes mellitus with proliferative diabetic retinopathy with traction retinal detachment not involving the macula, right eye	122	Proliferative Diabetic Retinopathy and Vitreous Hemorrhage		0.222	0.231	0.271	0.269	0.182	0.201	0.394
E09.3532	Drug or chemical induced diabetes mellitus with proliferative diabetic retinopathy with traction retinal detachment not involving the macula, left eye	18	Diabetes with Chronic Complications	19	0.302	0.351	0.340	0.423	0.326	0.373	0.440

ICD-10-CM Code	ICD-10-CM Code Description	V24 CMS-HCC	V24 CMS-HCC Disease Group	V24 CMS-HCC Hierarchies	Community, NonDual, Aged	Community, NonDual, Disabled	Community, FBDual, Aged	Community, FBDual, Disabled	Community, PBDual, Aged	Community, PBDual, Disabled	Institutional
E09.3532	Drug or chemical induced diabetes mellitus with proliferative diabetic retinopathy with traction retinal detachment not involving the macula, left eye	122	Proliferative Diabetic Retinopathy and Vitreous Hemorrhage		0.222	0.231	0.271	0.269	0.182	0.201	0.394
E09.3533	Drug or chemical induced diabetes mellitus with proliferative diabetic retinopathy with traction retinal detachment not involving the macula, bilateral	18	Diabetes with Chronic Complications	19	0.302	0.351	0.340	0.423	0.326	0.373	0.440
E09.3533	Drug or chemical induced diabetes mellitus with proliferative diabetic retinopathy with traction retinal detachment not involving the macula, bilateral	122	Proliferative Diabetic Retinopathy and Vitreous Hemorrhage		0.222	0.231	0.271	0.269	0.182	0.201	0.394
E09.3539	Drug or chemical induced diabetes mellitus with proliferative diabetic retinopathy with traction retinal detachment not involving the macula, unspecified eye	18	Diabetes with Chronic Complications	19	0.302	0.351	0.340	0.423	0.326	0.373	0.440
E09.3539	Drug or chemical induced diabetes mellitus with proliferative diabetic retinopathy with traction retinal detachment not involving the macula, unspecified eye	122	Proliferative Diabetic Retinopathy and Vitreous Hemorrhage		0.222	0.231	0.271	0.269	0.182	0.201	0.394
E09.3541	Drug or chemical induced diabetes mellitus with proliferative diabetic retinopathy with combined traction retinal detachment and rhegmatogenous retinal detachment, right eye	18	Diabetes with Chronic Complications	19	0.302	0.351	0.340	0.423	0.326	0.373	0.440
E09.3541	Drug or chemical induced diabetes mellitus with proliferative diabetic retinopathy with combined traction retinal detachment and rhegmatogenous retinal detachment, right eye	122	Proliferative Diabetic Retinopathy and Vitreous Hemorrhage		0.222	0.231	0.271	0.269	0.182	0.201	0.394
E09.3542	Drug or chemical induced diabetes mellitus with proliferative diabetic retinopathy with combined traction retinal detachment and rhegmatogenous retinal detachment, left eye	18	Diabetes with Chronic Complications	19	0.302	0.351	0.340	0.423	0.326	0.373	0.440
E09.3542	Drug or chemical induced diabetes mellitus with proliferative diabetic retinopathy with combined traction retinal detachment and rhegmatogenous retinal detachment, left eye	122	Proliferative Diabetic Retinopathy and Vitreous Hemorrhage		0.222	0.231	0.271	0.269	0.182	0.201	0.394
E09.3543	Drug or chemical induced diabetes mellitus with proliferative diabetic retinopathy with combined traction retinal detachment and rhegmatogenous retinal detachment, bilateral	18	Diabetes with Chronic Complications	19	0.302	0.351	0.340	0.423	0.326	0.373	0.440
E09.3543	Drug or chemical induced diabetes mellitus with proliferative diabetic retinopathy with combined traction retinal detachment and rhegmatogenous retinal detachment, bilateral	122	Proliferative Diabetic Retinopathy and Vitreous Hemorrhage		0.222	0.231	0.271	0.269	0.182	0.201	0.394

ICD-10-CM Code	ICD-10-CM Code Description	V24 CMS-HCC	V24 CMS-HCC Disease Group	V24 CMS-HCC Hierarchies	Community, NonDual, Aged	Community, NonDual, Disabled	Community, FBDual, Aged	Community, FBDual, Disabled	Community, PBDual, Aged	Community, PBDual, Disabled	Institutional
E09.3549	Drug or chemical induced diabetes mellitus with proliferative diabetic retinopathy with combined traction retinal detachment and rhegmatogenous retinal detachment, unspecified eye	18	Diabetes with Chronic Complications	19	0.302	0.351	0.340	0.423	0.326	0.373	0.440
E09.3549	Drug or chemical induced diabetes mellitus with proliferative diabetic retinopathy with combined traction retinal detachment and rhegmatogenous retinal detachment, unspecified eye	122	Proliferative Diabetic Retinopathy and Vitreous Hemorrhage		0.222	0.231	0.271	0.269	0.182	0.201	0.394
E09.3551	Drug or chemical induced diabetes mellitus with stable proliferative diabetic retinopathy, right eye	18	Diabetes with Chronic Complications	19	0.302	0.351	0.340	0.423	0.326	0.373	0.440
E09.3551	Drug or chemical induced diabetes mellitus with stable proliferative diabetic retinopathy, right eye	122	Proliferative Diabetic Retinopathy and Vitreous Hemorrhage		0.222	0.231	0.271	0.269	0.182	0.201	0.394
E09.3552	Drug or chemical induced diabetes mellitus with stable proliferative diabetic retinopathy, left eye	18	Diabetes with Chronic Complications	19	0.302	0.351	0.340	0.423	0.326	0.373	0.440
E09.3552	Drug or chemical induced diabetes mellitus with stable proliferative diabetic retinopathy, left eye	122	Proliferative Diabetic Retinopathy and Vitreous Hemorrhage		0.222	0.231	0.271	0.269	0.182	0.201	0.394
E09.3553	Drug or chemical induced diabetes mellitus with stable proliferative diabetic retinopathy, bilateral	18	Diabetes with Chronic Complications	19	0.302	0.351	0.340	0.423	0.326	0.373	0.440
E09.3553	Drug or chemical induced diabetes mellitus with stable proliferative diabetic retinopathy, bilateral	122	Proliferative Diabetic Retinopathy and Vitreous Hemorrhage		0.222	0.231	0.271	0.269	0.182	0.201	0.394
E09.3559	Drug or chemical induced diabetes mellitus with stable proliferative diabetic retinopathy, unspecified eye	18	Diabetes with Chronic Complications	19	0.302	0.351	0.340	0.423	0.326	0.373	0.440
E09.3559	Drug or chemical induced diabetes mellitus with stable proliferative diabetic retinopathy, unspecified eye	122	Proliferative Diabetic Retinopathy and Vitreous Hemorrhage		0.222	0.231	0.271	0.269	0.182	0.201	0.394
E09.3591	Drug or chemical induced diabetes mellitus with proliferative diabetic retinopathy without macular edema, right eye	18	Diabetes with Chronic Complications	19	0.302	0.351	0.340	0.423	0.326	0.373	0.440
E09.3591	Drug or chemical induced diabetes mellitus with proliferative diabetic retinopathy without macular edema, right eye	122	Proliferative Diabetic Retinopathy and Vitreous Hemorrhage		0.222	0.231	0.271	0.269	0.182	0.201	0.394
E09.3592	Drug or chemical induced diabetes mellitus with proliferative diabetic retinopathy without macular edema, left eye	18	Diabetes with Chronic Complications	19	0.302	0.351	0.340	0.423	0.326	0.373	0.440
E09.3592	Drug or chemical induced diabetes mellitus with proliferative diabetic retinopathy without macular edema, left eye	122	Proliferative Diabetic Retinopathy and Vitreous Hemorrhage		0.222	0.231	0.271	0.269	0.182	0.201	0.394
E09.3593	Drug or chemical induced diabetes mellitus with proliferative diabetic retinopathy without macular edema, bilateral	18	Diabetes with Chronic Complications	19	0.302	0.351	0.340	0.423	0.326	0.373	0.440
E09.3593	Drug or chemical induced diabetes mellitus with proliferative diabetic retinopathy without macular edema, bilateral	122	Proliferative Diabetic Retinopathy and Vitreous Hemorrhage		0.222	0.231	0.271	0.269	0.182	0.201	0.394

ICD-10-CM Code	ICD-10-CM Code Description	V24 CMS-HCC	V24 CMS-HCC Disease Group	V24 CMS-HCC Hierarchies	Community, NonDual, Aged	Community, NonDual, Disabled	Community, FBDual, Aged	Community, FBDual, Disabled	Community, PBDual, Aged	Community, PBDual, Disabled	Institutional
E09.3599	Drug or chemical induced diabetes mellitus with proliferative diabetic retinopathy without macular edema, unspecified eye	18	Diabetes with Chronic Complications	19	0.302	0.351	0.340	0.423	0.326	0.373	0.440
E09.3599	Drug or chemical induced diabetes mellitus with proliferative diabetic retinopathy without macular edema, unspecified eye	122	Proliferative Diabetic Retinopathy and Vitreous Hemorrhage		0.222	0.231	0.271	0.269	0.182	0.201	0.394
E09.36	Drug or chemical induced diabetes mellitus with diabetic cataract	18	Diabetes with Chronic Complications	19	0.302	0.351	0.340	0.423	0.326	0.373	0.440
E09.37X1	Drug or chemical induced diabetes mellitus with diabetic macular edema, resolved following treatment, right eye	18	Diabetes with Chronic Complications	19	0.302	0.351	0.340	0.423	0.326	0.373	0.440
E09.37X2	Drug or chemical induced diabetes mellitus with diabetic macular edema, resolved following treatment, left eye	18	Diabetes with Chronic Complications	19	0.302	0.351	0.340	0.423	0.326	0.373	0.440
E09.37X3	Drug or chemical induced diabetes mellitus with diabetic macular edema, resolved following treatment, bilateral	18	Diabetes with Chronic Complications	19	0.302	0.351	0.340	0.423	0.326	0.373	0.440
E09.37X9	Drug or chemical induced diabetes mellitus with diabetic macular edema, resolved following treatment, unspecified eye	18	Diabetes with Chronic Complications	19	0.302	0.351	0.340	0.423	0.326	0.373	0.440
E09.39	Drug or chemical induced diabetes mellitus with other diabetic ophthalmic complication	18	Diabetes with Chronic Complications	19	0.302	0.351	0.340	0.423	0.326	0.373	0.440
E09.40	Drug or chemical induced diabetes mellitus with neurological complications with diabetic neuropathy, unspecified	18	Diabetes with Chronic Complications	19	0.302	0.351	0.340	0.423	0.326	0.373	0.440
E09.41	Drug or chemical induced diabetes mellitus with neurological complications with diabetic mononeuropathy	18	Diabetes with Chronic Complications	19	0.302	0.351	0.340	0.423	0.326	0.373	0.440
E09.42	Drug or chemical induced diabetes mellitus with neurological complications with diabetic polyneuropathy	18	Diabetes with Chronic Complications	19	0.302	0.351	0.340	0.423	0.326	0.373	0.440
E09.43	Drug or chemical induced diabetes mellitus with neurological complications with diabetic autonomic (poly)neuropathy	18	Diabetes with Chronic Complications	19	0.302	0.351	0.340	0.423	0.326	0.373	0.440
E09.44	Drug or chemical induced diabetes mellitus with neurological complications with diabetic amyotrophy	18	Diabetes with Chronic Complications	19	0.302	0.351	0.340	0.423	0.326	0.373	0.440
E09.49	Drug or chemical induced diabetes mellitus with neurological complications with other diabetic neurological complication	18	Diabetes with Chronic Complications	19	0.302	0.351	0.340	0.423	0.326	0.373	0.440
E09.51	Drug or chemical induced diabetes mellitus with diabetic peripheral angiopathy without gangrene	18	Diabetes with Chronic Complications	19	0.302	0.351	0.340	0.423	0.326	0.373	0.440
E09.51	Drug or chemical induced diabetes mellitus with diabetic peripheral angiopathy without gangrene	108	Vascular Disease		0.288	0.301	0.294	0.267	0.297	0.314	0.093
E09.52	Drug or chemical induced diabetes mellitus with diabetic peripheral angiopathy with gangrene	18	Diabetes with Chronic Complications	19	0.302	0.351	0.340	0.423	0.326	0.373	0.440

ICD-10-CM Code	ICD-10-CM Code Description	V24 CMS-HCC	V24 CMS-HCC Disease Group	V24 CMS-HCC Hierarchies	Community, NonDual, Aged	Community, NonDual, Disabled	Community, FBDual, Aged	Community, FBDual, Disabled	Community, PBDual, Aged	Community, PBDual, Disabled	Institutional
E09.52	Drug or chemical induced diabetes mellitus with diabetic peripheral angiopathy with gangrene	106	Atherosclerosis of the Extremities with Ulceration or Gangrene	107,108, 161,189	1.488	1.521	1.724	1.748	1.504	1.525	0.867
E09.59	Drug or chemical induced diabetes mellitus with other circulatory complications	18	Diabetes with Chronic Complications	19	0.302	0.351	0.340	0.423	0.326	0.373	0.440
E09.610	Drug or chemical induced diabetes mellitus with diabetic neuropathic arthropathy	18	Diabetes with Chronic Complications	19	0.302	0.351	0.340	0.423	0.326	0.373	0.440
E09.618	Drug or chemical induced diabetes mellitus with other diabetic arthropathy	18	Diabetes with Chronic Complications	19	0.302	0.351	0.340	0.423	0.326	0.373	0.440
E09.620	Drug or chemical induced diabetes mellitus with diabetic dermatitis	18	Diabetes with Chronic Complications	19	0.302	0.351	0.340	0.423	0.326	0.373	0.440
E09.621	Drug or chemical induced diabetes mellitus with foot ulcer	18	Diabetes with Chronic Complications	19	0.302	0.351	0.340	0.423	0.326	0.373	0.440
E09.621	Drug or chemical induced diabetes mellitus with foot ulcer	161	Chronic Ulcer of Skin, Except Pressure		0.515	0.592	0.727	0.583	0.541	0.542	0.294
E09.622	Drug or chemical induced diabetes mellitus with other skin ulcer	18	Diabetes with Chronic Complications	19	0.302	0.351	0.340	0.423	0.326	0.373	0.440
E09.622	Drug or chemical induced diabetes mellitus with other skin ulcer	161	Chronic Ulcer of Skin, Except Pressure		0.515	0.592	0.727	0.583	0.541	0.542	0.294
E09.628	Drug or chemical induced diabetes mellitus with other skin complications	18	Diabetes with Chronic Complications	19	0.302	0.351	0.340	0.423	0.326	0.373	0.440
E09.630	Drug or chemical induced diabetes mellitus with periodontal disease	18	Diabetes with Chronic Complications	19	0.302	0.351	0.340	0.423	0.326	0.373	0.440
E09.638	Drug or chemical induced diabetes mellitus with other oral complications	18	Diabetes with Chronic Complications	19	0.302	0.351	0.340	0.423	0.326	0.373	0.440
E09.641	Drug or chemical induced diabetes mellitus with hypoglycemia with coma	17	Diabetes with Acute Complications	18,19	0.302	0.351	0.340	0.423	0.326	0.373	0.440
E09.649	Drug or chemical induced diabetes mellitus with hypoglycemia without coma	18	Diabetes with Chronic Complications	19	0.302	0.351	0.340	0.423	0.326	0.373	0.440
E09.65	Drug or chemical induced diabetes mellitus with hyperglycemia	18	Diabetes with Chronic Complications	19	0.302	0.351	0.340	0.423	0.326	0.373	0.440
E09.69	Drug or chemical induced diabetes mellitus with other specified complication	18	Diabetes with Chronic Complications	19	0.302	0.351	0.340	0.423	0.326	0.373	0.440
E09.8	Drug or chemical induced diabetes mellitus with unspecified complications	18	Diabetes with Chronic Complications	19	0.302	0.351	0.340	0.423	0.326	0.373	0.440
E09.9	Drug or chemical induced diabetes mellitus without complications	19	Diabetes without Complication		0.105	0.124	0.107	0.145	0.087	0.122	0.178
E10.10	Type 1 diabetes mellitus with ketoacidosis without coma	17	Diabetes with Acute Complications	18,19	0.302	0.351	0.340	0.423	0.326	0.373	0.440
E10.11	Type 1 diabetes mellitus with ketoacidosis with coma	17	Diabetes with Acute Complications	18,19	0.302	0.351	0.340	0.423	0.326	0.373	0.440
E10.21	Type 1 diabetes mellitus with diabetic nephropathy	18	Diabetes with Chronic Complications	19	0.302	0.351	0.340	0.423	0.326	0.373	0.440
E10.22	Type 1 diabetes mellitus with diabetic chronic kidney disease	18	Diabetes with Chronic Complications	19	0.302	0.351	0.340	0.423	0.326	0.373	0.440
E10.29	Type 1 diabetes mellitus with other diabetic kidney complication	18	Diabetes with Chronic Complications	19	0.302	0.351	0.340	0.423	0.326	0.373	0.440
E10.311	Type 1 diabetes mellitus with unspecified diabetic retinopathy with macular edema	18	Diabetes with Chronic Complications	19	0.302	0.351	0.340	0.423	0.326	0.373	0.440

ICD-10-CM Code	ICD-10-CM Code Description	V24 CMS-HCC	V24 CMS-HCC Disease Group	V24 CMS-HCC Hierarchies	Community, NonDual, Aged	Community, NonDual, Disabled	Community, FBDual, Aged	Community, FBDual, Disabled	Community, PBDual, Aged	Community, PBDual, Disabled	Institutional
E10.319	Type 1 diabetes mellitus with unspecified diabetic retinopathy without macular edema	18	Diabetes with Chronic Complications	19	0.302	0.351	0.340	0.423	0.326	0.373	0.440
E10.3211	Type 1 diabetes mellitus with mild nonproliferative diabetic retinopathy with macular edema, right eye	18	Diabetes with Chronic Complications	19	0.302	0.351	0.340	0.423	0.326	0.373	0.440
E10.3212	Type 1 diabetes mellitus with mild nonproliferative diabetic retinopathy with macular edema, left eye	18	Diabetes with Chronic Complications	19	0.302	0.351	0.340	0.423	0.326	0.373	0.440
E10.3213	Type 1 diabetes mellitus with mild nonproliferative diabetic retinopathy with macular edema, bilateral	18	Diabetes with Chronic Complications	19	0.302	0.351	0.340	0.423	0.326	0.373	0.440
E10.3219	Type 1 diabetes mellitus with mild nonproliferative diabetic retinopathy with macular edema, unspecified eye	18	Diabetes with Chronic Complications	19	0.302	0.351	0.340	0.423	0.326	0.373	0.440
E10.3291	Type 1 diabetes mellitus with mild nonproliferative diabetic retinopathy without macular edema, right eye	18	Diabetes with Chronic Complications	19	0.302	0.351	0.340	0.423	0.326	0.373	0.440
E10.3292	Type 1 diabetes mellitus with mild nonproliferative diabetic retinopathy without macular edema, left eye	18	Diabetes with Chronic Complications	19	0.302	0.351	0.340	0.423	0.326	0.373	0.440
E10.3293	Type 1 diabetes mellitus with mild nonproliferative diabetic retinopathy without macular edema, bilateral	18	Diabetes with Chronic Complications	19	0.302	0.351	0.340	0.423	0.326	0.373	0.440
E10.3299	Type 1 diabetes mellitus with mild nonproliferative diabetic retinopathy without macular edema, unspecified eye	18	Diabetes with Chronic Complications	19	0.302	0.351	0.340	0.423	0.326	0.373	0.440
E10.3311	Type 1 diabetes mellitus with moderate nonproliferative diabetic retinopathy with macular edema, right eye	18	Diabetes with Chronic Complications	19	0.302	0.351	0.340	0.423	0.326	0.373	0.440
E10.3312	Type 1 diabetes mellitus with moderate nonproliferative diabetic retinopathy with macular edema, left eye	18	Diabetes with Chronic Complications	19	0.302	0.351	0.340	0.423	0.326	0.373	0.440
E10.3313	Type 1 diabetes mellitus with moderate nonproliferative diabetic retinopathy with macular edema, bilateral	18	Diabetes with Chronic Complications	19	0.302	0.351	0.340	0.423	0.326	0.373	0.440
E10.3319	Type 1 diabetes mellitus with moderate nonproliferative diabetic retinopathy with macular edema, unspecified eye	18	Diabetes with Chronic Complications	19	0.302	0.351	0.340	0.423	0.326	0.373	0.440
E10.3391	Type 1 diabetes mellitus with moderate nonproliferative diabetic retinopathy without macular edema, right eye	18	Diabetes with Chronic Complications	19	0.302	0.351	0.340	0.423	0.326	0.373	0.440
E10.3392	Type 1 diabetes mellitus with moderate nonproliferative diabetic retinopathy without macular edema, left eye	18	Diabetes with Chronic Complications	19	0.302	0.351	0.340	0.423	0.326	0.373	0.440
E10.3393	Type 1 diabetes mellitus with moderate nonproliferative diabetic retinopathy without macular edema, bilateral	18	Diabetes with Chronic Complications	19	0.302	0.351	0.340	0.423	0.326	0.373	0.440
E10.3399	Type 1 diabetes mellitus with moderate nonproliferative diabetic retinopathy without macular edema, unspecified eye	18	Diabetes with Chronic Complications	19	0.302	0.351	0.340	0.423	0.326	0.373	0.440

ICD-10-CM Code	ICD-10-CM Code Description	V24 CMS-HCC	V24 CMS-HCC Disease Group	V24 CMS-HCC Hierarchies	Community, NonDual, Aged	Community, NonDual, Disabled	Community, FBDual, Aged	Community, FBDual, Disabled	Community, PBDual, Aged	Community, PBDual, Disabled	Institutional
E10.3411	Type 1 diabetes mellitus with severe nonproliferative diabetic retinopathy with macular edema, right eye	18	Diabetes with Chronic Complications	19	0.302	0.351	0.340	0.423	0.326	0.373	0.440
E10.3412	Type 1 diabetes mellitus with severe nonproliferative diabetic retinopathy with macular edema, left eye	18	Diabetes with Chronic Complications	19	0.302	0.351	0.340	0.423	0.326	0.373	0.440
E10.3413	Type 1 diabetes mellitus with severe nonproliferative diabetic retinopathy with macular edema, bilateral	18	Diabetes with Chronic Complications	19	0.302	0.351	0.340	0.423	0.326	0.373	0.440
E10.3419	Type 1 diabetes mellitus with severe nonproliferative diabetic retinopathy with macular edema, unspecified eye	18	Diabetes with Chronic Complications	19	0.302	0.351	0.340	0.423	0.326	0.373	0.440
E10.3491	Type 1 diabetes mellitus with severe nonproliferative diabetic retinopathy without macular edema, right eye	18	Diabetes with Chronic Complications	19	0.302	0.351	0.340	0.423	0.326	0.373	0.440
E10.3492	Type 1 diabetes mellitus with severe nonproliferative diabetic retinopathy without macular edema, left eye	18	Diabetes with Chronic Complications	19	0.302	0.351	0.340	0.423	0.326	0.373	0.440
E10.3493	Type 1 diabetes mellitus with severe nonproliferative diabetic retinopathy without macular edema, bilateral	18	Diabetes with Chronic Complications	19	0.302	0.351	0.340	0.423	0.326	0.373	0.440
E10.3499	Type 1 diabetes mellitus with severe nonproliferative diabetic retinopathy without macular edema, unspecified eye	18	Diabetes with Chronic Complications	19	0.302	0.351	0.340	0.423	0.326	0.373	0.440
E10.3511	Type 1 diabetes mellitus with proliferative diabetic retinopathy with macular edema, right eye	18	Diabetes with Chronic Complications	19	0.302	0.351	0.340	0.423	0.326	0.373	0.440
E10.3511	Type 1 diabetes mellitus with proliferative diabetic retinopathy with macular edema, right eye	122	Proliferative Diabetic Retinopathy and Vitreous Hemorrhage		0.222	0.231	0.271	0.269	0.182	0.201	0.394
E10.3512	Type 1 diabetes mellitus with proliferative diabetic retinopathy with macular edema, left eye	18	Diabetes with Chronic Complications	19	0.302	0.351	0.340	0.423	0.326	0.373	0.440
E10.3512	Type 1 diabetes mellitus with proliferative diabetic retinopathy with macular edema, left eye	122	Proliferative Diabetic Retinopathy and Vitreous Hemorrhage		0.222	0.231	0.271	0.269	0.182	0.201	0.394
E10.3513	Type 1 diabetes mellitus with proliferative diabetic retinopathy with macular edema, bilateral	18	Diabetes with Chronic Complications	19	0.302	0.351	0.340	0.423	0.326	0.373	0.440
E10.3513	Type 1 diabetes mellitus with proliferative diabetic retinopathy with macular edema, bilateral	122	Proliferative Diabetic Retinopathy and Vitreous Hemorrhage		0.222	0.231	0.271	0.269	0.182	0.201	0.394
E10.3519	Type 1 diabetes mellitus with proliferative diabetic retinopathy with macular edema, unspecified eye	18	Diabetes with Chronic Complications	19	0.302	0.351	0.340	0.423	0.326	0.373	0.440
E10.3519	Type 1 diabetes mellitus with proliferative diabetic retinopathy with macular edema, unspecified eye	122	Proliferative Diabetic Retinopathy and Vitreous Hemorrhage		0.222	0.231	0.271	0.269	0.182	0.201	0.394
E10.3521	Type 1 diabetes mellitus with proliferative diabetic retinopathy with traction retinal detachment involving the macula, right eye	18	Diabetes with Chronic Complications	19	0.302	0.351	0.340	0.423	0.326	0.373	0.440
E10.3521	Type 1 diabetes mellitus with proliferative diabetic retinopathy with traction retinal detachment involving the macula, right eye	122	Proliferative Diabetic Retinopathy and Vitreous Hemorrhage		0.222	0.231	0.271	0.269	0.182	0.201	0.394
E10.3522	Type 1 diabetes mellitus with proliferative diabetic retinopathy with traction retinal detachment involving the macula, left eye	18	Diabetes with Chronic Complications	19	0.302	0.351	0.340	0.423	0.326	0.373	0.440

ICD-10-CM Code	ICD-10-CM Code Description	V24 CMS-HCC	V24 CMS-HCC Disease Group	V24 CMS-HCC Hierarchies	Community, NonDual, Aged	Community, NonDual, Disabled	Community, FBDual, Aged	Community, FBDual, Disabled	Community, PBDual, Aged	Community, PBDual, Disabled	Institutional
E10.3522	Type 1 diabetes mellitus with proliferative diabetic retinopathy with traction retinal detachment involving the macula, left eye	122	Proliferative Diabetic Retinopathy and Vitreous Hemorrhage		0.222	0.231	0.271	0.269	0.182	0.201	0.394
E10.3523	Type 1 diabetes mellitus with proliferative diabetic retinopathy with traction retinal detachment involving the macula, bilateral	18	Diabetes with Chronic Complications	19	0.302	0.351	0.340	0.423	0.326	0.373	0.440
E10.3523	Type 1 diabetes mellitus with proliferative diabetic retinopathy with traction retinal detachment involving the macula, bilateral	122	Proliferative Diabetic Retinopathy and Vitreous Hemorrhage		0.222	0.231	0.271	0.269	0.182	0.201	0.394
E10.3529	Type 1 diabetes mellitus with proliferative diabetic retinopathy with traction retinal detachment involving the macula, unspecified eye	18	Diabetes with Chronic Complications	19	0.302	0.351	0.340	0.423	0.326	0.373	0.440
E10.3529	Type 1 diabetes mellitus with proliferative diabetic retinopathy with traction retinal detachment involving the macula, unspecified eye	122	Proliferative Diabetic Retinopathy and Vitreous Hemorrhage		0.222	0.231	0.271	0.269	0.182	0.201	0.394
E10.3531	Type 1 diabetes mellitus with proliferative diabetic retinopathy with traction retinal detachment not involving the macula, right eye	18	Diabetes with Chronic Complications	19	0.302	0.351	0.340	0.423	0.326	0.373	0.440
E10.3531	Type 1 diabetes mellitus with proliferative diabetic retinopathy with traction retinal detachment not involving the macula, right eye	122	Proliferative Diabetic Retinopathy and Vitreous Hemorrhage		0.222	0.231	0.271	0.269	0.182	0.201	0.394
E10.3532	Type 1 diabetes mellitus with proliferative diabetic retinopathy with traction retinal detachment not involving the macula, left eye	18	Diabetes with Chronic Complications	19	0.302	0.351	0.340	0.423	0.326	0.373	0.440
E10.3532	Type 1 diabetes mellitus with proliferative diabetic retinopathy with traction retinal detachment not involving the macula, left eye	122	Proliferative Diabetic Retinopathy and Vitreous Hemorrhage		0.222	0.231	0.271	0.269	0.182	0.201	0.394
E10.3533	Type 1 diabetes mellitus with proliferative diabetic retinopathy with traction retinal detachment not involving the macula, bilateral	18	Diabetes with Chronic Complications	19	0.302	0.351	0.340	0.423	0.326	0.373	0.440
E10.3533	Type 1 diabetes mellitus with proliferative diabetic retinopathy with traction retinal detachment not involving the macula, bilateral	122	Proliferative Diabetic Retinopathy and Vitreous Hemorrhage		0.222	0.231	0.271	0.269	0.182	0.201	0.394
E10.3539	Type 1 diabetes mellitus with proliferative diabetic retinopathy with traction retinal detachment not involving the macula, unspecified eye	18	Diabetes with Chronic Complications	19	0.302	0.351	0.340	0.423	0.326	0.373	0.440
E10.3539	Type 1 diabetes mellitus with proliferative diabetic retinopathy with traction retinal detachment not involving the macula, unspecified eye	122	Proliferative Diabetic Retinopathy and Vitreous Hemorrhage		0.222	0.231	0.271	0.269	0.182	0.201	0.394
E10.3541	Type 1 diabetes mellitus with proliferative diabetic retinopathy with combined traction retinal detachment and rhegmatogenous retinal detachment, right eye	18	Diabetes with Chronic Complications	19	0.302	0.351	0.340	0.423	0.326	0.373	0.440
E10.3541	Type 1 diabetes mellitus with proliferative diabetic retinopathy with combined traction retinal detachment and rhegmatogenous retinal detachment, right eye	122	Proliferative Diabetic Retinopathy and Vitreous Hemorrhage		0.222	0.231	0.271	0.269	0.182	0.201	0.394

2021 Optum360, LLC

ICD-10-CM Code	ICD-10-CM Code Description	V24 CMS-HCC	V24 CMS-HCC Disease Group	V24 CMS-HCC Hierarchies	Community, NonDual, Aged	Community, NonDual, Disabled	Community, FBDual, Aged	Community, FBDual, Disabled	Community, PBDual, Aged	Community, PBDual, Disabled	Institutional
E10.3542	Type 1 diabetes mellitus with proliferative diabetic retinopathy with combined traction retinal detachment and rhegmatogenous retinal detachment, left eye	18	Diabetes with Chronic Complications	19	0.302	0.351	0.340	0.423	0.326	0.373	0.440
E10.3542	Type 1 diabetes mellitus with proliferative diabetic retinopathy with combined traction retinal detachment and rhegmatogenous retinal detachment, left eye	122	Proliferative Diabetic Retinopathy and Vitreous Hemorrhage		0.222	0.231	0.271	0.269	0.182	0.201	0.394
E10.3543	Type 1 diabetes mellitus with proliferative diabetic retinopathy with combined traction retinal detachment and rhegmatogenous retinal detachment, bilateral	18	Diabetes with Chronic Complications	19	0.302	0.351	0.340	0.423	0.326	0.373	0.440
E10.3543	Type 1 diabetes mellitus with proliferative diabetic retinopathy with combined traction retinal detachment and rhegmatogenous retinal detachment, bilateral	122	Proliferative Diabetic Retinopathy and Vitreous Hemorrhage		0.222	0.231	0.271	0.269	0.182	0.201	0.394
E10.3549	Type 1 diabetes mellitus with proliferative diabetic retinopathy with combined traction retinal detachment and rhegmatogenous retinal detachment, unspecified eye	18	Diabetes with Chronic Complications	19	0.302	0.351	0.340	0.423	0.326	0.373	0.440
E10.3549	Type 1 diabetes mellitus with proliferative diabetic retinopathy with combined traction retinal detachment and rhegmatogenous retinal detachment, unspecified eye	122	Proliferative Diabetic Retinopathy and Vitreous Hemorrhage		0.222	0.231	0.271	0.269	0.182	0.201	0.394
E10.3551	Type 1 diabetes mellitus with stable proliferative diabetic retinopathy, right eye	18	Diabetes with Chronic Complications	19	0.302	0.351	0.340	0.423	0.326	0.373	0.440
E10.3551	Type 1 diabetes mellitus with stable proliferative diabetic retinopathy, right eye	122	Proliferative Diabetic Retinopathy and Vitreous Hemorrhage		0.222	0.231	0.271	0.269	0.182	0.201	0.394
E10.3552	Type 1 diabetes mellitus with stable proliferative diabetic retinopathy, left eye	18	Diabetes with Chronic Complications	19	0.302	0.351	0.340	0.423	0.326	0.373	0.440
E10.3552	Type 1 diabetes mellitus with stable proliferative diabetic retinopathy, left eye	122	Proliferative Diabetic Retinopathy and Vitreous Hemorrhage		0.222	0.231	0.271	0.269	0.182	0.201	0.394
E10.3553	Type 1 diabetes mellitus with stable proliferative diabetic retinopathy, bilateral	18	Diabetes with Chronic Complications	19	0.302	0.351	0.340	0.423	0.326	0.373	0.440
E10.3553	Type 1 diabetes mellitus with stable proliferative diabetic retinopathy, bilateral	122	Proliferative Diabetic Retinopathy and Vitreous Hemorrhage		0.222	0.231	0.271	0.269	0.182	0.201	0.394
E10.3559	Type 1 diabetes mellitus with stable proliferative diabetic retinopathy, unspecified eye	18	Diabetes with Chronic Complications	19	0.302	0.351	0.340	0.423	0.326	0.373	0.440
E10.3559	Type 1 diabetes mellitus with stable proliferative diabetic retinopathy, unspecified eye	122	Proliferative Diabetic Retinopathy and Vitreous Hemorrhage		0.222	0.231	0.271	0.269	0.182	0.201	0.394
E10.3591	Type 1 diabetes mellitus with proliferative diabetic retinopathy without macular edema, right eye	18	Diabetes with Chronic Complications	19	0.302	0.351	0.340	0.423	0.326	0.373	0.440
E10.3591	Type 1 diabetes mellitus with proliferative diabetic retinopathy without macular edema, right eye	122	Proliferative Diabetic Retinopathy and Vitreous Hemorrhage		0.222	0.231	0.271	0.269	0.182	0.201	0.394
E10.3592	Type 1 diabetes mellitus with proliferative diabetic retinopathy without macular edema, left eye	18	Diabetes with Chronic Complications	19	0.302	0.351	0.340	0.423	0.326	0.373	0.440

ICD-10-CM Code	ICD-10-CM Code Description	V24 CMS-HCC	V24 CMS-HCC Disease Group	V24 CMS-HCC Hierarchies	Community, NonDual, Aged	Community, NonDual, Disabled	Community, FBDual, Aged	Community, FBDual, Disabled	Community, PBDual, Aged	Community, PBDual, Disabled	Institutional
E10.3592	Type 1 diabetes mellitus with proliferative diabetic retinopathy without macular edema, left eye	122	Proliferative Diabetic Retinopathy and Vitreous Hemorrhage		0.222	0.231	0.271	0.269	0.182	0.201	0.394
E10.3593	Type 1 diabetes mellitus with proliferative diabetic retinopathy without macular edema, bilateral	18	Diabetes with Chronic Complications	19	0.302	0.351	0.340	0.423	0.326	0.373	0.440
E10.3593	Type 1 diabetes mellitus with proliferative diabetic retinopathy without macular edema, bilateral	122	Proliferative Diabetic Retinopathy and Vitreous Hemorrhage		0.222	0.231	0.271	0.269	0.182	0.201	0.394
E10.3599	Type 1 diabetes mellitus with proliferative diabetic retinopathy without macular edema, unspecified eye	18	Diabetes with Chronic Complications	19	0.302	0.351	0.340	0.423	0.326	0.373	0.440
E10.3599	Type 1 diabetes mellitus with proliferative diabetic retinopathy without macular edema, unspecified eye	122	Proliferative Diabetic Retinopathy and Vitreous Hemorrhage		0.222	0.231	0.271	0.269	0.182	0.201	0.394
E10.36	Type 1 diabetes mellitus with diabetic cataract	18	Diabetes with Chronic Complications	19	0.302	0.351	0.340	0.423	0.326	0.373	0.440
E10.37X1	Type 1 diabetes mellitus with diabetic macular edema, resolved following treatment, right eye	18	Diabetes with Chronic Complications	19	0.302	0.351	0.340	0.423	0.326	0.373	0.440
E10.37X2	Type 1 diabetes mellitus with diabetic macular edema, resolved following treatment, left eye	18	Diabetes with Chronic Complications	19	0.302	0.351	0.340	0.423	0.326	0.373	0.440
E10.37X3	Type 1 diabetes mellitus with diabetic macular edema, resolved following treatment, bilateral	18	Diabetes with Chronic Complications	19	0.302	0.351	0.340	0.423	0.326	0.373	0.440
E10.37X9	Type 1 diabetes mellitus with diabetic macular edema, resolved following treatment, unspecified eye	18	Diabetes with Chronic Complications	19	0.302	0.351	0.340	0.423	0.326	0.373	0.440
E10.39	Type 1 diabetes mellitus with other diabetic ophthalmic complication	18	Diabetes with Chronic Complications	19	0.302	0.351	0.340	0.423	0.326	0.373	0.440
E10.40	Type 1 diabetes mellitus with diabetic neuropathy, unspecified	18	Diabetes with Chronic Complications	19	0.302	0.351	0.340	0.423	0.326	0.373	0.440
E10.41	Type 1 diabetes mellitus with diabetic mononeuropathy	18	Diabetes with Chronic Complications	19	0.302	0.351	0.340	0.423	0.326	0.373	0.440
E10.42	Type 1 diabetes mellitus with diabetic polyneuropathy	18	Diabetes with Chronic Complications	19	0.302	0.351	0.340	0.423	0.326	0.373	0.440
E10.43	Type 1 diabetes mellitus with diabetic autonomic (poly)neuropathy	18	Diabetes with Chronic Complications	19	0.302	0.351	0.340	0.423	0.326	0.373	0.440
E10.44	Type 1 diabetes mellitus with diabetic amyotrophy	18	Diabetes with Chronic Complications	19	0.302	0.351	0.340	0.423	0.326	0.373	0.440
E10.49	Type 1 diabetes mellitus with other diabetic neurological complication	18	Diabetes with Chronic Complications	19	0.302	0.351	0.340	0.423	0.326	0.373	0.440
E10.51	Type 1 diabetes mellitus with diabetic peripheral angiopathy without gangrene	18	Diabetes with Chronic Complications	19	0.302	0.351	0.340	0.423	0.326	0.373	0.440
E10.51	Type 1 diabetes mellitus with diabetic peripheral angiopathy without gangrene	108	Vascular Disease		0.288	0.301	0.294	0.267	0.297	0.314	0.093
E10.52	Type 1 diabetes mellitus with diabetic peripheral angiopathy with gangrene	18	Diabetes with Chronic Complications	19	0.302	0.351	0.340	0.423	0.326	0.373	0.440
E10.52	Type 1 diabetes mellitus with diabetic peripheral angiopathy with gangrene	106	Atherosclerosis of the Extremities with Ulceration or Gangrene	107,108, 161,189	1.488	1.521	1.724	1.748	1.504	1.525	0.867
E10.59	Type 1 diabetes mellitus with other circulatory complications	18	Diabetes with Chronic Complications	19	0.302	0.351	0.340	0.423	0.326	0.373	0.440
E10.610	Type 1 diabetes mellitus with diabetic neuropathic arthropathy	18	Diabetes with Chronic Complications	19	0.302	0.351	0.340	0.423	0.326	0.373	0.440

ICD-10-CM Code	ICD-10-CM Code Description	V24 CMS-HCC	V24 CMS-HCC Disease Group	V24 CMS-HCC Hierarchies	Community, NonDual, Aged	Community, NonDual, Disabled	Community, FBDual, Aged	Community, FBDual, Disabled	Community, PBDual, Aged	Community, PBDual, Disabled	Institutional
E10.618	Type 1 diabetes mellitus with other diabetic arthropathy	18	Diabetes with Chronic Complications	19	0.302	0.351	0.340	0.423	0.326	0.373	0.440
E10.620	Type 1 diabetes mellitus with diabetic dermatitis	18	Diabetes with Chronic Complications	19	0.302	0.351	0.340	0.423	0.326	0.373	0.440
E10.621	Type 1 diabetes mellitus with foot ulcer	18	Diabetes with Chronic Complications	19	0.302	0.351	0.340	0.423	0.326	0.373	0.440
E10.621	Type 1 diabetes mellitus with foot ulcer	161	Chronic Ulcer of Skin, Except Pressure		0.515	0.592	0.727	0.583	0.541	0.542	0.294
E10.622	Type 1 diabetes mellitus with other skin ulcer	18	Diabetes with Chronic Complications	19	0.302	0.351	0.340	0.423	0.326	0.373	0.440
E10.622	Type 1 diabetes mellitus with other skin ulcer	161	Chronic Ulcer of Skin, Except Pressure		0.515	0.592	0.727	0.583	0.541	0.542	0.294
E10.628	Type 1 diabetes mellitus with other skin complications	18	Diabetes with Chronic Complications	19	0.302	0.351	0.340	0.423	0.326	0.373	0.440
E10.630	Type 1 diabetes mellitus with periodontal disease	18	Diabetes with Chronic Complications	19	0.302	0.351	0.340	0.423	0.326	0.373	0.440
E10.638	Type 1 diabetes mellitus with other oral complications	18	Diabetes with Chronic Complications	19	0.302	0.351	0.340	0.423	0.326	0.373	0.440
E10.641	Type 1 diabetes mellitus with hypoglycemia with coma	17	Diabetes with Acute Complications	18,19	0.302	0.351	0.340	0.423	0.326	0.373	0.440
E10.649	Type 1 diabetes mellitus with hypoglycemia without coma	18	Diabetes with Chronic Complications	19	0.302	0.351	0.340	0.423	0.326	0.373	0.440
E10.65	Type 1 diabetes mellitus with hyperglycemia	18	Diabetes with Chronic Complications	19	0.302	0.351	0.340	0.423	0.326	0.373	0.440
E10.69	Type 1 diabetes mellitus with other specified complication	18	Diabetes with Chronic Complications	19	0.302	0.351	0.340	0.423	0.326	0.373	0.440
E10.8	Type 1 diabetes mellitus with unspecified complications	18	Diabetes with Chronic Complications	19	0.302	0.351	0.340	0.423	0.326	0.373	0.440
E10.9	Type 1 diabetes mellitus without complications	19	Diabetes without Complication		0.105	0.124	0.107	0.145	0.087	0.122	0.178
E11.00	Type 2 diabetes mellitus with hyperosmolarity without nonketotic hyperglycemic-hyperosmolar coma (NKHHC)	17	Diabetes with Acute Complications	18,19	0.302	0.351	0.340	0.423	0.326	0.373	0.440
E11.01	Type 2 diabetes mellitus with hyperosmolarity with coma	17	Diabetes with Acute Complications	18,19	0.302	0.351	0.340	0.423	0.326	0.373	0.440
E11.10	Type 2 diabetes mellitus with ketoacidosis without coma	17	Diabetes with Acute Complications	18,19	0.302	0.351	0.340	0.423	0.326	0.373	0.440
E11.11	Type 2 diabetes mellitus with ketoacidosis with coma	17	Diabetes with Acute Complications	18,19	0.302	0.351	0.340	0.423	0.326	0.373	0.440
E11.21	Type 2 diabetes mellitus with diabetic nephropathy	18	Diabetes with Chronic Complications	19	0.302	0.351	0.340	0.423	0.326	0.373	0.440
E11.22	Type 2 diabetes mellitus with diabetic chronic kidney disease	18	Diabetes with Chronic Complications	19	0.302	0.351	0.340	0.423	0.326	0.373	0.440
E11.29	Type 2 diabetes mellitus with other diabetic kidney complication	18	Diabetes with Chronic Complications	19	0.302	0.351	0.340	0.423	0.326	0.373	0.440
E11.311	Type 2 diabetes mellitus with unspecified diabetic retinopathy with macular edema	18	Diabetes with Chronic Complications	19	0.302	0.351	0.340	0.423	0.326	0.373	0.440
E11.319	Type 2 diabetes mellitus with unspecified diabetic retinopathy without macular edema	18	Diabetes with Chronic Complications	19	0.302	0.351	0.340	0.423	0.326	0.373	0.440
E11.3211	Type 2 diabetes mellitus with mild nonproliferative diabetic retinopathy with macular edema, right eye	18	Diabetes with Chronic Complications	19	0.302	0.351	0.340	0.423	0.326	0.373	0.440
E11.3212	Type 2 diabetes mellitus with mild nonproliferative diabetic retinopathy with macular edema, left eye	18	Diabetes with Chronic Complications	19	0.302	0.351	0.340	0.423	0.326	0.373	0.440

ICD-10-CM Code	ICD-10-CM Code Description	V24 CMS-HCC	V24 CMS-HCC Disease Group	V24 CMS-HCC Hierarchies	Community, NonDual, Aged	Community, NonDual, Disabled	Community, FBDual, Aged	Community, FBDual, Disabled	Community, PBDual, Aged	Community, PBDual, Disabled	Institutional
E11.3213	Type 2 diabetes mellitus with mild nonproliferative diabetic retinopathy with macular edema, bilateral	18	Diabetes with Chronic Complications	19	0.302	0.351	0.340	0.423	0.326	0.373	0.440
E11.3219	Type 2 diabetes mellitus with mild nonproliferative diabetic retinopathy with macular edema, unspecified eye	18	Diabetes with Chronic Complications	19	0.302	0.351	0.340	0.423	0.326	0.373	0.440
E11.3291	Type 2 diabetes mellitus with mild nonproliferative diabetic retinopathy without macular edema, right eye	18	Diabetes with Chronic Complications	19	0.302	0.351	0.340	0.423	0.326	0.373	0.440
E11.3292	Type 2 diabetes mellitus with mild nonproliferative diabetic retinopathy without macular edema, left eye	18	Diabetes with Chronic Complications	19	0.302	0.351	0.340	0.423	0.326	0.373	0.440
E11.3293	Type 2 diabetes mellitus with mild nonproliferative diabetic retinopathy without macular edema, bilateral	18	Diabetes with Chronic Complications	19	0.302	0.351	0.340	0.423	0.326	0.373	0.440
E11.3299	Type 2 diabetes mellitus with mild nonproliferative diabetic retinopathy without macular edema, unspecified eye	18	Diabetes with Chronic Complications	19	0.302	0.351	0.340	0.423	0.326	0.373	0.440
E11.3311	Type 2 diabetes mellitus with moderate nonproliferative diabetic retinopathy with macular edema, right eye	18	Diabetes with Chronic Complications	19	0.302	0.351	0.340	0.423	0.326	0.373	0.440
E11.3312	Type 2 diabetes mellitus with moderate nonproliferative diabetic retinopathy with macular edema, left eye	18	Diabetes with Chronic Complications	19	0.302	0.351	0.340	0.423	0.326	0.373	0.440
E11.3313	Type 2 diabetes mellitus with moderate nonproliferative diabetic retinopathy with macular edema, bilateral	18	Diabetes with Chronic Complications	19	0.302	0.351	0.340	0.423	0.326	0.373	0.440
E11.3319	Type 2 diabetes mellitus with moderate nonproliferative diabetic retinopathy with macular edema, unspecified eye	18	Diabetes with Chronic Complications	19	0.302	0.351	0.340	0.423	0.326	0.373	0.440
E11.3391	Type 2 diabetes mellitus with moderate nonproliferative diabetic retinopathy without macular edema, right eye	18	Diabetes with Chronic Complications	19	0.302	0.351	0.340	0.423	0.326	0.373	0.440
E11.3392	Type 2 diabetes mellitus with moderate nonproliferative diabetic retinopathy without macular edema, left eye	18	Diabetes with Chronic Complications	19	0.302	0.351	0.340	0.423	0.326	0.373	0.440
E11.3393	Type 2 diabetes mellitus with moderate nonproliferative diabetic retinopathy without macular edema, bilateral	18	Diabetes with Chronic Complications	19	0.302	0.351	0.340	0.423	0.326	0.373	0.440
E11.3399	Type 2 diabetes mellitus with moderate nonproliferative diabetic retinopathy without macular edema, unspecified eye	18	Diabetes with Chronic Complications	19	0.302	0.351	0.340	0.423	0.326	0.373	0.440
E11.3411	Type 2 diabetes mellitus with severe nonproliferative diabetic retinopathy with macular edema, right eye	18	Diabetes with Chronic Complications	19	0.302	0.351	0.340	0.423	0.326	0.373	0.440
E11.3412	Type 2 diabetes mellitus with severe nonproliferative diabetic retinopathy with macular edema, left eye	18	Diabetes with Chronic Complications	19	0.302	0.351	0.340	0.423	0.326	0.373	0.440
E11.3413	Type 2 diabetes mellitus with severe nonproliferative diabetic retinopathy with macular edema, bilateral	18	Diabetes with Chronic Complications	19	0.302	0.351	0.340	0.423	0.326	0.373	0.440

ICD-10-CM Code	ICD-10-CM Code Description	V24 CMS-HCC	V24 CMS-HCC Disease Group	V24 CMS-HCC Hierarchies	Community, NonDual, Aged	Community, NonDual, Disabled	Community, FBDual, Aged	Community, FBDual, Disabled	Community, PBDual, Aged	Community, PBDual, Disabled	Institutional
E11.3419	Type 2 diabetes mellitus with severe nonproliferative diabetic retinopathy with macular edema, unspecified eye	18	Diabetes with Chronic Complications	19	0.302	0.351	0.340	0.423	0.326	0.373	0.440
E11.3491	Type 2 diabetes mellitus with severe nonproliferative diabetic retinopathy without macular edema, right eye	18	Diabetes with Chronic Complications	19	0.302	0.351	0.340	0.423	0.326	0.373	0.440
E11.3492	Type 2 diabetes mellitus with severe nonproliferative diabetic retinopathy without macular edema, left eye	18	Diabetes with Chronic Complications	19	0.302	0.351	0.340	0.423	0.326	0.373	0.440
E11.3493	Type 2 diabetes mellitus with severe nonproliferative diabetic retinopathy without macular edema, bilateral	18	Diabetes with Chronic Complications	19	0.302	0.351	0.340	0.423	0.326	0.373	0.440
E11.3499	Type 2 diabetes mellitus with severe nonproliferative diabetic retinopathy without macular edema, unspecified eye	18	Diabetes with Chronic Complications	19	0.302	0.351	0.340	0.423	0.326	0.373	0.440
E11.3511	Type 2 diabetes mellitus with proliferative diabetic retinopathy with macular edema, right eye	18	Diabetes with Chronic Complications	19	0.302	0.351	0.340	0.423	0.326	0.373	0.440
E11.3511	Type 2 diabetes mellitus with proliferative diabetic retinopathy with macular edema, right eye	122	Proliferative Diabetic Retinopathy and Vitreous Hemorrhage		0.222	0.231	0.271	0.269	0.182	0.201	0.394
E11.3512	Type 2 diabetes mellitus with proliferative diabetic retinopathy with macular edema, left eye	18	Diabetes with Chronic Complications	19	0.302	0.351	0.340	0.423	0.326	0.373	0.440
E11.3512	Type 2 diabetes mellitus with proliferative diabetic retinopathy with macular edema, left eye	122	Proliferative Diabetic Retinopathy and Vitreous Hemorrhage		0.222	0.231	0.271	0.269	0.182	0.201	0.394
E11.3513	Type 2 diabetes mellitus with proliferative diabetic retinopathy with macular edema, bilateral	18	Diabetes with Chronic Complications	19	0.302	0.351	0.340	0.423	0.326	0.373	0.440
E11.3513	Type 2 diabetes mellitus with proliferative diabetic retinopathy with macular edema, bilateral	122	Proliferative Diabetic Retinopathy and Vitreous Hemorrhage		0.222	0.231	0.271	0.269	0.182	0.201	0.394
E11.3519	Type 2 diabetes mellitus with proliferative diabetic retinopathy with macular edema, unspecified eye	18	Diabetes with Chronic Complications	19	0.302	0.351	0.340	0.423	0.326	0.373	0.440
E11.3519	Type 2 diabetes mellitus with proliferative diabetic retinopathy with macular edema, unspecified eye	122	Proliferative Diabetic Retinopathy and Vitreous Hemorrhage		0.222	0.231	0.271	0.269	0.182	0.201	0.394
E11.3521	Type 2 diabetes mellitus with proliferative diabetic retinopathy with traction retinal detachment involving the macula, right eye	18	Diabetes with Chronic Complications	19	0.302	0.351	0.340	0.423	0.326	0.373	0.440
E11.3521	Type 2 diabetes mellitus with proliferative diabetic retinopathy with traction retinal detachment involving the macula, right eye	122	Proliferative Diabetic Retinopathy and Vitreous Hemorrhage		0.222	0.231	0.271	0.269	0.182	0.201	0.394
E11.3522	Type 2 diabetes mellitus with proliferative diabetic retinopathy with traction retinal detachment involving the macula, left eye	18	Diabetes with Chronic Complications	19	0.302	0.351	0.340	0.423	0.326	0.373	0.440
E11.3522	Type 2 diabetes mellitus with proliferative diabetic retinopathy with traction retinal detachment involving the macula, left eye	122	Proliferative Diabetic Retinopathy and Vitreous Hemorrhage		0.222	0.231	0.271	0.269	0.182	0.201	0.394
E11.3523	Type 2 diabetes mellitus with proliferative diabetic retinopathy with traction retinal detachment involving the macula, bilateral	18	Diabetes with Chronic Complications	19	0.302	0.351	0.340	0.423	0.326	0.373	0.440

ICD-10-CM Code	ICD-10-CM Code Description	V24 CMS-HCC	V24 CMS-HCC Disease Group	V24 CMS-HCC Hierarchies	Community, NonDual, Aged	Community, NonDual, Disabled	Community, FBDual, Aged	Community, FBDual, Disabled	Community, PBDual, Aged	Community, PBDual, Disabled	Institutional
E11.3523	Type 2 diabetes mellitus with proliferative diabetic retinopathy with traction retinal detachment involving the macula, bilateral	122	Proliferative Diabetic Retinopathy and Vitreous Hemorrhage		0.222	0.231	0.271	0.269	0.182	0.201	0.394
E11.3529	Type 2 diabetes mellitus with proliferative diabetic retinopathy with traction retinal detachment involving the macula, unspecified eye	18	Diabetes with Chronic Complications	19	0.302	0.351	0.340	0.423	0.326	0.373	0.440
E11.3529	Type 2 diabetes mellitus with proliferative diabetic retinopathy with traction retinal detachment involving the macula, unspecified eye	122	Proliferative Diabetic Retinopathy and Vitreous Hemorrhage		0.222	0.231	0.271	0.269	0.182	0.201	0.394
E11.3531	Type 2 diabetes mellitus with proliferative diabetic retinopathy with traction retinal detachment not involving the macula, right eye	18	Diabetes with Chronic Complications	19	0.302	0.351	0.340	0.423	0.326	0.373	0.440
E11.3531	Type 2 diabetes mellitus with proliferative diabetic retinopathy with traction retinal detachment not involving the macula, right eye	122	Proliferative Diabetic Retinopathy and Vitreous Hemorrhage		0.222	0.231	0.271	0.269	0.182	0.201	0.394
E11.3532	Type 2 diabetes mellitus with proliferative diabetic retinopathy with traction retinal detachment not involving the macula, left eye	18	Diabetes with Chronic Complications	19	0.302	0.351	0.340	0.423	0.326	0.373	0.440
E11.3532	Type 2 diabetes mellitus with proliferative diabetic retinopathy with traction retinal detachment not involving the macula, left eye	122	Proliferative Diabetic Retinopathy and Vitreous Hemorrhage		0.222	0.231	0.271	0.269	0.182	0.201	0.394
E11.3533	Type 2 diabetes mellitus with proliferative diabetic retinopathy with traction retinal detachment not involving the macula, bilateral	18	Diabetes with Chronic Complications	19	0.302	0.351	0.340	0.423	0.326	0.373	0.440
E11.3533	Type 2 diabetes mellitus with proliferative diabetic retinopathy with traction retinal detachment not involving the macula, bilateral	122	Proliferative Diabetic Retinopathy and Vitreous Hemorrhage		0.222	0.231	0.271	0.269	0.182	0.201	0.394
E11.3539	Type 2 diabetes mellitus with proliferative diabetic retinopathy with traction retinal detachment not involving the macula, unspecified eye	18	Diabetes with Chronic Complications	19	0.302	0.351	0.340	0.423	0.326	0.373	0.440
E11.3539	Type 2 diabetes mellitus with proliferative diabetic retinopathy with traction retinal detachment not involving the macula, unspecified eye	122	Proliferative Diabetic Retinopathy and Vitreous Hemorrhage		0.222	0.231	0.271	0.269	0.182	0.201	0.394
E11.3541	Type 2 diabetes mellitus with proliferative diabetic retinopathy with combined traction retinal detachment and rhegmatogenous retinal detachment, right eye	18	Diabetes with Chronic Complications	19	0.302	0.351	0.340	0.423	0.326	0.373	0.440
E11.3541	Type 2 diabetes mellitus with proliferative diabetic retinopathy with combined traction retinal detachment and rhegmatogenous retinal detachment, right eye	122	Proliferative Diabetic Retinopathy and Vitreous Hemorrhage		0.222	0.231	0.271	0.269	0.182	0.201	0.394
E11.3542	Type 2 diabetes mellitus with proliferative diabetic retinopathy with combined traction retinal detachment and rhegmatogenous retinal detachment, left eye	18	Diabetes with Chronic Complications	19	0.302	0.351	0.340	0.423	0.326	0.373	0.440

ICD-10-CM Code	ICD-10-CM Code Description	V24 CMS-HCC	V24 CMS-HCC Disease Group	V24 CMS-HCC Hierarchies	Community, NonDual, Aged	Community, NonDual, Disabled	Community, FBDual, Aged	Community, FBDual, Disabled	Community, PBDual, Aged	Community, PBDual, Disabled	Institutional
E11.3542	Type 2 diabetes mellitus with proliferative diabetic retinopathy with combined traction retinal detachment and rhegmatogenous retinal detachment, left eye	122	Proliferative Diabetic Retinopathy and Vitreous Hemorrhage		0.222	0.231	0.271	0.269	0.182	0.201	0.394
E11.3543	Type 2 diabetes mellitus with proliferative diabetic retinopathy with combined traction retinal detachment and rhegmatogenous retinal detachment, bilateral	18	Diabetes with Chronic Complications	19	0.302	0.351	0.340	0.423	0.326	0.373	0.440
E11.3543	Type 2 diabetes mellitus with proliferative diabetic retinopathy with combined traction retinal detachment and rhegmatogenous retinal detachment, bilateral	122	Proliferative Diabetic Retinopathy and Vitreous Hemorrhage		0.222	0.231	0.271	0.269	0.182	0.201	0.394
E11.3549	Type 2 diabetes mellitus with proliferative diabetic retinopathy with combined traction retinal detachment and rhegmatogenous retinal detachment, unspecified eye	18	Diabetes with Chronic Complications	19	0.302	0.351	0.340	0.423	0.326	0.373	0.440
E11.3549	Type 2 diabetes mellitus with proliferative diabetic retinopathy with combined traction retinal detachment and rhegmatogenous retinal detachment, unspecified eye	122	Proliferative Diabetic Retinopathy and Vitreous Hemorrhage		0.222	0.231	0.271	0.269	0.182	0.201	0.394
E11.3551	Type 2 diabetes mellitus with stable proliferative diabetic retinopathy, right eye	18	Diabetes with Chronic Complications	19	0.302	0.351	0.340	0.423	0.326	0.373	0.440
E11.3551	Type 2 diabetes mellitus with stable proliferative diabetic retinopathy, right eye	122	Proliferative Diabetic Retinopathy and Vitreous Hemorrhage		0.222	0.231	0.271	0.269	0.182	0.201	0.394
E11.3552	Type 2 diabetes mellitus with stable proliferative diabetic retinopathy, left eye	18	Diabetes with Chronic Complications	19	0.302	0.351	0.340	0.423	0.326	0.373	0.440
E11.3552	Type 2 diabetes mellitus with stable proliferative diabetic retinopathy, left eye	122	Proliferative Diabetic Retinopathy and Vitreous Hemorrhage		0.222	0.231	0.271	0.269	0.182	0.201	0.394
E11.3553	Type 2 diabetes mellitus with stable proliferative diabetic retinopathy, bilateral	18	Diabetes with Chronic Complications	19	0.302	0.351	0.340	0.423	0.326	0.373	0.440
E11.3553	Type 2 diabetes mellitus with stable proliferative diabetic retinopathy, bilateral	122	Proliferative Diabetic Retinopathy and Vitreous Hemorrhage		0.222	0.231	0.271	0.269	0.182	0.201	0.394
E11.3559	Type 2 diabetes mellitus with stable proliferative diabetic retinopathy, unspecified eye	18	Diabetes with Chronic Complications	19	0.302	0.351	0.340	0.423	0.326	0.373	0.440
E11.3559	Type 2 diabetes mellitus with stable proliferative diabetic retinopathy, unspecified eye	122	Proliferative Diabetic Retinopathy and Vitreous Hemorrhage		0.222	0.231	0.271	0.269	0.182	0.201	0.394
E11.3591	Type 2 diabetes mellitus with proliferative diabetic retinopathy without macular edema, right eye	18	Diabetes with Chronic Complications	19	0.302	0.351	0.340	0.423	0.326	0.373	0.440
E11.3591	Type 2 diabetes mellitus with proliferative diabetic retinopathy without macular edema, right eye	122	Proliferative Diabetic Retinopathy and Vitreous Hemorrhage		0.222	0.231	0.271	0.269	0.182	0.201	0.394
E11.3592	Type 2 diabetes mellitus with proliferative diabetic retinopathy without macular edema, left eye	18	Diabetes with Chronic Complications	19	0.302	0.351	0.340	0.423	0.326	0.373	0.440
E11.3592	Type 2 diabetes mellitus with proliferative diabetic retinopathy without macular edema, left eye	122	Proliferative Diabetic Retinopathy and Vitreous Hemorrhage		0.222	0.231	0.271	0.269	0.182	0.201	0.394

ICD-10-CM Code	ICD-10-CM Code Description	V24 CMS-HCC	V24 CMS-HCC Disease Group	V24 CMS-HCC Hierarchies	Community, NonDual, Aged	Community, NonDual, Disabled	Community, FBDual, Aged	Community, FBDual, Disabled	Community, PBDual, Aged	Community, PBDual, Disabled	Institutional
E11.3593	Type 2 diabetes mellitus with proliferative diabetic retinopathy without macular edema, bilateral	18	Diabetes with Chronic Complications	19	0.302	0.351	0.340	0.423	0.326	0.373	0.440
E11.3593	Type 2 diabetes mellitus with proliferative diabetic retinopathy without macular edema, bilateral	122	Proliferative Diabetic Retinopathy and Vitreous Hemorrhage		0.222	0.231	0.271	0.269	0.182	0.201	0.394
E11.3599	Type 2 diabetes mellitus with proliferative diabetic retinopathy without macular edema, unspecified eye	18	Diabetes with Chronic Complications	19	0.302	0.351	0.340	0.423	0.326	0.373	0.440
E11.3599	Type 2 diabetes mellitus with proliferative diabetic retinopathy without macular edema, unspecified eye	122	Proliferative Diabetic Retinopathy and Vitreous Hemorrhage		0.222	0.231	0.271	0.269	0.182	0.201	0.394
E11.36	Type 2 diabetes mellitus with diabetic cataract	18	Diabetes with Chronic Complications	19	0.302	0.351	0.340	0.423	0.326	0.373	0.440
E11.37X1	Type 2 diabetes mellitus with diabetic macular edema, resolved following treatment, right eye	18	Diabetes with Chronic Complications	19	0.302	0.351	0.340	0.423	0.326	0.373	0.440
E11.37X2	Type 2 diabetes mellitus with diabetic macular edema, resolved following treatment, left eye	18	Diabetes with Chronic Complications	19	0.302	0.351	0.340	0.423	0.326	0.373	0.440
E11.37X3	Type 2 diabetes mellitus with diabetic macular edema, resolved following treatment, bilateral	18	Diabetes with Chronic Complications	19	0.302	0.351	0.340	0.423	0.326	0.373	0.440
E11.37X9	Type 2 diabetes mellitus with diabetic macular edema, resolved following treatment, unspecified eye	18	Diabetes with Chronic Complications	19	0.302	0.351	0.340	0.423	0.326	0.373	0.440
E11.39	Type 2 diabetes mellitus with other diabetic ophthalmic complication	18	Diabetes with Chronic Complications	19	0.302	0.351	0.340	0.423	0.326	0.373	0.440
E11.40	Type 2 diabetes mellitus with diabetic neuropathy, unspecified	18	Diabetes with Chronic Complications	19	0.302	0.351	0.340	0.423	0.326	0.373	0.440
E11.41	Type 2 diabetes mellitus with diabetic mononeuropathy	18	Diabetes with Chronic Complications	19	0.302	0.351	0.340	0.423	0.326	0.373	0.440
E11.42	Type 2 diabetes mellitus with diabetic polyneuropathy	18	Diabetes with Chronic Complications	19	0.302	0.351	0.340	0.423	0.326	0.373	0.440
E11.43	Type 2 diabetes mellitus with diabetic autonomic (poly)neuropathy	18	Diabetes with Chronic Complications	19	0.302	0.351	0.340	0.423	0.326	0.373	0.440
E11.44	Type 2 diabetes mellitus with diabetic amyotrophy	18	Diabetes with Chronic Complications	19	0.302	0.351	0.340	0.423	0.326	0.373	0.440
E11.49	Type 2 diabetes mellitus with other diabetic neurological complication	18	Diabetes with Chronic Complications	19	0.302	0.351	0.340	0.423	0.326	0.373	0.440
E11.51	Type 2 diabetes mellitus with diabetic peripheral angiopathy without gangrene	18	Diabetes with Chronic Complications	19	0.302	0.351	0.340	0.423	0.326	0.373	0.440
E11.51	Type 2 diabetes mellitus with diabetic peripheral angiopathy without gangrene	108	Vascular Disease		0.288	0.301	0.294	0.267	0.297	0.314	0.093
E11.52	Type 2 diabetes mellitus with diabetic peripheral angiopathy with gangrene	18	Diabetes with Chronic Complications	19	0.302	0.351	0.340	0.423	0.326	0.373	0.440
E11.52	Type 2 diabetes mellitus with diabetic peripheral angiopathy with gangrene	106	Atherosclerosis of the Extremities with Ulceration or Gangrene	107,108, 161,189	1.488	1.521	1.724	1.748	1.504	1.525	0.867
E11.59	Type 2 diabetes mellitus with other circulatory complications	18	Diabetes with Chronic Complications	19	0.302	0.351	0.340	0.423	0.326	0.373	0.440
E11.610	Type 2 diabetes mellitus with diabetic neuropathic arthropathy	18	Diabetes with Chronic Complications	19	0.302	0.351	0.340	0.423	0.326	0.373	0.440
E11.618	Type 2 diabetes mellitus with other diabetic arthropathy	18	Diabetes with Chronic Complications	19	0.302	0.351	0.340	0.423	0.326	0.373	0.440
E11.620	Type 2 diabetes mellitus with diabetic dermatitis	18	Diabetes with Chronic Complications	19	0.302	0.351	0.340	0.423	0.326	0.373	0.440

ICD-10-CM Code	ICD-10-CM Code Description	V24 CMS-HCC	V24 CMS-HCC Disease Group	V24 CMS-HCC Hierarchies	Community, NonDual, Aged	Community, NonDual, Disabled	Community, FBDual, Aged	Community, FBDual, Disabled	Community, PBDual, Aged	Community, PBDual, Disabled	Institutional
E11.621	Type 2 diabetes mellitus with foot ulcer	18	Diabetes with Chronic Complications	19	0.302	0.351	0.340	0.423	0.326	0.373	0.440
E11.621	Type 2 diabetes mellitus with foot ulcer	161	Chronic Ulcer of Skin, Except Pressure		0.515	0.592	0.727	0.583	0.541	0.542	0.294
E11.622	Type 2 diabetes mellitus with other skin ulcer	18	Diabetes with Chronic Complications	19	0.302	0.351	0.340	0.423	0.326	0.373	0.440
E11.622	Type 2 diabetes mellitus with other skin ulcer	161	Chronic Ulcer of Skin, Except Pressure		0.515	0.592	0.727	0.583	0.541	0.542	0.294
E11.628	Type 2 diabetes mellitus with other skin complications	18	Diabetes with Chronic Complications	19	0.302	0.351	0.340	0.423	0.326	0.373	0.440
E11.630	Type 2 diabetes mellitus with periodontal disease	18	Diabetes with Chronic Complications	19	0.302	0.351	0.340	0.423	0.326	0.373	0.440
E11.638	Type 2 diabetes mellitus with other oral complications	18	Diabetes with Chronic Complications	19	0.302	0.351	0.340	0.423	0.326	0.373	0.440
E11.641	Type 2 diabetes mellitus with hypoglycemia with coma	17	Diabetes with Acute Complications	18,19	0.302	0.351	0.340	0.423	0.326	0.373	0.440
E11.649	Type 2 diabetes mellitus with hypoglycemia without coma	18	Diabetes with Chronic Complications	19	0.302	0.351	0.340	0.423	0.326	0.373	0.440
E11.65	Type 2 diabetes mellitus with hyperglycemia	18	Diabetes with Chronic Complications	19	0.302	0.351	0.340	0.423	0.326	0.373	0.440
E11.69	Type 2 diabetes mellitus with other specified complication	18	Diabetes with Chronic Complications	19	0.302	0.351	0.340	0.423	0.326	0.373	0.440
E11.8	Type 2 diabetes mellitus with unspecified complications	18	Diabetes with Chronic Complications	19	0.302	0.351	0.340	0.423	0.326	0.373	0.440
E11.9	Type 2 diabetes mellitus without complications	19	Diabetes without Complication		0.105	0.124	0.107	0.145	0.087	0.122	0.178
E13.00	Other specified diabetes mellitus with hyperosmolarity without nonketotic hyperglycemic-hyperosmolar coma (NKHHC)	17	Diabetes with Acute Complications	18,19	0.302	0.351	0.340	0.423	0.326	0.373	0.440
E13.01	Other specified diabetes mellitus with hyperosmolarity with coma	17	Diabetes with Acute Complications	18,19	0.302	0.351	0.340	0.423	0.326	0.373	0.440
E13.10	Other specified diabetes mellitus with ketoacidosis without coma	17	Diabetes with Acute Complications	18,19	0.302	0.351	0.340	0.423	0.326	0.373	0.440
E13.11	Other specified diabetes mellitus with ketoacidosis with coma	17	Diabetes with Acute Complications	18,19	0.302	0.351	0.340	0.423	0.326	0.373	0.440
E13.21	Other specified diabetes mellitus with diabetic nephropathy	18	Diabetes with Chronic Complications	19	0.302	0.351	0.340	0.423	0.326	0.373	0.440
E13.22	Other specified diabetes mellitus with diabetic chronic kidney disease	18	Diabetes with Chronic Complications	19	0.302	0.351	0.340	0.423	0.326	0.373	0.440
E13.29	Other specified diabetes mellitus with other diabetic kidney complication	18	Diabetes with Chronic Complications	19	0.302	0.351	0.340	0.423	0.326	0.373	0.440
E13.311	Other specified diabetes mellitus with unspecified diabetic retinopathy with macular edema	18	Diabetes with Chronic Complications	19	0.302	0.351	0.340	0.423	0.326	0.373	0.440
E13.319	Other specified diabetes mellitus with unspecified diabetic retinopathy without macular edema	18	Diabetes with Chronic Complications	19	0.302	0.351	0.340	0.423	0.326	0.373	0.440
E13.3211	Other specified diabetes mellitus with mild nonproliferative diabetic retinopathy with macular edema, right eye	18	Diabetes with Chronic Complications	19	0.302	0.351	0.340	0.423	0.326	0.373	0.440
E13.3212	Other specified diabetes mellitus with mild nonproliferative diabetic retinopathy with macular edema, left eye	18	Diabetes with Chronic Complications	19	0.302	0.351	0.340	0.423	0.326	0.373	0.440
E13.3213	Other specified diabetes mellitus with mild nonproliferative diabetic retinopathy with macular edema, bilateral	18	Diabetes with Chronic Complications	19	0.302	0.351	0.340	0.423	0.326	0.373	0.440

ICD-10-CM Code	ICD-10-CM Code Description	V24 CMS-HCC	V24 CMS-HCC Disease Group	V24 CMS-HCC Hierarchies	Community, NonDual, Aged	Community, NonDual, Disabled	Community, FBDual, Aged	Community, FBDual, Disabled	Community, PBDual, Aged	Community, PBDual, Disabled	Institutional
E13.3219	Other specified diabetes mellitus with mild nonproliferative diabetic retinopathy with macular edema, unspecified eye	18	Diabetes with Chronic Complications	19	0.302	0.351	0.340	0.423	0.326	0.373	0.440
E13.3291	Other specified diabetes mellitus with mild nonproliferative diabetic retinopathy without macular edema, right eye	18	Diabetes with Chronic Complications	19	0.302	0.351	0.340	0.423	0.326	0.373	0.440
E13.3292	Other specified diabetes mellitus with mild nonproliferative diabetic retinopathy without macular edema, left eye	18	Diabetes with Chronic Complications	19	0.302	0.351	0.340	0.423	0.326	0.373	0.440
E13.3293	Other specified diabetes mellitus with mild nonproliferative diabetic retinopathy without macular edema, bilateral	18	Diabetes with Chronic Complications	19	0.302	0.351	0.340	0.423	0.326	0.373	0.440
E13.3299	Other specified diabetes mellitus with mild nonproliferative diabetic retinopathy without macular edema, unspecified eye	18	Diabetes with Chronic Complications	19	0.302	0.351	0.340	0.423	0.326	0.373	0.440
E13.3311	Other specified diabetes mellitus with moderate nonproliferative diabetic retinopathy with macular edema, right eye	18	Diabetes with Chronic Complications	19	0.302	0.351	0.340	0.423	0.326	0.373	0.440
E13.3312	Other specified diabetes mellitus with moderate nonproliferative diabetic retinopathy with macular edema, left eye	18	Diabetes with Chronic Complications	19	0.302	0.351	0.340	0.423	0.326	0.373	0.440
E13.3313	Other specified diabetes mellitus with moderate nonproliferative diabetic retinopathy with macular edema, bilateral	18	Diabetes with Chronic Complications	19	0.302	0.351	0.340	0.423	0.326	0.373	0.440
E13.3319	Other specified diabetes mellitus with moderate nonproliferative diabetic retinopathy with macular edema, unspecified eye	18	Diabetes with Chronic Complications	19	0.302	0.351	0.340	0.423	0.326	0.373	0.440
E13.3391	Other specified diabetes mellitus with moderate nonproliferative diabetic retinopathy without macular edema, right eye	18	Diabetes with Chronic Complications	19	0.302	0.351	0.340	0.423	0.326	0.373	0.440
E13.3392	Other specified diabetes mellitus with moderate nonproliferative diabetic retinopathy without macular edema, left eye	18	Diabetes with Chronic Complications	19	0.302	0.351	0.340	0.423	0.326	0.373	0.440
E13.3393	Other specified diabetes mellitus with moderate nonproliferative diabetic retinopathy without macular edema, bilateral	18	Diabetes with Chronic Complications	19	0.302	0.351	0.340	0.423	0.326	0.373	0.440
E13.3399	Other specified diabetes mellitus with moderate nonproliferative diabetic retinopathy without macular edema, unspecified eye	18	Diabetes with Chronic Complications	19	0.302	0.351	0.340	0.423	0.326	0.373	0.440
E13.3411	Other specified diabetes mellitus with severe nonproliferative diabetic retinopathy with macular edema, right eye	18	Diabetes with Chronic Complications	19	0.302	0.351	0.340	0.423	0.326	0.373	0.440
E13.3412	Other specified diabetes mellitus with severe nonproliferative diabetic retinopathy with macular edema, left eye	18	Diabetes with Chronic Complications	19	0.302	0.351	0.340	0.423	0.326	0.373	0.440

ICD-10-CM Code	ICD-10-CM Code Description	V24 CMS-HCC	V24 CMS-HCC Disease Group	V24 CMS-HCC Hierarchies	Community, NonDual, Aged	Community, NonDual, Disabled	Community, FBDual, Aged	Community, FBDual, Disabled	Community, PBDual, Aged	Community, PBDual, Disabled	Institutional
E13.3413	Other specified diabetes mellitus with severe nonproliferative diabetic retinopathy with macular edema, bilateral	18	Diabetes with Chronic Complications	19	0.302	0.351	0.340	0.423	0.326	0.373	0.440
E13.3419	Other specified diabetes mellitus with severe nonproliferative diabetic retinopathy with macular edema, unspecified eye	18	Diabetes with Chronic Complications	19	0.302	0.351	0.340	0.423	0.326	0.373	0.440
E13.3491	Other specified diabetes mellitus with severe nonproliferative diabetic retinopathy without macular edema, right eye	18	Diabetes with Chronic Complications	19	0.302	0.351	0.340	0.423	0.326	0.373	0.440
E13.3492	Other specified diabetes mellitus with severe nonproliferative diabetic retinopathy without macular edema, left eye	18	Diabetes with Chronic Complications	19	0.302	0.351	0.340	0.423	0.326	0.373	0.440
E13.3493	Other specified diabetes mellitus with severe nonproliferative diabetic retinopathy without macular edema, bilateral	18	Diabetes with Chronic Complications	19	0.302	0.351	0.340	0.423	0.326	0.373	0.440
E13.3499	Other specified diabetes mellitus with severe nonproliferative diabetic retinopathy without macular edema, unspecified eye	18	Diabetes with Chronic Complications	19	0.302	0.351	0.340	0.423	0.326	0.373	0.440
E13.3511	Other specified diabetes mellitus with proliferative diabetic retinopathy with macular edema, right eye	18	Diabetes with Chronic Complications	19	0.302	0.351	0.340	0.423	0.326	0.373	0.440
E13.3511	Other specified diabetes mellitus with proliferative diabetic retinopathy with macular edema, right eye	122	Proliferative Diabetic Retinopathy and Vitreous Hemorrhage		0.222	0.231	0.271	0.269	0.182	0.201	0.394
E13.3512	Other specified diabetes mellitus with proliferative diabetic retinopathy with macular edema, left eye	18	Diabetes with Chronic Complications	19	0.302	0.351	0.340	0.423	0.326	0.373	0.440
E13.3512	Other specified diabetes mellitus with proliferative diabetic retinopathy with macular edema, left eye	122	Proliferative Diabetic Retinopathy and Vitreous Hemorrhage		0.222	0.231	0.271	0.269	0.182	0.201	0.394
E13.3513	Other specified diabetes mellitus with proliferative diabetic retinopathy with macular edema, bilateral	18	Diabetes with Chronic Complications	19	0.302	0.351	0.340	0.423	0.326	0.373	0.440
E13.3513	Other specified diabetes mellitus with proliferative diabetic retinopathy with macular edema, bilateral	122	Proliferative Diabetic Retinopathy and Vitreous Hemorrhage		0.222	0.231	0.271	0.269	0.182	0.201	0.394
E13.3519	Other specified diabetes mellitus with proliferative diabetic retinopathy with macular edema, unspecified eye	18	Diabetes with Chronic Complications	19	0.302	0.351	0.340	0.423	0.326	0.373	0.440
E13.3519	Other specified diabetes mellitus with proliferative diabetic retinopathy with macular edema, unspecified eye	122	Proliferative Diabetic Retinopathy and Vitreous Hemorrhage		0.222	0.231	0.271	0.269	0.182	0.201	0.394
E13.3521	Other specified diabetes mellitus with proliferative diabetic retinopathy with traction retinal detachment involving the macula, right eye	18	Diabetes with Chronic Complications	19	0.302	0.351	0.340	0.423	0.326	0.373	0.440
E13.3521	Other specified diabetes mellitus with proliferative diabetic retinopathy with traction retinal detachment involving the macula, right eye	122	Proliferative Diabetic Retinopathy and Vitreous Hemorrhage		0.222	0.231	0.271	0.269	0.182	0.201	0.394
E13.3522	Other specified diabetes mellitus with proliferative diabetic retinopathy with traction retinal detachment involving the macula, left eye	18	Diabetes with Chronic Complications	19	0.302	0.351	0.340	0.423	0.326	0.373	0.440

ICD-10-CM Code	ICD-10-CM Code Description	V24 CMS-HCC	V24 CMS-HCC Disease Group	V24 CMS-HCC Hierarchies	Community, NonDual, Aged	Community, NonDual, Disabled	Community, FBDual, Aged	Community, FBDual, Disabled	Community, PBDual, Aged	Community, PBDual, Disabled	Institutional
E13.3522	Other specified diabetes mellitus with proliferative diabetic retinopathy with traction retinal detachment involving the macula, left eye	122	Proliferative Diabetic Retinopathy and Vitreous Hemorrhage		0.222	0.231	0.271	0.269	0.182	0.201	0.394
E13.3523	Other specified diabetes mellitus with proliferative diabetic retinopathy with traction retinal detachment involving the macula, bilateral	18	Diabetes with Chronic Complications	19	0.302	0.351	0.340	0.423	0.326	0.373	0.440
E13.3523	Other specified diabetes mellitus with proliferative diabetic retinopathy with traction retinal detachment involving the macula, bilateral	122	Proliferative Diabetic Retinopathy and Vitreous Hemorrhage		0.222	0.231	0.271	0.269	0.182	0.201	0.394
E13.3529	Other specified diabetes mellitus with proliferative diabetic retinopathy with traction retinal detachment involving the macula, unspecified eye	18	Diabetes with Chronic Complications	19	0.302	0.351	0.340	0.423	0.326	0.373	0.440
E13.3529	Other specified diabetes mellitus with proliferative diabetic retinopathy with traction retinal detachment involving the macula, unspecified eye	122	Proliferative Diabetic Retinopathy and Vitreous Hemorrhage		0.222	0.231	0.271	0.269	0.182	0.201	0.394
E13.3531	Other specified diabetes mellitus with proliferative diabetic retinopathy with traction retinal detachment not involving the macula, right eye	18	Diabetes with Chronic Complications	19	0.302	0.351	0.340	0.423	0.326	0.373	0.440
E13.3531	Other specified diabetes mellitus with proliferative diabetic retinopathy with traction retinal detachment not involving the macula, right eye	122	Proliferative Diabetic Retinopathy and Vitreous Hemorrhage		0.222	0.231	0.271	0.269	0.182	0.201	0.394
E13.3532	Other specified diabetes mellitus with proliferative diabetic retinopathy with traction retinal detachment not involving the macula, left eye	18	Diabetes with Chronic Complications	19	0.302	0.351	0.340	0.423	0.326	0.373	0.440
E13.3532	Other specified diabetes mellitus with proliferative diabetic retinopathy with traction retinal detachment not involving the macula, left eye	122	Proliferative Diabetic Retinopathy and Vitreous Hemorrhage		0.222	0.231	0.271	0.269	0.182	0.201	0.394
E13.3533	Other specified diabetes mellitus with proliferative diabetic retinopathy with traction retinal detachment not involving the macula, bilateral	18	Diabetes with Chronic Complications	19	0.302	0.351	0.340	0.423	0.326	0.373	0.440
E13.3533	Other specified diabetes mellitus with proliferative diabetic retinopathy with traction retinal detachment not involving the macula, bilateral	122	Proliferative Diabetic Retinopathy and Vitreous Hemorrhage		0.222	0.231	0.271	0.269	0.182	0.201	0.394
E13.3539	Other specified diabetes mellitus with proliferative diabetic retinopathy with traction retinal detachment not involving the macula, unspecified eye	18	Diabetes with Chronic Complications	19	0.302	0.351	0.340	0.423	0.326	0.373	0.440
E13.3539	Other specified diabetes mellitus with proliferative diabetic retinopathy with traction retinal detachment not involving the macula, unspecified eye	122	Proliferative Diabetic Retinopathy and Vitreous Hemorrhage		0.222	0.231	0.271	0.269	0.182	0.201	0.394
E13.3541	Other specified diabetes mellitus with proliferative diabetic retinopathy with combined traction retinal detachment and rhegmatogenous retinal detachment, right eye	18	Diabetes with Chronic Complications	19	0.302	0.351	0.340	0.423	0.326	0.373	0.440
E13.3541	Other specified diabetes mellitus with proliferative diabetic retinopathy with combined traction retinal detachment and rhegmatogenous retinal detachment, right eye	122	Proliferative Diabetic Retinopathy and Vitreous Hemorrhage		0.222	0.231	0.271	0.269	0.182	0.201	0.394

ICD-10-CM Code	ICD-10-CM Code Description	V24 CMS-HCC	V24 CMS-HCC Disease Group	V24 CMS-HCC Hierarchies	Community, NonDual, Aged	Community, NonDual, Disabled	Community, FBDual, Aged	Community, FBDual, Disabled	Community, PBDual, Aged	Community, PBDual, Disabled	Institutional
E13.3542	Other specified diabetes mellitus with proliferative diabetic retinopathy with combined traction retinal detachment and rhegmatogenous retinal detachment, left eye	18	Diabetes with Chronic Complications	19	0.302	0.351	0.340	0.423	0.326	0.373	0.440
E13.3542	Other specified diabetes mellitus with proliferative diabetic retinopathy with combined traction retinal detachment and rhegmatogenous retinal detachment, left eye	122	Proliferative Diabetic Retinopathy and Vitreous Hemorrhage		0.222	0.231	0.271	0.269	0.182	0.201	0.394
E13.3543	Other specified diabetes mellitus with proliferative diabetic retinopathy with combined traction retinal detachment and rhegmatogenous retinal detachment, bilateral	18	Diabetes with Chronic Complications	19	0.302	0.351	0.340	0.423	0.326	0.373	0.440
E13.3543	Other specified diabetes mellitus with proliferative diabetic retinopathy with combined traction retinal detachment and rhegmatogenous retinal detachment, bilateral	122	Proliferative Diabetic Retinopathy and Vitreous Hemorrhage		0.222	0.231	0.271	0.269	0.182	0.201	0.394
E13.3549	Other specified diabetes mellitus with proliferative diabetic retinopathy with combined traction retinal detachment and rhegmatogenous retinal detachment, unspecified eye	18	Diabetes with Chronic Complications	19	0.302	0.351	0.340	0.423	0.326	0.373	0.440
E13.3549	Other specified diabetes mellitus with proliferative diabetic retinopathy with combined traction retinal detachment and rhegmatogenous retinal detachment, unspecified eye	122	Proliferative Diabetic Retinopathy and Vitreous Hemorrhage		0.222	0.231	0.271	0.269	0.182	0.201	0.394
E13.3551	Other specified diabetes mellitus with stable proliferative diabetic retinopathy, right eye	18	Diabetes with Chronic Complications	19	0.302	0.351	0.340	0.423	0.326	0.373	0.440
E13.3551	Other specified diabetes mellitus with stable proliferative diabetic retinopathy, right eye	122	Proliferative Diabetic Retinopathy and Vitreous Hemorrhage		0.222	0.231	0.271	0.269	0.182	0.201	0.394
E13.3552	Other specified diabetes mellitus with stable proliferative diabetic retinopathy, left eye	18	Diabetes with Chronic Complications	19	0.302	0.351	0.340	0.423	0.326	0.373	0.440
E13.3552	Other specified diabetes mellitus with stable proliferative diabetic retinopathy, left eye	122	Proliferative Diabetic Retinopathy and Vitreous Hemorrhage		0.222	0.231	0.271	0.269	0.182	0.201	0.394
E13.3553	Other specified diabetes mellitus with stable proliferative diabetic retinopathy, bilateral	18	Diabetes with Chronic Complications	19	0.302	0.351	0.340	0.423	0.326	0.373	0.440
E13.3553	Other specified diabetes mellitus with stable proliferative diabetic retinopathy, bilateral	122	Proliferative Diabetic Retinopathy and Vitreous Hemorrhage		0.222	0.231	0.271	0.269	0.182	0.201	0.394
E13.3559	Other specified diabetes mellitus with stable proliferative diabetic retinopathy, unspecified eye	18	Diabetes with Chronic Complications	19	0.302	0.351	0.340	0.423	0.326	0.373	0.440
E13.3559	Other specified diabetes mellitus with stable proliferative diabetic retinopathy, unspecified eye	122	Proliferative Diabetic Retinopathy and Vitreous Hemorrhage		0.222	0.231	0.271	0.269	0.182	0.201	0.394
E13.3591	Other specified diabetes mellitus with proliferative diabetic retinopathy without macular edema, right eye	18	Diabetes with Chronic Complications	19	0.302	0.351	0.340	0.423	0.326	0.373	0.440
E13.3591	Other specified diabetes mellitus with proliferative diabetic retinopathy without macular edema, right eye	122	Proliferative Diabetic Retinopathy and Vitreous Hemorrhage		0.222	0.231	0.271	0.269	0.182	0.201	0.394
E13.3592	Other specified diabetes mellitus with proliferative diabetic retinopathy without macular edema, left eye	18	Diabetes with Chronic Complications	19	0.302	0.351	0.340	0.423	0.326	0.373	0.440

ICD-10-CM Code	ICD-10-CM Code Description	V24 CMS-HCC	V24 CMS-HCC Disease Group	V24 CMS-HCC Hierarchies	Community, NonDual, Aged	Community, NonDual, Disabled	Community, FBDual, Aged	Community, FBDual, Disabled	Community, PBDual, Aged	Community, PBDual, Disabled	Institutional
E13.3592	Other specified diabetes mellitus with proliferative diabetic retinopathy without macular edema, left eye	122	Proliferative Diabetic Retinopathy and Vitreous Hemorrhage		0.222	0.231	0.271	0.269	0.182	0.201	0.394
E13.3593	Other specified diabetes mellitus with proliferative diabetic retinopathy without macular edema, bilateral	18	Diabetes with Chronic Complications	19	0.302	0.351	0.340	0.423	0.326	0.373	0.440
E13.3593	Other specified diabetes mellitus with proliferative diabetic retinopathy without macular edema, bilateral	122	Proliferative Diabetic Retinopathy and Vitreous Hemorrhage		0.222	0.231	0.271	0.269	0.182	0.201	0.394
E13.3599	Other specified diabetes mellitus with proliferative diabetic retinopathy without macular edema, unspecified eye	18	Diabetes with Chronic Complications	19	0.302	0.351	0.340	0.423	0.326	0.373	0.440
E13.3599	Other specified diabetes mellitus with proliferative diabetic retinopathy without macular edema, unspecified eye	122	Proliferative Diabetic Retinopathy and Vitreous Hemorrhage		0.222	0.231	0.271	0.269	0.182	0.201	0.394
E13.36	Other specified diabetes mellitus with diabetic cataract	18	Diabetes with Chronic Complications	19	0.302	0.351	0.340	0.423	0.326	0.373	0.440
E13.37X1	Other specified diabetes mellitus with diabetic macular edema, resolved following treatment, right eye	18	Diabetes with Chronic Complications	19	0.302	0.351	0.340	0.423	0.326	0.373	0.440
E13.37X2	Other specified diabetes mellitus with diabetic macular edema, resolved following treatment, left eye	18	Diabetes with Chronic Complications	19	0.302	0.351	0.340	0.423	0.326	0.373	0.440
E13.37X3	Other specified diabetes mellitus with diabetic macular edema, resolved following treatment, bilateral	18	Diabetes with Chronic Complications	19	0.302	0.351	0.340	0.423	0.326	0.373	0.440
E13.37X9	Other specified diabetes mellitus with diabetic macular edema, resolved following treatment, unspecified eye	18	Diabetes with Chronic Complications	19	0.302	0.351	0.340	0.423	0.326	0.373	0.440
E13.39	Other specified diabetes mellitus with other diabetic ophthalmic complication	18	Diabetes with Chronic Complications	19	0.302	0.351	0.340	0.423	0.326	0.373	0.440
E13.40	Other specified diabetes mellitus with diabetic neuropathy, unspecified	18	Diabetes with Chronic Complications	19	0.302	0.351	0.340	0.423	0.326	0.373	0.440
E13.41	Other specified diabetes mellitus with diabetic mononeuropathy	18	Diabetes with Chronic Complications	19	0.302	0.351	0.340	0.423	0.326	0.373	0.440
E13.42	Other specified diabetes mellitus with diabetic polyneuropathy	18	Diabetes with Chronic Complications	19	0.302	0.351	0.340	0.423	0.326	0.373	0.440
E13.43	Other specified diabetes mellitus with diabetic autonomic (poly)neuropathy	18	Diabetes with Chronic Complications	19	0.302	0.351	0.340	0.423	0.326	0.373	0.440
E13.44	Other specified diabetes mellitus with diabetic amyotrophy	18	Diabetes with Chronic Complications	19	0.302	0.351	0.340	0.423	0.326	0.373	0.440
E13.49	Other specified diabetes mellitus with other diabetic neurological complication	18	Diabetes with Chronic Complications	19	0.302	0.351	0.340	0.423	0.326	0.373	0.440
E13.51	Other specified diabetes mellitus with diabetic peripheral angiopathy without gangrene	18	Diabetes with Chronic Complications	19	0.302	0.351	0.340	0.423	0.326	0.373	0.440
E13.51	Other specified diabetes mellitus with diabetic peripheral angiopathy without gangrene	108	Vascular Disease		0.288	0.301	0.294	0.267	0.297	0.314	0.093
E13.52	Other specified diabetes mellitus with diabetic peripheral angiopathy with gangrene	18	Diabetes with Chronic Complications	19	0.302	0.351	0.340	0.423	0.326	0.373	0.440
E13.52	Other specified diabetes mellitus with diabetic peripheral angiopathy with gangrene	106	Atherosclerosis of the Extremities with Ulceration or Gangrene	107,108, 161,189	1.488	1.521	1.724	1.748	1.504	1.525	0.867
E13.59	Other specified diabetes mellitus with other circulatory complications	18	Diabetes with Chronic Complications	19	0.302	0.351	0.340	0.423	0.326	0.373	0.440

ICD-10-CM Code	ICD-10-CM Code Description	V24 CMS-HCC	V24 CMS-HCC Disease Group	V24 CMS-HCC Hierarchies	Community, NonDual, Aged	Community, NonDual, Disabled	Community, FBDual, Aged	Community, FBDual, Disabled	Community, PBDual, Aged	Community, PBDual, Disabled	Institutional
E13.610	Other specified diabetes mellitus with diabetic neuropathic arthropathy	18	Diabetes with Chronic Complications	19	0.302	0.351	0.340	0.423	0.326	0.373	0.440
E13.618	Other specified diabetes mellitus with other diabetic arthropathy	18	Diabetes with Chronic Complications	19	0.302	0.351	0.340	0.423	0.326	0.373	0.440
E13.620	Other specified diabetes mellitus with diabetic dermatitis	18	Diabetes with Chronic Complications	19	0.302	0.351	0.340	0.423	0.326	0.373	0.440
E13.621	Other specified diabetes mellitus with foot ulcer	18	Diabetes with Chronic Complications	19	0.302	0.351	0.340	0.423	0.326	0.373	0.440
E13.621	Other specified diabetes mellitus with foot ulcer	161	Chronic Ulcer of Skin, Except Pressure		0.515	0.592	0.727	0.583	0.541	0.542	0.294
E13.622	Other specified diabetes mellitus with other skin ulcer	18	Diabetes with Chronic Complications	19	0.302	0.351	0.340	0.423	0.326	0.373	0.440
E13.622	Other specified diabetes mellitus with other skin ulcer	161	Chronic Ulcer of Skin, Except Pressure		0.515	0.592	0.727	0.583	0.541	0.542	0.294
E13.628	Other specified diabetes mellitus with other skin complications	18	Diabetes with Chronic Complications	19	0.302	0.351	0.340	0.423	0.326	0.373	0.440
E13.630	Other specified diabetes mellitus with periodontal disease	18	Diabetes with Chronic Complications	19	0.302	0.351	0.340	0.423	0.326	0.373	0.440
E13.638	Other specified diabetes mellitus with other oral complications	18	Diabetes with Chronic Complications	19	0.302	0.351	0.340	0.423	0.326	0.373	0.440
E13.641	Other specified diabetes mellitus with hypoglycemia with coma	17	Diabetes with Acute Complications	18,19	0.302	0.351	0.340	0.423	0.326	0.373	0.440
E13.649	Other specified diabetes mellitus with hypoglycemia without coma	18	Diabetes with Chronic Complications	19	0.302	0.351	0.340	0.423	0.326	0.373	0.440
E13.65	Other specified diabetes mellitus with hyperglycemia	18	Diabetes with Chronic Complications	19	0.302	0.351	0.340	0.423	0.326	0.373	0.440
E13.69	Other specified diabetes mellitus with other specified complication	18	Diabetes with Chronic Complications	19	0.302	0.351	0.340	0.423	0.326	0.373	0.440
E13.8	Other specified diabetes mellitus with unspecified complications	18	Diabetes with Chronic Complications	19	0.302	0.351	0.340	0.423	0.326	0.373	0.440
E13.9	Other specified diabetes mellitus without complications	19	Diabetes without Complication		0.105	0.124	0.107	0.145	0.087	0.122	0.178
E15	Nondiabetic hypoglycemic coma	23	Other Significant Endocrine and Metabolic Disorders		0.194	0.378	0.211	0.299	0.174	0.319	0.379
E20.0	Idiopathic hypoparathyroidism	23	Other Significant Endocrine and Metabolic Disorders		0.194	0.378	0.211	0.299	0.174	0.319	0.379
E20.8	Other hypoparathyroidism	23	Other Significant Endocrine and Metabolic Disorders		0.194	0.378	0.211	0.299	0.174	0.319	0.379
E20.9	Hypoparathyroidism, unspecified	23	Other Significant Endocrine and Metabolic Disorders		0.194	0.378	0.211	0.299	0.174	0.319	0.379
E21.0	Primary hyperparathyroidism	23	Other Significant Endocrine and Metabolic Disorders		0.194	0.378	0.211	0.299	0.174	0.319	0.379
E21.1	Secondary hyperparathyroidism, not elsewhere classified	23	Other Significant Endocrine and Metabolic Disorders		0.194	0.378	0.211	0.299	0.174	0.319	0.379
E21.2	Other hyperparathyroidism	23	Other Significant Endocrine and Metabolic Disorders		0.194	0.378	0.211	0.299	0.174	0.319	0.379
E21.3	Hyperparathyroidism, unspecified	23	Other Significant Endocrine and Metabolic Disorders		0.194	0.378	0.211	0.299	0.174	0.319	0.379
E21.4	Other specified disorders of parathyroid gland	23	Other Significant Endocrine and Metabolic Disorders		0.194	0.378	0.211	0.299	0.174	0.319	0.379
E21.5	Disorder of parathyroid gland, unspecified	23	Other Significant Endocrine and Metabolic Disorders		0.194	0.378	0.211	0.299	0.174	0.319	0.379
E22.0	Acromegaly and pituitary gigantism	23	Other Significant Endocrine and Metabolic Disorders		0.194	0.378	0.211	0.299	0.174	0.319	0.379
E22.1	Hyperprolactinemia	23	Other Significant Endocrine and Metabolic Disorders		0.194	0.378	0.211	0.299	0.174	0.319	0.379
E22.2	Syndrome of inappropriate secretion of antidiuretic hormone	23	Other Significant Endocrine and Metabolic Disorders		0.194	0.378	0.211	0.299	0.174	0.319	0.379

ICD-10-CM Code	ICD-10-CM Code Description	V24 CMS-HCC	V24 CMS-HCC Disease Group	V24 CMS-HCC Hierarchies	Community, NonDual, Aged	Community, NonDual, Disabled	Community, FBDual, Aged	Community, FBDual, Disabled	Community, PBDual, Aged	Community, PBDual, Disabled	Institutional
E22.8	Other hyperfunction of pituitary gland	23	Other Significant Endocrine and Metabolic Disorders		0.194	0.378	0.211	0.299	0.174	0.319	0.379
E22.9	Hyperfunction of pituitary gland, unspecified	23	Other Significant Endocrine and Metabolic Disorders		0.194	0.378	0.211	0.299	0.174	0.319	0.379
E23.0	Hypopituitarism	23	Other Significant Endocrine and Metabolic Disorders		0.194	0.378	0.211	0.299	0.174	0.319	0.379
E23.1	Drug-induced hypopituitarism	23	Other Significant Endocrine and Metabolic Disorders		0.194	0.378	0.211	0.299	0.174	0.319	0.379
E23.2	Diabetes insipidus	23	Other Significant Endocrine and Metabolic Disorders		0.194	0.378	0.211	0.299	0.174	0.319	0.379
E23.3	Hypothalamic dysfunction, not elsewhere classified	23	Other Significant Endocrine and Metabolic Disorders		0.194	0.378	0.211	0.299	0.174	0.319	0.379
E23.6	Other disorders of pituitary gland	23	Other Significant Endocrine and Metabolic Disorders		0.194	0.378	0.211	0.299	0.174	0.319	0.379
E23.7	Disorder of pituitary gland, unspecified	23	Other Significant Endocrine and Metabolic Disorders		0.194	0.378	0.211	0.299	0.174	0.319	0.379
E24.0	Pituitary-dependent Cushing's disease	23	Other Significant Endocrine and Metabolic Disorders		0.194	0.378	0.211	0.299	0.174	0.319	0.379
E24.1	Nelson's syndrome	23	Other Significant Endocrine and Metabolic Disorders		0.194	0.378	0.211	0.299	0.174	0.319	0.379
E24.2	Drug-induced Cushing's syndrome	23	Other Significant Endocrine and Metabolic Disorders		0.194	0.378	0.211	0.299	0.174	0.319	0.379
E24.3	Ectopic ACTH syndrome	23	Other Significant Endocrine and Metabolic Disorders		0.194	0.378	0.211	0.299	0.174	0.319	0.379
E24.4	Alcohol-induced pseudo-Cushing's syndrome	23	Other Significant Endocrine and Metabolic Disorders		0.194	0.378	0.211	0.299	0.174	0.319	0.379
E24.8	Other Cushing's syndrome	23	Other Significant Endocrine and Metabolic Disorders		0.194	0.378	0.211	0.299	0.174	0.319	0.379
E24.9	Cushing's syndrome, unspecified	23	Other Significant Endocrine and Metabolic Disorders		0.194	0.378	0.211	0.299	0.174	0.319	0.379
E25.0	Congenital adrenogenital disorders associated with enzyme deficiency	23	Other Significant Endocrine and Metabolic Disorders		0.194	0.378	0.211	0.299	0.174	0.319	0.379
E25.8	Other adrenogenital disorders	23	Other Significant Endocrine and Metabolic Disorders		0.194	0.378	0.211	0.299	0.174	0.319	0.379
E25.9	Adrenogenital disorder, unspecified	23	Other Significant Endocrine and Metabolic Disorders		0.194	0.378	0.211	0.299	0.174	0.319	0.379
E26.01	Conn's syndrome	23	Other Significant Endocrine and Metabolic Disorders		0.194	0.378	0.211	0.299	0.174	0.319	0.379
E26.02	Glucocorticoid-remediable aldosteronism	23	Other Significant Endocrine and Metabolic Disorders		0.194	0.378	0.211	0.299	0.174	0.319	0.379
E26.09	Other primary hyperaldosteronism	23	Other Significant Endocrine and Metabolic Disorders		0.194	0.378	0.211	0.299	0.174	0.319	0.379
E26.1	Secondary hyperaldosteronism	23	Other Significant Endocrine and Metabolic Disorders		0.194	0.378	0.211	0.299	0.174	0.319	0.379
E26.81	Bartter's syndrome	23	Other Significant Endocrine and Metabolic Disorders		0.194	0.378	0.211	0.299	0.174	0.319	0.379
E26.89	Other hyperaldosteronism	23	Other Significant Endocrine and Metabolic Disorders		0.194	0.378	0.211	0.299	0.174	0.319	0.379
E26.9	Hyperaldosteronism, unspecified	23	Other Significant Endocrine and Metabolic Disorders		0.194	0.378	0.211	0.299	0.174	0.319	0.379
E27.0	Other adrenocortical overactivity	23	Other Significant Endocrine and Metabolic Disorders		0.194	0.378	0.211	0.299	0.174	0.319	0.379
E27.1	Primary adrenocortical insufficiency	23	Other Significant Endocrine and Metabolic Disorders		0.194	0.378	0.211	0.299	0.174	0.319	0.379
E27.2	Addisonian crisis	23	Other Significant Endocrine and Metabolic Disorders		0.194	0.378	0.211	0.299	0.174	0.319	0.379
E27.3	Drug-induced adrenocortical insufficiency	23	Other Significant Endocrine and Metabolic Disorders		0.194	0.378	0.211	0.299	0.174	0.319	0.379

ICD-10-CM Code	ICD-10-CM Code Description	V24 CMS-HCC	V24 CMS-HCC Disease Group	V24 CMS-HCC Hierarchies	Community, NonDual, Aged	Community, NonDual, Disabled	Community, FBDual, Aged	Community, FBDual, Disabled	Community, PBDual, Aged	Community, PBDual, Disabled	Institutional
E27.40	Unspecified adrenocortical insufficiency	23	Other Significant Endocrine and Metabolic Disorders		0.194	0.378	0.211	0.299	0.174	0.319	0.379
E27.49	Other adrenocortical insufficiency	23	Other Significant Endocrine and Metabolic Disorders		0.194	0.378	0.211	0.299	0.174	0.319	0.379
E27.5	Adrenomedullary hyperfunction	23	Other Significant Endocrine and Metabolic Disorders		0.194	0.378	0.211	0.299	0.174	0.319	0.379
E27.8	Other specified disorders of adrenal gland	23	Other Significant Endocrine and Metabolic Disorders		0.194	0.378	0.211	0.299	0.174	0.319	0.379
E27.9	Disorder of adrenal gland, unspecified	23	Other Significant Endocrine and Metabolic Disorders		0.194	0.378	0.211	0.299	0.174	0.319	0.379
E31.0	Autoimmune polyglandular failure	23	Other Significant Endocrine and Metabolic Disorders		0.194	0.378	0.211	0.299	0.174	0.319	0.379
E31.1	Polyglandular hyperfunction	23	Other Significant Endocrine and Metabolic Disorders		0.194	0.378	0.211	0.299	0.174	0.319	0.379
E31.20	Multiple endocrine neoplasia [MEN] syndrome, unspecified	23	Other Significant Endocrine and Metabolic Disorders		0.194	0.378	0.211	0.299	0.174	0.319	0.379
E31.21	Multiple endocrine neoplasia [MEN] type I	23	Other Significant Endocrine and Metabolic Disorders		0.194	0.378	0.211	0.299	0.174	0.319	0.379
E31.22	Multiple endocrine neoplasia [MEN] type IIA	23	Other Significant Endocrine and Metabolic Disorders		0.194	0.378	0.211	0.299	0.174	0.319	0.379
E31.23	Multiple endocrine neoplasia [MEN] type IIB	23	Other Significant Endocrine and Metabolic Disorders		0.194	0.378	0.211	0.299	0.174	0.319	0.379
E31.8	Other polyglandular dysfunction	23	Other Significant Endocrine and Metabolic Disorders		0.194	0.378	0.211	0.299	0.174	0.319	0.379
E31.9	Polyglandular dysfunction, unspecified	23	Other Significant Endocrine and Metabolic Disorders		0.194	0.378	0.211	0.299	0.174	0.319	0.379
E32.0	Persistent hyperplasia of thymus	23	Other Significant Endocrine and Metabolic Disorders		0.194	0.378	0.211	0.299	0.174	0.319	0.379
E32.1	Abscess of thymus	23	Other Significant Endocrine and Metabolic Disorders		0.194	0.378	0.211	0.299	0.174	0.319	0.379
E32.8	Other diseases of thymus	23	Other Significant Endocrine and Metabolic Disorders		0.194	0.378	0.211	0.299	0.174	0.319	0.379
E32.9	Disease of thymus, unspecified	23	Other Significant Endocrine and Metabolic Disorders		0.194	0.378	0.211	0.299	0.174	0.319	0.379
E34.0	Carcinoid syndrome	12	Breast, Prostate, and Other Cancers and Tumors		0.150	0.212	0.158	0.212	0.154	0.181	0.210
E34.4	Constitutional tall stature	23	Other Significant Endocrine and Metabolic Disorders		0.194	0.378	0.211	0.299	0.174	0.319	0.379
E40	Kwashiorkor	21	Protein-Calorie Malnutrition		0.455	0.674	0.693	0.723	0.457	0.679	0.267
E41	Nutritional marasmus	21	Protein-Calorie Malnutrition		0.455	0.674	0.693	0.723	0.457	0.679	0.267
E42	Marasmic kwashiorkor	21	Protein-Calorie Malnutrition		0.455	0.674	0.693	0.723	0.457	0.679	0.267
E43	Unspecified severe protein-calorie malnutrition	21	Protein-Calorie Malnutrition		0.455	0.674	0.693	0.723	0.457	0.679	0.267
E44.0	Moderate protein-calorie malnutrition	21	Protein-Calorie Malnutrition		0.455	0.674	0.693	0.723	0.457	0.679	0.267
E44.1	Mild protein-calorie malnutrition	21	Protein-Calorie Malnutrition		0.455	0.674	0.693	0.723	0.457	0.679	0.267
E45	Retarded development following protein-calorie malnutrition	21	Protein-Calorie Malnutrition		0.455	0.674	0.693	0.723	0.457	0.679	0.267
E46	Unspecified protein-calorie malnutrition	21	Protein-Calorie Malnutrition		0.455	0.674	0.693	0.723	0.457	0.679	0.267
E64.0	Sequelae of protein-calorie malnutrition	21	Protein-Calorie Malnutrition		0.455	0.674	0.693	0.723	0.457	0.679	0.267
E66.01	Morbid (severe) obesity due to excess calories	22	Morbid Obesity		0.250	0.183	0.383	0.297	0.233	0.204	0.455
E66.2	Morbid (severe) obesity with alveolar hypoventilation	22	Morbid Obesity		0.250	0.183	0.383	0.297	0.233	0.204	0.455
E70.0	Classical phenylketonuria	23	Other Significant Endocrine and Metabolic Disorders		0.194	0.378	0.211	0.299	0.174	0.319	0.379

ICD-10-CM Code	ICD-10-CM Code Description	V24 CMS-HCC	V24 CMS-HCC Disease Group	V24 CMS-HCC Hierarchies	Community, NonDual, Aged	Community, NonDual, Disabled	Community, FBDual, Aged	Community, FBDual, Disabled	Community, PBDual, Aged	Community, PBDual, Disabled	Institutional
E70.1	Other hyperphenylalaninemias	23	Other Significant Endocrine and Metabolic Disorders		0.194	0.378	0.211	0.299	0.174	0.319	0.379
E70.20	Disorder of tyrosine metabolism, unspecified	23	Other Significant Endocrine and Metabolic Disorders		0.194	0.378	0.211	0.299	0.174	0.319	0.379
E70.21	Tyrosinemia	23	Other Significant Endocrine and Metabolic Disorders		0.194	0.378	0.211	0.299	0.174	0.319	0.379
E70.29	Other disorders of tyrosine metabolism	23	Other Significant Endocrine and Metabolic Disorders		0.194	0.378	0.211	0.299	0.174	0.319	0.379
E70.30	Albinism, unspecified	23	Other Significant Endocrine and Metabolic Disorders		0.194	0.378	0.211	0.299	0.174	0.319	0.379
E70.310	X-linked ocular albinism	23	Other Significant Endocrine and Metabolic Disorders		0.194	0.378	0.211	0.299	0.174	0.319	0.379
E70.311	Autosomal recessive ocular albinism	23	Other Significant Endocrine and Metabolic Disorders		0.194	0.378	0.211	0.299	0.174	0.319	0.379
E70.318	Other ocular albinism	23	Other Significant Endocrine and Metabolic Disorders		0.194	0.378	0.211	0.299	0.174	0.319	0.379
E70.319	Ocular albinism, unspecified	23	Other Significant Endocrine and Metabolic Disorders		0.194	0.378	0.211	0.299	0.174	0.319	0.379
E70.320	Tyrosinase negative oculocutaneous albinism	23	Other Significant Endocrine and Metabolic Disorders		0.194	0.378	0.211	0.299	0.174	0.319	0.379
E70.321	Tyrosinase positive oculocutaneous albinism	23	Other Significant Endocrine and Metabolic Disorders		0.194	0.378	0.211	0.299	0.174	0.319	0.379
E70.328	Other oculocutaneous albinism	23	Other Significant Endocrine and Metabolic Disorders		0.194	0.378	0.211	0.299	0.174	0.319	0.379
E70.329	Oculocutaneous albinism, unspecified	23	Other Significant Endocrine and Metabolic Disorders		0.194	0.378	0.211	0.299	0.174	0.319	0.379
E70.330	Chediak-Higashi syndrome	23	Other Significant Endocrine and Metabolic Disorders		0.194	0.378	0.211	0.299	0.174	0.319	0.379
E70.331	Hermansky-Pudlak syndrome	23	Other Significant Endocrine and Metabolic Disorders		0.194	0.378	0.211	0.299	0.174	0.319	0.379
E70.338	Other albinism with hematologic abnormality	23	Other Significant Endocrine and Metabolic Disorders		0.194	0.378	0.211	0.299	0.174	0.319	0.379
E70.339	Albinism with hematologic abnormality, unspecified	23	Other Significant Endocrine and Metabolic Disorders		0.194	0.378	0.211	0.299	0.174	0.319	0.379
E70.39	Other specified albinism	23	Other Significant Endocrine and Metabolic Disorders		0.194	0.378	0.211	0.299	0.174	0.319	0.379
E70.40	Disorders of histidine metabolism, unspecified	23	Other Significant Endocrine and Metabolic Disorders		0.194	0.378	0.211	0.299	0.174	0.319	0.379
E70.41	Histidinemia	23	Other Significant Endocrine and Metabolic Disorders		0.194	0.378	0.211	0.299	0.174	0.319	0.379
E70.49	Other disorders of histidine metabolism	23	Other Significant Endocrine and Metabolic Disorders		0.194	0.378	0.211	0.299	0.174	0.319	0.379
E70.5	Disorders of tryptophan metabolism	23	Other Significant Endocrine and Metabolic Disorders		0.194	0.378	0.211	0.299	0.174	0.319	0.379
E70.81	Aromatic L-amino acid decarboxylase deficiency	23	Other Significant Endocrine and Metabolic Disorders		0.194	0.378	0.211	0.299	0.174	0.319	0.379
E70.89	Other disorders of aromatic amino-acid metabolism	23	Other Significant Endocrine and Metabolic Disorders		0.194	0.378	0.211	0.299	0.174	0.319	0.379
E70.9	Disorder of aromatic amino-acid metabolism, unspecified	23	Other Significant Endocrine and Metabolic Disorders		0.194	0.378	0.211	0.299	0.174	0.319	0.379
E71.0	Maple-syrup-urine disease	23	Other Significant Endocrine and Metabolic Disorders		0.194	0.378	0.211	0.299	0.174	0.319	0.379
E71.110	Isovaleric acidemia	23	Other Significant Endocrine and Metabolic Disorders		0.194	0.378	0.211	0.299	0.174	0.319	0.379
E71.111	3-methylglutaconic aciduria	23	Other Significant Endocrine and Metabolic Disorders		0.194	0.378	0.211	0.299	0.174	0.319	0.379
E71.118	Other branched-chain organic acidurias	23	Other Significant Endocrine and Metabolic Disorders		0.194	0.378	0.211	0.299	0.174	0.319	0.379

2021 Optum360, LLC

ICD-10-CM Code	ICD-10-CM Code Description	V24 CMS-HCC	V24 CMS-HCC Disease Group	V24 CMS-HCC Hierarchies	Community, NonDual, Aged	Community, NonDual, Disabled	Community, FBDual, Aged	Community, FBDual, Disabled	Community, PBDual, Aged	Community, PBDual, Disabled	Institutional
E71.120	Methylmalonic acidemia	23	Other Significant Endocrine and Metabolic Disorders		0.194	0.378	0.211	0.299	0.174	0.319	0.379
E71.121	Propionic acidemia	23	Other Significant Endocrine and Metabolic Disorders		0.194	0.378	0.211	0.299	0.174	0.319	0.379
E71.128	Other disorders of propionate metabolism	23	Other Significant Endocrine and Metabolic Disorders		0.194	0.378	0.211	0.299	0.174	0.319	0.379
E71.19	Other disorders of branched-chain amino-acid metabolism	23	Other Significant Endocrine and Metabolic Disorders		0.194	0.378	0.211	0.299	0.174	0.319	0.379
E71.2	Disorder of branched-chain amino-acid metabolism, unspecified	23	Other Significant Endocrine and Metabolic Disorders		0.194	0.378	0.211	0.299	0.174	0.319	0.379
E71.310	Long chain/very long chain acyl CoA dehydrogenase deficiency	23	Other Significant Endocrine and Metabolic Disorders		0.194	0.378	0.211	0.299	0.174	0.319	0.379
E71.311	Medium chain acyl CoA dehydrogenase deficiency	23	Other Significant Endocrine and Metabolic Disorders		0.194	0.378	0.211	0.299	0.174	0.319	0.379
E71.312	Short chain acyl CoA dehydrogenase deficiency	23	Other Significant Endocrine and Metabolic Disorders		0.194	0.378	0.211	0.299	0.174	0.319	0.379
E71.313	Glutaric aciduria type II	23	Other Significant Endocrine and Metabolic Disorders		0.194	0.378	0.211	0.299	0.174	0.319	0.379
E71.314	Muscle carnitine palmitoyltransferase deficiency	23	Other Significant Endocrine and Metabolic Disorders		0.194	0.378	0.211	0.299	0.174	0.319	0.379
E71.318	Other disorders of fatty-acid oxidation	23	Other Significant Endocrine and Metabolic Disorders		0.194	0.378	0.211	0.299	0.174	0.319	0.379
E71.32	Disorders of ketone metabolism	23	Other Significant Endocrine and Metabolic Disorders		0.194	0.378	0.211	0.299	0.174	0.319	0.379
E71.39	Other disorders of fatty-acid metabolism	23	Other Significant Endocrine and Metabolic Disorders		0.194	0.378	0.211	0.299	0.174	0.319	0.379
E71.40	Disorder of carnitine metabolism, unspecified	23	Other Significant Endocrine and Metabolic Disorders		0.194	0.378	0.211	0.299	0.174	0.319	0.379
E71.41	Primary carnitine deficiency	23	Other Significant Endocrine and Metabolic Disorders		0.194	0.378	0.211	0.299	0.174	0.319	0.379
E71.42	Carnitine deficiency due to inborn errors of metabolism	23	Other Significant Endocrine and Metabolic Disorders		0.194	0.378	0.211	0.299	0.174	0.319	0.379
E71.43	Iatrogenic carnitine deficiency	23	Other Significant Endocrine and Metabolic Disorders		0.194	0.378	0.211	0.299	0.174	0.319	0.379
E71.440	Ruvalcaba-Myhre-Smith syndrome	23	Other Significant Endocrine and Metabolic Disorders		0.194	0.378	0.211	0.299	0.174	0.319	0.379
E71.448	Other secondary carnitine deficiency	23	Other Significant Endocrine and Metabolic Disorders		0.194	0.378	0.211	0.299	0.174	0.319	0.379
E71.50	Peroxisomal disorder, unspecified	23	Other Significant Endocrine and Metabolic Disorders		0.194	0.378	0.211	0.299	0.174	0.319	0.379
E71.510	Zellweger syndrome	23	Other Significant Endocrine and Metabolic Disorders		0.194	0.378	0.211	0.299	0.174	0.319	0.379
E71.511	Neonatal adrenoleukodystrophy	23	Other Significant Endocrine and Metabolic Disorders		0.194	0.378	0.211	0.299	0.174	0.319	0.379
E71.518	Other disorders of peroxisome biogenesis	23	Other Significant Endocrine and Metabolic Disorders		0.194	0.378	0.211	0.299	0.174	0.319	0.379
E71.520	Childhood cerebral X-linked adrenoleukodystrophy	23	Other Significant Endocrine and Metabolic Disorders		0.194	0.378	0.211	0.299	0.174	0.319	0.379
E71.521	Adolescent X-linked adrenoleukodystrophy	23	Other Significant Endocrine and Metabolic Disorders		0.194	0.378	0.211	0.299	0.174	0.319	0.379
E71.522	Adrenomyeloneuropathy	23	Other Significant Endocrine and Metabolic Disorders		0.194	0.378	0.211	0.299	0.174	0.319	0.379
E71.528	Other X-linked adrenoleukodystrophy	23	Other Significant Endocrine and Metabolic Disorders		0.194	0.378	0.211	0.299	0.174	0.319	0.379
E71.529	X-linked adrenoleukodystrophy, unspecified type	23	Other Significant Endocrine and Metabolic Disorders		0.194	0.378	0.211	0.299	0.174	0.319	0.379
E71.53	Other group 2 peroxisomal disorders	23	Other Significant Endocrine and Metabolic Disorders		0.194	0.378	0.211	0.299	0.174	0.319	0.379

ICD-10-CM Code	ICD-10-CM Code Description	V24 CMS-HCC	V24 CMS-HCC Disease Group	V24 CMS-HCC Hierarchies	Community, NonDual, Aged	Community, NonDual, Disabled	Community, FBDual, Aged	Community, FBDual, Disabled	Community, PBDual, Aged	Community, PBDual, Disabled	Institutional
E71.540	Rhizomelic chondrodysplasia punctata	23	Other Significant Endocrine and Metabolic Disorders		0.194	0.378	0.211	0.299	0.174	0.319	0.379
E71.541	Zellweger-like syndrome	23	Other Significant Endocrine and Metabolic Disorders		0.194	0.378	0.211	0.299	0.174	0.319	0.379
E71.542	Other group 3 peroxisomal disorders	23	Other Significant Endocrine and Metabolic Disorders		0.194	0.378	0.211	0.299	0.174	0.319	0.379
E71.548	Other peroxisomal disorders	23	Other Significant Endocrine and Metabolic Disorders		0.194	0.378	0.211	0.299	0.174	0.319	0.379
E72.00	Disorders of amino-acid transport, unspecified	23	Other Significant Endocrine and Metabolic Disorders		0.194	0.378	0.211	0.299	0.174	0.319	0.379
E72.01	Cystinuria	23	Other Significant Endocrine and Metabolic Disorders		0.194	0.378	0.211	0.299	0.174	0.319	0.379
E72.02	Hartnup's disease	23	Other Significant Endocrine and Metabolic Disorders		0.194	0.378	0.211	0.299	0.174	0.319	0.379
E72.03	Lowe's syndrome	23	Other Significant Endocrine and Metabolic Disorders		0.194	0.378	0.211	0.299	0.174	0.319	0.379
E72.04	Cystinosis	23	Other Significant Endocrine and Metabolic Disorders		0.194	0.378	0.211	0.299	0.174	0.319	0.379
E72.09	Other disorders of amino-acid transport	23	Other Significant Endocrine and Metabolic Disorders		0.194	0.378	0.211	0.299	0.174	0.319	0.379
E72.10	Disorders of sulfur-bearing amino-acid metabolism, unspecified	23	Other Significant Endocrine and Metabolic Disorders		0.194	0.378	0.211	0.299	0.174	0.319	0.379
E72.11	Homocystinuria	23	Other Significant Endocrine and Metabolic Disorders		0.194	0.378	0.211	0.299	0.174	0.319	0.379
E72.12	Methylenetetrahydrofolate reductase deficiency	23	Other Significant Endocrine and Metabolic Disorders		0.194	0.378	0.211	0.299	0.174	0.319	0.379
E72.19	Other disorders of sulfur-bearing amino-acid metabolism	23	Other Significant Endocrine and Metabolic Disorders		0.194	0.378	0.211	0.299	0.174	0.319	0.379
E72.20	Disorder of urea cycle metabolism, unspecified	23	Other Significant Endocrine and Metabolic Disorders		0.194	0.378	0.211	0.299	0.174	0.319	0.379
E72.21	Argininemia	23	Other Significant Endocrine and Metabolic Disorders		0.194	0.378	0.211	0.299	0.174	0.319	0.379
E72.22	Arginosuccinic aciduria	23	Other Significant Endocrine and Metabolic Disorders		0.194	0.378	0.211	0.299	0.174	0.319	0.379
E72.23	Citrullinemia	23	Other Significant Endocrine and Metabolic Disorders		0.194	0.378	0.211	0.299	0.174	0.319	0.379
E72.29	Other disorders of urea cycle metabolism	23	Other Significant Endocrine and Metabolic Disorders		0.194	0.378	0.211	0.299	0.174	0.319	0.379
E72.3	Disorders of lysine and hydroxylysine metabolism	23	Other Significant Endocrine and Metabolic Disorders		0.194	0.378	0.211	0.299	0.174	0.319	0.379
E72.4	Disorders of ornithine metabolism	23	Other Significant Endocrine and Metabolic Disorders		0.194	0.378	0.211	0.299	0.174	0.319	0.379
E72.50	Disorder of glycine metabolism, unspecified	23	Other Significant Endocrine and Metabolic Disorders		0.194	0.378	0.211	0.299	0.174	0.319	0.379
E72.51	Non-ketotic hyperglycinemia	23	Other Significant Endocrine and Metabolic Disorders		0.194	0.378	0.211	0.299	0.174	0.319	0.379
E72.52	Trimethylaminuria	23	Other Significant Endocrine and Metabolic Disorders		0.194	0.378	0.211	0.299	0.174	0.319	0.379
E72.53	Primary hyperoxaluria	23	Other Significant Endocrine and Metabolic Disorders		0.194	0.378	0.211	0.299	0.174	0.319	0.379
E72.59	Other disorders of glycine metabolism	23	Other Significant Endocrine and Metabolic Disorders		0.194	0.378	0.211	0.299	0.174	0.319	0.379
E72.81	Disorders of gamma aminobutyric acid metabolism	23	Other Significant Endocrine and Metabolic Disorders		0.194	0.378	0.211	0.299	0.174	0.319	0.379
E72.89	Other specified disorders of amino-acid metabolism	23	Other Significant Endocrine and Metabolic Disorders		0.194	0.378	0.211	0.299	0.174	0.319	0.379
E72.9	Disorder of amino-acid metabolism, unspecified	23	Other Significant Endocrine and Metabolic Disorders		0.194	0.378	0.211	0.299	0.174	0.319	0.379

ICD-10-CM Code	ICD-10-CM Code Description	V24 CMS-HCC	V24 CMS-HCC Disease Group	V24 CMS-HCC Hierarchies	Community, NonDual, Aged	Community, NonDual, Disabled	Community, FBDual, Aged	Community, FBDual, Disabled	Community, PBDual, Aged	Community, PBDual, Disabled	Institutional
E74.00	Glycogen storage disease, unspecified	23	Other Significant Endocrine and Metabolic Disorders		0.194	0.378	0.211	0.299	0.174	0.319	0.379
E74.01	von Gierke disease	23	Other Significant Endocrine and Metabolic Disorders		0.194	0.378	0.211	0.299	0.174	0.319	0.379
E74.02	Pompe disease	23	Other Significant Endocrine and Metabolic Disorders		0.194	0.378	0.211	0.299	0.174	0.319	0.379
E74.03	Cori disease	23	Other Significant Endocrine and Metabolic Disorders		0.194	0.378	0.211	0.299	0.174	0.319	0.379
E74.04	McArdle disease	23	Other Significant Endocrine and Metabolic Disorders		0.194	0.378	0.211	0.299	0.174	0.319	0.379
E74.09	Other glycogen storage disease	23	Other Significant Endocrine and Metabolic Disorders		0.194	0.378	0.211	0.299	0.174	0.319	0.379
E74.20	Disorders of galactose metabolism, unspecified	23	Other Significant Endocrine and Metabolic Disorders		0.194	0.378	0.211	0.299	0.174	0.319	0.379
E74.21	Galactosemia	23	Other Significant Endocrine and Metabolic Disorders		0.194	0.378	0.211	0.299	0.174	0.319	0.379
E74.29	Other disorders of galactose metabolism	23	Other Significant Endocrine and Metabolic Disorders		0.194	0.378	0.211	0.299	0.174	0.319	0.379
E74.4	Disorders of pyruvate metabolism and gluconeogenesis	23	Other Significant Endocrine and Metabolic Disorders		0.194	0.378	0.211	0.299	0.174	0.319	0.379
E74.810	Glucose transporter protein type 1 deficiency	23	Other Significant Endocrine and Metabolic Disorders		0.194	0.378	0.211	0.299	0.174	0.319	0.379
E74.818	Other disorders of glucose transport	23	Other Significant Endocrine and Metabolic Disorders		0.194	0.378	0.211	0.299	0.174	0.319	0.379
E74.819	Disorders of glucose transport, unspecified	23	Other Significant Endocrine and Metabolic Disorders		0.194	0.378	0.211	0.299	0.174	0.319	0.379
E74.89	Other specified disorders of carbohydrate metabolism	23	Other Significant Endocrine and Metabolic Disorders		0.194	0.378	0.211	0.299	0.174	0.319	0.379
E74.9	Disorder of carbohydrate metabolism, unspecified	23	Other Significant Endocrine and Metabolic Disorders		0.194	0.378	0.211	0.299	0.174	0.319	0.379
E75.00	GM2 gangliosidosis, unspecified	52	Dementia Without Complication		0.346	0.224	0.453	0.256	0.420	0.257	—
E75.01	Sandhoff disease	52	Dementia Without Complication		0.346	0.224	0.453	0.256	0.420	0.257	—
E75.02	Tay-Sachs disease	52	Dementia Without Complication		0.346	0.224	0.453	0.256	0.420	0.257	—
E75.09	Other GM2 gangliosidosis	52	Dementia Without Complication		0.346	0.224	0.453	0.256	0.420	0.257	—
E75.10	Unspecified gangliosidosis	52	Dementia Without Complication		0.346	0.224	0.453	0.256	0.420	0.257	—
E75.11	Mucolipidosis IV	52	Dementia Without Complication		0.346	0.224	0.453	0.256	0.420	0.257	—
E75.19	Other gangliosidosis	52	Dementia Without Complication		0.346	0.224	0.453	0.256	0.420	0.257	—
E75.21	Fabry (-Anderson) disease	23	Other Significant Endocrine and Metabolic Disorders		0.194	0.378	0.211	0.299	0.174	0.319	0.379
E75.22	Gaucher disease	23	Other Significant Endocrine and Metabolic Disorders		0.194	0.378	0.211	0.299	0.174	0.319	0.379
E75.23	Krabbe disease	52	Dementia Without Complication		0.346	0.224	0.453	0.256	0.420	0.257	—
E75.240	Niemann-Pick disease type A	23	Other Significant Endocrine and Metabolic Disorders		0.194	0.378	0.211	0.299	0.174	0.319	0.379
E75.241	Niemann-Pick disease type B	23	Other Significant Endocrine and Metabolic Disorders		0.194	0.378	0.211	0.299	0.174	0.319	0.379
E75.242	Niemann-Pick disease type C	23	Other Significant Endocrine and Metabolic Disorders		0.194	0.378	0.211	0.299	0.174	0.319	0.379
E75.243	Niemann-Pick disease type D	23	Other Significant Endocrine and Metabolic Disorders		0.194	0.378	0.211	0.299	0.174	0.319	0.379
E75.244	Niemann-Pick disease type A/B	23	Other Significant Endocrine and Metabolic Disorders		0.194	0.378	0.211	0.299	0.174	0.319	0.379
E75.248	Other Niemann-Pick disease	23	Other Significant Endocrine and Metabolic Disorders		0.194	0.378	0.211	0.299	0.174	0.319	0.379
E75.249	Niemann-Pick disease, unspecified	23	Other Significant Endocrine and Metabolic Disorders		0.194	0.378	0.211	0.299	0.174	0.319	0.379
E75.25	Metachromatic leukodystrophy	52	Dementia Without Complication		0.346	0.224	0.453	0.256	0.420	0.257	—

ICD-10-CM Code	ICD-10-CM Code Description	V24 CMS-HCC	V24 CMS-HCC Disease Group	V24 CMS-HCC Hierarchies	Community, NonDual, Aged	Community, NonDual, Disabled	Community, FBDual, Aged	Community, FBDual, Disabled	Community, PBDual, Aged	Community, PBDual, Disabled	Institutional
E75.26	Sulfatase deficiency	52	Dementia Without Complication		0.346	0.224	0.453	0.256	0.420	0.257	—
E75.29	Other sphingolipidosis	52	Dementia Without Complication		0.346	0.224	0.453	0.256	0.420	0.257	—
E75.3	Sphingolipidosis, unspecified	23	Other Significant Endocrine and Metabolic Disorders		0.194	0.378	0.211	0.299	0.174	0.319	0.379
E75.4	Neuronal ceroid lipofuscinosis	52	Dementia Without Complication		0.346	0.224	0.453	0.256	0.420	0.257	—
E76.01	Hurler's syndrome	23	Other Significant Endocrine and Metabolic Disorders		0.194	0.378	0.211	0.299	0.174	0.319	0.379
E76.02	Hurler-Scheie syndrome	23	Other Significant Endocrine and Metabolic Disorders		0.194	0.378	0.211	0.299	0.174	0.319	0.379
E76.03	Scheie's syndrome	23	Other Significant Endocrine and Metabolic Disorders		0.194	0.378	0.211	0.299	0.174	0.319	0.379
E76.1	Mucopolysaccharidosis, type II	23	Other Significant Endocrine and Metabolic Disorders		0.194	0.378	0.211	0.299	0.174	0.319	0.379
E76.210	Morquio A mucopolysaccharidoses	23	Other Significant Endocrine and Metabolic Disorders		0.194	0.378	0.211	0.299	0.174	0.319	0.379
E76.211	Morquio B mucopolysaccharidoses	23	Other Significant Endocrine and Metabolic Disorders		0.194	0.378	0.211	0.299	0.174	0.319	0.379
E76.219	Morquio mucopolysaccharidoses, unspecified	23	Other Significant Endocrine and Metabolic Disorders		0.194	0.378	0.211	0.299	0.174	0.319	0.379
E76.22	Sanfilippo mucopolysaccharidoses	23	Other Significant Endocrine and Metabolic Disorders		0.194	0.378	0.211	0.299	0.174	0.319	0.379
E76.29	Other mucopolysaccharidoses	23	Other Significant Endocrine and Metabolic Disorders		0.194	0.378	0.211	0.299	0.174	0.319	0.379
E76.3	Mucopolysaccharidosis, unspecified	23	Other Significant Endocrine and Metabolic Disorders		0.194	0.378	0.211	0.299	0.174	0.319	0.379
E76.8	Other disorders of glucosaminoglycan metabolism	23	Other Significant Endocrine and Metabolic Disorders		0.194	0.378	0.211	0.299	0.174	0.319	0.379
E76.9	Glucosaminoglycan metabolism disorder, unspecified	23	Other Significant Endocrine and Metabolic Disorders		0.194	0.378	0.211	0.299	0.174	0.319	0.379
E77.0	Defects in post-translational modification of lysosomal enzymes	23	Other Significant Endocrine and Metabolic Disorders		0.194	0.378	0.211	0.299	0.174	0.319	0.379
E77.1	Defects in glycoprotein degradation	23	Other Significant Endocrine and Metabolic Disorders		0.194	0.378	0.211	0.299	0.174	0.319	0.379
E77.8	Other disorders of glycoprotein metabolism	23	Other Significant Endocrine and Metabolic Disorders		0.194	0.378	0.211	0.299	0.174	0.319	0.379
E77.9	Disorder of glycoprotein metabolism, unspecified	23	Other Significant Endocrine and Metabolic Disorders		0.194	0.378	0.211	0.299	0.174	0.319	0.379
E79.1	Lesch-Nyhan syndrome	23	Other Significant Endocrine and Metabolic Disorders		0.194	0.378	0.211	0.299	0.174	0.319	0.379
E79.2	Myoadenylate deaminase deficiency	23	Other Significant Endocrine and Metabolic Disorders		0.194	0.378	0.211	0.299	0.174	0.319	0.379
E79.8	Other disorders of purine and pyrimidine metabolism	23	Other Significant Endocrine and Metabolic Disorders		0.194	0.378	0.211	0.299	0.174	0.319	0.379
E79.9	Disorder of purine and pyrimidine metabolism, unspecified	23	Other Significant Endocrine and Metabolic Disorders		0.194	0.378	0.211	0.299	0.174	0.319	0.379
E80.0	Hereditary erythropoietic porphyria	23	Other Significant Endocrine and Metabolic Disorders		0.194	0.378	0.211	0.299	0.174	0.319	0.379
E80.1	Porphyria cutanea tarda	23	Other Significant Endocrine and Metabolic Disorders		0.194	0.378	0.211	0.299	0.174	0.319	0.379
E80.20	Unspecified porphyria	23	Other Significant Endocrine and Metabolic Disorders		0.194	0.378	0.211	0.299	0.174	0.319	0.379
E80.21	Acute intermittent (hepatic) porphyria	23	Other Significant Endocrine and Metabolic Disorders		0.194	0.378	0.211	0.299	0.174	0.319	0.379
E80.29	Other porphyria	23	Other Significant Endocrine and Metabolic Disorders		0.194	0.378	0.211	0.299	0.174	0.319	0.379
E80.3	Defects of catalase and peroxidase	23	Other Significant Endocrine and Metabolic Disorders		0.194	0.378	0.211	0.299	0.174	0.319	0.379

ICD-10-CM Code	ICD-10-CM Code Description	V24 CMS-HCC	V24 CMS-HCC Disease Group	V24 CMS-HCC Hierarchies	Community, NonDual, Aged	Community, NonDual, Disabled	Community, FBDual, Aged	Community, FBDual, Disabled	Community, PBDual, Aged	Community, PBDual, Disabled	Institutional
E83.110	Hereditary hemochromatosis	23	Other Significant Endocrine and Metabolic Disorders		0.194	0.378	0.211	0.299	0.174	0.319	0.379
E84.0	Cystic fibrosis with pulmonary manifestations	110	Cystic Fibrosis	111,112	0.510	2.676	0.509	3.516	0.392	3.051	0.593
E84.11	Meconium ileus in cystic fibrosis	110	Cystic Fibrosis	111,112	0.510	2.676	0.509	3.516	0.392	3.051	0.593
E84.19	Cystic fibrosis with other intestinal manifestations	110	Cystic Fibrosis	111,112	0.510	2.676	0.509	3.516	0.392	3.051	0.593
E84.8	Cystic fibrosis with other manifestations	110	Cystic Fibrosis	111,112	0.510	2.676	0.509	3.516	0.392	3.051	0.593
E84.9	Cystic fibrosis, unspecified	110	Cystic Fibrosis	111,112	0.510	2.676	0.509	3.516	0.392	3.051	0.593
E85.0	Non-neuropathic heredofamilial amyloidosis	23	Other Significant Endocrine and Metabolic Disorders		0.194	0.378	0.211	0.299	0.174	0.319	0.379
E85.1	Neuropathic heredofamilial amyloidosis	23	Other Significant Endocrine and Metabolic Disorders		0.194	0.378	0.211	0.299	0.174	0.319	0.379
E85.2	Heredofamilial amyloidosis, unspecified	23	Other Significant Endocrine and Metabolic Disorders		0.194	0.378	0.211	0.299	0.174	0.319	0.379
E85.3	Secondary systemic amyloidosis	23	Other Significant Endocrine and Metabolic Disorders		0.194	0.378	0.211	0.299	0.174	0.319	0.379
E85.4	Organ-limited amyloidosis	23	Other Significant Endocrine and Metabolic Disorders		0.194	0.378	0.211	0.299	0.174	0.319	0.379
E85.81	Light chain (AL) amyloidosis	23	Other Significant Endocrine and Metabolic Disorders		0.194	0.378	0.211	0.299	0.174	0.319	0.379
E85.82	Wild-type transthyretin-related (ATTR) amyloidosis	23	Other Significant Endocrine and Metabolic Disorders		0.194	0.378	0.211	0.299	0.174	0.319	0.379
E85.89	Other amyloidosis	23	Other Significant Endocrine and Metabolic Disorders		0.194	0.378	0.211	0.299	0.174	0.319	0.379
E85.9	Amyloidosis, unspecified	23	Other Significant Endocrine and Metabolic Disorders		0.194	0.378	0.211	0.299	0.174	0.319	0.379
E88.01	Alpha-1-antitrypsin deficiency	23	Other Significant Endocrine and Metabolic Disorders		0.194	0.378	0.211	0.299	0.174	0.319	0.379
E88.40	Mitochondrial metabolism disorder, unspecified	23	Other Significant Endocrine and Metabolic Disorders		0.194	0.378	0.211	0.299	0.174	0.319	0.379
E88.41	MELAS syndrome	23	Other Significant Endocrine and Metabolic Disorders		0.194	0.378	0.211	0.299	0.174	0.319	0.379
E88.42	MERRF syndrome	23	Other Significant Endocrine and Metabolic Disorders		0.194	0.378	0.211	0.299	0.174	0.319	0.379
E88.49	Other mitochondrial metabolism disorders	23	Other Significant Endocrine and Metabolic Disorders		0.194	0.378	0.211	0.299	0.174	0.319	0.379
E88.89	Other specified metabolic disorders	23	Other Significant Endocrine and Metabolic Disorders		0.194	0.378	0.211	0.299	0.174	0.319	0.379
E89.2	Postprocedural hypoparathyroidism	23	Other Significant Endocrine and Metabolic Disorders		0.194	0.378	0.211	0.299	0.174	0.319	0.379
E89.3	Postprocedural hypopituitarism	23	Other Significant Endocrine and Metabolic Disorders		0.194	0.378	0.211	0.299	0.174	0.319	0.379
E89.6	Postprocedural adrenocortical (-medullary) hypofunction	23	Other Significant Endocrine and Metabolic Disorders		0.194	0.378	0.211	0.299	0.174	0.319	0.379
F01.50	Vascular dementia without behavioral disturbance	52	Dementia Without Complication		0.346	0.224	0.453	0.256	0.420	0.257	—
F01.51	Vascular dementia with behavioral disturbance	51	Dementia With Complications	52	0.346	0.224	0.453	0.256	0.420	0.257	—
F02.80	Dementia in other diseases classified elsewhere without behavioral disturbance	52	Dementia Without Complication		0.346	0.224	0.453	0.256	0.420	0.257	—
F02.81	Dementia in other diseases classified elsewhere with behavioral disturbance	51	Dementia With Complications	52	0.346	0.224	0.453	0.256	0.420	0.257	—
F03.90	Unspecified dementia without behavioral disturbance	52	Dementia Without Complication		0.346	0.224	0.453	0.256	0.420	0.257	—

ICD-10-CM Code	ICD-10-CM Code Description	V24 CMS-HCC	V24 CMS-HCC Disease Group	V24 CMS-HCC Hierarchies	Community, NonDual, Aged	Community, NonDual, Disabled	Community, FBDual, Aged	Community, FBDual, Disabled	Community, PBDual, Aged	Community, PBDual, Disabled	Institutional
F03.91	Unspecified dementia with behavioral disturbance	51	Dementia With Complications	52	0.346	0.224	0.453	0.256	0.420	0.257	—
F04	Amnestic disorder due to known physiological condition	52	Dementia Without Complication		0.346	0.224	0.453	0.256	0.420	0.257	—
F10.120	Alcohol abuse with intoxication, uncomplicated	55	Substance Use Disorder, Moderate/Severe, or Substance Use with Complications	56	0.329	0.279	0.538	0.356	0.372	0.275	0.178
F10.121	Alcohol abuse with intoxication delirium	55	Substance Use Disorder, Moderate/Severe, or Substance Use with Complications	56	0.329	0.279	0.538	0.356	0.372	0.275	0.178
F10.129	Alcohol abuse with intoxication, unspecified	55	Substance Use Disorder, Moderate/Severe, or Substance Use with Complications	56	0.329	0.279	0.538	0.356	0.372	0.275	0.178
F10.130	Alcohol abuse with withdrawal, uncomplicated	55	Substance Use Disorder, Moderate/Severe, or Substance Use with Complications	56	0.329	0.279	0.538	0.356	0.372	0.275	0.178
F10.131	Alcohol abuse with withdrawal delirium	54	Substance Use with Psychotic Complications	55,56	0.329	0.543	0.538	0.896	0.372	0.679	0.178
F10.132	Alcohol abuse with withdrawal with perceptual disturbance	54	Substance Use with Psychotic Complications	55,56	0.329	0.543	0.538	0.896	0.372	0.679	0.178
F10.139	Alcohol abuse with withdrawal, unspecified	55	Substance Use Disorder, Moderate/Severe, or Substance Use with Complications	56	0.329	0.279	0.538	0.356	0.372	0.275	0.178
F10.14	Alcohol abuse with alcohol-induced mood disorder	55	Substance Use Disorder, Moderate/Severe, or Substance Use with Complications	56	0.329	0.279	0.538	0.356	0.372	0.275	0.178
F10.150	Alcohol abuse with alcohol-induced psychotic disorder with delusions	54	Substance Use with Psychotic Complications	55,56	0.329	0.543	0.538	0.896	0.372	0.679	0.178
F10.151	Alcohol abuse with alcohol-induced psychotic disorder with hallucinations	54	Substance Use with Psychotic Complications	55,56	0.329	0.543	0.538	0.896	0.372	0.679	0.178
F10.159	Alcohol abuse with alcohol-induced psychotic disorder, unspecified	54	Substance Use with Psychotic Complications	55,56	0.329	0.543	0.538	0.896	0.372	0.679	0.178
F10.180	Alcohol abuse with alcohol-induced anxiety disorder	55	Substance Use Disorder, Moderate/Severe, or Substance Use with Complications	56	0.329	0.279	0.538	0.356	0.372	0.275	0.178
F10.181	Alcohol abuse with alcohol-induced sexual dysfunction	55	Substance Use Disorder, Moderate/Severe, or Substance Use with Complications	56	0.329	0.279	0.538	0.356	0.372	0.275	0.178
F10.182	Alcohol abuse with alcohol-induced sleep disorder	55	Substance Use Disorder, Moderate/Severe, or Substance Use with Complications	56	0.329	0.279	0.538	0.356	0.372	0.275	0.178
F10.188	Alcohol abuse with other alcohol-induced disorder	55	Substance Use Disorder, Moderate/Severe, or Substance Use with Complications	56	0.329	0.279	0.538	0.356	0.372	0.275	0.178
F10.19	Alcohol abuse with unspecified alcohol-induced disorder	55	Substance Use Disorder, Moderate/Severe, or Substance Use with Complications	56	0.329	0.279	0.538	0.356	0.372	0.275	0.178
F10.20	Alcohol dependence, uncomplicated	55	Substance Use Disorder, Moderate/Severe, or Substance Use with Complications	56	0.329	0.279	0.538	0.356	0.372	0.275	0.178
F10.21	Alcohol dependence, in remission	55	Substance Use Disorder, Moderate/Severe, or Substance Use with Complications	56	0.329	0.279	0.538	0.356	0.372	0.275	0.178
F10.220	Alcohol dependence with intoxication, uncomplicated	55	Substance Use Disorder, Moderate/Severe, or Substance Use with Complications	56	0.329	0.279	0.538	0.356	0.372	0.275	0.178
F10.221	Alcohol dependence with intoxication delirium	55	Substance Use Disorder, Moderate/Severe, or Substance Use with Complications	56	0.329	0.279	0.538	0.356	0.372	0.275	0.178

ICD-10-CM Code	ICD-10-CM Code Description	V24 CMS-HCC	V24 CMS-HCC Disease Group	V24 CMS-HCC Hierarchies	Community, NonDual, Aged	Community, NonDual, Disabled	Community, FBDual, Aged	Community, FBDual, Disabled	Community, PBDual, Aged	Community, PBDual, Disabled	Institutional
F10.229	Alcohol dependence with intoxication, unspecified	55	Substance Use Disorder, Moderate/Severe, or Substance Use with Complications	56	0.329	0.279	0.538	0.356	0.372	0.275	0.178
F10.230	Alcohol dependence with withdrawal, uncomplicated	55	Substance Use Disorder, Moderate/Severe, or Substance Use with Complications	56	0.329	0.279	0.538	0.356	0.372	0.275	0.178
F10.231	Alcohol dependence with withdrawal delirium	54	Substance Use with Psychotic Complications	55,56	0.329	0.543	0.538	0.896	0.372	0.679	0.178
F10.232	Alcohol dependence with withdrawal with perceptual disturbance	54	Substance Use with Psychotic Complications	55,56	0.329	0.543	0.538	0.896	0.372	0.679	0.178
F10.239	Alcohol dependence with withdrawal, unspecified	55	Substance Use Disorder, Moderate/Severe, or Substance Use with Complications	56	0.329	0.279	0.538	0.356	0.372	0.275	0.178
F10.24	Alcohol dependence with alcohol-induced mood disorder	55	Substance Use Disorder, Moderate/Severe, or Substance Use with Complications	56	0.329	0.279	0.538	0.356	0.372	0.275	0.178
F10.250	Alcohol dependence with alcohol-induced psychotic disorder with delusions	54	Substance Use with Psychotic Complications	55,56	0.329	0.543	0.538	0.896	0.372	0.679	0.178
F10.251	Alcohol dependence with alcohol-induced psychotic disorder with hallucinations	54	Substance Use with Psychotic Complications	55,56	0.329	0.543	0.538	0.896	0.372	0.679	0.178
F10.259	Alcohol dependence with alcohol-induced psychotic disorder, unspecified	54	Substance Use with Psychotic Complications	55,56	0.329	0.543	0.538	0.896	0.372	0.679	0.178
F10.26	Alcohol dependence with alcohol-induced persisting amnestic disorder	54	Substance Use with Psychotic Complications	55,56	0.329	0.543	0.538	0.896	0.372	0.679	0.178
F10.27	Alcohol dependence with alcohol-induced persisting dementia	54	Substance Use with Psychotic Complications	55,56	0.329	0.543	0.538	0.896	0.372	0.679	0.178
F10.280	Alcohol dependence with alcohol-induced anxiety disorder	55	Substance Use Disorder, Moderate/Severe, or Substance Use with Complications	56	0.329	0.279	0.538	0.356	0.372	0.275	0.178
F10.281	Alcohol dependence with alcohol-induced sexual dysfunction	55	Substance Use Disorder, Moderate/Severe, or Substance Use with Complications	56	0.329	0.279	0.538	0.356	0.372	0.275	0.178
F10.282	Alcohol dependence with alcohol-induced sleep disorder	55	Substance Use Disorder, Moderate/Severe, or Substance Use with Complications	56	0.329	0.279	0.538	0.356	0.372	0.275	0.178
F10.288	Alcohol dependence with other alcohol-induced disorder	55	Substance Use Disorder, Moderate/Severe, or Substance Use with Complications	56	0.329	0.279	0.538	0.356	0.372	0.275	0.178
F10.29	Alcohol dependence with unspecified alcohol-induced disorder	55	Substance Use Disorder, Moderate/Severe, or Substance Use with Complications	56	0.329	0.279	0.538	0.356	0.372	0.275	0.178
F10.920	Alcohol use, unspecified with intoxication, uncomplicated	55	Substance Use Disorder, Moderate/Severe, or Substance Use with Complications	56	0.329	0.279	0.538	0.356	0.372	0.275	0.178
F10.921	Alcohol use, unspecified with intoxication delirium	55	Substance Use Disorder, Moderate/Severe, or Substance Use with Complications	56	0.329	0.279	0.538	0.356	0.372	0.275	0.178
F10.929	Alcohol use, unspecified with intoxication, unspecified	55	Substance Use Disorder, Moderate/Severe, or Substance Use with Complications	56	0.329	0.279	0.538	0.356	0.372	0.275	0.178
F10.930	Alcohol use, unspecified with withdrawal, uncomplicated	55	Substance Use Disorder, Moderate/Severe, or Substance Use with Complications	56	0.329	0.279	0.538	0.356	0.372	0.275	0.178
F10.931	Alcohol use, unspecified with withdrawal delirium	54	Substance Use with Psychotic Complications	55,56	0.329	0.543	0.538	0.896	0.372	0.679	0.178

ICD-10-CM Code	ICD-10-CM Code Description	V24 CMS-HCC	V24 CMS-HCC Disease Group	V24 CMS-HCC Hierarchies	Community, NonDual, Aged	Community, NonDual, Disabled	Community, FBDual, Aged	Community, FBDual, Disabled	Community, PBDual, Aged	Community, PBDual, Disabled	Institutional
F10.932	Alcohol use, unspecified with withdrawal with perceptual disturbance	54	Substance Use with Psychotic Complications	55,56	0.329	0.543	0.538	0.896	0.372	0.679	0.178
F10.939	Alcohol use, unspecified with withdrawal, unspecified	55	Substance Use Disorder, Moderate/Severe, or Substance Use with Complications	56	0.329	0.279	0.538	0.356	0.372	0.275	0.178
F10.94	Alcohol use, unspecified with alcohol-induced mood disorder	55	Substance Use Disorder, Moderate/Severe, or Substance Use with Complications	56	0.329	0.279	0.538	0.356	0.372	0.275	0.178
F10.950	Alcohol use, unspecified with alcohol-induced psychotic disorder with delusions	54	Substance Use with Psychotic Complications	55,56	0.329	0.543	0.538	0.896	0.372	0.679	0.178
F10.951	Alcohol use, unspecified with alcohol-induced psychotic disorder with hallucinations	54	Substance Use with Psychotic Complications	55,56	0.329	0.543	0.538	0.896	0.372	0.679	0.178
F10.959	Alcohol use, unspecified with alcohol-induced psychotic disorder, unspecified	54	Substance Use with Psychotic Complications	55,56	0.329	0.543	0.538	0.896	0.372	0.679	0.178
F10.96	Alcohol use, unspecified with alcohol-induced persisting amnestic disorder	54	Substance Use with Psychotic Complications	55,56	0.329	0.543	0.538	0.896	0.372	0.679	0.178
F10.97	Alcohol use, unspecified with alcohol-induced persisting dementia	54	Substance Use with Psychotic Complications	55,56	0.329	0.543	0.538	0.896	0.372	0.679	0.178
F10.980	Alcohol use, unspecified with alcohol-induced anxiety disorder	55	Substance Use Disorder, Moderate/Severe, or Substance Use with Complications	56	0.329	0.279	0.538	0.356	0.372	0.275	0.178
F10.981	Alcohol use, unspecified with alcohol-induced sexual dysfunction	55	Substance Use Disorder, Moderate/Severe, or Substance Use with Complications	56	0.329	0.279	0.538	0.356	0.372	0.275	0.178
F10.982	Alcohol use, unspecified with alcohol-induced sleep disorder	55	Substance Use Disorder, Moderate/Severe, or Substance Use with Complications	56	0.329	0.279	0.538	0.356	0.372	0.275	0.178
F10.988	Alcohol use, unspecified with other alcohol-induced disorder	55	Substance Use Disorder, Moderate/Severe, or Substance Use with Complications	56	0.329	0.279	0.538	0.356	0.372	0.275	0.178
F10.99	Alcohol use, unspecified with unspecified alcohol-induced disorder	55	Substance Use Disorder, Moderate/Severe, or Substance Use with Complications	56	0.329	0.279	0.538	0.356	0.372	0.275	0.178
F11.10	Opioid abuse, uncomplicated	56	Substance Use Disorder, Mild, Except Alcohol and Cannabis		0.329	0.247	0.538	0.348	0.372	0.275	0.178
F11.11	Opioid abuse, in remission	56	Substance Use Disorder, Mild, Except Alcohol and Cannabis		0.329	0.247	0.538	0.348	0.372	0.275	0.178
F11.120	Opioid abuse with intoxication, uncomplicated	55	Substance Use Disorder, Moderate/Severe, or Substance Use with Complications	56	0.329	0.279	0.538	0.356	0.372	0.275	0.178
F11.121	Opioid abuse with intoxication delirium	55	Substance Use Disorder, Moderate/Severe, or Substance Use with Complications	56	0.329	0.279	0.538	0.356	0.372	0.275	0.178
F11.122	Opioid abuse with intoxication with perceptual disturbance	55	Substance Use Disorder, Moderate/Severe, or Substance Use with Complications	56	0.329	0.279	0.538	0.356	0.372	0.275	0.178
F11.129	Opioid abuse with intoxication, unspecified	55	Substance Use Disorder, Moderate/Severe, or Substance Use with Complications	56	0.329	0.279	0.538	0.356	0.372	0.275	0.178
F11.13	Opioid abuse with withdrawal	55	Substance Use Disorder, Moderate/Severe, or Substance Use with Complications	56	0.329	0.279	0.538	0.356	0.372	0.275	0.178
F11.14	Opioid abuse with opioid-induced mood disorder	55	Substance Use Disorder, Moderate/Severe, or Substance Use with Complications	56	0.329	0.279	0.538	0.356	0.372	0.275	0.178

ICD-10-CM Code	ICD-10-CM Code Description	V24 CMS-HCC	V24 CMS-HCC Disease Group	V24 CMS-HCC Hierarchies	Community, NonDual, Aged	Community, NonDual, Disabled	Community, FBDual, Aged	Community, FBDual, Disabled	Community, PBDual, Aged	Community, PBDual, Disabled	Institutional
F11.150	Opioid abuse with opioid-induced psychotic disorder with delusions	54	Substance Use with Psychotic Complications	55,56	0.329	0.543	0.538	0.896	0.372	0.679	0.178
F11.151	Opioid abuse with opioid-induced psychotic disorder with hallucinations	54	Substance Use with Psychotic Complications	55,56	0.329	0.543	0.538	0.896	0.372	0.679	0.178
F11.159	Opioid abuse with opioid-induced psychotic disorder, unspecified	54	Substance Use with Psychotic Complications	55,56	0.329	0.543	0.538	0.896	0.372	0.679	0.178
F11.181	Opioid abuse with opioid-induced sexual dysfunction	55	Substance Use Disorder, Moderate/Severe, or Substance Use with Complications	56	0.329	0.279	0.538	0.356	0.372	0.275	0.178
F11.182	Opioid abuse with opioid-induced sleep disorder	55	Substance Use Disorder, Moderate/Severe, or Substance Use with Complications	56	0.329	0.279	0.538	0.356	0.372	0.275	0.178
F11.188	Opioid abuse with other opioid-induced disorder	55	Substance Use Disorder, Moderate/Severe, or Substance Use with Complications	56	0.329	0.279	0.538	0.356	0.372	0.275	0.178
F11.19	Opioid abuse with unspecified opioid-induced disorder	55	Substance Use Disorder, Moderate/Severe, or Substance Use with Complications	56	0.329	0.279	0.538	0.356	0.372	0.275	0.178
F11.20	Opioid dependence, uncomplicated	55	Substance Use Disorder, Moderate/Severe, or Substance Use with Complications	56	0.329	0.279	0.538	0.356	0.372	0.275	0.178
F11.21	Opioid dependence, in remission	55	Substance Use Disorder, Moderate/Severe, or Substance Use with Complications	56	0.329	0.279	0.538	0.356	0.372	0.275	0.178
F11.220	Opioid dependence with intoxication, uncomplicated	55	Substance Use Disorder, Moderate/Severe, or Substance Use with Complications	56	0.329	0.279	0.538	0.356	0.372	0.275	0.178
F11.221	Opioid dependence with intoxication delirium	55	Substance Use Disorder, Moderate/Severe, or Substance Use with Complications	56	0.329	0.279	0.538	0.356	0.372	0.275	0.178
F11.222	Opioid dependence with intoxication with perceptual disturbance	55	Substance Use Disorder, Moderate/Severe, or Substance Use with Complications	56	0.329	0.279	0.538	0.356	0.372	0.275	0.178
F11.229	Opioid dependence with intoxication, unspecified	55	Substance Use Disorder, Moderate/Severe, or Substance Use with Complications	56	0.329	0.279	0.538	0.356	0.372	0.275	0.178
F11.23	Opioid dependence with withdrawal	55	Substance Use Disorder, Moderate/Severe, or Substance Use with Complications	56	0.329	0.279	0.538	0.356	0.372	0.275	0.178
F11.24	Opioid dependence with opioid-induced mood disorder	55	Substance Use Disorder, Moderate/Severe, or Substance Use with Complications	56	0.329	0.279	0.538	0.356	0.372	0.275	0.178
F11.250	Opioid dependence with opioid-induced psychotic disorder with delusions	54	Substance Use with Psychotic Complications	55,56	0.329	0.543	0.538	0.896	0.372	0.679	0.178
F11.251	Opioid dependence with opioid-induced psychotic disorder with hallucinations	54	Substance Use with Psychotic Complications	55,56	0.329	0.543	0.538	0.896	0.372	0.679	0.178
F11.259	Opioid dependence with opioid-induced psychotic disorder, unspecified	54	Substance Use with Psychotic Complications	55,56	0.329	0.543	0.538	0.896	0.372	0.679	0.178
F11.281	Opioid dependence with opioid-induced sexual dysfunction	55	Substance Use Disorder, Moderate/Severe, or Substance Use with Complications	56	0.329	0.279	0.538	0.356	0.372	0.275	0.178
F11.282	Opioid dependence with opioid-induced sleep disorder	55	Substance Use Disorder, Moderate/Severe, or Substance Use with Complications	56	0.329	0.279	0.538	0.356	0.372	0.275	0.178
F11.288	Opioid dependence with other opioid-induced disorder	55	Substance Use Disorder, Moderate/Severe, or Substance Use with Complications	56	0.329	0.279	0.538	0.356	0.372	0.275	0.178

ICD-10-CM Code	ICD-10-CM Code Description	V24 CMS-HCC	V24 CMS-HCC Disease Group	V24 CMS-HCC Hierarchies	Community, NonDual, Aged	Community, NonDual, Disabled	Community, FBDual, Aged	Community, FBDual, Disabled	Community, PBDual, Aged	Community, PBDual, Disabled	Institutional
F11.29	Opioid dependence with unspecified opioid-induced disorder	55	Substance Use Disorder, Moderate/Severe, or Substance Use with Complications	56	0.329	0.279	0.538	0.356	0.372	0.275	0.178
F11.920	Opioid use, unspecified with intoxication, uncomplicated	55	Substance Use Disorder, Moderate/Severe, or Substance Use with Complications	56	0.329	0.279	0.538	0.356	0.372	0.275	0.178
F11.921	Opioid use, unspecified with intoxication delirium	55	Substance Use Disorder, Moderate/Severe, or Substance Use with Complications	56	0.329	0.279	0.538	0.356	0.372	0.275	0.178
F11.922	Opioid use, unspecified with intoxication with perceptual disturbance	55	Substance Use Disorder, Moderate/Severe, or Substance Use with Complications	56	0.329	0.279	0.538	0.356	0.372	0.275	0.178
F11.929	Opioid use, unspecified with intoxication, unspecified	55	Substance Use Disorder, Moderate/Severe, or Substance Use with Complications	56	0.329	0.279	0.538	0.356	0.372	0.275	0.178
F11.93	Opioid use, unspecified with withdrawal	55	Substance Use Disorder, Moderate/Severe, or Substance Use with Complications	56	0.329	0.279	0.538	0.356	0.372	0.275	0.178
F11.94	Opioid use, unspecified with opioid-induced mood disorder	55	Substance Use Disorder, Moderate/Severe, or Substance Use with Complications	56	0.329	0.279	0.538	0.356	0.372	0.275	0.178
F11.950	Opioid use, unspecified with opioid-induced psychotic disorder with delusions	54	Substance Use with Psychotic Complications	55,56	0.329	0.543	0.538	0.896	0.372	0.679	0.178
F11.951	Opioid use, unspecified with opioid-induced psychotic disorder with hallucinations	54	Substance Use with Psychotic Complications	55,56	0.329	0.543	0.538	0.896	0.372	0.679	0.178
F11.959	Opioid use, unspecified with opioid-induced psychotic disorder, unspecified	54	Substance Use with Psychotic Complications	55,56	0.329	0.543	0.538	0.896	0.372	0.679	0.178
F11.981	Opioid use, unspecified with opioid-induced sexual dysfunction	55	Substance Use Disorder, Moderate/Severe, or Substance Use with Complications	56	0.329	0.279	0.538	0.356	0.372	0.275	0.178
F11.982	Opioid use, unspecified with opioid-induced sleep disorder	55	Substance Use Disorder, Moderate/Severe, or Substance Use with Complications	56	0.329	0.279	0.538	0.356	0.372	0.275	0.178
F11.988	Opioid use, unspecified with other opioid-induced disorder	55	Substance Use Disorder, Moderate/Severe, or Substance Use with Complications	56	0.329	0.279	0.538	0.356	0.372	0.275	0.178
F11.99	Opioid use, unspecified with unspecified opioid-induced disorder	55	Substance Use Disorder, Moderate/Severe, or Substance Use with Complications	56	0.329	0.279	0.538	0.356	0.372	0.275	0.178
F12.120	Cannabis abuse with intoxication, uncomplicated	55	Substance Use Disorder, Moderate/Severe, or Substance Use with Complications	56	0.329	0.279	0.538	0.356	0.372	0.275	0.178
F12.121	Cannabis abuse with intoxication delirium	55	Substance Use Disorder, Moderate/Severe, or Substance Use with Complications	56	0.329	0.279	0.538	0.356	0.372	0.275	0.178
F12.122	Cannabis abuse with intoxication with perceptual disturbance	55	Substance Use Disorder, Moderate/Severe, or Substance Use with Complications	56	0.329	0.279	0.538	0.356	0.372	0.275	0.178
F12.129	Cannabis abuse with intoxication, unspecified	55	Substance Use Disorder, Moderate/Severe, or Substance Use with Complications	56	0.329	0.279	0.538	0.356	0.372	0.275	0.178
F12.13	Cannabis abuse with withdrawal	55	Substance Use Disorder, Moderate/Severe, or Substance Use with Complications	56	0.329	0.279	0.538	0.356	0.372	0.275	0.178
F12.150	Cannabis abuse with psychotic disorder with delusions	54	Substance Use with Psychotic Complications	55,56	0.329	0.543	0.538	0.896	0.372	0.679	0.178
F12.151	Cannabis abuse with psychotic disorder with hallucinations	54	Substance Use with Psychotic Complications	55,56	0.329	0.543	0.538	0.896	0.372	0.679	0.178

ICD-10-CM Code	ICD-10-CM Code Description	V24 CMS-HCC	V24 CMS-HCC Disease Group	V24 CMS-HCC Hierarchies	Community, NonDual, Aged	Community, NonDual, Disabled	Community, FBDual, Aged	Community, FBDual, Disabled	Community, PBDual, Aged	Community, PBDual, Disabled	Institutional
F12.159	Cannabis abuse with psychotic disorder, unspecified	54	Substance Use with Psychotic Complications	55,56	0.329	0.543	0.538	0.896	0.372	0.679	0.178
F12.180	Cannabis abuse with cannabis-induced anxiety disorder	55	Substance Use Disorder, Moderate/Severe, or Substance Use with Complications	56	0.329	0.279	0.538	0.356	0.372	0.275	0.178
F12.188	Cannabis abuse with other cannabis-induced disorder	55	Substance Use Disorder, Moderate/Severe, or Substance Use with Complications	56	0.329	0.279	0.538	0.356	0.372	0.275	0.178
F12.19	Cannabis abuse with unspecified cannabis-induced disorder	55	Substance Use Disorder, Moderate/Severe, or Substance Use with Complications	56	0.329	0.279	0.538	0.356	0.372	0.275	0.178
F12.20	Cannabis dependence, uncomplicated	55	Substance Use Disorder, Moderate/Severe, or Substance Use with Complications	56	0.329	0.279	0.538	0.356	0.372	0.275	0.178
F12.21	Cannabis dependence, in remission	55	Substance Use Disorder, Moderate/Severe, or Substance Use with Complications	56	0.329	0.279	0.538	0.356	0.372	0.275	0.178
F12.220	Cannabis dependence with intoxication, uncomplicated	55	Substance Use Disorder, Moderate/Severe, or Substance Use with Complications	56	0.329	0.279	0.538	0.356	0.372	0.275	0.178
F12.221	Cannabis dependence with intoxication delirium	55	Substance Use Disorder, Moderate/Severe, or Substance Use with Complications	56	0.329	0.279	0.538	0.356	0.372	0.275	0.178
F12.222	Cannabis dependence with intoxication with perceptual disturbance	55	Substance Use Disorder, Moderate/Severe, or Substance Use with Complications	56	0.329	0.279	0.538	0.356	0.372	0.275	0.178
F12.229	Cannabis dependence with intoxication, unspecified	55	Substance Use Disorder, Moderate/Severe, or Substance Use with Complications	56	0.329	0.279	0.538	0.356	0.372	0.275	0.178
F12.23	Cannabis dependence with withdrawal	55	Substance Use Disorder, Moderate/Severe, or Substance Use with Complications	56	0.329	0.279	0.538	0.356	0.372	0.275	0.178
F12.250	Cannabis dependence with psychotic disorder with delusions	54	Substance Use with Psychotic Complications	55,56	0.329	0.543	0.538	0.896	0.372	0.679	0.178
F12.251	Cannabis dependence with psychotic disorder with hallucinations	54	Substance Use with Psychotic Complications	55,56	0.329	0.543	0.538	0.896	0.372	0.679	0.178
F12.259	Cannabis dependence with psychotic disorder, unspecified	54	Substance Use with Psychotic Complications	55,56	0.329	0.543	0.538	0.896	0.372	0.679	0.178
F12.280	Cannabis dependence with cannabis-induced anxiety disorder	55	Substance Use Disorder, Moderate/Severe, or Substance Use with Complications	56	0.329	0.279	0.538	0.356	0.372	0.275	0.178
F12.288	Cannabis dependence with other cannabis-induced disorder	55	Substance Use Disorder, Moderate/Severe, or Substance Use with Complications	56	0.329	0.279	0.538	0.356	0.372	0.275	0.178
F12.29	Cannabis dependence with unspecified cannabis-induced disorder	55	Substance Use Disorder, Moderate/Severe, or Substance Use with Complications	56	0.329	0.279	0.538	0.356	0.372	0.275	0.178
F12.920	Cannabis use, unspecified with intoxication, uncomplicated	55	Substance Use Disorder, Moderate/Severe, or Substance Use with Complications	56	0.329	0.279	0.538	0.356	0.372	0.275	0.178
F12.921	Cannabis use, unspecified with intoxication delirium	55	Substance Use Disorder, Moderate/Severe, or Substance Use with Complications	56	0.329	0.279	0.538	0.356	0.372	0.275	0.178
F12.922	Cannabis use, unspecified with intoxication with perceptual disturbance	55	Substance Use Disorder, Moderate/Severe, or Substance Use with Complications	56	0.329	0.279	0.538	0.356	0.372	0.275	0.178
F12.929	Cannabis use, unspecified with intoxication, unspecified	55	Substance Use Disorder, Moderate/Severe, or Substance Use with Complications	56	0.329	0.279	0.538	0.356	0.372	0.275	0.178

ICD-10-CM Code	ICD-10-CM Code Description	V24 CMS-HCC	V24 CMS-HCC Disease Group	V24 CMS-HCC Hierarchies	Community, NonDual, Aged	Community, NonDual, Disabled	Community, FBDual, Aged	Community, FBDual, Disabled	Community, PBDual, Aged	Community, PBDual, Disabled	Institutional
F12.93	Cannabis use, unspecified with withdrawal	55	Substance Use Disorder, Moderate/ Severe, or Substance Use with Complications	56	0.329	0.279	0.538	0.356	0.372	0.275	0.178
F12.950	Cannabis use, unspecified with psychotic disorder with delusions	54	Substance Use with Psychotic Complications	55,56	0.329	0.543	0.538	0.896	0.372	0.679	0.178
F12.951	Cannabis use, unspecified with psychotic disorder with hallucinations	54	Substance Use with Psychotic Complications	55,56	0.329	0.543	0.538	0.896	0.372	0.679	0.178
F12.959	Cannabis use, unspecified with psychotic disorder, unspecified	54	Substance Use with Psychotic Complications	55,56	0.329	0.543	0.538	0.896	0.372	0.679	0.178
F12.980	Cannabis use, unspecified with anxiety disorder	55	Substance Use Disorder, Moderate/ Severe, or Substance Use with Complications	56	0.329	0.279	0.538	0.356	0.372	0.275	0.178
F12.988	Cannabis use, unspecified with other cannabis-induced disorder	55	Substance Use Disorder, Moderate/ Severe, or Substance Use with Complications	56	0.329	0.279	0.538	0.356	0.372	0.275	0.178
F12.99	Cannabis use, unspecified with unspecified cannabis-induced disorder	55	Substance Use Disorder, Moderate/ Severe, or Substance Use with Complications	56	0.329	0.279	0.538	0.356	0.372	0.275	0.178
F13.10	Sedative, hypnotic or anxiolytic abuse, uncomplicated	56	Substance Use Disorder, Mild, Except Alcohol and Cannabis		0.329	0.247	0.538	0.348	0.372	0.275	0.178
F13.11	Sedative, hypnotic or anxiolytic abuse, in remission	56	Substance Use Disorder, Mild, Except Alcohol and Cannabis		0.329	0.247	0.538	0.348	0.372	0.275	0.178
F13.120	Sedative, hypnotic or anxiolytic abuse with intoxication, uncomplicated	55	Substance Use Disorder, Moderate/ Severe, or Substance Use with Complications	56	0.329	0.279	0.538	0.356	0.372	0.275	0.178
F13.121	Sedative, hypnotic or anxiolytic abuse with intoxication delirium	55	Substance Use Disorder, Moderate/ Severe, or Substance Use with Complications	56	0.329	0.279	0.538	0.356	0.372	0.275	0.178
F13.129	Sedative, hypnotic or anxiolytic abuse with intoxication, unspecified	55	Substance Use Disorder, Moderate/ Severe, or Substance Use with Complications	56	0.329	0.279	0.538	0.356	0.372	0.275	0.178
F13.130	Sedative, hypnotic or anxiolytic abuse with withdrawal, uncomplicated	55	Substance Use Disorder, Moderate/ Severe, or Substance Use with Complications	56	0.329	0.279	0.538	0.356	0.372	0.275	0.178
F13.131	Sedative, hypnotic or anxiolytic abuse with withdrawal delirium	54	Substance Use with Psychotic Complications	55,56	0.329	0.543	0.538	0.896	0.372	0.679	0.178
F13.132	Sedative, hypnotic or anxiolytic abuse with withdrawal with perceptual disturbance	54	Substance Use with Psychotic Complications	55,56	0.329	0.543	0.538	0.896	0.372	0.679	0.178
F13.139	Sedative, hypnotic or anxiolytic abuse with withdrawal, unspecified	55	Substance Use Disorder, Moderate/ Severe, or Substance Use with Complications	56	0.329	0.279	0.538	0.356	0.372	0.275	0.178
F13.14	Sedative, hypnotic or anxiolytic abuse with sedative, hypnotic or anxiolytic-induced mood disorder	55	Substance Use Disorder, Moderate/ Severe, or Substance Use with Complications	56	0.329	0.279	0.538	0.356	0.372	0.275	0.178
F13.150	Sedative, hypnotic or anxiolytic abuse with sedative, hypnotic or anxiolytic-induced psychotic disorder with delusions	54	Substance Use with Psychotic Complications	55,56	0.329	0.543	0.538	0.896	0.372	0.679	0.178
F13.151	Sedative, hypnotic or anxiolytic abuse with sedative, hypnotic or anxiolytic-induced psychotic disorder with hallucinations	54	Substance Use with Psychotic Complications	55,56	0.329	0.543	0.538	0.896	0.372	0.679	0.178
F13.159	Sedative, hypnotic or anxiolytic abuse with sedative, hypnotic or anxiolytic-induced psychotic disorder, unspecified	54	Substance Use with Psychotic Complications	55,56	0.329	0.543	0.538	0.896	0.372	0.679	0.178
F13.180	Sedative, hypnotic or anxiolytic abuse with sedative, hypnotic or anxiolytic-induced anxiety disorder	55	Substance Use Disorder, Moderate/ Severe, or Substance Use with Complications	56	0.329	0.279	0.538	0.356	0.372	0.275	0.178

ICD-10-CM Code	ICD-10-CM Code Description	V24 CMS-HCC	V24 CMS-HCC Disease Group	V24 CMS-HCC Hierarchies	Community, NonDual, Aged	Community, NonDual, Disabled	Community, FBDual, Aged	Community, FBDual, Disabled	Community, PBDual, Aged	Community, PBDual, Disabled	Institutional
F13.181	Sedative, hypnotic or anxiolytic abuse with sedative, hypnotic or anxiolytic-induced sexual dysfunction	55	Substance Use Disorder, Moderate/Severe, or Substance Use with Complications	56	0.329	0.279	0.538	0.356	0.372	0.275	0.178
F13.182	Sedative, hypnotic or anxiolytic abuse with sedative, hypnotic or anxiolytic-induced sleep disorder	55	Substance Use Disorder, Moderate/Severe, or Substance Use with Complications	56	0.329	0.279	0.538	0.356	0.372	0.275	0.178
F13.188	Sedative, hypnotic or anxiolytic abuse with other sedative, hypnotic or anxiolytic-induced disorder	55	Substance Use Disorder, Moderate/Severe, or Substance Use with Complications	56	0.329	0.279	0.538	0.356	0.372	0.275	0.178
F13.19	Sedative, hypnotic or anxiolytic abuse with unspecified sedative, hypnotic or anxiolytic-induced disorder	55	Substance Use Disorder, Moderate/Severe, or Substance Use with Complications	56	0.329	0.279	0.538	0.356	0.372	0.275	0.178
F13.20	Sedative, hypnotic or anxiolytic dependence, uncomplicated	55	Substance Use Disorder, Moderate/Severe, or Substance Use with Complications	56	0.329	0.279	0.538	0.356	0.372	0.275	0.178
F13.21	Sedative, hypnotic or anxiolytic dependence, in remission	55	Substance Use Disorder, Moderate/Severe, or Substance Use with Complications	56	0.329	0.279	0.538	0.356	0.372	0.275	0.178
F13.220	Sedative, hypnotic or anxiolytic dependence with intoxication, uncomplicated	55	Substance Use Disorder, Moderate/Severe, or Substance Use with Complications	56	0.329	0.279	0.538	0.356	0.372	0.275	0.178
F13.221	Sedative, hypnotic or anxiolytic dependence with intoxication delirium	55	Substance Use Disorder, Moderate/Severe, or Substance Use with Complications	56	0.329	0.279	0.538	0.356	0.372	0.275	0.178
F13.229	Sedative, hypnotic or anxiolytic dependence with intoxication, unspecified	55	Substance Use Disorder, Moderate/Severe, or Substance Use with Complications	56	0.329	0.279	0.538	0.356	0.372	0.275	0.178
F13.230	Sedative, hypnotic or anxiolytic dependence with withdrawal, uncomplicated	55	Substance Use Disorder, Moderate/Severe, or Substance Use with Complications	56	0.329	0.279	0.538	0.356	0.372	0.275	0.178
F13.231	Sedative, hypnotic or anxiolytic dependence with withdrawal delirium	54	Substance Use with Psychotic Complications	55,56	0.329	0.543	0.538	0.896	0.372	0.679	0.178
F13.232	Sedative, hypnotic or anxiolytic dependence with withdrawal with perceptual disturbance	54	Substance Use with Psychotic Complications	55,56	0.329	0.543	0.538	0.896	0.372	0.679	0.178
F13.239	Sedative, hypnotic or anxiolytic dependence with withdrawal, unspecified	55	Substance Use Disorder, Moderate/Severe, or Substance Use with Complications	56	0.329	0.279	0.538	0.356	0.372	0.275	0.178
F13.24	Sedative, hypnotic or anxiolytic dependence with sedative, hypnotic or anxiolytic-induced mood disorder	55	Substance Use Disorder, Moderate/Severe, or Substance Use with Complications	56	0.329	0.279	0.538	0.356	0.372	0.275	0.178
F13.250	Sedative, hypnotic or anxiolytic dependence with sedative, hypnotic or anxiolytic-induced psychotic disorder with delusions	54	Substance Use with Psychotic Complications	55,56	0.329	0.543	0.538	0.896	0.372	0.679	0.178
F13.251	Sedative, hypnotic or anxiolytic dependence with sedative, hypnotic or anxiolytic-induced psychotic disorder with hallucinations	54	Substance Use with Psychotic Complications	55,56	0.329	0.543	0.538	0.896	0.372	0.679	0.178
F13.259	Sedative, hypnotic or anxiolytic dependence with sedative, hypnotic or anxiolytic-induced psychotic disorder, unspecified	54	Substance Use with Psychotic Complications	55,56	0.329	0.543	0.538	0.896	0.372	0.679	0.178
F13.26	Sedative, hypnotic or anxiolytic dependence with sedative, hypnotic or anxiolytic-induced persisting amnestic disorder	54	Substance Use with Psychotic Complications	55,56	0.329	0.543	0.538	0.896	0.372	0.679	0.178

ICD-10-CM Code	ICD-10-CM Code Description	V24 CMS-HCC	V24 CMS-HCC Disease Group	V24 CMS-HCC Hierarchies	Community, NonDual, Aged	Community, NonDual, Disabled	Community, FBDual, Aged	Community, FBDual, Disabled	Community, PBDual, Aged	Community, PBDual, Disabled	Institutional
F13.27	Sedative, hypnotic or anxiolytic dependence with sedative, hypnotic or anxiolytic-induced persisting dementia	54	Substance Use with Psychotic Complications	55,56	0.329	0.543	0.538	0.896	0.372	0.679	0.178
F13.280	Sedative, hypnotic or anxiolytic dependence with sedative, hypnotic or anxiolytic-induced anxiety disorder	55	Substance Use Disorder, Moderate/ Severe, or Substance Use with Complications	56	0.329	0.279	0.538	0.356	0.372	0.275	0.178
F13.281	Sedative, hypnotic or anxiolytic dependence with sedative, hypnotic or anxiolytic-induced sexual dysfunction	55	Substance Use Disorder, Moderate/ Severe, or Substance Use with Complications	56	0.329	0.279	0.538	0.356	0.372	0.275	0.178
F13.282	Sedative, hypnotic or anxiolytic dependence with sedative, hypnotic or anxiolytic-induced sleep disorder	55	Substance Use Disorder, Moderate/ Severe, or Substance Use with Complications	56	0.329	0.279	0.538	0.356	0.372	0.275	0.178
F13.288	Sedative, hypnotic or anxiolytic dependence with other sedative, hypnotic or anxiolytic-induced disorder	55	Substance Use Disorder, Moderate/ Severe, or Substance Use with Complications	56	0.329	0.279	0.538	0.356	0.372	0.275	0.178
F13.29	Sedative, hypnotic or anxiolytic dependence with unspecified sedative, hypnotic or anxiolytic-induced disorder	55	Substance Use Disorder, Moderate/ Severe, or Substance Use with Complications	56	0.329	0.279	0.538	0.356	0.372	0.275	0.178
F13.920	Sedative, hypnotic or anxiolytic use, unspecified with intoxication, uncomplicated	55	Substance Use Disorder, Moderate/ Severe, or Substance Use with Complications	56	0.329	0.279	0.538	0.356	0.372	0.275	0.178
F13.921	Sedative, hypnotic or anxiolytic use, unspecified with intoxication delirium	55	Substance Use Disorder, Moderate/ Severe, or Substance Use with Complications	56	0.329	0.279	0.538	0.356	0.372	0.275	0.178
F13.929	Sedative, hypnotic or anxiolytic use, unspecified with intoxication, unspecified	55	Substance Use Disorder, Moderate/ Severe, or Substance Use with Complications	56	0.329	0.279	0.538	0.356	0.372	0.275	0.178
F13.930	Sedative, hypnotic or anxiolytic use, unspecified with withdrawal, uncomplicated	55	Substance Use Disorder, Moderate/ Severe, or Substance Use with Complications	56	0.329	0.279	0.538	0.356	0.372	0.275	0.178
F13.931	Sedative, hypnotic or anxiolytic use, unspecified with withdrawal delirium	54	Substance Use with Psychotic Complications	55,56	0.329	0.543	0.538	0.896	0.372	0.679	0.178
F13.932	Sedative, hypnotic or anxiolytic use, unspecified with withdrawal with perceptual disturbances	54	Substance Use with Psychotic Complications	55,56	0.329	0.543	0.538	0.896	0.372	0.679	0.178
F13.939	Sedative, hypnotic or anxiolytic use, unspecified with withdrawal, unspecified	55	Substance Use Disorder, Moderate/ Severe, or Substance Use with Complications	56	0.329	0.279	0.538	0.356	0.372	0.275	0.178
F13.94	Sedative, hypnotic or anxiolytic use, unspecified with sedative, hypnotic or anxiolytic-induced mood disorder	55	Substance Use Disorder, Moderate/ Severe, or Substance Use with Complications	56	0.329	0.279	0.538	0.356	0.372	0.275	0.178
F13.950	Sedative, hypnotic or anxiolytic use, unspecified with sedative, hypnotic or anxiolytic-induced psychotic disorder with delusions	54	Substance Use with Psychotic Complications	55,56	0.329	0.543	0.538	0.896	0.372	0.679	0.178
F13.951	Sedative, hypnotic or anxiolytic use, unspecified with sedative, hypnotic or anxiolytic-induced psychotic disorder with hallucinations	54	Substance Use with Psychotic Complications	55,56	0.329	0.543	0.538	0.896	0.372	0.679	0.178
F13.959	Sedative, hypnotic or anxiolytic use, unspecified with sedative, hypnotic or anxiolytic-induced psychotic disorder, unspecified	54	Substance Use with Psychotic Complications	55,56	0.329	0.543	0.538	0.896	0.372	0.679	0.178
F13.96	Sedative, hypnotic or anxiolytic use, unspecified with sedative, hypnotic or anxiolytic-induced persisting amnestic disorder	54	Substance Use with Psychotic Complications	55,56	0.329	0.543	0.538	0.896	0.372	0.679	0.178

ICD-10-CM Code	ICD-10-CM Code Description	V24 CMS-HCC	V24 CMS-HCC Disease Group	V24 CMS-HCC Hierarchies	Community, NonDual, Aged	Community, NonDual, Disabled	Community, FBDual, Aged	Community, FBDual, Disabled	Community, PBDual, Aged	Community, PBDual, Disabled	Institutional
F13.97	Sedative, hypnotic or anxiolytic use, unspecified with sedative, hypnotic or anxiolytic-induced persisting dementia	54	Substance Use with Psychotic Complications	55,56	0.329	0.543	0.538	0.896	0.372	0.679	0.178
F13.980	Sedative, hypnotic or anxiolytic use, unspecified with sedative, hypnotic or anxiolytic-induced anxiety disorder	55	Substance Use Disorder, Moderate/Severe, or Substance Use with Complications	56	0.329	0.279	0.538	0.356	0.372	0.275	0.178
F13.981	Sedative, hypnotic or anxiolytic use, unspecified with sedative, hypnotic or anxiolytic-induced sexual dysfunction	55	Substance Use Disorder, Moderate/Severe, or Substance Use with Complications	56	0.329	0.279	0.538	0.356	0.372	0.275	0.178
F13.982	Sedative, hypnotic or anxiolytic use, unspecified with sedative, hypnotic or anxiolytic-induced sleep disorder	55	Substance Use Disorder, Moderate/Severe, or Substance Use with Complications	56	0.329	0.279	0.538	0.356	0.372	0.275	0.178
F13.988	Sedative, hypnotic or anxiolytic use, unspecified with other sedative, hypnotic or anxiolytic-induced disorder	55	Substance Use Disorder, Moderate/Severe, or Substance Use with Complications	56	0.329	0.279	0.538	0.356	0.372	0.275	0.178
F13.99	Sedative, hypnotic or anxiolytic use, unspecified with unspecified sedative, hypnotic or anxiolytic-induced disorder	55	Substance Use Disorder, Moderate/Severe, or Substance Use with Complications	56	0.329	0.279	0.538	0.356	0.372	0.275	0.178
F14.10	Cocaine abuse, uncomplicated	56	Substance Use Disorder, Mild, Except Alcohol and Cannabis		0.329	0.247	0.538	0.348	0.372	0.275	0.178
F14.11	Cocaine abuse, in remission	56	Substance Use Disorder, Mild, Except Alcohol and Cannabis		0.329	0.247	0.538	0.348	0.372	0.275	0.178
F14.120	Cocaine abuse with intoxication, uncomplicated	55	Substance Use Disorder, Moderate/Severe, or Substance Use with Complications	56	0.329	0.279	0.538	0.356	0.372	0.275	0.178
F14.121	Cocaine abuse with intoxication with delirium	55	Substance Use Disorder, Moderate/Severe, or Substance Use with Complications	56	0.329	0.279	0.538	0.356	0.372	0.275	0.178
F14.122	Cocaine abuse with intoxication with perceptual disturbance	55	Substance Use Disorder, Moderate/Severe, or Substance Use with Complications	56	0.329	0.279	0.538	0.356	0.372	0.275	0.178
F14.129	Cocaine abuse with intoxication, unspecified	55	Substance Use Disorder, Moderate/Severe, or Substance Use with Complications	56	0.329	0.279	0.538	0.356	0.372	0.275	0.178
F14.13	Cocaine abuse, unspecified with withdrawal	55	Substance Use Disorder, Moderate/Severe, or Substance Use with Complications	56	0.329	0.279	0.538	0.356	0.372	0.275	0.178
F14.14	Cocaine abuse with cocaine-induced mood disorder	55	Substance Use Disorder, Moderate/Severe, or Substance Use with Complications	56	0.329	0.279	0.538	0.356	0.372	0.275	0.178
F14.150	Cocaine abuse with cocaine-induced psychotic disorder with delusions	54	Substance Use with Psychotic Complications	55,56	0.329	0.543	0.538	0.896	0.372	0.679	0.178
F14.151	Cocaine abuse with cocaine-induced psychotic disorder with hallucinations	54	Substance Use with Psychotic Complications	55,56	0.329	0.543	0.538	0.896	0.372	0.679	0.178
F14.159	Cocaine abuse with cocaine-induced psychotic disorder, unspecified	54	Substance Use with Psychotic Complications	55,56	0.329	0.543	0.538	0.896	0.372	0.679	0.178
F14.180	Cocaine abuse with cocaine-induced anxiety disorder	55	Substance Use Disorder, Moderate/Severe, or Substance Use with Complications	56	0.329	0.279	0.538	0.356	0.372	0.275	0.178
F14.181	Cocaine abuse with cocaine-induced sexual dysfunction	55	Substance Use Disorder, Moderate/Severe, or Substance Use with Complications	56	0.329	0.279	0.538	0.356	0.372	0.275	0.178
F14.182	Cocaine abuse with cocaine-induced sleep disorder	55	Substance Use Disorder, Moderate/Severe, or Substance Use with Complications	56	0.329	0.279	0.538	0.356	0.372	0.275	0.178

ICD-10-CM Code	ICD-10-CM Code Description	V24 CMS-HCC	V24 CMS-HCC Disease Group	V24 CMS-HCC Hierarchies	Community, NonDual, Aged	Community, NonDual, Disabled	Community, FBDual, Aged	Community, FBDual, Disabled	Community, PBDual, Aged	Community, PBDual, Disabled	Institutional
F14.188	Cocaine abuse with other cocaine-induced disorder	55	Substance Use Disorder, Moderate/Severe, or Substance Use with Complications	56	0.329	0.279	0.538	0.356	0.372	0.275	0.178
F14.19	Cocaine abuse with unspecified cocaine-induced disorder	55	Substance Use Disorder, Moderate/Severe, or Substance Use with Complications	56	0.329	0.279	0.538	0.356	0.372	0.275	0.178
F14.20	Cocaine dependence, uncomplicated	55	Substance Use Disorder, Moderate/Severe, or Substance Use with Complications	56	0.329	0.279	0.538	0.356	0.372	0.275	0.178
F14.21	Cocaine dependence, in remission	55	Substance Use Disorder, Moderate/Severe, or Substance Use with Complications	56	0.329	0.279	0.538	0.356	0.372	0.275	0.178
F14.220	Cocaine dependence with intoxication, uncomplicated	55	Substance Use Disorder, Moderate/Severe, or Substance Use with Complications	56	0.329	0.279	0.538	0.356	0.372	0.275	0.178
F14.221	Cocaine dependence with intoxication delirium	55	Substance Use Disorder, Moderate/Severe, or Substance Use with Complications	56	0.329	0.279	0.538	0.356	0.372	0.275	0.178
F14.222	Cocaine dependence with intoxication with perceptual disturbance	55	Substance Use Disorder, Moderate/Severe, or Substance Use with Complications	56	0.329	0.279	0.538	0.356	0.372	0.275	0.178
F14.229	Cocaine dependence with intoxication, unspecified	55	Substance Use Disorder, Moderate/Severe, or Substance Use with Complications	56	0.329	0.279	0.538	0.356	0.372	0.275	0.178
F14.23	Cocaine dependence with withdrawal	55	Substance Use Disorder, Moderate/Severe, or Substance Use with Complications	56	0.329	0.279	0.538	0.356	0.372	0.275	0.178
F14.24	Cocaine dependence with cocaine-induced mood disorder	55	Substance Use Disorder, Moderate/Severe, or Substance Use with Complications	56	0.329	0.279	0.538	0.356	0.372	0.275	0.178
F14.250	Cocaine dependence with cocaine-induced psychotic disorder with delusions	54	Substance Use with Psychotic Complications	55,56	0.329	0.543	0.538	0.896	0.372	0.679	0.178
F14.251	Cocaine dependence with cocaine-induced psychotic disorder with hallucinations	54	Substance Use with Psychotic Complications	55,56	0.329	0.543	0.538	0.896	0.372	0.679	0.178
F14.259	Cocaine dependence with cocaine-induced psychotic disorder, unspecified	54	Substance Use with Psychotic Complications	55,56	0.329	0.543	0.538	0.896	0.372	0.679	0.178
F14.280	Cocaine dependence with cocaine-induced anxiety disorder	55	Substance Use Disorder, Moderate/Severe, or Substance Use with Complications	56	0.329	0.279	0.538	0.356	0.372	0.275	0.178
F14.281	Cocaine dependence with cocaine-induced sexual dysfunction	55	Substance Use Disorder, Moderate/Severe, or Substance Use with Complications	56	0.329	0.279	0.538	0.356	0.372	0.275	0.178
F14.282	Cocaine dependence with cocaine-induced sleep disorder	55	Substance Use Disorder, Moderate/Severe, or Substance Use with Complications	56	0.329	0.279	0.538	0.356	0.372	0.275	0.178
F14.288	Cocaine dependence with other cocaine-induced disorder	55	Substance Use Disorder, Moderate/Severe, or Substance Use with Complications	56	0.329	0.279	0.538	0.356	0.372	0.275	0.178
F14.29	Cocaine dependence with unspecified cocaine-induced disorder	55	Substance Use Disorder, Moderate/Severe, or Substance Use with Complications	56	0.329	0.279	0.538	0.356	0.372	0.275	0.178
F14.920	Cocaine use, unspecified with intoxication, uncomplicated	55	Substance Use Disorder, Moderate/Severe, or Substance Use with Complications	56	0.329	0.279	0.538	0.356	0.372	0.275	0.178
F14.921	Cocaine use, unspecified with intoxication delirium	55	Substance Use Disorder, Moderate/Severe, or Substance Use with Complications	56	0.329	0.279	0.538	0.356	0.372	0.275	0.178

ICD-10-CM Code	ICD-10-CM Code Description	V24 CMS-HCC	V24 CMS-HCC Disease Group	V24 CMS-HCC Hierarchies	Community, NonDual, Aged	Community, NonDual, Disabled	Community, FBDual, Aged	Community, FBDual, Disabled	Community, PBDual, Aged	Community, PBDual, Disabled	Institutional
F14.922	Cocaine use, unspecified with intoxication with perceptual disturbance	55	Substance Use Disorder, Moderate/Severe, or Substance Use with Complications	56	0.329	0.279	0.538	0.356	0.372	0.275	0.178
F14.929	Cocaine use, unspecified with intoxication, unspecified	55	Substance Use Disorder, Moderate/Severe, or Substance Use with Complications	56	0.329	0.279	0.538	0.356	0.372	0.275	0.178
F14.93	Cocaine use, unspecified with withdrawal	55	Substance Use Disorder, Moderate/Severe, or Substance Use with Complications	56	0.329	0.279	0.538	0.356	0.372	0.275	0.178
F14.94	Cocaine use, unspecified with cocaine-induced mood disorder	55	Substance Use Disorder, Moderate/Severe, or Substance Use with Complications	56	0.329	0.279	0.538	0.356	0.372	0.275	0.178
F14.950	Cocaine use, unspecified with cocaine-induced psychotic disorder with delusions	54	Substance Use with Psychotic Complications	55,56	0.329	0.543	0.538	0.896	0.372	0.679	0.178
F14.951	Cocaine use, unspecified with cocaine-induced psychotic disorder with hallucinations	54	Substance Use with Psychotic Complications	55,56	0.329	0.543	0.538	0.896	0.372	0.679	0.178
F14.959	Cocaine use, unspecified with cocaine-induced psychotic disorder, unspecified	54	Substance Use with Psychotic Complications	55,56	0.329	0.543	0.538	0.896	0.372	0.679	0.178
F14.980	Cocaine use, unspecified with cocaine-induced anxiety disorder	55	Substance Use Disorder, Moderate/Severe, or Substance Use with Complications	56	0.329	0.279	0.538	0.356	0.372	0.275	0.178
F14.981	Cocaine use, unspecified with cocaine-induced sexual dysfunction	55	Substance Use Disorder, Moderate/Severe, or Substance Use with Complications	56	0.329	0.279	0.538	0.356	0.372	0.275	0.178
F14.982	Cocaine use, unspecified with cocaine-induced sleep disorder	55	Substance Use Disorder, Moderate/Severe, or Substance Use with Complications	56	0.329	0.279	0.538	0.356	0.372	0.275	0.178
F14.988	Cocaine use, unspecified with other cocaine-induced disorder	55	Substance Use Disorder, Moderate/Severe, or Substance Use with Complications	56	0.329	0.279	0.538	0.356	0.372	0.275	0.178
F14.99	Cocaine use, unspecified with unspecified cocaine-induced disorder	55	Substance Use Disorder, Moderate/Severe, or Substance Use with Complications	56	0.329	0.279	0.538	0.356	0.372	0.275	0.178
F15.10	Other stimulant abuse, uncomplicated	56	Substance Use Disorder, Mild, Except Alcohol and Cannabis		0.329	0.247	0.538	0.348	0.372	0.275	0.178
F15.11	Other stimulant abuse, in remission	56	Substance Use Disorder, Mild, Except Alcohol and Cannabis		0.329	0.247	0.538	0.348	0.372	0.275	0.178
F15.120	Other stimulant abuse with intoxication, uncomplicated	55	Substance Use Disorder, Moderate/Severe, or Substance Use with Complications	56	0.329	0.279	0.538	0.356	0.372	0.275	0.178
F15.121	Other stimulant abuse with intoxication delirium	55	Substance Use Disorder, Moderate/Severe, or Substance Use with Complications	56	0.329	0.279	0.538	0.356	0.372	0.275	0.178
F15.122	Other stimulant abuse with intoxication with perceptual disturbance	55	Substance Use Disorder, Moderate/Severe, or Substance Use with Complications	56	0.329	0.279	0.538	0.356	0.372	0.275	0.178
F15.129	Other stimulant abuse with intoxication, unspecified	55	Substance Use Disorder, Moderate/Severe, or Substance Use with Complications	56	0.329	0.279	0.538	0.356	0.372	0.275	0.178
F15.13	Other stimulant abuse with withdrawal	55	Substance Use Disorder, Moderate/Severe, or Substance Use with Complications	56	0.329	0.279	0.538	0.356	0.372	0.275	0.178
F15.14	Other stimulant abuse with stimulant-induced mood disorder	55	Substance Use Disorder, Moderate/Severe, or Substance Use with Complications	56	0.329	0.279	0.538	0.356	0.372	0.275	0.178
F15.150	Other stimulant abuse with stimulant-induced psychotic disorder with delusions	54	Substance Use with Psychotic Complications	55,56	0.329	0.543	0.538	0.896	0.372	0.679	0.178

ICD-10-CM Code	ICD-10-CM Code Description	V24 CMS-HCC	V24 CMS-HCC Disease Group	V24 CMS-HCC Hierarchies	Community, NonDual, Aged	Community, NonDual, Disabled	Community, FBDual, Aged	Community, FBDual, Disabled	Community, PBDual, Aged	Community, PBDual, Disabled	Institutional
F15.151	Other stimulant abuse with stimulant-induced psychotic disorder with hallucinations	54	Substance Use with Psychotic Complications	55,56	0.329	0.543	0.538	0.896	0.372	0.679	0.178
F15.159	Other stimulant abuse with stimulant-induced psychotic disorder, unspecified	54	Substance Use with Psychotic Complications	55,56	0.329	0.543	0.538	0.896	0.372	0.679	0.178
F15.18Ø	Other stimulant abuse with stimulant-induced anxiety disorder	55	Substance Use Disorder, Moderate/Severe, or Substance Use with Complications	56	0.329	0.279	0.538	0.356	0.372	0.275	0.178
F15.181	Other stimulant abuse with stimulant-induced sexual dysfunction	55	Substance Use Disorder, Moderate/Severe, or Substance Use with Complications	56	0.329	0.279	0.538	0.356	0.372	0.275	0.178
F15.182	Other stimulant abuse with stimulant-induced sleep disorder	55	Substance Use Disorder, Moderate/Severe, or Substance Use with Complications	56	0.329	0.279	0.538	0.356	0.372	0.275	0.178
F15.188	Other stimulant abuse with other stimulant-induced disorder	55	Substance Use Disorder, Moderate/Severe, or Substance Use with Complications	56	0.329	0.279	0.538	0.356	0.372	0.275	0.178
F15.19	Other stimulant abuse with unspecified stimulant-induced disorder	55	Substance Use Disorder, Moderate/Severe, or Substance Use with Complications	56	0.329	0.279	0.538	0.356	0.372	0.275	0.178
F15.2Ø	Other stimulant dependence, uncomplicated	55	Substance Use Disorder, Moderate/Severe, or Substance Use with Complications	56	0.329	0.279	0.538	0.356	0.372	0.275	0.178
F15.21	Other stimulant dependence, in remission	55	Substance Use Disorder, Moderate/Severe, or Substance Use with Complications	56	0.329	0.279	0.538	0.356	0.372	0.275	0.178
F15.22Ø	Other stimulant dependence with intoxication, uncomplicated	55	Substance Use Disorder, Moderate/Severe, or Substance Use with Complications	56	0.329	0.279	0.538	0.356	0.372	0.275	0.178
F15.221	Other stimulant dependence with intoxication delirium	55	Substance Use Disorder, Moderate/Severe, or Substance Use with Complications	56	0.329	0.279	0.538	0.356	0.372	0.275	0.178
F15.222	Other stimulant dependence with intoxication with perceptual disturbance	55	Substance Use Disorder, Moderate/Severe, or Substance Use with Complications	56	0.329	0.279	0.538	0.356	0.372	0.275	0.178
F15.229	Other stimulant dependence with intoxication, unspecified	55	Substance Use Disorder, Moderate/Severe, or Substance Use with Complications	56	0.329	0.279	0.538	0.356	0.372	0.275	0.178
F15.23	Other stimulant dependence with withdrawal	55	Substance Use Disorder, Moderate/Severe, or Substance Use with Complications	56	0.329	0.279	0.538	0.356	0.372	0.275	0.178
F15.24	Other stimulant dependence with stimulant-induced mood disorder	55	Substance Use Disorder, Moderate/Severe, or Substance Use with Complications	56	0.329	0.279	0.538	0.356	0.372	0.275	0.178
F15.25Ø	Other stimulant dependence with stimulant-induced psychotic disorder with delusions	54	Substance Use with Psychotic Complications	55,56	0.329	0.543	0.538	0.896	0.372	0.679	0.178
F15.251	Other stimulant dependence with stimulant-induced psychotic disorder with hallucinations	54	Substance Use with Psychotic Complications	55,56	0.329	0.543	0.538	0.896	0.372	0.679	0.178
F15.259	Other stimulant dependence with stimulant-induced psychotic disorder, unspecified	54	Substance Use with Psychotic Complications	55,56	0.329	0.543	0.538	0.896	0.372	0.679	0.178
F15.28Ø	Other stimulant dependence with stimulant-induced anxiety disorder	55	Substance Use Disorder, Moderate/Severe, or Substance Use with Complications	56	0.329	0.279	0.538	0.356	0.372	0.275	0.178
F15.281	Other stimulant dependence with stimulant-induced sexual dysfunction	55	Substance Use Disorder, Moderate/Severe, or Substance Use with Complications	56	0.329	0.279	0.538	0.356	0.372	0.275	0.178

ICD-10-CM Code	ICD-10-CM Code Description	V24 CMS-HCC	V24 CMS-HCC Disease Group	V24 CMS-HCC Hierarchies	Community, NonDual, Aged	Community, NonDual, Disabled	Community, FBDual, Aged	Community, FBDual, Disabled	Community, PBDual, Aged	Community, PBDual, Disabled	Institutional
F15.282	Other stimulant dependence with stimulant-induced sleep disorder	55	Substance Use Disorder, Moderate/Severe, or Substance Use with Complications	56	0.329	0.279	0.538	0.356	0.372	0.275	0.178
F15.288	Other stimulant dependence with other stimulant-induced disorder	55	Substance Use Disorder, Moderate/Severe, or Substance Use with Complications	56	0.329	0.279	0.538	0.356	0.372	0.275	0.178
F15.29	Other stimulant dependence with unspecified stimulant-induced disorder	55	Substance Use Disorder, Moderate/Severe, or Substance Use with Complications	56	0.329	0.279	0.538	0.356	0.372	0.275	0.178
F15.920	Other stimulant use, unspecified with intoxication, uncomplicated	55	Substance Use Disorder, Moderate/Severe, or Substance Use with Complications	56	0.329	0.279	0.538	0.356	0.372	0.275	0.178
F15.921	Other stimulant use, unspecified with intoxication delirium	55	Substance Use Disorder, Moderate/Severe, or Substance Use with Complications	56	0.329	0.279	0.538	0.356	0.372	0.275	0.178
F15.922	Other stimulant use, unspecified with intoxication with perceptual disturbance	55	Substance Use Disorder, Moderate/Severe, or Substance Use with Complications	56	0.329	0.279	0.538	0.356	0.372	0.275	0.178
F15.929	Other stimulant use, unspecified with intoxication, unspecified	55	Substance Use Disorder, Moderate/Severe, or Substance Use with Complications	56	0.329	0.279	0.538	0.356	0.372	0.275	0.178
F15.93	Other stimulant use, unspecified with withdrawal	55	Substance Use Disorder, Moderate/Severe, or Substance Use with Complications	56	0.329	0.279	0.538	0.356	0.372	0.275	0.178
F15.94	Other stimulant use, unspecified with stimulant-induced mood disorder	55	Substance Use Disorder, Moderate/Severe, or Substance Use with Complications	56	0.329	0.279	0.538	0.356	0.372	0.275	0.178
F15.950	Other stimulant use, unspecified with stimulant-induced psychotic disorder with delusions	54	Substance Use with Psychotic Complications	55,56	0.329	0.543	0.538	0.896	0.372	0.679	0.178
F15.951	Other stimulant use, unspecified with stimulant-induced psychotic disorder with hallucinations	54	Substance Use with Psychotic Complications	55,56	0.329	0.543	0.538	0.896	0.372	0.679	0.178
F15.959	Other stimulant use, unspecified with stimulant-induced psychotic disorder, unspecified	54	Substance Use with Psychotic Complications	55,56	0.329	0.543	0.538	0.896	0.372	0.679	0.178
F15.980	Other stimulant use, unspecified with stimulant-induced anxiety disorder	55	Substance Use Disorder, Moderate/Severe, or Substance Use with Complications	56	0.329	0.279	0.538	0.356	0.372	0.275	0.178
F15.981	Other stimulant use, unspecified with stimulant-induced sexual dysfunction	55	Substance Use Disorder, Moderate/Severe, or Substance Use with Complications	56	0.329	0.279	0.538	0.356	0.372	0.275	0.178
F15.982	Other stimulant use, unspecified with stimulant-induced sleep disorder	55	Substance Use Disorder, Moderate/Severe, or Substance Use with Complications	56	0.329	0.279	0.538	0.356	0.372	0.275	0.178
F15.988	Other stimulant use, unspecified with other stimulant-induced disorder	55	Substance Use Disorder, Moderate/Severe, or Substance Use with Complications	56	0.329	0.279	0.538	0.356	0.372	0.275	0.178
F15.99	Other stimulant use, unspecified with unspecified stimulant-induced disorder	55	Substance Use Disorder, Moderate/Severe, or Substance Use with Complications	56	0.329	0.279	0.538	0.356	0.372	0.275	0.178
F16.10	Hallucinogen abuse, uncomplicated	56	Substance Use Disorder, Mild, Except Alcohol and Cannabis		0.329	0.247	0.538	0.348	0.372	0.275	0.178
F16.11	Hallucinogen abuse, in remission	56	Substance Use Disorder, Mild, Except Alcohol and Cannabis		0.329	0.247	0.538	0.348	0.372	0.275	0.178
F16.120	Hallucinogen abuse with intoxication, uncomplicated	55	Substance Use Disorder, Moderate/Severe, or Substance Use with Complications	56	0.329	0.279	0.538	0.356	0.372	0.275	0.178
F16.121	Hallucinogen abuse with intoxication with delirium	55	Substance Use Disorder, Moderate/Severe, or Substance Use with Complications	56	0.329	0.279	0.538	0.356	0.372	0.275	0.178

ICD-10-CM Code	ICD-10-CM Code Description	V24 CMS-HCC	V24 CMS-HCC Disease Group	V24 CMS-HCC Hierarchies	Community, NonDual, Aged	Community, NonDual, Disabled	Community, FBDual, Aged	Community, FBDual, Disabled	Community, PBDual, Aged	Community, PBDual, Disabled	Institutional
F16.122	Hallucinogen abuse with intoxication with perceptual disturbance	55	Substance Use Disorder, Moderate/Severe, or Substance Use with Complications	56	0.329	0.279	0.538	0.356	0.372	0.275	0.178
F16.129	Hallucinogen abuse with intoxication, unspecified	55	Substance Use Disorder, Moderate/Severe, or Substance Use with Complications	56	0.329	0.279	0.538	0.356	0.372	0.275	0.178
F16.14	Hallucinogen abuse with hallucinogen-induced mood disorder	55	Substance Use Disorder, Moderate/Severe, or Substance Use with Complications	56	0.329	0.279	0.538	0.356	0.372	0.275	0.178
F16.15Ø	Hallucinogen abuse with hallucinogen-induced psychotic disorder with delusions	54	Substance Use with Psychotic Complications	55,56	0.329	0.543	0.538	0.896	0.372	0.679	0.178
F16.151	Hallucinogen abuse with hallucinogen-induced psychotic disorder with hallucinations	54	Substance Use with Psychotic Complications	55,56	0.329	0.543	0.538	0.896	0.372	0.679	0.178
F16.159	Hallucinogen abuse with hallucinogen-induced psychotic disorder, unspecified	54	Substance Use with Psychotic Complications	55,56	0.329	0.543	0.538	0.896	0.372	0.679	0.178
F16.18Ø	Hallucinogen abuse with hallucinogen-induced anxiety disorder	55	Substance Use Disorder, Moderate/Severe, or Substance Use with Complications	56	0.329	0.279	0.538	0.356	0.372	0.275	0.178
F16.183	Hallucinogen abuse with hallucinogen persisting perception disorder (flashbacks)	55	Substance Use Disorder, Moderate/Severe, or Substance Use with Complications	56	0.329	0.279	0.538	0.356	0.372	0.275	0.178
F16.188	Hallucinogen abuse with other hallucinogen-induced disorder	55	Substance Use Disorder, Moderate/Severe, or Substance Use with Complications	56	0.329	0.279	0.538	0.356	0.372	0.275	0.178
F16.19	Hallucinogen abuse with unspecified hallucinogen-induced disorder	55	Substance Use Disorder, Moderate/Severe, or Substance Use with Complications	56	0.329	0.279	0.538	0.356	0.372	0.275	0.178
F16.2Ø	Hallucinogen dependence, uncomplicated	55	Substance Use Disorder, Moderate/Severe, or Substance Use with Complications	56	0.329	0.279	0.538	0.356	0.372	0.275	0.178
F16.21	Hallucinogen dependence, in remission	55	Substance Use Disorder, Moderate/Severe, or Substance Use with Complications	56	0.329	0.279	0.538	0.356	0.372	0.275	0.178
F16.22Ø	Hallucinogen dependence with intoxication, uncomplicated	55	Substance Use Disorder, Moderate/Severe, or Substance Use with Complications	56	0.329	0.279	0.538	0.356	0.372	0.275	0.178
F16.221	Hallucinogen dependence with intoxication with delirium	55	Substance Use Disorder, Moderate/Severe, or Substance Use with Complications	56	0.329	0.279	0.538	0.356	0.372	0.275	0.178
F16.229	Hallucinogen dependence with intoxication, unspecified	55	Substance Use Disorder, Moderate/Severe, or Substance Use with Complications	56	0.329	0.279	0.538	0.356	0.372	0.275	0.178
F16.24	Hallucinogen dependence with hallucinogen-induced mood disorder	55	Substance Use Disorder, Moderate/Severe, or Substance Use with Complications	56	0.329	0.279	0.538	0.356	0.372	0.275	0.178
F16.25Ø	Hallucinogen dependence with hallucinogen-induced psychotic disorder with delusions	54	Substance Use with Psychotic Complications	55,56	0.329	0.543	0.538	0.896	0.372	0.679	0.178
F16.251	Hallucinogen dependence with hallucinogen-induced psychotic disorder with hallucinations	54	Substance Use with Psychotic Complications	55,56	0.329	0.543	0.538	0.896	0.372	0.679	0.178
F16.259	Hallucinogen dependence with hallucinogen-induced psychotic disorder, unspecified	54	Substance Use with Psychotic Complications	55,56	0.329	0.543	0.538	0.896	0.372	0.679	0.178
F16.28Ø	Hallucinogen dependence with hallucinogen-induced anxiety disorder	55	Substance Use Disorder, Moderate/Severe, or Substance Use with Complications	56	0.329	0.279	0.538	0.356	0.372	0.275	0.178

ICD-10-CM Code	ICD-10-CM Code Description	V24 CMS-HCC	V24 CMS-HCC Disease Group	V24 CMS-HCC Hierarchies	Community, NonDual, Aged	Community, NonDual, Disabled	Community, FBDual, Aged	Community, FBDual, Disabled	Community, PBDual, Aged	Community, PBDual, Disabled	Institutional
F16.283	Hallucinogen dependence with hallucinogen persisting perception disorder (flashbacks)	55	Substance Use Disorder, Moderate/Severe, or Substance Use with Complications	56	0.329	0.279	0.538	0.356	0.372	0.275	0.178
F16.288	Hallucinogen dependence with other hallucinogen-induced disorder	55	Substance Use Disorder, Moderate/Severe, or Substance Use with Complications	56	0.329	0.279	0.538	0.356	0.372	0.275	0.178
F16.29	Hallucinogen dependence with unspecified hallucinogen-induced disorder	55	Substance Use Disorder, Moderate/Severe, or Substance Use with Complications	56	0.329	0.279	0.538	0.356	0.372	0.275	0.178
F16.920	Hallucinogen use, unspecified with intoxication, uncomplicated	55	Substance Use Disorder, Moderate/Severe, or Substance Use with Complications	56	0.329	0.279	0.538	0.356	0.372	0.275	0.178
F16.921	Hallucinogen use, unspecified with intoxication with delirium	55	Substance Use Disorder, Moderate/Severe, or Substance Use with Complications	56	0.329	0.279	0.538	0.356	0.372	0.275	0.178
F16.929	Hallucinogen use, unspecified with intoxication, unspecified	55	Substance Use Disorder, Moderate/Severe, or Substance Use with Complications	56	0.329	0.279	0.538	0.356	0.372	0.275	0.178
F16.94	Hallucinogen use, unspecified with hallucinogen-induced mood disorder	55	Substance Use Disorder, Moderate/Severe, or Substance Use with Complications	56	0.329	0.279	0.538	0.356	0.372	0.275	0.178
F16.950	Hallucinogen use, unspecified with hallucinogen-induced psychotic disorder with delusions	54	Substance Use with Psychotic Complications	55,56	0.329	0.543	0.538	0.896	0.372	0.679	0.178
F16.951	Hallucinogen use, unspecified with hallucinogen-induced psychotic disorder with hallucinations	54	Substance Use with Psychotic Complications	55,56	0.329	0.543	0.538	0.896	0.372	0.679	0.178
F16.959	Hallucinogen use, unspecified with hallucinogen-induced psychotic disorder, unspecified	54	Substance Use with Psychotic Complications	55,56	0.329	0.543	0.538	0.896	0.372	0.679	0.178
F16.980	Hallucinogen use, unspecified with hallucinogen-induced anxiety disorder	55	Substance Use Disorder, Moderate/Severe, or Substance Use with Complications	56	0.329	0.279	0.538	0.356	0.372	0.275	0.178
F16.983	Hallucinogen use, unspecified with hallucinogen persisting perception disorder (flashbacks)	55	Substance Use Disorder, Moderate/Severe, or Substance Use with Complications	56	0.329	0.279	0.538	0.356	0.372	0.275	0.178
F16.988	Hallucinogen use, unspecified with other hallucinogen-induced disorder	55	Substance Use Disorder, Moderate/Severe, or Substance Use with Complications	56	0.329	0.279	0.538	0.356	0.372	0.275	0.178
F16.99	Hallucinogen use, unspecified with unspecified hallucinogen-induced disorder	55	Substance Use Disorder, Moderate/Severe, or Substance Use with Complications	56	0.329	0.279	0.538	0.356	0.372	0.275	0.178
F18.10	Inhalant abuse, uncomplicated	56	Substance Use Disorder, Mild, Except Alcohol and Cannabis		0.329	0.247	0.538	0.348	0.372	0.275	0.178
F18.11	Inhalant abuse, in remission	56	Substance Use Disorder, Mild, Except Alcohol and Cannabis		0.329	0.247	0.538	0.348	0.372	0.275	0.178
F18.120	Inhalant abuse with intoxication, uncomplicated	55	Substance Use Disorder, Moderate/Severe, or Substance Use with Complications	56	0.329	0.279	0.538	0.356	0.372	0.275	0.178
F18.121	Inhalant abuse with intoxication delirium	55	Substance Use Disorder, Moderate/Severe, or Substance Use with Complications	56	0.329	0.279	0.538	0.356	0.372	0.275	0.178
F18.129	Inhalant abuse with intoxication, unspecified	55	Substance Use Disorder, Moderate/Severe, or Substance Use with Complications	56	0.329	0.279	0.538	0.356	0.372	0.275	0.178
F18.14	Inhalant abuse with inhalant-induced mood disorder	55	Substance Use Disorder, Moderate/Severe, or Substance Use with Complications	56	0.329	0.279	0.538	0.356	0.372	0.275	0.178
F18.150	Inhalant abuse with inhalant-induced psychotic disorder with delusions	54	Substance Use with Psychotic Complications	55,56	0.329	0.543	0.538	0.896	0.372	0.679	0.178

ICD-10-CM Code	ICD-10-CM Code Description	V24 CMS-HCC	V24 CMS-HCC Disease Group	V24 CMS-HCC Hierarchies	Community, NonDual, Aged	Community, NonDual, Disabled	Community, FBDual, Aged	Community, FBDual, Disabled	Community, PBDual, Aged	Community, PBDual, Disabled	Institutional
F18.151	Inhalant abuse with inhalant-induced psychotic disorder with hallucinations	54	Substance Use with Psychotic Complications	55,56	0.329	0.543	0.538	0.896	0.372	0.679	0.178
F18.159	Inhalant abuse with inhalant-induced psychotic disorder, unspecified	54	Substance Use with Psychotic Complications	55,56	0.329	0.543	0.538	0.896	0.372	0.679	0.178
F18.17	Inhalant abuse with inhalant-induced dementia	54	Substance Use with Psychotic Complications	55,56	0.329	0.543	0.538	0.896	0.372	0.679	0.178
F18.180	Inhalant abuse with inhalant-induced anxiety disorder	55	Substance Use Disorder, Moderate/Severe, or Substance Use with Complications	56	0.329	0.279	0.538	0.356	0.372	0.275	0.178
F18.188	Inhalant abuse with other inhalant-induced disorder	55	Substance Use Disorder, Moderate/Severe, or Substance Use with Complications	56	0.329	0.279	0.538	0.356	0.372	0.275	0.178
F18.19	Inhalant abuse with unspecified inhalant-induced disorder	55	Substance Use Disorder, Moderate/Severe, or Substance Use with Complications	56	0.329	0.279	0.538	0.356	0.372	0.275	0.178
F18.20	Inhalant dependence, uncomplicated	55	Substance Use Disorder, Moderate/Severe, or Substance Use with Complications	56	0.329	0.279	0.538	0.356	0.372	0.275	0.178
F18.21	Inhalant dependence, in remission	55	Substance Use Disorder, Moderate/Severe, or Substance Use with Complications	56	0.329	0.279	0.538	0.356	0.372	0.275	0.178
F18.220	Inhalant dependence with intoxication, uncomplicated	55	Substance Use Disorder, Moderate/Severe, or Substance Use with Complications	56	0.329	0.279	0.538	0.356	0.372	0.275	0.178
F18.221	Inhalant dependence with intoxication delirium	55	Substance Use Disorder, Moderate/Severe, or Substance Use with Complications	56	0.329	0.279	0.538	0.356	0.372	0.275	0.178
F18.229	Inhalant dependence with intoxication, unspecified	55	Substance Use Disorder, Moderate/Severe, or Substance Use with Complications	56	0.329	0.279	0.538	0.356	0.372	0.275	0.178
F18.24	Inhalant dependence with inhalant-induced mood disorder	55	Substance Use Disorder, Moderate/Severe, or Substance Use with Complications	56	0.329	0.279	0.538	0.356	0.372	0.275	0.178
F18.250	Inhalant dependence with inhalant-induced psychotic disorder with delusions	54	Substance Use with Psychotic Complications	55,56	0.329	0.543	0.538	0.896	0.372	0.679	0.178
F18.251	Inhalant dependence with inhalant-induced psychotic disorder with hallucinations	54	Substance Use with Psychotic Complications	55,56	0.329	0.543	0.538	0.896	0.372	0.679	0.178
F18.259	Inhalant dependence with inhalant-induced psychotic disorder, unspecified	54	Substance Use with Psychotic Complications	55,56	0.329	0.543	0.538	0.896	0.372	0.679	0.178
F18.27	Inhalant dependence with inhalant-induced dementia	54	Substance Use with Psychotic Complications	55,56	0.329	0.543	0.538	0.896	0.372	0.679	0.178
F18.280	Inhalant dependence with inhalant-induced anxiety disorder	55	Substance Use Disorder, Moderate/Severe, or Substance Use with Complications	56	0.329	0.279	0.538	0.356	0.372	0.275	0.178
F18.288	Inhalant dependence with other inhalant-induced disorder	55	Substance Use Disorder, Moderate/Severe, or Substance Use with Complications	56	0.329	0.279	0.538	0.356	0.372	0.275	0.178
F18.29	Inhalant dependence with unspecified inhalant-induced disorder	55	Substance Use Disorder, Moderate/Severe, or Substance Use with Complications	56	0.329	0.279	0.538	0.356	0.372	0.275	0.178
F18.920	Inhalant use, unspecified with intoxication, uncomplicated	55	Substance Use Disorder, Moderate/Severe, or Substance Use with Complications	56	0.329	0.279	0.538	0.356	0.372	0.275	0.178
F18.921	Inhalant use, unspecified with intoxication with delirium	55	Substance Use Disorder, Moderate/Severe, or Substance Use with Complications	56	0.329	0.279	0.538	0.356	0.372	0.275	0.178

ICD-10-CM Code	ICD-10-CM Code Description	V24 CMS-HCC	V24 CMS-HCC Disease Group	V24 CMS-HCC Hierarchies	Community, NonDual, Aged	Community, NonDual, Disabled	Community, FBDual, Aged	Community, FBDual, Disabled	Community, PBDual, Aged	Community, PBDual, Disabled	Institutional
F18.929	Inhalant use, unspecified with intoxication, unspecified	55	Substance Use Disorder, Moderate/Severe, or Substance Use with Complications	56	0.329	0.279	0.538	0.356	0.372	0.275	0.178
F18.94	Inhalant use, unspecified with inhalant-induced mood disorder	55	Substance Use Disorder, Moderate/Severe, or Substance Use with Complications	56	0.329	0.279	0.538	0.356	0.372	0.275	0.178
F18.950	Inhalant use, unspecified with inhalant-induced psychotic disorder with delusions	54	Substance Use with Psychotic Complications	55,56	0.329	0.543	0.538	0.896	0.372	0.679	0.178
F18.951	Inhalant use, unspecified with inhalant-induced psychotic disorder with hallucinations	54	Substance Use with Psychotic Complications	55,56	0.329	0.543	0.538	0.896	0.372	0.679	0.178
F18.959	Inhalant use, unspecified with inhalant-induced psychotic disorder, unspecified	54	Substance Use with Psychotic Complications	55,56	0.329	0.543	0.538	0.896	0.372	0.679	0.178
F18.97	Inhalant use, unspecified with inhalant-induced persisting dementia	54	Substance Use with Psychotic Complications	55,56	0.329	0.543	0.538	0.896	0.372	0.679	0.178
F18.980	Inhalant use, unspecified with inhalant-induced anxiety disorder	55	Substance Use Disorder, Moderate/Severe, or Substance Use with Complications	56	0.329	0.279	0.538	0.356	0.372	0.275	0.178
F18.988	Inhalant use, unspecified with other inhalant-induced disorder	55	Substance Use Disorder, Moderate/Severe, or Substance Use with Complications	56	0.329	0.279	0.538	0.356	0.372	0.275	0.178
F18.99	Inhalant use, unspecified with unspecified inhalant-induced disorder	55	Substance Use Disorder, Moderate/Severe, or Substance Use with Complications	56	0.329	0.279	0.538	0.356	0.372	0.275	0.178
F19.10	Other psychoactive substance abuse, uncomplicated	56	Substance Use Disorder, Mild, Except Alcohol and Cannabis		0.329	0.247	0.538	0.348	0.372	0.275	0.178
F19.11	Other psychoactive substance abuse, in remission	56	Substance Use Disorder, Mild, Except Alcohol and Cannabis		0.329	0.247	0.538	0.348	0.372	0.275	0.178
F19.120	Other psychoactive substance abuse with intoxication, uncomplicated	55	Substance Use Disorder, Moderate/Severe, or Substance Use with Complications	56	0.329	0.279	0.538	0.356	0.372	0.275	0.178
F19.121	Other psychoactive substance abuse with intoxication delirium	55	Substance Use Disorder, Moderate/Severe, or Substance Use with Complications	56	0.329	0.279	0.538	0.356	0.372	0.275	0.178
F19.122	Other psychoactive substance abuse with intoxication with perceptual disturbances	55	Substance Use Disorder, Moderate/Severe, or Substance Use with Complications	56	0.329	0.279	0.538	0.356	0.372	0.275	0.178
F19.129	Other psychoactive substance abuse with intoxication, unspecified	55	Substance Use Disorder, Moderate/Severe, or Substance Use with Complications	56	0.329	0.279	0.538	0.356	0.372	0.275	0.178
F19.130	Other psychoactive substance abuse with withdrawal, uncomplicated	55	Substance Use Disorder, Moderate/Severe, or Substance Use with Complications	56	0.329	0.279	0.538	0.356	0.372	0.275	0.178
F19.131	Other psychoactive substance abuse with withdrawal delirium	54	Substance Use with Psychotic Complications	55,56	0.329	0.543	0.538	0.896	0.372	0.679	0.178
F19.132	Other psychoactive substance abuse with withdrawal with perceptual disturbance	54	Substance Use with Psychotic Complications	55,56	0.329	0.543	0.538	0.896	0.372	0.679	0.178
F19.139	Other psychoactive substance abuse with withdrawal, unspecified	55	Substance Use Disorder, Moderate/Severe, or Substance Use with Complications	56	0.329	0.279	0.538	0.356	0.372	0.275	0.178
F19.14	Other psychoactive substance abuse with psychoactive substance-induced mood disorder	55	Substance Use Disorder, Moderate/Severe, or Substance Use with Complications	56	0.329	0.279	0.538	0.356	0.372	0.275	0.178
F19.150	Other psychoactive substance abuse with psychoactive substance-induced psychotic disorder with delusions	54	Substance Use with Psychotic Complications	55,56	0.329	0.543	0.538	0.896	0.372	0.679	0.178

ICD-10-CM Code	ICD-10-CM Code Description	V24 CMS-HCC	V24 CMS-HCC Disease Group	V24 CMS-HCC Hierarchies	Community, NonDual, Aged	Community, NonDual, Disabled	Community, FBDual, Aged	Community, FBDual, Disabled	Community, PBDual, Aged	Community, PBDual, Disabled	Institutional
F19.151	Other psychoactive substance abuse with psychoactive substance-induced psychotic disorder with hallucinations	54	Substance Use with Psychotic Complications	55,56	0.329	0.543	0.538	0.896	0.372	0.679	0.178
F19.159	Other psychoactive substance abuse with psychoactive substance-induced psychotic disorder, unspecified	54	Substance Use with Psychotic Complications	55,56	0.329	0.543	0.538	0.896	0.372	0.679	0.178
F19.16	Other psychoactive substance abuse with psychoactive substance-induced persisting amnestic disorder	54	Substance Use with Psychotic Complications	55,56	0.329	0.543	0.538	0.896	0.372	0.679	0.178
F19.17	Other psychoactive substance abuse with psychoactive substance-induced persisting dementia	54	Substance Use with Psychotic Complications	55,56	0.329	0.543	0.538	0.896	0.372	0.679	0.178
F19.180	Other psychoactive substance abuse with psychoactive substance-induced anxiety disorder	55	Substance Use Disorder, Moderate/Severe, or Substance Use with Complications	56	0.329	0.279	0.538	0.356	0.372	0.275	0.178
F19.181	Other psychoactive substance abuse with psychoactive substance-induced sexual dysfunction	55	Substance Use Disorder, Moderate/Severe, or Substance Use with Complications	56	0.329	0.279	0.538	0.356	0.372	0.275	0.178
F19.182	Other psychoactive substance abuse with psychoactive substance-induced sleep disorder	55	Substance Use Disorder, Moderate/Severe, or Substance Use with Complications	56	0.329	0.279	0.538	0.356	0.372	0.275	0.178
F19.188	Other psychoactive substance abuse with other psychoactive substance-induced disorder	55	Substance Use Disorder, Moderate/Severe, or Substance Use with Complications	56	0.329	0.279	0.538	0.356	0.372	0.275	0.178
F19.19	Other psychoactive substance abuse with unspecified psychoactive substance-induced disorder	55	Substance Use Disorder, Moderate/Severe, or Substance Use with Complications	56	0.329	0.279	0.538	0.356	0.372	0.275	0.178
F19.20	Other psychoactive substance dependence, uncomplicated	55	Substance Use Disorder, Moderate/Severe, or Substance Use with Complications	56	0.329	0.279	0.538	0.356	0.372	0.275	0.178
F19.21	Other psychoactive substance dependence, in remission	55	Substance Use Disorder, Moderate/Severe, or Substance Use with Complications	56	0.329	0.279	0.538	0.356	0.372	0.275	0.178
F19.220	Other psychoactive substance dependence with intoxication, uncomplicated	55	Substance Use Disorder, Moderate/Severe, or Substance Use with Complications	56	0.329	0.279	0.538	0.356	0.372	0.275	0.178
F19.221	Other psychoactive substance dependence with intoxication delirium	55	Substance Use Disorder, Moderate/Severe, or Substance Use with Complications	56	0.329	0.279	0.538	0.356	0.372	0.275	0.178
F19.222	Other psychoactive substance dependence with intoxication with perceptual disturbance	55	Substance Use Disorder, Moderate/Severe, or Substance Use with Complications	56	0.329	0.279	0.538	0.356	0.372	0.275	0.178
F19.229	Other psychoactive substance dependence with intoxication, unspecified	55	Substance Use Disorder, Moderate/Severe, or Substance Use with Complications	56	0.329	0.279	0.538	0.356	0.372	0.275	0.178
F19.230	Other psychoactive substance dependence with withdrawal, uncomplicated	55	Substance Use Disorder, Moderate/Severe, or Substance Use with Complications	56	0.329	0.279	0.538	0.356	0.372	0.275	0.178
F19.231	Other psychoactive substance dependence with withdrawal delirium	54	Substance Use with Psychotic Complications	55,56	0.329	0.543	0.538	0.896	0.372	0.679	0.178
F19.232	Other psychoactive substance dependence with withdrawal with perceptual disturbance	54	Substance Use with Psychotic Complications	55,56	0.329	0.543	0.538	0.896	0.372	0.679	0.178
F19.239	Other psychoactive substance dependence with withdrawal, unspecified	55	Substance Use Disorder, Moderate/Severe, or Substance Use with Complications	56	0.329	0.279	0.538	0.356	0.372	0.275	0.178
F19.24	Other psychoactive substance dependence with psychoactive substance-induced mood disorder	55	Substance Use Disorder, Moderate/Severe, or Substance Use with Complications	56	0.329	0.279	0.538	0.356	0.372	0.275	0.178

ICD-10-CM Code	ICD-10-CM Code Description	V24 CMS-HCC	V24 CMS-HCC Disease Group	V24 CMS-HCC Hierarchies	Community, NonDual, Aged	Community, NonDual, Disabled	Community, FBDual, Aged	Community, FBDual, Disabled	Community, PBDual, Aged	Community, PBDual, Disabled	Institutional
F19.250	Other psychoactive substance dependence with psychoactive substance-induced psychotic disorder with delusions	54	Substance Use with Psychotic Complications	55,56	0.329	0.543	0.538	0.896	0.372	0.679	0.178
F19.251	Other psychoactive substance dependence with psychoactive substance-induced psychotic disorder with hallucinations	54	Substance Use with Psychotic Complications	55,56	0.329	0.543	0.538	0.896	0.372	0.679	0.178
F19.259	Other psychoactive substance dependence with psychoactive substance-induced psychotic disorder, unspecified	54	Substance Use with Psychotic Complications	55,56	0.329	0.543	0.538	0.896	0.372	0.679	0.178
F19.26	Other psychoactive substance dependence with psychoactive substance-induced persisting amnestic disorder	54	Substance Use with Psychotic Complications	55,56	0.329	0.543	0.538	0.896	0.372	0.679	0.178
F19.27	Other psychoactive substance dependence with psychoactive substance-induced persisting dementia	54	Substance Use with Psychotic Complications	55,56	0.329	0.543	0.538	0.896	0.372	0.679	0.178
F19.280	Other psychoactive substance dependence with psychoactive substance-induced anxiety disorder	55	Substance Use Disorder, Moderate/Severe, or Substance Use with Complications	56	0.329	0.279	0.538	0.356	0.372	0.275	0.178
F19.281	Other psychoactive substance dependence with psychoactive substance-induced sexual dysfunction	55	Substance Use Disorder, Moderate/Severe, or Substance Use with Complications	56	0.329	0.279	0.538	0.356	0.372	0.275	0.178
F19.282	Other psychoactive substance dependence with psychoactive substance-induced sleep disorder	55	Substance Use Disorder, Moderate/Severe, or Substance Use with Complications	56	0.329	0.279	0.538	0.356	0.372	0.275	0.178
F19.288	Other psychoactive substance dependence with other psychoactive substance-induced disorder	55	Substance Use Disorder, Moderate/Severe, or Substance Use with Complications	56	0.329	0.279	0.538	0.356	0.372	0.275	0.178
F19.29	Other psychoactive substance dependence with unspecified psychoactive substance-induced disorder	55	Substance Use Disorder, Moderate/Severe, or Substance Use with Complications	56	0.329	0.279	0.538	0.356	0.372	0.275	0.178
F19.920	Other psychoactive substance use, unspecified with intoxication, uncomplicated	55	Substance Use Disorder, Moderate/Severe, or Substance Use with Complications	56	0.329	0.279	0.538	0.356	0.372	0.275	0.178
F19.921	Other psychoactive substance use, unspecified with intoxication with delirium	55	Substance Use Disorder, Moderate/Severe, or Substance Use with Complications	56	0.329	0.279	0.538	0.356	0.372	0.275	0.178
F19.922	Other psychoactive substance use, unspecified with intoxication with perceptual disturbance	55	Substance Use Disorder, Moderate/Severe, or Substance Use with Complications	56	0.329	0.279	0.538	0.356	0.372	0.275	0.178
F19.929	Other psychoactive substance use, unspecified with intoxication, unspecified	55	Substance Use Disorder, Moderate/Severe, or Substance Use with Complications	56	0.329	0.279	0.538	0.356	0.372	0.275	0.178
F19.930	Other psychoactive substance use, unspecified with withdrawal, uncomplicated	55	Substance Use Disorder, Moderate/Severe, or Substance Use with Complications	56	0.329	0.279	0.538	0.356	0.372	0.275	0.178
F19.931	Other psychoactive substance use, unspecified with withdrawal delirium	54	Substance Use with Psychotic Complications	55,56	0.329	0.543	0.538	0.896	0.372	0.679	0.178
F19.932	Other psychoactive substance use, unspecified with withdrawal with perceptual disturbance	54	Substance Use with Psychotic Complications	55,56	0.329	0.543	0.538	0.896	0.372	0.679	0.178
F19.939	Other psychoactive substance use, unspecified with withdrawal, unspecified	55	Substance Use Disorder, Moderate/Severe, or Substance Use with Complications	56	0.329	0.279	0.538	0.356	0.372	0.275	0.178

ICD-10-CM Code	ICD-10-CM Code Description	V24 CMS-HCC	V24 CMS-HCC Disease Group	V24 CMS-HCC Hierarchies	Community, NonDual, Aged	Community, NonDual, Disabled	Community, FBDual, Aged	Community, FBDual, Disabled	Community, PBDual, Aged	Community, PBDual, Disabled	Institutional
F19.94	Other psychoactive substance use, unspecified with psychoactive substance-induced mood disorder	55	Substance Use Disorder, Moderate/Severe, or Substance Use with Complications	56	0.329	0.279	0.538	0.356	0.372	0.275	0.178
F19.950	Other psychoactive substance use, unspecified with psychoactive substance-induced psychotic disorder with delusions	54	Substance Use with Psychotic Complications	55,56	0.329	0.543	0.538	0.896	0.372	0.679	0.178
F19.951	Other psychoactive substance use, unspecified with psychoactive substance-induced psychotic disorder with hallucinations	54	Substance Use with Psychotic Complications	55,56	0.329	0.543	0.538	0.896	0.372	0.679	0.178
F19.959	Other psychoactive substance use, unspecified with psychoactive substance-induced psychotic disorder, unspecified	54	Substance Use with Psychotic Complications	55,56	0.329	0.543	0.538	0.896	0.372	0.679	0.178
F19.96	Other psychoactive substance use, unspecified with psychoactive substance-induced persisting amnestic disorder	54	Substance Use with Psychotic Complications	55,56	0.329	0.543	0.538	0.896	0.372	0.679	0.178
F19.97	Other psychoactive substance use, unspecified with psychoactive substance-induced persisting dementia	54	Substance Use with Psychotic Complications	55,56	0.329	0.543	0.538	0.896	0.372	0.679	0.178
F19.980	Other psychoactive substance use, unspecified with psychoactive substance-induced anxiety disorder	55	Substance Use Disorder, Moderate/Severe, or Substance Use with Complications	56	0.329	0.279	0.538	0.356	0.372	0.275	0.178
F19.981	Other psychoactive substance use, unspecified with psychoactive substance-induced sexual dysfunction	55	Substance Use Disorder, Moderate/Severe, or Substance Use with Complications	56	0.329	0.279	0.538	0.356	0.372	0.275	0.178
F19.982	Other psychoactive substance use, unspecified with psychoactive substance-induced sleep disorder	55	Substance Use Disorder, Moderate/Severe, or Substance Use with Complications	56	0.329	0.279	0.538	0.356	0.372	0.275	0.178
F19.988	Other psychoactive substance use, unspecified with other psychoactive substance-induced disorder	55	Substance Use Disorder, Moderate/Severe, or Substance Use with Complications	56	0.329	0.279	0.538	0.356	0.372	0.275	0.178
F19.99	Other psychoactive substance use, unspecified with unspecified psychoactive substance-induced disorder	55	Substance Use Disorder, Moderate/Severe, or Substance Use with Complications	56	0.329	0.279	0.538	0.356	0.372	0.275	0.178
F20.0	Paranoid schizophrenia	57	Schizophrenia	58,59,60	0.524	0.352	0.570	0.381	0.495	0.309	0.187
F20.1	Disorganized schizophrenia	57	Schizophrenia	58,59,60	0.524	0.352	0.570	0.381	0.495	0.309	0.187
F20.2	Catatonic schizophrenia	57	Schizophrenia	58,59,60	0.524	0.352	0.570	0.381	0.495	0.309	0.187
F20.3	Undifferentiated schizophrenia	57	Schizophrenia	58,59,60	0.524	0.352	0.570	0.381	0.495	0.309	0.187
F20.5	Residual schizophrenia	57	Schizophrenia	58,59,60	0.524	0.352	0.570	0.381	0.495	0.309	0.187
F20.81	Schizophreniform disorder	57	Schizophrenia	58,59,60	0.524	0.352	0.570	0.381	0.495	0.309	0.187
F20.89	Other schizophrenia	57	Schizophrenia	58,59,60	0.524	0.352	0.570	0.381	0.495	0.309	0.187
F20.9	Schizophrenia, unspecified	57	Schizophrenia	58,59,60	0.524	0.352	0.570	0.381	0.495	0.309	0.187
F21	Schizotypal disorder	60	Personality Disorders		0.309	0.108	0.299	0.100	0.255	0.065	—
F22	Delusional disorders	59	Major Depressive, Bipolar, and Paranoid Disorders	60	0.309	0.164	0.299	0.127	0.306	0.109	0.187
F23	Brief psychotic disorder	58	Reactive and Unspecified Psychosis	59,60	0.393	0.352	0.570	0.231	0.449	0.239	0.187
F24	Shared psychotic disorder	59	Major Depressive, Bipolar, and Paranoid Disorders	60	0.309	0.164	0.299	0.127	0.306	0.109	0.187
F25.0	Schizoaffective disorder, bipolar type	57	Schizophrenia	58,59,60	0.524	0.352	0.570	0.381	0.495	0.309	0.187
F25.1	Schizoaffective disorder, depressive type	57	Schizophrenia	58,59,60	0.524	0.352	0.570	0.381	0.495	0.309	0.187
F25.8	Other schizoaffective disorders	57	Schizophrenia	58,59,60	0.524	0.352	0.570	0.381	0.495	0.309	0.187
F25.9	Schizoaffective disorder, unspecified	57	Schizophrenia	58,59,60	0.524	0.352	0.570	0.381	0.495	0.309	0.187

ICD-10-CM Code	ICD-10-CM Code Description	V24 CMS-HCC	V24 CMS-HCC Disease Group	V24 CMS-HCC Hierarchies	Community, NonDual, Aged	Community, NonDual, Disabled	Community, FBDual, Aged	Community, FBDual, Disabled	Community, PBDual, Aged	Community, PBDual, Disabled	Institutional
F28	Other psychotic disorder not due to a substance or known physiological condition	58	Reactive and Unspecified Psychosis	59,60	0.393	0.352	0.570	0.231	0.449	0.239	0.187
F29	Unspecified psychosis not due to a substance or known physiological condition	58	Reactive and Unspecified Psychosis	59,60	0.393	0.352	0.570	0.231	0.449	0.239	0.187
F30.10	Manic episode without psychotic symptoms, unspecified	59	Major Depressive, Bipolar, and Paranoid Disorders	60	0.309	0.164	0.299	0.127	0.306	0.109	0.187
F30.11	Manic episode without psychotic symptoms, mild	59	Major Depressive, Bipolar, and Paranoid Disorders	60	0.309	0.164	0.299	0.127	0.306	0.109	0.187
F30.12	Manic episode without psychotic symptoms, moderate	59	Major Depressive, Bipolar, and Paranoid Disorders	60	0.309	0.164	0.299	0.127	0.306	0.109	0.187
F30.13	Manic episode, severe, without psychotic symptoms	59	Major Depressive, Bipolar, and Paranoid Disorders	60	0.309	0.164	0.299	0.127	0.306	0.109	0.187
F30.2	Manic episode, severe with psychotic symptoms	59	Major Depressive, Bipolar, and Paranoid Disorders	60	0.309	0.164	0.299	0.127	0.306	0.109	0.187
F30.3	Manic episode in partial remission	59	Major Depressive, Bipolar, and Paranoid Disorders	60	0.309	0.164	0.299	0.127	0.306	0.109	0.187
F30.4	Manic episode in full remission	59	Major Depressive, Bipolar, and Paranoid Disorders	60	0.309	0.164	0.299	0.127	0.306	0.109	0.187
F30.8	Other manic episodes	59	Major Depressive, Bipolar, and Paranoid Disorders	60	0.309	0.164	0.299	0.127	0.306	0.109	0.187
F30.9	Manic episode, unspecified	59	Major Depressive, Bipolar, and Paranoid Disorders	60	0.309	0.164	0.299	0.127	0.306	0.109	0.187
F31.0	Bipolar disorder, current episode hypomanic	59	Major Depressive, Bipolar, and Paranoid Disorders	60	0.309	0.164	0.299	0.127	0.306	0.109	0.187
F31.10	Bipolar disorder, current episode manic without psychotic features, unspecified	59	Major Depressive, Bipolar, and Paranoid Disorders	60	0.309	0.164	0.299	0.127	0.306	0.109	0.187
F31.11	Bipolar disorder, current episode manic without psychotic features, mild	59	Major Depressive, Bipolar, and Paranoid Disorders	60	0.309	0.164	0.299	0.127	0.306	0.109	0.187
F31.12	Bipolar disorder, current episode manic without psychotic features, moderate	59	Major Depressive, Bipolar, and Paranoid Disorders	60	0.309	0.164	0.299	0.127	0.306	0.109	0.187
F31.13	Bipolar disorder, current episode manic without psychotic features, severe	59	Major Depressive, Bipolar, and Paranoid Disorders	60	0.309	0.164	0.299	0.127	0.306	0.109	0.187
F31.2	Bipolar disorder, current episode manic severe with psychotic features	59	Major Depressive, Bipolar, and Paranoid Disorders	60	0.309	0.164	0.299	0.127	0.306	0.109	0.187
F31.30	Bipolar disorder, current episode depressed, mild or moderate severity, unspecified	59	Major Depressive, Bipolar, and Paranoid Disorders	60	0.309	0.164	0.299	0.127	0.306	0.109	0.187
F31.31	Bipolar disorder, current episode depressed, mild	59	Major Depressive, Bipolar, and Paranoid Disorders	60	0.309	0.164	0.299	0.127	0.306	0.109	0.187
F31.32	Bipolar disorder, current episode depressed, moderate	59	Major Depressive, Bipolar, and Paranoid Disorders	60	0.309	0.164	0.299	0.127	0.306	0.109	0.187
F31.4	Bipolar disorder, current episode depressed, severe, without psychotic features	59	Major Depressive, Bipolar, and Paranoid Disorders	60	0.309	0.164	0.299	0.127	0.306	0.109	0.187
F31.5	Bipolar disorder, current episode depressed, severe, with psychotic features	59	Major Depressive, Bipolar, and Paranoid Disorders	60	0.309	0.164	0.299	0.127	0.306	0.109	0.187
F31.60	Bipolar disorder, current episode mixed, unspecified	59	Major Depressive, Bipolar, and Paranoid Disorders	60	0.309	0.164	0.299	0.127	0.306	0.109	0.187
F31.61	Bipolar disorder, current episode mixed, mild	59	Major Depressive, Bipolar, and Paranoid Disorders	60	0.309	0.164	0.299	0.127	0.306	0.109	0.187
F31.62	Bipolar disorder, current episode mixed, moderate	59	Major Depressive, Bipolar, and Paranoid Disorders	60	0.309	0.164	0.299	0.127	0.306	0.109	0.187

ICD-10-CM Code	ICD-10-CM Code Description	V24 CMS-HCC	V24 CMS-HCC Disease Group	V24 CMS-HCC Hierarchies	Community, NonDual, Aged	Community, NonDual, Disabled	Community, FBDual, Aged	Community, FBDual, Disabled	Community, PBDual, Aged	Community, PBDual, Disabled	Institutional
F31.63	Bipolar disorder, current episode mixed, severe, without psychotic features	59	Major Depressive, Bipolar, and Paranoid Disorders	60	0.309	0.164	0.299	0.127	0.306	0.109	0.187
F31.64	Bipolar disorder, current episode mixed, severe, with psychotic features	59	Major Depressive, Bipolar, and Paranoid Disorders	60	0.309	0.164	0.299	0.127	0.306	0.109	0.187
F31.70	Bipolar disorder, currently in remission, most recent episode unspecified	59	Major Depressive, Bipolar, and Paranoid Disorders	60	0.309	0.164	0.299	0.127	0.306	0.109	0.187
F31.71	Bipolar disorder, in partial remission, most recent episode hypomanic	59	Major Depressive, Bipolar, and Paranoid Disorders	60	0.309	0.164	0.299	0.127	0.306	0.109	0.187
F31.72	Bipolar disorder, in full remission, most recent episode hypomanic	59	Major Depressive, Bipolar, and Paranoid Disorders	60	0.309	0.164	0.299	0.127	0.306	0.109	0.187
F31.73	Bipolar disorder, in partial remission, most recent episode manic	59	Major Depressive, Bipolar, and Paranoid Disorders	60	0.309	0.164	0.299	0.127	0.306	0.109	0.187
F31.74	Bipolar disorder, in full remission, most recent episode manic	59	Major Depressive, Bipolar, and Paranoid Disorders	60	0.309	0.164	0.299	0.127	0.306	0.109	0.187
F31.75	Bipolar disorder, in partial remission, most recent episode depressed	59	Major Depressive, Bipolar, and Paranoid Disorders	60	0.309	0.164	0.299	0.127	0.306	0.109	0.187
F31.76	Bipolar disorder, in full remission, most recent episode depressed	59	Major Depressive, Bipolar, and Paranoid Disorders	60	0.309	0.164	0.299	0.127	0.306	0.109	0.187
F31.77	Bipolar disorder, in partial remission, most recent episode mixed	59	Major Depressive, Bipolar, and Paranoid Disorders	60	0.309	0.164	0.299	0.127	0.306	0.109	0.187
F31.78	Bipolar disorder, in full remission, most recent episode mixed	59	Major Depressive, Bipolar, and Paranoid Disorders	60	0.309	0.164	0.299	0.127	0.306	0.109	0.187
F31.81	Bipolar II disorder	59	Major Depressive, Bipolar, and Paranoid Disorders	60	0.309	0.164	0.299	0.127	0.306	0.109	0.187
F31.89	Other bipolar disorder	59	Major Depressive, Bipolar, and Paranoid Disorders	60	0.309	0.164	0.299	0.127	0.306	0.109	0.187
F31.9	Bipolar disorder, unspecified	59	Major Depressive, Bipolar, and Paranoid Disorders	60	0.309	0.164	0.299	0.127	0.306	0.109	0.187
F32.0	Major depressive disorder, single episode, mild	59	Major Depressive, Bipolar, and Paranoid Disorders	60	0.309	0.164	0.299	0.127	0.306	0.109	0.187
F32.1	Major depressive disorder, single episode, moderate	59	Major Depressive, Bipolar, and Paranoid Disorders	60	0.309	0.164	0.299	0.127	0.306	0.109	0.187
F32.2	Major depressive disorder, single episode, severe without psychotic features	59	Major Depressive, Bipolar, and Paranoid Disorders	60	0.309	0.164	0.299	0.127	0.306	0.109	0.187
F32.3	Major depressive disorder, single episode, severe with psychotic features	59	Major Depressive, Bipolar, and Paranoid Disorders	60	0.309	0.164	0.299	0.127	0.306	0.109	0.187
F32.4	Major depressive disorder, single episode, in partial remission	59	Major Depressive, Bipolar, and Paranoid Disorders	60	0.309	0.164	0.299	0.127	0.306	0.109	0.187
F32.5	Major depressive disorder, single episode, in full remission	59	Major Depressive, Bipolar, and Paranoid Disorders	60	0.309	0.164	0.299	0.127	0.306	0.109	0.187
F33.0	Major depressive disorder, recurrent, mild	59	Major Depressive, Bipolar, and Paranoid Disorders	60	0.309	0.164	0.299	0.127	0.306	0.109	0.187
F33.1	Major depressive disorder, recurrent, moderate	59	Major Depressive, Bipolar, and Paranoid Disorders	60	0.309	0.164	0.299	0.127	0.306	0.109	0.187
F33.2	Major depressive disorder, recurrent severe without psychotic features	59	Major Depressive, Bipolar, and Paranoid Disorders	60	0.309	0.164	0.299	0.127	0.306	0.109	0.187
F33.3	Major depressive disorder, recurrent, severe with psychotic symptoms	59	Major Depressive, Bipolar, and Paranoid Disorders	60	0.309	0.164	0.299	0.127	0.306	0.109	0.187
F33.40	Major depressive disorder, recurrent, in remission, unspecified	59	Major Depressive, Bipolar, and Paranoid Disorders	60	0.309	0.164	0.299	0.127	0.306	0.109	0.187
F33.41	Major depressive disorder, recurrent, in partial remission	59	Major Depressive, Bipolar, and Paranoid Disorders	60	0.309	0.164	0.299	0.127	0.306	0.109	0.187
F33.42	Major depressive disorder, recurrent, in full remission	59	Major Depressive, Bipolar, and Paranoid Disorders	60	0.309	0.164	0.299	0.127	0.306	0.109	0.187

ICD-10-CM Code	ICD-10-CM Code Description	V24 CMS-HCC	V24 CMS-HCC Disease Group	V24 CMS-HCC Hierarchies	Community, NonDual, Aged	Community, NonDual, Disabled	Community, FBDual, Aged	Community, FBDual, Disabled	Community, PBDual, Aged	Community, PBDual, Disabled	Institutional
F33.8	Other recurrent depressive disorders	59	Major Depressive, Bipolar, and Paranoid Disorders	60	0.309	0.164	0.299	0.127	0.306	0.109	0.187
F33.9	Major depressive disorder, recurrent, unspecified	59	Major Depressive, Bipolar, and Paranoid Disorders	60	0.309	0.164	0.299	0.127	0.306	0.109	0.187
F34.81	Disruptive mood dysregulation disorder	59	Major Depressive, Bipolar, and Paranoid Disorders	60	0.309	0.164	0.299	0.127	0.306	0.109	0.187
F34.89	Other specified persistent mood disorders	59	Major Depressive, Bipolar, and Paranoid Disorders	60	0.309	0.164	0.299	0.127	0.306	0.109	0.187
F34.9	Persistent mood [affective] disorder, unspecified	59	Major Depressive, Bipolar, and Paranoid Disorders	60	0.309	0.164	0.299	0.127	0.306	0.109	0.187
F39	Unspecified mood [affective] disorder	59	Major Depressive, Bipolar, and Paranoid Disorders	60	0.309	0.164	0.299	0.127	0.306	0.109	0.187
F44.0	Dissociative amnesia	60	Personality Disorders		0.309	0.108	0.299	0.100	0.255	0.065	—
F44.1	Dissociative fugue	60	Personality Disorders		0.309	0.108	0.299	0.100	0.255	0.065	—
F44.81	Dissociative identity disorder	60	Personality Disorders		0.309	0.108	0.299	0.100	0.255	0.065	—
F48.1	Depersonalization-derealization syndrome	60	Personality Disorders		0.309	0.108	0.299	0.100	0.255	0.065	—
F53.1	Puerperal psychosis	58	Reactive and Unspecified Psychosis	59,60	0.393	0.352	0.570	0.231	0.449	0.239	0.187
F60.0	Paranoid personality disorder	60	Personality Disorders		0.309	0.108	0.299	0.100	0.255	0.065	—
F60.1	Schizoid personality disorder	60	Personality Disorders		0.309	0.108	0.299	0.100	0.255	0.065	—
F60.2	Antisocial personality disorder	60	Personality Disorders		0.309	0.108	0.299	0.100	0.255	0.065	—
F60.3	Borderline personality disorder	60	Personality Disorders		0.309	0.108	0.299	0.100	0.255	0.065	—
F60.4	Histrionic personality disorder	60	Personality Disorders		0.309	0.108	0.299	0.100	0.255	0.065	—
F60.5	Obsessive-compulsive personality disorder	60	Personality Disorders		0.309	0.108	0.299	0.100	0.255	0.065	—
F60.6	Avoidant personality disorder	60	Personality Disorders		0.309	0.108	0.299	0.100	0.255	0.065	—
F60.7	Dependent personality disorder	60	Personality Disorders		0.309	0.108	0.299	0.100	0.255	0.065	—
F60.81	Narcissistic personality disorder	60	Personality Disorders		0.309	0.108	0.299	0.100	0.255	0.065	—
F60.89	Other specific personality disorders	60	Personality Disorders		0.309	0.108	0.299	0.100	0.255	0.065	—
F60.9	Personality disorder, unspecified	60	Personality Disorders		0.309	0.108	0.299	0.100	0.255	0.065	—
G04.1	Tropical spastic paraplegia	72	Spinal Cord Disorders/Injuries	169	0.481	0.369	0.532	0.377	0.512	0.336	0.289
G04.82	Acute flaccid myelitis	72	Spinal Cord Disorders/Injuries	169	0.481	0.369	0.532	0.377	0.512	0.336	0.289
G04.89	Other myelitis	72	Spinal Cord Disorders/Injuries	169	0.481	0.369	0.532	0.377	0.512	0.336	0.289
G04.91	Myelitis, unspecified	72	Spinal Cord Disorders/Injuries	169	0.481	0.369	0.532	0.377	0.512	0.336	0.289
G05.4	Myelitis in diseases classified elsewhere	72	Spinal Cord Disorders/Injuries	169	0.481	0.369	0.532	0.377	0.512	0.336	0.289
G10	Huntington's disease	78	Parkinson's and Huntington's Diseases		0.606	0.501	0.601	0.443	0.536	0.430	0.159
G11.0	Congenital nonprogressive ataxia	72	Spinal Cord Disorders/Injuries	169	0.481	0.369	0.532	0.377	0.512	0.336	0.289
G11.10	Early-onset cerebellar ataxia, unspecified	72	Spinal Cord Disorders/Injuries	169	0.481	0.369	0.532	0.377	0.512	0.336	0.289
G11.11	Friedreich ataxia	72	Spinal Cord Disorders/Injuries	169	0.481	0.369	0.532	0.377	0.512	0.336	0.289
G11.19	Other early-onset cerebellar ataxia	72	Spinal Cord Disorders/Injuries	169	0.481	0.369	0.532	0.377	0.512	0.336	0.289
G11.2	Late-onset cerebellar ataxia	72	Spinal Cord Disorders/Injuries	169	0.481	0.369	0.532	0.377	0.512	0.336	0.289
G11.3	Cerebellar ataxia with defective DNA repair	72	Spinal Cord Disorders/Injuries	169	0.481	0.369	0.532	0.377	0.512	0.336	0.289
G11.4	Hereditary spastic paraplegia	72	Spinal Cord Disorders/Injuries	169	0.481	0.369	0.532	0.377	0.512	0.336	0.289
G11.8	Other hereditary ataxias	72	Spinal Cord Disorders/Injuries	169	0.481	0.369	0.532	0.377	0.512	0.336	0.289
G11.9	Hereditary ataxia, unspecified	72	Spinal Cord Disorders/Injuries	169	0.481	0.369	0.532	0.377	0.512	0.336	0.289
G12.0	Infantile spinal muscular atrophy, type I [Werdnig-Hoffman]	72	Spinal Cord Disorders/Injuries	169	0.481	0.369	0.532	0.377	0.512	0.336	0.289
G12.1	Other inherited spinal muscular atrophy	72	Spinal Cord Disorders/Injuries	169	0.481	0.369	0.532	0.377	0.512	0.336	0.289
G12.20	Motor neuron disease, unspecified	73	Amyotrophic Lateral Sclerosis and Other Motor Neuron Disease		0.999	1.132	1.101	1.245	0.687	0.933	0.476

ICD-10-CM Code	ICD-10-CM Code Description	V24 CMS-HCC	V24 CMS-HCC Disease Group	V24 CMS-HCC Hierarchies	Community, NonDual, Aged	Community, NonDual, Disabled	Community, FBDual, Aged	Community, FBDual, Disabled	Community, PBDual, Aged	Community, PBDual, Disabled	Institutional
G12.21	Amyotrophic lateral sclerosis	73	Amyotrophic Lateral Sclerosis and Other Motor Neuron Disease		0.999	1.132	1.101	1.245	0.687	0.933	0.476
G12.22	Progressive bulbar palsy	73	Amyotrophic Lateral Sclerosis and Other Motor Neuron Disease		0.999	1.132	1.101	1.245	0.687	0.933	0.476
G12.23	Primary lateral sclerosis	73	Amyotrophic Lateral Sclerosis and Other Motor Neuron Disease		0.999	1.132	1.101	1.245	0.687	0.933	0.476
G12.24	Familial motor neuron disease	73	Amyotrophic Lateral Sclerosis and Other Motor Neuron Disease		0.999	1.132	1.101	1.245	0.687	0.933	0.476
G12.25	Progressive spinal muscle atrophy	73	Amyotrophic Lateral Sclerosis and Other Motor Neuron Disease		0.999	1.132	1.101	1.245	0.687	0.933	0.476
G12.29	Other motor neuron disease	73	Amyotrophic Lateral Sclerosis and Other Motor Neuron Disease		0.999	1.132	1.101	1.245	0.687	0.933	0.476
G12.8	Other spinal muscular atrophies and related syndromes	72	Spinal Cord Disorders/Injuries	169	0.481	0.369	0.532	0.377	0.512	0.336	0.289
G12.9	Spinal muscular atrophy, unspecified	72	Spinal Cord Disorders/Injuries	169	0.481	0.369	0.532	0.377	0.512	0.336	0.289
G13.0	Paraneoplastic neuromyopathy and neuropathy	75	Myasthenia Gravis/Myoneural Disorders and Guillain-Barre Syndrome/Inflammatory and Toxic Neuropathy		0.472	0.481	0.407	0.404	0.287	0.314	0.332
G13.1	Other systemic atrophy primarily affecting central nervous system in neoplastic disease	75	Myasthenia Gravis/Myoneural Disorders and Guillain-Barre Syndrome/Inflammatory and Toxic Neuropathy		0.472	0.481	0.407	0.404	0.287	0.314	0.332
G13.2	Systemic atrophy primarily affecting the central nervous system in myxedema	52	Dementia Without Complication		0.346	0.224	0.453	0.256	0.420	0.257	—
G13.8	Systemic atrophy primarily affecting central nervous system in other diseases classified elsewhere	52	Dementia Without Complication		0.346	0.224	0.453	0.256	0.420	0.257	—
G20	Parkinson's disease	78	Parkinson's and Huntington's Diseases		0.606	0.501	0.601	0.443	0.536	0.430	0.159
G21.11	Neuroleptic induced parkinsonism	78	Parkinson's and Huntington's Diseases		0.606	0.501	0.601	0.443	0.536	0.430	0.159
G21.19	Other drug induced secondary parkinsonism	78	Parkinson's and Huntington's Diseases		0.606	0.501	0.601	0.443	0.536	0.430	0.159
G21.2	Secondary parkinsonism due to other external agents	78	Parkinson's and Huntington's Diseases		0.606	0.501	0.601	0.443	0.536	0.430	0.159
G21.3	Postencephalitic parkinsonism	78	Parkinson's and Huntington's Diseases		0.606	0.501	0.601	0.443	0.536	0.430	0.159
G21.4	Vascular parkinsonism	78	Parkinson's and Huntington's Diseases		0.606	0.501	0.601	0.443	0.536	0.430	0.159
G21.8	Other secondary parkinsonism	78	Parkinson's and Huntington's Diseases		0.606	0.501	0.601	0.443	0.536	0.430	0.159
G21.9	Secondary parkinsonism, unspecified	78	Parkinson's and Huntington's Diseases		0.606	0.501	0.601	0.443	0.536	0.430	0.159
G23.0	Hallervorden-Spatz disease	78	Parkinson's and Huntington's Diseases		0.606	0.501	0.601	0.443	0.536	0.430	0.159
G23.1	Progressive supranuclear ophthalmoplegia [Steele-Richardson-Olszewski]	78	Parkinson's and Huntington's Diseases		0.606	0.501	0.601	0.443	0.536	0.430	0.159
G23.2	Striatonigral degeneration	78	Parkinson's and Huntington's Diseases		0.606	0.501	0.601	0.443	0.536	0.430	0.159
G23.8	Other specified degenerative diseases of basal ganglia	78	Parkinson's and Huntington's Diseases		0.606	0.501	0.601	0.443	0.536	0.430	0.159
G23.9	Degenerative disease of basal ganglia, unspecified	78	Parkinson's and Huntington's Diseases		0.606	0.501	0.601	0.443	0.536	0.430	0.159
G30.0	Alzheimer's disease with early onset	52	Dementia Without Complication		0.346	0.224	0.453	0.256	0.420	0.257	—
G30.1	Alzheimer's disease with late onset	52	Dementia Without Complication		0.346	0.224	0.453	0.256	0.420	0.257	—
G30.8	Other Alzheimer's disease	52	Dementia Without Complication		0.346	0.224	0.453	0.256	0.420	0.257	—
G30.9	Alzheimer's disease, unspecified	52	Dementia Without Complication		0.346	0.224	0.453	0.256	0.420	0.257	—
G31.01	Pick's disease	52	Dementia Without Complication		0.346	0.224	0.453	0.256	0.420	0.257	—
G31.09	Other frontotemporal dementia	52	Dementia Without Complication		0.346	0.224	0.453	0.256	0.420	0.257	—
G31.1	Senile degeneration of brain, not elsewhere classified	52	Dementia Without Complication		0.346	0.224	0.453	0.256	0.420	0.257	—

2021 Optum360, LLC

ICD-10-CM Code	ICD-10-CM Code Description	V24 CMS-HCC	V24 CMS-HCC Disease Group	V24 CMS-HCC Hierarchies	Community, NonDual, Aged	Community, NonDual, Disabled	Community, FBDual, Aged	Community, FBDual, Disabled	Community, PBDual, Aged	Community, PBDual, Disabled	Institutional
G31.2	Degeneration of nervous system due to alcohol	52	Dementia Without Complication		0.346	0.224	0.453	0.256	0.420	0.257	—
G31.81	Alpers disease	52	Dementia Without Complication		0.346	0.224	0.453	0.256	0.420	0.257	—
G31.82	Leigh's disease	52	Dementia Without Complication		0.346	0.224	0.453	0.256	0.420	0.257	—
G31.83	Dementia with Lewy bodies	52	Dementia Without Complication		0.346	0.224	0.453	0.256	0.420	0.257	—
G31.85	Corticobasal degeneration	52	Dementia Without Complication		0.346	0.224	0.453	0.256	0.420	0.257	—
G31.89	Other specified degenerative diseases of nervous system	52	Dementia Without Complication		0.346	0.224	0.453	0.256	0.420	0.257	—
G31.9	Degenerative disease of nervous system, unspecified	52	Dementia Without Complication		0.346	0.224	0.453	0.256	0.420	0.257	—
G32.0	Subacute combined degeneration of spinal cord in diseases classified elsewhere	72	Spinal Cord Disorders/Injuries	169	0.481	0.369	0.532	0.377	0.512	0.336	0.289
G32.81	Cerebellar ataxia in diseases classified elsewhere	72	Spinal Cord Disorders/Injuries	169	0.481	0.369	0.532	0.377	0.512	0.336	0.289
G35	Multiple sclerosis	77	Multiple Sclerosis		0.423	0.566	0.742	0.789	0.276	0.460	—
G36.0	Neuromyelitis optica [Devic]	77	Multiple Sclerosis		0.423	0.566	0.742	0.789	0.276	0.460	—
G36.1	Acute and subacute hemorrhagic leukoencephalitis [Hurst]	77	Multiple Sclerosis		0.423	0.566	0.742	0.789	0.276	0.460	—
G36.8	Other specified acute disseminated demyelination	77	Multiple Sclerosis		0.423	0.566	0.742	0.789	0.276	0.460	—
G36.9	Acute disseminated demyelination, unspecified	77	Multiple Sclerosis		0.423	0.566	0.742	0.789	0.276	0.460	—
G37.0	Diffuse sclerosis of central nervous system	77	Multiple Sclerosis		0.423	0.566	0.742	0.789	0.276	0.460	—
G37.1	Central demyelination of corpus callosum	77	Multiple Sclerosis		0.423	0.566	0.742	0.789	0.276	0.460	—
G37.2	Central pontine myelinolysis	77	Multiple Sclerosis		0.423	0.566	0.742	0.789	0.276	0.460	—
G37.3	Acute transverse myelitis in demyelinating disease of central nervous system	72	Spinal Cord Disorders/Injuries	169	0.481	0.369	0.532	0.377	0.512	0.336	0.289
G37.4	Subacute necrotizing myelitis of central nervous system	72	Spinal Cord Disorders/Injuries	169	0.481	0.369	0.532	0.377	0.512	0.336	0.289
G37.5	Concentric sclerosis [Balo] of central nervous system	77	Multiple Sclerosis		0.423	0.566	0.742	0.789	0.276	0.460	—
G37.8	Other specified demyelinating diseases of central nervous system	77	Multiple Sclerosis		0.423	0.566	0.742	0.789	0.276	0.460	—
G37.9	Demyelinating disease of central nervous system, unspecified	77	Multiple Sclerosis		0.423	0.566	0.742	0.789	0.276	0.460	—
G40.001	Localization-related (focal) (partial) idiopathic epilepsy and epileptic syndromes with seizures of localized onset, not intractable, with status epilepticus	79	Seizure Disorders and Convulsions		0.220	0.196	0.237	0.139	0.257	0.169	0.065
G40.009	Localization-related (focal) (partial) idiopathic epilepsy and epileptic syndromes with seizures of localized onset, not intractable, without status epilepticus	79	Seizure Disorders and Convulsions		0.220	0.196	0.237	0.139	0.257	0.169	0.065
G40.011	Localization-related (focal) (partial) idiopathic epilepsy and epileptic syndromes with seizures of localized onset, intractable, with status epilepticus	79	Seizure Disorders and Convulsions		0.220	0.196	0.237	0.139	0.257	0.169	0.065
G40.019	Localization-related (focal) (partial) idiopathic epilepsy and epileptic syndromes with seizures of localized onset, intractable, without status epilepticus	79	Seizure Disorders and Convulsions		0.220	0.196	0.237	0.139	0.257	0.169	0.065

ICD-10-CM Code	ICD-10-CM Code Description	V24 CMS-HCC	V24 CMS-HCC Disease Group	V24 CMS-HCC Hierarchies	Community, NonDual, Aged	Community, NonDual, Disabled	Community, FBDual, Aged	Community, FBDual, Disabled	Community, PBDual, Aged	Community, PBDual, Disabled	Institutional
G40.101	Localization-related (focal) (partial) symptomatic epilepsy and epileptic syndromes with simple partial seizures, not intractable, with status epilepticus	79	Seizure Disorders and Convulsions		0.220	0.196	0.237	0.139	0.257	0.169	0.065
G40.109	Localization-related (focal) (partial) symptomatic epilepsy and epileptic syndromes with simple partial seizures, not intractable, without status epilepticus	79	Seizure Disorders and Convulsions		0.220	0.196	0.237	0.139	0.257	0.169	0.065
G40.111	Localization-related (focal) (partial) symptomatic epilepsy and epileptic syndromes with simple partial seizures, intractable, with status epilepticus	79	Seizure Disorders and Convulsions		0.220	0.196	0.237	0.139	0.257	0.169	0.065
G40.119	Localization-related (focal) (partial) symptomatic epilepsy and epileptic syndromes with simple partial seizures, intractable, without status epilepticus	79	Seizure Disorders and Convulsions		0.220	0.196	0.237	0.139	0.257	0.169	0.065
G40.201	Localization-related (focal) (partial) symptomatic epilepsy and epileptic syndromes with complex partial seizures, not intractable, with status epilepticus	79	Seizure Disorders and Convulsions		0.220	0.196	0.237	0.139	0.257	0.169	0.065
G40.209	Localization-related (focal) (partial) symptomatic epilepsy and epileptic syndromes with complex partial seizures, not intractable, without status epilepticus	79	Seizure Disorders and Convulsions		0.220	0.196	0.237	0.139	0.257	0.169	0.065
G40.211	Localization-related (focal) (partial) symptomatic epilepsy and epileptic syndromes with complex partial seizures, intractable, with status epilepticus	79	Seizure Disorders and Convulsions		0.220	0.196	0.237	0.139	0.257	0.169	0.065
G40.219	Localization-related (focal) (partial) symptomatic epilepsy and epileptic syndromes with complex partial seizures, intractable, without status epilepticus	79	Seizure Disorders and Convulsions		0.220	0.196	0.237	0.139	0.257	0.169	0.065
G40.301	Generalized idiopathic epilepsy and epileptic syndromes, not intractable, with status epilepticus	79	Seizure Disorders and Convulsions		0.220	0.196	0.237	0.139	0.257	0.169	0.065
G40.309	Generalized idiopathic epilepsy and epileptic syndromes, not intractable, without status epilepticus	79	Seizure Disorders and Convulsions		0.220	0.196	0.237	0.139	0.257	0.169	0.065
G40.311	Generalized idiopathic epilepsy and epileptic syndromes, intractable, with status epilepticus	79	Seizure Disorders and Convulsions		0.220	0.196	0.237	0.139	0.257	0.169	0.065
G40.319	Generalized idiopathic epilepsy and epileptic syndromes, intractable, without status epilepticus	79	Seizure Disorders and Convulsions		0.220	0.196	0.237	0.139	0.257	0.169	0.065
G40.401	Other generalized epilepsy and epileptic syndromes, not intractable, with status epilepticus	79	Seizure Disorders and Convulsions		0.220	0.196	0.237	0.139	0.257	0.169	0.065
G40.409	Other generalized epilepsy and epileptic syndromes, not intractable, without status epilepticus	79	Seizure Disorders and Convulsions		0.220	0.196	0.237	0.139	0.257	0.169	0.065
G40.411	Other generalized epilepsy and epileptic syndromes, intractable, with status epilepticus	79	Seizure Disorders and Convulsions		0.220	0.196	0.237	0.139	0.257	0.169	0.065

ICD-10-CM Code	ICD-10-CM Code Description	V24 CMS-HCC	V24 CMS-HCC Disease Group	V24 CMS-HCC Hierarchies	Community, NonDual, Aged	Community, NonDual, Disabled	Community, FBDual, Aged	Community, FBDual, Disabled	Community, PBDual, Aged	Community, PBDual, Disabled	Institutional
G40.419	Other generalized epilepsy and epileptic syndromes, intractable, without status epilepticus	79	Seizure Disorders and Convulsions		0.220	0.196	0.237	0.139	0.257	0.169	0.065
G40.42	Cyclin-Dependent Kinase-Like 5 Deficiency Disorder	79	Seizure Disorders and Convulsions		0.220	0.196	0.237	0.139	0.257	0.169	0.065
G40.501	Epileptic seizures related to external causes, not intractable, with status epilepticus	79	Seizure Disorders and Convulsions		0.220	0.196	0.237	0.139	0.257	0.169	0.065
G40.509	Epileptic seizures related to external causes, not intractable, without status epilepticus	79	Seizure Disorders and Convulsions		0.220	0.196	0.237	0.139	0.257	0.169	0.065
G40.801	Other epilepsy, not intractable, with status epilepticus	79	Seizure Disorders and Convulsions		0.220	0.196	0.237	0.139	0.257	0.169	0.065
G40.802	Other epilepsy, not intractable, without status epilepticus	79	Seizure Disorders and Convulsions		0.220	0.196	0.237	0.139	0.257	0.169	0.065
G40.803	Other epilepsy, intractable, with status epilepticus	79	Seizure Disorders and Convulsions		0.220	0.196	0.237	0.139	0.257	0.169	0.065
G40.804	Other epilepsy, intractable, without status epilepticus	79	Seizure Disorders and Convulsions		0.220	0.196	0.237	0.139	0.257	0.169	0.065
G40.811	Lennox-Gastaut syndrome, not intractable, with status epilepticus	79	Seizure Disorders and Convulsions		0.220	0.196	0.237	0.139	0.257	0.169	0.065
G40.812	Lennox-Gastaut syndrome, not intractable, without status epilepticus	79	Seizure Disorders and Convulsions		0.220	0.196	0.237	0.139	0.257	0.169	0.065
G40.813	Lennox-Gastaut syndrome, intractable, with status epilepticus	79	Seizure Disorders and Convulsions		0.220	0.196	0.237	0.139	0.257	0.169	0.065
G40.814	Lennox-Gastaut syndrome, intractable, without status epilepticus	79	Seizure Disorders and Convulsions		0.220	0.196	0.237	0.139	0.257	0.169	0.065
G40.821	Epileptic spasms, not intractable, with status epilepticus	79	Seizure Disorders and Convulsions		0.220	0.196	0.237	0.139	0.257	0.169	0.065
G40.822	Epileptic spasms, not intractable, without status epilepticus	79	Seizure Disorders and Convulsions		0.220	0.196	0.237	0.139	0.257	0.169	0.065
G40.823	Epileptic spasms, intractable, with status epilepticus	79	Seizure Disorders and Convulsions		0.220	0.196	0.237	0.139	0.257	0.169	0.065
G40.824	Epileptic spasms, intractable, without status epilepticus	79	Seizure Disorders and Convulsions		0.220	0.196	0.237	0.139	0.257	0.169	0.065
G40.833	Dravet syndrome, intractable, with status epilepticus	79	Seizure Disorders and Convulsions		0.220	0.196	0.237	0.139	0.257	0.169	0.065
G40.834	Dravet syndrome, intractable, without status epilepticus	79	Seizure Disorders and Convulsions		0.220	0.196	0.237	0.139	0.257	0.169	0.065
G40.89	Other seizures	79	Seizure Disorders and Convulsions		0.220	0.196	0.237	0.139	0.257	0.169	0.065
G40.901	Epilepsy, unspecified, not intractable, with status epilepticus	79	Seizure Disorders and Convulsions		0.220	0.196	0.237	0.139	0.257	0.169	0.065
G40.909	Epilepsy, unspecified, not intractable, without status epilepticus	79	Seizure Disorders and Convulsions		0.220	0.196	0.237	0.139	0.257	0.169	0.065
G40.911	Epilepsy, unspecified, intractable, with status epilepticus	79	Seizure Disorders and Convulsions		0.220	0.196	0.237	0.139	0.257	0.169	0.065
G40.919	Epilepsy, unspecified, intractable, without status epilepticus	79	Seizure Disorders and Convulsions		0.220	0.196	0.237	0.139	0.257	0.169	0.065
G40.A01	Absence epileptic syndrome, not intractable, with status epilepticus	79	Seizure Disorders and Convulsions		0.220	0.196	0.237	0.139	0.257	0.169	0.065
G40.A09	Absence epileptic syndrome, not intractable, without status epilepticus	79	Seizure Disorders and Convulsions		0.220	0.196	0.237	0.139	0.257	0.169	0.065
G40.A11	Absence epileptic syndrome, intractable, with status epilepticus	79	Seizure Disorders and Convulsions		0.220	0.196	0.237	0.139	0.257	0.169	0.065
G40.A19	Absence epileptic syndrome, intractable, without status epilepticus	79	Seizure Disorders and Convulsions		0.220	0.196	0.237	0.139	0.257	0.169	0.065
G40.B01	Juvenile myoclonic epilepsy, not intractable, with status epilepticus	79	Seizure Disorders and Convulsions		0.220	0.196	0.237	0.139	0.257	0.169	0.065

ICD-10-CM Code	ICD-10-CM Code Description	V24 CMS-HCC	V24 CMS-HCC Disease Group	V24 CMS-HCC Hierarchies	Community, NonDual, Aged	Community, NonDual, Disabled	Community, FBDual, Aged	Community, FBDual, Disabled	Community, PBDual, Aged	Community, PBDual, Disabled	Institutional
G40.B09	Juvenile myoclonic epilepsy, not intractable, without status epilepticus	79	Seizure Disorders and Convulsions		0.220	0.196	0.237	0.139	0.257	0.169	0.065
G40.B11	Juvenile myoclonic epilepsy, intractable, with status epilepticus	79	Seizure Disorders and Convulsions		0.220	0.196	0.237	0.139	0.257	0.169	0.065
G40.B19	Juvenile myoclonic epilepsy, intractable, without status epilepticus	79	Seizure Disorders and Convulsions		0.220	0.196	0.237	0.139	0.257	0.169	0.065
G54.6	Phantom limb syndrome with pain	189	Amputation Status, Lower Limb/ Amputation Complications		0.519	0.437	0.795	0.934	0.697	0.626	0.357
G54.7	Phantom limb syndrome without pain	189	Amputation Status, Lower Limb/ Amputation Complications		0.519	0.437	0.795	0.934	0.697	0.626	0.357
G61.0	Guillain-Barre syndrome	75	Myasthenia Gravis/Myoneural Disorders and Guillain-Barre Syndrome/Inflammatory and Toxic Neuropathy		0.472	0.481	0.407	0.404	0.287	0.314	0.332
G61.1	Serum neuropathy	75	Myasthenia Gravis/Myoneural Disorders and Guillain-Barre Syndrome/Inflammatory and Toxic Neuropathy		0.472	0.481	0.407	0.404	0.287	0.314	0.332
G61.81	Chronic inflammatory demyelinating polyneuritis	75	Myasthenia Gravis/Myoneural Disorders and Guillain-Barre Syndrome/Inflammatory and Toxic Neuropathy		0.472	0.481	0.407	0.404	0.287	0.314	0.332
G61.82	Multifocal motor neuropathy	75	Myasthenia Gravis/Myoneural Disorders and Guillain-Barre Syndrome/Inflammatory and Toxic Neuropathy		0.472	0.481	0.407	0.404	0.287	0.314	0.332
G61.89	Other inflammatory polyneuropathies	75	Myasthenia Gravis/Myoneural Disorders and Guillain-Barre Syndrome/Inflammatory and Toxic Neuropathy		0.472	0.481	0.407	0.404	0.287	0.314	0.332
G61.9	Inflammatory polyneuropathy, unspecified	75	Myasthenia Gravis/Myoneural Disorders and Guillain-Barre Syndrome/Inflammatory and Toxic Neuropathy		0.472	0.481	0.407	0.404	0.287	0.314	0.332
G62.0	Drug-induced polyneuropathy	75	Myasthenia Gravis/Myoneural Disorders and Guillain-Barre Syndrome/Inflammatory and Toxic Neuropathy		0.472	0.481	0.407	0.404	0.287	0.314	0.332
G62.1	Alcoholic polyneuropathy	75	Myasthenia Gravis/Myoneural Disorders and Guillain-Barre Syndrome/Inflammatory and Toxic Neuropathy		0.472	0.481	0.407	0.404	0.287	0.314	0.332
G62.2	Polyneuropathy due to other toxic agents	75	Myasthenia Gravis/Myoneural Disorders and Guillain-Barre Syndrome/Inflammatory and Toxic Neuropathy		0.472	0.481	0.407	0.404	0.287	0.314	0.332
G62.81	Critical illness polyneuropathy	75	Myasthenia Gravis/Myoneural Disorders and Guillain-Barre Syndrome/Inflammatory and Toxic Neuropathy		0.472	0.481	0.407	0.404	0.287	0.314	0.332
G62.82	Radiation-induced polyneuropathy	75	Myasthenia Gravis/Myoneural Disorders and Guillain-Barre Syndrome/Inflammatory and Toxic Neuropathy		0.472	0.481	0.407	0.404	0.287	0.314	0.332
G63	Polyneuropathy in diseases classified elsewhere	75	Myasthenia Gravis/Myoneural Disorders and Guillain-Barre Syndrome/Inflammatory and Toxic Neuropathy		0.472	0.481	0.407	0.404	0.287	0.314	0.332
G65.0	Sequelae of Guillain-Barre syndrome	75	Myasthenia Gravis/Myoneural Disorders and Guillain-Barre Syndrome/Inflammatory and Toxic Neuropathy		0.472	0.481	0.407	0.404	0.287	0.314	0.332

ICD-10-CM Code	ICD-10-CM Code Description	V24 CMS-HCC	V24 CMS-HCC Disease Group	V24 CMS-HCC Hierarchies	Community, NonDual, Aged	Community, NonDual, Disabled	Community, FBDual, Aged	Community, FBDual, Disabled	Community, PBDual, Aged	Community, PBDual, Disabled	Institutional
G65.1	Sequelae of other inflammatory polyneuropathy	75	Myasthenia Gravis/Myoneural Disorders and Guillain-Barre Syndrome/Inflammatory and Toxic Neuropathy		0.472	0.481	0.407	0.404	0.287	0.314	0.332
G65.2	Sequelae of toxic polyneuropathy	75	Myasthenia Gravis/Myoneural Disorders and Guillain-Barre Syndrome/Inflammatory and Toxic Neuropathy		0.472	0.481	0.407	0.404	0.287	0.314	0.332
G70.00	Myasthenia gravis without (acute) exacerbation	75	Myasthenia Gravis/Myoneural Disorders and Guillain-Barre Syndrome/Inflammatory and Toxic Neuropathy		0.472	0.481	0.407	0.404	0.287	0.314	0.332
G70.01	Myasthenia gravis with (acute) exacerbation	75	Myasthenia Gravis/Myoneural Disorders and Guillain-Barre Syndrome/Inflammatory and Toxic Neuropathy		0.472	0.481	0.407	0.404	0.287	0.314	0.332
G70.1	Toxic myoneural disorders	75	Myasthenia Gravis/Myoneural Disorders and Guillain-Barre Syndrome/Inflammatory and Toxic Neuropathy		0.472	0.481	0.407	0.404	0.287	0.314	0.332
G70.2	Congenital and developmental myasthenia	75	Myasthenia Gravis/Myoneural Disorders and Guillain-Barre Syndrome/Inflammatory and Toxic Neuropathy		0.472	0.481	0.407	0.404	0.287	0.314	0.332
G70.80	Lambert-Eaton syndrome, unspecified	75	Myasthenia Gravis/Myoneural Disorders and Guillain-Barre Syndrome/Inflammatory and Toxic Neuropathy		0.472	0.481	0.407	0.404	0.287	0.314	0.332
G70.81	Lambert-Eaton syndrome in disease classified elsewhere	75	Myasthenia Gravis/Myoneural Disorders and Guillain-Barre Syndrome/Inflammatory and Toxic Neuropathy		0.472	0.481	0.407	0.404	0.287	0.314	0.332
G70.89	Other specified myoneural disorders	75	Myasthenia Gravis/Myoneural Disorders and Guillain-Barre Syndrome/Inflammatory and Toxic Neuropathy		0.472	0.481	0.407	0.404	0.287	0.314	0.332
G70.9	Myoneural disorder, unspecified	75	Myasthenia Gravis/Myoneural Disorders and Guillain-Barre Syndrome/Inflammatory and Toxic Neuropathy		0.472	0.481	0.407	0.404	0.287	0.314	0.332
G71.00	Muscular dystrophy, unspecified	76	Muscular Dystrophy		0.518	0.621	0.413	0.597	—	0.286	0.356
G71.01	Duchenne or Becker muscular dystrophy	76	Muscular Dystrophy		0.518	0.621	0.413	0.597	—	0.286	0.356
G71.02	Facioscapulohumeral muscular dystrophy	76	Muscular Dystrophy		0.518	0.621	0.413	0.597	—	0.286	0.356
G71.09	Other specified muscular dystrophies	76	Muscular Dystrophy		0.518	0.621	0.413	0.597	—	0.286	0.356
G71.11	Myotonic muscular dystrophy	76	Muscular Dystrophy		0.518	0.621	0.413	0.597	—	0.286	0.356
G71.20	Congenital myopathy, unspecified	76	Muscular Dystrophy		0.518	0.621	0.413	0.597	—	0.286	0.356
G71.21	Nemaline myopathy	76	Muscular Dystrophy		0.518	0.621	0.413	0.597	—	0.286	0.356
G71.220	X-linked myotubular myopathy	76	Muscular Dystrophy		0.518	0.621	0.413	0.597	—	0.286	0.356
G71.228	Other centronuclear myopathy	76	Muscular Dystrophy		0.518	0.621	0.413	0.597	—	0.286	0.356
G71.29	Other congenital myopathy	76	Muscular Dystrophy		0.518	0.621	0.413	0.597	—	0.286	0.356
G73.1	Lambert-Eaton syndrome in neoplastic disease	75	Myasthenia Gravis/Myoneural Disorders and Guillain-Barre Syndrome/Inflammatory and Toxic Neuropathy		0.472	0.481	0.407	0.404	0.287	0.314	0.332
G73.3	Myasthenic syndromes in other diseases classified elsewhere	75	Myasthenia Gravis/Myoneural Disorders and Guillain-Barre Syndrome/Inflammatory and Toxic Neuropathy		0.472	0.481	0.407	0.404	0.287	0.314	0.332
G80.0	Spastic quadriplegic cerebral palsy	74	Cerebral Palsy		0.339	0.098	—	—	0.114	—	—

ICD-10-CM Code	ICD-10-CM Code Description	V24 CMS-HCC	V24 CMS-HCC Disease Group	V24 CMS-HCC Hierarchies	Community, NonDual, Aged	Community, NonDual, Disabled	Community, FBDual, Aged	Community, FBDual, Disabled	Community, PBDual, Aged	Community, PBDual, Disabled	Institutional
G80.1	Spastic diplegic cerebral palsy	74	Cerebral Palsy		0.339	0.098	—	—	0.114	—	—
G80.2	Spastic hemiplegic cerebral palsy	74	Cerebral Palsy		0.339	0.098	—	—	0.114	—	—
G80.3	Athetoid cerebral palsy	74	Cerebral Palsy		0.339	0.098	—	—	0.114	—	—
G80.4	Ataxic cerebral palsy	74	Cerebral Palsy		0.339	0.098	—	—	0.114	—	—
G80.8	Other cerebral palsy	74	Cerebral Palsy		0.339	0.098	—	—	0.114	—	—
G80.9	Cerebral palsy, unspecified	74	Cerebral Palsy		0.339	0.098	—	—	0.114	—	—
G81.00	Flaccid hemiplegia affecting unspecified side	103	Hemiplegia/Hemiparesis	104	0.437	0.281	0.487	0.296	0.438	0.310	—
G81.01	Flaccid hemiplegia affecting right dominant side	103	Hemiplegia/Hemiparesis	104	0.437	0.281	0.487	0.296	0.438	0.310	—
G81.02	Flaccid hemiplegia affecting left dominant side	103	Hemiplegia/Hemiparesis	104	0.437	0.281	0.487	0.296	0.438	0.310	—
G81.03	Flaccid hemiplegia affecting right nondominant side	103	Hemiplegia/Hemiparesis	104	0.437	0.281	0.487	0.296	0.438	0.310	—
G81.04	Flaccid hemiplegia affecting left nondominant side	103	Hemiplegia/Hemiparesis	104	0.437	0.281	0.487	0.296	0.438	0.310	—
G81.10	Spastic hemiplegia affecting unspecified side	103	Hemiplegia/Hemiparesis	104	0.437	0.281	0.487	0.296	0.438	0.310	—
G81.11	Spastic hemiplegia affecting right dominant side	103	Hemiplegia/Hemiparesis	104	0.437	0.281	0.487	0.296	0.438	0.310	—
G81.12	Spastic hemiplegia affecting left dominant side	103	Hemiplegia/Hemiparesis	104	0.437	0.281	0.487	0.296	0.438	0.310	—
G81.13	Spastic hemiplegia affecting right nondominant side	103	Hemiplegia/Hemiparesis	104	0.437	0.281	0.487	0.296	0.438	0.310	—
G81.14	Spastic hemiplegia affecting left nondominant side	103	Hemiplegia/Hemiparesis	104	0.437	0.281	0.487	0.296	0.438	0.310	—
G81.90	Hemiplegia, unspecified affecting unspecified side	103	Hemiplegia/Hemiparesis	104	0.437	0.281	0.487	0.296	0.438	0.310	—
G81.91	Hemiplegia, unspecified affecting right dominant side	103	Hemiplegia/Hemiparesis	104	0.437	0.281	0.487	0.296	0.438	0.310	—
G81.92	Hemiplegia, unspecified affecting left dominant side	103	Hemiplegia/Hemiparesis	104	0.437	0.281	0.487	0.296	0.438	0.310	—
G81.93	Hemiplegia, unspecified affecting right nondominant side	103	Hemiplegia/Hemiparesis	104	0.437	0.281	0.487	0.296	0.438	0.310	—
G81.94	Hemiplegia, unspecified affecting left nondominant side	103	Hemiplegia/Hemiparesis	104	0.437	0.281	0.487	0.296	0.438	0.310	—
G82.20	Paraplegia, unspecified	71	Paraplegia	72,104, 169	1.068	0.739	0.921	0.957	1.000	0.933	0.492
G82.21	Paraplegia, complete	71	Paraplegia	72,104, 169	1.068	0.739	0.921	0.957	1.000	0.933	0.492
G82.22	Paraplegia, incomplete	71	Paraplegia	72,104, 169	1.068	0.739	0.921	0.957	1.000	0.933	0.492
G82.50	Quadriplegia, unspecified	70	Quadriplegia	71,72, 103,104, 169	1.242	1.001	1.038	1.000	1.000	1.134	0.549
G82.51	Quadriplegia, C1-C4 complete	70	Quadriplegia	71,72, 103,104, 169	1.242	1.001	1.038	1.000	1.000	1.134	0.549
G82.52	Quadriplegia, C1-C4 incomplete	70	Quadriplegia	71,72, 103,104, 169	1.242	1.001	1.038	1.000	1.000	1.134	0.549
G82.53	Quadriplegia, C5-C7 complete	70	Quadriplegia	71,72, 103,104, 169	1.242	1.001	1.038	1.000	1.000	1.134	0.549
G82.54	Quadriplegia, C5-C7 incomplete	70	Quadriplegia	71,72, 103,104, 169	1.242	1.001	1.038	1.000	1.000	1.134	0.549

ICD-10-CM Code	ICD-10-CM Code Description	V24 CMS-HCC	V24 CMS-HCC Disease Group	V24 CMS-HCC Hierarchies	Community, NonDual, Aged	Community, NonDual, Disabled	Community, FBDual, Aged	Community, FBDual, Disabled	Community, PBDual, Aged	Community, PBDual, Disabled	Institutional
G83.0	Diplegia of upper limbs	104	Monoplegia, Other Paralytic Syndromes		0.331	0.270	0.345	0.258	0.300	0.164	—
G83.10	Monoplegia of lower limb affecting unspecified side	104	Monoplegia, Other Paralytic Syndromes		0.331	0.270	0.345	0.258	0.300	0.164	—
G83.11	Monoplegia of lower limb affecting right dominant side	104	Monoplegia, Other Paralytic Syndromes		0.331	0.270	0.345	0.258	0.300	0.164	—
G83.12	Monoplegia of lower limb affecting left dominant side	104	Monoplegia, Other Paralytic Syndromes		0.331	0.270	0.345	0.258	0.300	0.164	—
G83.13	Monoplegia of lower limb affecting right nondominant side	104	Monoplegia, Other Paralytic Syndromes		0.331	0.270	0.345	0.258	0.300	0.164	—
G83.14	Monoplegia of lower limb affecting left nondominant side	104	Monoplegia, Other Paralytic Syndromes		0.331	0.270	0.345	0.258	0.300	0.164	—
G83.20	Monoplegia of upper limb affecting unspecified side	104	Monoplegia, Other Paralytic Syndromes		0.331	0.270	0.345	0.258	0.300	0.164	—
G83.21	Monoplegia of upper limb affecting right dominant side	104	Monoplegia, Other Paralytic Syndromes		0.331	0.270	0.345	0.258	0.300	0.164	—
G83.22	Monoplegia of upper limb affecting left dominant side	104	Monoplegia, Other Paralytic Syndromes		0.331	0.270	0.345	0.258	0.300	0.164	—
G83.23	Monoplegia of upper limb affecting right nondominant side	104	Monoplegia, Other Paralytic Syndromes		0.331	0.270	0.345	0.258	0.300	0.164	—
G83.24	Monoplegia of upper limb affecting left nondominant side	104	Monoplegia, Other Paralytic Syndromes		0.331	0.270	0.345	0.258	0.300	0.164	—
G83.30	Monoplegia, unspecified affecting unspecified side	104	Monoplegia, Other Paralytic Syndromes		0.331	0.270	0.345	0.258	0.300	0.164	—
G83.31	Monoplegia, unspecified affecting right dominant side	104	Monoplegia, Other Paralytic Syndromes		0.331	0.270	0.345	0.258	0.300	0.164	—
G83.32	Monoplegia, unspecified affecting left dominant side	104	Monoplegia, Other Paralytic Syndromes		0.331	0.270	0.345	0.258	0.300	0.164	—
G83.33	Monoplegia, unspecified affecting right nondominant side	104	Monoplegia, Other Paralytic Syndromes		0.331	0.270	0.345	0.258	0.300	0.164	—
G83.34	Monoplegia, unspecified affecting left nondominant side	104	Monoplegia, Other Paralytic Syndromes		0.331	0.270	0.345	0.258	0.300	0.164	—
G83.4	Cauda equina syndrome	72	Spinal Cord Disorders/Injuries	169	0.481	0.369	0.532	0.377	0.512	0.336	0.289
G83.5	Locked-in state	104	Monoplegia, Other Paralytic Syndromes		0.331	0.270	0.345	0.258	0.300	0.164	—
G83.81	Brown-Sequard syndrome	104	Monoplegia, Other Paralytic Syndromes		0.331	0.270	0.345	0.258	0.300	0.164	—
G83.82	Anterior cord syndrome	104	Monoplegia, Other Paralytic Syndromes		0.331	0.270	0.345	0.258	0.300	0.164	—
G83.83	Posterior cord syndrome	104	Monoplegia, Other Paralytic Syndromes		0.331	0.270	0.345	0.258	0.300	0.164	—
G83.84	Todd's paralysis (postepileptic)	104	Monoplegia, Other Paralytic Syndromes		0.331	0.270	0.345	0.258	0.300	0.164	—
G83.89	Other specified paralytic syndromes	104	Monoplegia, Other Paralytic Syndromes		0.331	0.270	0.345	0.258	0.300	0.164	—
G83.9	Paralytic syndrome, unspecified	104	Monoplegia, Other Paralytic Syndromes		0.331	0.270	0.345	0.258	0.300	0.164	—
G90.1	Familial dysautonomia [Riley-Day]	72	Spinal Cord Disorders/Injuries	169	0.481	0.369	0.532	0.377	0.512	0.336	0.289
G90.3	Multi-system degeneration of the autonomic nervous system	78	Parkinson's and Huntington's Diseases		0.606	0.501	0.601	0.443	0.536	0.430	0.159
G91.0	Communicating hydrocephalus	51	Dementia With Complications	52	0.346	0.224	0.453	0.256	0.420	0.257	—
G91.1	Obstructive hydrocephalus	51	Dementia With Complications	52	0.346	0.224	0.453	0.256	0.420	0.257	—
G91.2	(Idiopathic) normal pressure hydrocephalus	51	Dementia With Complications	52	0.346	0.224	0.453	0.256	0.420	0.257	—
G91.3	Post-traumatic hydrocephalus, unspecified	51	Dementia With Complications	52	0.346	0.224	0.453	0.256	0.420	0.257	—
G91.4	Hydrocephalus in diseases classified elsewhere	51	Dementia With Complications	52	0.346	0.224	0.453	0.256	0.420	0.257	—

ICD-10-CM Code	ICD-10-CM Code Description	V24 CMS-HCC	V24 CMS-HCC Disease Group	V24 CMS-HCC Hierarchies	Community, NonDual, Aged	Community, NonDual, Disabled	Community, FBDual, Aged	Community, FBDual, Disabled	Community, PBDual, Aged	Community, PBDual, Disabled	Institutional
G91.8	Other hydrocephalus	51	Dementia With Complications	52	0.346	0.224	0.453	0.256	0.420	0.257	—
G91.9	Hydrocephalus, unspecified	51	Dementia With Complications	52	0.346	0.224	0.453	0.256	0.420	0.257	—
G93.1	Anoxic brain damage, not elsewhere classified	80	Coma, Brain Compression/Anoxic Damage		0.486	0.274	0.511	0.105	0.729	0.134	—
G93.5	Compression of brain	80	Coma, Brain Compression/Anoxic Damage		0.486	0.274	0.511	0.105	0.729	0.134	—
G93.6	Cerebral edema	80	Coma, Brain Compression/Anoxic Damage		0.486	0.274	0.511	0.105	0.729	0.134	—
G93.7	Reye's syndrome	52	Dementia Without Complication		0.346	0.224	0.453	0.256	0.420	0.257	—
G95.0	Syringomyelia and syringobulbia	72	Spinal Cord Disorders/Injuries	169	0.481	0.369	0.532	0.377	0.512	0.336	0.289
G95.11	Acute infarction of spinal cord (embolic) (nonembolic)	72	Spinal Cord Disorders/Injuries	169	0.481	0.369	0.532	0.377	0.512	0.336	0.289
G95.19	Other vascular myelopathies	72	Spinal Cord Disorders/Injuries	169	0.481	0.369	0.532	0.377	0.512	0.336	0.289
G95.20	Unspecified cord compression	72	Spinal Cord Disorders/Injuries	169	0.481	0.369	0.532	0.377	0.512	0.336	0.289
G95.29	Other cord compression	72	Spinal Cord Disorders/Injuries	169	0.481	0.369	0.532	0.377	0.512	0.336	0.289
G95.81	Conus medullaris syndrome	72	Spinal Cord Disorders/Injuries	169	0.481	0.369	0.532	0.377	0.512	0.336	0.289
G95.89	Other specified diseases of spinal cord	72	Spinal Cord Disorders/Injuries	169	0.481	0.369	0.532	0.377	0.512	0.336	0.289
G95.9	Disease of spinal cord, unspecified	72	Spinal Cord Disorders/Injuries	169	0.481	0.369	0.532	0.377	0.512	0.336	0.289
G99.2	Myelopathy in diseases classified elsewhere	72	Spinal Cord Disorders/Injuries	169	0.481	0.369	0.532	0.377	0.512	0.336	0.289
H35.3210	Exudative age-related macular degeneration, right eye, stage unspecified	124	Exudative Macular Degeneration		0.521	0.314	0.298	0.145	0.393	0.158	0.217
H35.3211	Exudative age-related macular degeneration, right eye, with active choroidal neovascularization	124	Exudative Macular Degeneration		0.521	0.314	0.298	0.145	0.393	0.158	0.217
H35.3212	Exudative age-related macular degeneration, right eye, with inactive choroidal neovascularization	124	Exudative Macular Degeneration		0.521	0.314	0.298	0.145	0.393	0.158	0.217
H35.3213	Exudative age-related macular degeneration, right eye, with inactive scar	124	Exudative Macular Degeneration		0.521	0.314	0.298	0.145	0.393	0.158	0.217
H35.3220	Exudative age-related macular degeneration, left eye, stage unspecified	124	Exudative Macular Degeneration		0.521	0.314	0.298	0.145	0.393	0.158	0.217
H35.3221	Exudative age-related macular degeneration, left eye, with active choroidal neovascularization	124	Exudative Macular Degeneration		0.521	0.314	0.298	0.145	0.393	0.158	0.217
H35.3222	Exudative age-related macular degeneration, left eye, with inactive choroidal neovascularization	124	Exudative Macular Degeneration		0.521	0.314	0.298	0.145	0.393	0.158	0.217
H35.3223	Exudative age-related macular degeneration, left eye, with inactive scar	124	Exudative Macular Degeneration		0.521	0.314	0.298	0.145	0.393	0.158	0.217
H35.3230	Exudative age-related macular degeneration, bilateral, stage unspecified	124	Exudative Macular Degeneration		0.521	0.314	0.298	0.145	0.393	0.158	0.217
H35.3231	Exudative age-related macular degeneration, bilateral, with active choroidal neovascularization	124	Exudative Macular Degeneration		0.521	0.314	0.298	0.145	0.393	0.158	0.217
H35.3232	Exudative age-related macular degeneration, bilateral, with inactive choroidal neovascularization	124	Exudative Macular Degeneration		0.521	0.314	0.298	0.145	0.393	0.158	0.217
H35.3233	Exudative age-related macular degeneration, bilateral, with inactive scar	124	Exudative Macular Degeneration		0.521	0.314	0.298	0.145	0.393	0.158	0.217

ICD-10-CM Code	ICD-10-CM Code Description	V24 CMS-HCC	V24 CMS-HCC Disease Group	V24 CMS-HCC Hierarchies	Community, NonDual, Aged	Community, NonDual, Disabled	Community, FBDual, Aged	Community, FBDual, Disabled	Community, PBDual, Aged	Community, PBDual, Disabled	Institutional
H35.3290	Exudative age-related macular degeneration, unspecified eye, stage unspecified	124	Exudative Macular Degeneration		0.521	0.314	0.298	0.145	0.393	0.158	0.217
H35.3291	Exudative age-related macular degeneration, unspecified eye, with active choroidal neovascularization	124	Exudative Macular Degeneration		0.521	0.314	0.298	0.145	0.393	0.158	0.217
H35.3292	Exudative age-related macular degeneration, unspecified eye, with inactive choroidal neovascularization	124	Exudative Macular Degeneration		0.521	0.314	0.298	0.145	0.393	0.158	0.217
H35.3293	Exudative age-related macular degeneration, unspecified eye, with inactive scar	124	Exudative Macular Degeneration		0.521	0.314	0.298	0.145	0.393	0.158	0.217
H43.10	Vitreous hemorrhage, unspecified eye	122	Proliferative Diabetic Retinopathy and Vitreous Hemorrhage		0.222	0.231	0.271	0.269	0.182	0.201	0.394
H43.11	Vitreous hemorrhage, right eye	122	Proliferative Diabetic Retinopathy and Vitreous Hemorrhage		0.222	0.231	0.271	0.269	0.182	0.201	0.394
H43.12	Vitreous hemorrhage, left eye	122	Proliferative Diabetic Retinopathy and Vitreous Hemorrhage		0.222	0.231	0.271	0.269	0.182	0.201	0.394
H43.13	Vitreous hemorrhage, bilateral	122	Proliferative Diabetic Retinopathy and Vitreous Hemorrhage		0.222	0.231	0.271	0.269	0.182	0.201	0.394
H49.811	Kearns-Sayre syndrome, right eye	23	Other Significant Endocrine and Metabolic Disorders		0.194	0.378	0.211	0.299	0.174	0.319	0.379
H49.812	Kearns-Sayre syndrome, left eye	23	Other Significant Endocrine and Metabolic Disorders		0.194	0.378	0.211	0.299	0.174	0.319	0.379
H49.813	Kearns-Sayre syndrome, bilateral	23	Other Significant Endocrine and Metabolic Disorders		0.194	0.378	0.211	0.299	0.174	0.319	0.379
H49.819	Kearns-Sayre syndrome, unspecified eye	23	Other Significant Endocrine and Metabolic Disorders		0.194	0.378	0.211	0.299	0.174	0.319	0.379
I09.81	Rheumatic heart failure	85	Congestive Heart Failure		0.331	0.447	0.371	0.486	0.336	0.422	0.203
I11.0	Hypertensive heart disease with heart failure	85	Congestive Heart Failure		0.331	0.447	0.371	0.486	0.336	0.422	0.203
I12.0	Hypertensive chronic kidney disease with stage 5 chronic kidney disease or end stage renal disease	136	Chronic Kidney Disease, Stage 5	137,138	0.289	0.231	0.260	0.323	0.280	0.261	0.245
I13.0	Hypertensive heart and chronic kidney disease with heart failure and stage 1 through stage 4 chronic kidney disease, or unspecified chronic kidney disease	85	Congestive Heart Failure		0.331	0.447	0.371	0.486	0.336	0.422	0.203
I13.11	Hypertensive heart and chronic kidney disease without heart failure, with stage 5 chronic kidney disease, or end stage renal disease	136	Chronic Kidney Disease, Stage 5	137,138	0.289	0.231	0.260	0.323	0.280	0.261	0.245
I13.2	Hypertensive heart and chronic kidney disease with heart failure and with stage 5 chronic kidney disease, or end stage renal disease	85	Congestive Heart Failure		0.331	0.447	0.371	0.486	0.336	0.422	0.203
I13.2	Hypertensive heart and chronic kidney disease with heart failure and with stage 5 chronic kidney disease, or end stage renal disease	136	Chronic Kidney Disease, Stage 5	137,138	0.289	0.231	0.260	0.323	0.280	0.261	0.245
I20.0	Unstable angina	87	Unstable Angina and Other Acute Ischemic Heart Disease	88	0.195	0.264	0.302	0.425	0.276	0.379	0.366
I20.1	Angina pectoris with documented spasm	88	Angina Pectoris		0.135	0.111	0.034	0.152	0.149	0.149	0.366
I20.8	Other forms of angina pectoris	88	Angina Pectoris		0.135	0.111	0.034	0.152	0.149	0.149	0.366
I20.9	Angina pectoris, unspecified	88	Angina Pectoris		0.135	0.111	0.034	0.152	0.149	0.149	0.366
I21.01	ST elevation (STEMI) myocardial infarction involving left main coronary artery	86	Acute Myocardial Infarction	87,88	0.195	0.264	0.377	0.425	0.293	0.379	0.366

ICD-10-CM Code	ICD-10-CM Code Description	V24 CMS-HCC	V24 CMS-HCC Disease Group	V24 CMS-HCC Hierarchies	Community, NonDual, Aged	Community, NonDual, Disabled	Community, FBDual, Aged	Community, FBDual, Disabled	Community, PBDual, Aged	Community, PBDual, Disabled	Institutional
I21.02	ST elevation (STEMI) myocardial infarction involving left anterior descending coronary artery	86	Acute Myocardial Infarction	87,88	0.195	0.264	0.377	0.425	0.293	0.379	0.366
I21.09	ST elevation (STEMI) myocardial infarction involving other coronary artery of anterior wall	86	Acute Myocardial Infarction	87,88	0.195	0.264	0.377	0.425	0.293	0.379	0.366
I21.11	ST elevation (STEMI) myocardial infarction involving right coronary artery	86	Acute Myocardial Infarction	87,88	0.195	0.264	0.377	0.425	0.293	0.379	0.366
I21.19	ST elevation (STEMI) myocardial infarction involving other coronary artery of inferior wall	86	Acute Myocardial Infarction	87,88	0.195	0.264	0.377	0.425	0.293	0.379	0.366
I21.21	ST elevation (STEMI) myocardial infarction involving left circumflex coronary artery	86	Acute Myocardial Infarction	87,88	0.195	0.264	0.377	0.425	0.293	0.379	0.366
I21.29	ST elevation (STEMI) myocardial infarction involving other sites	86	Acute Myocardial Infarction	87,88	0.195	0.264	0.377	0.425	0.293	0.379	0.366
I21.3	ST elevation (STEMI) myocardial infarction of unspecified site	86	Acute Myocardial Infarction	87,88	0.195	0.264	0.377	0.425	0.293	0.379	0.366
I21.4	Non-ST elevation (NSTEMI) myocardial infarction	86	Acute Myocardial Infarction	87,88	0.195	0.264	0.377	0.425	0.293	0.379	0.366
I21.9	Acute myocardial infarction, unspecified	86	Acute Myocardial Infarction	87,88	0.195	0.264	0.377	0.425	0.293	0.379	0.366
I21.A1	Myocardial infarction type 2	86	Acute Myocardial Infarction	87,88	0.195	0.264	0.377	0.425	0.293	0.379	0.366
I21.A9	Other myocardial infarction type	86	Acute Myocardial Infarction	87,88	0.195	0.264	0.377	0.425	0.293	0.379	0.366
I22.0	Subsequent ST elevation (STEMI) myocardial infarction of anterior wall	86	Acute Myocardial Infarction	87,88	0.195	0.264	0.377	0.425	0.293	0.379	0.366
I22.1	Subsequent ST elevation (STEMI) myocardial infarction of inferior wall	86	Acute Myocardial Infarction	87,88	0.195	0.264	0.377	0.425	0.293	0.379	0.366
I22.2	Subsequent non-ST elevation (NSTEMI) myocardial infarction	86	Acute Myocardial Infarction	87,88	0.195	0.264	0.377	0.425	0.293	0.379	0.366
I22.8	Subsequent ST elevation (STEMI) myocardial infarction of other sites	86	Acute Myocardial Infarction	87,88	0.195	0.264	0.377	0.425	0.293	0.379	0.366
I22.9	Subsequent ST elevation (STEMI) myocardial infarction of unspecified site	86	Acute Myocardial Infarction	87,88	0.195	0.264	0.377	0.425	0.293	0.379	0.366
I23.0	Hemopericardium as current complication following acute myocardial infarction	87	Unstable Angina and Other Acute Ischemic Heart Disease	88	0.195	0.264	0.302	0.425	0.276	0.379	0.366
I23.1	Atrial septal defect as current complication following acute myocardial infarction	87	Unstable Angina and Other Acute Ischemic Heart Disease	88	0.195	0.264	0.302	0.425	0.276	0.379	0.366
I23.2	Ventricular septal defect as current complication following acute myocardial infarction	87	Unstable Angina and Other Acute Ischemic Heart Disease	88	0.195	0.264	0.302	0.425	0.276	0.379	0.366
I23.3	Rupture of cardiac wall without hemopericardium as current complication following acute myocardial infarction	87	Unstable Angina and Other Acute Ischemic Heart Disease	88	0.195	0.264	0.302	0.425	0.276	0.379	0.366
I23.4	Rupture of chordae tendineae as current complication following acute myocardial infarction	86	Acute Myocardial Infarction	87,88	0.195	0.264	0.377	0.425	0.293	0.379	0.366
I23.5	Rupture of papillary muscle as current complication following acute myocardial infarction	86	Acute Myocardial Infarction	87,88	0.195	0.264	0.377	0.425	0.293	0.379	0.366
I23.6	Thrombosis of atrium, auricular appendage, and ventricle as current complications following acute myocardial infarction	87	Unstable Angina and Other Acute Ischemic Heart Disease	88	0.195	0.264	0.302	0.425	0.276	0.379	0.366

ICD-10-CM Code	ICD-10-CM Code Description	V24 CMS-HCC	V24 CMS-HCC Disease Group	V24 CMS-HCC Hierarchies	Community, NonDual, Aged	Community, NonDual, Disabled	Community, FBDual, Aged	Community, FBDual, Disabled	Community, PBDual, Aged	Community, PBDual, Disabled	Institutional
I23.7	Postinfarction angina	87	Unstable Angina and Other Acute Ischemic Heart Disease	88	0.195	0.264	0.302	0.425	0.276	0.379	0.366
I23.8	Other current complications following acute myocardial infarction	87	Unstable Angina and Other Acute Ischemic Heart Disease	88	0.195	0.264	0.302	0.425	0.276	0.379	0.366
I24.0	Acute coronary thrombosis not resulting in myocardial infarction	87	Unstable Angina and Other Acute Ischemic Heart Disease	88	0.195	0.264	0.302	0.425	0.276	0.379	0.366
I24.1	Dressler's syndrome	87	Unstable Angina and Other Acute Ischemic Heart Disease	88	0.195	0.264	0.302	0.425	0.276	0.379	0.366
I24.8	Other forms of acute ischemic heart disease	87	Unstable Angina and Other Acute Ischemic Heart Disease	88	0.195	0.264	0.302	0.425	0.276	0.379	0.366
I24.9	Acute ischemic heart disease, unspecified	87	Unstable Angina and Other Acute Ischemic Heart Disease	88	0.195	0.264	0.302	0.425	0.276	0.379	0.366
I25.110	Atherosclerotic heart disease of native coronary artery with unstable angina pectoris	87	Unstable Angina and Other Acute Ischemic Heart Disease	88	0.195	0.264	0.302	0.425	0.276	0.379	0.366
I25.111	Atherosclerotic heart disease of native coronary artery with angina pectoris with documented spasm	88	Angina Pectoris		0.135	0.111	0.034	0.152	0.149	0.149	0.366
I25.118	Atherosclerotic heart disease of native coronary artery with other forms of angina pectoris	88	Angina Pectoris		0.135	0.111	0.034	0.152	0.149	0.149	0.366
I25.119	Atherosclerotic heart disease of native coronary artery with unspecified angina pectoris	88	Angina Pectoris		0.135	0.111	0.034	0.152	0.149	0.149	0.366
I25.700	Atherosclerosis of coronary artery bypass graft(s), unspecified, with unstable angina pectoris	87	Unstable Angina and Other Acute Ischemic Heart Disease	88	0.195	0.264	0.302	0.425	0.276	0.379	0.366
I25.701	Atherosclerosis of coronary artery bypass graft(s), unspecified, with angina pectoris with documented spasm	88	Angina Pectoris		0.135	0.111	0.034	0.152	0.149	0.149	0.366
I25.708	Atherosclerosis of coronary artery bypass graft(s), unspecified, with other forms of angina pectoris	88	Angina Pectoris		0.135	0.111	0.034	0.152	0.149	0.149	0.366
I25.709	Atherosclerosis of coronary artery bypass graft(s), unspecified, with unspecified angina pectoris	88	Angina Pectoris		0.135	0.111	0.034	0.152	0.149	0.149	0.366
I25.710	Atherosclerosis of autologous vein coronary artery bypass graft(s) with unstable angina pectoris	87	Unstable Angina and Other Acute Ischemic Heart Disease	88	0.195	0.264	0.302	0.425	0.276	0.379	0.366
I25.711	Atherosclerosis of autologous vein coronary artery bypass graft(s) with angina pectoris with documented spasm	88	Angina Pectoris		0.135	0.111	0.034	0.152	0.149	0.149	0.366
I25.718	Atherosclerosis of autologous vein coronary artery bypass graft(s) with other forms of angina pectoris	88	Angina Pectoris		0.135	0.111	0.034	0.152	0.149	0.149	0.366
I25.719	Atherosclerosis of autologous vein coronary artery bypass graft(s) with unspecified angina pectoris	88	Angina Pectoris		0.135	0.111	0.034	0.152	0.149	0.149	0.366
I25.720	Atherosclerosis of autologous artery coronary artery bypass graft(s) with unstable angina pectoris	87	Unstable Angina and Other Acute Ischemic Heart Disease	88	0.195	0.264	0.302	0.425	0.276	0.379	0.366
I25.721	Atherosclerosis of autologous artery coronary artery bypass graft(s) with angina pectoris with documented spasm	88	Angina Pectoris		0.135	0.111	0.034	0.152	0.149	0.149	0.366
I25.728	Atherosclerosis of autologous artery coronary artery bypass graft(s) with other forms of angina pectoris	88	Angina Pectoris		0.135	0.111	0.034	0.152	0.149	0.149	0.366

ICD-10-CM Code	ICD-10-CM Code Description	V24 CMS-HCC	V24 CMS-HCC Disease Group	V24 CMS-HCC Hierarchies	Community, NonDual, Aged	Community, NonDual, Disabled	Community, FBDual, Aged	Community, FBDual, Disabled	Community, PBDual, Aged	Community, PBDual, Disabled	Institutional
I25.729	Atherosclerosis of autologous artery coronary artery bypass graft(s) with unspecified angina pectoris	88	Angina Pectoris		0.135	0.111	0.034	0.152	0.149	0.149	0.366
I25.730	Atherosclerosis of nonautologous biological coronary artery bypass graft(s) with unstable angina pectoris	87	Unstable Angina and Other Acute Ischemic Heart Disease	88	0.195	0.264	0.302	0.425	0.276	0.379	0.366
I25.731	Atherosclerosis of nonautologous biological coronary artery bypass graft(s) with angina pectoris with documented spasm	88	Angina Pectoris		0.135	0.111	0.034	0.152	0.149	0.149	0.366
I25.738	Atherosclerosis of nonautologous biological coronary artery bypass graft(s) with other forms of angina pectoris	88	Angina Pectoris		0.135	0.111	0.034	0.152	0.149	0.149	0.366
I25.739	Atherosclerosis of nonautologous biological coronary artery bypass graft(s) with unspecified angina pectoris	88	Angina Pectoris		0.135	0.111	0.034	0.152	0.149	0.149	0.366
I25.750	Atherosclerosis of native coronary artery of transplanted heart with unstable angina	87	Unstable Angina and Other Acute Ischemic Heart Disease	88	0.195	0.264	0.302	0.425	0.276	0.379	0.366
I25.751	Atherosclerosis of native coronary artery of transplanted heart with angina pectoris with documented spasm	88	Angina Pectoris		0.135	0.111	0.034	0.152	0.149	0.149	0.366
I25.758	Atherosclerosis of native coronary artery of transplanted heart with other forms of angina pectoris	88	Angina Pectoris		0.135	0.111	0.034	0.152	0.149	0.149	0.366
I25.759	Atherosclerosis of native coronary artery of transplanted heart with unspecified angina pectoris	88	Angina Pectoris		0.135	0.111	0.034	0.152	0.149	0.149	0.366
I25.760	Atherosclerosis of bypass graft of coronary artery of transplanted heart with unstable angina	87	Unstable Angina and Other Acute Ischemic Heart Disease	88	0.195	0.264	0.302	0.425	0.276	0.379	0.366
I25.761	Atherosclerosis of bypass graft of coronary artery of transplanted heart with angina pectoris with documented spasm	88	Angina Pectoris		0.135	0.111	0.034	0.152	0.149	0.149	0.366
I25.768	Atherosclerosis of bypass graft of coronary artery of transplanted heart with other forms of angina pectoris	88	Angina Pectoris		0.135	0.111	0.034	0.152	0.149	0.149	0.366
I25.769	Atherosclerosis of bypass graft of coronary artery of transplanted heart with unspecified angina pectoris	88	Angina Pectoris		0.135	0.111	0.034	0.152	0.149	0.149	0.366
I25.790	Atherosclerosis of other coronary artery bypass graft(s) with unstable angina pectoris	87	Unstable Angina and Other Acute Ischemic Heart Disease	88	0.195	0.264	0.302	0.425	0.276	0.379	0.366
I25.791	Atherosclerosis of other coronary artery bypass graft(s) with angina pectoris with documented spasm	88	Angina Pectoris		0.135	0.111	0.034	0.152	0.149	0.149	0.366
I25.798	Atherosclerosis of other coronary artery bypass graft(s) with other forms of angina pectoris	88	Angina Pectoris		0.135	0.111	0.034	0.152	0.149	0.149	0.366
I25.799	Atherosclerosis of other coronary artery bypass graft(s) with unspecified angina pectoris	88	Angina Pectoris		0.135	0.111	0.034	0.152	0.149	0.149	0.366
I26.01	Septic pulmonary embolism with acute cor pulmonale	85	Congestive Heart Failure		0.331	0.447	0.371	0.486	0.336	0.422	0.203
I26.01	Septic pulmonary embolism with acute cor pulmonale	107	Vascular Disease with Complications	108	0.383	0.464	0.565	0.653	0.463	0.450	0.299
I26.02	Saddle embolus of pulmonary artery with acute cor pulmonale	85	Congestive Heart Failure		0.331	0.447	0.371	0.486	0.336	0.422	0.203

ICD-10-CM Code	ICD-10-CM Code Description	V24 CMS-HCC	V24 CMS-HCC Disease Group	V24 CMS-HCC Hierarchies	Community, NonDual, Aged	Community, NonDual, Disabled	Community, FBDual, Aged	Community, FBDual, Disabled	Community, PBDual, Aged	Community, PBDual, Disabled	Institutional
I26.02	Saddle embolus of pulmonary artery with acute cor pulmonale	107	Vascular Disease with Complications	108	0.383	0.464	0.565	0.653	0.463	0.450	0.299
I26.09	Other pulmonary embolism with acute cor pulmonale	85	Congestive Heart Failure		0.331	0.447	0.371	0.486	0.336	0.422	0.203
I26.09	Other pulmonary embolism with acute cor pulmonale	107	Vascular Disease with Complications	108	0.383	0.464	0.565	0.653	0.463	0.450	0.299
I26.90	Septic pulmonary embolism without acute cor pulmonale	107	Vascular Disease with Complications	108	0.383	0.464	0.565	0.653	0.463	0.450	0.299
I26.92	Saddle embolus of pulmonary artery without acute cor pulmonale	107	Vascular Disease with Complications	108	0.383	0.464	0.565	0.653	0.463	0.450	0.299
I26.93	Single subsegmental pulmonary embolism without acute cor pulmonale	107	Vascular Disease with Complications	108	0.383	0.464	0.565	0.653	0.463	0.450	0.299
I26.94	Multiple subsegmental pulmonary emboli without acute cor pulmonale	107	Vascular Disease with Complications	108	0.383	0.464	0.565	0.653	0.463	0.450	0.299
I26.99	Other pulmonary embolism without acute cor pulmonale	107	Vascular Disease with Complications	108	0.383	0.464	0.565	0.653	0.463	0.450	0.299
I27.0	Primary pulmonary hypertension	85	Congestive Heart Failure		0.331	0.447	0.371	0.486	0.336	0.422	0.203
I27.1	Kyphoscoliotic heart disease	85	Congestive Heart Failure		0.331	0.447	0.371	0.486	0.336	0.422	0.203
I27.20	Pulmonary hypertension, unspecified	85	Congestive Heart Failure		0.331	0.447	0.371	0.486	0.336	0.422	0.203
I27.21	Secondary pulmonary arterial hypertension	85	Congestive Heart Failure		0.331	0.447	0.371	0.486	0.336	0.422	0.203
I27.22	Pulmonary hypertension due to left heart disease	85	Congestive Heart Failure		0.331	0.447	0.371	0.486	0.336	0.422	0.203
I27.23	Pulmonary hypertension due to lung diseases and hypoxia	85	Congestive Heart Failure		0.331	0.447	0.371	0.486	0.336	0.422	0.203
I27.24	Chronic thromboembolic pulmonary hypertension	85	Congestive Heart Failure		0.331	0.447	0.371	0.486	0.336	0.422	0.203
I27.29	Other secondary pulmonary hypertension	85	Congestive Heart Failure		0.331	0.447	0.371	0.486	0.336	0.422	0.203
I27.81	Cor pulmonale (chronic)	85	Congestive Heart Failure		0.331	0.447	0.371	0.486	0.336	0.422	0.203
I27.82	Chronic pulmonary embolism	107	Vascular Disease with Complications	108	0.383	0.464	0.565	0.653	0.463	0.450	0.299
I27.83	Eisenmenger's syndrome	85	Congestive Heart Failure		0.331	0.447	0.371	0.486	0.336	0.422	0.203
I27.89	Other specified pulmonary heart diseases	85	Congestive Heart Failure		0.331	0.447	0.371	0.486	0.336	0.422	0.203
I27.9	Pulmonary heart disease, unspecified	85	Congestive Heart Failure		0.331	0.447	0.371	0.486	0.336	0.422	0.203
I28.0	Arteriovenous fistula of pulmonary vessels	85	Congestive Heart Failure		0.331	0.447	0.371	0.486	0.336	0.422	0.203
I28.1	Aneurysm of pulmonary artery	85	Congestive Heart Failure		0.331	0.447	0.371	0.486	0.336	0.422	0.203
I28.8	Other diseases of pulmonary vessels	85	Congestive Heart Failure		0.331	0.447	0.371	0.486	0.336	0.422	0.203
I28.9	Disease of pulmonary vessels, unspecified	85	Congestive Heart Failure		0.331	0.447	0.371	0.486	0.336	0.422	0.203
I42.0	Dilated cardiomyopathy	85	Congestive Heart Failure		0.331	0.447	0.371	0.486	0.336	0.422	0.203
I42.1	Obstructive hypertrophic cardiomyopathy	85	Congestive Heart Failure		0.331	0.447	0.371	0.486	0.336	0.422	0.203
I42.2	Other hypertrophic cardiomyopathy	85	Congestive Heart Failure		0.331	0.447	0.371	0.486	0.336	0.422	0.203
I42.3	Endomyocardial (eosinophilic) disease	85	Congestive Heart Failure		0.331	0.447	0.371	0.486	0.336	0.422	0.203
I42.4	Endocardial fibroelastosis	85	Congestive Heart Failure		0.331	0.447	0.371	0.486	0.336	0.422	0.203
I42.5	Other restrictive cardiomyopathy	85	Congestive Heart Failure		0.331	0.447	0.371	0.486	0.336	0.422	0.203
I42.6	Alcoholic cardiomyopathy	85	Congestive Heart Failure		0.331	0.447	0.371	0.486	0.336	0.422	0.203
I42.7	Cardiomyopathy due to drug and external agent	85	Congestive Heart Failure		0.331	0.447	0.371	0.486	0.336	0.422	0.203
I42.8	Other cardiomyopathies	85	Congestive Heart Failure		0.331	0.447	0.371	0.486	0.336	0.422	0.203
I42.9	Cardiomyopathy, unspecified	85	Congestive Heart Failure		0.331	0.447	0.371	0.486	0.336	0.422	0.203

ICD-10-CM Code	ICD-10-CM Code Description	V24 CMS-HCC	V24 CMS-HCC Disease Group	V24 CMS-HCC Hierarchies	Community, NonDual, Aged	Community, NonDual, Disabled	Community, FBDual, Aged	Community, FBDual, Disabled	Community, PBDual, Aged	Community, PBDual, Disabled	Institutional
I43	Cardiomyopathy in diseases classified elsewhere	85	Congestive Heart Failure		0.331	0.447	0.371	0.486	0.336	0.422	0.203
I44.2	Atrioventricular block, complete	96	Specified Heart Arrhythmias		0.268	0.262	0.384	0.308	0.264	0.281	0.252
I46.2	Cardiac arrest due to underlying cardiac condition	84	Cardio-Respiratory Failure and Shock		0.282	0.385	0.492	0.531	0.361	0.343	0.313
I46.8	Cardiac arrest due to other underlying condition	84	Cardio-Respiratory Failure and Shock		0.282	0.385	0.492	0.531	0.361	0.343	0.313
I46.9	Cardiac arrest, cause unspecified	84	Cardio-Respiratory Failure and Shock		0.282	0.385	0.492	0.531	0.361	0.343	0.313
I47.0	Re-entry ventricular arrhythmia	96	Specified Heart Arrhythmias		0.268	0.262	0.384	0.308	0.264	0.281	0.252
I47.1	Supraventricular tachycardia	96	Specified Heart Arrhythmias		0.268	0.262	0.384	0.308	0.264	0.281	0.252
I47.2	Ventricular tachycardia	96	Specified Heart Arrhythmias		0.268	0.262	0.384	0.308	0.264	0.281	0.252
I47.9	Paroxysmal tachycardia, unspecified	96	Specified Heart Arrhythmias		0.268	0.262	0.384	0.308	0.264	0.281	0.252
I48.0	Paroxysmal atrial fibrillation	96	Specified Heart Arrhythmias		0.268	0.262	0.384	0.308	0.264	0.281	0.252
I48.11	Longstanding persistent atrial fibrillation	96	Specified Heart Arrhythmias		0.268	0.262	0.384	0.308	0.264	0.281	0.252
I48.19	Other persistent atrial fibrillation	96	Specified Heart Arrhythmias		0.268	0.262	0.384	0.308	0.264	0.281	0.252
I48.20	Chronic atrial fibrillation, unspecified	96	Specified Heart Arrhythmias		0.268	0.262	0.384	0.308	0.264	0.281	0.252
I48.21	Permanent atrial fibrillation	96	Specified Heart Arrhythmias		0.268	0.262	0.384	0.308	0.264	0.281	0.252
I48.3	Typical atrial flutter	96	Specified Heart Arrhythmias		0.268	0.262	0.384	0.308	0.264	0.281	0.252
I48.4	Atypical atrial flutter	96	Specified Heart Arrhythmias		0.268	0.262	0.384	0.308	0.264	0.281	0.252
I48.91	Unspecified atrial fibrillation	96	Specified Heart Arrhythmias		0.268	0.262	0.384	0.308	0.264	0.281	0.252
I48.92	Unspecified atrial flutter	96	Specified Heart Arrhythmias		0.268	0.262	0.384	0.308	0.264	0.281	0.252
I49.01	Ventricular fibrillation	84	Cardio-Respiratory Failure and Shock		0.282	0.385	0.492	0.531	0.361	0.343	0.313
I49.02	Ventricular flutter	84	Cardio-Respiratory Failure and Shock		0.282	0.385	0.492	0.531	0.361	0.343	0.313
I49.2	Junctional premature depolarization	96	Specified Heart Arrhythmias		0.268	0.262	0.384	0.308	0.264	0.281	0.252
I49.5	Sick sinus syndrome	96	Specified Heart Arrhythmias		0.268	0.262	0.384	0.308	0.264	0.281	0.252
I50.1	Left ventricular failure, unspecified	85	Congestive Heart Failure		0.331	0.447	0.371	0.486	0.336	0.422	0.203
I50.20	Unspecified systolic (congestive) heart failure	85	Congestive Heart Failure		0.331	0.447	0.371	0.486	0.336	0.422	0.203
I50.21	Acute systolic (congestive) heart failure	85	Congestive Heart Failure		0.331	0.447	0.371	0.486	0.336	0.422	0.203
I50.22	Chronic systolic (congestive) heart failure	85	Congestive Heart Failure		0.331	0.447	0.371	0.486	0.336	0.422	0.203
I50.23	Acute on chronic systolic (congestive) heart failure	85	Congestive Heart Failure		0.331	0.447	0.371	0.486	0.336	0.422	0.203
I50.30	Unspecified diastolic (congestive) heart failure	85	Congestive Heart Failure		0.331	0.447	0.371	0.486	0.336	0.422	0.203
I50.31	Acute diastolic (congestive) heart failure	85	Congestive Heart Failure		0.331	0.447	0.371	0.486	0.336	0.422	0.203
I50.32	Chronic diastolic (congestive) heart failure	85	Congestive Heart Failure		0.331	0.447	0.371	0.486	0.336	0.422	0.203
I50.33	Acute on chronic diastolic (congestive) heart failure	85	Congestive Heart Failure		0.331	0.447	0.371	0.486	0.336	0.422	0.203
I50.40	Unspecified combined systolic (congestive) and diastolic (congestive) heart failure	85	Congestive Heart Failure		0.331	0.447	0.371	0.486	0.336	0.422	0.203
I50.41	Acute combined systolic (congestive) and diastolic (congestive) heart failure	85	Congestive Heart Failure		0.331	0.447	0.371	0.486	0.336	0.422	0.203
I50.42	Chronic combined systolic (congestive) and diastolic (congestive) heart failure	85	Congestive Heart Failure		0.331	0.447	0.371	0.486	0.336	0.422	0.203
I50.43	Acute on chronic combined systolic (congestive) and diastolic (congestive) heart failure	85	Congestive Heart Failure		0.331	0.447	0.371	0.486	0.336	0.422	0.203
I50.810	Right heart failure, unspecified	85	Congestive Heart Failure		0.331	0.447	0.371	0.486	0.336	0.422	0.203

ICD-10-CM Code	ICD-10-CM Code Description	V24 CMS-HCC	V24 CMS-HCC Disease Group	V24 CMS-HCC Hierarchies	Community, NonDual, Aged	Community, NonDual, Disabled	Community, FBDual, Aged	Community, FBDual, Disabled	Community, PBDual, Aged	Community, PBDual, Disabled	Institutional
I50.811	Acute right heart failure	85	Congestive Heart Failure		0.331	0.447	0.371	0.486	0.336	0.422	0.203
I50.812	Chronic right heart failure	85	Congestive Heart Failure		0.331	0.447	0.371	0.486	0.336	0.422	0.203
I50.813	Acute on chronic right heart failure	85	Congestive Heart Failure		0.331	0.447	0.371	0.486	0.336	0.422	0.203
I50.814	Right heart failure due to left heart failure	85	Congestive Heart Failure		0.331	0.447	0.371	0.486	0.336	0.422	0.203
I50.82	Biventricular heart failure	85	Congestive Heart Failure		0.331	0.447	0.371	0.486	0.336	0.422	0.203
I50.83	High output heart failure	85	Congestive Heart Failure		0.331	0.447	0.371	0.486	0.336	0.422	0.203
I50.84	End stage heart failure	85	Congestive Heart Failure		0.331	0.447	0.371	0.486	0.336	0.422	0.203
I50.89	Other heart failure	85	Congestive Heart Failure		0.331	0.447	0.371	0.486	0.336	0.422	0.203
I50.9	Heart failure, unspecified	85	Congestive Heart Failure		0.331	0.447	0.371	0.486	0.336	0.422	0.203
I51.1	Rupture of chordae tendineae, not elsewhere classified	86	Acute Myocardial Infarction	87,88	0.195	0.264	0.377	0.425	0.293	0.379	0.366
I51.2	Rupture of papillary muscle, not elsewhere classified	86	Acute Myocardial Infarction	87,88	0.195	0.264	0.377	0.425	0.293	0.379	0.366
I51.4	Myocarditis, unspecified	85	Congestive Heart Failure		0.331	0.447	0.371	0.486	0.336	0.422	0.203
I51.5	Myocardial degeneration	85	Congestive Heart Failure		0.331	0.447	0.371	0.486	0.336	0.422	0.203
I60.00	Nontraumatic subarachnoid hemorrhage from unspecified carotid siphon and bifurcation	99	Intracranial Hemorrhage	100	0.230	0.170	0.380	0.486	0.230	0.163	0.111
I60.01	Nontraumatic subarachnoid hemorrhage from right carotid siphon and bifurcation	99	Intracranial Hemorrhage	100	0.230	0.170	0.380	0.486	0.230	0.163	0.111
I60.02	Nontraumatic subarachnoid hemorrhage from left carotid siphon and bifurcation	99	Intracranial Hemorrhage	100	0.230	0.170	0.380	0.486	0.230	0.163	0.111
I60.10	Nontraumatic subarachnoid hemorrhage from unspecified middle cerebral artery	99	Intracranial Hemorrhage	100	0.230	0.170	0.380	0.486	0.230	0.163	0.111
I60.11	Nontraumatic subarachnoid hemorrhage from right middle cerebral artery	99	Intracranial Hemorrhage	100	0.230	0.170	0.380	0.486	0.230	0.163	0.111
I60.12	Nontraumatic subarachnoid hemorrhage from left middle cerebral artery	99	Intracranial Hemorrhage	100	0.230	0.170	0.380	0.486	0.230	0.163	0.111
I60.2	Nontraumatic subarachnoid hemorrhage from anterior communicating artery	99	Intracranial Hemorrhage	100	0.230	0.170	0.380	0.486	0.230	0.163	0.111
I60.30	Nontraumatic subarachnoid hemorrhage from unspecified posterior communicating artery	99	Intracranial Hemorrhage	100	0.230	0.170	0.380	0.486	0.230	0.163	0.111
I60.31	Nontraumatic subarachnoid hemorrhage from right posterior communicating artery	99	Intracranial Hemorrhage	100	0.230	0.170	0.380	0.486	0.230	0.163	0.111
I60.32	Nontraumatic subarachnoid hemorrhage from left posterior communicating artery	99	Intracranial Hemorrhage	100	0.230	0.170	0.380	0.486	0.230	0.163	0.111
I60.4	Nontraumatic subarachnoid hemorrhage from basilar artery	99	Intracranial Hemorrhage	100	0.230	0.170	0.380	0.486	0.230	0.163	0.111
I60.50	Nontraumatic subarachnoid hemorrhage from unspecified vertebral artery	99	Intracranial Hemorrhage	100	0.230	0.170	0.380	0.486	0.230	0.163	0.111
I60.51	Nontraumatic subarachnoid hemorrhage from right vertebral artery	99	Intracranial Hemorrhage	100	0.230	0.170	0.380	0.486	0.230	0.163	0.111
I60.52	Nontraumatic subarachnoid hemorrhage from left vertebral artery	99	Intracranial Hemorrhage	100	0.230	0.170	0.380	0.486	0.230	0.163	0.111
I60.6	Nontraumatic subarachnoid hemorrhage from other intracranial arteries	99	Intracranial Hemorrhage	100	0.230	0.170	0.380	0.486	0.230	0.163	0.111

ICD-10-CM Code	ICD-10-CM Code Description	V24 CMS-HCC	V24 CMS-HCC Disease Group	V24 CMS-HCC Hierarchies	Community, NonDual, Aged	Community, NonDual, Disabled	Community, FBDual, Aged	Community, FBDual, Disabled	Community, PBDual, Aged	Community, PBDual, Disabled	Institutional
I60.7	Nontraumatic subarachnoid hemorrhage from unspecified intracranial artery	99	Intracranial Hemorrhage	100	0.230	0.170	0.380	0.486	0.230	0.163	0.111
I60.8	Other nontraumatic subarachnoid hemorrhage	99	Intracranial Hemorrhage	100	0.230	0.170	0.380	0.486	0.230	0.163	0.111
I60.9	Nontraumatic subarachnoid hemorrhage, unspecified	99	Intracranial Hemorrhage	100	0.230	0.170	0.380	0.486	0.230	0.163	0.111
I61.0	Nontraumatic intracerebral hemorrhage in hemisphere, subcortical	99	Intracranial Hemorrhage	100	0.230	0.170	0.380	0.486	0.230	0.163	0.111
I61.1	Nontraumatic intracerebral hemorrhage in hemisphere, cortical	99	Intracranial Hemorrhage	100	0.230	0.170	0.380	0.486	0.230	0.163	0.111
I61.2	Nontraumatic intracerebral hemorrhage in hemisphere, unspecified	99	Intracranial Hemorrhage	100	0.230	0.170	0.380	0.486	0.230	0.163	0.111
I61.3	Nontraumatic intracerebral hemorrhage in brain stem	99	Intracranial Hemorrhage	100	0.230	0.170	0.380	0.486	0.230	0.163	0.111
I61.4	Nontraumatic intracerebral hemorrhage in cerebellum	99	Intracranial Hemorrhage	100	0.230	0.170	0.380	0.486	0.230	0.163	0.111
I61.5	Nontraumatic intracerebral hemorrhage, intraventricular	99	Intracranial Hemorrhage	100	0.230	0.170	0.380	0.486	0.230	0.163	0.111
I61.6	Nontraumatic intracerebral hemorrhage, multiple localized	99	Intracranial Hemorrhage	100	0.230	0.170	0.380	0.486	0.230	0.163	0.111
I61.8	Other nontraumatic intracerebral hemorrhage	99	Intracranial Hemorrhage	100	0.230	0.170	0.380	0.486	0.230	0.163	0.111
I61.9	Nontraumatic intracerebral hemorrhage, unspecified	99	Intracranial Hemorrhage	100	0.230	0.170	0.380	0.486	0.230	0.163	0.111
I62.00	Nontraumatic subdural hemorrhage, unspecified	99	Intracranial Hemorrhage	100	0.230	0.170	0.380	0.486	0.230	0.163	0.111
I62.01	Nontraumatic acute subdural hemorrhage	99	Intracranial Hemorrhage	100	0.230	0.170	0.380	0.486	0.230	0.163	0.111
I62.02	Nontraumatic subacute subdural hemorrhage	99	Intracranial Hemorrhage	100	0.230	0.170	0.380	0.486	0.230	0.163	0.111
I62.03	Nontraumatic chronic subdural hemorrhage	99	Intracranial Hemorrhage	100	0.230	0.170	0.380	0.486	0.230	0.163	0.111
I62.1	Nontraumatic extradural hemorrhage	99	Intracranial Hemorrhage	100	0.230	0.170	0.380	0.486	0.230	0.163	0.111
I62.9	Nontraumatic intracranial hemorrhage, unspecified	99	Intracranial Hemorrhage	100	0.230	0.170	0.380	0.486	0.230	0.163	0.111
I63.00	Cerebral infarction due to thrombosis of unspecified precerebral artery	100	Ischemic or Unspecified Stroke		0.230	0.146	0.380	0.324	0.230	0.163	0.111
I63.011	Cerebral infarction due to thrombosis of right vertebral artery	100	Ischemic or Unspecified Stroke		0.230	0.146	0.380	0.324	0.230	0.163	0.111
I63.012	Cerebral infarction due to thrombosis of left vertebral artery	100	Ischemic or Unspecified Stroke		0.230	0.146	0.380	0.324	0.230	0.163	0.111
I63.013	Cerebral infarction due to thrombosis of bilateral vertebral arteries	100	Ischemic or Unspecified Stroke		0.230	0.146	0.380	0.324	0.230	0.163	0.111
I63.019	Cerebral infarction due to thrombosis of unspecified vertebral artery	100	Ischemic or Unspecified Stroke		0.230	0.146	0.380	0.324	0.230	0.163	0.111
I63.02	Cerebral infarction due to thrombosis of basilar artery	100	Ischemic or Unspecified Stroke		0.230	0.146	0.380	0.324	0.230	0.163	0.111
I63.031	Cerebral infarction due to thrombosis of right carotid artery	100	Ischemic or Unspecified Stroke		0.230	0.146	0.380	0.324	0.230	0.163	0.111
I63.032	Cerebral infarction due to thrombosis of left carotid artery	100	Ischemic or Unspecified Stroke		0.230	0.146	0.380	0.324	0.230	0.163	0.111
I63.033	Cerebral infarction due to thrombosis of bilateral carotid arteries	100	Ischemic or Unspecified Stroke		0.230	0.146	0.380	0.324	0.230	0.163	0.111
I63.039	Cerebral infarction due to thrombosis of unspecified carotid artery	100	Ischemic or Unspecified Stroke		0.230	0.146	0.380	0.324	0.230	0.163	0.111

ICD-10-CM Code	ICD-10-CM Code Description	V24 CMS-HCC	V24 CMS-HCC Disease Group	V24 CMS-HCC Hierarchies	Community, NonDual, Aged	Community, NonDual, Disabled	Community, FBDual, Aged	Community, FBDual, Disabled	Community, PBDual, Aged	Community, PBDual, Disabled	Institutional
I63.09	Cerebral infarction due to thrombosis of other precerebral artery	100	Ischemic or Unspecified Stroke		0.230	0.146	0.380	0.324	0.230	0.163	0.111
I63.10	Cerebral infarction due to embolism of unspecified precerebral artery	100	Ischemic or Unspecified Stroke		0.230	0.146	0.380	0.324	0.230	0.163	0.111
I63.111	Cerebral infarction due to embolism of right vertebral artery	100	Ischemic or Unspecified Stroke		0.230	0.146	0.380	0.324	0.230	0.163	0.111
I63.112	Cerebral infarction due to embolism of left vertebral artery	100	Ischemic or Unspecified Stroke		0.230	0.146	0.380	0.324	0.230	0.163	0.111
I63.113	Cerebral infarction due to embolism of bilateral vertebral arteries	100	Ischemic or Unspecified Stroke		0.230	0.146	0.380	0.324	0.230	0.163	0.111
I63.119	Cerebral infarction due to embolism of unspecified vertebral artery	100	Ischemic or Unspecified Stroke		0.230	0.146	0.380	0.324	0.230	0.163	0.111
I63.12	Cerebral infarction due to embolism of basilar artery	100	Ischemic or Unspecified Stroke		0.230	0.146	0.380	0.324	0.230	0.163	0.111
I63.131	Cerebral infarction due to embolism of right carotid artery	100	Ischemic or Unspecified Stroke		0.230	0.146	0.380	0.324	0.230	0.163	0.111
I63.132	Cerebral infarction due to embolism of left carotid artery	100	Ischemic or Unspecified Stroke		0.230	0.146	0.380	0.324	0.230	0.163	0.111
I63.133	Cerebral infarction due to embolism of bilateral carotid arteries	100	Ischemic or Unspecified Stroke		0.230	0.146	0.380	0.324	0.230	0.163	0.111
I63.139	Cerebral infarction due to embolism of unspecified carotid artery	100	Ischemic or Unspecified Stroke		0.230	0.146	0.380	0.324	0.230	0.163	0.111
I63.19	Cerebral infarction due to embolism of other precerebral artery	100	Ischemic or Unspecified Stroke		0.230	0.146	0.380	0.324	0.230	0.163	0.111
I63.20	Cerebral infarction due to unspecified occlusion or stenosis of unspecified precerebral arteries	100	Ischemic or Unspecified Stroke		0.230	0.146	0.380	0.324	0.230	0.163	0.111
I63.211	Cerebral infarction due to unspecified occlusion or stenosis of right vertebral artery	100	Ischemic or Unspecified Stroke		0.230	0.146	0.380	0.324	0.230	0.163	0.111
I63.212	Cerebral infarction due to unspecified occlusion or stenosis of left vertebral artery	100	Ischemic or Unspecified Stroke		0.230	0.146	0.380	0.324	0.230	0.163	0.111
I63.213	Cerebral infarction due to unspecified occlusion or stenosis of bilateral vertebral arteries	100	Ischemic or Unspecified Stroke		0.230	0.146	0.380	0.324	0.230	0.163	0.111
I63.219	Cerebral infarction due to unspecified occlusion or stenosis of unspecified vertebral artery	100	Ischemic or Unspecified Stroke		0.230	0.146	0.380	0.324	0.230	0.163	0.111
I63.22	Cerebral infarction due to unspecified occlusion or stenosis of basilar artery	100	Ischemic or Unspecified Stroke		0.230	0.146	0.380	0.324	0.230	0.163	0.111
I63.231	Cerebral infarction due to unspecified occlusion or stenosis of right carotid arteries	100	Ischemic or Unspecified Stroke		0.230	0.146	0.380	0.324	0.230	0.163	0.111
I63.232	Cerebral infarction due to unspecified occlusion or stenosis of left carotid arteries	100	Ischemic or Unspecified Stroke		0.230	0.146	0.380	0.324	0.230	0.163	0.111
I63.233	Cerebral infarction due to unspecified occlusion or stenosis of bilateral carotid arteries	100	Ischemic or Unspecified Stroke		0.230	0.146	0.380	0.324	0.230	0.163	0.111
I63.239	Cerebral infarction due to unspecified occlusion or stenosis of unspecified carotid artery	100	Ischemic or Unspecified Stroke		0.230	0.146	0.380	0.324	0.230	0.163	0.111
I63.29	Cerebral infarction due to unspecified occlusion or stenosis of other precerebral arteries	100	Ischemic or Unspecified Stroke		0.230	0.146	0.380	0.324	0.230	0.163	0.111
I63.30	Cerebral infarction due to thrombosis of unspecified cerebral artery	100	Ischemic or Unspecified Stroke		0.230	0.146	0.380	0.324	0.230	0.163	0.111
I63.311	Cerebral infarction due to thrombosis of right middle cerebral artery	100	Ischemic or Unspecified Stroke		0.230	0.146	0.380	0.324	0.230	0.163	0.111

ICD-10-CM Code	ICD-10-CM Code Description	V24 CMS-HCC	V24 CMS-HCC Disease Group	V24 CMS-HCC Hierarchies	Community, NonDual, Aged	Community, NonDual, Disabled	Community, FBDual, Aged	Community, FBDual, Disabled	Community, PBDual, Aged	Community, PBDual, Disabled	Institutional
I63.312	Cerebral infarction due to thrombosis of left middle cerebral artery	100	Ischemic or Unspecified Stroke		0.230	0.146	0.380	0.324	0.230	0.163	0.111
I63.313	Cerebral infarction due to thrombosis of bilateral middle cerebral arteries	100	Ischemic or Unspecified Stroke		0.230	0.146	0.380	0.324	0.230	0.163	0.111
I63.319	Cerebral infarction due to thrombosis of unspecified middle cerebral artery	100	Ischemic or Unspecified Stroke		0.230	0.146	0.380	0.324	0.230	0.163	0.111
I63.321	Cerebral infarction due to thrombosis of right anterior cerebral artery	100	Ischemic or Unspecified Stroke		0.230	0.146	0.380	0.324	0.230	0.163	0.111
I63.322	Cerebral infarction due to thrombosis of left anterior cerebral artery	100	Ischemic or Unspecified Stroke		0.230	0.146	0.380	0.324	0.230	0.163	0.111
I63.323	Cerebral infarction due to thrombosis of bilateral anterior cerebral arteries	100	Ischemic or Unspecified Stroke		0.230	0.146	0.380	0.324	0.230	0.163	0.111
I63.329	Cerebral infarction due to thrombosis of unspecified anterior cerebral artery	100	Ischemic or Unspecified Stroke		0.230	0.146	0.380	0.324	0.230	0.163	0.111
I63.331	Cerebral infarction due to thrombosis of right posterior cerebral artery	100	Ischemic or Unspecified Stroke		0.230	0.146	0.380	0.324	0.230	0.163	0.111
I63.332	Cerebral infarction due to thrombosis of left posterior cerebral artery	100	Ischemic or Unspecified Stroke		0.230	0.146	0.380	0.324	0.230	0.163	0.111
I63.333	Cerebral infarction due to thrombosis of bilateral posterior cerebral arteries	100	Ischemic or Unspecified Stroke		0.230	0.146	0.380	0.324	0.230	0.163	0.111
I63.339	Cerebral infarction due to thrombosis of unspecified posterior cerebral artery	100	Ischemic or Unspecified Stroke		0.230	0.146	0.380	0.324	0.230	0.163	0.111
I63.341	Cerebral infarction due to thrombosis of right cerebellar artery	100	Ischemic or Unspecified Stroke		0.230	0.146	0.380	0.324	0.230	0.163	0.111
I63.342	Cerebral infarction due to thrombosis of left cerebellar artery	100	Ischemic or Unspecified Stroke		0.230	0.146	0.380	0.324	0.230	0.163	0.111
I63.343	Cerebral infarction due to thrombosis of bilateral cerebellar arteries	100	Ischemic or Unspecified Stroke		0.230	0.146	0.380	0.324	0.230	0.163	0.111
I63.349	Cerebral infarction due to thrombosis of unspecified cerebellar artery	100	Ischemic or Unspecified Stroke		0.230	0.146	0.380	0.324	0.230	0.163	0.111
I63.39	Cerebral infarction due to thrombosis of other cerebral artery	100	Ischemic or Unspecified Stroke		0.230	0.146	0.380	0.324	0.230	0.163	0.111
I63.40	Cerebral infarction due to embolism of unspecified cerebral artery	100	Ischemic or Unspecified Stroke		0.230	0.146	0.380	0.324	0.230	0.163	0.111
I63.411	Cerebral infarction due to embolism of right middle cerebral artery	100	Ischemic or Unspecified Stroke		0.230	0.146	0.380	0.324	0.230	0.163	0.111
I63.412	Cerebral infarction due to embolism of left middle cerebral artery	100	Ischemic or Unspecified Stroke		0.230	0.146	0.380	0.324	0.230	0.163	0.111
I63.413	Cerebral infarction due to embolism of bilateral middle cerebral arteries	100	Ischemic or Unspecified Stroke		0.230	0.146	0.380	0.324	0.230	0.163	0.111
I63.419	Cerebral infarction due to embolism of unspecified middle cerebral artery	100	Ischemic or Unspecified Stroke		0.230	0.146	0.380	0.324	0.230	0.163	0.111
I63.421	Cerebral infarction due to embolism of right anterior cerebral artery	100	Ischemic or Unspecified Stroke		0.230	0.146	0.380	0.324	0.230	0.163	0.111
I63.422	Cerebral infarction due to embolism of left anterior cerebral artery	100	Ischemic or Unspecified Stroke		0.230	0.146	0.380	0.324	0.230	0.163	0.111
I63.423	Cerebral infarction due to embolism of bilateral anterior cerebral arteries	100	Ischemic or Unspecified Stroke		0.230	0.146	0.380	0.324	0.230	0.163	0.111
I63.429	Cerebral infarction due to embolism of unspecified anterior cerebral artery	100	Ischemic or Unspecified Stroke		0.230	0.146	0.380	0.324	0.230	0.163	0.111
I63.431	Cerebral infarction due to embolism of right posterior cerebral artery	100	Ischemic or Unspecified Stroke		0.230	0.146	0.380	0.324	0.230	0.163	0.111
I63.432	Cerebral infarction due to embolism of left posterior cerebral artery	100	Ischemic or Unspecified Stroke		0.230	0.146	0.380	0.324	0.230	0.163	0.111
I63.433	Cerebral infarction due to embolism of bilateral posterior cerebral arteries	100	Ischemic or Unspecified Stroke		0.230	0.146	0.380	0.324	0.230	0.163	0.111

2021 Optum360, LLC

ICD-10-CM Code	ICD-10-CM Code Description	V24 CMS-HCC	V24 CMS-HCC Disease Group	V24 CMS-HCC Hierarchies	Community, NonDual, Aged	Community, NonDual, Disabled	Community, FBDual, Aged	Community, FBDual, Disabled	Community, PBDual, Aged	Community, PBDual, Disabled	Institutional
I63.439	Cerebral infarction due to embolism of unspecified posterior cerebral artery	100	Ischemic or Unspecified Stroke		0.230	0.146	0.380	0.324	0.230	0.163	0.111
I63.441	Cerebral infarction due to embolism of right cerebellar artery	100	Ischemic or Unspecified Stroke		0.230	0.146	0.380	0.324	0.230	0.163	0.111
I63.442	Cerebral infarction due to embolism of left cerebellar artery	100	Ischemic or Unspecified Stroke		0.230	0.146	0.380	0.324	0.230	0.163	0.111
I63.443	Cerebral infarction due to embolism of bilateral cerebellar arteries	100	Ischemic or Unspecified Stroke		0.230	0.146	0.380	0.324	0.230	0.163	0.111
I63.449	Cerebral infarction due to embolism of unspecified cerebellar artery	100	Ischemic or Unspecified Stroke		0.230	0.146	0.380	0.324	0.230	0.163	0.111
I63.49	Cerebral infarction due to embolism of other cerebral artery	100	Ischemic or Unspecified Stroke		0.230	0.146	0.380	0.324	0.230	0.163	0.111
I63.50	Cerebral infarction due to unspecified occlusion or stenosis of unspecified cerebral artery	100	Ischemic or Unspecified Stroke		0.230	0.146	0.380	0.324	0.230	0.163	0.111
I63.511	Cerebral infarction due to unspecified occlusion or stenosis of right middle cerebral artery	100	Ischemic or Unspecified Stroke		0.230	0.146	0.380	0.324	0.230	0.163	0.111
I63.512	Cerebral infarction due to unspecified occlusion or stenosis of left middle cerebral artery	100	Ischemic or Unspecified Stroke		0.230	0.146	0.380	0.324	0.230	0.163	0.111
I63.513	Cerebral infarction due to unspecified occlusion or stenosis of bilateral middle cerebral arteries	100	Ischemic or Unspecified Stroke		0.230	0.146	0.380	0.324	0.230	0.163	0.111
I63.519	Cerebral infarction due to unspecified occlusion or stenosis of unspecified middle cerebral artery	100	Ischemic or Unspecified Stroke		0.230	0.146	0.380	0.324	0.230	0.163	0.111
I63.521	Cerebral infarction due to unspecified occlusion or stenosis of right anterior cerebral artery	100	Ischemic or Unspecified Stroke		0.230	0.146	0.380	0.324	0.230	0.163	0.111
I63.522	Cerebral infarction due to unspecified occlusion or stenosis of left anterior cerebral artery	100	Ischemic or Unspecified Stroke		0.230	0.146	0.380	0.324	0.230	0.163	0.111
I63.523	Cerebral infarction due to unspecified occlusion or stenosis of bilateral anterior cerebral arteries	100	Ischemic or Unspecified Stroke		0.230	0.146	0.380	0.324	0.230	0.163	0.111
I63.529	Cerebral infarction due to unspecified occlusion or stenosis of unspecified anterior cerebral artery	100	Ischemic or Unspecified Stroke		0.230	0.146	0.380	0.324	0.230	0.163	0.111
I63.531	Cerebral infarction due to unspecified occlusion or stenosis of right posterior cerebral artery	100	Ischemic or Unspecified Stroke		0.230	0.146	0.380	0.324	0.230	0.163	0.111
I63.532	Cerebral infarction due to unspecified occlusion or stenosis of left posterior cerebral artery	100	Ischemic or Unspecified Stroke		0.230	0.146	0.380	0.324	0.230	0.163	0.111
I63.533	Cerebral infarction due to unspecified occlusion or stenosis of bilateral posterior cerebral arteries	100	Ischemic or Unspecified Stroke		0.230	0.146	0.380	0.324	0.230	0.163	0.111
I63.539	Cerebral infarction due to unspecified occlusion or stenosis of unspecified posterior cerebral artery	100	Ischemic or Unspecified Stroke		0.230	0.146	0.380	0.324	0.230	0.163	0.111
I63.541	Cerebral infarction due to unspecified occlusion or stenosis of right cerebellar artery	100	Ischemic or Unspecified Stroke		0.230	0.146	0.380	0.324	0.230	0.163	0.111
I63.542	Cerebral infarction due to unspecified occlusion or stenosis of left cerebellar artery	100	Ischemic or Unspecified Stroke		0.230	0.146	0.380	0.324	0.230	0.163	0.111
I63.543	Cerebral infarction due to unspecified occlusion or stenosis of bilateral cerebellar arteries	100	Ischemic or Unspecified Stroke		0.230	0.146	0.380	0.324	0.230	0.163	0.111

ICD-10-CM Code	ICD-10-CM Code Description	V24 CMS-HCC	V24 CMS-HCC Disease Group	V24 CMS-HCC Hierarchies	Community, NonDual, Aged	Community, NonDual, Disabled	Community, FBDual, Aged	Community, FBDual, Disabled	Community, PBDual, Aged	Community, PBDual, Disabled	Institutional
I63.549	Cerebral infarction due to unspecified occlusion or stenosis of unspecified cerebellar artery	100	Ischemic or Unspecified Stroke		0.230	0.146	0.380	0.324	0.230	0.163	0.111
I63.59	Cerebral infarction due to unspecified occlusion or stenosis of other cerebral artery	100	Ischemic or Unspecified Stroke		0.230	0.146	0.380	0.324	0.230	0.163	0.111
I63.6	Cerebral infarction due to cerebral venous thrombosis, nonpyogenic	100	Ischemic or Unspecified Stroke		0.230	0.146	0.380	0.324	0.230	0.163	0.111
I63.81	Other cerebral infarction due to occlusion or stenosis of small artery	100	Ischemic or Unspecified Stroke		0.230	0.146	0.380	0.324	0.230	0.163	0.111
I63.89	Other cerebral infarction	100	Ischemic or Unspecified Stroke		0.230	0.146	0.380	0.324	0.230	0.163	0.111
I63.9	Cerebral infarction, unspecified	100	Ischemic or Unspecified Stroke		0.230	0.146	0.380	0.324	0.230	0.163	0.111
I67.0	Dissection of cerebral arteries, nonruptured	107	Vascular Disease with Complications	108	0.383	0.464	0.565	0.653	0.463	0.450	0.299
I67.3	Progressive vascular leukoencephalopathy	52	Dementia Without Complication		0.346	0.224	0.453	0.256	0.420	0.257	—
I69.031	Monoplegia of upper limb following nontraumatic subarachnoid hemorrhage affecting right dominant side	104	Monoplegia, Other Paralytic Syndromes		0.331	0.270	0.345	0.258	0.300	0.164	—
I69.032	Monoplegia of upper limb following nontraumatic subarachnoid hemorrhage affecting left dominant side	104	Monoplegia, Other Paralytic Syndromes		0.331	0.270	0.345	0.258	0.300	0.164	—
I69.033	Monoplegia of upper limb following nontraumatic subarachnoid hemorrhage affecting right non-dominant side	104	Monoplegia, Other Paralytic Syndromes		0.331	0.270	0.345	0.258	0.300	0.164	—
I69.034	Monoplegia of upper limb following nontraumatic subarachnoid hemorrhage affecting left non-dominant side	104	Monoplegia, Other Paralytic Syndromes		0.331	0.270	0.345	0.258	0.300	0.164	—
I69.039	Monoplegia of upper limb following nontraumatic subarachnoid hemorrhage affecting unspecified side	104	Monoplegia, Other Paralytic Syndromes		0.331	0.270	0.345	0.258	0.300	0.164	—
I69.041	Monoplegia of lower limb following nontraumatic subarachnoid hemorrhage affecting right dominant side	104	Monoplegia, Other Paralytic Syndromes		0.331	0.270	0.345	0.258	0.300	0.164	—
I69.042	Monoplegia of lower limb following nontraumatic subarachnoid hemorrhage affecting left dominant side	104	Monoplegia, Other Paralytic Syndromes		0.331	0.270	0.345	0.258	0.300	0.164	—
I69.043	Monoplegia of lower limb following nontraumatic subarachnoid hemorrhage affecting right non-dominant side	104	Monoplegia, Other Paralytic Syndromes		0.331	0.270	0.345	0.258	0.300	0.164	—
I69.044	Monoplegia of lower limb following nontraumatic subarachnoid hemorrhage affecting left non-dominant side	104	Monoplegia, Other Paralytic Syndromes		0.331	0.270	0.345	0.258	0.300	0.164	—
I69.049	Monoplegia of lower limb following nontraumatic subarachnoid hemorrhage affecting unspecified side	104	Monoplegia, Other Paralytic Syndromes		0.331	0.270	0.345	0.258	0.300	0.164	—
I69.051	Hemiplegia and hemiparesis following nontraumatic subarachnoid hemorrhage affecting right dominant side	103	Hemiplegia/Hemiparesis	104	0.437	0.281	0.487	0.296	0.438	0.310	—

ICD-10-CM Code	ICD-10-CM Code Description	V24 CMS-HCC	V24 CMS-HCC Disease Group	V24 CMS-HCC Hierarchies	Community, NonDual, Aged	Community, NonDual, Disabled	Community, FBDual, Aged	Community, FBDual, Disabled	Community, PBDual, Aged	Community, PBDual, Disabled	Institutional
I69.052	Hemiplegia and hemiparesis following nontraumatic subarachnoid hemorrhage affecting left dominant side	103	Hemiplegia/Hemiparesis	104	0.437	0.281	0.487	0.296	0.438	0.310	—
I69.053	Hemiplegia and hemiparesis following nontraumatic subarachnoid hemorrhage affecting right non-dominant side	103	Hemiplegia/Hemiparesis	104	0.437	0.281	0.487	0.296	0.438	0.310	—
I69.054	Hemiplegia and hemiparesis following nontraumatic subarachnoid hemorrhage affecting left non-dominant side	103	Hemiplegia/Hemiparesis	104	0.437	0.281	0.487	0.296	0.438	0.310	—
I69.059	Hemiplegia and hemiparesis following nontraumatic subarachnoid hemorrhage affecting unspecified side	103	Hemiplegia/Hemiparesis	104	0.437	0.281	0.487	0.296	0.438	0.310	—
I69.061	Other paralytic syndrome following nontraumatic subarachnoid hemorrhage affecting right dominant side	104	Monoplegia, Other Paralytic Syndromes		0.331	0.270	0.345	0.258	0.300	0.164	—
I69.062	Other paralytic syndrome following nontraumatic subarachnoid hemorrhage affecting left dominant side	104	Monoplegia, Other Paralytic Syndromes		0.331	0.270	0.345	0.258	0.300	0.164	—
I69.063	Other paralytic syndrome following nontraumatic subarachnoid hemorrhage affecting right non-dominant side	104	Monoplegia, Other Paralytic Syndromes		0.331	0.270	0.345	0.258	0.300	0.164	—
I69.064	Other paralytic syndrome following nontraumatic subarachnoid hemorrhage affecting left non-dominant side	104	Monoplegia, Other Paralytic Syndromes		0.331	0.270	0.345	0.258	0.300	0.164	—
I69.065	Other paralytic syndrome following nontraumatic subarachnoid hemorrhage, bilateral	104	Monoplegia, Other Paralytic Syndromes		0.331	0.270	0.345	0.258	0.300	0.164	—
I69.069	Other paralytic syndrome following nontraumatic subarachnoid hemorrhage affecting unspecified side	104	Monoplegia, Other Paralytic Syndromes		0.331	0.270	0.345	0.258	0.300	0.164	—
I69.131	Monoplegia of upper limb following nontraumatic intracerebral hemorrhage affecting right dominant side	104	Monoplegia, Other Paralytic Syndromes		0.331	0.270	0.345	0.258	0.300	0.164	—
I69.132	Monoplegia of upper limb following nontraumatic intracerebral hemorrhage affecting left dominant side	104	Monoplegia, Other Paralytic Syndromes		0.331	0.270	0.345	0.258	0.300	0.164	—
I69.133	Monoplegia of upper limb following nontraumatic intracerebral hemorrhage affecting right non-dominant side	104	Monoplegia, Other Paralytic Syndromes		0.331	0.270	0.345	0.258	0.300	0.164	—
I69.134	Monoplegia of upper limb following nontraumatic intracerebral hemorrhage affecting left non-dominant side	104	Monoplegia, Other Paralytic Syndromes		0.331	0.270	0.345	0.258	0.300	0.164	—
I69.139	Monoplegia of upper limb following nontraumatic intracerebral hemorrhage affecting unspecified side	104	Monoplegia, Other Paralytic Syndromes		0.331	0.270	0.345	0.258	0.300	0.164	—
I69.141	Monoplegia of lower limb following nontraumatic intracerebral hemorrhage affecting right dominant side	104	Monoplegia, Other Paralytic Syndromes		0.331	0.270	0.345	0.258	0.300	0.164	—

ICD-10-CM Code	ICD-10-CM Code Description	V24 CMS-HCC	V24 CMS-HCC Disease Group	V24 CMS-HCC Hierarchies	Community, NonDual, Aged	Community, NonDual, Disabled	Community, FBDual, Aged	Community, FBDual, Disabled	Community, PBDual, Aged	Community, PBDual, Disabled	Institutional
I69.142	Monoplegia of lower limb following nontraumatic intracerebral hemorrhage affecting left dominant side	104	Monoplegia, Other Paralytic Syndromes		0.331	0.270	0.345	0.258	0.300	0.164	—
I69.143	Monoplegia of lower limb following nontraumatic intracerebral hemorrhage affecting right non-dominant side	104	Monoplegia, Other Paralytic Syndromes		0.331	0.270	0.345	0.258	0.300	0.164	—
I69.144	Monoplegia of lower limb following nontraumatic intracerebral hemorrhage affecting left non-dominant side	104	Monoplegia, Other Paralytic Syndromes		0.331	0.270	0.345	0.258	0.300	0.164	—
I69.149	Monoplegia of lower limb following nontraumatic intracerebral hemorrhage affecting unspecified side	104	Monoplegia, Other Paralytic Syndromes		0.331	0.270	0.345	0.258	0.300	0.164	—
I69.151	Hemiplegia and hemiparesis following nontraumatic intracerebral hemorrhage affecting right dominant side	103	Hemiplegia/Hemiparesis	104	0.437	0.281	0.487	0.296	0.438	0.310	—
I69.152	Hemiplegia and hemiparesis following nontraumatic intracerebral hemorrhage affecting left dominant side	103	Hemiplegia/Hemiparesis	104	0.437	0.281	0.487	0.296	0.438	0.310	—
I69.153	Hemiplegia and hemiparesis following nontraumatic intracerebral hemorrhage affecting right non-dominant side	103	Hemiplegia/Hemiparesis	104	0.437	0.281	0.487	0.296	0.438	0.310	—
I69.154	Hemiplegia and hemiparesis following nontraumatic intracerebral hemorrhage affecting left non-dominant side	103	Hemiplegia/Hemiparesis	104	0.437	0.281	0.487	0.296	0.438	0.310	—
I69.159	Hemiplegia and hemiparesis following nontraumatic intracerebral hemorrhage affecting unspecified side	103	Hemiplegia/Hemiparesis	104	0.437	0.281	0.487	0.296	0.438	0.310	—
I69.161	Other paralytic syndrome following nontraumatic intracerebral hemorrhage affecting right dominant side	104	Monoplegia, Other Paralytic Syndromes		0.331	0.270	0.345	0.258	0.300	0.164	—
I69.162	Other paralytic syndrome following nontraumatic intracerebral hemorrhage affecting left dominant side	104	Monoplegia, Other Paralytic Syndromes		0.331	0.270	0.345	0.258	0.300	0.164	—
I69.163	Other paralytic syndrome following nontraumatic intracerebral hemorrhage affecting right non-dominant side	104	Monoplegia, Other Paralytic Syndromes		0.331	0.270	0.345	0.258	0.300	0.164	—
I69.164	Other paralytic syndrome following nontraumatic intracerebral hemorrhage affecting left non-dominant side	104	Monoplegia, Other Paralytic Syndromes		0.331	0.270	0.345	0.258	0.300	0.164	—
I69.165	Other paralytic syndrome following nontraumatic intracerebral hemorrhage, bilateral	104	Monoplegia, Other Paralytic Syndromes		0.331	0.270	0.345	0.258	0.300	0.164	—
I69.169	Other paralytic syndrome following nontraumatic intracerebral hemorrhage affecting unspecified side	104	Monoplegia, Other Paralytic Syndromes		0.331	0.270	0.345	0.258	0.300	0.164	—
I69.231	Monoplegia of upper limb following other nontraumatic intracranial hemorrhage affecting right dominant side	104	Monoplegia, Other Paralytic Syndromes		0.331	0.270	0.345	0.258	0.300	0.164	—

ICD-10-CM Code	ICD-10-CM Code Description	V24 CMS-HCC	V24 CMS-HCC Disease Group	V24 CMS-HCC Hierarchies	Community, NonDual, Aged	Community, NonDual, Disabled	Community, FBDual, Aged	Community, FBDual, Disabled	Community, PBDual, Aged	Community, PBDual, Disabled	Institutional
I69.232	Monoplegia of upper limb following other nontraumatic intracranial hemorrhage affecting left dominant side	104	Monoplegia, Other Paralytic Syndromes		0.331	0.270	0.345	0.258	0.300	0.164	—
I69.233	Monoplegia of upper limb following other nontraumatic intracranial hemorrhage affecting right non-dominant side	104	Monoplegia, Other Paralytic Syndromes		0.331	0.270	0.345	0.258	0.300	0.164	—
I69.234	Monoplegia of upper limb following other nontraumatic intracranial hemorrhage affecting left non-dominant side	104	Monoplegia, Other Paralytic Syndromes		0.331	0.270	0.345	0.258	0.300	0.164	—
I69.239	Monoplegia of upper limb following other nontraumatic intracranial hemorrhage affecting unspecified side	104	Monoplegia, Other Paralytic Syndromes		0.331	0.270	0.345	0.258	0.300	0.164	—
I69.241	Monoplegia of lower limb following other nontraumatic intracranial hemorrhage affecting right dominant side	104	Monoplegia, Other Paralytic Syndromes		0.331	0.270	0.345	0.258	0.300	0.164	—
I69.242	Monoplegia of lower limb following other nontraumatic intracranial hemorrhage affecting left dominant side	104	Monoplegia, Other Paralytic Syndromes		0.331	0.270	0.345	0.258	0.300	0.164	—
I69.243	Monoplegia of lower limb following other nontraumatic intracranial hemorrhage affecting right non-dominant side	104	Monoplegia, Other Paralytic Syndromes		0.331	0.270	0.345	0.258	0.300	0.164	—
I69.244	Monoplegia of lower limb following other nontraumatic intracranial hemorrhage affecting left non-dominant side	104	Monoplegia, Other Paralytic Syndromes		0.331	0.270	0.345	0.258	0.300	0.164	—
I69.249	Monoplegia of lower limb following other nontraumatic intracranial hemorrhage affecting unspecified side	104	Monoplegia, Other Paralytic Syndromes		0.331	0.270	0.345	0.258	0.300	0.164	—
I69.251	Hemiplegia and hemiparesis following other nontraumatic intracranial hemorrhage affecting right dominant side	103	Hemiplegia/Hemiparesis	104	0.437	0.281	0.487	0.296	0.438	0.310	—
I69.252	Hemiplegia and hemiparesis following other nontraumatic intracranial hemorrhage affecting left dominant side	103	Hemiplegia/Hemiparesis	104	0.437	0.281	0.487	0.296	0.438	0.310	—
I69.253	Hemiplegia and hemiparesis following other nontraumatic intracranial hemorrhage affecting right non-dominant side	103	Hemiplegia/Hemiparesis	104	0.437	0.281	0.487	0.296	0.438	0.310	—
I69.254	Hemiplegia and hemiparesis following other nontraumatic intracranial hemorrhage affecting left non-dominant side	103	Hemiplegia/Hemiparesis	104	0.437	0.281	0.487	0.296	0.438	0.310	—
I69.259	Hemiplegia and hemiparesis following other nontraumatic intracranial hemorrhage affecting unspecified side	103	Hemiplegia/Hemiparesis	104	0.437	0.281	0.487	0.296	0.438	0.310	—
I69.261	Other paralytic syndrome following other nontraumatic intracranial hemorrhage affecting right dominant side	104	Monoplegia, Other Paralytic Syndromes		0.331	0.270	0.345	0.258	0.300	0.164	—

ICD-10-CM Code	ICD-10-CM Code Description	V24 CMS-HCC	V24 CMS-HCC Disease Group	V24 CMS-HCC Hierarchies	Community, NonDual, Aged	Community, NonDual, Disabled	Community, FBDual, Aged	Community, FBDual, Disabled	Community, PBDual, Aged	Community, PBDual, Disabled	Institutional
I69.262	Other paralytic syndrome following other nontraumatic intracranial hemorrhage affecting left dominant side	104	Monoplegia, Other Paralytic Syndromes		0.331	0.270	0.345	0.258	0.300	0.164	—
I69.263	Other paralytic syndrome following other nontraumatic intracranial hemorrhage affecting right non-dominant side	104	Monoplegia, Other Paralytic Syndromes		0.331	0.270	0.345	0.258	0.300	0.164	—
I69.264	Other paralytic syndrome following other nontraumatic intracranial hemorrhage affecting left non-dominant side	104	Monoplegia, Other Paralytic Syndromes		0.331	0.270	0.345	0.258	0.300	0.164	—
I69.265	Other paralytic syndrome following other nontraumatic intracranial hemorrhage, bilateral	104	Monoplegia, Other Paralytic Syndromes		0.331	0.270	0.345	0.258	0.300	0.164	—
I69.269	Other paralytic syndrome following other nontraumatic intracranial hemorrhage affecting unspecified side	104	Monoplegia, Other Paralytic Syndromes		0.331	0.270	0.345	0.258	0.300	0.164	—
I69.331	Monoplegia of upper limb following cerebral infarction affecting right dominant side	104	Monoplegia, Other Paralytic Syndromes		0.331	0.270	0.345	0.258	0.300	0.164	—
I69.332	Monoplegia of upper limb following cerebral infarction affecting left dominant side	104	Monoplegia, Other Paralytic Syndromes		0.331	0.270	0.345	0.258	0.300	0.164	—
I69.333	Monoplegia of upper limb following cerebral infarction affecting right non-dominant side	104	Monoplegia, Other Paralytic Syndromes		0.331	0.270	0.345	0.258	0.300	0.164	—
I69.334	Monoplegia of upper limb following cerebral infarction affecting left non-dominant side	104	Monoplegia, Other Paralytic Syndromes		0.331	0.270	0.345	0.258	0.300	0.164	—
I69.339	Monoplegia of upper limb following cerebral infarction affecting unspecified side	104	Monoplegia, Other Paralytic Syndromes		0.331	0.270	0.345	0.258	0.300	0.164	—
I69.341	Monoplegia of lower limb following cerebral infarction affecting right dominant side	104	Monoplegia, Other Paralytic Syndromes		0.331	0.270	0.345	0.258	0.300	0.164	—
I69.342	Monoplegia of lower limb following cerebral infarction affecting left dominant side	104	Monoplegia, Other Paralytic Syndromes		0.331	0.270	0.345	0.258	0.300	0.164	—
I69.343	Monoplegia of lower limb following cerebral infarction affecting right non-dominant side	104	Monoplegia, Other Paralytic Syndromes		0.331	0.270	0.345	0.258	0.300	0.164	—
I69.344	Monoplegia of lower limb following cerebral infarction affecting left non-dominant side	104	Monoplegia, Other Paralytic Syndromes		0.331	0.270	0.345	0.258	0.300	0.164	—
I69.349	Monoplegia of lower limb following cerebral infarction affecting unspecified side	104	Monoplegia, Other Paralytic Syndromes		0.331	0.270	0.345	0.258	0.300	0.164	—
I69.351	Hemiplegia and hemiparesis following cerebral infarction affecting right dominant side	103	Hemiplegia/Hemiparesis	104	0.437	0.281	0.487	0.296	0.438	0.310	—
I69.352	Hemiplegia and hemiparesis following cerebral infarction affecting left dominant side	103	Hemiplegia/Hemiparesis	104	0.437	0.281	0.487	0.296	0.438	0.310	—
I69.353	Hemiplegia and hemiparesis following cerebral infarction affecting right non-dominant side	103	Hemiplegia/Hemiparesis	104	0.437	0.281	0.487	0.296	0.438	0.310	—
I69.354	Hemiplegia and hemiparesis following cerebral infarction affecting left non-dominant side	103	Hemiplegia/Hemiparesis	104	0.437	0.281	0.487	0.296	0.438	0.310	—

ICD-10-CM Code	ICD-10-CM Code Description	V24 CMS-HCC	V24 CMS-HCC Disease Group	V24 CMS-HCC Hierarchies	Community, NonDual, Aged	Community, NonDual, Disabled	Community, FBDual, Aged	Community, FBDual, Disabled	Community, PBDual, Aged	Community, PBDual, Disabled	Institutional
I69.359	Hemiplegia and hemiparesis following cerebral infarction affecting unspecified side	103	Hemiplegia/Hemiparesis	104	0.437	0.281	0.487	0.296	0.438	0.310	—
I69.361	Other paralytic syndrome following cerebral infarction affecting right dominant side	104	Monoplegia, Other Paralytic Syndromes		0.331	0.270	0.345	0.258	0.300	0.164	—
I69.362	Other paralytic syndrome following cerebral infarction affecting left dominant side	104	Monoplegia, Other Paralytic Syndromes		0.331	0.270	0.345	0.258	0.300	0.164	—
I69.363	Other paralytic syndrome following cerebral infarction affecting right non-dominant side	104	Monoplegia, Other Paralytic Syndromes		0.331	0.270	0.345	0.258	0.300	0.164	—
I69.364	Other paralytic syndrome following cerebral infarction affecting left non-dominant side	104	Monoplegia, Other Paralytic Syndromes		0.331	0.270	0.345	0.258	0.300	0.164	—
I69.365	Other paralytic syndrome following cerebral infarction, bilateral	104	Monoplegia, Other Paralytic Syndromes		0.331	0.270	0.345	0.258	0.300	0.164	—
I69.369	Other paralytic syndrome following cerebral infarction affecting unspecified side	104	Monoplegia, Other Paralytic Syndromes		0.331	0.270	0.345	0.258	0.300	0.164	—
I69.831	Monoplegia of upper limb following other cerebrovascular disease affecting right dominant side	104	Monoplegia, Other Paralytic Syndromes		0.331	0.270	0.345	0.258	0.300	0.164	—
I69.832	Monoplegia of upper limb following other cerebrovascular disease affecting left dominant side	104	Monoplegia, Other Paralytic Syndromes		0.331	0.270	0.345	0.258	0.300	0.164	—
I69.833	Monoplegia of upper limb following other cerebrovascular disease affecting right non-dominant side	104	Monoplegia, Other Paralytic Syndromes		0.331	0.270	0.345	0.258	0.300	0.164	—
I69.834	Monoplegia of upper limb following other cerebrovascular disease affecting left non-dominant side	104	Monoplegia, Other Paralytic Syndromes		0.331	0.270	0.345	0.258	0.300	0.164	—
I69.839	Monoplegia of upper limb following other cerebrovascular disease affecting unspecified side	104	Monoplegia, Other Paralytic Syndromes		0.331	0.270	0.345	0.258	0.300	0.164	—
I69.841	Monoplegia of lower limb following other cerebrovascular disease affecting right dominant side	104	Monoplegia, Other Paralytic Syndromes		0.331	0.270	0.345	0.258	0.300	0.164	—
I69.842	Monoplegia of lower limb following other cerebrovascular disease affecting left dominant side	104	Monoplegia, Other Paralytic Syndromes		0.331	0.270	0.345	0.258	0.300	0.164	—
I69.843	Monoplegia of lower limb following other cerebrovascular disease affecting right non-dominant side	104	Monoplegia, Other Paralytic Syndromes		0.331	0.270	0.345	0.258	0.300	0.164	—
I69.844	Monoplegia of lower limb following other cerebrovascular disease affecting left non-dominant side	104	Monoplegia, Other Paralytic Syndromes		0.331	0.270	0.345	0.258	0.300	0.164	—
I69.849	Monoplegia of lower limb following other cerebrovascular disease affecting unspecified side	104	Monoplegia, Other Paralytic Syndromes		0.331	0.270	0.345	0.258	0.300	0.164	—
I69.851	Hemiplegia and hemiparesis following other cerebrovascular disease affecting right dominant side	103	Hemiplegia/Hemiparesis	104	0.437	0.281	0.487	0.296	0.438	0.310	—
I69.852	Hemiplegia and hemiparesis following other cerebrovascular disease affecting left dominant side	103	Hemiplegia/Hemiparesis	104	0.437	0.281	0.487	0.296	0.438	0.310	—
I69.853	Hemiplegia and hemiparesis following other cerebrovascular disease affecting right non-dominant side	103	Hemiplegia/Hemiparesis	104	0.437	0.281	0.487	0.296	0.438	0.310	—

ICD-10-CM Code	ICD-10-CM Code Description	V24 CMS-HCC	V24 CMS-HCC Disease Group	V24 CMS-HCC Hierarchies	Community, NonDual, Aged	Community, NonDual, Disabled	Community, FBDual, Aged	Community, FBDual, Disabled	Community, PBDual, Aged	Community, PBDual, Disabled	Institutional
I69.854	Hemiplegia and hemiparesis following other cerebrovascular disease affecting left non-dominant side	103	Hemiplegia/Hemiparesis	104	0.437	0.281	0.487	0.296	0.438	0.310	—
I69.859	Hemiplegia and hemiparesis following other cerebrovascular disease affecting unspecified side	103	Hemiplegia/Hemiparesis	104	0.437	0.281	0.487	0.296	0.438	0.310	—
I69.861	Other paralytic syndrome following other cerebrovascular disease affecting right dominant side	104	Monoplegia, Other Paralytic Syndromes		0.331	0.270	0.345	0.258	0.300	0.164	—
I69.862	Other paralytic syndrome following other cerebrovascular disease affecting left dominant side	104	Monoplegia, Other Paralytic Syndromes		0.331	0.270	0.345	0.258	0.300	0.164	—
I69.863	Other paralytic syndrome following other cerebrovascular disease affecting right non-dominant side	104	Monoplegia, Other Paralytic Syndromes		0.331	0.270	0.345	0.258	0.300	0.164	—
I69.864	Other paralytic syndrome following other cerebrovascular disease affecting left non-dominant side	104	Monoplegia, Other Paralytic Syndromes		0.331	0.270	0.345	0.258	0.300	0.164	—
I69.865	Other paralytic syndrome following other cerebrovascular disease, bilateral	104	Monoplegia, Other Paralytic Syndromes		0.331	0.270	0.345	0.258	0.300	0.164	—
I69.869	Other paralytic syndrome following other cerebrovascular disease affecting unspecified side	104	Monoplegia, Other Paralytic Syndromes		0.331	0.270	0.345	0.258	0.300	0.164	—
I69.931	Monoplegia of upper limb following unspecified cerebrovascular disease affecting right dominant side	104	Monoplegia, Other Paralytic Syndromes		0.331	0.270	0.345	0.258	0.300	0.164	—
I69.932	Monoplegia of upper limb following unspecified cerebrovascular disease affecting left dominant side	104	Monoplegia, Other Paralytic Syndromes		0.331	0.270	0.345	0.258	0.300	0.164	—
I69.933	Monoplegia of upper limb following unspecified cerebrovascular disease affecting right non-dominant side	104	Monoplegia, Other Paralytic Syndromes		0.331	0.270	0.345	0.258	0.300	0.164	—
I69.934	Monoplegia of upper limb following unspecified cerebrovascular disease affecting left non-dominant side	104	Monoplegia, Other Paralytic Syndromes		0.331	0.270	0.345	0.258	0.300	0.164	—
I69.939	Monoplegia of upper limb following unspecified cerebrovascular disease affecting unspecified side	104	Monoplegia, Other Paralytic Syndromes		0.331	0.270	0.345	0.258	0.300	0.164	—
I69.941	Monoplegia of lower limb following unspecified cerebrovascular disease affecting right dominant side	104	Monoplegia, Other Paralytic Syndromes		0.331	0.270	0.345	0.258	0.300	0.164	—
I69.942	Monoplegia of lower limb following unspecified cerebrovascular disease affecting left dominant side	104	Monoplegia, Other Paralytic Syndromes		0.331	0.270	0.345	0.258	0.300	0.164	—
I69.943	Monoplegia of lower limb following unspecified cerebrovascular disease affecting right non-dominant side	104	Monoplegia, Other Paralytic Syndromes		0.331	0.270	0.345	0.258	0.300	0.164	—
I69.944	Monoplegia of lower limb following unspecified cerebrovascular disease affecting left non-dominant side	104	Monoplegia, Other Paralytic Syndromes		0.331	0.270	0.345	0.258	0.300	0.164	—
I69.949	Monoplegia of lower limb following unspecified cerebrovascular disease affecting unspecified side	104	Monoplegia, Other Paralytic Syndromes		0.331	0.270	0.345	0.258	0.300	0.164	—
I69.951	Hemiplegia and hemiparesis following unspecified cerebrovascular disease affecting right dominant side	103	Hemiplegia/Hemiparesis	104	0.437	0.281	0.487	0.296	0.438	0.310	—

ICD-10-CM Code	ICD-10-CM Code Description	V24 CMS-HCC	V24 CMS-HCC Disease Group	V24 CMS-HCC Hierarchies	Community, NonDual, Aged	Community, NonDual, Disabled	Community, FBDual, Aged	Community, FBDual, Disabled	Community, PBDual, Aged	Community, PBDual, Disabled	Institutional
I69.952	Hemiplegia and hemiparesis following unspecified cerebrovascular disease affecting left dominant side	103	Hemiplegia/Hemiparesis	104	0.437	0.281	0.487	0.296	0.438	0.310	—
I69.953	Hemiplegia and hemiparesis following unspecified cerebrovascular disease affecting right non-dominant side	103	Hemiplegia/Hemiparesis	104	0.437	0.281	0.487	0.296	0.438	0.310	—
I69.954	Hemiplegia and hemiparesis following unspecified cerebrovascular disease affecting left non-dominant side	103	Hemiplegia/Hemiparesis	104	0.437	0.281	0.487	0.296	0.438	0.310	—
I69.959	Hemiplegia and hemiparesis following unspecified cerebrovascular disease affecting unspecified side	103	Hemiplegia/Hemiparesis	104	0.437	0.281	0.487	0.296	0.438	0.310	—
I69.961	Other paralytic syndrome following unspecified cerebrovascular disease affecting right dominant side	104	Monoplegia, Other Paralytic Syndromes		0.331	0.270	0.345	0.258	0.300	0.164	—
I69.962	Other paralytic syndrome following unspecified cerebrovascular disease affecting left dominant side	104	Monoplegia, Other Paralytic Syndromes		0.331	0.270	0.345	0.258	0.300	0.164	—
I69.963	Other paralytic syndrome following unspecified cerebrovascular disease affecting right non-dominant side	104	Monoplegia, Other Paralytic Syndromes		0.331	0.270	0.345	0.258	0.300	0.164	—
I69.964	Other paralytic syndrome following unspecified cerebrovascular disease affecting left non-dominant side	104	Monoplegia, Other Paralytic Syndromes		0.331	0.270	0.345	0.258	0.300	0.164	—
I69.965	Other paralytic syndrome following unspecified cerebrovascular disease, bilateral	104	Monoplegia, Other Paralytic Syndromes		0.331	0.270	0.345	0.258	0.300	0.164	—
I69.969	Other paralytic syndrome following unspecified cerebrovascular disease affecting unspecified side	104	Monoplegia, Other Paralytic Syndromes		0.331	0.270	0.345	0.258	0.300	0.164	—
I70.0	Atherosclerosis of aorta	108	Vascular Disease		0.288	0.301	0.294	0.267	0.297	0.314	0.093
I70.1	Atherosclerosis of renal artery	108	Vascular Disease		0.288	0.301	0.294	0.267	0.297	0.314	0.093
I70.201	Unspecified atherosclerosis of native arteries of extremities, right leg	108	Vascular Disease		0.288	0.301	0.294	0.267	0.297	0.314	0.093
I70.202	Unspecified atherosclerosis of native arteries of extremities, left leg	108	Vascular Disease		0.288	0.301	0.294	0.267	0.297	0.314	0.093
I70.203	Unspecified atherosclerosis of native arteries of extremities, bilateral legs	108	Vascular Disease		0.288	0.301	0.294	0.267	0.297	0.314	0.093
I70.208	Unspecified atherosclerosis of native arteries of extremities, other extremity	108	Vascular Disease		0.288	0.301	0.294	0.267	0.297	0.314	0.093
I70.209	Unspecified atherosclerosis of native arteries of extremities, unspecified extremity	108	Vascular Disease		0.288	0.301	0.294	0.267	0.297	0.314	0.093
I70.211	Atherosclerosis of native arteries of extremities with intermittent claudication, right leg	108	Vascular Disease		0.288	0.301	0.294	0.267	0.297	0.314	0.093
I70.212	Atherosclerosis of native arteries of extremities with intermittent claudication, left leg	108	Vascular Disease		0.288	0.301	0.294	0.267	0.297	0.314	0.093
I70.213	Atherosclerosis of native arteries of extremities with intermittent claudication, bilateral legs	108	Vascular Disease		0.288	0.301	0.294	0.267	0.297	0.314	0.093
I70.218	Atherosclerosis of native arteries of extremities with intermittent claudication, other extremity	108	Vascular Disease		0.288	0.301	0.294	0.267	0.297	0.314	0.093

ICD-10-CM Code	ICD-10-CM Code Description	V24 CMS-HCC	V24 CMS-HCC Disease Group	V24 CMS-HCC Hierarchies	Community, NonDual, Aged	Community, NonDual, Disabled	Community, FBDual, Aged	Community, FBDual, Disabled	Community, PBDual, Aged	Community, PBDual, Disabled	Institutional
I70.219	Atherosclerosis of native arteries of extremities with intermittent claudication, unspecified extremity	108	Vascular Disease		0.288	0.301	0.294	0.267	0.297	0.314	0.093
I70.221	Atherosclerosis of native arteries of extremities with rest pain, right leg	108	Vascular Disease		0.288	0.301	0.294	0.267	0.297	0.314	0.093
I70.222	Atherosclerosis of native arteries of extremities with rest pain, left leg	108	Vascular Disease		0.288	0.301	0.294	0.267	0.297	0.314	0.093
I70.223	Atherosclerosis of native arteries of extremities with rest pain, bilateral legs	108	Vascular Disease		0.288	0.301	0.294	0.267	0.297	0.314	0.093
I70.228	Atherosclerosis of native arteries of extremities with rest pain, other extremity	108	Vascular Disease		0.288	0.301	0.294	0.267	0.297	0.314	0.093
I70.229	Atherosclerosis of native arteries of extremities with rest pain, unspecified extremity	108	Vascular Disease		0.288	0.301	0.294	0.267	0.297	0.314	0.093
I70.231	Atherosclerosis of native arteries of right leg with ulceration of thigh	106	Atherosclerosis of the Extremities with Ulceration or Gangrene	107,108, 161,189	1.488	1.521	1.724	1.748	1.504	1.525	0.867
I70.231	Atherosclerosis of native arteries of right leg with ulceration of thigh	161	Chronic Ulcer of Skin, Except Pressure		0.515	0.592	0.727	0.583	0.541	0.542	0.294
I70.232	Atherosclerosis of native arteries of right leg with ulceration of calf	106	Atherosclerosis of the Extremities with Ulceration or Gangrene	107,108, 161,189	1.488	1.521	1.724	1.748	1.504	1.525	0.867
I70.232	Atherosclerosis of native arteries of right leg with ulceration of calf	161	Chronic Ulcer of Skin, Except Pressure		0.515	0.592	0.727	0.583	0.541	0.542	0.294
I70.233	Atherosclerosis of native arteries of right leg with ulceration of ankle	106	Atherosclerosis of the Extremities with Ulceration or Gangrene	107,108, 161,189	1.488	1.521	1.724	1.748	1.504	1.525	0.867
I70.233	Atherosclerosis of native arteries of right leg with ulceration of ankle	161	Chronic Ulcer of Skin, Except Pressure		0.515	0.592	0.727	0.583	0.541	0.542	0.294
I70.234	Atherosclerosis of native arteries of right leg with ulceration of heel and midfoot	106	Atherosclerosis of the Extremities with Ulceration or Gangrene	107,108, 161,189	1.488	1.521	1.724	1.748	1.504	1.525	0.867
I70.234	Atherosclerosis of native arteries of right leg with ulceration of heel and midfoot	161	Chronic Ulcer of Skin, Except Pressure		0.515	0.592	0.727	0.583	0.541	0.542	0.294
I70.235	Atherosclerosis of native arteries of right leg with ulceration of other part of foot	106	Atherosclerosis of the Extremities with Ulceration or Gangrene	107,108, 161,189	1.488	1.521	1.724	1.748	1.504	1.525	0.867
I70.235	Atherosclerosis of native arteries of right leg with ulceration of other part of foot	161	Chronic Ulcer of Skin, Except Pressure		0.515	0.592	0.727	0.583	0.541	0.542	0.294
I70.238	Atherosclerosis of native arteries of right leg with ulceration of other part of lower leg	106	Atherosclerosis of the Extremities with Ulceration or Gangrene	107,108, 161,189	1.488	1.521	1.724	1.748	1.504	1.525	0.867
I70.238	Atherosclerosis of native arteries of right leg with ulceration of other part of lower leg	161	Chronic Ulcer of Skin, Except Pressure		0.515	0.592	0.727	0.583	0.541	0.542	0.294
I70.239	Atherosclerosis of native arteries of right leg with ulceration of unspecified site	106	Atherosclerosis of the Extremities with Ulceration or Gangrene	107,108, 161,189	1.488	1.521	1.724	1.748	1.504	1.525	0.867
I70.239	Atherosclerosis of native arteries of right leg with ulceration of unspecified site	161	Chronic Ulcer of Skin, Except Pressure		0.515	0.592	0.727	0.583	0.541	0.542	0.294
I70.241	Atherosclerosis of native arteries of left leg with ulceration of thigh	106	Atherosclerosis of the Extremities with Ulceration or Gangrene	107,108, 161,189	1.488	1.521	1.724	1.748	1.504	1.525	0.867
I70.241	Atherosclerosis of native arteries of left leg with ulceration of thigh	161	Chronic Ulcer of Skin, Except Pressure		0.515	0.592	0.727	0.583	0.541	0.542	0.294
I70.242	Atherosclerosis of native arteries of left leg with ulceration of calf	106	Atherosclerosis of the Extremities with Ulceration or Gangrene	107,108, 161,189	1.488	1.521	1.724	1.748	1.504	1.525	0.867
I70.242	Atherosclerosis of native arteries of left leg with ulceration of calf	161	Chronic Ulcer of Skin, Except Pressure		0.515	0.592	0.727	0.583	0.541	0.542	0.294

ICD-10-CM Code	ICD-10-CM Code Description	V24 CMS-HCC	V24 CMS-HCC Disease Group	V24 CMS-HCC Hierarchies	Community, NonDual, Aged	Community, NonDual, Disabled	Community, FBDual, Aged	Community, FBDual, Disabled	Community, PBDual, Aged	Community, PBDual, Disabled	Institutional
I70.243	Atherosclerosis of native arteries of left leg with ulceration of ankle	106	Atherosclerosis of the Extremities with Ulceration or Gangrene	107,108, 161,189	1.488	1.521	1.724	1.748	1.504	1.525	0.867
I70.243	Atherosclerosis of native arteries of left leg with ulceration of ankle	161	Chronic Ulcer of Skin, Except Pressure		0.515	0.592	0.727	0.583	0.541	0.542	0.294
I70.244	Atherosclerosis of native arteries of left leg with ulceration of heel and midfoot	106	Atherosclerosis of the Extremities with Ulceration or Gangrene	107,108, 161,189	1.488	1.521	1.724	1.748	1.504	1.525	0.867
I70.244	Atherosclerosis of native arteries of left leg with ulceration of heel and midfoot	161	Chronic Ulcer of Skin, Except Pressure		0.515	0.592	0.727	0.583	0.541	0.542	0.294
I70.245	Atherosclerosis of native arteries of left leg with ulceration of other part of foot	106	Atherosclerosis of the Extremities with Ulceration or Gangrene	107,108, 161,189	1.488	1.521	1.724	1.748	1.504	1.525	0.867
I70.245	Atherosclerosis of native arteries of left leg with ulceration of other part of foot	161	Chronic Ulcer of Skin, Except Pressure		0.515	0.592	0.727	0.583	0.541	0.542	0.294
I70.248	Atherosclerosis of native arteries of left leg with ulceration of other part of lower leg	106	Atherosclerosis of the Extremities with Ulceration or Gangrene	107,108, 161,189	1.488	1.521	1.724	1.748	1.504	1.525	0.867
I70.248	Atherosclerosis of native arteries of left leg with ulceration of other part of lower leg	161	Chronic Ulcer of Skin, Except Pressure		0.515	0.592	0.727	0.583	0.541	0.542	0.294
I70.249	Atherosclerosis of native arteries of left leg with ulceration of unspecified site	106	Atherosclerosis of the Extremities with Ulceration or Gangrene	107,108, 161,189	1.488	1.521	1.724	1.748	1.504	1.525	0.867
I70.249	Atherosclerosis of native arteries of left leg with ulceration of unspecified site	161	Chronic Ulcer of Skin, Except Pressure		0.515	0.592	0.727	0.583	0.541	0.542	0.294
I70.25	Atherosclerosis of native arteries of other extremities with ulceration	106	Atherosclerosis of the Extremities with Ulceration or Gangrene	107,108, 161,189	1.488	1.521	1.724	1.748	1.504	1.525	0.867
I70.25	Atherosclerosis of native arteries of other extremities with ulceration	161	Chronic Ulcer of Skin, Except Pressure		0.515	0.592	0.727	0.583	0.541	0.542	0.294
I70.261	Atherosclerosis of native arteries of extremities with gangrene, right leg	106	Atherosclerosis of the Extremities with Ulceration or Gangrene	107,108, 161,189	1.488	1.521	1.724	1.748	1.504	1.525	0.867
I70.262	Atherosclerosis of native arteries of extremities with gangrene, left leg	106	Atherosclerosis of the Extremities with Ulceration or Gangrene	107,108, 161,189	1.488	1.521	1.724	1.748	1.504	1.525	0.867
I70.263	Atherosclerosis of native arteries of extremities with gangrene, bilateral legs	106	Atherosclerosis of the Extremities with Ulceration or Gangrene	107,108, 161,189	1.488	1.521	1.724	1.748	1.504	1.525	0.867
I70.268	Atherosclerosis of native arteries of extremities with gangrene, other extremity	106	Atherosclerosis of the Extremities with Ulceration or Gangrene	107,108, 161,189	1.488	1.521	1.724	1.748	1.504	1.525	0.867
I70.269	Atherosclerosis of native arteries of extremities with gangrene, unspecified extremity	106	Atherosclerosis of the Extremities with Ulceration or Gangrene	107,108, 161,189	1.488	1.521	1.724	1.748	1.504	1.525	0.867
I70.291	Other atherosclerosis of native arteries of extremities, right leg	108	Vascular Disease		0.288	0.301	0.294	0.267	0.297	0.314	0.093
I70.292	Other atherosclerosis of native arteries of extremities, left leg	108	Vascular Disease		0.288	0.301	0.294	0.267	0.297	0.314	0.093
I70.293	Other atherosclerosis of native arteries of extremities, bilateral legs	108	Vascular Disease		0.288	0.301	0.294	0.267	0.297	0.314	0.093
I70.298	Other atherosclerosis of native arteries of extremities, other extremity	108	Vascular Disease		0.288	0.301	0.294	0.267	0.297	0.314	0.093
I70.299	Other atherosclerosis of native arteries of extremities, unspecified extremity	108	Vascular Disease		0.288	0.301	0.294	0.267	0.297	0.314	0.093
I70.301	Unspecified atherosclerosis of unspecified type of bypass graft(s) of the extremities, right leg	108	Vascular Disease		0.288	0.301	0.294	0.267	0.297	0.314	0.093

ICD-10-CM Code	ICD-10-CM Code Description	V24 CMS-HCC	V24 CMS-HCC Disease Group	V24 CMS-HCC Hierarchies	Community, NonDual, Aged	Community, NonDual, Disabled	Community, FBDual, Aged	Community, FBDual, Disabled	Community, PBDual, Aged	Community, PBDual, Disabled	Institutional
I70.302	Unspecified atherosclerosis of unspecified type of bypass graft(s) of the extremities, left leg	108	Vascular Disease		0.288	0.301	0.294	0.267	0.297	0.314	0.093
I70.303	Unspecified atherosclerosis of unspecified type of bypass graft(s) of the extremities, bilateral legs	108	Vascular Disease		0.288	0.301	0.294	0.267	0.297	0.314	0.093
I70.308	Unspecified atherosclerosis of unspecified type of bypass graft(s) of the extremities, other extremity	108	Vascular Disease		0.288	0.301	0.294	0.267	0.297	0.314	0.093
I70.309	Unspecified atherosclerosis of unspecified type of bypass graft(s) of the extremities, unspecified extremity	108	Vascular Disease		0.288	0.301	0.294	0.267	0.297	0.314	0.093
I70.311	Atherosclerosis of unspecified type of bypass graft(s) of the extremities with intermittent claudication, right leg	108	Vascular Disease		0.288	0.301	0.294	0.267	0.297	0.314	0.093
I70.312	Atherosclerosis of unspecified type of bypass graft(s) of the extremities with intermittent claudication, left leg	108	Vascular Disease		0.288	0.301	0.294	0.267	0.297	0.314	0.093
I70.313	Atherosclerosis of unspecified type of bypass graft(s) of the extremities with intermittent claudication, bilateral legs	108	Vascular Disease		0.288	0.301	0.294	0.267	0.297	0.314	0.093
I70.318	Atherosclerosis of unspecified type of bypass graft(s) of the extremities with intermittent claudication, other extremity	108	Vascular Disease		0.288	0.301	0.294	0.267	0.297	0.314	0.093
I70.319	Atherosclerosis of unspecified type of bypass graft(s) of the extremities with intermittent claudication, unspecified extremity	108	Vascular Disease		0.288	0.301	0.294	0.267	0.297	0.314	0.093
I70.321	Atherosclerosis of unspecified type of bypass graft(s) of the extremities with rest pain, right leg	108	Vascular Disease		0.288	0.301	0.294	0.267	0.297	0.314	0.093
I70.322	Atherosclerosis of unspecified type of bypass graft(s) of the extremities with rest pain, left leg	108	Vascular Disease		0.288	0.301	0.294	0.267	0.297	0.314	0.093
I70.323	Atherosclerosis of unspecified type of bypass graft(s) of the extremities with rest pain, bilateral legs	108	Vascular Disease		0.288	0.301	0.294	0.267	0.297	0.314	0.093
I70.328	Atherosclerosis of unspecified type of bypass graft(s) of the extremities with rest pain, other extremity	108	Vascular Disease		0.288	0.301	0.294	0.267	0.297	0.314	0.093
I70.329	Atherosclerosis of unspecified type of bypass graft(s) of the extremities with rest pain, unspecified extremity	108	Vascular Disease		0.288	0.301	0.294	0.267	0.297	0.314	0.093
I70.331	Atherosclerosis of unspecified type of bypass graft(s) of the right leg with ulceration of thigh	106	Atherosclerosis of the Extremities with Ulceration or Gangrene	107,108, 161,189	1.488	1.521	1.724	1.748	1.504	1.525	0.867
I70.331	Atherosclerosis of unspecified type of bypass graft(s) of the right leg with ulceration of thigh	161	Chronic Ulcer of Skin, Except Pressure		0.515	0.592	0.727	0.583	0.541	0.542	0.294
I70.332	Atherosclerosis of unspecified type of bypass graft(s) of the right leg with ulceration of calf	106	Atherosclerosis of the Extremities with Ulceration or Gangrene	107,108, 161,189	1.488	1.521	1.724	1.748	1.504	1.525	0.867
I70.332	Atherosclerosis of unspecified type of bypass graft(s) of the right leg with ulceration of calf	161	Chronic Ulcer of Skin, Except Pressure		0.515	0.592	0.727	0.583	0.541	0.542	0.294
I70.333	Atherosclerosis of unspecified type of bypass graft(s) of the right leg with ulceration of ankle	106	Atherosclerosis of the Extremities with Ulceration or Gangrene	107,108, 161,189	1.488	1.521	1.724	1.748	1.504	1.525	0.867

ICD-10-CM Code	ICD-10-CM Code Description	V24 CMS-HCC	V24 CMS-HCC Disease Group	V24 CMS-HCC Hierarchies	Community, NonDual, Aged	Community, NonDual, Disabled	Community, FBDual, Aged	Community, FBDual, Disabled	Community, PBDual, Aged	Community, PBDual, Disabled	Institutional
I70.333	Atherosclerosis of unspecified type of bypass graft(s) of the right leg with ulceration of ankle	161	Chronic Ulcer of Skin, Except Pressure		0.515	0.592	0.727	0.583	0.541	0.542	0.294
I70.334	Atherosclerosis of unspecified type of bypass graft(s) of the right leg with ulceration of heel and midfoot	106	Atherosclerosis of the Extremities with Ulceration or Gangrene	107,108, 161,189	1.488	1.521	1.724	1.748	1.504	1.525	0.867
I70.334	Atherosclerosis of unspecified type of bypass graft(s) of the right leg with ulceration of heel and midfoot	161	Chronic Ulcer of Skin, Except Pressure		0.515	0.592	0.727	0.583	0.541	0.542	0.294
I70.335	Atherosclerosis of unspecified type of bypass graft(s) of the right leg with ulceration of other part of foot	106	Atherosclerosis of the Extremities with Ulceration or Gangrene	107,108, 161,189	1.488	1.521	1.724	1.748	1.504	1.525	0.867
I70.335	Atherosclerosis of unspecified type of bypass graft(s) of the right leg with ulceration of other part of foot	161	Chronic Ulcer of Skin, Except Pressure		0.515	0.592	0.727	0.583	0.541	0.542	0.294
I70.338	Atherosclerosis of unspecified type of bypass graft(s) of the right leg with ulceration of other part of lower leg	106	Atherosclerosis of the Extremities with Ulceration or Gangrene	107,108, 161,189	1.488	1.521	1.724	1.748	1.504	1.525	0.867
I70.338	Atherosclerosis of unspecified type of bypass graft(s) of the right leg with ulceration of other part of lower leg	161	Chronic Ulcer of Skin, Except Pressure		0.515	0.592	0.727	0.583	0.541	0.542	0.294
I70.339	Atherosclerosis of unspecified type of bypass graft(s) of the right leg with ulceration of unspecified site	106	Atherosclerosis of the Extremities with Ulceration or Gangrene	107,108, 161,189	1.488	1.521	1.724	1.748	1.504	1.525	0.867
I70.339	Atherosclerosis of unspecified type of bypass graft(s) of the right leg with ulceration of unspecified site	161	Chronic Ulcer of Skin, Except Pressure		0.515	0.592	0.727	0.583	0.541	0.542	0.294
I70.341	Atherosclerosis of unspecified type of bypass graft(s) of the left leg with ulceration of thigh	106	Atherosclerosis of the Extremities with Ulceration or Gangrene	107,108, 161,189	1.488	1.521	1.724	1.748	1.504	1.525	0.867
I70.341	Atherosclerosis of unspecified type of bypass graft(s) of the left leg with ulceration of thigh	161	Chronic Ulcer of Skin, Except Pressure		0.515	0.592	0.727	0.583	0.541	0.542	0.294
I70.342	Atherosclerosis of unspecified type of bypass graft(s) of the left leg with ulceration of calf	106	Atherosclerosis of the Extremities with Ulceration or Gangrene	107,108, 161,189	1.488	1.521	1.724	1.748	1.504	1.525	0.867
I70.342	Atherosclerosis of unspecified type of bypass graft(s) of the left leg with ulceration of calf	161	Chronic Ulcer of Skin, Except Pressure		0.515	0.592	0.727	0.583	0.541	0.542	0.294
I70.343	Atherosclerosis of unspecified type of bypass graft(s) of the left leg with ulceration of ankle	106	Atherosclerosis of the Extremities with Ulceration or Gangrene	107,108, 161,189	1.488	1.521	1.724	1.748	1.504	1.525	0.867
I70.343	Atherosclerosis of unspecified type of bypass graft(s) of the left leg with ulceration of ankle	161	Chronic Ulcer of Skin, Except Pressure		0.515	0.592	0.727	0.583	0.541	0.542	0.294
I70.344	Atherosclerosis of unspecified type of bypass graft(s) of the left leg with ulceration of heel and midfoot	106	Atherosclerosis of the Extremities with Ulceration or Gangrene	107,108, 161,189	1.488	1.521	1.724	1.748	1.504	1.525	0.867
I70.344	Atherosclerosis of unspecified type of bypass graft(s) of the left leg with ulceration of heel and midfoot	161	Chronic Ulcer of Skin, Except Pressure		0.515	0.592	0.727	0.583	0.541	0.542	0.294
I70.345	Atherosclerosis of unspecified type of bypass graft(s) of the left leg with ulceration of other part of foot	106	Atherosclerosis of the Extremities with Ulceration or Gangrene	107,108, 161,189	1.488	1.521	1.724	1.748	1.504	1.525	0.867
I70.345	Atherosclerosis of unspecified type of bypass graft(s) of the left leg with ulceration of other part of foot	161	Chronic Ulcer of Skin, Except Pressure		0.515	0.592	0.727	0.583	0.541	0.542	0.294
I70.348	Atherosclerosis of unspecified type of bypass graft(s) of the left leg with ulceration of other part of lower leg	106	Atherosclerosis of the Extremities with Ulceration or Gangrene	107,108, 161,189	1.488	1.521	1.724	1.748	1.504	1.525	0.867

ICD-10-CM Code	ICD-10-CM Code Description	V24 CMS-HCC	V24 CMS-HCC Disease Group	V24 CMS-HCC Hierarchies	Community, NonDual, Aged	Community, NonDual, Disabled	Community, FBDual, Aged	Community, FBDual, Disabled	Community, PBDual, Aged	Community, PBDual, Disabled	Institutional
I70.348	Atherosclerosis of unspecified type of bypass graft(s) of the left leg with ulceration of other part of lower leg	161	Chronic Ulcer of Skin, Except Pressure		0.515	0.592	0.727	0.583	0.541	0.542	0.294
I70.349	Atherosclerosis of unspecified type of bypass graft(s) of the left leg with ulceration of unspecified site	106	Atherosclerosis of the Extremities with Ulceration or Gangrene	107,108, 161,189	1.488	1.521	1.724	1.748	1.504	1.525	0.867
I70.349	Atherosclerosis of unspecified type of bypass graft(s) of the left leg with ulceration of unspecified site	161	Chronic Ulcer of Skin, Except Pressure		0.515	0.592	0.727	0.583	0.541	0.542	0.294
I70.35	Atherosclerosis of unspecified type of bypass graft(s) of other extremity with ulceration	106	Atherosclerosis of the Extremities with Ulceration or Gangrene	107,108, 161,189	1.488	1.521	1.724	1.748	1.504	1.525	0.867
I70.35	Atherosclerosis of unspecified type of bypass graft(s) of other extremity with ulceration	161	Chronic Ulcer of Skin, Except Pressure		0.515	0.592	0.727	0.583	0.541	0.542	0.294
I70.361	Atherosclerosis of unspecified type of bypass graft(s) of the extremities with gangrene, right leg	106	Atherosclerosis of the Extremities with Ulceration or Gangrene	107,108, 161,189	1.488	1.521	1.724	1.748	1.504	1.525	0.867
I70.362	Atherosclerosis of unspecified type of bypass graft(s) of the extremities with gangrene, left leg	106	Atherosclerosis of the Extremities with Ulceration or Gangrene	107,108, 161,189	1.488	1.521	1.724	1.748	1.504	1.525	0.867
I70.363	Atherosclerosis of unspecified type of bypass graft(s) of the extremities with gangrene, bilateral legs	106	Atherosclerosis of the Extremities with Ulceration or Gangrene	107,108, 161,189	1.488	1.521	1.724	1.748	1.504	1.525	0.867
I70.368	Atherosclerosis of unspecified type of bypass graft(s) of the extremities with gangrene, other extremity	106	Atherosclerosis of the Extremities with Ulceration or Gangrene	107,108, 161,189	1.488	1.521	1.724	1.748	1.504	1.525	0.867
I70.369	Atherosclerosis of unspecified type of bypass graft(s) of the extremities with gangrene, unspecified extremity	106	Atherosclerosis of the Extremities with Ulceration or Gangrene	107,108, 161,189	1.488	1.521	1.724	1.748	1.504	1.525	0.867
I70.391	Other atherosclerosis of unspecified type of bypass graft(s) of the extremities, right leg	108	Vascular Disease		0.288	0.301	0.294	0.267	0.297	0.314	0.093
I70.392	Other atherosclerosis of unspecified type of bypass graft(s) of the extremities, left leg	108	Vascular Disease		0.288	0.301	0.294	0.267	0.297	0.314	0.093
I70.393	Other atherosclerosis of unspecified type of bypass graft(s) of the extremities, bilateral legs	108	Vascular Disease		0.288	0.301	0.294	0.267	0.297	0.314	0.093
I70.398	Other atherosclerosis of unspecified type of bypass graft(s) of the extremities, other extremity	108	Vascular Disease		0.288	0.301	0.294	0.267	0.297	0.314	0.093
I70.399	Other atherosclerosis of unspecified type of bypass graft(s) of the extremities, unspecified extremity	108	Vascular Disease		0.288	0.301	0.294	0.267	0.297	0.314	0.093
I70.401	Unspecified atherosclerosis of autologous vein bypass graft(s) of the extremities, right leg	108	Vascular Disease		0.288	0.301	0.294	0.267	0.297	0.314	0.093
I70.402	Unspecified atherosclerosis of autologous vein bypass graft(s) of the extremities, left leg	108	Vascular Disease		0.288	0.301	0.294	0.267	0.297	0.314	0.093
I70.403	Unspecified atherosclerosis of autologous vein bypass graft(s) of the extremities, bilateral legs	108	Vascular Disease		0.288	0.301	0.294	0.267	0.297	0.314	0.093
I70.408	Unspecified atherosclerosis of autologous vein bypass graft(s) of the extremities, other extremity	108	Vascular Disease		0.288	0.301	0.294	0.267	0.297	0.314	0.093
I70.409	Unspecified atherosclerosis of autologous vein bypass graft(s) of the extremities, unspecified extremity	108	Vascular Disease		0.288	0.301	0.294	0.267	0.297	0.314	0.093

ICD-10-CM Code	ICD-10-CM Code Description	V24 CMS-HCC	V24 CMS-HCC Disease Group	V24 CMS-HCC Hierarchies	Community, NonDual, Aged	Community, NonDual, Disabled	Community, FBDual, Aged	Community, FBDual, Disabled	Community, PBDual, Aged	Community, PBDual, Disabled	Institutional
I70.411	Atherosclerosis of autologous vein bypass graft(s) of the extremities with intermittent claudication, right leg	108	Vascular Disease		0.288	0.301	0.294	0.267	0.297	0.314	0.093
I70.412	Atherosclerosis of autologous vein bypass graft(s) of the extremities with intermittent claudication, left leg	108	Vascular Disease		0.288	0.301	0.294	0.267	0.297	0.314	0.093
I70.413	Atherosclerosis of autologous vein bypass graft(s) of the extremities with intermittent claudication, bilateral legs	108	Vascular Disease		0.288	0.301	0.294	0.267	0.297	0.314	0.093
I70.418	Atherosclerosis of autologous vein bypass graft(s) of the extremities with intermittent claudication, other extremity	108	Vascular Disease		0.288	0.301	0.294	0.267	0.297	0.314	0.093
I70.419	Atherosclerosis of autologous vein bypass graft(s) of the extremities with intermittent claudication, unspecified extremity	108	Vascular Disease		0.288	0.301	0.294	0.267	0.297	0.314	0.093
I70.421	Atherosclerosis of autologous vein bypass graft(s) of the extremities with rest pain, right leg	108	Vascular Disease		0.288	0.301	0.294	0.267	0.297	0.314	0.093
I70.422	Atherosclerosis of autologous vein bypass graft(s) of the extremities with rest pain, left leg	108	Vascular Disease		0.288	0.301	0.294	0.267	0.297	0.314	0.093
I70.423	Atherosclerosis of autologous vein bypass graft(s) of the extremities with rest pain, bilateral legs	108	Vascular Disease		0.288	0.301	0.294	0.267	0.297	0.314	0.093
I70.428	Atherosclerosis of autologous vein bypass graft(s) of the extremities with rest pain, other extremity	108	Vascular Disease		0.288	0.301	0.294	0.267	0.297	0.314	0.093
I70.429	Atherosclerosis of autologous vein bypass graft(s) of the extremities with rest pain, unspecified extremity	108	Vascular Disease		0.288	0.301	0.294	0.267	0.297	0.314	0.093
I70.431	Atherosclerosis of autologous vein bypass graft(s) of the right leg with ulceration of thigh	106	Atherosclerosis of the Extremities with Ulceration or Gangrene	107,108, 161,189	1.488	1.521	1.724	1.748	1.504	1.525	0.867
I70.431	Atherosclerosis of autologous vein bypass graft(s) of the right leg with ulceration of thigh	161	Chronic Ulcer of Skin, Except Pressure		0.515	0.592	0.727	0.583	0.541	0.542	0.294
I70.432	Atherosclerosis of autologous vein bypass graft(s) of the right leg with ulceration of calf	106	Atherosclerosis of the Extremities with Ulceration or Gangrene	107,108, 161,189	1.488	1.521	1.724	1.748	1.504	1.525	0.867
I70.432	Atherosclerosis of autologous vein bypass graft(s) of the right leg with ulceration of calf	161	Chronic Ulcer of Skin, Except Pressure		0.515	0.592	0.727	0.583	0.541	0.542	0.294
I70.433	Atherosclerosis of autologous vein bypass graft(s) of the right leg with ulceration of ankle	106	Atherosclerosis of the Extremities with Ulceration or Gangrene	107,108, 161,189	1.488	1.521	1.724	1.748	1.504	1.525	0.867
I70.433	Atherosclerosis of autologous vein bypass graft(s) of the right leg with ulceration of ankle	161	Chronic Ulcer of Skin, Except Pressure		0.515	0.592	0.727	0.583	0.541	0.542	0.294
I70.434	Atherosclerosis of autologous vein bypass graft(s) of the right leg with ulceration of heel and midfoot	106	Atherosclerosis of the Extremities with Ulceration or Gangrene	107,108, 161,189	1.488	1.521	1.724	1.748	1.504	1.525	0.867
I70.434	Atherosclerosis of autologous vein bypass graft(s) of the right leg with ulceration of heel and midfoot	161	Chronic Ulcer of Skin, Except Pressure		0.515	0.592	0.727	0.583	0.541	0.542	0.294
I70.435	Atherosclerosis of autologous vein bypass graft(s) of the right leg with ulceration of other part of foot	106	Atherosclerosis of the Extremities with Ulceration or Gangrene	107,108, 161,189	1.488	1.521	1.724	1.748	1.504	1.525	0.867

ICD-10-CM Code	ICD-10-CM Code Description	V24 CMS-HCC	V24 CMS-HCC Disease Group	V24 CMS-HCC Hierarchies	Community, NonDual, Aged	Community, NonDual, Disabled	Community, FBDual, Aged	Community, FBDual, Disabled	Community, PBDual, Aged	Community, PBDual, Disabled	Institutional
I70.435	Atherosclerosis of autologous vein bypass graft(s) of the right leg with ulceration of other part of foot	161	Chronic Ulcer of Skin, Except Pressure		0.515	0.592	0.727	0.583	0.541	0.542	0.294
I70.438	Atherosclerosis of autologous vein bypass graft(s) of the right leg with ulceration of other part of lower leg	106	Atherosclerosis of the Extremities with Ulceration or Gangrene	107,108, 161,189	1.488	1.521	1.724	1.748	1.504	1.525	0.867
I70.438	Atherosclerosis of autologous vein bypass graft(s) of the right leg with ulceration of other part of lower leg	161	Chronic Ulcer of Skin, Except Pressure		0.515	0.592	0.727	0.583	0.541	0.542	0.294
I70.439	Atherosclerosis of autologous vein bypass graft(s) of the right leg with ulceration of unspecified site	106	Atherosclerosis of the Extremities with Ulceration or Gangrene	107,108, 161,189	1.488	1.521	1.724	1.748	1.504	1.525	0.867
I70.439	Atherosclerosis of autologous vein bypass graft(s) of the right leg with ulceration of unspecified site	161	Chronic Ulcer of Skin, Except Pressure		0.515	0.592	0.727	0.583	0.541	0.542	0.294
I70.441	Atherosclerosis of autologous vein bypass graft(s) of the left leg with ulceration of thigh	106	Atherosclerosis of the Extremities with Ulceration or Gangrene	107,108, 161,189	1.488	1.521	1.724	1.748	1.504	1.525	0.867
I70.441	Atherosclerosis of autologous vein bypass graft(s) of the left leg with ulceration of thigh	161	Chronic Ulcer of Skin, Except Pressure		0.515	0.592	0.727	0.583	0.541	0.542	0.294
I70.442	Atherosclerosis of autologous vein bypass graft(s) of the left leg with ulceration of calf	106	Atherosclerosis of the Extremities with Ulceration or Gangrene	107,108, 161,189	1.488	1.521	1.724	1.748	1.504	1.525	0.867
I70.442	Atherosclerosis of autologous vein bypass graft(s) of the left leg with ulceration of calf	161	Chronic Ulcer of Skin, Except Pressure		0.515	0.592	0.727	0.583	0.541	0.542	0.294
I70.443	Atherosclerosis of autologous vein bypass graft(s) of the left leg with ulceration of ankle	106	Atherosclerosis of the Extremities with Ulceration or Gangrene	107,108, 161,189	1.488	1.521	1.724	1.748	1.504	1.525	0.867
I70.443	Atherosclerosis of autologous vein bypass graft(s) of the left leg with ulceration of ankle	161	Chronic Ulcer of Skin, Except Pressure		0.515	0.592	0.727	0.583	0.541	0.542	0.294
I70.444	Atherosclerosis of autologous vein bypass graft(s) of the left leg with ulceration of heel and midfoot	106	Atherosclerosis of the Extremities with Ulceration or Gangrene	107,108, 161,189	1.488	1.521	1.724	1.748	1.504	1.525	0.867
I70.444	Atherosclerosis of autologous vein bypass graft(s) of the left leg with ulceration of heel and midfoot	161	Chronic Ulcer of Skin, Except Pressure		0.515	0.592	0.727	0.583	0.541	0.542	0.294
I70.445	Atherosclerosis of autologous vein bypass graft(s) of the left leg with ulceration of other part of foot	106	Atherosclerosis of the Extremities with Ulceration or Gangrene	107,108, 161,189	1.488	1.521	1.724	1.748	1.504	1.525	0.867
I70.445	Atherosclerosis of autologous vein bypass graft(s) of the left leg with ulceration of other part of foot	161	Chronic Ulcer of Skin, Except Pressure		0.515	0.592	0.727	0.583	0.541	0.542	0.294
I70.448	Atherosclerosis of autologous vein bypass graft(s) of the left leg with ulceration of other part of lower leg	106	Atherosclerosis of the Extremities with Ulceration or Gangrene	107,108, 161,189	1.488	1.521	1.724	1.748	1.504	1.525	0.867
I70.448	Atherosclerosis of autologous vein bypass graft(s) of the left leg with ulceration of other part of lower leg	161	Chronic Ulcer of Skin, Except Pressure		0.515	0.592	0.727	0.583	0.541	0.542	0.294
I70.449	Atherosclerosis of autologous vein bypass graft(s) of the left leg with ulceration of unspecified site	106	Atherosclerosis of the Extremities with Ulceration or Gangrene	107,108, 161,189	1.488	1.521	1.724	1.748	1.504	1.525	0.867
I70.449	Atherosclerosis of autologous vein bypass graft(s) of the left leg with ulceration of unspecified site	161	Chronic Ulcer of Skin, Except Pressure		0.515	0.592	0.727	0.583	0.541	0.542	0.294
I70.45	Atherosclerosis of autologous vein bypass graft(s) of other extremity with ulceration	106	Atherosclerosis of the Extremities with Ulceration or Gangrene	107,108, 161,189	1.488	1.521	1.724	1.748	1.504	1.525	0.867

ICD-10-CM Code	ICD-10-CM Code Description	V24 CMS-HCC	V24 CMS-HCC Disease Group	V24 CMS-HCC Hierarchies	Community, NonDual, Aged	Community, NonDual, Disabled	Community, FBDual, Aged	Community, FBDual, Disabled	Community, PBDual, Aged	Community, PBDual, Disabled	Institutional
I70.45	Atherosclerosis of autologous vein bypass graft(s) of other extremity with ulceration	161	Chronic Ulcer of Skin, Except Pressure		0.515	0.592	0.727	0.583	0.541	0.542	0.294
I70.461	Atherosclerosis of autologous vein bypass graft(s) of the extremities with gangrene, right leg	106	Atherosclerosis of the Extremities with Ulceration or Gangrene	107,108, 161,189	1.488	1.521	1.724	1.748	1.504	1.525	0.867
I70.462	Atherosclerosis of autologous vein bypass graft(s) of the extremities with gangrene, left leg	106	Atherosclerosis of the Extremities with Ulceration or Gangrene	107,108, 161,189	1.488	1.521	1.724	1.748	1.504	1.525	0.867
I70.463	Atherosclerosis of autologous vein bypass graft(s) of the extremities with gangrene, bilateral legs	106	Atherosclerosis of the Extremities with Ulceration or Gangrene	107,108, 161,189	1.488	1.521	1.724	1.748	1.504	1.525	0.867
I70.468	Atherosclerosis of autologous vein bypass graft(s) of the extremities with gangrene, other extremity	106	Atherosclerosis of the Extremities with Ulceration or Gangrene	107,108, 161,189	1.488	1.521	1.724	1.748	1.504	1.525	0.867
I70.469	Atherosclerosis of autologous vein bypass graft(s) of the extremities with gangrene, unspecified extremity	106	Atherosclerosis of the Extremities with Ulceration or Gangrene	107,108, 161,189	1.488	1.521	1.724	1.748	1.504	1.525	0.867
I70.491	Other atherosclerosis of autologous vein bypass graft(s) of the extremities, right leg	108	Vascular Disease		0.288	0.301	0.294	0.267	0.297	0.314	0.093
I70.492	Other atherosclerosis of autologous vein bypass graft(s) of the extremities, left leg	108	Vascular Disease		0.288	0.301	0.294	0.267	0.297	0.314	0.093
I70.493	Other atherosclerosis of autologous vein bypass graft(s) of the extremities, bilateral legs	108	Vascular Disease		0.288	0.301	0.294	0.267	0.297	0.314	0.093
I70.498	Other atherosclerosis of autologous vein bypass graft(s) of the extremities, other extremity	108	Vascular Disease		0.288	0.301	0.294	0.267	0.297	0.314	0.093
I70.499	Other atherosclerosis of autologous vein bypass graft(s) of the extremities, unspecified extremity	108	Vascular Disease		0.288	0.301	0.294	0.267	0.297	0.314	0.093
I70.501	Unspecified atherosclerosis of nonautologous biological bypass graft(s) of the extremities, right leg	108	Vascular Disease		0.288	0.301	0.294	0.267	0.297	0.314	0.093
I70.502	Unspecified atherosclerosis of nonautologous biological bypass graft(s) of the extremities, left leg	108	Vascular Disease		0.288	0.301	0.294	0.267	0.297	0.314	0.093
I70.503	Unspecified atherosclerosis of nonautologous biological bypass graft(s) of the extremities, bilateral legs	108	Vascular Disease		0.288	0.301	0.294	0.267	0.297	0.314	0.093
I70.508	Unspecified atherosclerosis of nonautologous biological bypass graft(s) of the extremities, other extremity	108	Vascular Disease		0.288	0.301	0.294	0.267	0.297	0.314	0.093
I70.509	Unspecified atherosclerosis of nonautologous biological bypass graft(s) of the extremities, unspecified extremity	108	Vascular Disease		0.288	0.301	0.294	0.267	0.297	0.314	0.093
I70.511	Atherosclerosis of nonautologous biological bypass graft(s) of the extremities with intermittent claudication, right leg	108	Vascular Disease		0.288	0.301	0.294	0.267	0.297	0.314	0.093
I70.512	Atherosclerosis of nonautologous biological bypass graft(s) of the extremities with intermittent claudication, left leg	108	Vascular Disease		0.288	0.301	0.294	0.267	0.297	0.314	0.093

ICD-10-CM Code	ICD-10-CM Code Description	V24 CMS-HCC	V24 CMS-HCC Disease Group	V24 CMS-HCC Hierarchies	Community, NonDual, Aged	Community, NonDual, Disabled	Community, FBDual, Aged	Community, FBDual, Disabled	Community, PBDual, Aged	Community, PBDual, Disabled	Institutional
I70.513	Atherosclerosis of nonautologous biological bypass graft(s) of the extremities with intermittent claudication, bilateral legs	108	Vascular Disease		0.288	0.301	0.294	0.267	0.297	0.314	0.093
I70.518	Atherosclerosis of nonautologous biological bypass graft(s) of the extremities with intermittent claudication, other extremity	108	Vascular Disease		0.288	0.301	0.294	0.267	0.297	0.314	0.093
I70.519	Atherosclerosis of nonautologous biological bypass graft(s) of the extremities with intermittent claudication, unspecified extremity	108	Vascular Disease		0.288	0.301	0.294	0.267	0.297	0.314	0.093
I70.521	Atherosclerosis of nonautologous biological bypass graft(s) of the extremities with rest pain, right leg	108	Vascular Disease		0.288	0.301	0.294	0.267	0.297	0.314	0.093
I70.522	Atherosclerosis of nonautologous biological bypass graft(s) of the extremities with rest pain, left leg	108	Vascular Disease		0.288	0.301	0.294	0.267	0.297	0.314	0.093
I70.523	Atherosclerosis of nonautologous biological bypass graft(s) of the extremities with rest pain, bilateral legs	108	Vascular Disease		0.288	0.301	0.294	0.267	0.297	0.314	0.093
I70.528	Atherosclerosis of nonautologous biological bypass graft(s) of the extremities with rest pain, other extremity	108	Vascular Disease		0.288	0.301	0.294	0.267	0.297	0.314	0.093
I70.529	Atherosclerosis of nonautologous biological bypass graft(s) of the extremities with rest pain, unspecified extremity	108	Vascular Disease		0.288	0.301	0.294	0.267	0.297	0.314	0.093
I70.531	Atherosclerosis of nonautologous biological bypass graft(s) of the right leg with ulceration of thigh	106	Atherosclerosis of the Extremities with Ulceration or Gangrene	107,108, 161,189	1.488	1.521	1.724	1.748	1.504	1.525	0.867
I70.531	Atherosclerosis of nonautologous biological bypass graft(s) of the right leg with ulceration of thigh	161	Chronic Ulcer of Skin, Except Pressure		0.515	0.592	0.727	0.583	0.541	0.542	0.294
I70.532	Atherosclerosis of nonautologous biological bypass graft(s) of the right leg with ulceration of calf	106	Atherosclerosis of the Extremities with Ulceration or Gangrene	107,108, 161,189	1.488	1.521	1.724	1.748	1.504	1.525	0.867
I70.532	Atherosclerosis of nonautologous biological bypass graft(s) of the right leg with ulceration of calf	161	Chronic Ulcer of Skin, Except Pressure		0.515	0.592	0.727	0.583	0.541	0.542	0.294
I70.533	Atherosclerosis of nonautologous biological bypass graft(s) of the right leg with ulceration of ankle	106	Atherosclerosis of the Extremities with Ulceration or Gangrene	107,108, 161,189	1.488	1.521	1.724	1.748	1.504	1.525	0.867
I70.533	Atherosclerosis of nonautologous biological bypass graft(s) of the right leg with ulceration of ankle	161	Chronic Ulcer of Skin, Except Pressure		0.515	0.592	0.727	0.583	0.541	0.542	0.294
I70.534	Atherosclerosis of nonautologous biological bypass graft(s) of the right leg with ulceration of heel and midfoot	106	Atherosclerosis of the Extremities with Ulceration or Gangrene	107,108, 161,189	1.488	1.521	1.724	1.748	1.504	1.525	0.867
I70.534	Atherosclerosis of nonautologous biological bypass graft(s) of the right leg with ulceration of heel and midfoot	161	Chronic Ulcer of Skin, Except Pressure		0.515	0.592	0.727	0.583	0.541	0.542	0.294
I70.535	Atherosclerosis of nonautologous biological bypass graft(s) of the right leg with ulceration of other part of foot	106	Atherosclerosis of the Extremities with Ulceration or Gangrene	107,108, 161,189	1.488	1.521	1.724	1.748	1.504	1.525	0.867

ICD-10-CM Code	ICD-10-CM Code Description	V24 CMS-HCC	V24 CMS-HCC Disease Group	V24 CMS-HCC Hierarchies	Community, NonDual, Aged	Community, NonDual, Disabled	Community, FBDual, Aged	Community, FBDual, Disabled	Community, PBDual, Aged	Community, PBDual, Disabled	Institutional
I70.535	Atherosclerosis of nonautologous biological bypass graft(s) of the right leg with ulceration of other part of foot	161	Chronic Ulcer of Skin, Except Pressure		0.515	0.592	0.727	0.583	0.541	0.542	0.294
I70.538	Atherosclerosis of nonautologous biological bypass graft(s) of the right leg with ulceration of other part of lower leg	106	Atherosclerosis of the Extremities with Ulceration or Gangrene	107,108, 161,189	1.488	1.521	1.724	1.748	1.504	1.525	0.867
I70.538	Atherosclerosis of nonautologous biological bypass graft(s) of the right leg with ulceration of other part of lower leg	161	Chronic Ulcer of Skin, Except Pressure		0.515	0.592	0.727	0.583	0.541	0.542	0.294
I70.539	Atherosclerosis of nonautologous biological bypass graft(s) of the right leg with ulceration of unspecified site	106	Atherosclerosis of the Extremities with Ulceration or Gangrene	107,108, 161,189	1.488	1.521	1.724	1.748	1.504	1.525	0.867
I70.539	Atherosclerosis of nonautologous biological bypass graft(s) of the right leg with ulceration of unspecified site	161	Chronic Ulcer of Skin, Except Pressure		0.515	0.592	0.727	0.583	0.541	0.542	0.294
I70.541	Atherosclerosis of nonautologous biological bypass graft(s) of the left leg with ulceration of thigh	106	Atherosclerosis of the Extremities with Ulceration or Gangrene	107,108, 161,189	1.488	1.521	1.724	1.748	1.504	1.525	0.867
I70.541	Atherosclerosis of nonautologous biological bypass graft(s) of the left leg with ulceration of thigh	161	Chronic Ulcer of Skin, Except Pressure		0.515	0.592	0.727	0.583	0.541	0.542	0.294
I70.542	Atherosclerosis of nonautologous biological bypass graft(s) of the left leg with ulceration of calf	106	Atherosclerosis of the Extremities with Ulceration or Gangrene	107,108, 161,189	1.488	1.521	1.724	1.748	1.504	1.525	0.867
I70.542	Atherosclerosis of nonautologous biological bypass graft(s) of the left leg with ulceration of calf	161	Chronic Ulcer of Skin, Except Pressure		0.515	0.592	0.727	0.583	0.541	0.542	0.294
I70.543	Atherosclerosis of nonautologous biological bypass graft(s) of the left leg with ulceration of ankle	106	Atherosclerosis of the Extremities with Ulceration or Gangrene	107,108, 161,189	1.488	1.521	1.724	1.748	1.504	1.525	0.867
I70.543	Atherosclerosis of nonautologous biological bypass graft(s) of the left leg with ulceration of ankle	161	Chronic Ulcer of Skin, Except Pressure		0.515	0.592	0.727	0.583	0.541	0.542	0.294
I70.544	Atherosclerosis of nonautologous biological bypass graft(s) of the left leg with ulceration of heel and midfoot	106	Atherosclerosis of the Extremities with Ulceration or Gangrene	107,108, 161,189	1.488	1.521	1.724	1.748	1.504	1.525	0.867
I70.544	Atherosclerosis of nonautologous biological bypass graft(s) of the left leg with ulceration of heel and midfoot	161	Chronic Ulcer of Skin, Except Pressure		0.515	0.592	0.727	0.583	0.541	0.542	0.294
I70.545	Atherosclerosis of nonautologous biological bypass graft(s) of the left leg with ulceration of other part of foot	106	Atherosclerosis of the Extremities with Ulceration or Gangrene	107,108, 161,189	1.488	1.521	1.724	1.748	1.504	1.525	0.867
I70.545	Atherosclerosis of nonautologous biological bypass graft(s) of the left leg with ulceration of other part of foot	161	Chronic Ulcer of Skin, Except Pressure		0.515	0.592	0.727	0.583	0.541	0.542	0.294
I70.548	Atherosclerosis of nonautologous biological bypass graft(s) of the left leg with ulceration of other part of lower leg	106	Atherosclerosis of the Extremities with Ulceration or Gangrene	107,108, 161,189	1.488	1.521	1.724	1.748	1.504	1.525	0.867
I70.548	Atherosclerosis of nonautologous biological bypass graft(s) of the left leg with ulceration of other part of lower leg	161	Chronic Ulcer of Skin, Except Pressure		0.515	0.592	0.727	0.583	0.541	0.542	0.294

ICD-10-CM Code	ICD-10-CM Code Description	V24 CMS-HCC	V24 CMS-HCC Disease Group	V24 CMS-HCC Hierarchies	Community, NonDual, Aged	Community, NonDual, Disabled	Community, FBDual, Aged	Community, FBDual, Disabled	Community, PBDual, Aged	Community, PBDual, Disabled	Institutional
I70.549	Atherosclerosis of nonautologous biological bypass graft(s) of the left leg with ulceration of unspecified site	106	Atherosclerosis of the Extremities with Ulceration or Gangrene	107,108, 161,189	1.488	1.521	1.724	1.748	1.504	1.525	0.867
I70.549	Atherosclerosis of nonautologous biological bypass graft(s) of the left leg with ulceration of unspecified site	161	Chronic Ulcer of Skin, Except Pressure		0.515	0.592	0.727	0.583	0.541	0.542	0.294
I70.55	Atherosclerosis of nonautologous biological bypass graft(s) of other extremity with ulceration	106	Atherosclerosis of the Extremities with Ulceration or Gangrene	107,108, 161,189	1.488	1.521	1.724	1.748	1.504	1.525	0.867
I70.55	Atherosclerosis of nonautologous biological bypass graft(s) of other extremity with ulceration	161	Chronic Ulcer of Skin, Except Pressure		0.515	0.592	0.727	0.583	0.541	0.542	0.294
I70.561	Atherosclerosis of nonautologous biological bypass graft(s) of the extremities with gangrene, right leg	106	Atherosclerosis of the Extremities with Ulceration or Gangrene	107,108, 161,189	1.488	1.521	1.724	1.748	1.504	1.525	0.867
I70.562	Atherosclerosis of nonautologous biological bypass graft(s) of the extremities with gangrene, left leg	106	Atherosclerosis of the Extremities with Ulceration or Gangrene	107,108, 161,189	1.488	1.521	1.724	1.748	1.504	1.525	0.867
I70.563	Atherosclerosis of nonautologous biological bypass graft(s) of the extremities with gangrene, bilateral legs	106	Atherosclerosis of the Extremities with Ulceration or Gangrene	107,108, 161,189	1.488	1.521	1.724	1.748	1.504	1.525	0.867
I70.568	Atherosclerosis of nonautologous biological bypass graft(s) of the extremities with gangrene, other extremity	106	Atherosclerosis of the Extremities with Ulceration or Gangrene	107,108, 161,189	1.488	1.521	1.724	1.748	1.504	1.525	0.867
I70.569	Atherosclerosis of nonautologous biological bypass graft(s) of the extremities with gangrene, unspecified extremity	106	Atherosclerosis of the Extremities with Ulceration or Gangrene	107,108, 161,189	1.488	1.521	1.724	1.748	1.504	1.525	0.867
I70.591	Other atherosclerosis of nonautologous biological bypass graft(s) of the extremities, right leg	108	Vascular Disease		0.288	0.301	0.294	0.267	0.297	0.314	0.093
I70.592	Other atherosclerosis of nonautologous biological bypass graft(s) of the extremities, left leg	108	Vascular Disease		0.288	0.301	0.294	0.267	0.297	0.314	0.093
I70.593	Other atherosclerosis of nonautologous biological bypass graft(s) of the extremities, bilateral legs	108	Vascular Disease		0.288	0.301	0.294	0.267	0.297	0.314	0.093
I70.598	Other atherosclerosis of nonautologous biological bypass graft(s) of the extremities, other extremity	108	Vascular Disease		0.288	0.301	0.294	0.267	0.297	0.314	0.093
I70.599	Other atherosclerosis of nonautologous biological bypass graft(s) of the extremities, unspecified extremity	108	Vascular Disease		0.288	0.301	0.294	0.267	0.297	0.314	0.093
I70.601	Unspecified atherosclerosis of nonbiological bypass graft(s) of the extremities, right leg	108	Vascular Disease		0.288	0.301	0.294	0.267	0.297	0.314	0.093
I70.602	Unspecified atherosclerosis of nonbiological bypass graft(s) of the extremities, left leg	108	Vascular Disease		0.288	0.301	0.294	0.267	0.297	0.314	0.093
I70.603	Unspecified atherosclerosis of nonbiological bypass graft(s) of the extremities, bilateral legs	108	Vascular Disease		0.288	0.301	0.294	0.267	0.297	0.314	0.093
I70.608	Unspecified atherosclerosis of nonbiological bypass graft(s) of the extremities, other extremity	108	Vascular Disease		0.288	0.301	0.294	0.267	0.297	0.314	0.093

ICD-10-CM Code	ICD-10-CM Code Description	V24 CMS-HCC	V24 CMS-HCC Disease Group	V24 CMS-HCC Hierarchies	Community, NonDual, Aged	Community, NonDual, Disabled	Community, FBDual, Aged	Community, FBDual, Disabled	Community, PBDual, Aged	Community, PBDual, Disabled	Institutional
I70.609	Unspecified atherosclerosis of nonbiological bypass graft(s) of the extremities, unspecified extremity	108	Vascular Disease		0.288	0.301	0.294	0.267	0.297	0.314	0.093
I70.611	Atherosclerosis of nonbiological bypass graft(s) of the extremities with intermittent claudication, right leg	108	Vascular Disease		0.288	0.301	0.294	0.267	0.297	0.314	0.093
I70.612	Atherosclerosis of nonbiological bypass graft(s) of the extremities with intermittent claudication, left leg	108	Vascular Disease		0.288	0.301	0.294	0.267	0.297	0.314	0.093
I70.613	Atherosclerosis of nonbiological bypass graft(s) of the extremities with intermittent claudication, bilateral legs	108	Vascular Disease		0.288	0.301	0.294	0.267	0.297	0.314	0.093
I70.618	Atherosclerosis of nonbiological bypass graft(s) of the extremities with intermittent claudication, other extremity	108	Vascular Disease		0.288	0.301	0.294	0.267	0.297	0.314	0.093
I70.619	Atherosclerosis of nonbiological bypass graft(s) of the extremities with intermittent claudication, unspecified extremity	108	Vascular Disease		0.288	0.301	0.294	0.267	0.297	0.314	0.093
I70.621	Atherosclerosis of nonbiological bypass graft(s) of the extremities with rest pain, right leg	108	Vascular Disease		0.288	0.301	0.294	0.267	0.297	0.314	0.093
I70.622	Atherosclerosis of nonbiological bypass graft(s) of the extremities with rest pain, left leg	108	Vascular Disease		0.288	0.301	0.294	0.267	0.297	0.314	0.093
I70.623	Atherosclerosis of nonbiological bypass graft(s) of the extremities with rest pain, bilateral legs	108	Vascular Disease		0.288	0.301	0.294	0.267	0.297	0.314	0.093
I70.628	Atherosclerosis of nonbiological bypass graft(s) of the extremities with rest pain, other extremity	108	Vascular Disease		0.288	0.301	0.294	0.267	0.297	0.314	0.093
I70.629	Atherosclerosis of nonbiological bypass graft(s) of the extremities with rest pain, unspecified extremity	108	Vascular Disease		0.288	0.301	0.294	0.267	0.297	0.314	0.093
I70.631	Atherosclerosis of nonbiological bypass graft(s) of the right leg with ulceration of thigh	106	Atherosclerosis of the Extremities with Ulceration or Gangrene	107,108, 161,189	1.488	1.521	1.724	1.748	1.504	1.525	0.867
I70.631	Atherosclerosis of nonbiological bypass graft(s) of the right leg with ulceration of thigh	161	Chronic Ulcer of Skin, Except Pressure		0.515	0.592	0.727	0.583	0.541	0.542	0.294
I70.632	Atherosclerosis of nonbiological bypass graft(s) of the right leg with ulceration of calf	106	Atherosclerosis of the Extremities with Ulceration or Gangrene	107,108, 161,189	1.488	1.521	1.724	1.748	1.504	1.525	0.867
I70.632	Atherosclerosis of nonbiological bypass graft(s) of the right leg with ulceration of calf	161	Chronic Ulcer of Skin, Except Pressure		0.515	0.592	0.727	0.583	0.541	0.542	0.294
I70.633	Atherosclerosis of nonbiological bypass graft(s) of the right leg with ulceration of ankle	106	Atherosclerosis of the Extremities with Ulceration or Gangrene	107,108, 161,189	1.488	1.521	1.724	1.748	1.504	1.525	0.867
I70.633	Atherosclerosis of nonbiological bypass graft(s) of the right leg with ulceration of ankle	161	Chronic Ulcer of Skin, Except Pressure		0.515	0.592	0.727	0.583	0.541	0.542	0.294
I70.634	Atherosclerosis of nonbiological bypass graft(s) of the right leg with ulceration of heel and midfoot	106	Atherosclerosis of the Extremities with Ulceration or Gangrene	107,108, 161,189	1.488	1.521	1.724	1.748	1.504	1.525	0.867
I70.634	Atherosclerosis of nonbiological bypass graft(s) of the right leg with ulceration of heel and midfoot	161	Chronic Ulcer of Skin, Except Pressure		0.515	0.592	0.727	0.583	0.541	0.542	0.294

ICD-10-CM Code	ICD-10-CM Code Description	V24 CMS-HCC	V24 CMS-HCC Disease Group	V24 CMS-HCC Hierarchies	Community, NonDual, Aged	Community, NonDual, Disabled	Community, FBDual, Aged	Community, FBDual, Disabled	Community, PBDual, Aged	Community, PBDual, Disabled	Institutional
I70.635	Atherosclerosis of nonbiological bypass graft(s) of the right leg with ulceration of other part of foot	106	Atherosclerosis of the Extremities with Ulceration or Gangrene	107,108, 161,189	1.488	1.521	1.724	1.748	1.504	1.525	0.867
I70.635	Atherosclerosis of nonbiological bypass graft(s) of the right leg with ulceration of other part of foot	161	Chronic Ulcer of Skin, Except Pressure		0.515	0.592	0.727	0.583	0.541	0.542	0.294
I70.638	Atherosclerosis of nonbiological bypass graft(s) of the right leg with ulceration of other part of lower leg	106	Atherosclerosis of the Extremities with Ulceration or Gangrene	107,108, 161,189	1.488	1.521	1.724	1.748	1.504	1.525	0.867
I70.638	Atherosclerosis of nonbiological bypass graft(s) of the right leg with ulceration of other part of lower leg	161	Chronic Ulcer of Skin, Except Pressure		0.515	0.592	0.727	0.583	0.541	0.542	0.294
I70.639	Atherosclerosis of nonbiological bypass graft(s) of the right leg with ulceration of unspecified site	106	Atherosclerosis of the Extremities with Ulceration or Gangrene	107,108, 161,189	1.488	1.521	1.724	1.748	1.504	1.525	0.867
I70.639	Atherosclerosis of nonbiological bypass graft(s) of the right leg with ulceration of unspecified site	161	Chronic Ulcer of Skin, Except Pressure		0.515	0.592	0.727	0.583	0.541	0.542	0.294
I70.641	Atherosclerosis of nonbiological bypass graft(s) of the left leg with ulceration of thigh	106	Atherosclerosis of the Extremities with Ulceration or Gangrene	107,108, 161,189	1.488	1.521	1.724	1.748	1.504	1.525	0.867
I70.641	Atherosclerosis of nonbiological bypass graft(s) of the left leg with ulceration of thigh	161	Chronic Ulcer of Skin, Except Pressure		0.515	0.592	0.727	0.583	0.541	0.542	0.294
I70.642	Atherosclerosis of nonbiological bypass graft(s) of the left leg with ulceration of calf	106	Atherosclerosis of the Extremities with Ulceration or Gangrene	107,108, 161,189	1.488	1.521	1.724	1.748	1.504	1.525	0.867
I70.642	Atherosclerosis of nonbiological bypass graft(s) of the left leg with ulceration of calf	161	Chronic Ulcer of Skin, Except Pressure		0.515	0.592	0.727	0.583	0.541	0.542	0.294
I70.643	Atherosclerosis of nonbiological bypass graft(s) of the left leg with ulceration of ankle	106	Atherosclerosis of the Extremities with Ulceration or Gangrene	107,108, 161,189	1.488	1.521	1.724	1.748	1.504	1.525	0.867
I70.643	Atherosclerosis of nonbiological bypass graft(s) of the left leg with ulceration of ankle	161	Chronic Ulcer of Skin, Except Pressure		0.515	0.592	0.727	0.583	0.541	0.542	0.294
I70.644	Atherosclerosis of nonbiological bypass graft(s) of the left leg with ulceration of heel and midfoot	106	Atherosclerosis of the Extremities with Ulceration or Gangrene	107,108, 161,189	1.488	1.521	1.724	1.748	1.504	1.525	0.867
I70.644	Atherosclerosis of nonbiological bypass graft(s) of the left leg with ulceration of heel and midfoot	161	Chronic Ulcer of Skin, Except Pressure		0.515	0.592	0.727	0.583	0.541	0.542	0.294
I70.645	Atherosclerosis of nonbiological bypass graft(s) of the left leg with ulceration of other part of foot	106	Atherosclerosis of the Extremities with Ulceration or Gangrene	107,108, 161,189	1.488	1.521	1.724	1.748	1.504	1.525	0.867
I70.645	Atherosclerosis of nonbiological bypass graft(s) of the left leg with ulceration of other part of foot	161	Chronic Ulcer of Skin, Except Pressure		0.515	0.592	0.727	0.583	0.541	0.542	0.294
I70.648	Atherosclerosis of nonbiological bypass graft(s) of the left leg with ulceration of other part of lower leg	106	Atherosclerosis of the Extremities with Ulceration or Gangrene	107,108, 161,189	1.488	1.521	1.724	1.748	1.504	1.525	0.867
I70.648	Atherosclerosis of nonbiological bypass graft(s) of the left leg with ulceration of other part of lower leg	161	Chronic Ulcer of Skin, Except Pressure		0.515	0.592	0.727	0.583	0.541	0.542	0.294
I70.649	Atherosclerosis of nonbiological bypass graft(s) of the left leg with ulceration of unspecified site	106	Atherosclerosis of the Extremities with Ulceration or Gangrene	107,108, 161,189	1.488	1.521	1.724	1.748	1.504	1.525	0.867
I70.649	Atherosclerosis of nonbiological bypass graft(s) of the left leg with ulceration of unspecified site	161	Chronic Ulcer of Skin, Except Pressure		0.515	0.592	0.727	0.583	0.541	0.542	0.294

ICD-10-CM Code	ICD-10-CM Code Description	V24 CMS-HCC	V24 CMS-HCC Disease Group	V24 CMS-HCC Hierarchies	Community, NonDual, Aged	Community, NonDual, Disabled	Community, FBDual, Aged	Community, FBDual, Disabled	Community, PBDual, Aged	Community, PBDual, Disabled	Institutional
I70.65	Atherosclerosis of nonbiological bypass graft(s) of other extremity with ulceration	106	Atherosclerosis of the Extremities with Ulceration or Gangrene	107,108, 161,189	1.488	1.521	1.724	1.748	1.504	1.525	0.867
I70.65	Atherosclerosis of nonbiological bypass graft(s) of other extremity with ulceration	161	Chronic Ulcer of Skin, Except Pressure		0.515	0.592	0.727	0.583	0.541	0.542	0.294
I70.661	Atherosclerosis of nonbiological bypass graft(s) of the extremities with gangrene, right leg	106	Atherosclerosis of the Extremities with Ulceration or Gangrene	107,108, 161,189	1.488	1.521	1.724	1.748	1.504	1.525	0.867
I70.662	Atherosclerosis of nonbiological bypass graft(s) of the extremities with gangrene, left leg	106	Atherosclerosis of the Extremities with Ulceration or Gangrene	107,108, 161,189	1.488	1.521	1.724	1.748	1.504	1.525	0.867
I70.663	Atherosclerosis of nonbiological bypass graft(s) of the extremities with gangrene, bilateral legs	106	Atherosclerosis of the Extremities with Ulceration or Gangrene	107,108, 161,189	1.488	1.521	1.724	1.748	1.504	1.525	0.867
I70.668	Atherosclerosis of nonbiological bypass graft(s) of the extremities with gangrene, other extremity	106	Atherosclerosis of the Extremities with Ulceration or Gangrene	107,108, 161,189	1.488	1.521	1.724	1.748	1.504	1.525	0.867
I70.669	Atherosclerosis of nonbiological bypass graft(s) of the extremities with gangrene, unspecified extremity	106	Atherosclerosis of the Extremities with Ulceration or Gangrene	107,108, 161,189	1.488	1.521	1.724	1.748	1.504	1.525	0.867
I70.691	Other atherosclerosis of nonbiological bypass graft(s) of the extremities, right leg	108	Vascular Disease		0.288	0.301	0.294	0.267	0.297	0.314	0.093
I70.692	Other atherosclerosis of nonbiological bypass graft(s) of the extremities, left leg	108	Vascular Disease		0.288	0.301	0.294	0.267	0.297	0.314	0.093
I70.693	Other atherosclerosis of nonbiological bypass graft(s) of the extremities, bilateral legs	108	Vascular Disease		0.288	0.301	0.294	0.267	0.297	0.314	0.093
I70.698	Other atherosclerosis of nonbiological bypass graft(s) of the extremities, other extremity	108	Vascular Disease		0.288	0.301	0.294	0.267	0.297	0.314	0.093
I70.699	Other atherosclerosis of nonbiological bypass graft(s) of the extremities, unspecified extremity	108	Vascular Disease		0.288	0.301	0.294	0.267	0.297	0.314	0.093
I70.701	Unspecified atherosclerosis of other type of bypass graft(s) of the extremities, right leg	108	Vascular Disease		0.288	0.301	0.294	0.267	0.297	0.314	0.093
I70.702	Unspecified atherosclerosis of other type of bypass graft(s) of the extremities, left leg	108	Vascular Disease		0.288	0.301	0.294	0.267	0.297	0.314	0.093
I70.703	Unspecified atherosclerosis of other type of bypass graft(s) of the extremities, bilateral legs	108	Vascular Disease		0.288	0.301	0.294	0.267	0.297	0.314	0.093
I70.708	Unspecified atherosclerosis of other type of bypass graft(s) of the extremities, other extremity	108	Vascular Disease		0.288	0.301	0.294	0.267	0.297	0.314	0.093
I70.709	Unspecified atherosclerosis of other type of bypass graft(s) of the extremities, unspecified extremity	108	Vascular Disease		0.288	0.301	0.294	0.267	0.297	0.314	0.093
I70.711	Atherosclerosis of other type of bypass graft(s) of the extremities with intermittent claudication, right leg	108	Vascular Disease		0.288	0.301	0.294	0.267	0.297	0.314	0.093
I70.712	Atherosclerosis of other type of bypass graft(s) of the extremities with intermittent claudication, left leg	108	Vascular Disease		0.288	0.301	0.294	0.267	0.297	0.314	0.093
I70.713	Atherosclerosis of other type of bypass graft(s) of the extremities with intermittent claudication, bilateral legs	108	Vascular Disease		0.288	0.301	0.294	0.267	0.297	0.314	0.093

ICD-10-CM Code	ICD-10-CM Code Description	V24 CMS-HCC	V24 CMS-HCC Disease Group	V24 CMS-HCC Hierarchies	Community, NonDual, Aged	Community, NonDual, Disabled	Community, FBDual, Aged	Community, FBDual, Disabled	Community, PBDual, Aged	Community, PBDual, Disabled	Institutional
I70.718	Atherosclerosis of other type of bypass graft(s) of the extremities with intermittent claudication, other extremity	108	Vascular Disease		0.288	0.301	0.294	0.267	0.297	0.314	0.093
I70.719	Atherosclerosis of other type of bypass graft(s) of the extremities with intermittent claudication, unspecified extremity	108	Vascular Disease		0.288	0.301	0.294	0.267	0.297	0.314	0.093
I70.721	Atherosclerosis of other type of bypass graft(s) of the extremities with rest pain, right leg	108	Vascular Disease		0.288	0.301	0.294	0.267	0.297	0.314	0.093
I70.722	Atherosclerosis of other type of bypass graft(s) of the extremities with rest pain, left leg	108	Vascular Disease		0.288	0.301	0.294	0.267	0.297	0.314	0.093
I70.723	Atherosclerosis of other type of bypass graft(s) of the extremities with rest pain, bilateral legs	108	Vascular Disease		0.288	0.301	0.294	0.267	0.297	0.314	0.093
I70.728	Atherosclerosis of other type of bypass graft(s) of the extremities with rest pain, other extremity	108	Vascular Disease		0.288	0.301	0.294	0.267	0.297	0.314	0.093
I70.729	Atherosclerosis of other type of bypass graft(s) of the extremities with rest pain, unspecified extremity	108	Vascular Disease		0.288	0.301	0.294	0.267	0.297	0.314	0.093
I70.731	Atherosclerosis of other type of bypass graft(s) of the right leg with ulceration of thigh	106	Atherosclerosis of the Extremities with Ulceration or Gangrene	107,108, 161,189	1.488	1.521	1.724	1.748	1.504	1.525	0.867
I70.731	Atherosclerosis of other type of bypass graft(s) of the right leg with ulceration of thigh	161	Chronic Ulcer of Skin, Except Pressure		0.515	0.592	0.727	0.583	0.541	0.542	0.294
I70.732	Atherosclerosis of other type of bypass graft(s) of the right leg with ulceration of calf	106	Atherosclerosis of the Extremities with Ulceration or Gangrene	107,108, 161,189	1.488	1.521	1.724	1.748	1.504	1.525	0.867
I70.732	Atherosclerosis of other type of bypass graft(s) of the right leg with ulceration of calf	161	Chronic Ulcer of Skin, Except Pressure		0.515	0.592	0.727	0.583	0.541	0.542	0.294
I70.733	Atherosclerosis of other type of bypass graft(s) of the right leg with ulceration of ankle	106	Atherosclerosis of the Extremities with Ulceration or Gangrene	107,108, 161,189	1.488	1.521	1.724	1.748	1.504	1.525	0.867
I70.733	Atherosclerosis of other type of bypass graft(s) of the right leg with ulceration of ankle	161	Chronic Ulcer of Skin, Except Pressure		0.515	0.592	0.727	0.583	0.541	0.542	0.294
I70.734	Atherosclerosis of other type of bypass graft(s) of the right leg with ulceration of heel and midfoot	106	Atherosclerosis of the Extremities with Ulceration or Gangrene	107,108, 161,189	1.488	1.521	1.724	1.748	1.504	1.525	0.867
I70.734	Atherosclerosis of other type of bypass graft(s) of the right leg with ulceration of heel and midfoot	161	Chronic Ulcer of Skin, Except Pressure		0.515	0.592	0.727	0.583	0.541	0.542	0.294
I70.735	Atherosclerosis of other type of bypass graft(s) of the right leg with ulceration of other part of foot	106	Atherosclerosis of the Extremities with Ulceration or Gangrene	107,108, 161,189	1.488	1.521	1.724	1.748	1.504	1.525	0.867
I70.735	Atherosclerosis of other type of bypass graft(s) of the right leg with ulceration of other part of foot	161	Chronic Ulcer of Skin, Except Pressure		0.515	0.592	0.727	0.583	0.541	0.542	0.294
I70.738	Atherosclerosis of other type of bypass graft(s) of the right leg with ulceration of other part of lower leg	106	Atherosclerosis of the Extremities with Ulceration or Gangrene	107,108, 161,189	1.488	1.521	1.724	1.748	1.504	1.525	0.867
I70.738	Atherosclerosis of other type of bypass graft(s) of the right leg with ulceration of other part of lower leg	161	Chronic Ulcer of Skin, Except Pressure		0.515	0.592	0.727	0.583	0.541	0.542	0.294
I70.739	Atherosclerosis of other type of bypass graft(s) of the right leg with ulceration of unspecified site	106	Atherosclerosis of the Extremities with Ulceration or Gangrene	107,108, 161,189	1.488	1.521	1.724	1.748	1.504	1.525	0.867

ICD-10-CM Code	ICD-10-CM Code Description	V24 CMS-HCC	V24 CMS-HCC Disease Group	V24 CMS-HCC Hierarchies	Community, NonDual, Aged	Community, NonDual, Disabled	Community, FBDual, Aged	Community, FBDual, Disabled	Community, PBDual, Aged	Community, PBDual, Disabled	Institutional
I70.739	Atherosclerosis of other type of bypass graft(s) of the right leg with ulceration of unspecified site	161	Chronic Ulcer of Skin, Except Pressure		0.515	0.592	0.727	0.583	0.541	0.542	0.294
I70.741	Atherosclerosis of other type of bypass graft(s) of the left leg with ulceration of thigh	106	Atherosclerosis of the Extremities with Ulceration or Gangrene	107,108, 161,189	1.488	1.521	1.724	1.748	1.504	1.525	0.867
I70.741	Atherosclerosis of other type of bypass graft(s) of the left leg with ulceration of thigh	161	Chronic Ulcer of Skin, Except Pressure		0.515	0.592	0.727	0.583	0.541	0.542	0.294
I70.742	Atherosclerosis of other type of bypass graft(s) of the left leg with ulceration of calf	106	Atherosclerosis of the Extremities with Ulceration or Gangrene	107,108, 161,189	1.488	1.521	1.724	1.748	1.504	1.525	0.867
I70.742	Atherosclerosis of other type of bypass graft(s) of the left leg with ulceration of calf	161	Chronic Ulcer of Skin, Except Pressure		0.515	0.592	0.727	0.583	0.541	0.542	0.294
I70.743	Atherosclerosis of other type of bypass graft(s) of the left leg with ulceration of ankle	106	Atherosclerosis of the Extremities with Ulceration or Gangrene	107,108, 161,189	1.488	1.521	1.724	1.748	1.504	1.525	0.867
I70.743	Atherosclerosis of other type of bypass graft(s) of the left leg with ulceration of ankle	161	Chronic Ulcer of Skin, Except Pressure		0.515	0.592	0.727	0.583	0.541	0.542	0.294
I70.744	Atherosclerosis of other type of bypass graft(s) of the left leg with ulceration of heel and midfoot	106	Atherosclerosis of the Extremities with Ulceration or Gangrene	107,108, 161,189	1.488	1.521	1.724	1.748	1.504	1.525	0.867
I70.744	Atherosclerosis of other type of bypass graft(s) of the left leg with ulceration of heel and midfoot	161	Chronic Ulcer of Skin, Except Pressure		0.515	0.592	0.727	0.583	0.541	0.542	0.294
I70.745	Atherosclerosis of other type of bypass graft(s) of the left leg with ulceration of other part of foot	106	Atherosclerosis of the Extremities with Ulceration or Gangrene	107,108, 161,189	1.488	1.521	1.724	1.748	1.504	1.525	0.867
I70.745	Atherosclerosis of other type of bypass graft(s) of the left leg with ulceration of other part of foot	161	Chronic Ulcer of Skin, Except Pressure		0.515	0.592	0.727	0.583	0.541	0.542	0.294
I70.748	Atherosclerosis of other type of bypass graft(s) of the left leg with ulceration of other part of lower leg	106	Atherosclerosis of the Extremities with Ulceration or Gangrene	107,108, 161,189	1.488	1.521	1.724	1.748	1.504	1.525	0.867
I70.748	Atherosclerosis of other type of bypass graft(s) of the left leg with ulceration of other part of lower leg	161	Chronic Ulcer of Skin, Except Pressure		0.515	0.592	0.727	0.583	0.541	0.542	0.294
I70.749	Atherosclerosis of other type of bypass graft(s) of the left leg with ulceration of unspecified site	106	Atherosclerosis of the Extremities with Ulceration or Gangrene	107,108, 161,189	1.488	1.521	1.724	1.748	1.504	1.525	0.867
I70.749	Atherosclerosis of other type of bypass graft(s) of the left leg with ulceration of unspecified site	161	Chronic Ulcer of Skin, Except Pressure		0.515	0.592	0.727	0.583	0.541	0.542	0.294
I70.75	Atherosclerosis of other type of bypass graft(s) of other extremity with ulceration	106	Atherosclerosis of the Extremities with Ulceration or Gangrene	107,108, 161,189	1.488	1.521	1.724	1.748	1.504	1.525	0.867
I70.75	Atherosclerosis of other type of bypass graft(s) of other extremity with ulceration	161	Chronic Ulcer of Skin, Except Pressure		0.515	0.592	0.727	0.583	0.541	0.542	0.294
I70.761	Atherosclerosis of other type of bypass graft(s) of the extremities with gangrene, right leg	106	Atherosclerosis of the Extremities with Ulceration or Gangrene	107,108, 161,189	1.488	1.521	1.724	1.748	1.504	1.525	0.867
I70.762	Atherosclerosis of other type of bypass graft(s) of the extremities with gangrene, left leg	106	Atherosclerosis of the Extremities with Ulceration or Gangrene	107,108, 161,189	1.488	1.521	1.724	1.748	1.504	1.525	0.867
I70.763	Atherosclerosis of other type of bypass graft(s) of the extremities with gangrene, bilateral legs	106	Atherosclerosis of the Extremities with Ulceration or Gangrene	107,108, 161,189	1.488	1.521	1.724	1.748	1.504	1.525	0.867

ICD-10-CM Code	ICD-10-CM Code Description	V24 CMS-HCC	V24 CMS-HCC Disease Group	V24 CMS-HCC Hierarchies	Community, NonDual, Aged	Community, NonDual, Disabled	Community, FBDual, Aged	Community, FBDual, Disabled	Community, PBDual, Aged	Community, PBDual, Disabled	Institutional
I70.768	Atherosclerosis of other type of bypass graft(s) of the extremities with gangrene, other extremity	106	Atherosclerosis of the Extremities with Ulceration or Gangrene	107,108, 161,189	1.488	1.521	1.724	1.748	1.504	1.525	0.867
I70.769	Atherosclerosis of other type of bypass graft(s) of the extremities with gangrene, unspecified extremity	106	Atherosclerosis of the Extremities with Ulceration or Gangrene	107,108, 161,189	1.488	1.521	1.724	1.748	1.504	1.525	0.867
I70.791	Other atherosclerosis of other type of bypass graft(s) of the extremities, right leg	108	Vascular Disease		0.288	0.301	0.294	0.267	0.297	0.314	0.093
I70.792	Other atherosclerosis of other type of bypass graft(s) of the extremities, left leg	108	Vascular Disease		0.288	0.301	0.294	0.267	0.297	0.314	0.093
I70.793	Other atherosclerosis of other type of bypass graft(s) of the extremities, bilateral legs	108	Vascular Disease		0.288	0.301	0.294	0.267	0.297	0.314	0.093
I70.798	Other atherosclerosis of other type of bypass graft(s) of the extremities, other extremity	108	Vascular Disease		0.288	0.301	0.294	0.267	0.297	0.314	0.093
I70.799	Other atherosclerosis of other type of bypass graft(s) of the extremities, unspecified extremity	108	Vascular Disease		0.288	0.301	0.294	0.267	0.297	0.314	0.093
I70.92	Chronic total occlusion of artery of the extremities	108	Vascular Disease		0.288	0.301	0.294	0.267	0.297	0.314	0.093
I71.00	Dissection of unspecified site of aorta	107	Vascular Disease with Complications	108	0.383	0.464	0.565	0.653	0.463	0.450	0.299
I71.01	Dissection of thoracic aorta	107	Vascular Disease with Complications	108	0.383	0.464	0.565	0.653	0.463	0.450	0.299
I71.02	Dissection of abdominal aorta	107	Vascular Disease with Complications	108	0.383	0.464	0.565	0.653	0.463	0.450	0.299
I71.03	Dissection of thoracoabdominal aorta	107	Vascular Disease with Complications	108	0.383	0.464	0.565	0.653	0.463	0.450	0.299
I71.1	Thoracic aortic aneurysm, ruptured	107	Vascular Disease with Complications	108	0.383	0.464	0.565	0.653	0.463	0.450	0.299
I71.2	Thoracic aortic aneurysm, without rupture	108	Vascular Disease		0.288	0.301	0.294	0.267	0.297	0.314	0.093
I71.3	Abdominal aortic aneurysm, ruptured	107	Vascular Disease with Complications	108	0.383	0.464	0.565	0.653	0.463	0.450	0.299
I71.4	Abdominal aortic aneurysm, without rupture	108	Vascular Disease		0.288	0.301	0.294	0.267	0.297	0.314	0.093
I71.5	Thoracoabdominal aortic aneurysm, ruptured	107	Vascular Disease with Complications	108	0.383	0.464	0.565	0.653	0.463	0.450	0.299
I71.6	Thoracoabdominal aortic aneurysm, without rupture	108	Vascular Disease		0.288	0.301	0.294	0.267	0.297	0.314	0.093
I71.8	Aortic aneurysm of unspecified site, ruptured	107	Vascular Disease with Complications	108	0.383	0.464	0.565	0.653	0.463	0.450	0.299
I71.9	Aortic aneurysm of unspecified site, without rupture	108	Vascular Disease		0.288	0.301	0.294	0.267	0.297	0.314	0.093
I72.0	Aneurysm of carotid artery	108	Vascular Disease		0.288	0.301	0.294	0.267	0.297	0.314	0.093
I72.1	Aneurysm of artery of upper extremity	108	Vascular Disease		0.288	0.301	0.294	0.267	0.297	0.314	0.093
I72.2	Aneurysm of renal artery	108	Vascular Disease		0.288	0.301	0.294	0.267	0.297	0.314	0.093
I72.3	Aneurysm of iliac artery	108	Vascular Disease		0.288	0.301	0.294	0.267	0.297	0.314	0.093
I72.4	Aneurysm of artery of lower extremity	108	Vascular Disease		0.288	0.301	0.294	0.267	0.297	0.314	0.093
I72.5	Aneurysm of other precerebral arteries	108	Vascular Disease		0.288	0.301	0.294	0.267	0.297	0.314	0.093
I72.6	Aneurysm of vertebral artery	108	Vascular Disease		0.288	0.301	0.294	0.267	0.297	0.314	0.093
I72.8	Aneurysm of other specified arteries	108	Vascular Disease		0.288	0.301	0.294	0.267	0.297	0.314	0.093
I72.9	Aneurysm of unspecified site	108	Vascular Disease		0.288	0.301	0.294	0.267	0.297	0.314	0.093
I73.01	Raynaud's syndrome with gangrene	106	Atherosclerosis of the Extremities with Ulceration or Gangrene	107,108, 161,189	1.488	1.521	1.724	1.748	1.504	1.525	0.867
I73.1	Thromboangiitis obliterans [Buerger's disease]	108	Vascular Disease		0.288	0.301	0.294	0.267	0.297	0.314	0.093
I73.81	Erythromelalgia	108	Vascular Disease		0.288	0.301	0.294	0.267	0.297	0.314	0.093

ICD-10-CM Code	ICD-10-CM Code Description	V24 CMS-HCC	V24 CMS-HCC Disease Group	V24 CMS-HCC Hierarchies	Community, NonDual, Aged	Community, NonDual, Disabled	Community, FBDual, Aged	Community, FBDual, Disabled	Community, PBDual, Aged	Community, PBDual, Disabled	Institutional
I73.89	Other specified peripheral vascular diseases	108	Vascular Disease		0.288	0.301	0.294	0.267	0.297	0.314	0.093
I73.9	Peripheral vascular disease, unspecified	108	Vascular Disease		0.288	0.301	0.294	0.267	0.297	0.314	0.093
I74.01	Saddle embolus of abdominal aorta	107	Vascular Disease with Complications	108	0.383	0.464	0.565	0.653	0.463	0.450	0.299
I74.09	Other arterial embolism and thrombosis of abdominal aorta	107	Vascular Disease with Complications	108	0.383	0.464	0.565	0.653	0.463	0.450	0.299
I74.10	Embolism and thrombosis of unspecified parts of aorta	107	Vascular Disease with Complications	108	0.383	0.464	0.565	0.653	0.463	0.450	0.299
I74.11	Embolism and thrombosis of thoracic aorta	107	Vascular Disease with Complications	108	0.383	0.464	0.565	0.653	0.463	0.450	0.299
I74.19	Embolism and thrombosis of other parts of aorta	107	Vascular Disease with Complications	108	0.383	0.464	0.565	0.653	0.463	0.450	0.299
I74.2	Embolism and thrombosis of arteries of the upper extremities	107	Vascular Disease with Complications	108	0.383	0.464	0.565	0.653	0.463	0.450	0.299
I74.3	Embolism and thrombosis of arteries of the lower extremities	107	Vascular Disease with Complications	108	0.383	0.464	0.565	0.653	0.463	0.450	0.299
I74.4	Embolism and thrombosis of arteries of extremities, unspecified	107	Vascular Disease with Complications	108	0.383	0.464	0.565	0.653	0.463	0.450	0.299
I74.5	Embolism and thrombosis of iliac artery	107	Vascular Disease with Complications	108	0.383	0.464	0.565	0.653	0.463	0.450	0.299
I74.8	Embolism and thrombosis of other arteries	107	Vascular Disease with Complications	108	0.383	0.464	0.565	0.653	0.463	0.450	0.299
I74.9	Embolism and thrombosis of unspecified artery	107	Vascular Disease with Complications	108	0.383	0.464	0.565	0.653	0.463	0.450	0.299
I75.011	Atheroembolism of right upper extremity	107	Vascular Disease with Complications	108	0.383	0.464	0.565	0.653	0.463	0.450	0.299
I75.012	Atheroembolism of left upper extremity	107	Vascular Disease with Complications	108	0.383	0.464	0.565	0.653	0.463	0.450	0.299
I75.013	Atheroembolism of bilateral upper extremities	107	Vascular Disease with Complications	108	0.383	0.464	0.565	0.653	0.463	0.450	0.299
I75.019	Atheroembolism of unspecified upper extremity	107	Vascular Disease with Complications	108	0.383	0.464	0.565	0.653	0.463	0.450	0.299
I75.021	Atheroembolism of right lower extremity	107	Vascular Disease with Complications	108	0.383	0.464	0.565	0.653	0.463	0.450	0.299
I75.022	Atheroembolism of left lower extremity	107	Vascular Disease with Complications	108	0.383	0.464	0.565	0.653	0.463	0.450	0.299
I75.023	Atheroembolism of bilateral lower extremities	107	Vascular Disease with Complications	108	0.383	0.464	0.565	0.653	0.463	0.450	0.299
I75.029	Atheroembolism of unspecified lower extremity	107	Vascular Disease with Complications	108	0.383	0.464	0.565	0.653	0.463	0.450	0.299
I75.81	Atheroembolism of kidney	107	Vascular Disease with Complications	108	0.383	0.464	0.565	0.653	0.463	0.450	0.299
I75.89	Atheroembolism of other site	107	Vascular Disease with Complications	108	0.383	0.464	0.565	0.653	0.463	0.450	0.299
I76	Septic arterial embolism	107	Vascular Disease with Complications	108	0.383	0.464	0.565	0.653	0.463	0.450	0.299
I77.0	Arteriovenous fistula, acquired	108	Vascular Disease		0.288	0.301	0.294	0.267	0.297	0.314	0.093
I77.1	Stricture of artery	108	Vascular Disease		0.288	0.301	0.294	0.267	0.297	0.314	0.093
I77.2	Rupture of artery	108	Vascular Disease		0.288	0.301	0.294	0.267	0.297	0.314	0.093
I77.3	Arterial fibromuscular dysplasia	108	Vascular Disease		0.288	0.301	0.294	0.267	0.297	0.314	0.093
I77.4	Celiac artery compression syndrome	108	Vascular Disease		0.288	0.301	0.294	0.267	0.297	0.314	0.093
I77.5	Necrosis of artery	108	Vascular Disease		0.288	0.301	0.294	0.267	0.297	0.314	0.093
I77.6	Arteritis, unspecified	108	Vascular Disease		0.288	0.301	0.294	0.267	0.297	0.314	0.093
I77.70	Dissection of unspecified artery	107	Vascular Disease with Complications	108	0.383	0.464	0.565	0.653	0.463	0.450	0.299
I77.71	Dissection of carotid artery	107	Vascular Disease with Complications	108	0.383	0.464	0.565	0.653	0.463	0.450	0.299
I77.72	Dissection of iliac artery	107	Vascular Disease with Complications	108	0.383	0.464	0.565	0.653	0.463	0.450	0.299
I77.73	Dissection of renal artery	107	Vascular Disease with Complications	108	0.383	0.464	0.565	0.653	0.463	0.450	0.299
I77.74	Dissection of vertebral artery	107	Vascular Disease with Complications	108	0.383	0.464	0.565	0.653	0.463	0.450	0.299

ICD-10-CM Code	ICD-10-CM Code Description	V24 CMS-HCC	V24 CMS-HCC Disease Group	V24 CMS-HCC Hierarchies	Community, NonDual, Aged	Community, NonDual, Disabled	Community, FBDual, Aged	Community, FBDual, Disabled	Community, PBDual, Aged	Community, PBDual, Disabled	Institutional
I77.75	Dissection of other precerebral arteries	107	Vascular Disease with Complications	108	0.383	0.464	0.565	0.653	0.463	0.450	0.299
I77.76	Dissection of artery of upper extremity	107	Vascular Disease with Complications	108	0.383	0.464	0.565	0.653	0.463	0.450	0.299
I77.77	Dissection of artery of lower extremity	107	Vascular Disease with Complications	108	0.383	0.464	0.565	0.653	0.463	0.450	0.299
I77.79	Dissection of other specified artery	107	Vascular Disease with Complications	108	0.383	0.464	0.565	0.653	0.463	0.450	0.299
I77.810	Thoracic aortic ectasia	108	Vascular Disease		0.288	0.301	0.294	0.267	0.297	0.314	0.093
I77.811	Abdominal aortic ectasia	108	Vascular Disease		0.288	0.301	0.294	0.267	0.297	0.314	0.093
I77.812	Thoracoabdominal aortic ectasia	108	Vascular Disease		0.288	0.301	0.294	0.267	0.297	0.314	0.093
I77.819	Aortic ectasia, unspecified site	108	Vascular Disease		0.288	0.301	0.294	0.267	0.297	0.314	0.093
I77.89	Other specified disorders of arteries and arterioles	108	Vascular Disease		0.288	0.301	0.294	0.267	0.297	0.314	0.093
I77.9	Disorder of arteries and arterioles, unspecified	108	Vascular Disease		0.288	0.301	0.294	0.267	0.297	0.314	0.093
I78.0	Hereditary hemorrhagic telangiectasia	108	Vascular Disease		0.288	0.301	0.294	0.267	0.297	0.314	0.093
I79.0	Aneurysm of aorta in diseases classified elsewhere	108	Vascular Disease		0.288	0.301	0.294	0.267	0.297	0.314	0.093
I79.1	Aortitis in diseases classified elsewhere	108	Vascular Disease		0.288	0.301	0.294	0.267	0.297	0.314	0.093
I79.8	Other disorders of arteries, arterioles and capillaries in diseases classified elsewhere	108	Vascular Disease		0.288	0.301	0.294	0.267	0.297	0.314	0.093
I80.10	Phlebitis and thrombophlebitis of unspecified femoral vein	108	Vascular Disease		0.288	0.301	0.294	0.267	0.297	0.314	0.093
I80.11	Phlebitis and thrombophlebitis of right femoral vein	108	Vascular Disease		0.288	0.301	0.294	0.267	0.297	0.314	0.093
I80.12	Phlebitis and thrombophlebitis of left femoral vein	108	Vascular Disease		0.288	0.301	0.294	0.267	0.297	0.314	0.093
I80.13	Phlebitis and thrombophlebitis of femoral vein, bilateral	108	Vascular Disease		0.288	0.301	0.294	0.267	0.297	0.314	0.093
I80.201	Phlebitis and thrombophlebitis of unspecified deep vessels of right lower extremity	108	Vascular Disease		0.288	0.301	0.294	0.267	0.297	0.314	0.093
I80.202	Phlebitis and thrombophlebitis of unspecified deep vessels of left lower extremity	108	Vascular Disease		0.288	0.301	0.294	0.267	0.297	0.314	0.093
I80.203	Phlebitis and thrombophlebitis of unspecified deep vessels of lower extremities, bilateral	108	Vascular Disease		0.288	0.301	0.294	0.267	0.297	0.314	0.093
I80.209	Phlebitis and thrombophlebitis of unspecified deep vessels of unspecified lower extremity	108	Vascular Disease		0.288	0.301	0.294	0.267	0.297	0.314	0.093
I80.211	Phlebitis and thrombophlebitis of right iliac vein	108	Vascular Disease		0.288	0.301	0.294	0.267	0.297	0.314	0.093
I80.212	Phlebitis and thrombophlebitis of left iliac vein	108	Vascular Disease		0.288	0.301	0.294	0.267	0.297	0.314	0.093
I80.213	Phlebitis and thrombophlebitis of iliac vein, bilateral	108	Vascular Disease		0.288	0.301	0.294	0.267	0.297	0.314	0.093
I80.219	Phlebitis and thrombophlebitis of unspecified iliac vein	108	Vascular Disease		0.288	0.301	0.294	0.267	0.297	0.314	0.093
I80.221	Phlebitis and thrombophlebitis of right popliteal vein	108	Vascular Disease		0.288	0.301	0.294	0.267	0.297	0.314	0.093
I80.222	Phlebitis and thrombophlebitis of left popliteal vein	108	Vascular Disease		0.288	0.301	0.294	0.267	0.297	0.314	0.093
I80.223	Phlebitis and thrombophlebitis of popliteal vein, bilateral	108	Vascular Disease		0.288	0.301	0.294	0.267	0.297	0.314	0.093

ICD-10-CM Code	ICD-10-CM Code Description	V24 CMS-HCC	V24 CMS-HCC Disease Group	V24 CMS-HCC Hierarchies	Community, NonDual, Aged	Community, NonDual, Disabled	Community, FBDual, Aged	Community, FBDual, Disabled	Community, PBDual, Aged	Community, PBDual, Disabled	Institutional
I80.229	Phlebitis and thrombophlebitis of unspecified popliteal vein	108	Vascular Disease		0.288	0.301	0.294	0.267	0.297	0.314	0.093
I80.231	Phlebitis and thrombophlebitis of right tibial vein	108	Vascular Disease		0.288	0.301	0.294	0.267	0.297	0.314	0.093
I80.232	Phlebitis and thrombophlebitis of left tibial vein	108	Vascular Disease		0.288	0.301	0.294	0.267	0.297	0.314	0.093
I80.233	Phlebitis and thrombophlebitis of tibial vein, bilateral	108	Vascular Disease		0.288	0.301	0.294	0.267	0.297	0.314	0.093
I80.239	Phlebitis and thrombophlebitis of unspecified tibial vein	108	Vascular Disease		0.288	0.301	0.294	0.267	0.297	0.314	0.093
I80.241	Phlebitis and thrombophlebitis of right peroneal vein	108	Vascular Disease		0.288	0.301	0.294	0.267	0.297	0.314	0.093
I80.242	Phlebitis and thrombophlebitis of left peroneal vein	108	Vascular Disease		0.288	0.301	0.294	0.267	0.297	0.314	0.093
I80.243	Phlebitis and thrombophlebitis of peroneal vein, bilateral	108	Vascular Disease		0.288	0.301	0.294	0.267	0.297	0.314	0.093
I80.249	Phlebitis and thrombophlebitis of unspecified peroneal vein	108	Vascular Disease		0.288	0.301	0.294	0.267	0.297	0.314	0.093
I80.251	Phlebitis and thrombophlebitis of right calf muscular vein	108	Vascular Disease		0.288	0.301	0.294	0.267	0.297	0.314	0.093
I80.252	Phlebitis and thrombophlebitis of left calf muscular vein	108	Vascular Disease		0.288	0.301	0.294	0.267	0.297	0.314	0.093
I80.253	Phlebitis and thrombophlebitis of calf muscular vein, bilateral	108	Vascular Disease		0.288	0.301	0.294	0.267	0.297	0.314	0.093
I80.259	Phlebitis and thrombophlebitis of unspecified calf muscular vein	108	Vascular Disease		0.288	0.301	0.294	0.267	0.297	0.314	0.093
I80.291	Phlebitis and thrombophlebitis of other deep vessels of right lower extremity	108	Vascular Disease		0.288	0.301	0.294	0.267	0.297	0.314	0.093
I80.292	Phlebitis and thrombophlebitis of other deep vessels of left lower extremity	108	Vascular Disease		0.288	0.301	0.294	0.267	0.297	0.314	0.093
I80.293	Phlebitis and thrombophlebitis of other deep vessels of lower extremity, bilateral	108	Vascular Disease		0.288	0.301	0.294	0.267	0.297	0.314	0.093
I80.299	Phlebitis and thrombophlebitis of other deep vessels of unspecified lower extremity	108	Vascular Disease		0.288	0.301	0.294	0.267	0.297	0.314	0.093
I82.0	Budd-Chiari syndrome	108	Vascular Disease		0.288	0.301	0.294	0.267	0.297	0.314	0.093
I82.210	Acute embolism and thrombosis of superior vena cava	108	Vascular Disease		0.288	0.301	0.294	0.267	0.297	0.314	0.093
I82.211	Chronic embolism and thrombosis of superior vena cava	108	Vascular Disease		0.288	0.301	0.294	0.267	0.297	0.314	0.093
I82.220	Acute embolism and thrombosis of inferior vena cava	108	Vascular Disease		0.288	0.301	0.294	0.267	0.297	0.314	0.093
I82.221	Chronic embolism and thrombosis of inferior vena cava	108	Vascular Disease		0.288	0.301	0.294	0.267	0.297	0.314	0.093
I82.290	Acute embolism and thrombosis of other thoracic veins	108	Vascular Disease		0.288	0.301	0.294	0.267	0.297	0.314	0.093
I82.291	Chronic embolism and thrombosis of other thoracic veins	108	Vascular Disease		0.288	0.301	0.294	0.267	0.297	0.314	0.093
I82.3	Embolism and thrombosis of renal vein	108	Vascular Disease		0.288	0.301	0.294	0.267	0.297	0.314	0.093
I82.401	Acute embolism and thrombosis of unspecified deep veins of right lower extremity	108	Vascular Disease		0.288	0.301	0.294	0.267	0.297	0.314	0.093
I82.402	Acute embolism and thrombosis of unspecified deep veins of left lower extremity	108	Vascular Disease		0.288	0.301	0.294	0.267	0.297	0.314	0.093

ICD-10-CM Code	ICD-10-CM Code Description	V24 CMS-HCC	V24 CMS-HCC Disease Group	V24 CMS-HCC Hierarchies	Community, NonDual, Aged	Community, NonDual, Disabled	Community, FBDual, Aged	Community, FBDual, Disabled	Community, PBDual, Aged	Community, PBDual, Disabled	Institutional
I82.403	Acute embolism and thrombosis of unspecified deep veins of lower extremity, bilateral	108	Vascular Disease		0.288	0.301	0.294	0.267	0.297	0.314	0.093
I82.409	Acute embolism and thrombosis of unspecified deep veins of unspecified lower extremity	108	Vascular Disease		0.288	0.301	0.294	0.267	0.297	0.314	0.093
I82.411	Acute embolism and thrombosis of right femoral vein	108	Vascular Disease		0.288	0.301	0.294	0.267	0.297	0.314	0.093
I82.412	Acute embolism and thrombosis of left femoral vein	108	Vascular Disease		0.288	0.301	0.294	0.267	0.297	0.314	0.093
I82.413	Acute embolism and thrombosis of femoral vein, bilateral	108	Vascular Disease		0.288	0.301	0.294	0.267	0.297	0.314	0.093
I82.419	Acute embolism and thrombosis of unspecified femoral vein	108	Vascular Disease		0.288	0.301	0.294	0.267	0.297	0.314	0.093
I82.421	Acute embolism and thrombosis of right iliac vein	108	Vascular Disease		0.288	0.301	0.294	0.267	0.297	0.314	0.093
I82.422	Acute embolism and thrombosis of left iliac vein	108	Vascular Disease		0.288	0.301	0.294	0.267	0.297	0.314	0.093
I82.423	Acute embolism and thrombosis of iliac vein, bilateral	108	Vascular Disease		0.288	0.301	0.294	0.267	0.297	0.314	0.093
I82.429	Acute embolism and thrombosis of unspecified iliac vein	108	Vascular Disease		0.288	0.301	0.294	0.267	0.297	0.314	0.093
I82.431	Acute embolism and thrombosis of right popliteal vein	108	Vascular Disease		0.288	0.301	0.294	0.267	0.297	0.314	0.093
I82.432	Acute embolism and thrombosis of left popliteal vein	108	Vascular Disease		0.288	0.301	0.294	0.267	0.297	0.314	0.093
I82.433	Acute embolism and thrombosis of popliteal vein, bilateral	108	Vascular Disease		0.288	0.301	0.294	0.267	0.297	0.314	0.093
I82.439	Acute embolism and thrombosis of unspecified popliteal vein	108	Vascular Disease		0.288	0.301	0.294	0.267	0.297	0.314	0.093
I82.441	Acute embolism and thrombosis of right tibial vein	108	Vascular Disease		0.288	0.301	0.294	0.267	0.297	0.314	0.093
I82.442	Acute embolism and thrombosis of left tibial vein	108	Vascular Disease		0.288	0.301	0.294	0.267	0.297	0.314	0.093
I82.443	Acute embolism and thrombosis of tibial vein, bilateral	108	Vascular Disease		0.288	0.301	0.294	0.267	0.297	0.314	0.093
I82.449	Acute embolism and thrombosis of unspecified tibial vein	108	Vascular Disease		0.288	0.301	0.294	0.267	0.297	0.314	0.093
I82.451	Acute embolism and thrombosis of right peroneal vein	108	Vascular Disease		0.288	0.301	0.294	0.267	0.297	0.314	0.093
I82.452	Acute embolism and thrombosis of left peroneal vein	108	Vascular Disease		0.288	0.301	0.294	0.267	0.297	0.314	0.093
I82.453	Acute embolism and thrombosis of peroneal vein, bilateral	108	Vascular Disease		0.288	0.301	0.294	0.267	0.297	0.314	0.093
I82.459	Acute embolism and thrombosis of unspecified peroneal vein	108	Vascular Disease		0.288	0.301	0.294	0.267	0.297	0.314	0.093
I82.461	Acute embolism and thrombosis of right calf muscular vein	108	Vascular Disease		0.288	0.301	0.294	0.267	0.297	0.314	0.093
I82.462	Acute embolism and thrombosis of left calf muscular vein	108	Vascular Disease		0.288	0.301	0.294	0.267	0.297	0.314	0.093
I82.463	Acute embolism and thrombosis of calf muscular vein, bilateral	108	Vascular Disease		0.288	0.301	0.294	0.267	0.297	0.314	0.093
I82.469	Acute embolism and thrombosis of unspecified calf muscular vein	108	Vascular Disease		0.288	0.301	0.294	0.267	0.297	0.314	0.093
I82.491	Acute embolism and thrombosis of other specified deep vein of right lower extremity	108	Vascular Disease		0.288	0.301	0.294	0.267	0.297	0.314	0.093

ICD-10-CM Code	ICD-10-CM Code Description	V24 CMS-HCC	V24 CMS-HCC Disease Group	V24 CMS-HCC Hierarchies	Community, NonDual, Aged	Community, NonDual, Disabled	Community, FBDual, Aged	Community, FBDual, Disabled	Community, PBDual, Aged	Community, PBDual, Disabled	Institutional
I82.492	Acute embolism and thrombosis of other specified deep vein of left lower extremity	108	Vascular Disease		0.288	0.301	0.294	0.267	0.297	0.314	0.093
I82.493	Acute embolism and thrombosis of other specified deep vein of lower extremity, bilateral	108	Vascular Disease		0.288	0.301	0.294	0.267	0.297	0.314	0.093
I82.499	Acute embolism and thrombosis of other specified deep vein of unspecified lower extremity	108	Vascular Disease		0.288	0.301	0.294	0.267	0.297	0.314	0.093
I82.4Y1	Acute embolism and thrombosis of unspecified deep veins of right proximal lower extremity	108	Vascular Disease		0.288	0.301	0.294	0.267	0.297	0.314	0.093
I82.4Y2	Acute embolism and thrombosis of unspecified deep veins of left proximal lower extremity	108	Vascular Disease		0.288	0.301	0.294	0.267	0.297	0.314	0.093
I82.4Y3	Acute embolism and thrombosis of unspecified deep veins of proximal lower extremity, bilateral	108	Vascular Disease		0.288	0.301	0.294	0.267	0.297	0.314	0.093
I82.4Y9	Acute embolism and thrombosis of unspecified deep veins of unspecified proximal lower extremity	108	Vascular Disease		0.288	0.301	0.294	0.267	0.297	0.314	0.093
I82.4Z1	Acute embolism and thrombosis of unspecified deep veins of right distal lower extremity	108	Vascular Disease		0.288	0.301	0.294	0.267	0.297	0.314	0.093
I82.4Z2	Acute embolism and thrombosis of unspecified deep veins of left distal lower extremity	108	Vascular Disease		0.288	0.301	0.294	0.267	0.297	0.314	0.093
I82.4Z3	Acute embolism and thrombosis of unspecified deep veins of distal lower extremity, bilateral	108	Vascular Disease		0.288	0.301	0.294	0.267	0.297	0.314	0.093
I82.4Z9	Acute embolism and thrombosis of unspecified deep veins of unspecified distal lower extremity	108	Vascular Disease		0.288	0.301	0.294	0.267	0.297	0.314	0.093
I82.501	Chronic embolism and thrombosis of unspecified deep veins of right lower extremity	108	Vascular Disease		0.288	0.301	0.294	0.267	0.297	0.314	0.093
I82.502	Chronic embolism and thrombosis of unspecified deep veins of left lower extremity	108	Vascular Disease		0.288	0.301	0.294	0.267	0.297	0.314	0.093
I82.503	Chronic embolism and thrombosis of unspecified deep veins of lower extremity, bilateral	108	Vascular Disease		0.288	0.301	0.294	0.267	0.297	0.314	0.093
I82.509	Chronic embolism and thrombosis of unspecified deep veins of unspecified lower extremity	108	Vascular Disease		0.288	0.301	0.294	0.267	0.297	0.314	0.093
I82.511	Chronic embolism and thrombosis of right femoral vein	108	Vascular Disease		0.288	0.301	0.294	0.267	0.297	0.314	0.093
I82.512	Chronic embolism and thrombosis of left femoral vein	108	Vascular Disease		0.288	0.301	0.294	0.267	0.297	0.314	0.093
I82.513	Chronic embolism and thrombosis of femoral vein, bilateral	108	Vascular Disease		0.288	0.301	0.294	0.267	0.297	0.314	0.093
I82.519	Chronic embolism and thrombosis of unspecified femoral vein	108	Vascular Disease		0.288	0.301	0.294	0.267	0.297	0.314	0.093
I82.521	Chronic embolism and thrombosis of right iliac vein	108	Vascular Disease		0.288	0.301	0.294	0.267	0.297	0.314	0.093
I82.522	Chronic embolism and thrombosis of left iliac vein	108	Vascular Disease		0.288	0.301	0.294	0.267	0.297	0.314	0.093
I82.523	Chronic embolism and thrombosis of iliac vein, bilateral	108	Vascular Disease		0.288	0.301	0.294	0.267	0.297	0.314	0.093
I82.529	Chronic embolism and thrombosis of unspecified iliac vein	108	Vascular Disease		0.288	0.301	0.294	0.267	0.297	0.314	0.093

ICD-10-CM Code	ICD-10-CM Code Description	V24 CMS-HCC	V24 CMS-HCC Disease Group	V24 CMS-HCC Hierarchies	Community, NonDual, Aged	Community, NonDual, Disabled	Community, FBDual, Aged	Community, FBDual, Disabled	Community, PBDual, Aged	Community, PBDual, Disabled	Institutional
I82.531	Chronic embolism and thrombosis of right popliteal vein	108	Vascular Disease		0.288	0.301	0.294	0.267	0.297	0.314	0.093
I82.532	Chronic embolism and thrombosis of left popliteal vein	108	Vascular Disease		0.288	0.301	0.294	0.267	0.297	0.314	0.093
I82.533	Chronic embolism and thrombosis of popliteal vein, bilateral	108	Vascular Disease		0.288	0.301	0.294	0.267	0.297	0.314	0.093
I82.539	Chronic embolism and thrombosis of unspecified popliteal vein	108	Vascular Disease		0.288	0.301	0.294	0.267	0.297	0.314	0.093
I82.541	Chronic embolism and thrombosis of right tibial vein	108	Vascular Disease		0.288	0.301	0.294	0.267	0.297	0.314	0.093
I82.542	Chronic embolism and thrombosis of left tibial vein	108	Vascular Disease		0.288	0.301	0.294	0.267	0.297	0.314	0.093
I82.543	Chronic embolism and thrombosis of tibial vein, bilateral	108	Vascular Disease		0.288	0.301	0.294	0.267	0.297	0.314	0.093
I82.549	Chronic embolism and thrombosis of unspecified tibial vein	108	Vascular Disease		0.288	0.301	0.294	0.267	0.297	0.314	0.093
I82.551	Chronic embolism and thrombosis of right peroneal vein	108	Vascular Disease		0.288	0.301	0.294	0.267	0.297	0.314	0.093
I82.552	Chronic embolism and thrombosis of left peroneal vein	108	Vascular Disease		0.288	0.301	0.294	0.267	0.297	0.314	0.093
I82.553	Chronic embolism and thrombosis of peroneal vein, bilateral	108	Vascular Disease		0.288	0.301	0.294	0.267	0.297	0.314	0.093
I82.559	Chronic embolism and thrombosis of unspecified peroneal vein	108	Vascular Disease		0.288	0.301	0.294	0.267	0.297	0.314	0.093
I82.561	Chronic embolism and thrombosis of right calf muscular vein	108	Vascular Disease		0.288	0.301	0.294	0.267	0.297	0.314	0.093
I82.562	Chronic embolism and thrombosis of left calf muscular vein	108	Vascular Disease		0.288	0.301	0.294	0.267	0.297	0.314	0.093
I82.563	Chronic embolism and thrombosis of calf muscular vein, bilateral	108	Vascular Disease		0.288	0.301	0.294	0.267	0.297	0.314	0.093
I82.569	Chronic embolism and thrombosis of unspecified calf muscular vein	108	Vascular Disease		0.288	0.301	0.294	0.267	0.297	0.314	0.093
I82.591	Chronic embolism and thrombosis of other specified deep vein of right lower extremity	108	Vascular Disease		0.288	0.301	0.294	0.267	0.297	0.314	0.093
I82.592	Chronic embolism and thrombosis of other specified deep vein of left lower extremity	108	Vascular Disease		0.288	0.301	0.294	0.267	0.297	0.314	0.093
I82.593	Chronic embolism and thrombosis of other specified deep vein of lower extremity, bilateral	108	Vascular Disease		0.288	0.301	0.294	0.267	0.297	0.314	0.093
I82.599	Chronic embolism and thrombosis of other specified deep vein of unspecified lower extremity	108	Vascular Disease		0.288	0.301	0.294	0.267	0.297	0.314	0.093
I82.5Y1	Chronic embolism and thrombosis of unspecified deep veins of right proximal lower extremity	108	Vascular Disease		0.288	0.301	0.294	0.267	0.297	0.314	0.093
I82.5Y2	Chronic embolism and thrombosis of unspecified deep veins of left proximal lower extremity	108	Vascular Disease		0.288	0.301	0.294	0.267	0.297	0.314	0.093
I82.5Y3	Chronic embolism and thrombosis of unspecified deep veins of proximal lower extremity, bilateral	108	Vascular Disease		0.288	0.301	0.294	0.267	0.297	0.314	0.093
I82.5Y9	Chronic embolism and thrombosis of unspecified deep veins of unspecified proximal lower extremity	108	Vascular Disease		0.288	0.301	0.294	0.267	0.297	0.314	0.093
I82.5Z1	Chronic embolism and thrombosis of unspecified deep veins of right distal lower extremity	108	Vascular Disease		0.288	0.301	0.294	0.267	0.297	0.314	0.093

ICD-10-CM Code	ICD-10-CM Code Description	V24 CMS-HCC	V24 CMS-HCC Disease Group	V24 CMS-HCC Hierarchies	Community, NonDual, Aged	Community, NonDual, Disabled	Community, FBDual, Aged	Community, FBDual, Disabled	Community, PBDual, Aged	Community, PBDual, Disabled	Institutional
I82.5Z2	Chronic embolism and thrombosis of unspecified deep veins of left distal lower extremity	108	Vascular Disease		0.288	0.301	0.294	0.267	0.297	0.314	0.093
I82.5Z3	Chronic embolism and thrombosis of unspecified deep veins of distal lower extremity, bilateral	108	Vascular Disease		0.288	0.301	0.294	0.267	0.297	0.314	0.093
I82.5Z9	Chronic embolism and thrombosis of unspecified deep veins of unspecified distal lower extremity	108	Vascular Disease		0.288	0.301	0.294	0.267	0.297	0.314	0.093
I82.621	Acute embolism and thrombosis of deep veins of right upper extremity	108	Vascular Disease		0.288	0.301	0.294	0.267	0.297	0.314	0.093
I82.622	Acute embolism and thrombosis of deep veins of left upper extremity	108	Vascular Disease		0.288	0.301	0.294	0.267	0.297	0.314	0.093
I82.623	Acute embolism and thrombosis of deep veins of upper extremity, bilateral	108	Vascular Disease		0.288	0.301	0.294	0.267	0.297	0.314	0.093
I82.629	Acute embolism and thrombosis of deep veins of unspecified upper extremity	108	Vascular Disease		0.288	0.301	0.294	0.267	0.297	0.314	0.093
I82.721	Chronic embolism and thrombosis of deep veins of right upper extremity	108	Vascular Disease		0.288	0.301	0.294	0.267	0.297	0.314	0.093
I82.722	Chronic embolism and thrombosis of deep veins of left upper extremity	108	Vascular Disease		0.288	0.301	0.294	0.267	0.297	0.314	0.093
I82.723	Chronic embolism and thrombosis of deep veins of upper extremity, bilateral	108	Vascular Disease		0.288	0.301	0.294	0.267	0.297	0.314	0.093
I82.729	Chronic embolism and thrombosis of deep veins of unspecified upper extremity	108	Vascular Disease		0.288	0.301	0.294	0.267	0.297	0.314	0.093
I82.A11	Acute embolism and thrombosis of right axillary vein	108	Vascular Disease		0.288	0.301	0.294	0.267	0.297	0.314	0.093
I82.A12	Acute embolism and thrombosis of left axillary vein	108	Vascular Disease		0.288	0.301	0.294	0.267	0.297	0.314	0.093
I82.A13	Acute embolism and thrombosis of axillary vein, bilateral	108	Vascular Disease		0.288	0.301	0.294	0.267	0.297	0.314	0.093
I82.A19	Acute embolism and thrombosis of unspecified axillary vein	108	Vascular Disease		0.288	0.301	0.294	0.267	0.297	0.314	0.093
I82.A21	Chronic embolism and thrombosis of right axillary vein	108	Vascular Disease		0.288	0.301	0.294	0.267	0.297	0.314	0.093
I82.A22	Chronic embolism and thrombosis of left axillary vein	108	Vascular Disease		0.288	0.301	0.294	0.267	0.297	0.314	0.093
I82.A23	Chronic embolism and thrombosis of axillary vein, bilateral	108	Vascular Disease		0.288	0.301	0.294	0.267	0.297	0.314	0.093
I82.A29	Chronic embolism and thrombosis of unspecified axillary vein	108	Vascular Disease		0.288	0.301	0.294	0.267	0.297	0.314	0.093
I82.B11	Acute embolism and thrombosis of right subclavian vein	108	Vascular Disease		0.288	0.301	0.294	0.267	0.297	0.314	0.093
I82.B12	Acute embolism and thrombosis of left subclavian vein	108	Vascular Disease		0.288	0.301	0.294	0.267	0.297	0.314	0.093
I82.B13	Acute embolism and thrombosis of subclavian vein, bilateral	108	Vascular Disease		0.288	0.301	0.294	0.267	0.297	0.314	0.093
I82.B19	Acute embolism and thrombosis of unspecified subclavian vein	108	Vascular Disease		0.288	0.301	0.294	0.267	0.297	0.314	0.093
I82.B21	Chronic embolism and thrombosis of right subclavian vein	108	Vascular Disease		0.288	0.301	0.294	0.267	0.297	0.314	0.093
I82.B22	Chronic embolism and thrombosis of left subclavian vein	108	Vascular Disease		0.288	0.301	0.294	0.267	0.297	0.314	0.093
I82.B23	Chronic embolism and thrombosis of subclavian vein, bilateral	108	Vascular Disease		0.288	0.301	0.294	0.267	0.297	0.314	0.093

ICD-10-CM Code	ICD-10-CM Code Description	V24 CMS-HCC	V24 CMS-HCC Disease Group	V24 CMS-HCC Hierarchies	Community, NonDual, Aged	Community, NonDual, Disabled	Community, FBDual, Aged	Community, FBDual, Disabled	Community, PBDual, Aged	Community, PBDual, Disabled	Institutional
I82.B29	Chronic embolism and thrombosis of unspecified subclavian vein	108	Vascular Disease		0.288	0.301	0.294	0.267	0.297	0.314	0.093
I82.C11	Acute embolism and thrombosis of right internal jugular vein	108	Vascular Disease		0.288	0.301	0.294	0.267	0.297	0.314	0.093
I82.C12	Acute embolism and thrombosis of left internal jugular vein	108	Vascular Disease		0.288	0.301	0.294	0.267	0.297	0.314	0.093
I82.C13	Acute embolism and thrombosis of internal jugular vein, bilateral	108	Vascular Disease		0.288	0.301	0.294	0.267	0.297	0.314	0.093
I82.C19	Acute embolism and thrombosis of unspecified internal jugular vein	108	Vascular Disease		0.288	0.301	0.294	0.267	0.297	0.314	0.093
I82.C21	Chronic embolism and thrombosis of right internal jugular vein	108	Vascular Disease		0.288	0.301	0.294	0.267	0.297	0.314	0.093
I82.C22	Chronic embolism and thrombosis of left internal jugular vein	108	Vascular Disease		0.288	0.301	0.294	0.267	0.297	0.314	0.093
I82.C23	Chronic embolism and thrombosis of internal jugular vein, bilateral	108	Vascular Disease		0.288	0.301	0.294	0.267	0.297	0.314	0.093
I82.C29	Chronic embolism and thrombosis of unspecified internal jugular vein	108	Vascular Disease		0.288	0.301	0.294	0.267	0.297	0.314	0.093
I83.001	Varicose veins of unspecified lower extremity with ulcer of thigh	107	Vascular Disease with Complications	108	0.383	0.464	0.565	0.653	0.463	0.450	0.299
I83.002	Varicose veins of unspecified lower extremity with ulcer of calf	107	Vascular Disease with Complications	108	0.383	0.464	0.565	0.653	0.463	0.450	0.299
I83.003	Varicose veins of unspecified lower extremity with ulcer of ankle	107	Vascular Disease with Complications	108	0.383	0.464	0.565	0.653	0.463	0.450	0.299
I83.004	Varicose veins of unspecified lower extremity with ulcer of heel and midfoot	107	Vascular Disease with Complications	108	0.383	0.464	0.565	0.653	0.463	0.450	0.299
I83.005	Varicose veins of unspecified lower extremity with ulcer other part of foot	107	Vascular Disease with Complications	108	0.383	0.464	0.565	0.653	0.463	0.450	0.299
I83.008	Varicose veins of unspecified lower extremity with ulcer other part of lower leg	107	Vascular Disease with Complications	108	0.383	0.464	0.565	0.653	0.463	0.450	0.299
I83.009	Varicose veins of unspecified lower extremity with ulcer of unspecified site	107	Vascular Disease with Complications	108	0.383	0.464	0.565	0.653	0.463	0.450	0.299
I83.011	Varicose veins of right lower extremity with ulcer of thigh	107	Vascular Disease with Complications	108	0.383	0.464	0.565	0.653	0.463	0.450	0.299
I83.012	Varicose veins of right lower extremity with ulcer of calf	107	Vascular Disease with Complications	108	0.383	0.464	0.565	0.653	0.463	0.450	0.299
I83.013	Varicose veins of right lower extremity with ulcer of ankle	107	Vascular Disease with Complications	108	0.383	0.464	0.565	0.653	0.463	0.450	0.299
I83.014	Varicose veins of right lower extremity with ulcer of heel and midfoot	107	Vascular Disease with Complications	108	0.383	0.464	0.565	0.653	0.463	0.450	0.299
I83.015	Varicose veins of right lower extremity with ulcer other part of foot	107	Vascular Disease with Complications	108	0.383	0.464	0.565	0.653	0.463	0.450	0.299
I83.018	Varicose veins of right lower extremity with ulcer other part of lower leg	107	Vascular Disease with Complications	108	0.383	0.464	0.565	0.653	0.463	0.450	0.299
I83.019	Varicose veins of right lower extremity with ulcer of unspecified site	107	Vascular Disease with Complications	108	0.383	0.464	0.565	0.653	0.463	0.450	0.299
I83.021	Varicose veins of left lower extremity with ulcer of thigh	107	Vascular Disease with Complications	108	0.383	0.464	0.565	0.653	0.463	0.450	0.299
I83.022	Varicose veins of left lower extremity with ulcer of calf	107	Vascular Disease with Complications	108	0.383	0.464	0.565	0.653	0.463	0.450	0.299
I83.023	Varicose veins of left lower extremity with ulcer of ankle	107	Vascular Disease with Complications	108	0.383	0.464	0.565	0.653	0.463	0.450	0.299

ICD-10-CM Code	ICD-10-CM Code Description	V24 CMS-HCC	V24 CMS-HCC Disease Group	V24 CMS-HCC Hierarchies	Community, NonDual, Aged	Community, NonDual, Disabled	Community, FBDual, Aged	Community, FBDual, Disabled	Community, PBDual, Aged	Community, PBDual, Disabled	Institutional
I83.024	Varicose veins of left lower extremity with ulcer of heel and midfoot	107	Vascular Disease with Complications	108	0.383	0.464	0.565	0.653	0.463	0.450	0.299
I83.025	Varicose veins of left lower extremity with ulcer other part of foot	107	Vascular Disease with Complications	108	0.383	0.464	0.565	0.653	0.463	0.450	0.299
I83.028	Varicose veins of left lower extremity with ulcer other part of lower leg	107	Vascular Disease with Complications	108	0.383	0.464	0.565	0.653	0.463	0.450	0.299
I83.029	Varicose veins of left lower extremity with ulcer of unspecified site	107	Vascular Disease with Complications	108	0.383	0.464	0.565	0.653	0.463	0.450	0.299
I83.201	Varicose veins of unspecified lower extremity with both ulcer of thigh and inflammation	107	Vascular Disease with Complications	108	0.383	0.464	0.565	0.653	0.463	0.450	0.299
I83.202	Varicose veins of unspecified lower extremity with both ulcer of calf and inflammation	107	Vascular Disease with Complications	108	0.383	0.464	0.565	0.653	0.463	0.450	0.299
I83.203	Varicose veins of unspecified lower extremity with both ulcer of ankle and inflammation	107	Vascular Disease with Complications	108	0.383	0.464	0.565	0.653	0.463	0.450	0.299
I83.204	Varicose veins of unspecified lower extremity with both ulcer of heel and midfoot and inflammation	107	Vascular Disease with Complications	108	0.383	0.464	0.565	0.653	0.463	0.450	0.299
I83.205	Varicose veins of unspecified lower extremity with both ulcer other part of foot and inflammation	107	Vascular Disease with Complications	108	0.383	0.464	0.565	0.653	0.463	0.450	0.299
I83.208	Varicose veins of unspecified lower extremity with both ulcer of other part of lower extremity and inflammation	107	Vascular Disease with Complications	108	0.383	0.464	0.565	0.653	0.463	0.450	0.299
I83.209	Varicose veins of unspecified lower extremity with both ulcer of unspecified site and inflammation	107	Vascular Disease with Complications	108	0.383	0.464	0.565	0.653	0.463	0.450	0.299
I83.211	Varicose veins of right lower extremity with both ulcer of thigh and inflammation	107	Vascular Disease with Complications	108	0.383	0.464	0.565	0.653	0.463	0.450	0.299
I83.212	Varicose veins of right lower extremity with both ulcer of calf and inflammation	107	Vascular Disease with Complications	108	0.383	0.464	0.565	0.653	0.463	0.450	0.299
I83.213	Varicose veins of right lower extremity with both ulcer of ankle and inflammation	107	Vascular Disease with Complications	108	0.383	0.464	0.565	0.653	0.463	0.450	0.299
I83.214	Varicose veins of right lower extremity with both ulcer of heel and midfoot and inflammation	107	Vascular Disease with Complications	108	0.383	0.464	0.565	0.653	0.463	0.450	0.299
I83.215	Varicose veins of right lower extremity with both ulcer other part of foot and inflammation	107	Vascular Disease with Complications	108	0.383	0.464	0.565	0.653	0.463	0.450	0.299
I83.218	Varicose veins of right lower extremity with both ulcer of other part of lower extremity and inflammation	107	Vascular Disease with Complications	108	0.383	0.464	0.565	0.653	0.463	0.450	0.299
I83.219	Varicose veins of right lower extremity with both ulcer of unspecified site and inflammation	107	Vascular Disease with Complications	108	0.383	0.464	0.565	0.653	0.463	0.450	0.299
I83.221	Varicose veins of left lower extremity with both ulcer of thigh and inflammation	107	Vascular Disease with Complications	108	0.383	0.464	0.565	0.653	0.463	0.450	0.299
I83.222	Varicose veins of left lower extremity with both ulcer of calf and inflammation	107	Vascular Disease with Complications	108	0.383	0.464	0.565	0.653	0.463	0.450	0.299
I83.223	Varicose veins of left lower extremity with both ulcer of ankle and inflammation	107	Vascular Disease with Complications	108	0.383	0.464	0.565	0.653	0.463	0.450	0.299

ICD-10-CM Code	ICD-10-CM Code Description	V24 CMS-HCC	V24 CMS-HCC Disease Group	V24 CMS-HCC Hierarchies	Community, NonDual, Aged	Community, NonDual, Disabled	Community, FBDual, Aged	Community, FBDual, Disabled	Community, PBDual, Aged	Community, PBDual, Disabled	Institutional
I83.224	Varicose veins of left lower extremity with both ulcer of heel and midfoot and inflammation	107	Vascular Disease with Complications	108	0.383	0.464	0.565	0.653	0.463	0.450	0.299
I83.225	Varicose veins of left lower extremity with both ulcer other part of foot and inflammation	107	Vascular Disease with Complications	108	0.383	0.464	0.565	0.653	0.463	0.450	0.299
I83.228	Varicose veins of left lower extremity with both ulcer of other part of lower extremity and inflammation	107	Vascular Disease with Complications	108	0.383	0.464	0.565	0.653	0.463	0.450	0.299
I83.229	Varicose veins of left lower extremity with both ulcer of unspecified site and inflammation	107	Vascular Disease with Complications	108	0.383	0.464	0.565	0.653	0.463	0.450	0.299
I85.00	Esophageal varices without bleeding	27	End-Stage Liver Disease	28,29,80	0.882	1.065	1.111	1.101	0.729	0.887	0.874
I85.01	Esophageal varices with bleeding	27	End-Stage Liver Disease	28,29,80	0.882	1.065	1.111	1.101	0.729	0.887	0.874
I85.10	Secondary esophageal varices without bleeding	27	End-Stage Liver Disease	28,29,80	0.882	1.065	1.111	1.101	0.729	0.887	0.874
I85.11	Secondary esophageal varices with bleeding	27	End-Stage Liver Disease	28,29,80	0.882	1.065	1.111	1.101	0.729	0.887	0.874
I87.011	Postthrombotic syndrome with ulcer of right lower extremity	107	Vascular Disease with Complications	108	0.383	0.464	0.565	0.653	0.463	0.450	0.299
I87.012	Postthrombotic syndrome with ulcer of left lower extremity	107	Vascular Disease with Complications	108	0.383	0.464	0.565	0.653	0.463	0.450	0.299
I87.013	Postthrombotic syndrome with ulcer of bilateral lower extremity	107	Vascular Disease with Complications	108	0.383	0.464	0.565	0.653	0.463	0.450	0.299
I87.019	Postthrombotic syndrome with ulcer of unspecified lower extremity	107	Vascular Disease with Complications	108	0.383	0.464	0.565	0.653	0.463	0.450	0.299
I87.031	Postthrombotic syndrome with ulcer and inflammation of right lower extremity	107	Vascular Disease with Complications	108	0.383	0.464	0.565	0.653	0.463	0.450	0.299
I87.032	Postthrombotic syndrome with ulcer and inflammation of left lower extremity	107	Vascular Disease with Complications	108	0.383	0.464	0.565	0.653	0.463	0.450	0.299
I87.033	Postthrombotic syndrome with ulcer and inflammation of bilateral lower extremity	107	Vascular Disease with Complications	108	0.383	0.464	0.565	0.653	0.463	0.450	0.299
I87.039	Postthrombotic syndrome with ulcer and inflammation of unspecified lower extremity	107	Vascular Disease with Complications	108	0.383	0.464	0.565	0.653	0.463	0.450	0.299
I87.311	Chronic venous hypertension (idiopathic) with ulcer of right lower extremity	107	Vascular Disease with Complications	108	0.383	0.464	0.565	0.653	0.463	0.450	0.299
I87.312	Chronic venous hypertension (idiopathic) with ulcer of left lower extremity	107	Vascular Disease with Complications	108	0.383	0.464	0.565	0.653	0.463	0.450	0.299
I87.313	Chronic venous hypertension (idiopathic) with ulcer of bilateral lower extremity	107	Vascular Disease with Complications	108	0.383	0.464	0.565	0.653	0.463	0.450	0.299
I87.319	Chronic venous hypertension (idiopathic) with ulcer of unspecified lower extremity	107	Vascular Disease with Complications	108	0.383	0.464	0.565	0.653	0.463	0.450	0.299
I87.331	Chronic venous hypertension (idiopathic) with ulcer and inflammation of right lower extremity	107	Vascular Disease with Complications	108	0.383	0.464	0.565	0.653	0.463	0.450	0.299
I87.332	Chronic venous hypertension (idiopathic) with ulcer and inflammation of left lower extremity	107	Vascular Disease with Complications	108	0.383	0.464	0.565	0.653	0.463	0.450	0.299
I87.333	Chronic venous hypertension (idiopathic) with ulcer and inflammation of bilateral lower extremity	107	Vascular Disease with Complications	108	0.383	0.464	0.565	0.653	0.463	0.450	0.299

ICD-10-CM Code	ICD-10-CM Code Description	V24 CMS-HCC	V24 CMS-HCC Disease Group	V24 CMS-HCC Hierarchies	Community, NonDual, Aged	Community, NonDual, Disabled	Community, FBDual, Aged	Community, FBDual, Disabled	Community, PBDual, Aged	Community, PBDual, Disabled	Institutional
I87.339	Chronic venous hypertension (idiopathic) with ulcer and inflammation of unspecified lower extremity	107	Vascular Disease with Complications	108	0.383	0.464	0.565	0.653	0.463	0.450	0.299
I96	Gangrene, not elsewhere classified	106	Atherosclerosis of the Extremities with Ulceration or Gangrene	107,108, 161,189	1.488	1.521	1.724	1.748	1.504	1.525	0.867
I97.810	Intraoperative cerebrovascular infarction during cardiac surgery	100	Ischemic or Unspecified Stroke		0.230	0.146	0.380	0.324	0.230	0.163	0.111
I97.811	Intraoperative cerebrovascular infarction during other surgery	100	Ischemic or Unspecified Stroke		0.230	0.146	0.380	0.324	0.230	0.163	0.111
I97.820	Postprocedural cerebrovascular infarction following cardiac surgery	100	Ischemic or Unspecified Stroke		0.230	0.146	0.380	0.324	0.230	0.163	0.111
I97.821	Postprocedural cerebrovascular infarction following other surgery	100	Ischemic or Unspecified Stroke		0.230	0.146	0.380	0.324	0.230	0.163	0.111
J13	Pneumonia due to Streptococcus pneumoniae	115	Pneumococcal Pneumonia, Empyema, Lung Abscess		0.130	—	0.258	—	0.093	0.082	0.156
J14	Pneumonia due to Hemophilus influenzae	115	Pneumococcal Pneumonia, Empyema, Lung Abscess		0.130	—	0.258	—	0.093	0.082	0.156
J15.0	Pneumonia due to Klebsiella pneumoniae	114	Aspiration and Specified Bacterial Pneumonias	115	0.517	0.236	0.641	0.375	0.514	0.198	0.156
J15.1	Pneumonia due to Pseudomonas	114	Aspiration and Specified Bacterial Pneumonias	115	0.517	0.236	0.641	0.375	0.514	0.198	0.156
J15.20	Pneumonia due to staphylococcus, unspecified	114	Aspiration and Specified Bacterial Pneumonias	115	0.517	0.236	0.641	0.375	0.514	0.198	0.156
J15.211	Pneumonia due to Methicillin susceptible Staphylococcus aureus	114	Aspiration and Specified Bacterial Pneumonias	115	0.517	0.236	0.641	0.375	0.514	0.198	0.156
J15.212	Pneumonia due to Methicillin resistant Staphylococcus aureus	114	Aspiration and Specified Bacterial Pneumonias	115	0.517	0.236	0.641	0.375	0.514	0.198	0.156
J15.29	Pneumonia due to other staphylococcus	114	Aspiration and Specified Bacterial Pneumonias	115	0.517	0.236	0.641	0.375	0.514	0.198	0.156
J15.3	Pneumonia due to streptococcus, group B	115	Pneumococcal Pneumonia, Empyema, Lung Abscess		0.130	—	0.258	—	0.093	0.082	0.156
J15.4	Pneumonia due to other streptococci	115	Pneumococcal Pneumonia, Empyema, Lung Abscess		0.130	—	0.258	—	0.093	0.082	0.156
J15.5	Pneumonia due to Escherichia coli	114	Aspiration and Specified Bacterial Pneumonias	115	0.517	0.236	0.641	0.375	0.514	0.198	0.156
J15.6	Pneumonia due to other Gram-negative bacteria	114	Aspiration and Specified Bacterial Pneumonias	115	0.517	0.236	0.641	0.375	0.514	0.198	0.156
J15.8	Pneumonia due to other specified bacteria	114	Aspiration and Specified Bacterial Pneumonias	115	0.517	0.236	0.641	0.375	0.514	0.198	0.156
J18.1	Lobar pneumonia, unspecified organism	115	Pneumococcal Pneumonia, Empyema, Lung Abscess		0.130	—	0.258	—	0.093	0.082	0.156
J41.0	Simple chronic bronchitis	111	Chronic Obstructive Pulmonary Disease	112	0.335	0.246	0.430	0.331	0.358	0.267	0.311
J41.1	Mucopurulent chronic bronchitis	111	Chronic Obstructive Pulmonary Disease	112	0.335	0.246	0.430	0.331	0.358	0.267	0.311
J41.8	Mixed simple and mucopurulent chronic bronchitis	111	Chronic Obstructive Pulmonary Disease	112	0.335	0.246	0.430	0.331	0.358	0.267	0.311
J42	Unspecified chronic bronchitis	111	Chronic Obstructive Pulmonary Disease	112	0.335	0.246	0.430	0.331	0.358	0.267	0.311
J43.0	Unilateral pulmonary emphysema [MacLeod's syndrome]	111	Chronic Obstructive Pulmonary Disease	112	0.335	0.246	0.430	0.331	0.358	0.267	0.311
J43.1	Panlobular emphysema	111	Chronic Obstructive Pulmonary Disease	112	0.335	0.246	0.430	0.331	0.358	0.267	0.311
J43.2	Centrilobular emphysema	111	Chronic Obstructive Pulmonary Disease	112	0.335	0.246	0.430	0.331	0.358	0.267	0.311
J43.8	Other emphysema	111	Chronic Obstructive Pulmonary Disease	112	0.335	0.246	0.430	0.331	0.358	0.267	0.311

ICD-10-CM Code	ICD-10-CM Code Description	V24 CMS-HCC	V24 CMS-HCC Disease Group	V24 CMS-HCC Hierarchies	Community, NonDual, Aged	Community, NonDual, Disabled	Community, FBDual, Aged	Community, FBDual, Disabled	Community, PBDual, Aged	Community, PBDual, Disabled	Institutional
J43.9	Emphysema, unspecified	111	Chronic Obstructive Pulmonary Disease	112	0.335	0.246	0.430	0.331	0.358	0.267	0.311
J44.0	Chronic obstructive pulmonary disease with (acute) lower respiratory infection	111	Chronic Obstructive Pulmonary Disease	112	0.335	0.246	0.430	0.331	0.358	0.267	0.311
J44.1	Chronic obstructive pulmonary disease with (acute) exacerbation	111	Chronic Obstructive Pulmonary Disease	112	0.335	0.246	0.430	0.331	0.358	0.267	0.311
J44.9	Chronic obstructive pulmonary disease, unspecified	111	Chronic Obstructive Pulmonary Disease	112	0.335	0.246	0.430	0.331	0.358	0.267	0.311
J47.0	Bronchiectasis with acute lower respiratory infection	112	Fibrosis of Lung and Other Chronic Lung Disorders		0.219	0.237	0.161	0.275	0.200	0.229	0.110
J47.1	Bronchiectasis with (acute) exacerbation	112	Fibrosis of Lung and Other Chronic Lung Disorders		0.219	0.237	0.161	0.275	0.200	0.229	0.110
J47.9	Bronchiectasis, uncomplicated	112	Fibrosis of Lung and Other Chronic Lung Disorders		0.219	0.237	0.161	0.275	0.200	0.229	0.110
J60	Coalworker's pneumoconiosis	112	Fibrosis of Lung and Other Chronic Lung Disorders		0.219	0.237	0.161	0.275	0.200	0.229	0.110
J61	Pneumoconiosis due to asbestos and other mineral fibers	112	Fibrosis of Lung and Other Chronic Lung Disorders		0.219	0.237	0.161	0.275	0.200	0.229	0.110
J62.0	Pneumoconiosis due to talc dust	112	Fibrosis of Lung and Other Chronic Lung Disorders		0.219	0.237	0.161	0.275	0.200	0.229	0.110
J62.8	Pneumoconiosis due to other dust containing silica	112	Fibrosis of Lung and Other Chronic Lung Disorders		0.219	0.237	0.161	0.275	0.200	0.229	0.110
J63.0	Aluminosis (of lung)	112	Fibrosis of Lung and Other Chronic Lung Disorders		0.219	0.237	0.161	0.275	0.200	0.229	0.110
J63.1	Bauxite fibrosis (of lung)	112	Fibrosis of Lung and Other Chronic Lung Disorders		0.219	0.237	0.161	0.275	0.200	0.229	0.110
J63.2	Berylliosis	112	Fibrosis of Lung and Other Chronic Lung Disorders		0.219	0.237	0.161	0.275	0.200	0.229	0.110
J63.3	Graphite fibrosis (of lung)	112	Fibrosis of Lung and Other Chronic Lung Disorders		0.219	0.237	0.161	0.275	0.200	0.229	0.110
J63.4	Siderosis	112	Fibrosis of Lung and Other Chronic Lung Disorders		0.219	0.237	0.161	0.275	0.200	0.229	0.110
J63.5	Stannosis	112	Fibrosis of Lung and Other Chronic Lung Disorders		0.219	0.237	0.161	0.275	0.200	0.229	0.110
J63.6	Pneumoconiosis due to other specified inorganic dusts	112	Fibrosis of Lung and Other Chronic Lung Disorders		0.219	0.237	0.161	0.275	0.200	0.229	0.110
J64	Unspecified pneumoconiosis	112	Fibrosis of Lung and Other Chronic Lung Disorders		0.219	0.237	0.161	0.275	0.200	0.229	0.110
J65	Pneumoconiosis associated with tuberculosis	112	Fibrosis of Lung and Other Chronic Lung Disorders		0.219	0.237	0.161	0.275	0.200	0.229	0.110
J66.0	Byssinosis	112	Fibrosis of Lung and Other Chronic Lung Disorders		0.219	0.237	0.161	0.275	0.200	0.229	0.110
J66.1	Flax-dressers' disease	112	Fibrosis of Lung and Other Chronic Lung Disorders		0.219	0.237	0.161	0.275	0.200	0.229	0.110
J66.2	Cannabinosis	112	Fibrosis of Lung and Other Chronic Lung Disorders		0.219	0.237	0.161	0.275	0.200	0.229	0.110
J66.8	Airway disease due to other specific organic dusts	112	Fibrosis of Lung and Other Chronic Lung Disorders		0.219	0.237	0.161	0.275	0.200	0.229	0.110
J67.0	Farmer's lung	112	Fibrosis of Lung and Other Chronic Lung Disorders		0.219	0.237	0.161	0.275	0.200	0.229	0.110
J67.1	Bagassosis	112	Fibrosis of Lung and Other Chronic Lung Disorders		0.219	0.237	0.161	0.275	0.200	0.229	0.110
J67.2	Bird fancier's lung	112	Fibrosis of Lung and Other Chronic Lung Disorders		0.219	0.237	0.161	0.275	0.200	0.229	0.110
J67.3	Suberosis	112	Fibrosis of Lung and Other Chronic Lung Disorders		0.219	0.237	0.161	0.275	0.200	0.229	0.110
J67.4	Maltworker's lung	112	Fibrosis of Lung and Other Chronic Lung Disorders		0.219	0.237	0.161	0.275	0.200	0.229	0.110

ICD-10-CM Code	ICD-10-CM Code Description	V24 CMS-HCC	V24 CMS-HCC Disease Group	V24 CMS-HCC Hierarchies	Community, NonDual, Aged	Community, NonDual, Disabled	Community, FBDual, Aged	Community, FBDual, Disabled	Community, PBDual, Aged	Community, PBDual, Disabled	Institutional
J67.5	Mushroom-worker's lung	112	Fibrosis of Lung and Other Chronic Lung Disorders		0.219	0.237	0.161	0.275	0.200	0.229	0.110
J67.6	Maple-bark-stripper's lung	112	Fibrosis of Lung and Other Chronic Lung Disorders		0.219	0.237	0.161	0.275	0.200	0.229	0.110
J67.7	Air conditioner and humidifier lung	112	Fibrosis of Lung and Other Chronic Lung Disorders		0.219	0.237	0.161	0.275	0.200	0.229	0.110
J67.8	Hypersensitivity pneumonitis due to other organic dusts	112	Fibrosis of Lung and Other Chronic Lung Disorders		0.219	0.237	0.161	0.275	0.200	0.229	0.110
J67.9	Hypersensitivity pneumonitis due to unspecified organic dust	112	Fibrosis of Lung and Other Chronic Lung Disorders		0.219	0.237	0.161	0.275	0.200	0.229	0.110
J68.Ø	Bronchitis and pneumonitis due to chemicals, gases, fumes and vapors	112	Fibrosis of Lung and Other Chronic Lung Disorders		0.219	0.237	0.161	0.275	0.200	0.229	0.110
J68.1	Pulmonary edema due to chemicals, gases, fumes and vapors	112	Fibrosis of Lung and Other Chronic Lung Disorders		0.219	0.237	0.161	0.275	0.200	0.229	0.110
J68.2	Upper respiratory inflammation due to chemicals, gases, fumes and vapors, not elsewhere classified	112	Fibrosis of Lung and Other Chronic Lung Disorders		0.219	0.237	0.161	0.275	0.200	0.229	0.110
J68.3	Other acute and subacute respiratory conditions due to chemicals, gases, fumes and vapors	112	Fibrosis of Lung and Other Chronic Lung Disorders		0.219	0.237	0.161	0.275	0.200	0.229	0.110
J68.4	Chronic respiratory conditions due to chemicals, gases, fumes and vapors	112	Fibrosis of Lung and Other Chronic Lung Disorders		0.219	0.237	0.161	0.275	0.200	0.229	0.110
J68.8	Other respiratory conditions due to chemicals, gases, fumes and vapors	112	Fibrosis of Lung and Other Chronic Lung Disorders		0.219	0.237	0.161	0.275	0.200	0.229	0.110
J68.9	Unspecified respiratory condition due to chemicals, gases, fumes and vapors	112	Fibrosis of Lung and Other Chronic Lung Disorders		0.219	0.237	0.161	0.275	0.200	0.229	0.110
J69.Ø	Pneumonitis due to inhalation of food and vomit	114	Aspiration and Specified Bacterial Pneumonias	115	0.517	0.236	0.641	0.375	0.514	0.198	0.156
J69.1	Pneumonitis due to inhalation of oils and essences	114	Aspiration and Specified Bacterial Pneumonias	115	0.517	0.236	0.641	0.375	0.514	0.198	0.156
J69.8	Pneumonitis due to inhalation of other solids and liquids	114	Aspiration and Specified Bacterial Pneumonias	115	0.517	0.236	0.641	0.375	0.514	0.198	0.156
J70.Ø	Acute pulmonary manifestations due to radiation	112	Fibrosis of Lung and Other Chronic Lung Disorders		0.219	0.237	0.161	0.275	0.200	0.229	0.110
J70.1	Chronic and other pulmonary manifestations due to radiation	112	Fibrosis of Lung and Other Chronic Lung Disorders		0.219	0.237	0.161	0.275	0.200	0.229	0.110
J70.2	Acute drug-induced interstitial lung disorders	112	Fibrosis of Lung and Other Chronic Lung Disorders		0.219	0.237	0.161	0.275	0.200	0.229	0.110
J70.3	Chronic drug-induced interstitial lung disorders	112	Fibrosis of Lung and Other Chronic Lung Disorders		0.219	0.237	0.161	0.275	0.200	0.229	0.110
J70.4	Drug-induced interstitial lung disorders, unspecified	112	Fibrosis of Lung and Other Chronic Lung Disorders		0.219	0.237	0.161	0.275	0.200	0.229	0.110
J70.5	Respiratory conditions due to smoke inhalation	112	Fibrosis of Lung and Other Chronic Lung Disorders		0.219	0.237	0.161	0.275	0.200	0.229	0.110
J70.8	Respiratory conditions due to other specified external agents	112	Fibrosis of Lung and Other Chronic Lung Disorders		0.219	0.237	0.161	0.275	0.200	0.229	0.110
J70.9	Respiratory conditions due to unspecified external agent	112	Fibrosis of Lung and Other Chronic Lung Disorders		0.219	0.237	0.161	0.275	0.200	0.229	0.110
J8Ø	Acute respiratory distress syndrome	84	Cardio-Respiratory Failure and Shock		0.282	0.385	0.492	0.531	0.361	0.343	0.313
J81.Ø	Acute pulmonary edema	84	Cardio-Respiratory Failure and Shock		0.282	0.385	0.492	0.531	0.361	0.343	0.313
J82.81	Chronic eosinophilic pneumonia	111	Chronic Obstructive Pulmonary Disease	112	0.335	0.246	0.430	0.331	0.358	0.267	0.311
J82.89	Other pulmonary eosinophilia, not elsewhere classified	112	Fibrosis of Lung and Other Chronic Lung Disorders		0.219	0.237	0.161	0.275	0.200	0.229	0.110
J84.Ø1	Alveolar proteinosis	112	Fibrosis of Lung and Other Chronic Lung Disorders		0.219	0.237	0.161	0.275	0.200	0.229	0.110
J84.Ø2	Pulmonary alveolar microlithiasis	112	Fibrosis of Lung and Other Chronic Lung Disorders		0.219	0.237	0.161	0.275	0.200	0.229	0.110

ICD-10-CM Code	ICD-10-CM Code Description	V24 CMS-HCC	V24 CMS-HCC Disease Group	V24 CMS-HCC Hierarchies	Community, NonDual, Aged	Community, NonDual, Disabled	Community, FBDual, Aged	Community, FBDual, Disabled	Community, PBDual, Aged	Community, PBDual, Disabled	Institutional
J84.Ø3	Idiopathic pulmonary hemosiderosis	112	Fibrosis of Lung and Other Chronic Lung Disorders		0.219	0.237	0.161	0.275	0.200	0.229	0.110
J84.Ø9	Other alveolar and parieto-alveolar conditions	112	Fibrosis of Lung and Other Chronic Lung Disorders		0.219	0.237	0.161	0.275	0.200	0.229	0.110
J84.1Ø	Pulmonary fibrosis, unspecified	112	Fibrosis of Lung and Other Chronic Lung Disorders		0.219	0.237	0.161	0.275	0.200	0.229	0.110
J84.111	Idiopathic interstitial pneumonia, not otherwise specified	112	Fibrosis of Lung and Other Chronic Lung Disorders		0.219	0.237	0.161	0.275	0.200	0.229	0.110
J84.112	Idiopathic pulmonary fibrosis	112	Fibrosis of Lung and Other Chronic Lung Disorders		0.219	0.237	0.161	0.275	0.200	0.229	0.110
J84.113	Idiopathic non-specific interstitial pneumonitis	112	Fibrosis of Lung and Other Chronic Lung Disorders		0.219	0.237	0.161	0.275	0.200	0.229	0.110
J84.114	Acute interstitial pneumonitis	112	Fibrosis of Lung and Other Chronic Lung Disorders		0.219	0.237	0.161	0.275	0.200	0.229	0.110
J84.115	Respiratory bronchiolitis interstitial lung disease	112	Fibrosis of Lung and Other Chronic Lung Disorders		0.219	0.237	0.161	0.275	0.200	0.229	0.110
J84.116	Cryptogenic organizing pneumonia	112	Fibrosis of Lung and Other Chronic Lung Disorders		0.219	0.237	0.161	0.275	0.200	0.229	0.110
J84.117	Desquamative interstitial pneumonia	112	Fibrosis of Lung and Other Chronic Lung Disorders		0.219	0.237	0.161	0.275	0.200	0.229	0.110
J84.17Ø	Interstitial lung disease with progressive fibrotic phenotype in diseases classified elsewhere	112	Fibrosis of Lung and Other Chronic Lung Disorders		0.219	0.237	0.161	0.275	0.200	0.229	0.110
J84.178	Other interstitial pulmonary diseases with fibrosis in diseases classified elsewhere	112	Fibrosis of Lung and Other Chronic Lung Disorders		0.219	0.237	0.161	0.275	0.200	0.229	0.110
J84.2	Lymphoid interstitial pneumonia	112	Fibrosis of Lung and Other Chronic Lung Disorders		0.219	0.237	0.161	0.275	0.200	0.229	0.110
J84.81	Lymphangioleiomyomatosis	112	Fibrosis of Lung and Other Chronic Lung Disorders		0.219	0.237	0.161	0.275	0.200	0.229	0.110
J84.82	Adult pulmonary Langerhans cell histiocytosis	112	Fibrosis of Lung and Other Chronic Lung Disorders		0.219	0.237	0.161	0.275	0.200	0.229	0.110
J84.83	Surfactant mutations of the lung	112	Fibrosis of Lung and Other Chronic Lung Disorders		0.219	0.237	0.161	0.275	0.200	0.229	0.110
J84.841	Neuroendocrine cell hyperplasia of infancy	112	Fibrosis of Lung and Other Chronic Lung Disorders		0.219	0.237	0.161	0.275	0.200	0.229	0.110
J84.842	Pulmonary interstitial glycogenosis	112	Fibrosis of Lung and Other Chronic Lung Disorders		0.219	0.237	0.161	0.275	0.200	0.229	0.110
J84.843	Alveolar capillary dysplasia with vein misalignment	112	Fibrosis of Lung and Other Chronic Lung Disorders		0.219	0.237	0.161	0.275	0.200	0.229	0.110
J84.848	Other interstitial lung diseases of childhood	112	Fibrosis of Lung and Other Chronic Lung Disorders		0.219	0.237	0.161	0.275	0.200	0.229	0.110
J84.89	Other specified interstitial pulmonary diseases	112	Fibrosis of Lung and Other Chronic Lung Disorders		0.219	0.237	0.161	0.275	0.200	0.229	0.110
J84.9	Interstitial pulmonary disease, unspecified	112	Fibrosis of Lung and Other Chronic Lung Disorders		0.219	0.237	0.161	0.275	0.200	0.229	0.110
J85.Ø	Gangrene and necrosis of lung	115	Pneumococcal Pneumonia, Empyema, Lung Abscess		0.130	—	0.258	—	0.093	0.082	0.156
J85.1	Abscess of lung with pneumonia	115	Pneumococcal Pneumonia, Empyema, Lung Abscess		0.130	—	0.258	—	0.093	0.082	0.156
J85.2	Abscess of lung without pneumonia	115	Pneumococcal Pneumonia, Empyema, Lung Abscess		0.130	—	0.258	—	0.093	0.082	0.156
J85.3	Abscess of mediastinum	115	Pneumococcal Pneumonia, Empyema, Lung Abscess		0.130	—	0.258	—	0.093	0.082	0.156
J86.Ø	Pyothorax with fistula	115	Pneumococcal Pneumonia, Empyema, Lung Abscess		0.130	—	0.258	—	0.093	0.082	0.156
J86.9	Pyothorax without fistula	115	Pneumococcal Pneumonia, Empyema, Lung Abscess		0.130	—	0.258	—	0.093	0.082	0.156

ICD-10-CM Code	ICD-10-CM Code Description	V24 CMS-HCC	V24 CMS-HCC Disease Group	V24 CMS-HCC Hierarchies	Community, NonDual, Aged	Community, NonDual, Disabled	Community, FBDual, Aged	Community, FBDual, Disabled	Community, PBDual, Aged	Community, PBDual, Disabled	Institutional
J95.00	Unspecified tracheostomy complication	82	Respirator Dependence/Tracheostomy Status	83,84	1.000	0.781	2.183	1.465	0.836	0.769	1.622
J95.01	Hemorrhage from tracheostomy stoma	82	Respirator Dependence/Tracheostomy Status	83,84	1.000	0.781	2.183	1.465	0.836	0.769	1.622
J95.02	Infection of tracheostomy stoma	82	Respirator Dependence/Tracheostomy Status	83,84	1.000	0.781	2.183	1.465	0.836	0.769	1.622
J95.03	Malfunction of tracheostomy stoma	82	Respirator Dependence/Tracheostomy Status	83,84	1.000	0.781	2.183	1.465	0.836	0.769	1.622
J95.04	Tracheo-esophageal fistula following tracheostomy	82	Respirator Dependence/Tracheostomy Status	83,84	1.000	0.781	2.183	1.465	0.836	0.769	1.622
J95.09	Other tracheostomy complication	82	Respirator Dependence/Tracheostomy Status	83,84	1.000	0.781	2.183	1.465	0.836	0.769	1.622
J95.1	Acute pulmonary insufficiency following thoracic surgery	84	Cardio-Respiratory Failure and Shock		0.282	0.385	0.492	0.531	0.361	0.343	0.313
J95.2	Acute pulmonary insufficiency following nonthoracic surgery	84	Cardio-Respiratory Failure and Shock		0.282	0.385	0.492	0.531	0.361	0.343	0.313
J95.3	Chronic pulmonary insufficiency following surgery	84	Cardio-Respiratory Failure and Shock		0.282	0.385	0.492	0.531	0.361	0.343	0.313
J95.821	Acute postprocedural respiratory failure	84	Cardio-Respiratory Failure and Shock		0.282	0.385	0.492	0.531	0.361	0.343	0.313
J95.822	Acute and chronic postprocedural respiratory failure	84	Cardio-Respiratory Failure and Shock		0.282	0.385	0.492	0.531	0.361	0.343	0.313
J95.850	Mechanical complication of respirator	82	Respirator Dependence/Tracheostomy Status	83,84	1.000	0.781	2.183	1.465	0.836	0.769	1.622
J95.851	Ventilator associated pneumonia	114	Aspiration and Specified Bacterial Pneumonias	115	0.517	0.236	0.641	0.375	0.514	0.198	0.156
J95.859	Other complication of respirator [ventilator]	82	Respirator Dependence/Tracheostomy Status	83,84	1.000	0.781	2.183	1.465	0.836	0.769	1.622
J96.00	Acute respiratory failure, unspecified whether with hypoxia or hypercapnia	84	Cardio-Respiratory Failure and Shock		0.282	0.385	0.492	0.531	0.361	0.343	0.313
J96.01	Acute respiratory failure with hypoxia	84	Cardio-Respiratory Failure and Shock		0.282	0.385	0.492	0.531	0.361	0.343	0.313
J96.02	Acute respiratory failure with hypercapnia	84	Cardio-Respiratory Failure and Shock		0.282	0.385	0.492	0.531	0.361	0.343	0.313
J96.10	Chronic respiratory failure, unspecified whether with hypoxia or hypercapnia	84	Cardio-Respiratory Failure and Shock		0.282	0.385	0.492	0.531	0.361	0.343	0.313
J96.11	Chronic respiratory failure with hypoxia	84	Cardio-Respiratory Failure and Shock		0.282	0.385	0.492	0.531	0.361	0.343	0.313
J96.12	Chronic respiratory failure with hypercapnia	84	Cardio-Respiratory Failure and Shock		0.282	0.385	0.492	0.531	0.361	0.343	0.313
J96.20	Acute and chronic respiratory failure, unspecified whether with hypoxia or hypercapnia	84	Cardio-Respiratory Failure and Shock		0.282	0.385	0.492	0.531	0.361	0.343	0.313
J96.21	Acute and chronic respiratory failure with hypoxia	84	Cardio-Respiratory Failure and Shock		0.282	0.385	0.492	0.531	0.361	0.343	0.313
J96.22	Acute and chronic respiratory failure with hypercapnia	84	Cardio-Respiratory Failure and Shock		0.282	0.385	0.492	0.531	0.361	0.343	0.313
J96.90	Respiratory failure, unspecified, unspecified whether with hypoxia or hypercapnia	84	Cardio-Respiratory Failure and Shock		0.282	0.385	0.492	0.531	0.361	0.343	0.313
J96.91	Respiratory failure, unspecified with hypoxia	84	Cardio-Respiratory Failure and Shock		0.282	0.385	0.492	0.531	0.361	0.343	0.313
J96.92	Respiratory failure, unspecified with hypercapnia	84	Cardio-Respiratory Failure and Shock		0.282	0.385	0.492	0.531	0.361	0.343	0.313
J98.2	Interstitial emphysema	111	Chronic Obstructive Pulmonary Disease	112	0.335	0.246	0.430	0.331	0.358	0.267	0.311
J98.3	Compensatory emphysema	111	Chronic Obstructive Pulmonary Disease	112	0.335	0.246	0.430	0.331	0.358	0.267	0.311

ICD-10-CM Code	ICD-10-CM Code Description	V24 CMS-HCC	V24 CMS-HCC Disease Group	V24 CMS-HCC Hierarchies	Community, NonDual, Aged	Community, NonDual, Disabled	Community, FBDual, Aged	Community, FBDual, Disabled	Community, PBDual, Aged	Community, PBDual, Disabled	Institutional
J99	Respiratory disorders in diseases classified elsewhere	112	Fibrosis of Lung and Other Chronic Lung Disorders		0.219	0.237	0.161	0.275	0.200	0.229	0.110
K25.1	Acute gastric ulcer with perforation	33	Intestinal Obstruction/Perforation		0.219	0.503	0.258	0.538	0.232	0.552	0.352
K25.2	Acute gastric ulcer with both hemorrhage and perforation	33	Intestinal Obstruction/Perforation		0.219	0.503	0.258	0.538	0.232	0.552	0.352
K25.5	Chronic or unspecified gastric ulcer with perforation	33	Intestinal Obstruction/Perforation		0.219	0.503	0.258	0.538	0.232	0.552	0.352
K25.6	Chronic or unspecified gastric ulcer with both hemorrhage and perforation	33	Intestinal Obstruction/Perforation		0.219	0.503	0.258	0.538	0.232	0.552	0.352
K26.1	Acute duodenal ulcer with perforation	33	Intestinal Obstruction/Perforation		0.219	0.503	0.258	0.538	0.232	0.552	0.352
K26.2	Acute duodenal ulcer with both hemorrhage and perforation	33	Intestinal Obstruction/Perforation		0.219	0.503	0.258	0.538	0.232	0.552	0.352
K26.5	Chronic or unspecified duodenal ulcer with perforation	33	Intestinal Obstruction/Perforation		0.219	0.503	0.258	0.538	0.232	0.552	0.352
K26.6	Chronic or unspecified duodenal ulcer with both hemorrhage and perforation	33	Intestinal Obstruction/Perforation		0.219	0.503	0.258	0.538	0.232	0.552	0.352
K27.1	Acute peptic ulcer, site unspecified, with perforation	33	Intestinal Obstruction/Perforation		0.219	0.503	0.258	0.538	0.232	0.552	0.352
K27.2	Acute peptic ulcer, site unspecified, with both hemorrhage and perforation	33	Intestinal Obstruction/Perforation		0.219	0.503	0.258	0.538	0.232	0.552	0.352
K27.5	Chronic or unspecified peptic ulcer, site unspecified, with perforation	33	Intestinal Obstruction/Perforation		0.219	0.503	0.258	0.538	0.232	0.552	0.352
K27.6	Chronic or unspecified peptic ulcer, site unspecified, with both hemorrhage and perforation	33	Intestinal Obstruction/Perforation		0.219	0.503	0.258	0.538	0.232	0.552	0.352
K28.1	Acute gastrojejunal ulcer with perforation	33	Intestinal Obstruction/Perforation		0.219	0.503	0.258	0.538	0.232	0.552	0.352
K28.2	Acute gastrojejunal ulcer with both hemorrhage and perforation	33	Intestinal Obstruction/Perforation		0.219	0.503	0.258	0.538	0.232	0.552	0.352
K28.5	Chronic or unspecified gastrojejunal ulcer with perforation	33	Intestinal Obstruction/Perforation		0.219	0.503	0.258	0.538	0.232	0.552	0.352
K28.6	Chronic or unspecified gastrojejunal ulcer with both hemorrhage and perforation	33	Intestinal Obstruction/Perforation		0.219	0.503	0.258	0.538	0.232	0.552	0.352
K50.00	Crohn's disease of small intestine without complications	35	Inflammatory Bowel Disease		0.308	0.523	0.275	0.551	0.275	0.543	0.355
K50.011	Crohn's disease of small intestine with rectal bleeding	35	Inflammatory Bowel Disease		0.308	0.523	0.275	0.551	0.275	0.543	0.355
K50.012	Crohn's disease of small intestine with intestinal obstruction	33	Intestinal Obstruction/Perforation		0.219	0.503	0.258	0.538	0.232	0.552	0.352
K50.012	Crohn's disease of small intestine with intestinal obstruction	35	Inflammatory Bowel Disease		0.308	0.523	0.275	0.551	0.275	0.543	0.355
K50.013	Crohn's disease of small intestine with fistula	35	Inflammatory Bowel Disease		0.308	0.523	0.275	0.551	0.275	0.543	0.355
K50.014	Crohn's disease of small intestine with abscess	35	Inflammatory Bowel Disease		0.308	0.523	0.275	0.551	0.275	0.543	0.355
K50.018	Crohn's disease of small intestine with other complication	35	Inflammatory Bowel Disease		0.308	0.523	0.275	0.551	0.275	0.543	0.355
K50.019	Crohn's disease of small intestine with unspecified complications	35	Inflammatory Bowel Disease		0.308	0.523	0.275	0.551	0.275	0.543	0.355
K50.10	Crohn's disease of large intestine without complications	35	Inflammatory Bowel Disease		0.308	0.523	0.275	0.551	0.275	0.543	0.355
K50.111	Crohn's disease of large intestine with rectal bleeding	35	Inflammatory Bowel Disease		0.308	0.523	0.275	0.551	0.275	0.543	0.355

ICD-10-CM Code	ICD-10-CM Code Description	V24 CMS-HCC	V24 CMS-HCC Disease Group	V24 CMS-HCC Hierarchies	Community, NonDual, Aged	Community, NonDual, Disabled	Community, FBDual, Aged	Community, FBDual, Disabled	Community, PBDual, Aged	Community, PBDual, Disabled	Institutional
K50.112	Crohn's disease of large intestine with intestinal obstruction	33	Intestinal Obstruction/Perforation		0.219	0.503	0.258	0.538	0.232	0.552	0.352
K50.112	Crohn's disease of large intestine with intestinal obstruction	35	Inflammatory Bowel Disease		0.308	0.523	0.275	0.551	0.275	0.543	0.355
K50.113	Crohn's disease of large intestine with fistula	35	Inflammatory Bowel Disease		0.308	0.523	0.275	0.551	0.275	0.543	0.355
K50.114	Crohn's disease of large intestine with abscess	35	Inflammatory Bowel Disease		0.308	0.523	0.275	0.551	0.275	0.543	0.355
K50.118	Crohn's disease of large intestine with other complication	35	Inflammatory Bowel Disease		0.308	0.523	0.275	0.551	0.275	0.543	0.355
K50.119	Crohn's disease of large intestine with unspecified complications	35	Inflammatory Bowel Disease		0.308	0.523	0.275	0.551	0.275	0.543	0.355
K50.80	Crohn's disease of both small and large intestine without complications	35	Inflammatory Bowel Disease		0.308	0.523	0.275	0.551	0.275	0.543	0.355
K50.811	Crohn's disease of both small and large intestine with rectal bleeding	35	Inflammatory Bowel Disease		0.308	0.523	0.275	0.551	0.275	0.543	0.355
K50.812	Crohn's disease of both small and large intestine with intestinal obstruction	33	Intestinal Obstruction/Perforation		0.219	0.503	0.258	0.538	0.232	0.552	0.352
K50.812	Crohn's disease of both small and large intestine with intestinal obstruction	35	Inflammatory Bowel Disease		0.308	0.523	0.275	0.551	0.275	0.543	0.355
K50.813	Crohn's disease of both small and large intestine with fistula	35	Inflammatory Bowel Disease		0.308	0.523	0.275	0.551	0.275	0.543	0.355
K50.814	Crohn's disease of both small and large intestine with abscess	35	Inflammatory Bowel Disease		0.308	0.523	0.275	0.551	0.275	0.543	0.355
K50.818	Crohn's disease of both small and large intestine with other complication	35	Inflammatory Bowel Disease		0.308	0.523	0.275	0.551	0.275	0.543	0.355
K50.819	Crohn's disease of both small and large intestine with unspecified complications	35	Inflammatory Bowel Disease		0.308	0.523	0.275	0.551	0.275	0.543	0.355
K50.90	Crohn's disease, unspecified, without complications	35	Inflammatory Bowel Disease		0.308	0.523	0.275	0.551	0.275	0.543	0.355
K50.911	Crohn's disease, unspecified, with rectal bleeding	35	Inflammatory Bowel Disease		0.308	0.523	0.275	0.551	0.275	0.543	0.355
K50.912	Crohn's disease, unspecified, with intestinal obstruction	33	Intestinal Obstruction/Perforation		0.219	0.503	0.258	0.538	0.232	0.552	0.352
K50.912	Crohn's disease, unspecified, with intestinal obstruction	35	Inflammatory Bowel Disease		0.308	0.523	0.275	0.551	0.275	0.543	0.355
K50.913	Crohn's disease, unspecified, with fistula	35	Inflammatory Bowel Disease		0.308	0.523	0.275	0.551	0.275	0.543	0.355
K50.914	Crohn's disease, unspecified, with abscess	35	Inflammatory Bowel Disease		0.308	0.523	0.275	0.551	0.275	0.543	0.355
K50.918	Crohn's disease, unspecified, with other complication	35	Inflammatory Bowel Disease		0.308	0.523	0.275	0.551	0.275	0.543	0.355
K50.919	Crohn's disease, unspecified, with unspecified complications	35	Inflammatory Bowel Disease		0.308	0.523	0.275	0.551	0.275	0.543	0.355
K51.00	Ulcerative (chronic) pancolitis without complications	35	Inflammatory Bowel Disease		0.308	0.523	0.275	0.551	0.275	0.543	0.355
K51.011	Ulcerative (chronic) pancolitis with rectal bleeding	35	Inflammatory Bowel Disease		0.308	0.523	0.275	0.551	0.275	0.543	0.355
K51.012	Ulcerative (chronic) pancolitis with intestinal obstruction	33	Intestinal Obstruction/Perforation		0.219	0.503	0.258	0.538	0.232	0.552	0.352
K51.012	Ulcerative (chronic) pancolitis with intestinal obstruction	35	Inflammatory Bowel Disease		0.308	0.523	0.275	0.551	0.275	0.543	0.355
K51.013	Ulcerative (chronic) pancolitis with fistula	35	Inflammatory Bowel Disease		0.308	0.523	0.275	0.551	0.275	0.543	0.355

ICD-10-CM Code	ICD-10-CM Code Description	V24 CMS-HCC	V24 CMS-HCC Disease Group	V24 CMS-HCC Hierarchies	Community, NonDual, Aged	Community, NonDual, Disabled	Community, FBDual, Aged	Community, FBDual, Disabled	Community, PBDual, Aged	Community, PBDual, Disabled	Institutional
K51.014	Ulcerative (chronic) pancolitis with abscess	35	Inflammatory Bowel Disease		0.308	0.523	0.275	0.551	0.275	0.543	0.355
K51.018	Ulcerative (chronic) pancolitis with other complication	35	Inflammatory Bowel Disease		0.308	0.523	0.275	0.551	0.275	0.543	0.355
K51.019	Ulcerative (chronic) pancolitis with unspecified complications	35	Inflammatory Bowel Disease		0.308	0.523	0.275	0.551	0.275	0.543	0.355
K51.20	Ulcerative (chronic) proctitis without complications	35	Inflammatory Bowel Disease		0.308	0.523	0.275	0.551	0.275	0.543	0.355
K51.211	Ulcerative (chronic) proctitis with rectal bleeding	35	Inflammatory Bowel Disease		0.308	0.523	0.275	0.551	0.275	0.543	0.355
K51.212	Ulcerative (chronic) proctitis with intestinal obstruction	33	Intestinal Obstruction/Perforation		0.219	0.503	0.258	0.538	0.232	0.552	0.352
K51.212	Ulcerative (chronic) proctitis with intestinal obstruction	35	Inflammatory Bowel Disease		0.308	0.523	0.275	0.551	0.275	0.543	0.355
K51.213	Ulcerative (chronic) proctitis with fistula	35	Inflammatory Bowel Disease		0.308	0.523	0.275	0.551	0.275	0.543	0.355
K51.214	Ulcerative (chronic) proctitis with abscess	35	Inflammatory Bowel Disease		0.308	0.523	0.275	0.551	0.275	0.543	0.355
K51.218	Ulcerative (chronic) proctitis with other complication	35	Inflammatory Bowel Disease		0.308	0.523	0.275	0.551	0.275	0.543	0.355
K51.219	Ulcerative (chronic) proctitis with unspecified complications	35	Inflammatory Bowel Disease		0.308	0.523	0.275	0.551	0.275	0.543	0.355
K51.30	Ulcerative (chronic) rectosigmoiditis without complications	35	Inflammatory Bowel Disease		0.308	0.523	0.275	0.551	0.275	0.543	0.355
K51.311	Ulcerative (chronic) rectosigmoiditis with rectal bleeding	35	Inflammatory Bowel Disease		0.308	0.523	0.275	0.551	0.275	0.543	0.355
K51.312	Ulcerative (chronic) rectosigmoiditis with intestinal obstruction	33	Intestinal Obstruction/Perforation		0.219	0.503	0.258	0.538	0.232	0.552	0.352
K51.312	Ulcerative (chronic) rectosigmoiditis with intestinal obstruction	35	Inflammatory Bowel Disease		0.308	0.523	0.275	0.551	0.275	0.543	0.355
K51.313	Ulcerative (chronic) rectosigmoiditis with fistula	35	Inflammatory Bowel Disease		0.308	0.523	0.275	0.551	0.275	0.543	0.355
K51.314	Ulcerative (chronic) rectosigmoiditis with abscess	35	Inflammatory Bowel Disease		0.308	0.523	0.275	0.551	0.275	0.543	0.355
K51.318	Ulcerative (chronic) rectosigmoiditis with other complication	35	Inflammatory Bowel Disease		0.308	0.523	0.275	0.551	0.275	0.543	0.355
K51.319	Ulcerative (chronic) rectosigmoiditis with unspecified complications	35	Inflammatory Bowel Disease		0.308	0.523	0.275	0.551	0.275	0.543	0.355
K51.40	Inflammatory polyps of colon without complications	35	Inflammatory Bowel Disease		0.308	0.523	0.275	0.551	0.275	0.543	0.355
K51.411	Inflammatory polyps of colon with rectal bleeding	35	Inflammatory Bowel Disease		0.308	0.523	0.275	0.551	0.275	0.543	0.355
K51.412	Inflammatory polyps of colon with intestinal obstruction	33	Intestinal Obstruction/Perforation		0.219	0.503	0.258	0.538	0.232	0.552	0.352
K51.412	Inflammatory polyps of colon with intestinal obstruction	35	Inflammatory Bowel Disease		0.308	0.523	0.275	0.551	0.275	0.543	0.355
K51.413	Inflammatory polyps of colon with fistula	35	Inflammatory Bowel Disease		0.308	0.523	0.275	0.551	0.275	0.543	0.355
K51.414	Inflammatory polyps of colon with abscess	35	Inflammatory Bowel Disease		0.308	0.523	0.275	0.551	0.275	0.543	0.355
K51.418	Inflammatory polyps of colon with other complication	35	Inflammatory Bowel Disease		0.308	0.523	0.275	0.551	0.275	0.543	0.355
K51.419	Inflammatory polyps of colon with unspecified complications	35	Inflammatory Bowel Disease		0.308	0.523	0.275	0.551	0.275	0.543	0.355
K51.50	Left sided colitis without complications	35	Inflammatory Bowel Disease		0.308	0.523	0.275	0.551	0.275	0.543	0.355
K51.511	Left sided colitis with rectal bleeding	35	Inflammatory Bowel Disease		0.308	0.523	0.275	0.551	0.275	0.543	0.355

ICD-10-CM Code	ICD-10-CM Code Description	V24 CMS-HCC	V24 CMS-HCC Disease Group	V24 CMS-HCC Hierarchies	Community, NonDual, Aged	Community, NonDual, Disabled	Community, FBDual, Aged	Community, FBDual, Disabled	Community, PBDual, Aged	Community, PBDual, Disabled	Institutional
K51.512	Left sided colitis with intestinal obstruction	33	Intestinal Obstruction/Perforation		0.219	0.503	0.258	0.538	0.232	0.552	0.352
K51.512	Left sided colitis with intestinal obstruction	35	Inflammatory Bowel Disease		0.308	0.523	0.275	0.551	0.275	0.543	0.355
K51.513	Left sided colitis with fistula	35	Inflammatory Bowel Disease		0.308	0.523	0.275	0.551	0.275	0.543	0.355
K51.514	Left sided colitis with abscess	35	Inflammatory Bowel Disease		0.308	0.523	0.275	0.551	0.275	0.543	0.355
K51.518	Left sided colitis with other complication	35	Inflammatory Bowel Disease		0.308	0.523	0.275	0.551	0.275	0.543	0.355
K51.519	Left sided colitis with unspecified complications	35	Inflammatory Bowel Disease		0.308	0.523	0.275	0.551	0.275	0.543	0.355
K51.80	Other ulcerative colitis without complications	35	Inflammatory Bowel Disease		0.308	0.523	0.275	0.551	0.275	0.543	0.355
K51.811	Other ulcerative colitis with rectal bleeding	35	Inflammatory Bowel Disease		0.308	0.523	0.275	0.551	0.275	0.543	0.355
K51.812	Other ulcerative colitis with intestinal obstruction	33	Intestinal Obstruction/Perforation		0.219	0.503	0.258	0.538	0.232	0.552	0.352
K51.812	Other ulcerative colitis with intestinal obstruction	35	Inflammatory Bowel Disease		0.308	0.523	0.275	0.551	0.275	0.543	0.355
K51.813	Other ulcerative colitis with fistula	35	Inflammatory Bowel Disease		0.308	0.523	0.275	0.551	0.275	0.543	0.355
K51.814	Other ulcerative colitis with abscess	35	Inflammatory Bowel Disease		0.308	0.523	0.275	0.551	0.275	0.543	0.355
K51.818	Other ulcerative colitis with other complication	35	Inflammatory Bowel Disease		0.308	0.523	0.275	0.551	0.275	0.543	0.355
K51.819	Other ulcerative colitis with unspecified complications	35	Inflammatory Bowel Disease		0.308	0.523	0.275	0.551	0.275	0.543	0.355
K51.90	Ulcerative colitis, unspecified, without complications	35	Inflammatory Bowel Disease		0.308	0.523	0.275	0.551	0.275	0.543	0.355
K51.911	Ulcerative colitis, unspecified with rectal bleeding	35	Inflammatory Bowel Disease		0.308	0.523	0.275	0.551	0.275	0.543	0.355
K51.912	Ulcerative colitis, unspecified with intestinal obstruction	33	Intestinal Obstruction/Perforation		0.219	0.503	0.258	0.538	0.232	0.552	0.352
K51.912	Ulcerative colitis, unspecified with intestinal obstruction	35	Inflammatory Bowel Disease		0.308	0.523	0.275	0.551	0.275	0.543	0.355
K51.913	Ulcerative colitis, unspecified with fistula	35	Inflammatory Bowel Disease		0.308	0.523	0.275	0.551	0.275	0.543	0.355
K51.914	Ulcerative colitis, unspecified with abscess	35	Inflammatory Bowel Disease		0.308	0.523	0.275	0.551	0.275	0.543	0.355
K51.918	Ulcerative colitis, unspecified with other complication	35	Inflammatory Bowel Disease		0.308	0.523	0.275	0.551	0.275	0.543	0.355
K51.919	Ulcerative colitis, unspecified with unspecified complications	35	Inflammatory Bowel Disease		0.308	0.523	0.275	0.551	0.275	0.543	0.355
K55.011	Focal (segmental) acute (reversible) ischemia of small intestine	107	Vascular Disease with Complications	108	0.383	0.464	0.565	0.653	0.463	0.450	0.299
K55.012	Diffuse acute (reversible) ischemia of small intestine	107	Vascular Disease with Complications	108	0.383	0.464	0.565	0.653	0.463	0.450	0.299
K55.019	Acute (reversible) ischemia of small intestine, extent unspecified	107	Vascular Disease with Complications	108	0.383	0.464	0.565	0.653	0.463	0.450	0.299
K55.021	Focal (segmental) acute infarction of small intestine	107	Vascular Disease with Complications	108	0.383	0.464	0.565	0.653	0.463	0.450	0.299
K55.022	Diffuse acute infarction of small intestine	107	Vascular Disease with Complications	108	0.383	0.464	0.565	0.653	0.463	0.450	0.299
K55.029	Acute infarction of small intestine, extent unspecified	107	Vascular Disease with Complications	108	0.383	0.464	0.565	0.653	0.463	0.450	0.299
K55.031	Focal (segmental) acute (reversible) ischemia of large intestine	107	Vascular Disease with Complications	108	0.383	0.464	0.565	0.653	0.463	0.450	0.299
K55.032	Diffuse acute (reversible) ischemia of large intestine	107	Vascular Disease with Complications	108	0.383	0.464	0.565	0.653	0.463	0.450	0.299
K55.039	Acute (reversible) ischemia of large intestine, extent unspecified	107	Vascular Disease with Complications	108	0.383	0.464	0.565	0.653	0.463	0.450	0.299

ICD-10-CM Code	ICD-10-CM Code Description	V24 CMS-HCC	V24 CMS-HCC Disease Group	V24 CMS-HCC Hierarchies	Community, NonDual, Aged	Community, NonDual, Disabled	Community, FBDual, Aged	Community, FBDual, Disabled	Community, PBDual, Aged	Community, PBDual, Disabled	Institutional
K55.041	Focal (segmental) acute infarction of large intestine	107	Vascular Disease with Complications	108	0.383	0.464	0.565	0.653	0.463	0.450	0.299
K55.042	Diffuse acute infarction of large intestine	107	Vascular Disease with Complications	108	0.383	0.464	0.565	0.653	0.463	0.450	0.299
K55.049	Acute infarction of large intestine, extent unspecified	107	Vascular Disease with Complications	108	0.383	0.464	0.565	0.653	0.463	0.450	0.299
K55.051	Focal (segmental) acute (reversible) ischemia of intestine, part unspecified	107	Vascular Disease with Complications	108	0.383	0.464	0.565	0.653	0.463	0.450	0.299
K55.052	Diffuse acute (reversible) ischemia of intestine, part unspecified	107	Vascular Disease with Complications	108	0.383	0.464	0.565	0.653	0.463	0.450	0.299
K55.059	Acute (reversible) ischemia of intestine, part and extent unspecified	107	Vascular Disease with Complications	108	0.383	0.464	0.565	0.653	0.463	0.450	0.299
K55.061	Focal (segmental) acute infarction of intestine, part unspecified	107	Vascular Disease with Complications	108	0.383	0.464	0.565	0.653	0.463	0.450	0.299
K55.062	Diffuse acute infarction of intestine, part unspecified	107	Vascular Disease with Complications	108	0.383	0.464	0.565	0.653	0.463	0.450	0.299
K55.069	Acute infarction of intestine, part and extent unspecified	107	Vascular Disease with Complications	108	0.383	0.464	0.565	0.653	0.463	0.450	0.299
K55.1	Chronic vascular disorders of intestine	108	Vascular Disease		0.288	0.301	0.294	0.267	0.297	0.314	0.093
K55.30	Necrotizing enterocolitis, unspecified	107	Vascular Disease with Complications	108	0.383	0.464	0.565	0.653	0.463	0.450	0.299
K55.31	Stage 1 necrotizing enterocolitis	107	Vascular Disease with Complications	108	0.383	0.464	0.565	0.653	0.463	0.450	0.299
K55.32	Stage 2 necrotizing enterocolitis	107	Vascular Disease with Complications	108	0.383	0.464	0.565	0.653	0.463	0.450	0.299
K55.33	Stage 3 necrotizing enterocolitis	107	Vascular Disease with Complications	108	0.383	0.464	0.565	0.653	0.463	0.450	0.299
K55.8	Other vascular disorders of intestine	108	Vascular Disease		0.288	0.301	0.294	0.267	0.297	0.314	0.093
K55.9	Vascular disorder of intestine, unspecified	108	Vascular Disease		0.288	0.301	0.294	0.267	0.297	0.314	0.093
K56.0	Paralytic ileus	33	Intestinal Obstruction/Perforation		0.219	0.503	0.258	0.538	0.232	0.552	0.352
K56.1	Intussusception	33	Intestinal Obstruction/Perforation		0.219	0.503	0.258	0.538	0.232	0.552	0.352
K56.2	Volvulus	33	Intestinal Obstruction/Perforation		0.219	0.503	0.258	0.538	0.232	0.552	0.352
K56.3	Gallstone ileus	33	Intestinal Obstruction/Perforation		0.219	0.503	0.258	0.538	0.232	0.552	0.352
K56.41	Fecal impaction	33	Intestinal Obstruction/Perforation		0.219	0.503	0.258	0.538	0.232	0.552	0.352
K56.49	Other impaction of intestine	33	Intestinal Obstruction/Perforation		0.219	0.503	0.258	0.538	0.232	0.552	0.352
K56.50	Intestinal adhesions [bands], unspecified as to partial versus complete obstruction	33	Intestinal Obstruction/Perforation		0.219	0.503	0.258	0.538	0.232	0.552	0.352
K56.51	Intestinal adhesions [bands], with partial obstruction	33	Intestinal Obstruction/Perforation		0.219	0.503	0.258	0.538	0.232	0.552	0.352
K56.52	Intestinal adhesions [bands] with complete obstruction	33	Intestinal Obstruction/Perforation		0.219	0.503	0.258	0.538	0.232	0.552	0.352
K56.600	Partial intestinal obstruction, unspecified as to cause	33	Intestinal Obstruction/Perforation		0.219	0.503	0.258	0.538	0.232	0.552	0.352
K56.601	Complete intestinal obstruction, unspecified as to cause	33	Intestinal Obstruction/Perforation		0.219	0.503	0.258	0.538	0.232	0.552	0.352
K56.609	Unspecified intestinal obstruction, unspecified as to partial versus complete obstruction	33	Intestinal Obstruction/Perforation		0.219	0.503	0.258	0.538	0.232	0.552	0.352
K56.690	Other partial intestinal obstruction	33	Intestinal Obstruction/Perforation		0.219	0.503	0.258	0.538	0.232	0.552	0.352
K56.691	Other complete intestinal obstruction	33	Intestinal Obstruction/Perforation		0.219	0.503	0.258	0.538	0.232	0.552	0.352
K56.699	Other intestinal obstruction unspecified as to partial versus complete obstruction	33	Intestinal Obstruction/Perforation		0.219	0.503	0.258	0.538	0.232	0.552	0.352
K56.7	Ileus, unspecified	33	Intestinal Obstruction/Perforation		0.219	0.503	0.258	0.538	0.232	0.552	0.352
K59.31	Toxic megacolon	33	Intestinal Obstruction/Perforation		0.219	0.503	0.258	0.538	0.232	0.552	0.352
K63.1	Perforation of intestine (nontraumatic)	33	Intestinal Obstruction/Perforation		0.219	0.503	0.258	0.538	0.232	0.552	0.352

ICD-10-CM Code	ICD-10-CM Code Description	V24 CMS-HCC	V24 CMS-HCC Disease Group	V24 CMS-HCC Hierarchies	Community, NonDual, Aged	Community, NonDual, Disabled	Community, FBDual, Aged	Community, FBDual, Disabled	Community, PBDual, Aged	Community, PBDual, Disabled	Institutional
K65.0	Generalized (acute) peritonitis	33	Intestinal Obstruction/Perforation		0.219	0.503	0.258	0.538	0.232	0.552	0.352
K65.1	Peritoneal abscess	33	Intestinal Obstruction/Perforation		0.219	0.503	0.258	0.538	0.232	0.552	0.352
K65.2	Spontaneous bacterial peritonitis	33	Intestinal Obstruction/Perforation		0.219	0.503	0.258	0.538	0.232	0.552	0.352
K65.3	Choleperitonitis	33	Intestinal Obstruction/Perforation		0.219	0.503	0.258	0.538	0.232	0.552	0.352
K65.4	Sclerosing mesenteritis	33	Intestinal Obstruction/Perforation		0.219	0.503	0.258	0.538	0.232	0.552	0.352
K65.8	Other peritonitis	33	Intestinal Obstruction/Perforation		0.219	0.503	0.258	0.538	0.232	0.552	0.352
K65.9	Peritonitis, unspecified	33	Intestinal Obstruction/Perforation		0.219	0.503	0.258	0.538	0.232	0.552	0.352
K67	Disorders of peritoneum in infectious diseases classified elsewhere	33	Intestinal Obstruction/Perforation		0.219	0.503	0.258	0.538	0.232	0.552	0.352
K68.12	Psoas muscle abscess	33	Intestinal Obstruction/Perforation		0.219	0.503	0.258	0.538	0.232	0.552	0.352
K68.19	Other retroperitoneal abscess	33	Intestinal Obstruction/Perforation		0.219	0.503	0.258	0.538	0.232	0.552	0.352
K70.30	Alcoholic cirrhosis of liver without ascites	28	Cirrhosis of Liver	29	0.363	0.334	0.411	0.365	0.403	0.341	0.485
K70.31	Alcoholic cirrhosis of liver with ascites	28	Cirrhosis of Liver	29	0.363	0.334	0.411	0.365	0.403	0.341	0.485
K70.40	Alcoholic hepatic failure without coma	28	Cirrhosis of Liver	29	0.363	0.334	0.411	0.365	0.403	0.341	0.485
K70.41	Alcoholic hepatic failure with coma	27	End-Stage Liver Disease	28,29,80	0.882	1.065	1.111	1.101	0.729	0.887	0.874
K70.41	Alcoholic hepatic failure with coma	28	Cirrhosis of Liver	29	0.363	0.334	0.411	0.365	0.403	0.341	0.485
K70.9	Alcoholic liver disease, unspecified	28	Cirrhosis of Liver	29	0.363	0.334	0.411	0.365	0.403	0.341	0.485
K71.11	Toxic liver disease with hepatic necrosis, with coma	27	End-Stage Liver Disease	28,29,80	0.882	1.065	1.111	1.101	0.729	0.887	0.874
K72.01	Acute and subacute hepatic failure with coma	27	End-Stage Liver Disease	28,29,80	0.882	1.065	1.111	1.101	0.729	0.887	0.874
K72.10	Chronic hepatic failure without coma	27	End-Stage Liver Disease	28,29,80	0.882	1.065	1.111	1.101	0.729	0.887	0.874
K72.11	Chronic hepatic failure with coma	27	End-Stage Liver Disease	28,29,80	0.882	1.065	1.111	1.101	0.729	0.887	0.874
K72.90	Hepatic failure, unspecified without coma	27	End-Stage Liver Disease	28,29,80	0.882	1.065	1.111	1.101	0.729	0.887	0.874
K72.91	Hepatic failure, unspecified with coma	27	End-Stage Liver Disease	28,29,80	0.882	1.065	1.111	1.101	0.729	0.887	0.874
K73.0	Chronic persistent hepatitis, not elsewhere classified	29	Chronic Hepatitis		0.147	0.314	0.042	0.292	0.181	0.238	0.485
K73.1	Chronic lobular hepatitis, not elsewhere classified	29	Chronic Hepatitis		0.147	0.314	0.042	0.292	0.181	0.238	0.485
K73.2	Chronic active hepatitis, not elsewhere classified	29	Chronic Hepatitis		0.147	0.314	0.042	0.292	0.181	0.238	0.485
K73.8	Other chronic hepatitis, not elsewhere classified	29	Chronic Hepatitis		0.147	0.314	0.042	0.292	0.181	0.238	0.485
K73.9	Chronic hepatitis, unspecified	29	Chronic Hepatitis		0.147	0.314	0.042	0.292	0.181	0.238	0.485
K74.3	Primary biliary cirrhosis	28	Cirrhosis of Liver	29	0.363	0.334	0.411	0.365	0.403	0.341	0.485
K74.4	Secondary biliary cirrhosis	28	Cirrhosis of Liver	29	0.363	0.334	0.411	0.365	0.403	0.341	0.485
K74.5	Biliary cirrhosis, unspecified	28	Cirrhosis of Liver	29	0.363	0.334	0.411	0.365	0.403	0.341	0.485
K74.60	Unspecified cirrhosis of liver	28	Cirrhosis of Liver	29	0.363	0.334	0.411	0.365	0.403	0.341	0.485
K74.69	Other cirrhosis of liver	28	Cirrhosis of Liver	29	0.363	0.334	0.411	0.365	0.403	0.341	0.485
K75.4	Autoimmune hepatitis	29	Chronic Hepatitis		0.147	0.314	0.042	0.292	0.181	0.238	0.485
K76.6	Portal hypertension	27	End-Stage Liver Disease	28,29,80	0.882	1.065	1.111	1.101	0.729	0.887	0.874
K76.7	Hepatorenal syndrome	27	End-Stage Liver Disease	28,29,80	0.882	1.065	1.111	1.101	0.729	0.887	0.874
K76.81	Hepatopulmonary syndrome	27	End-Stage Liver Disease	28,29,80	0.882	1.065	1.111	1.101	0.729	0.887	0.874
K86.0	Alcohol-induced chronic pancreatitis	34	Chronic Pancreatitis		0.287	0.580	0.349	0.762	0.371	0.597	0.422
K86.1	Other chronic pancreatitis	34	Chronic Pancreatitis		0.287	0.580	0.349	0.762	0.371	0.597	0.422
K91.850	Pouchitis	188	Artificial Openings for Feeding or Elimination		0.534	0.755	0.742	0.770	0.520	0.732	0.514
K91.858	Other complications of intestinal pouch	188	Artificial Openings for Feeding or Elimination		0.534	0.755	0.742	0.770	0.520	0.732	0.514
K94.00	Colostomy complication, unspecified	188	Artificial Openings for Feeding or Elimination		0.534	0.755	0.742	0.770	0.520	0.732	0.514

ICD-10-CM Code	ICD-10-CM Code Description	V24 CMS-HCC	V24 CMS-HCC Disease Group	V24 CMS-HCC Hierarchies	Community, NonDual, Aged	Community, NonDual, Disabled	Community, FBDual, Aged	Community, FBDual, Disabled	Community, PBDual, Aged	Community, PBDual, Disabled	Institutional
K94.Ø1	Colostomy hemorrhage	188	Artificial Openings for Feeding or Elimination		0.534	0.755	0.742	0.770	0.520	0.732	0.514
K94.Ø2	Colostomy infection	188	Artificial Openings for Feeding or Elimination		0.534	0.755	0.742	0.770	0.520	0.732	0.514
K94.Ø3	Colostomy malfunction	188	Artificial Openings for Feeding or Elimination		0.534	0.755	0.742	0.770	0.520	0.732	0.514
K94.Ø9	Other complications of colostomy	188	Artificial Openings for Feeding or Elimination		0.534	0.755	0.742	0.770	0.520	0.732	0.514
K94.10	Enterostomy complication, unspecified	188	Artificial Openings for Feeding or Elimination		0.534	0.755	0.742	0.770	0.520	0.732	0.514
K94.11	Enterostomy hemorrhage	188	Artificial Openings for Feeding or Elimination		0.534	0.755	0.742	0.770	0.520	0.732	0.514
K94.12	Enterostomy infection	188	Artificial Openings for Feeding or Elimination		0.534	0.755	0.742	0.770	0.520	0.732	0.514
K94.13	Enterostomy malfunction	188	Artificial Openings for Feeding or Elimination		0.534	0.755	0.742	0.770	0.520	0.732	0.514
K94.19	Other complications of enterostomy	188	Artificial Openings for Feeding or Elimination		0.534	0.755	0.742	0.770	0.520	0.732	0.514
K94.2Ø	Gastrostomy complication, unspecified	188	Artificial Openings for Feeding or Elimination		0.534	0.755	0.742	0.770	0.520	0.732	0.514
K94.21	Gastrostomy hemorrhage	188	Artificial Openings for Feeding or Elimination		0.534	0.755	0.742	0.770	0.520	0.732	0.514
K94.22	Gastrostomy infection	188	Artificial Openings for Feeding or Elimination		0.534	0.755	0.742	0.770	0.520	0.732	0.514
K94.23	Gastrostomy malfunction	188	Artificial Openings for Feeding or Elimination		0.534	0.755	0.742	0.770	0.520	0.732	0.514
K94.29	Other complications of gastrostomy	188	Artificial Openings for Feeding or Elimination		0.534	0.755	0.742	0.770	0.520	0.732	0.514
K94.3Ø	Esophagostomy complications, unspecified	188	Artificial Openings for Feeding or Elimination		0.534	0.755	0.742	0.770	0.520	0.732	0.514
K94.31	Esophagostomy hemorrhage	188	Artificial Openings for Feeding or Elimination		0.534	0.755	0.742	0.770	0.520	0.732	0.514
K94.32	Esophagostomy infection	188	Artificial Openings for Feeding or Elimination		0.534	0.755	0.742	0.770	0.520	0.732	0.514
K94.33	Esophagostomy malfunction	188	Artificial Openings for Feeding or Elimination		0.534	0.755	0.742	0.770	0.520	0.732	0.514
K94.39	Other complications of esophagostomy	188	Artificial Openings for Feeding or Elimination		0.534	0.755	0.742	0.770	0.520	0.732	0.514
L12.3Ø	Acquired epidermolysis bullosa, unspecified	162	Severe Skin Burn or Condition		0.224	0.506	0.162	0.308	—	0.324	—
L12.31	Epidermolysis bullosa due to drug	162	Severe Skin Burn or Condition		0.224	0.506	0.162	0.308	—	0.324	—
L12.35	Other acquired epidermolysis bullosa	162	Severe Skin Burn or Condition		0.224	0.506	0.162	0.308	—	0.324	—
L40.5Ø	Arthropathic psoriasis, unspecified	40	Rheumatoid Arthritis and Inflammatory Connective Tissue Disease		0.421	0.367	0.371	0.328	0.347	0.264	0.292
L40.51	Distal interphalangeal psoriatic arthropathy	40	Rheumatoid Arthritis and Inflammatory Connective Tissue Disease		0.421	0.367	0.371	0.328	0.347	0.264	0.292
L40.52	Psoriatic arthritis mutilans	40	Rheumatoid Arthritis and Inflammatory Connective Tissue Disease		0.421	0.367	0.371	0.328	0.347	0.264	0.292
L40.53	Psoriatic spondylitis	40	Rheumatoid Arthritis and Inflammatory Connective Tissue Disease		0.421	0.367	0.371	0.328	0.347	0.264	0.292
L40.54	Psoriatic juvenile arthropathy	40	Rheumatoid Arthritis and Inflammatory Connective Tissue Disease		0.421	0.367	0.371	0.328	0.347	0.264	0.292

ICD-10-CM Code	ICD-10-CM Code Description	V24 CMS-HCC	V24 CMS-HCC Disease Group	V24 CMS-HCC Hierarchies	Community, NonDual, Aged	Community, NonDual, Disabled	Community, FBDual, Aged	Community, FBDual, Disabled	Community, PBDual, Aged	Community, PBDual, Disabled	Institutional
L40.59	Other psoriatic arthropathy	40	Rheumatoid Arthritis and Inflammatory Connective Tissue Disease		0.421	0.367	0.371	0.328	0.347	0.264	0.292
L51.1	Stevens-Johnson syndrome	162	Severe Skin Burn or Condition		0.224	0.506	0.162	0.308	—	0.324	—
L51.2	Toxic epidermal necrolysis [Lyell]	162	Severe Skin Burn or Condition		0.224	0.506	0.162	0.308	—	0.324	—
L51.3	Stevens-Johnson syndrome-toxic epidermal necrolysis overlap syndrome	162	Severe Skin Burn or Condition		0.224	0.506	0.162	0.308	—	0.324	—
L89.000	Pressure ulcer of unspecified elbow, unstageable	158	Pressure Ulcer of Skin with Full Thickness Skin Loss	159,161	1.069	1.212	1.471	1.380	1.162	0.925	0.322
L89.002	Pressure ulcer of unspecified elbow, stage 2	159	Pressure Ulcer of Skin with Partial Thickness Skin Loss	161	0.656	0.628	0.863	0.467	0.649	0.824	0.322
L89.003	Pressure ulcer of unspecified elbow, stage 3	158	Pressure Ulcer of Skin with Full Thickness Skin Loss	159,161	1.069	1.212	1.471	1.380	1.162	0.925	0.322
L89.004	Pressure ulcer of unspecified elbow, stage 4	157	Pressure Ulcer of Skin with Necrosis Through to Muscle, Tendon, or Bone	158,159, 161	2.028	2.097	2.463	2.582	2.028	2.512	0.854
L89.010	Pressure ulcer of right elbow, unstageable	158	Pressure Ulcer of Skin with Full Thickness Skin Loss	159,161	1.069	1.212	1.471	1.380	1.162	0.925	0.322
L89.012	Pressure ulcer of right elbow, stage 2	159	Pressure Ulcer of Skin with Partial Thickness Skin Loss	161	0.656	0.628	0.863	0.467	0.649	0.824	0.322
L89.013	Pressure ulcer of right elbow, stage 3	158	Pressure Ulcer of Skin with Full Thickness Skin Loss	159,161	1.069	1.212	1.471	1.380	1.162	0.925	0.322
L89.014	Pressure ulcer of right elbow, stage 4	157	Pressure Ulcer of Skin with Necrosis Through to Muscle, Tendon, or Bone	158,159, 161	2.028	2.097	2.463	2.582	2.028	2.512	0.854
L89.020	Pressure ulcer of left elbow, unstageable	158	Pressure Ulcer of Skin with Full Thickness Skin Loss	159,161	1.069	1.212	1.471	1.380	1.162	0.925	0.322
L89.022	Pressure ulcer of left elbow, stage 2	159	Pressure Ulcer of Skin with Partial Thickness Skin Loss	161	0.656	0.628	0.863	0.467	0.649	0.824	0.322
L89.023	Pressure ulcer of left elbow, stage 3	158	Pressure Ulcer of Skin with Full Thickness Skin Loss	159,161	1.069	1.212	1.471	1.380	1.162	0.925	0.322
L89.024	Pressure ulcer of left elbow, stage 4	157	Pressure Ulcer of Skin with Necrosis Through to Muscle, Tendon, or Bone	158,159, 161	2.028	2.097	2.463	2.582	2.028	2.512	0.854
L89.100	Pressure ulcer of unspecified part of back, unstageable	158	Pressure Ulcer of Skin with Full Thickness Skin Loss	159,161	1.069	1.212	1.471	1.380	1.162	0.925	0.322
L89.102	Pressure ulcer of unspecified part of back, stage 2	159	Pressure Ulcer of Skin with Partial Thickness Skin Loss	161	0.656	0.628	0.863	0.467	0.649	0.824	0.322
L89.103	Pressure ulcer of unspecified part of back, stage 3	158	Pressure Ulcer of Skin with Full Thickness Skin Loss	159,161	1.069	1.212	1.471	1.380	1.162	0.925	0.322
L89.104	Pressure ulcer of unspecified part of back, stage 4	157	Pressure Ulcer of Skin with Necrosis Through to Muscle, Tendon, or Bone	158,159, 161	2.028	2.097	2.463	2.582	2.028	2.512	0.854
L89.110	Pressure ulcer of right upper back, unstageable	158	Pressure Ulcer of Skin with Full Thickness Skin Loss	159,161	1.069	1.212	1.471	1.380	1.162	0.925	0.322
L89.112	Pressure ulcer of right upper back, stage 2	159	Pressure Ulcer of Skin with Partial Thickness Skin Loss	161	0.656	0.628	0.863	0.467	0.649	0.824	0.322
L89.113	Pressure ulcer of right upper back, stage 3	158	Pressure Ulcer of Skin with Full Thickness Skin Loss	159,161	1.069	1.212	1.471	1.380	1.162	0.925	0.322
L89.114	Pressure ulcer of right upper back, stage 4	157	Pressure Ulcer of Skin with Necrosis Through to Muscle, Tendon, or Bone	158,159, 161	2.028	2.097	2.463	2.582	2.028	2.512	0.854
L89.120	Pressure ulcer of left upper back, unstageable	158	Pressure Ulcer of Skin with Full Thickness Skin Loss	159,161	1.069	1.212	1.471	1.380	1.162	0.925	0.322
L89.122	Pressure ulcer of left upper back, stage 2	159	Pressure Ulcer of Skin with Partial Thickness Skin Loss	161	0.656	0.628	0.863	0.467	0.649	0.824	0.322
L89.123	Pressure ulcer of left upper back, stage 3	158	Pressure Ulcer of Skin with Full Thickness Skin Loss	159,161	1.069	1.212	1.471	1.380	1.162	0.925	0.322
L89.124	Pressure ulcer of left upper back, stage 4	157	Pressure Ulcer of Skin with Necrosis Through to Muscle, Tendon, or Bone	158,159, 161	2.028	2.097	2.463	2.582	2.028	2.512	0.854
L89.130	Pressure ulcer of right lower back, unstageable	158	Pressure Ulcer of Skin with Full Thickness Skin Loss	159,161	1.069	1.212	1.471	1.380	1.162	0.925	0.322

ICD-10-CM Code	ICD-10-CM Code Description	V24 CMS-HCC	V24 CMS-HCC Disease Group	V24 CMS-HCC Hierarchies	Community, NonDual, Aged	Community, NonDual, Disabled	Community, FBDual, Aged	Community, FBDual, Disabled	Community, PBDual, Aged	Community, PBDual, Disabled	Institutional
L89.132	Pressure ulcer of right lower back, stage 2	159	Pressure Ulcer of Skin with Partial Thickness Skin Loss	161	0.656	0.628	0.863	0.467	0.649	0.824	0.322
L89.133	Pressure ulcer of right lower back, stage 3	158	Pressure Ulcer of Skin with Full Thickness Skin Loss	159,161	1.069	1.212	1.471	1.380	1.162	0.925	0.322
L89.134	Pressure ulcer of right lower back, stage 4	157	Pressure Ulcer of Skin with Necrosis Through to Muscle, Tendon, or Bone	158,159, 161	2.028	2.097	2.463	2.582	2.028	2.512	0.854
L89.140	Pressure ulcer of left lower back, unstageable	158	Pressure Ulcer of Skin with Full Thickness Skin Loss	159,161	1.069	1.212	1.471	1.380	1.162	0.925	0.322
L89.142	Pressure ulcer of left lower back, stage 2	159	Pressure Ulcer of Skin with Partial Thickness Skin Loss	161	0.656	0.628	0.863	0.467	0.649	0.824	0.322
L89.143	Pressure ulcer of left lower back, stage 3	158	Pressure Ulcer of Skin with Full Thickness Skin Loss	159,161	1.069	1.212	1.471	1.380	1.162	0.925	0.322
L89.144	Pressure ulcer of left lower back, stage 4	157	Pressure Ulcer of Skin with Necrosis Through to Muscle, Tendon, or Bone	158,159, 161	2.028	2.097	2.463	2.582	2.028	2.512	0.854
L89.150	Pressure ulcer of sacral region, unstageable	158	Pressure Ulcer of Skin with Full Thickness Skin Loss	159,161	1.069	1.212	1.471	1.380	1.162	0.925	0.322
L89.152	Pressure ulcer of sacral region, stage 2	159	Pressure Ulcer of Skin with Partial Thickness Skin Loss	161	0.656	0.628	0.863	0.467	0.649	0.824	0.322
L89.153	Pressure ulcer of sacral region, stage 3	158	Pressure Ulcer of Skin with Full Thickness Skin Loss	159,161	1.069	1.212	1.471	1.380	1.162	0.925	0.322
L89.154	Pressure ulcer of sacral region, stage 4	157	Pressure Ulcer of Skin with Necrosis Through to Muscle, Tendon, or Bone	158,159, 161	2.028	2.097	2.463	2.582	2.028	2.512	0.854
L89.200	Pressure ulcer of unspecified hip, unstageable	158	Pressure Ulcer of Skin with Full Thickness Skin Loss	159,161	1.069	1.212	1.471	1.380	1.162	0.925	0.322
L89.202	Pressure ulcer of unspecified hip, stage 2	159	Pressure Ulcer of Skin with Partial Thickness Skin Loss	161	0.656	0.628	0.863	0.467	0.649	0.824	0.322
L89.203	Pressure ulcer of unspecified hip, stage 3	158	Pressure Ulcer of Skin with Full Thickness Skin Loss	159,161	1.069	1.212	1.471	1.380	1.162	0.925	0.322
L89.204	Pressure ulcer of unspecified hip, stage 4	157	Pressure Ulcer of Skin with Necrosis Through to Muscle, Tendon, or Bone	158,159, 161	2.028	2.097	2.463	2.582	2.028	2.512	0.854
L89.210	Pressure ulcer of right hip, unstageable	158	Pressure Ulcer of Skin with Full Thickness Skin Loss	159,161	1.069	1.212	1.471	1.380	1.162	0.925	0.322
L89.212	Pressure ulcer of right hip, stage 2	159	Pressure Ulcer of Skin with Partial Thickness Skin Loss	161	0.656	0.628	0.863	0.467	0.649	0.824	0.322
L89.213	Pressure ulcer of right hip, stage 3	158	Pressure Ulcer of Skin with Full Thickness Skin Loss	159,161	1.069	1.212	1.471	1.380	1.162	0.925	0.322
L89.214	Pressure ulcer of right hip, stage 4	157	Pressure Ulcer of Skin with Necrosis Through to Muscle, Tendon, or Bone	158,159, 161	2.028	2.097	2.463	2.582	2.028	2.512	0.854
L89.220	Pressure ulcer of left hip, unstageable	158	Pressure Ulcer of Skin with Full Thickness Skin Loss	159,161	1.069	1.212	1.471	1.380	1.162	0.925	0.322
L89.222	Pressure ulcer of left hip, stage 2	159	Pressure Ulcer of Skin with Partial Thickness Skin Loss	161	0.656	0.628	0.863	0.467	0.649	0.824	0.322
L89.223	Pressure ulcer of left hip, stage 3	158	Pressure Ulcer of Skin with Full Thickness Skin Loss	159,161	1.069	1.212	1.471	1.380	1.162	0.925	0.322
L89.224	Pressure ulcer of left hip, stage 4	157	Pressure Ulcer of Skin with Necrosis Through to Muscle, Tendon, or Bone	158,159, 161	2.028	2.097	2.463	2.582	2.028	2.512	0.854
L89.300	Pressure ulcer of unspecified buttock, unstageable	158	Pressure Ulcer of Skin with Full Thickness Skin Loss	159,161	1.069	1.212	1.471	1.380	1.162	0.925	0.322
L89.302	Pressure ulcer of unspecified buttock, stage 2	159	Pressure Ulcer of Skin with Partial Thickness Skin Loss	161	0.656	0.628	0.863	0.467	0.649	0.824	0.322
L89.303	Pressure ulcer of unspecified buttock, stage 3	158	Pressure Ulcer of Skin with Full Thickness Skin Loss	159,161	1.069	1.212	1.471	1.380	1.162	0.925	0.322
L89.304	Pressure ulcer of unspecified buttock, stage 4	157	Pressure Ulcer of Skin with Necrosis Through to Muscle, Tendon, or Bone	158,159, 161	2.028	2.097	2.463	2.582	2.028	2.512	0.854
L89.310	Pressure ulcer of right buttock, unstageable	158	Pressure Ulcer of Skin with Full Thickness Skin Loss	159,161	1.069	1.212	1.471	1.380	1.162	0.925	0.322
L89.312	Pressure ulcer of right buttock, stage 2	159	Pressure Ulcer of Skin with Partial Thickness Skin Loss	161	0.656	0.628	0.863	0.467	0.649	0.824	0.322

ICD-10-CM Code	ICD-10-CM Code Description	V24 CMS-HCC	V24 CMS-HCC Disease Group	V24 CMS-HCC Hierarchies	Community, NonDual, Aged	Community, NonDual, Disabled	Community, FBDual, Aged	Community, FBDual, Disabled	Community, PBDual, Aged	Community, PBDual, Disabled	Institutional
L89.313	Pressure ulcer of right buttock, stage 3	158	Pressure Ulcer of Skin with Full Thickness Skin Loss	159,161	1.069	1.212	1.471	1.380	1.162	0.925	0.322
L89.314	Pressure ulcer of right buttock, stage 4	157	Pressure Ulcer of Skin with Necrosis Through to Muscle, Tendon, or Bone	158,159, 161	2.028	2.097	2.463	2.582	2.028	2.512	0.854
L89.320	Pressure ulcer of left buttock, unstageable	158	Pressure Ulcer of Skin with Full Thickness Skin Loss	159,161	1.069	1.212	1.471	1.380	1.162	0.925	0.322
L89.322	Pressure ulcer of left buttock, stage 2	159	Pressure Ulcer of Skin with Partial Thickness Skin Loss	161	0.656	0.628	0.863	0.467	0.649	0.824	0.322
L89.323	Pressure ulcer of left buttock, stage 3	158	Pressure Ulcer of Skin with Full Thickness Skin Loss	159,161	1.069	1.212	1.471	1.380	1.162	0.925	0.322
L89.324	Pressure ulcer of left buttock, stage 4	157	Pressure Ulcer of Skin with Necrosis Through to Muscle, Tendon, or Bone	158,159, 161	2.028	2.097	2.463	2.582	2.028	2.512	0.854
L89.42	Pressure ulcer of contiguous site of back, buttock and hip, stage 2	159	Pressure Ulcer of Skin with Partial Thickness Skin Loss	161	0.656	0.628	0.863	0.467	0.649	0.824	0.322
L89.43	Pressure ulcer of contiguous site of back, buttock and hip, stage 3	158	Pressure Ulcer of Skin with Full Thickness Skin Loss	159,161	1.069	1.212	1.471	1.380	1.162	0.925	0.322
L89.44	Pressure ulcer of contiguous site of back, buttock and hip, stage 4	157	Pressure Ulcer of Skin with Necrosis Through to Muscle, Tendon, or Bone	158,159, 161	2.028	2.097	2.463	2.582	2.028	2.512	0.854
L89.45	Pressure ulcer of contiguous site of back, buttock and hip, unstageable	158	Pressure Ulcer of Skin with Full Thickness Skin Loss	159,161	1.069	1.212	1.471	1.380	1.162	0.925	0.322
L89.500	Pressure ulcer of unspecified ankle, unstageable	158	Pressure Ulcer of Skin with Full Thickness Skin Loss	159,161	1.069	1.212	1.471	1.380	1.162	0.925	0.322
L89.502	Pressure ulcer of unspecified ankle, stage 2	159	Pressure Ulcer of Skin with Partial Thickness Skin Loss	161	0.656	0.628	0.863	0.467	0.649	0.824	0.322
L89.503	Pressure ulcer of unspecified ankle, stage 3	158	Pressure Ulcer of Skin with Full Thickness Skin Loss	159,161	1.069	1.212	1.471	1.380	1.162	0.925	0.322
L89.504	Pressure ulcer of unspecified ankle, stage 4	157	Pressure Ulcer of Skin with Necrosis Through to Muscle, Tendon, or Bone	158,159, 161	2.028	2.097	2.463	2.582	2.028	2.512	0.854
L89.510	Pressure ulcer of right ankle, unstageable	158	Pressure Ulcer of Skin with Full Thickness Skin Loss	159,161	1.069	1.212	1.471	1.380	1.162	0.925	0.322
L89.512	Pressure ulcer of right ankle, stage 2	159	Pressure Ulcer of Skin with Partial Thickness Skin Loss	161	0.656	0.628	0.863	0.467	0.649	0.824	0.322
L89.513	Pressure ulcer of right ankle, stage 3	158	Pressure Ulcer of Skin with Full Thickness Skin Loss	159,161	1.069	1.212	1.471	1.380	1.162	0.925	0.322
L89.514	Pressure ulcer of right ankle, stage 4	157	Pressure Ulcer of Skin with Necrosis Through to Muscle, Tendon, or Bone	158,159, 161	2.028	2.097	2.463	2.582	2.028	2.512	0.854
L89.520	Pressure ulcer of left ankle, unstageable	158	Pressure Ulcer of Skin with Full Thickness Skin Loss	159,161	1.069	1.212	1.471	1.380	1.162	0.925	0.322
L89.522	Pressure ulcer of left ankle, stage 2	159	Pressure Ulcer of Skin with Partial Thickness Skin Loss	161	0.656	0.628	0.863	0.467	0.649	0.824	0.322
L89.523	Pressure ulcer of left ankle, stage 3	158	Pressure Ulcer of Skin with Full Thickness Skin Loss	159,161	1.069	1.212	1.471	1.380	1.162	0.925	0.322
L89.524	Pressure ulcer of left ankle, stage 4	157	Pressure Ulcer of Skin with Necrosis Through to Muscle, Tendon, or Bone	158,159, 161	2.028	2.097	2.463	2.582	2.028	2.512	0.854
L89.600	Pressure ulcer of unspecified heel, unstageable	158	Pressure Ulcer of Skin with Full Thickness Skin Loss	159,161	1.069	1.212	1.471	1.380	1.162	0.925	0.322
L89.602	Pressure ulcer of unspecified heel, stage 2	159	Pressure Ulcer of Skin with Partial Thickness Skin Loss	161	0.656	0.628	0.863	0.467	0.649	0.824	0.322
L89.603	Pressure ulcer of unspecified heel, stage 3	158	Pressure Ulcer of Skin with Full Thickness Skin Loss	159,161	1.069	1.212	1.471	1.380	1.162	0.925	0.322
L89.604	Pressure ulcer of unspecified heel, stage 4	157	Pressure Ulcer of Skin with Necrosis Through to Muscle, Tendon, or Bone	158,159, 161	2.028	2.097	2.463	2.582	2.028	2.512	0.854
L89.610	Pressure ulcer of right heel, unstageable	158	Pressure Ulcer of Skin with Full Thickness Skin Loss	159,161	1.069	1.212	1.471	1.380	1.162	0.925	0.322
L89.612	Pressure ulcer of right heel, stage 2	159	Pressure Ulcer of Skin with Partial Thickness Skin Loss	161	0.656	0.628	0.863	0.467	0.649	0.824	0.322
L89.613	Pressure ulcer of right heel, stage 3	158	Pressure Ulcer of Skin with Full Thickness Skin Loss	159,161	1.069	1.212	1.471	1.380	1.162	0.925	0.322

ICD-10-CM Code	ICD-10-CM Code Description	V24 CMS-HCC	V24 CMS-HCC Disease Group	V24 CMS-HCC Hierarchies	Community, NonDual, Aged	Community, NonDual, Disabled	Community, FBDual, Aged	Community, FBDual, Disabled	Community, PBDual, Aged	Community, PBDual, Disabled	Institutional
L89.614	Pressure ulcer of right heel, stage 4	157	Pressure Ulcer of Skin with Necrosis Through to Muscle, Tendon, or Bone	158,159, 161	2.028	2.097	2.463	2.582	2.028	2.512	0.854
L89.620	Pressure ulcer of left heel, unstageable	158	Pressure Ulcer of Skin with Full Thickness Skin Loss	159,161	1.069	1.212	1.471	1.380	1.162	0.925	0.322
L89.622	Pressure ulcer of left heel, stage 2	159	Pressure Ulcer of Skin with Partial Thickness Skin Loss	161	0.656	0.628	0.863	0.467	0.649	0.824	0.322
L89.623	Pressure ulcer of left heel, stage 3	158	Pressure Ulcer of Skin with Full Thickness Skin Loss	159,161	1.069	1.212	1.471	1.380	1.162	0.925	0.322
L89.624	Pressure ulcer of left heel, stage 4	157	Pressure Ulcer of Skin with Necrosis Through to Muscle, Tendon, or Bone	158,159, 161	2.028	2.097	2.463	2.582	2.028	2.512	0.854
L89.810	Pressure ulcer of head, unstageable	158	Pressure Ulcer of Skin with Full Thickness Skin Loss	159,161	1.069	1.212	1.471	1.380	1.162	0.925	0.322
L89.812	Pressure ulcer of head, stage 2	159	Pressure Ulcer of Skin with Partial Thickness Skin Loss	161	0.656	0.628	0.863	0.467	0.649	0.824	0.322
L89.813	Pressure ulcer of head, stage 3	158	Pressure Ulcer of Skin with Full Thickness Skin Loss	159,161	1.069	1.212	1.471	1.380	1.162	0.925	0.322
L89.814	Pressure ulcer of head, stage 4	157	Pressure Ulcer of Skin with Necrosis Through to Muscle, Tendon, or Bone	158,159, 161	2.028	2.097	2.463	2.582	2.028	2.512	0.854
L89.890	Pressure ulcer of other site, unstageable	158	Pressure Ulcer of Skin with Full Thickness Skin Loss	159,161	1.069	1.212	1.471	1.380	1.162	0.925	0.322
L89.892	Pressure ulcer of other site, stage 2	159	Pressure Ulcer of Skin with Partial Thickness Skin Loss	161	0.656	0.628	0.863	0.467	0.649	0.824	0.322
L89.893	Pressure ulcer of other site, stage 3	158	Pressure Ulcer of Skin with Full Thickness Skin Loss	159,161	1.069	1.212	1.471	1.380	1.162	0.925	0.322
L89.894	Pressure ulcer of other site, stage 4	157	Pressure Ulcer of Skin with Necrosis Through to Muscle, Tendon, or Bone	158,159, 161	2.028	2.097	2.463	2.582	2.028	2.512	0.854
L89.92	Pressure ulcer of unspecified site, stage 2	159	Pressure Ulcer of Skin with Partial Thickness Skin Loss	161	0.656	0.628	0.863	0.467	0.649	0.824	0.322
L89.93	Pressure ulcer of unspecified site, stage 3	158	Pressure Ulcer of Skin with Full Thickness Skin Loss	159,161	1.069	1.212	1.471	1.380	1.162	0.925	0.322
L89.94	Pressure ulcer of unspecified site, stage 4	157	Pressure Ulcer of Skin with Necrosis Through to Muscle, Tendon, or Bone	158,159, 161	2.028	2.097	2.463	2.582	2.028	2.512	0.854
L89.95	Pressure ulcer of unspecified site, unstageable	158	Pressure Ulcer of Skin with Full Thickness Skin Loss	159,161	1.069	1.212	1.471	1.380	1.162	0.925	0.322
L97.101	Non-pressure chronic ulcer of unspecified thigh limited to breakdown of skin	161	Chronic Ulcer of Skin, Except Pressure		0.515	0.592	0.727	0.583	0.541	0.542	0.294
L97.102	Non-pressure chronic ulcer of unspecified thigh with fat layer exposed	161	Chronic Ulcer of Skin, Except Pressure		0.515	0.592	0.727	0.583	0.541	0.542	0.294
L97.103	Non-pressure chronic ulcer of unspecified thigh with necrosis of muscle	161	Chronic Ulcer of Skin, Except Pressure		0.515	0.592	0.727	0.583	0.541	0.542	0.294
L97.104	Non-pressure chronic ulcer of unspecified thigh with necrosis of bone	161	Chronic Ulcer of Skin, Except Pressure		0.515	0.592	0.727	0.583	0.541	0.542	0.294
L97.105	Non-pressure chronic ulcer of unspecified thigh with muscle involvement without evidence of necrosis	161	Chronic Ulcer of Skin, Except Pressure		0.515	0.592	0.727	0.583	0.541	0.542	0.294
L97.106	Non-pressure chronic ulcer of unspecified thigh with bone involvement without evidence of necrosis	161	Chronic Ulcer of Skin, Except Pressure		0.515	0.592	0.727	0.583	0.541	0.542	0.294
L97.108	Non-pressure chronic ulcer of unspecified thigh with other specified severity	161	Chronic Ulcer of Skin, Except Pressure		0.515	0.592	0.727	0.583	0.541	0.542	0.294
L97.109	Non-pressure chronic ulcer of unspecified thigh with unspecified severity	161	Chronic Ulcer of Skin, Except Pressure		0.515	0.592	0.727	0.583	0.541	0.542	0.294

ICD-10-CM Code	ICD-10-CM Code Description	V24 CMS-HCC	V24 CMS-HCC Disease Group	V24 CMS-HCC Hierarchies	Community, NonDual, Aged	Community, NonDual, Disabled	Community, FBDual, Aged	Community, FBDual, Disabled	Community, PBDual, Aged	Community, PBDual, Disabled	Institutional
L97.111	Non-pressure chronic ulcer of right thigh limited to breakdown of skin	161	Chronic Ulcer of Skin, Except Pressure		0.515	0.592	0.727	0.583	0.541	0.542	0.294
L97.112	Non-pressure chronic ulcer of right thigh with fat layer exposed	161	Chronic Ulcer of Skin, Except Pressure		0.515	0.592	0.727	0.583	0.541	0.542	0.294
L97.113	Non-pressure chronic ulcer of right thigh with necrosis of muscle	161	Chronic Ulcer of Skin, Except Pressure		0.515	0.592	0.727	0.583	0.541	0.542	0.294
L97.114	Non-pressure chronic ulcer of right thigh with necrosis of bone	161	Chronic Ulcer of Skin, Except Pressure		0.515	0.592	0.727	0.583	0.541	0.542	0.294
L97.115	Non-pressure chronic ulcer of right thigh with muscle involvement without evidence of necrosis	161	Chronic Ulcer of Skin, Except Pressure		0.515	0.592	0.727	0.583	0.541	0.542	0.294
L97.116	Non-pressure chronic ulcer of right thigh with bone involvement without evidence of necrosis	161	Chronic Ulcer of Skin, Except Pressure		0.515	0.592	0.727	0.583	0.541	0.542	0.294
L97.118	Non-pressure chronic ulcer of right thigh with other specified severity	161	Chronic Ulcer of Skin, Except Pressure		0.515	0.592	0.727	0.583	0.541	0.542	0.294
L97.119	Non-pressure chronic ulcer of right thigh with unspecified severity	161	Chronic Ulcer of Skin, Except Pressure		0.515	0.592	0.727	0.583	0.541	0.542	0.294
L97.121	Non-pressure chronic ulcer of left thigh limited to breakdown of skin	161	Chronic Ulcer of Skin, Except Pressure		0.515	0.592	0.727	0.583	0.541	0.542	0.294
L97.122	Non-pressure chronic ulcer of left thigh with fat layer exposed	161	Chronic Ulcer of Skin, Except Pressure		0.515	0.592	0.727	0.583	0.541	0.542	0.294
L97.123	Non-pressure chronic ulcer of left thigh with necrosis of muscle	161	Chronic Ulcer of Skin, Except Pressure		0.515	0.592	0.727	0.583	0.541	0.542	0.294
L97.124	Non-pressure chronic ulcer of left thigh with necrosis of bone	161	Chronic Ulcer of Skin, Except Pressure		0.515	0.592	0.727	0.583	0.541	0.542	0.294
L97.125	Non-pressure chronic ulcer of left thigh with muscle involvement without evidence of necrosis	161	Chronic Ulcer of Skin, Except Pressure		0.515	0.592	0.727	0.583	0.541	0.542	0.294
L97.126	Non-pressure chronic ulcer of left thigh with bone involvement without evidence of necrosis	161	Chronic Ulcer of Skin, Except Pressure		0.515	0.592	0.727	0.583	0.541	0.542	0.294
L97.128	Non-pressure chronic ulcer of left thigh with other specified severity	161	Chronic Ulcer of Skin, Except Pressure		0.515	0.592	0.727	0.583	0.541	0.542	0.294
L97.129	Non-pressure chronic ulcer of left thigh with unspecified severity	161	Chronic Ulcer of Skin, Except Pressure		0.515	0.592	0.727	0.583	0.541	0.542	0.294
L97.201	Non-pressure chronic ulcer of unspecified calf limited to breakdown of skin	161	Chronic Ulcer of Skin, Except Pressure		0.515	0.592	0.727	0.583	0.541	0.542	0.294
L97.202	Non-pressure chronic ulcer of unspecified calf with fat layer exposed	161	Chronic Ulcer of Skin, Except Pressure		0.515	0.592	0.727	0.583	0.541	0.542	0.294
L97.203	Non-pressure chronic ulcer of unspecified calf with necrosis of muscle	161	Chronic Ulcer of Skin, Except Pressure		0.515	0.592	0.727	0.583	0.541	0.542	0.294
L97.204	Non-pressure chronic ulcer of unspecified calf with necrosis of bone	161	Chronic Ulcer of Skin, Except Pressure		0.515	0.592	0.727	0.583	0.541	0.542	0.294
L97.205	Non-pressure chronic ulcer of unspecified calf with muscle involvement without evidence of necrosis	161	Chronic Ulcer of Skin, Except Pressure		0.515	0.592	0.727	0.583	0.541	0.542	0.294
L97.206	Non-pressure chronic ulcer of unspecified calf with bone involvement without evidence of necrosis	161	Chronic Ulcer of Skin, Except Pressure		0.515	0.592	0.727	0.583	0.541	0.542	0.294
L97.208	Non-pressure chronic ulcer of unspecified calf with other specified severity	161	Chronic Ulcer of Skin, Except Pressure		0.515	0.592	0.727	0.583	0.541	0.542	0.294

ICD-10-CM Code	ICD-10-CM Code Description	V24 CMS-HCC	V24 CMS-HCC Disease Group	V24 CMS-HCC Hierarchies	Community, NonDual, Aged	Community, NonDual, Disabled	Community, FBDual, Aged	Community, FBDual, Disabled	Community, PBDual, Aged	Community, PBDual, Disabled	Institutional
L97.209	Non-pressure chronic ulcer of unspecified calf with unspecified severity	161	Chronic Ulcer of Skin, Except Pressure		0.515	0.592	0.727	0.583	0.541	0.542	0.294
L97.211	Non-pressure chronic ulcer of right calf limited to breakdown of skin	161	Chronic Ulcer of Skin, Except Pressure		0.515	0.592	0.727	0.583	0.541	0.542	0.294
L97.212	Non-pressure chronic ulcer of right calf with fat layer exposed	161	Chronic Ulcer of Skin, Except Pressure		0.515	0.592	0.727	0.583	0.541	0.542	0.294
L97.213	Non-pressure chronic ulcer of right calf with necrosis of muscle	161	Chronic Ulcer of Skin, Except Pressure		0.515	0.592	0.727	0.583	0.541	0.542	0.294
L97.214	Non-pressure chronic ulcer of right calf with necrosis of bone	161	Chronic Ulcer of Skin, Except Pressure		0.515	0.592	0.727	0.583	0.541	0.542	0.294
L97.215	Non-pressure chronic ulcer of right calf with muscle involvement without evidence of necrosis	161	Chronic Ulcer of Skin, Except Pressure		0.515	0.592	0.727	0.583	0.541	0.542	0.294
L97.216	Non-pressure chronic ulcer of right calf with bone involvement without evidence of necrosis	161	Chronic Ulcer of Skin, Except Pressure		0.515	0.592	0.727	0.583	0.541	0.542	0.294
L97.218	Non-pressure chronic ulcer of right calf with other specified severity	161	Chronic Ulcer of Skin, Except Pressure		0.515	0.592	0.727	0.583	0.541	0.542	0.294
L97.219	Non-pressure chronic ulcer of right calf with unspecified severity	161	Chronic Ulcer of Skin, Except Pressure		0.515	0.592	0.727	0.583	0.541	0.542	0.294
L97.221	Non-pressure chronic ulcer of left calf limited to breakdown of skin	161	Chronic Ulcer of Skin, Except Pressure		0.515	0.592	0.727	0.583	0.541	0.542	0.294
L97.222	Non-pressure chronic ulcer of left calf with fat layer exposed	161	Chronic Ulcer of Skin, Except Pressure		0.515	0.592	0.727	0.583	0.541	0.542	0.294
L97.223	Non-pressure chronic ulcer of left calf with necrosis of muscle	161	Chronic Ulcer of Skin, Except Pressure		0.515	0.592	0.727	0.583	0.541	0.542	0.294
L97.224	Non-pressure chronic ulcer of left calf with necrosis of bone	161	Chronic Ulcer of Skin, Except Pressure		0.515	0.592	0.727	0.583	0.541	0.542	0.294
L97.225	Non-pressure chronic ulcer of left calf with muscle involvement without evidence of necrosis	161	Chronic Ulcer of Skin, Except Pressure		0.515	0.592	0.727	0.583	0.541	0.542	0.294
L97.226	Non-pressure chronic ulcer of left calf with bone involvement without evidence of necrosis	161	Chronic Ulcer of Skin, Except Pressure		0.515	0.592	0.727	0.583	0.541	0.542	0.294
L97.228	Non-pressure chronic ulcer of left calf with other specified severity	161	Chronic Ulcer of Skin, Except Pressure		0.515	0.592	0.727	0.583	0.541	0.542	0.294
L97.229	Non-pressure chronic ulcer of left calf with unspecified severity	161	Chronic Ulcer of Skin, Except Pressure		0.515	0.592	0.727	0.583	0.541	0.542	0.294
L97.301	Non-pressure chronic ulcer of unspecified ankle limited to breakdown of skin	161	Chronic Ulcer of Skin, Except Pressure		0.515	0.592	0.727	0.583	0.541	0.542	0.294
L97.302	Non-pressure chronic ulcer of unspecified ankle with fat layer exposed	161	Chronic Ulcer of Skin, Except Pressure		0.515	0.592	0.727	0.583	0.541	0.542	0.294
L97.303	Non-pressure chronic ulcer of unspecified ankle with necrosis of muscle	161	Chronic Ulcer of Skin, Except Pressure		0.515	0.592	0.727	0.583	0.541	0.542	0.294
L97.304	Non-pressure chronic ulcer of unspecified ankle with necrosis of bone	161	Chronic Ulcer of Skin, Except Pressure		0.515	0.592	0.727	0.583	0.541	0.542	0.294
L97.305	Non-pressure chronic ulcer of unspecified ankle with muscle involvement without evidence of necrosis	161	Chronic Ulcer of Skin, Except Pressure		0.515	0.592	0.727	0.583	0.541	0.542	0.294
L97.306	Non-pressure chronic ulcer of unspecified ankle with bone involvement without evidence of necrosis	161	Chronic Ulcer of Skin, Except Pressure		0.515	0.592	0.727	0.583	0.541	0.542	0.294

ICD-10-CM Code	ICD-10-CM Code Description	V24 CMS-HCC	V24 CMS-HCC Disease Group	V24 CMS-HCC Hierarchies	Community, NonDual, Aged	Community, NonDual, Disabled	Community, FBDual, Aged	Community, FBDual, Disabled	Community, PBDual, Aged	Community, PBDual, Disabled	Institutional
L97.308	Non-pressure chronic ulcer of unspecified ankle with other specified severity	161	Chronic Ulcer of Skin, Except Pressure		0.515	0.592	0.727	0.583	0.541	0.542	0.294
L97.309	Non-pressure chronic ulcer of unspecified ankle with unspecified severity	161	Chronic Ulcer of Skin, Except Pressure		0.515	0.592	0.727	0.583	0.541	0.542	0.294
L97.311	Non-pressure chronic ulcer of right ankle limited to breakdown of skin	161	Chronic Ulcer of Skin, Except Pressure		0.515	0.592	0.727	0.583	0.541	0.542	0.294
L97.312	Non-pressure chronic ulcer of right ankle with fat layer exposed	161	Chronic Ulcer of Skin, Except Pressure		0.515	0.592	0.727	0.583	0.541	0.542	0.294
L97.313	Non-pressure chronic ulcer of right ankle with necrosis of muscle	161	Chronic Ulcer of Skin, Except Pressure		0.515	0.592	0.727	0.583	0.541	0.542	0.294
L97.314	Non-pressure chronic ulcer of right ankle with necrosis of bone	161	Chronic Ulcer of Skin, Except Pressure		0.515	0.592	0.727	0.583	0.541	0.542	0.294
L97.315	Non-pressure chronic ulcer of right ankle with muscle involvement without evidence of necrosis	161	Chronic Ulcer of Skin, Except Pressure		0.515	0.592	0.727	0.583	0.541	0.542	0.294
L97.316	Non-pressure chronic ulcer of right ankle with bone involvement without evidence of necrosis	161	Chronic Ulcer of Skin, Except Pressure		0.515	0.592	0.727	0.583	0.541	0.542	0.294
L97.318	Non-pressure chronic ulcer of right ankle with other specified severity	161	Chronic Ulcer of Skin, Except Pressure		0.515	0.592	0.727	0.583	0.541	0.542	0.294
L97.319	Non-pressure chronic ulcer of right ankle with unspecified severity	161	Chronic Ulcer of Skin, Except Pressure		0.515	0.592	0.727	0.583	0.541	0.542	0.294
L97.321	Non-pressure chronic ulcer of left ankle limited to breakdown of skin	161	Chronic Ulcer of Skin, Except Pressure		0.515	0.592	0.727	0.583	0.541	0.542	0.294
L97.322	Non-pressure chronic ulcer of left ankle with fat layer exposed	161	Chronic Ulcer of Skin, Except Pressure		0.515	0.592	0.727	0.583	0.541	0.542	0.294
L97.323	Non-pressure chronic ulcer of left ankle with necrosis of muscle	161	Chronic Ulcer of Skin, Except Pressure		0.515	0.592	0.727	0.583	0.541	0.542	0.294
L97.324	Non-pressure chronic ulcer of left ankle with necrosis of bone	161	Chronic Ulcer of Skin, Except Pressure		0.515	0.592	0.727	0.583	0.541	0.542	0.294
L97.325	Non-pressure chronic ulcer of left ankle with muscle involvement without evidence of necrosis	161	Chronic Ulcer of Skin, Except Pressure		0.515	0.592	0.727	0.583	0.541	0.542	0.294
L97.326	Non-pressure chronic ulcer of left ankle with bone involvement without evidence of necrosis	161	Chronic Ulcer of Skin, Except Pressure		0.515	0.592	0.727	0.583	0.541	0.542	0.294
L97.328	Non-pressure chronic ulcer of left ankle with other specified severity	161	Chronic Ulcer of Skin, Except Pressure		0.515	0.592	0.727	0.583	0.541	0.542	0.294
L97.329	Non-pressure chronic ulcer of left ankle with unspecified severity	161	Chronic Ulcer of Skin, Except Pressure		0.515	0.592	0.727	0.583	0.541	0.542	0.294
L97.401	Non-pressure chronic ulcer of unspecified heel and midfoot limited to breakdown of skin	161	Chronic Ulcer of Skin, Except Pressure		0.515	0.592	0.727	0.583	0.541	0.542	0.294
L97.402	Non-pressure chronic ulcer of unspecified heel and midfoot with fat layer exposed	161	Chronic Ulcer of Skin, Except Pressure		0.515	0.592	0.727	0.583	0.541	0.542	0.294
L97.403	Non-pressure chronic ulcer of unspecified heel and midfoot with necrosis of muscle	161	Chronic Ulcer of Skin, Except Pressure		0.515	0.592	0.727	0.583	0.541	0.542	0.294
L97.404	Non-pressure chronic ulcer of unspecified heel and midfoot with necrosis of bone	161	Chronic Ulcer of Skin, Except Pressure		0.515	0.592	0.727	0.583	0.541	0.542	0.294
L97.405	Non-pressure chronic ulcer of unspecified heel and midfoot with muscle involvement without evidence of necrosis	161	Chronic Ulcer of Skin, Except Pressure		0.515	0.592	0.727	0.583	0.541	0.542	0.294

ICD-10-CM Code	ICD-10-CM Code Description	V24 CMS-HCC	V24 CMS-HCC Disease Group	V24 CMS-HCC Hierarchies	Community, NonDual, Aged	Community, NonDual, Disabled	Community, FBDual, Aged	Community, FBDual, Disabled	Community, PBDual, Aged	Community, PBDual, Disabled	Institutional
L97.406	Non-pressure chronic ulcer of unspecified heel and midfoot with bone involvement without evidence of necrosis	161	Chronic Ulcer of Skin, Except Pressure		0.515	0.592	0.727	0.583	0.541	0.542	0.294
L97.408	Non-pressure chronic ulcer of unspecified heel and midfoot with other specified severity	161	Chronic Ulcer of Skin, Except Pressure		0.515	0.592	0.727	0.583	0.541	0.542	0.294
L97.409	Non-pressure chronic ulcer of unspecified heel and midfoot with unspecified severity	161	Chronic Ulcer of Skin, Except Pressure		0.515	0.592	0.727	0.583	0.541	0.542	0.294
L97.411	Non-pressure chronic ulcer of right heel and midfoot limited to breakdown of skin	161	Chronic Ulcer of Skin, Except Pressure		0.515	0.592	0.727	0.583	0.541	0.542	0.294
L97.412	Non-pressure chronic ulcer of right heel and midfoot with fat layer exposed	161	Chronic Ulcer of Skin, Except Pressure		0.515	0.592	0.727	0.583	0.541	0.542	0.294
L97.413	Non-pressure chronic ulcer of right heel and midfoot with necrosis of muscle	161	Chronic Ulcer of Skin, Except Pressure		0.515	0.592	0.727	0.583	0.541	0.542	0.294
L97.414	Non-pressure chronic ulcer of right heel and midfoot with necrosis of bone	161	Chronic Ulcer of Skin, Except Pressure		0.515	0.592	0.727	0.583	0.541	0.542	0.294
L97.415	Non-pressure chronic ulcer of right heel and midfoot with muscle involvement without evidence of necrosis	161	Chronic Ulcer of Skin, Except Pressure		0.515	0.592	0.727	0.583	0.541	0.542	0.294
L97.416	Non-pressure chronic ulcer of right heel and midfoot with bone involvement without evidence of necrosis	161	Chronic Ulcer of Skin, Except Pressure		0.515	0.592	0.727	0.583	0.541	0.542	0.294
L97.418	Non-pressure chronic ulcer of right heel and midfoot with other specified severity	161	Chronic Ulcer of Skin, Except Pressure		0.515	0.592	0.727	0.583	0.541	0.542	0.294
L97.419	Non-pressure chronic ulcer of right heel and midfoot with unspecified severity	161	Chronic Ulcer of Skin, Except Pressure		0.515	0.592	0.727	0.583	0.541	0.542	0.294
L97.421	Non-pressure chronic ulcer of left heel and midfoot limited to breakdown of skin	161	Chronic Ulcer of Skin, Except Pressure		0.515	0.592	0.727	0.583	0.541	0.542	0.294
L97.422	Non-pressure chronic ulcer of left heel and midfoot with fat layer exposed	161	Chronic Ulcer of Skin, Except Pressure		0.515	0.592	0.727	0.583	0.541	0.542	0.294
L97.423	Non-pressure chronic ulcer of left heel and midfoot with necrosis of muscle	161	Chronic Ulcer of Skin, Except Pressure		0.515	0.592	0.727	0.583	0.541	0.542	0.294
L97.424	Non-pressure chronic ulcer of left heel and midfoot with necrosis of bone	161	Chronic Ulcer of Skin, Except Pressure		0.515	0.592	0.727	0.583	0.541	0.542	0.294
L97.425	Non-pressure chronic ulcer of left heel and midfoot with muscle involvement without evidence of necrosis	161	Chronic Ulcer of Skin, Except Pressure		0.515	0.592	0.727	0.583	0.541	0.542	0.294
L97.426	Non-pressure chronic ulcer of left heel and midfoot with bone involvement without evidence of necrosis	161	Chronic Ulcer of Skin, Except Pressure		0.515	0.592	0.727	0.583	0.541	0.542	0.294
L97.428	Non-pressure chronic ulcer of left heel and midfoot with other specified severity	161	Chronic Ulcer of Skin, Except Pressure		0.515	0.592	0.727	0.583	0.541	0.542	0.294
L97.429	Non-pressure chronic ulcer of left heel and midfoot with unspecified severity	161	Chronic Ulcer of Skin, Except Pressure		0.515	0.592	0.727	0.583	0.541	0.542	0.294

ICD-10-CM Code	ICD-10-CM Code Description	V24 CMS-HCC	V24 CMS-HCC Disease Group	V24 CMS-HCC Hierarchies	Community, NonDual, Aged	Community, NonDual, Disabled	Community, FBDual, Aged	Community, FBDual, Disabled	Community, PBDual, Aged	Community, PBDual, Disabled	Institutional
L97.501	Non-pressure chronic ulcer of other part of unspecified foot limited to breakdown of skin	161	Chronic Ulcer of Skin, Except Pressure		0.515	0.592	0.727	0.583	0.541	0.542	0.294
L97.502	Non-pressure chronic ulcer of other part of unspecified foot with fat layer exposed	161	Chronic Ulcer of Skin, Except Pressure		0.515	0.592	0.727	0.583	0.541	0.542	0.294
L97.503	Non-pressure chronic ulcer of other part of unspecified foot with necrosis of muscle	161	Chronic Ulcer of Skin, Except Pressure		0.515	0.592	0.727	0.583	0.541*	0.542	0.294
L97.504	Non-pressure chronic ulcer of other part of unspecified foot with necrosis of bone	161	Chronic Ulcer of Skin, Except Pressure		0.515	0.592	0.727	0.583	0.541	0.542	0.294
L97.505	Non-pressure chronic ulcer of other part of unspecified foot with muscle involvement without evidence of necrosis	161	Chronic Ulcer of Skin, Except Pressure		0.515	0.592	0.727	0.583	0.541	0.542	0.294
L97.506	Non-pressure chronic ulcer of other part of unspecified foot with bone involvement without evidence of necrosis	161	Chronic Ulcer of Skin, Except Pressure		0.515	0.592	0.727	0.583	0.541	0.542	0.294
L97.508	Non-pressure chronic ulcer of other part of unspecified foot with other specified severity	161	Chronic Ulcer of Skin, Except Pressure		0.515	0.592	0.727	0.583	0.541	0.542	0.294
L97.509	Non-pressure chronic ulcer of other part of unspecified foot with unspecified severity	161	Chronic Ulcer of Skin, Except Pressure		0.515	0.592	0.727	0.583	0.541	0.542	0.294
L97.511	Non-pressure chronic ulcer of other part of right foot limited to breakdown of skin	161	Chronic Ulcer of Skin, Except Pressure		0.515	0.592	0.727	0.583	0.541	0.542	0.294
L97.512	Non-pressure chronic ulcer of other part of right foot with fat layer exposed	161	Chronic Ulcer of Skin, Except Pressure		0.515	0.592	0.727	0.583	0.541	0.542	0.294
L97.513	Non-pressure chronic ulcer of other part of right foot with necrosis of muscle	161	Chronic Ulcer of Skin, Except Pressure		0.515	0.592	0.727	0.583	0.541	0.542	0.294
L97.514	Non-pressure chronic ulcer of other part of right foot with necrosis of bone	161	Chronic Ulcer of Skin, Except Pressure		0.515	0.592	0.727	0.583	0.541	0.542	0.294
L97.515	Non-pressure chronic ulcer of other part of right foot with muscle involvement without evidence of necrosis	161	Chronic Ulcer of Skin, Except Pressure		0.515	0.592	0.727	0.583	0.541	0.542	0.294
L97.516	Non-pressure chronic ulcer of other part of right foot with bone involvement without evidence of necrosis	161	Chronic Ulcer of Skin, Except Pressure		0.515	0.592	0.727	0.583	0.541	0.542	0.294
L97.518	Non-pressure chronic ulcer of other part of right foot with other specified severity	161	Chronic Ulcer of Skin, Except Pressure		0.515	0.592	0.727	0.583	0.541	0.542	0.294
L97.519	Non-pressure chronic ulcer of other part of right foot with unspecified severity	161	Chronic Ulcer of Skin, Except Pressure		0.515	0.592	0.727	0.583	0.541	0.542	0.294
L97.521	Non-pressure chronic ulcer of other part of left foot limited to breakdown of skin	161	Chronic Ulcer of Skin, Except Pressure		0.515	0.592	0.727	0.583	0.541	0.542	0.294
L97.522	Non-pressure chronic ulcer of other part of left foot with fat layer exposed	161	Chronic Ulcer of Skin, Except Pressure		0.515	0.592	0.727	0.583	0.541	0.542	0.294
L97.523	Non-pressure chronic ulcer of other part of left foot with necrosis of muscle	161	Chronic Ulcer of Skin, Except Pressure		0.515	0.592	0.727	0.583	0.541	0.542	0.294
L97.524	Non-pressure chronic ulcer of other part of left foot with necrosis of bone	161	Chronic Ulcer of Skin, Except Pressure		0.515	0.592	0.727	0.583	0.541	0.542	0.294

ICD-10-CM Code	ICD-10-CM Code Description	V24 CMS-HCC	V24 CMS-HCC Disease Group	V24 CMS-HCC Hierarchies	Community, NonDual, Aged	Community, NonDual, Disabled	Community, FBDual, Aged	Community, FBDual, Disabled	Community, PBDual, Aged	Community, PBDual, Disabled	Institutional
L97.525	Non-pressure chronic ulcer of other part of left foot with muscle involvement without evidence of necrosis	161	Chronic Ulcer of Skin, Except Pressure		0.515	0.592	0.727	0.583	0.541	0.542	0.294
L97.526	Non-pressure chronic ulcer of other part of left foot with bone involvement without evidence of necrosis	161	Chronic Ulcer of Skin, Except Pressure		0.515	0.592	0.727	0.583	0.541	0.542	0.294
L97.528	Non-pressure chronic ulcer of other part of left foot with other specified severity	161	Chronic Ulcer of Skin, Except Pressure		0.515	0.592	0.727	0.583	0.541	0.542	0.294
L97.529	Non-pressure chronic ulcer of other part of left foot with unspecified severity	161	Chronic Ulcer of Skin, Except Pressure		0.515	0.592	0.727	0.583	0.541	0.542	0.294
L97.801	Non-pressure chronic ulcer of other part of unspecified lower leg limited to breakdown of skin	161	Chronic Ulcer of Skin, Except Pressure		0.515	0.592	0.727	0.583	0.541	0.542	0.294
L97.802	Non-pressure chronic ulcer of other part of unspecified lower leg with fat layer exposed	161	Chronic Ulcer of Skin, Except Pressure		0.515	0.592	0.727	0.583	0.541	0.542	0.294
L97.803	Non-pressure chronic ulcer of other part of unspecified lower leg with necrosis of muscle	161	Chronic Ulcer of Skin, Except Pressure		0.515	0.592	0.727	0.583	0.541	0.542	0.294
L97.804	Non-pressure chronic ulcer of other part of unspecified lower leg with necrosis of bone	161	Chronic Ulcer of Skin, Except Pressure		0.515	0.592	0.727	0.583	0.541	0.542	0.294
L97.805	Non-pressure chronic ulcer of other part of unspecified lower leg with muscle involvement without evidence of necrosis	161	Chronic Ulcer of Skin, Except Pressure		0.515	0.592	0.727	0.583	0.541	0.542	0.294
L97.806	Non-pressure chronic ulcer of other part of unspecified lower leg with bone involvement without evidence of necrosis	161	Chronic Ulcer of Skin, Except Pressure		0.515	0.592	0.727	0.583	0.541	0.542	0.294
L97.808	Non-pressure chronic ulcer of other part of unspecified lower leg with other specified severity	161	Chronic Ulcer of Skin, Except Pressure		0.515	0.592	0.727	0.583	0.541	0.542	0.294
L97.809	Non-pressure chronic ulcer of other part of unspecified lower leg with unspecified severity	161	Chronic Ulcer of Skin, Except Pressure		0.515	0.592	0.727	0.583	0.541	0.542	0.294
L97.811	Non-pressure chronic ulcer of other part of right lower leg limited to breakdown of skin	161	Chronic Ulcer of Skin, Except Pressure		0.515	0.592	0.727	0.583	0.541	0.542	0.294
L97.812	Non-pressure chronic ulcer of other part of right lower leg with fat layer exposed	161	Chronic Ulcer of Skin, Except Pressure		0.515	0.592	0.727	0.583	0.541	0.542	0.294
L97.813	Non-pressure chronic ulcer of other part of right lower leg with necrosis of muscle	161	Chronic Ulcer of Skin, Except Pressure		0.515	0.592	0.727	0.583	0.541	0.542	0.294
L97.814	Non-pressure chronic ulcer of other part of right lower leg with necrosis of bone	161	Chronic Ulcer of Skin, Except Pressure		0.515	0.592	0.727	0.583	0.541	0.542	0.294
L97.815	Non-pressure chronic ulcer of other part of right lower leg with muscle involvement without evidence of necrosis	161	Chronic Ulcer of Skin, Except Pressure		0.515	0.592	0.727	0.583	0.541	0.542	0.294
L97.816	Non-pressure chronic ulcer of other part of right lower leg with bone involvement without evidence of necrosis	161	Chronic Ulcer of Skin, Except Pressure		0.515	0.592	0.727	0.583	0.541	0.542	0.294

ICD-10-CM Code	ICD-10-CM Code Description	V24 CMS-HCC	V24 CMS-HCC Disease Group	V24 CMS-HCC Hierarchies	Community, NonDual, Aged	Community, NonDual, Disabled	Community, FBDual, Aged	Community, FBDual, Disabled	Community, PBDual, Aged	Community, PBDual, Disabled	Institutional
L97.818	Non-pressure chronic ulcer of other part of right lower leg with other specified severity	161	Chronic Ulcer of Skin, Except Pressure		0.515	0.592	0.727	0.583	0.541	0.542	0.294
L97.819	Non-pressure chronic ulcer of other part of right lower leg with unspecified severity	161	Chronic Ulcer of Skin, Except Pressure		0.515	0.592	0.727	0.583	0.541	0.542	0.294
L97.821	Non-pressure chronic ulcer of other part of left lower leg limited to breakdown of skin	161	Chronic Ulcer of Skin, Except Pressure		0.515	0.592	0.727	0.583	0.541	0.542	0.294
L97.822	Non-pressure chronic ulcer of other part of left lower leg with fat layer exposed	161	Chronic Ulcer of Skin, Except Pressure		0.515	0.592	0.727	0.583	0.541	0.542	0.294
L97.823	Non-pressure chronic ulcer of other part of left lower leg with necrosis of muscle	161	Chronic Ulcer of Skin, Except Pressure		0.515	0.592	0.727	0.583	0.541	0.542	0.294
L97.824	Non-pressure chronic ulcer of other part of left lower leg with necrosis of bone	161	Chronic Ulcer of Skin, Except Pressure		0.515	0.592	0.727	0.583	0.541	0.542	0.294
L97.825	Non-pressure chronic ulcer of other part of left lower leg with muscle involvement without evidence of necrosis	161	Chronic Ulcer of Skin, Except Pressure		0.515	0.592	0.727	0.583	0.541	0.542	0.294
L97.826	Non-pressure chronic ulcer of other part of left lower leg with bone involvement without evidence of necrosis	161	Chronic Ulcer of Skin, Except Pressure		0.515	0.592	0.727	0.583	0.541	0.542	0.294
L97.828	Non-pressure chronic ulcer of other part of left lower leg with other specified severity	161	Chronic Ulcer of Skin, Except Pressure		0.515	0.592	0.727	0.583	0.541	0.542	0.294
L97.829	Non-pressure chronic ulcer of other part of left lower leg with unspecified severity	161	Chronic Ulcer of Skin, Except Pressure		0.515	0.592	0.727	0.583	0.541	0.542	0.294
L97.901	Non-pressure chronic ulcer of unspecified part of unspecified lower leg limited to breakdown of skin	161	Chronic Ulcer of Skin, Except Pressure		0.515	0.592	0.727	0.583	0.541	0.542	0.294
L97.902	Non-pressure chronic ulcer of unspecified part of unspecified lower leg with fat layer exposed	161	Chronic Ulcer of Skin, Except Pressure		0.515	0.592	0.727	0.583	0.541	0.542	0.294
L97.903	Non-pressure chronic ulcer of unspecified part of unspecified lower leg with necrosis of muscle	161	Chronic Ulcer of Skin, Except Pressure		0.515	0.592	0.727	0.583	0.541	0.542	0.294
L97.904	Non-pressure chronic ulcer of unspecified part of unspecified lower leg with necrosis of bone	161	Chronic Ulcer of Skin, Except Pressure		0.515	0.592	0.727	0.583	0.541	0.542	0.294
L97.905	Non-pressure chronic ulcer of unspecified part of unspecified lower leg with muscle involvement without evidence of necrosis	161	Chronic Ulcer of Skin, Except Pressure		0.515	0.592	0.727	0.583	0.541	0.542	0.294
L97.906	Non-pressure chronic ulcer of unspecified part of unspecified lower leg with bone involvement without evidence of necrosis	161	Chronic Ulcer of Skin, Except Pressure		0.515	0.592	0.727	0.583	0.541	0.542	0.294
L97.908	Non-pressure chronic ulcer of unspecified part of unspecified lower leg with other specified severity	161	Chronic Ulcer of Skin, Except Pressure		0.515	0.592	0.727	0.583	0.541	0.542	0.294
L97.909	Non-pressure chronic ulcer of unspecified part of unspecified lower leg with unspecified severity	161	Chronic Ulcer of Skin, Except Pressure		0.515	0.592	0.727	0.583	0.541	0.542	0.294
L97.911	Non-pressure chronic ulcer of unspecified part of right lower leg limited to breakdown of skin	161	Chronic Ulcer of Skin, Except Pressure		0.515	0.592	0.727	0.583	0.541	0.542	0.294

ICD-10-CM Code	ICD-10-CM Code Description	V24 CMS-HCC	V24 CMS-HCC Disease Group	V24 CMS-HCC Hierarchies	Community, NonDual, Aged	Community, NonDual, Disabled	Community, FBDual, Aged	Community, FBDual, Disabled	Community, PBDual, Aged	Community, PBDual, Disabled	Institutional
L97.912	Non-pressure chronic ulcer of unspecified part of right lower leg with fat layer exposed	161	Chronic Ulcer of Skin, Except Pressure		0.515	0.592	0.727	0.583	0.541	0.542	0.294
L97.913	Non-pressure chronic ulcer of unspecified part of right lower leg with necrosis of muscle	161	Chronic Ulcer of Skin, Except Pressure		0.515	0.592	0.727	0.583	0.541	0.542	0.294
L97.914	Non-pressure chronic ulcer of unspecified part of right lower leg with necrosis of bone	161	Chronic Ulcer of Skin, Except Pressure		0.515	0.592	0.727	0.583	0.541	0.542	0.294
L97.915	Non-pressure chronic ulcer of unspecified part of right lower leg with muscle involvement without evidence of necrosis	161	Chronic Ulcer of Skin, Except Pressure		0.515	0.592	0.727	0.583	0.541	0.542	0.294
L97.916	Non-pressure chronic ulcer of unspecified part of right lower leg with bone involvement without evidence of necrosis	161	Chronic Ulcer of Skin, Except Pressure		0.515	0.592	0.727	0.583	0.541	0.542	0.294
L97.918	Non-pressure chronic ulcer of unspecified part of right lower leg with other specified severity	161	Chronic Ulcer of Skin, Except Pressure		0.515	0.592	0.727	0.583	0.541	0.542	0.294
L97.919	Non-pressure chronic ulcer of unspecified part of right lower leg with unspecified severity	161	Chronic Ulcer of Skin, Except Pressure		0.515	0.592	0.727	0.583	0.541	0.542	0.294
L97.921	Non-pressure chronic ulcer of unspecified part of left lower leg limited to breakdown of skin	161	Chronic Ulcer of Skin, Except Pressure		0.515	0.592	0.727	0.583	0.541	0.542	0.294
L97.922	Non-pressure chronic ulcer of unspecified part of left lower leg with fat layer exposed	161	Chronic Ulcer of Skin, Except Pressure		0.515	0.592	0.727	0.583	0.541	0.542	0.294
L97.923	Non-pressure chronic ulcer of unspecified part of left lower leg with necrosis of muscle	161	Chronic Ulcer of Skin, Except Pressure		0.515	0.592	0.727	0.583	0.541	0.542	0.294
L97.924	Non-pressure chronic ulcer of unspecified part of left lower leg with necrosis of bone	161	Chronic Ulcer of Skin, Except Pressure		0.515	0.592	0.727	0.583	0.541	0.542	0.294
L97.925	Non-pressure chronic ulcer of unspecified part of left lower leg with muscle involvement without evidence of necrosis	161	Chronic Ulcer of Skin, Except Pressure		0.515	0.592	0.727	0.583	0.541	0.542	0.294
L97.926	Non-pressure chronic ulcer of unspecified part of left lower leg with bone involvement without evidence of necrosis	161	Chronic Ulcer of Skin, Except Pressure		0.515	0.592	0.727	0.583	0.541	0.542	0.294
L97.928	Non-pressure chronic ulcer of unspecified part of left lower leg with other specified severity	161	Chronic Ulcer of Skin, Except Pressure		0.515	0.592	0.727	0.583	0.541	0.542	0.294
L97.929	Non-pressure chronic ulcer of unspecified part of left lower leg with unspecified severity	161	Chronic Ulcer of Skin, Except Pressure		0.515	0.592	0.727	0.583	0.541	0.542	0.294
L98.411	Non-pressure chronic ulcer of buttock limited to breakdown of skin	161	Chronic Ulcer of Skin, Except Pressure		0.515	0.592	0.727	0.583	0.541	0.542	0.294
L98.412	Non-pressure chronic ulcer of buttock with fat layer exposed	161	Chronic Ulcer of Skin, Except Pressure		0.515	0.592	0.727	0.583	0.541	0.542	0.294
L98.413	Non-pressure chronic ulcer of buttock with necrosis of muscle	161	Chronic Ulcer of Skin, Except Pressure		0.515	0.592	0.727	0.583	0.541	0.542	0.294
L98.414	Non-pressure chronic ulcer of buttock with necrosis of bone	161	Chronic Ulcer of Skin, Except Pressure		0.515	0.592	0.727	0.583	0.541	0.542	0.294
L98.415	Non-pressure chronic ulcer of buttock with muscle involvement without evidence of necrosis	161	Chronic Ulcer of Skin, Except Pressure		0.515	0.592	0.727	0.583	0.541	0.542	0.294

ICD-10-CM Code	ICD-10-CM Code Description	V24 CMS-HCC	V24 CMS-HCC Disease Group	V24 CMS-HCC Hierarchies	Community, NonDual, Aged	Community, NonDual, Disabled	Community, FBDual, Aged	Community, FBDual, Disabled	Community, PBDual, Aged	Community, PBDual, Disabled	Institutional
L98.416	Non-pressure chronic ulcer of buttock with bone involvement without evidence of necrosis	161	Chronic Ulcer of Skin, Except Pressure		0.515	0.592	0.727	0.583	0.541	0.542	0.294
L98.418	Non-pressure chronic ulcer of buttock with other specified severity	161	Chronic Ulcer of Skin, Except Pressure		0.515	0.592	0.727	0.583	0.541	0.542	0.294
L98.419	Non-pressure chronic ulcer of buttock with unspecified severity	161	Chronic Ulcer of Skin, Except Pressure		0.515	0.592	0.727	0.583	0.541	0.542	0.294
L98.421	Non-pressure chronic ulcer of back limited to breakdown of skin	161	Chronic Ulcer of Skin, Except Pressure		0.515	0.592	0.727	0.583	0.541	0.542	0.294
L98.422	Non-pressure chronic ulcer of back with fat layer exposed	161	Chronic Ulcer of Skin, Except Pressure		0.515	0.592	0.727	0.583	0.541	0.542	0.294
L98.423	Non-pressure chronic ulcer of back with necrosis of muscle	161	Chronic Ulcer of Skin, Except Pressure		0.515	0.592	0.727	0.583	0.541	0.542	0.294
L98.424	Non-pressure chronic ulcer of back with necrosis of bone	161	Chronic Ulcer of Skin, Except Pressure		0.515	0.592	0.727	0.583	0.541	0.542	0.294
L98.425	Non-pressure chronic ulcer of back with muscle involvement without evidence of necrosis	161	Chronic Ulcer of Skin, Except Pressure		0.515	0.592	0.727	0.583	0.541	0.542	0.294
L98.426	Non-pressure chronic ulcer of back with bone involvement without evidence of necrosis	161	Chronic Ulcer of Skin, Except Pressure		0.515	0.592	0.727	0.583	0.541	0.542	0.294
L98.428	Non-pressure chronic ulcer of back with other specified severity	161	Chronic Ulcer of Skin, Except Pressure		0.515	0.592	0.727	0.583	0.541	0.542	0.294
L98.429	Non-pressure chronic ulcer of back with unspecified severity	161	Chronic Ulcer of Skin, Except Pressure		0.515	0.592	0.727	0.583	0.541	0.542	0.294
L98.491	Non-pressure chronic ulcer of skin of other sites limited to breakdown of skin	161	Chronic Ulcer of Skin, Except Pressure		0.515	0.592	0.727	0.583	0.541	0.542	0.294
L98.492	Non-pressure chronic ulcer of skin of other sites with fat layer exposed	161	Chronic Ulcer of Skin, Except Pressure		0.515	0.592	0.727	0.583	0.541	0.542	0.294
L98.493	Non-pressure chronic ulcer of skin of other sites with necrosis of muscle	161	Chronic Ulcer of Skin, Except Pressure		0.515	0.592	0.727	0.583	0.541	0.542	0.294
L98.494	Non-pressure chronic ulcer of skin of other sites with necrosis of bone	161	Chronic Ulcer of Skin, Except Pressure		0.515	0.592	0.727	0.583	0.541	0.542	0.294
L98.495	Non-pressure chronic ulcer of skin of other sites with muscle involvement without evidence of necrosis	161	Chronic Ulcer of Skin, Except Pressure		0.515	0.592	0.727	0.583	0.541	0.542	0.294
L98.496	Non-pressure chronic ulcer of skin of other sites with bone involvement without evidence of necrosis	161	Chronic Ulcer of Skin, Except Pressure		0.515	0.592	0.727	0.583	0.541	0.542	0.294
L98.498	Non-pressure chronic ulcer of skin of other sites with other specified severity	161	Chronic Ulcer of Skin, Except Pressure		0.515	0.592	0.727	0.583	0.541	0.542	0.294
L98.499	Non-pressure chronic ulcer of skin of other sites with unspecified severity	161	Chronic Ulcer of Skin, Except Pressure		0.515	0.592	0.727	0.583	0.541	0.542	0.294
M00.00	Staphylococcal arthritis, unspecified joint	39	Bone/Joint/Muscle Infections/Necrosis		0.401	0.378	0.558	0.682	0.443	0.435	0.401
M00.011	Staphylococcal arthritis, right shoulder	39	Bone/Joint/Muscle Infections/Necrosis		0.401	0.378	0.558	0.682	0.443	0.435	0.401
M00.012	Staphylococcal arthritis, left shoulder	39	Bone/Joint/Muscle Infections/Necrosis		0.401	0.378	0.558	0.682	0.443	0.435	0.401
M00.019	Staphylococcal arthritis, unspecified shoulder	39	Bone/Joint/Muscle Infections/Necrosis		0.401	0.378	0.558	0.682	0.443	0.435	0.401
M00.021	Staphylococcal arthritis, right elbow	39	Bone/Joint/Muscle Infections/Necrosis		0.401	0.378	0.558	0.682	0.443	0.435	0.401
M00.022	Staphylococcal arthritis, left elbow	39	Bone/Joint/Muscle Infections/Necrosis		0.401	0.378	0.558	0.682	0.443	0.435	0.401
M00.029	Staphylococcal arthritis, unspecified elbow	39	Bone/Joint/Muscle Infections/Necrosis		0.401	0.378	0.558	0.682	0.443	0.435	0.401
M00.031	Staphylococcal arthritis, right wrist	39	Bone/Joint/Muscle Infections/Necrosis		0.401	0.378	0.558	0.682	0.443	0.435	0.401
M00.032	Staphylococcal arthritis, left wrist	39	Bone/Joint/Muscle Infections/Necrosis		0.401	0.378	0.558	0.682	0.443	0.435	0.401

ICD-10-CM Code	ICD-10-CM Code Description	V24 CMS-HCC	V24 CMS-HCC Disease Group	V24 CMS-HCC Hierarchies	Community, NonDual, Aged	Community, NonDual, Disabled	Community, FBDual, Aged	Community, FBDual, Disabled	Community, PBDual, Aged	Community, PBDual, Disabled	Institutional
M00.039	Staphylococcal arthritis, unspecified wrist	39	Bone/Joint/Muscle Infections/Necrosis		0.401	0.378	0.558	0.682	0.443	0.435	0.401
M00.041	Staphylococcal arthritis, right hand	39	Bone/Joint/Muscle Infections/Necrosis		0.401	0.378	0.558	0.682	0.443	0.435	0.401
M00.042	Staphylococcal arthritis, left hand	39	Bone/Joint/Muscle Infections/Necrosis		0.401	0.378	0.558	0.682	0.443	0.435	0.401
M00.049	Staphylococcal arthritis, unspecified hand	39	Bone/Joint/Muscle Infections/Necrosis		0.401	0.378	0.558	0.682	0.443	0.435	0.401
M00.051	Staphylococcal arthritis, right hip	39	Bone/Joint/Muscle Infections/Necrosis		0.401	0.378	0.558	0.682	0.443	0.435	0.401
M00.052	Staphylococcal arthritis, left hip	39	Bone/Joint/Muscle Infections/Necrosis		0.401	0.378	0.558	0.682	0.443	0.435	0.401
M00.059	Staphylococcal arthritis, unspecified hip	39	Bone/Joint/Muscle Infections/Necrosis		0.401	0.378	0.558	0.682	0.443	0.435	0.401
M00.061	Staphylococcal arthritis, right knee	39	Bone/Joint/Muscle Infections/Necrosis		0.401	0.378	0.558	0.682	0.443	0.435	0.401
M00.062	Staphylococcal arthritis, left knee	39	Bone/Joint/Muscle Infections/Necrosis		0.401	0.378	0.558	0.682	0.443	0.435	0.401
M00.069	Staphylococcal arthritis, unspecified knee	39	Bone/Joint/Muscle Infections/Necrosis		0.401	0.378	0.558	0.682	0.443	0.435	0.401
M00.071	Staphylococcal arthritis, right ankle and foot	39	Bone/Joint/Muscle Infections/Necrosis		0.401	0.378	0.558	0.682	0.443	0.435	0.401
M00.072	Staphylococcal arthritis, left ankle and foot	39	Bone/Joint/Muscle Infections/Necrosis		0.401	0.378	0.558	0.682	0.443	0.435	0.401
M00.079	Staphylococcal arthritis, unspecified ankle and foot	39	Bone/Joint/Muscle Infections/Necrosis		0.401	0.378	0.558	0.682	0.443	0.435	0.401
M00.08	Staphylococcal arthritis, vertebrae	39	Bone/Joint/Muscle Infections/Necrosis		0.401	0.378	0.558	0.682	0.443	0.435	0.401
M00.09	Staphylococcal polyarthritis	39	Bone/Joint/Muscle Infections/Necrosis		0.401	0.378	0.558	0.682	0.443	0.435	0.401
M00.10	Pneumococcal arthritis, unspecified joint	39	Bone/Joint/Muscle Infections/Necrosis		0.401	0.378	0.558	0.682	0.443	0.435	0.401
M00.111	Pneumococcal arthritis, right shoulder	39	Bone/Joint/Muscle Infections/Necrosis		0.401	0.378	0.558	0.682	0.443	0.435	0.401
M00.112	Pneumococcal arthritis, left shoulder	39	Bone/Joint/Muscle Infections/Necrosis		0.401	0.378	0.558	0.682	0.443	0.435	0.401
M00.119	Pneumococcal arthritis, unspecified shoulder	39	Bone/Joint/Muscle Infections/Necrosis		0.401	0.378	0.558	0.682	0.443	0.435	0.401
M00.121	Pneumococcal arthritis, right elbow	39	Bone/Joint/Muscle Infections/Necrosis		0.401	0.378	0.558	0.682	0.443	0.435	0.401
M00.122	Pneumococcal arthritis, left elbow	39	Bone/Joint/Muscle Infections/Necrosis		0.401	0.378	0.558	0.682	0.443	0.435	0.401
M00.129	Pneumococcal arthritis, unspecified elbow	39	Bone/Joint/Muscle Infections/Necrosis		0.401	0.378	0.558	0.682	0.443	0.435	0.401
M00.131	Pneumococcal arthritis, right wrist	39	Bone/Joint/Muscle Infections/Necrosis		0.401	0.378	0.558	0.682	0.443	0.435	0.401
M00.132	Pneumococcal arthritis, left wrist	39	Bone/Joint/Muscle Infections/Necrosis		0.401	0.378	0.558	0.682	0.443	0.435	0.401
M00.139	Pneumococcal arthritis, unspecified wrist	39	Bone/Joint/Muscle Infections/Necrosis		0.401	0.378	0.558	0.682	0.443	0.435	0.401
M00.141	Pneumococcal arthritis, right hand	39	Bone/Joint/Muscle Infections/Necrosis		0.401	0.378	0.558	0.682	0.443	0.435	0.401
M00.142	Pneumococcal arthritis, left hand	39	Bone/Joint/Muscle Infections/Necrosis		0.401	0.378	0.558	0.682	0.443	0.435	0.401
M00.149	Pneumococcal arthritis, unspecified hand	39	Bone/Joint/Muscle Infections/Necrosis		0.401	0.378	0.558	0.682	0.443	0.435	0.401
M00.151	Pneumococcal arthritis, right hip	39	Bone/Joint/Muscle Infections/Necrosis		0.401	0.378	0.558	0.682	0.443	0.435	0.401
M00.152	Pneumococcal arthritis, left hip	39	Bone/Joint/Muscle Infections/Necrosis		0.401	0.378	0.558	0.682	0.443	0.435	0.401
M00.159	Pneumococcal arthritis, unspecified hip	39	Bone/Joint/Muscle Infections/Necrosis		0.401	0.378	0.558	0.682	0.443	0.435	0.401
M00.161	Pneumococcal arthritis, right knee	39	Bone/Joint/Muscle Infections/Necrosis		0.401	0.378	0.558	0.682	0.443	0.435	0.401
M00.162	Pneumococcal arthritis, left knee	39	Bone/Joint/Muscle Infections/Necrosis		0.401	0.378	0.558	0.682	0.443	0.435	0.401
M00.169	Pneumococcal arthritis, unspecified knee	39	Bone/Joint/Muscle Infections/Necrosis		0.401	0.378	0.558	0.682	0.443	0.435	0.401
M00.171	Pneumococcal arthritis, right ankle and foot	39	Bone/Joint/Muscle Infections/Necrosis		0.401	0.378	0.558	0.682	0.443	0.435	0.401
M00.172	Pneumococcal arthritis, left ankle and foot	39	Bone/Joint/Muscle Infections/Necrosis		0.401	0.378	0.558	0.682	0.443	0.435	0.401
M00.179	Pneumococcal arthritis, unspecified ankle and foot	39	Bone/Joint/Muscle Infections/Necrosis		0.401	0.378	0.558	0.682	0.443	0.435	0.401
M00.18	Pneumococcal arthritis, vertebrae	39	Bone/Joint/Muscle Infections/Necrosis		0.401	0.378	0.558	0.682	0.443	0.435	0.401

ICD-10-CM Code	ICD-10-CM Code Description	V24 CMS-HCC	V24 CMS-HCC Disease Group	V24 CMS-HCC Hierarchies	Community, NonDual, Aged	Community, NonDual, Disabled	Community, FBDual, Aged	Community, FBDual, Disabled	Community, PBDual, Aged	Community, PBDual, Disabled	Institutional
M00.19	Pneumococcal polyarthritis	39	Bone/Joint/Muscle Infections/Necrosis		0.401	0.378	0.558	0.682	0.443	0.435	0.401
M00.20	Other streptococcal arthritis, unspecified joint	39	Bone/Joint/Muscle Infections/Necrosis		0.401	0.378	0.558	0.682	0.443	0.435	0.401
M00.211	Other streptococcal arthritis, right shoulder	39	Bone/Joint/Muscle Infections/Necrosis		0.401	0.378	0.558	0.682	0.443	0.435	0.401
M00.212	Other streptococcal arthritis, left shoulder	39	Bone/Joint/Muscle Infections/Necrosis		0.401	0.378	0.558	0.682	0.443	0.435	0.401
M00.219	Other streptococcal arthritis, unspecified shoulder	39	Bone/Joint/Muscle Infections/Necrosis		0.401	0.378	0.558	0.682	0.443	0.435	0.401
M00.221	Other streptococcal arthritis, right elbow	39	Bone/Joint/Muscle Infections/Necrosis		0.401	0.378	0.558	0.682	0.443	0.435	0.401
M00.222	Other streptococcal arthritis, left elbow	39	Bone/Joint/Muscle Infections/Necrosis		0.401	0.378	0.558	0.682	0.443	0.435	0.401
M00.229	Other streptococcal arthritis, unspecified elbow	39	Bone/Joint/Muscle Infections/Necrosis		0.401	0.378	0.558	0.682	0.443	0.435	0.401
M00.231	Other streptococcal arthritis, right wrist	39	Bone/Joint/Muscle Infections/Necrosis		0.401	0.378	0.558	0.682	0.443	0.435	0.401
M00.232	Other streptococcal arthritis, left wrist	39	Bone/Joint/Muscle Infections/Necrosis		0.401	0.378	0.558	0.682	0.443	0.435	0.401
M00.239	Other streptococcal arthritis, unspecified wrist	39	Bone/Joint/Muscle Infections/Necrosis		0.401	0.378	0.558	0.682	0.443	0.435	0.401
M00.241	Other streptococcal arthritis, right hand	39	Bone/Joint/Muscle Infections/Necrosis		0.401	0.378	0.558	0.682	0.443	0.435	0.401
M00.242	Other streptococcal arthritis, left hand	39	Bone/Joint/Muscle Infections/Necrosis		0.401	0.378	0.558	0.682	0.443	0.435	0.401
M00.249	Other streptococcal arthritis, unspecified hand	39	Bone/Joint/Muscle Infections/Necrosis		0.401	0.378	0.558	0.682	0.443	0.435	0.401
M00.251	Other streptococcal arthritis, right hip	39	Bone/Joint/Muscle Infections/Necrosis		0.401	0.378	0.558	0.682	0.443	0.435	0.401
M00.252	Other streptococcal arthritis, left hip	39	Bone/Joint/Muscle Infections/Necrosis		0.401	0.378	0.558	0.682	0.443	0.435	0.401
M00.259	Other streptococcal arthritis, unspecified hip	39	Bone/Joint/Muscle Infections/Necrosis		0.401	0.378	0.558	0.682	0.443	0.435	0.401
M00.261	Other streptococcal arthritis, right knee	39	Bone/Joint/Muscle Infections/Necrosis		0.401	0.378	0.558	0.682	0.443	0.435	0.401
M00.262	Other streptococcal arthritis, left knee	39	Bone/Joint/Muscle Infections/Necrosis		0.401	0.378	0.558	0.682	0.443	0.435	0.401
M00.269	Other streptococcal arthritis, unspecified knee	39	Bone/Joint/Muscle Infections/Necrosis		0.401	0.378	0.558	0.682	0.443	0.435	0.401
M00.271	Other streptococcal arthritis, right ankle and foot	39	Bone/Joint/Muscle Infections/Necrosis		0.401	0.378	0.558	0.682	0.443	0.435	0.401
M00.272	Other streptococcal arthritis, left ankle and foot	39	Bone/Joint/Muscle Infections/Necrosis		0.401	0.378	0.558	0.682	0.443	0.435	0.401
M00.279	Other streptococcal arthritis, unspecified ankle and foot	39	Bone/Joint/Muscle Infections/Necrosis		0.401	0.378	0.558	0.682	0.443	0.435	0.401
M00.28	Other streptococcal arthritis, vertebrae	39	Bone/Joint/Muscle Infections/Necrosis		0.401	0.378	0.558	0.682	0.443	0.435	0.401
M00.29	Other streptococcal polyarthritis	39	Bone/Joint/Muscle Infections/Necrosis		0.401	0.378	0.558	0.682	0.443	0.435	0.401
M00.80	Arthritis due to other bacteria, unspecified joint	39	Bone/Joint/Muscle Infections/Necrosis		0.401	0.378	0.558	0.682	0.443	0.435	0.401
M00.811	Arthritis due to other bacteria, right shoulder	39	Bone/Joint/Muscle Infections/Necrosis		0.401	0.378	0.558	0.682	0.443	0.435	0.401
M00.812	Arthritis due to other bacteria, left shoulder	39	Bone/Joint/Muscle Infections/Necrosis		0.401	0.378	0.558	0.682	0.443	0.435	0.401
M00.819	Arthritis due to other bacteria, unspecified shoulder	39	Bone/Joint/Muscle Infections/Necrosis		0.401	0.378	0.558	0.682	0.443	0.435	0.401
M00.821	Arthritis due to other bacteria, right elbow	39	Bone/Joint/Muscle Infections/Necrosis		0.401	0.378	0.558	0.682	0.443	0.435	0.401
M00.822	Arthritis due to other bacteria, left elbow	39	Bone/Joint/Muscle Infections/Necrosis		0.401	0.378	0.558	0.682	0.443	0.435	0.401
M00.829	Arthritis due to other bacteria, unspecified elbow	39	Bone/Joint/Muscle Infections/Necrosis		0.401	0.378	0.558	0.682	0.443	0.435	0.401

ICD-10-CM Code	ICD-10-CM Code Description	V24 CMS-HCC	V24 CMS-HCC Disease Group	V24 CMS-HCC Hierarchies	Community, NonDual, Aged	Community, NonDual, Disabled	Community, FBDual, Aged	Community, FBDual, Disabled	Community, PBDual, Aged	Community, PBDual, Disabled	Institutional
M00.831	Arthritis due to other bacteria, right wrist	39	Bone/Joint/Muscle Infections/Necrosis		0.401	0.378	0.558	0.682	0.443	0.435	0.401
M00.832	Arthritis due to other bacteria, left wrist	39	Bone/Joint/Muscle Infections/Necrosis		0.401	0.378	0.558	0.682	0.443	0.435	0.401
M00.839	Arthritis due to other bacteria, unspecified wrist	39	Bone/Joint/Muscle Infections/Necrosis		0.401	0.378	0.558	0.682	0.443	0.435	0.401
M00.841	Arthritis due to other bacteria, right hand	39	Bone/Joint/Muscle Infections/Necrosis		0.401	0.378	0.558	0.682	0.443	0.435	0.401
M00.842	Arthritis due to other bacteria, left hand	39	Bone/Joint/Muscle Infections/Necrosis		0.401	0.378	0.558	0.682	0.443	0.435	0.401
M00.849	Arthritis due to other bacteria, unspecified hand	39	Bone/Joint/Muscle Infections/Necrosis		0.401	0.378	0.558	0.682	0.443	0.435	0.401
M00.851	Arthritis due to other bacteria, right hip	39	Bone/Joint/Muscle Infections/Necrosis		0.401	0.378	0.558	0.682	0.443	0.435	0.401
M00.852	Arthritis due to other bacteria, left hip	39	Bone/Joint/Muscle Infections/Necrosis		0.401	0.378	0.558	0.682	0.443	0.435	0.401
M00.859	Arthritis due to other bacteria, unspecified hip	39	Bone/Joint/Muscle Infections/Necrosis		0.401	0.378	0.558	0.682	0.443	0.435	0.401
M00.861	Arthritis due to other bacteria, right knee	39	Bone/Joint/Muscle Infections/Necrosis		0.401	0.378	0.558	0.682	0.443	0.435	0.401
M00.862	Arthritis due to other bacteria, left knee	39	Bone/Joint/Muscle Infections/Necrosis		0.401	0.378	0.558	0.682	0.443	0.435	0.401
M00.869	Arthritis due to other bacteria, unspecified knee	39	Bone/Joint/Muscle Infections/Necrosis		0.401	0.378	0.558	0.682	0.443	0.435	0.401
M00.871	Arthritis due to other bacteria, right ankle and foot	39	Bone/Joint/Muscle Infections/Necrosis		0.401	0.378	0.558	0.682	0.443	0.435	0.401
M00.872	Arthritis due to other bacteria, left ankle and foot	39	Bone/Joint/Muscle Infections/Necrosis		0.401	0.378	0.558	0.682	0.443	0.435	0.401
M00.879	Arthritis due to other bacteria, unspecified ankle and foot	39	Bone/Joint/Muscle Infections/Necrosis		0.401	0.378	0.558	0.682	0.443	0.435	0.401
M00.88	Arthritis due to other bacteria, vertebrae	39	Bone/Joint/Muscle Infections/Necrosis		0.401	0.378	0.558	0.682	0.443	0.435	0.401
M00.89	Polyarthritis due to other bacteria	39	Bone/Joint/Muscle Infections/Necrosis		0.401	0.378	0.558	0.682	0.443	0.435	0.401
M00.9	Pyogenic arthritis, unspecified	39	Bone/Joint/Muscle Infections/Necrosis		0.401	0.378	0.558	0.682	0.443	0.435	0.401
M01.X0	Direct infection of unspecified joint in infectious and parasitic diseases classified elsewhere	39	Bone/Joint/Muscle Infections/Necrosis		0.401	0.378	0.558	0.682	0.443	0.435	0.401
M01.X11	Direct infection of right shoulder in infectious and parasitic diseases classified elsewhere	39	Bone/Joint/Muscle Infections/Necrosis		0.401	0.378	0.558	0.682	0.443	0.435	0.401
M01.X12	Direct infection of left shoulder in infectious and parasitic diseases classified elsewhere	39	Bone/Joint/Muscle Infections/Necrosis		0.401	0.378	0.558	0.682	0.443	0.435	0.401
M01.X19	Direct infection of unspecified shoulder in infectious and parasitic diseases classified elsewhere	39	Bone/Joint/Muscle Infections/Necrosis		0.401	0.378	0.558	0.682	0.443	0.435	0.401
M01.X21	Direct infection of right elbow in infectious and parasitic diseases classified elsewhere	39	Bone/Joint/Muscle Infections/Necrosis		0.401	0.378	0.558	0.682	0.443	0.435	0.401
M01.X22	Direct infection of left elbow in infectious and parasitic diseases classified elsewhere	39	Bone/Joint/Muscle Infections/Necrosis		0.401	0.378	0.558	0.682	0.443	0.435	0.401
M01.X29	Direct infection of unspecified elbow in infectious and parasitic diseases classified elsewhere	39	Bone/Joint/Muscle Infections/Necrosis		0.401	0.378	0.558	0.682	0.443	0.435	0.401
M01.X31	Direct infection of right wrist in infectious and parasitic diseases classified elsewhere	39	Bone/Joint/Muscle Infections/Necrosis		0.401	0.378	0.558	0.682	0.443	0.435	0.401

ICD-10-CM Code	ICD-10-CM Code Description	V24 CMS-HCC	V24 CMS-HCC Disease Group	V24 CMS-HCC Hierarchies	Community, NonDual, Aged	Community, NonDual, Disabled	Community, FBDual, Aged	Community, FBDual, Disabled	Community, PBDual, Aged	Community, PBDual, Disabled	Institutional
M01.X32	Direct infection of left wrist in infectious and parasitic diseases classified elsewhere	39	Bone/Joint/Muscle Infections/Necrosis		0.401	0.378	0.558	0.682	0.443	0.435	0.401
M01.X39	Direct infection of unspecified wrist in infectious and parasitic diseases classified elsewhere	39	Bone/Joint/Muscle Infections/Necrosis		0.401	0.378	0.558	0.682	0.443	0.435	0.401
M01.X41	Direct infection of right hand in infectious and parasitic diseases classified elsewhere	39	Bone/Joint/Muscle Infections/Necrosis		0.401	0.378	0.558	0.682	0.443	0.435	0.401
M01.X42	Direct infection of left hand in infectious and parasitic diseases classified elsewhere	39	Bone/Joint/Muscle Infections/Necrosis		0.401	0.378	0.558	0.682	0.443	0.435	0.401
M01.X49	Direct infection of unspecified hand in infectious and parasitic diseases classified elsewhere	39	Bone/Joint/Muscle Infections/Necrosis		0.401	0.378	0.558	0.682	0.443	0.435	0.401
M01.X51	Direct infection of right hip in infectious and parasitic diseases classified elsewhere	39	Bone/Joint/Muscle Infections/Necrosis		0.401	0.378	0.558	0.682	0.443	0.435	0.401
M01.X52	Direct infection of left hip in infectious and parasitic diseases classified elsewhere	39	Bone/Joint/Muscle Infections/Necrosis		0.401	0.378	0.558	0.682	0.443	0.435	0.401
M01.X59	Direct infection of unspecified hip in infectious and parasitic diseases classified elsewhere	39	Bone/Joint/Muscle Infections/Necrosis		0.401	0.378	0.558	0.682	0.443	0.435	0.401
M01.X61	Direct infection of right knee in infectious and parasitic diseases classified elsewhere	39	Bone/Joint/Muscle Infections/Necrosis		0.401	0.378	0.558	0.682	0.443	0.435	0.401
M01.X62	Direct infection of left knee in infectious and parasitic diseases classified elsewhere	39	Bone/Joint/Muscle Infections/Necrosis		0.401	0.378	0.558	0.682	0.443	0.435	0.401
M01.X69	Direct infection of unspecified knee in infectious and parasitic diseases classified elsewhere	39	Bone/Joint/Muscle Infections/Necrosis		0.401	0.378	0.558	0.682	0.443	0.435	0.401
M01.X71	Direct infection of right ankle and foot in infectious and parasitic diseases classified elsewhere	39	Bone/Joint/Muscle Infections/Necrosis		0.401	0.378	0.558	0.682	0.443	0.435	0.401
M01.X72	Direct infection of left ankle and foot in infectious and parasitic diseases classified elsewhere	39	Bone/Joint/Muscle Infections/Necrosis		0.401	0.378	0.558	0.682	0.443	0.435	0.401
M01.X79	Direct infection of unspecified ankle and foot in infectious and parasitic diseases classified elsewhere	39	Bone/Joint/Muscle Infections/Necrosis		0.401	0.378	0.558	0.682	0.443	0.435	0.401
M01.X8	Direct infection of vertebrae in infectious and parasitic diseases classified elsewhere	39	Bone/Joint/Muscle Infections/Necrosis		0.401	0.378	0.558	0.682	0.443	0.435	0.401
M01.X9	Direct infection of multiple joints in infectious and parasitic diseases classified elsewhere	39	Bone/Joint/Muscle Infections/Necrosis		0.401	0.378	0.558	0.682	0.443	0.435	0.401
M02.10	Postdysenteric arthropathy, unspecified site	39	Bone/Joint/Muscle Infections/Necrosis		0.401	0.378	0.558	0.682	0.443	0.435	0.401
M02.111	Postdysenteric arthropathy, right shoulder	39	Bone/Joint/Muscle Infections/Necrosis		0.401	0.378	0.558	0.682	0.443	0.435	0.401
M02.112	Postdysenteric arthropathy, left shoulder	39	Bone/Joint/Muscle Infections/Necrosis		0.401	0.378	0.558	0.682	0.443	0.435	0.401
M02.119	Postdysenteric arthropathy, unspecified shoulder	39	Bone/Joint/Muscle Infections/Necrosis		0.401	0.378	0.558	0.682	0.443	0.435	0.401
M02.121	Postdysenteric arthropathy, right elbow	39	Bone/Joint/Muscle Infections/Necrosis		0.401	0.378	0.558	0.682	0.443	0.435	0.401
M02.122	Postdysenteric arthropathy, left elbow	39	Bone/Joint/Muscle Infections/Necrosis		0.401	0.378	0.558	0.682	0.443	0.435	0.401

ICD-10-CM Code	ICD-10-CM Code Description	V24 CMS-HCC	V24 CMS-HCC Disease Group	V24 CMS-HCC Hierarchies	Community, NonDual, Aged	Community, NonDual, Disabled	Community, FBDual, Aged	Community, FBDual, Disabled	Community, PBDual, Aged	Community, PBDual, Disabled	Institutional
M02.129	Postdysenteric arthropathy, unspecified elbow	39	Bone/Joint/Muscle Infections/Necrosis		0.401	0.378	0.558	0.682	0.443	0.435	0.401
M02.131	Postdysenteric arthropathy, right wrist	39	Bone/Joint/Muscle Infections/Necrosis		0.401	0.378	0.558	0.682	0.443	0.435	0.401
M02.132	Postdysenteric arthropathy, left wrist	39	Bone/Joint/Muscle Infections/Necrosis		0.401	0.378	0.558	0.682	0.443	0.435	0.401
M02.139	Postdysenteric arthropathy, unspecified wrist	39	Bone/Joint/Muscle Infections/Necrosis		0.401	0.378	0.558	0.682	0.443	0.435	0.401
M02.141	Postdysenteric arthropathy, right hand	39	Bone/Joint/Muscle Infections/Necrosis		0.401	0.378	0.558	0.682	0.443	0.435	0.401
M02.142	Postdysenteric arthropathy, left hand	39	Bone/Joint/Muscle Infections/Necrosis		0.401	0.378	0.558	0.682	0.443	0.435	0.401
M02.149	Postdysenteric arthropathy, unspecified hand	39	Bone/Joint/Muscle Infections/Necrosis		0.401	0.378	0.558	0.682	0.443	0.435	0.401
M02.151	Postdysenteric arthropathy, right hip	39	Bone/Joint/Muscle Infections/Necrosis		0.401	0.378	0.558	0.682	0.443	0.435	0.401
M02.152	Postdysenteric arthropathy, left hip	39	Bone/Joint/Muscle Infections/Necrosis		0.401	0.378	0.558	0.682	0.443	0.435	0.401
M02.159	Postdysenteric arthropathy, unspecified hip	39	Bone/Joint/Muscle Infections/Necrosis		0.401	0.378	0.558	0.682	0.443	0.435	0.401
M02.161	Postdysenteric arthropathy, right knee	39	Bone/Joint/Muscle Infections/Necrosis		0.401	0.378	0.558	0.682	0.443	0.435	0.401
M02.162	Postdysenteric arthropathy, left knee	39	Bone/Joint/Muscle Infections/Necrosis		0.401	0.378	0.558	0.682	0.443	0.435	0.401
M02.169	Postdysenteric arthropathy, unspecified knee	39	Bone/Joint/Muscle Infections/Necrosis		0.401	0.378	0.558	0.682	0.443	0.435	0.401
M02.171	Postdysenteric arthropathy, right ankle and foot	39	Bone/Joint/Muscle Infections/Necrosis		0.401	0.378	0.558	0.682	0.443	0.435	0.401
M02.172	Postdysenteric arthropathy, left ankle and foot	39	Bone/Joint/Muscle Infections/Necrosis		0.401	0.378	0.558	0.682	0.443	0.435	0.401
M02.179	Postdysenteric arthropathy, unspecified ankle and foot	39	Bone/Joint/Muscle Infections/Necrosis		0.401	0.378	0.558	0.682	0.443	0.435	0.401
M02.18	Postdysenteric arthropathy, vertebrae	39	Bone/Joint/Muscle Infections/Necrosis		0.401	0.378	0.558	0.682	0.443	0.435	0.401
M02.19	Postdysenteric arthropathy, multiple sites	39	Bone/Joint/Muscle Infections/Necrosis		0.401	0.378	0.558	0.682	0.443	0.435	0.401
M02.30	Reiter's disease, unspecified site	40	Rheumatoid Arthritis and Inflammatory Connective Tissue Disease		0.421	0.367	0.371	0.328	0.347	0.264	0.292
M02.311	Reiter's disease, right shoulder	40	Rheumatoid Arthritis and Inflammatory Connective Tissue Disease		0.421	0.367	0.371	0.328	0.347	0.264	0.292
M02.312	Reiter's disease, left shoulder	40	Rheumatoid Arthritis and Inflammatory Connective Tissue Disease		0.421	0.367	0.371	0.328	0.347	0.264	0.292
M02.319	Reiter's disease, unspecified shoulder	40	Rheumatoid Arthritis and Inflammatory Connective Tissue Disease		0.421	0.367	0.371	0.328	0.347	0.264	0.292
M02.321	Reiter's disease, right elbow	40	Rheumatoid Arthritis and Inflammatory Connective Tissue Disease		0.421	0.367	0.371	0.328	0.347	0.264	0.292
M02.322	Reiter's disease, left elbow	40	Rheumatoid Arthritis and Inflammatory Connective Tissue Disease		0.421	0.367	0.371	0.328	0.347	0.264	0.292
M02.329	Reiter's disease, unspecified elbow	40	Rheumatoid Arthritis and Inflammatory Connective Tissue Disease		0.421	0.367	0.371	0.328	0.347	0.264	0.292
M02.331	Reiter's disease, right wrist	40	Rheumatoid Arthritis and Inflammatory Connective Tissue Disease		0.421	0.367	0.371	0.328	0.347	0.264	0.292
M02.332	Reiter's disease, left wrist	40	Rheumatoid Arthritis and Inflammatory Connective Tissue Disease		0.421	0.367	0.371	0.328	0.347	0.264	0.292

ICD-10-CM Code	ICD-10-CM Code Description	V24 CMS-HCC	V24 CMS-HCC Disease Group	V24 CMS-HCC Hierarchies	Community, NonDual, Aged	Community, NonDual, Disabled	Community, FBDual, Aged	Community, FBDual, Disabled	Community, PBDual, Aged	Community, PBDual, Disabled	Institutional
M02.339	Reiter's disease, unspecified wrist	40	Rheumatoid Arthritis and Inflammatory Connective Tissue Disease		0.421	0.367	0.371	0.328	0.347	0.264	0.292
M02.341	Reiter's disease, right hand	40	Rheumatoid Arthritis and Inflammatory Connective Tissue Disease		0.421	0.367	0.371	0.328	0.347	0.264	0.292
M02.342	Reiter's disease, left hand	40	Rheumatoid Arthritis and Inflammatory Connective Tissue Disease		0.421	0.367	0.371	0.328	0.347	0.264	0.292
M02.349	Reiter's disease, unspecified hand	40	Rheumatoid Arthritis and Inflammatory Connective Tissue Disease		0.421	0.367	0.371	0.328	0.347	0.264	0.292
M02.351	Reiter's disease, right hip	40	Rheumatoid Arthritis and Inflammatory Connective Tissue Disease		0.421	0.367	0.371	0.328	0.347	0.264	0.292
M02.352	Reiter's disease, left hip	40	Rheumatoid Arthritis and Inflammatory Connective Tissue Disease		0.421	0.367	0.371	0.328	0.347	0.264	0.292
M02.359	Reiter's disease, unspecified hip	40	Rheumatoid Arthritis and Inflammatory Connective Tissue Disease		0.421	0.367	0.371	0.328	0.347	0.264	0.292
M02.361	Reiter's disease, right knee	40	Rheumatoid Arthritis and Inflammatory Connective Tissue Disease		0.421	0.367	0.371	0.328	0.347	0.264	0.292
M02.362	Reiter's disease, left knee	40	Rheumatoid Arthritis and Inflammatory Connective Tissue Disease		0.421	0.367	0.371	0.328	0.347	0.264	0.292
M02.369	Reiter's disease, unspecified knee	40	Rheumatoid Arthritis and Inflammatory Connective Tissue Disease		0.421	0.367	0.371	0.328	0.347	0.264	0.292
M02.371	Reiter's disease, right ankle and foot	40	Rheumatoid Arthritis and Inflammatory Connective Tissue Disease		0.421	0.367	0.371	0.328	0.347	0.264	0.292
M02.372	Reiter's disease, left ankle and foot	40	Rheumatoid Arthritis and Inflammatory Connective Tissue Disease		0.421	0.367	0.371	0.328	0.347	0.264	0.292
M02.379	Reiter's disease, unspecified ankle and foot	40	Rheumatoid Arthritis and Inflammatory Connective Tissue Disease		0.421	0.367	0.371	0.328	0.347	0.264	0.292
M02.38	Reiter's disease, vertebrae	40	Rheumatoid Arthritis and Inflammatory Connective Tissue Disease		0.421	0.367	0.371	0.328	0.347	0.264	0.292
M02.39	Reiter's disease, multiple sites	40	Rheumatoid Arthritis and Inflammatory Connective Tissue Disease		0.421	0.367	0.371	0.328	0.347	0.264	0.292
M02.80	Other reactive arthropathies, unspecified site	39	Bone/Joint/Muscle Infections/Necrosis		0.401	0.378	0.558	0.682	0.443	0.435	0.401
M02.811	Other reactive arthropathies, right shoulder	39	Bone/Joint/Muscle Infections/Necrosis		0.401	0.378	0.558	0.682	0.443	0.435	0.401
M02.812	Other reactive arthropathies, left shoulder	39	Bone/Joint/Muscle Infections/Necrosis		0.401	0.378	0.558	0.682	0.443	0.435	0.401
M02.819	Other reactive arthropathies, unspecified shoulder	39	Bone/Joint/Muscle Infections/Necrosis		0.401	0.378	0.558	0.682	0.443	0.435	0.401
M02.821	Other reactive arthropathies, right elbow	39	Bone/Joint/Muscle Infections/Necrosis		0.401	0.378	0.558	0.682	0.443	0.435	0.401
M02.822	Other reactive arthropathies, left elbow	39	Bone/Joint/Muscle Infections/Necrosis		0.401	0.378	0.558	0.682	0.443	0.435	0.401
M02.829	Other reactive arthropathies, unspecified elbow	39	Bone/Joint/Muscle Infections/Necrosis		0.401	0.378	0.558	0.682	0.443	0.435	0.401
M02.831	Other reactive arthropathies, right wrist	39	Bone/Joint/Muscle Infections/Necrosis		0.401	0.378	0.558	0.682	0.443	0.435	0.401

ICD-10-CM Code	ICD-10-CM Code Description	V24 CMS-HCC	V24 CMS-HCC Disease Group	V24 CMS-HCC Hierarchies	Community, NonDual, Aged	Community, NonDual, Disabled	Community, FBDual, Aged	Community, FBDual, Disabled	Community, PBDual, Aged	Community, PBDual, Disabled	Institutional
M02.832	Other reactive arthropathies, left wrist	39	Bone/Joint/Muscle Infections/Necrosis		0.401	0.378	0.558	0.682	0.443	0.435	0.401
M02.839	Other reactive arthropathies, unspecified wrist	39	Bone/Joint/Muscle Infections/Necrosis		0.401	0.378	0.558	0.682	0.443	0.435	0.401
M02.841	Other reactive arthropathies, right hand	39	Bone/Joint/Muscle Infections/Necrosis		0.401	0.378	0.558	0.682	0.443	0.435	0.401
M02.842	Other reactive arthropathies, left hand	39	Bone/Joint/Muscle Infections/Necrosis		0.401	0.378	0.558	0.682	0.443	0.435	0.401
M02.849	Other reactive arthropathies, unspecified hand	39	Bone/Joint/Muscle Infections/Necrosis		0.401	0.378	0.558	0.682	0.443	0.435	0.401
M02.851	Other reactive arthropathies, right hip	39	Bone/Joint/Muscle Infections/Necrosis		0.401	0.378	0.558	0.682	0.443	0.435	0.401
M02.852	Other reactive arthropathies, left hip	39	Bone/Joint/Muscle Infections/Necrosis		0.401	0.378	0.558	0.682	0.443	0.435	0.401
M02.859	Other reactive arthropathies, unspecified hip	39	Bone/Joint/Muscle Infections/Necrosis		0.401	0.378	0.558	0.682	0.443	0.435	0.401
M02.861	Other reactive arthropathies, right knee	39	Bone/Joint/Muscle Infections/Necrosis		0.401	0.378	0.558	0.682	0.443	0.435	0.401
M02.862	Other reactive arthropathies, left knee	39	Bone/Joint/Muscle Infections/Necrosis		0.401	0.378	0.558	0.682	0.443	0.435	0.401
M02.869	Other reactive arthropathies, unspecified knee	39	Bone/Joint/Muscle Infections/Necrosis		0.401	0.378	0.558	0.682	0.443	0.435	0.401
M02.871	Other reactive arthropathies, right ankle and foot	39	Bone/Joint/Muscle Infections/Necrosis		0.401	0.378	0.558	0.682	0.443	0.435	0.401
M02.872	Other reactive arthropathies, left ankle and foot	39	Bone/Joint/Muscle Infections/Necrosis		0.401	0.378	0.558	0.682	0.443	0.435	0.401
M02.879	Other reactive arthropathies, unspecified ankle and foot	39	Bone/Joint/Muscle Infections/Necrosis		0.401	0.378	0.558	0.682	0.443	0.435	0.401
M02.88	Other reactive arthropathies, vertebrae	39	Bone/Joint/Muscle Infections/Necrosis		0.401	0.378	0.558	0.682	0.443	0.435	0.401
M02.89	Other reactive arthropathies, multiple sites	39	Bone/Joint/Muscle Infections/Necrosis		0.401	0.378	0.558	0.682	0.443	0.435	0.401
M02.9	Reactive arthropathy, unspecified	39	Bone/Joint/Muscle Infections/Necrosis		0.401	0.378	0.558	0.682	0.443	0.435	0.401
M04.1	Periodic fever syndromes	40	Rheumatoid Arthritis and Inflammatory Connective Tissue Disease		0.421	0.367	0.371	0.328	0.347	0.264	0.292
M04.2	Cryopyrin-associated periodic syndromes	40	Rheumatoid Arthritis and Inflammatory Connective Tissue Disease		0.421	0.367	0.371	0.328	0.347	0.264	0.292
M04.8	Other autoinflammatory syndromes	40	Rheumatoid Arthritis and Inflammatory Connective Tissue Disease		0.421	0.367	0.371	0.328	0.347	0.264	0.292
M04.9	Autoinflammatory syndrome, unspecified	40	Rheumatoid Arthritis and Inflammatory Connective Tissue Disease		0.421	0.367	0.371	0.328	0.347	0.264	0.292
M05.00	Felty's syndrome, unspecified site	40	Rheumatoid Arthritis and Inflammatory Connective Tissue Disease		0.421	0.367	0.371	0.328	0.347	0.264	0.292
M05.011	Felty's syndrome, right shoulder	40	Rheumatoid Arthritis and Inflammatory Connective Tissue Disease		0.421	0.367	0.371	0.328	0.347	0.264	0.292
M05.012	Felty's syndrome, left shoulder	40	Rheumatoid Arthritis and Inflammatory Connective Tissue Disease		0.421	0.367	0.371	0.328	0.347	0.264	0.292
M05.019	Felty's syndrome, unspecified shoulder	40	Rheumatoid Arthritis and Inflammatory Connective Tissue Disease		0.421	0.367	0.371	0.328	0.347	0.264	0.292
M05.021	Felty's syndrome, right elbow	40	Rheumatoid Arthritis and Inflammatory Connective Tissue Disease		0.421	0.367	0.371	0.328	0.347	0.264	0.292

ICD-10-CM Code	ICD-10-CM Code Description	V24 CMS-HCC	V24 CMS-HCC Disease Group	V24 CMS-HCC Hierarchies	Community, NonDual, Aged	Community, NonDual, Disabled	Community, FBDual, Aged	Community, FBDual, Disabled	Community, PBDual, Aged	Community, PBDual, Disabled	Institutional
M05.022	Felty's syndrome, left elbow	40	Rheumatoid Arthritis and Inflammatory Connective Tissue Disease		0.421	0.367	0.371	0.328	0.347	0.264	0.292
M05.029	Felty's syndrome, unspecified elbow	40	Rheumatoid Arthritis and Inflammatory Connective Tissue Disease		0.421	0.367	0.371	0.328	0.347	0.264	0.292
M05.031	Felty's syndrome, right wrist	40	Rheumatoid Arthritis and Inflammatory Connective Tissue Disease		0.421	0.367	0.371	0.328	0.347	0.264	0.292
M05.032	Felty's syndrome, left wrist	40	Rheumatoid Arthritis and Inflammatory Connective Tissue Disease		0.421	0.367	0.371	0.328	0.347	0.264	0.292
M05.039	Felty's syndrome, unspecified wrist	40	Rheumatoid Arthritis and Inflammatory Connective Tissue Disease		0.421	0.367	0.371	0.328	0.347	0.264	0.292
M05.041	Felty's syndrome, right hand	40	Rheumatoid Arthritis and Inflammatory Connective Tissue Disease		0.421	0.367	0.371	0.328	0.347	0.264	0.292
M05.042	Felty's syndrome, left hand	40	Rheumatoid Arthritis and Inflammatory Connective Tissue Disease		0.421	0.367	0.371	0.328	0.347	0.264	0.292
M05.049	Felty's syndrome, unspecified hand	40	Rheumatoid Arthritis and Inflammatory Connective Tissue Disease		0.421	0.367	0.371	0.328	0.347	0.264	0.292
M05.051	Felty's syndrome, right hip	40	Rheumatoid Arthritis and Inflammatory Connective Tissue Disease		0.421	0.367	0.371	0.328	0.347	0.264	0.292
M05.052	Felty's syndrome, left hip	40	Rheumatoid Arthritis and Inflammatory Connective Tissue Disease		0.421	0.367	0.371	0.328	0.347	0.264	0.292
M05.059	Felty's syndrome, unspecified hip	40	Rheumatoid Arthritis and Inflammatory Connective Tissue Disease		0.421	0.367	0.371	0.328	0.347	0.264	0.292
M05.061	Felty's syndrome, right knee	40	Rheumatoid Arthritis and Inflammatory Connective Tissue Disease		0.421	0.367	0.371	0.328	0.347	0.264	0.292
M05.062	Felty's syndrome, left knee	40	Rheumatoid Arthritis and Inflammatory Connective Tissue Disease		0.421	0.367	0.371	0.328	0.347	0.264	0.292
M05.069	Felty's syndrome, unspecified knee	40	Rheumatoid Arthritis and Inflammatory Connective Tissue Disease		0.421	0.367	0.371	0.328	0.347	0.264	0.292
M05.071	Felty's syndrome, right ankle and foot	40	Rheumatoid Arthritis and Inflammatory Connective Tissue Disease		0.421	0.367	0.371	0.328	0.347	0.264	0.292
M05.072	Felty's syndrome, left ankle and foot	40	Rheumatoid Arthritis and Inflammatory Connective Tissue Disease		0.421	0.367	0.371	0.328	0.347	0.264	0.292
M05.079	Felty's syndrome, unspecified ankle and foot	40	Rheumatoid Arthritis and Inflammatory Connective Tissue Disease		0.421	0.367	0.371	0.328	0.347	0.264	0.292
M05.09	Felty's syndrome, multiple sites	40	Rheumatoid Arthritis and Inflammatory Connective Tissue Disease		0.421	0.367	0.371	0.328	0.347	0.264	0.292
M05.10	Rheumatoid lung disease with rheumatoid arthritis of unspecified site	40	Rheumatoid Arthritis and Inflammatory Connective Tissue Disease		0.421	0.367	0.371	0.328	0.347	0.264	0.292
M05.111	Rheumatoid lung disease with rheumatoid arthritis of right shoulder	40	Rheumatoid Arthritis and Inflammatory Connective Tissue Disease		0.421	0.367	0.371	0.328	0.347	0.264	0.292

ICD-10-CM Code	ICD-10-CM Code Description	V24 CMS-HCC	V24 CMS-HCC Disease Group	V24 CMS-HCC Hierarchies	Community, NonDual, Aged	Community, NonDual, Disabled	Community, FBDual, Aged	Community, FBDual, Disabled	Community, PBDual, Aged	Community, PBDual, Disabled	Institutional
M05.112	Rheumatoid lung disease with rheumatoid arthritis of left shoulder	40	Rheumatoid Arthritis and Inflammatory Connective Tissue Disease		0.421	0.367	0.371	0.328	0.347	0.264	0.292
M05.119	Rheumatoid lung disease with rheumatoid arthritis of unspecified shoulder	40	Rheumatoid Arthritis and Inflammatory Connective Tissue Disease		0.421	0.367	0.371	0.328	0.347	0.264	0.292
M05.121	Rheumatoid lung disease with rheumatoid arthritis of right elbow	40	Rheumatoid Arthritis and Inflammatory Connective Tissue Disease		0.421	0.367	0.371	0.328	0.347	0.264	0.292
M05.122	Rheumatoid lung disease with rheumatoid arthritis of left elbow	40	Rheumatoid Arthritis and Inflammatory Connective Tissue Disease		0.421	0.367	0.371	0.328	0.347	0.264	0.292
M05.129	Rheumatoid lung disease with rheumatoid arthritis of unspecified elbow	40	Rheumatoid Arthritis and Inflammatory Connective Tissue Disease		0.421	0.367	0.371	0.328	0.347	0.264	0.292
M05.131	Rheumatoid lung disease with rheumatoid arthritis of right wrist	40	Rheumatoid Arthritis and Inflammatory Connective Tissue Disease		0.421	0.367	0.371	0.328	0.347	0.264	0.292
M05.132	Rheumatoid lung disease with rheumatoid arthritis of left wrist	40	Rheumatoid Arthritis and Inflammatory Connective Tissue Disease		0.421	0.367	0.371	0.328	0.347	0.264	0.292
M05.139	Rheumatoid lung disease with rheumatoid arthritis of unspecified wrist	40	Rheumatoid Arthritis and Inflammatory Connective Tissue Disease		0.421	0.367	0.371	0.328	0.347	0.264	0.292
M05.141	Rheumatoid lung disease with rheumatoid arthritis of right hand	40	Rheumatoid Arthritis and Inflammatory Connective Tissue Disease		0.421	0.367	0.371	0.328	0.347	0.264	0.292
M05.142	Rheumatoid lung disease with rheumatoid arthritis of left hand	40	Rheumatoid Arthritis and Inflammatory Connective Tissue Disease		0.421	0.367	0.371	0.328	0.347	0.264	0.292
M05.149	Rheumatoid lung disease with rheumatoid arthritis of unspecified hand	40	Rheumatoid Arthritis and Inflammatory Connective Tissue Disease		0.421	0.367	0.371	0.328	0.347	0.264	0.292
M05.151	Rheumatoid lung disease with rheumatoid arthritis of right hip	40	Rheumatoid Arthritis and Inflammatory Connective Tissue Disease		0.421	0.367	0.371	0.328	0.347	0.264	0.292
M05.152	Rheumatoid lung disease with rheumatoid arthritis of left hip	40	Rheumatoid Arthritis and Inflammatory Connective Tissue Disease		0.421	0.367	0.371	0.328	0.347	0.264	0.292
M05.159	Rheumatoid lung disease with rheumatoid arthritis of unspecified hip	40	Rheumatoid Arthritis and Inflammatory Connective Tissue Disease		0.421	0.367	0.371	0.328	0.347	0.264	0.292
M05.161	Rheumatoid lung disease with rheumatoid arthritis of right knee	40	Rheumatoid Arthritis and Inflammatory Connective Tissue Disease		0.421	0.367	0.371	0.328	0.347	0.264	0.292
M05.162	Rheumatoid lung disease with rheumatoid arthritis of left knee	40	Rheumatoid Arthritis and Inflammatory Connective Tissue Disease		0.421	0.367	0.371	0.328	0.347	0.264	0.292
M05.169	Rheumatoid lung disease with rheumatoid arthritis of unspecified knee	40	Rheumatoid Arthritis and Inflammatory Connective Tissue Disease		0.421	0.367	0.371	0.328	0.347	0.264	0.292
M05.171	Rheumatoid lung disease with rheumatoid arthritis of right ankle and foot	40	Rheumatoid Arthritis and Inflammatory Connective Tissue Disease		0.421	0.367	0.371	0.328	0.347	0.264	0.292
M05.172	Rheumatoid lung disease with rheumatoid arthritis of left ankle and foot	40	Rheumatoid Arthritis and Inflammatory Connective Tissue Disease		0.421	0.367	0.371	0.328	0.347	0.264	0.292
M05.179	Rheumatoid lung disease with rheumatoid arthritis of unspecified ankle and foot	40	Rheumatoid Arthritis and Inflammatory Connective Tissue Disease		0.421	0.367	0.371	0.328	0.347	0.264	0.292

ICD-10-CM Code	ICD-10-CM Code Description	V24 CMS-HCC	V24 CMS-HCC Disease Group	V24 CMS-HCC Hierarchies	Community, NonDual, Aged	Community, NonDual, Disabled	Community, FBDual, Aged	Community, FBDual, Disabled	Community, PBDual, Aged	Community, PBDual, Disabled	Institutional
MØ5.19	Rheumatoid lung disease with rheumatoid arthritis of multiple sites	40	Rheumatoid Arthritis and Inflammatory Connective Tissue Disease		0.421	0.367	0.371	0.328	0.347	0.264	0.292
MØ5.2Ø	Rheumatoid vasculitis with rheumatoid arthritis of unspecified site	40	Rheumatoid Arthritis and Inflammatory Connective Tissue Disease		0.421	0.367	0.371	0.328	0.347	0.264	0.292
MØ5.211	Rheumatoid vasculitis with rheumatoid arthritis of right shoulder	40	Rheumatoid Arthritis and Inflammatory Connective Tissue Disease		0.421	0.367	0.371	0.328	0.347	0.264	0.292
MØ5.212	Rheumatoid vasculitis with rheumatoid arthritis of left shoulder	40	Rheumatoid Arthritis and Inflammatory Connective Tissue Disease		0.421	0.367	0.371	0.328	0.347	0.264	0.292
MØ5.219	Rheumatoid vasculitis with rheumatoid arthritis of unspecified shoulder	40	Rheumatoid Arthritis and Inflammatory Connective Tissue Disease		0.421	0.367	0.371	0.328	0.347	0.264	0.292
MØ5.221	Rheumatoid vasculitis with rheumatoid arthritis of right elbow	40	Rheumatoid Arthritis and Inflammatory Connective Tissue Disease		0.421	0.367	0.371	0.328	0.347	0.264	0.292
MØ5.222	Rheumatoid vasculitis with rheumatoid arthritis of left elbow	40	Rheumatoid Arthritis and Inflammatory Connective Tissue Disease		0.421	0.367	0.371	0.328	0.347	0.264	0.292
MØ5.229	Rheumatoid vasculitis with rheumatoid arthritis of unspecified elbow	40	Rheumatoid Arthritis and Inflammatory Connective Tissue Disease		0.421	0.367	0.371	0.328	0.347	0.264	0.292
MØ5.231	Rheumatoid vasculitis with rheumatoid arthritis of right wrist	40	Rheumatoid Arthritis and Inflammatory Connective Tissue Disease		0.421	0.367	0.371	0.328	0.347	0.264	0.292
MØ5.232	Rheumatoid vasculitis with rheumatoid arthritis of left wrist	40	Rheumatoid Arthritis and Inflammatory Connective Tissue Disease		0.421	0.367	0.371	0.328	0.347	0.264	0.292
MØ5.239	Rheumatoid vasculitis with rheumatoid arthritis of unspecified wrist	40	Rheumatoid Arthritis and Inflammatory Connective Tissue Disease		0.421	0.367	0.371	0.328	0.347	0.264	0.292
MØ5.241	Rheumatoid vasculitis with rheumatoid arthritis of right hand	40	Rheumatoid Arthritis and Inflammatory Connective Tissue Disease		0.421	0.367	0.371	0.328	0.347	0.264	0.292
MØ5.242	Rheumatoid vasculitis with rheumatoid arthritis of left hand	40	Rheumatoid Arthritis and Inflammatory Connective Tissue Disease		0.421	0.367	0.371	0.328	0.347	0.264	0.292
MØ5.249	Rheumatoid vasculitis with rheumatoid arthritis of unspecified hand	40	Rheumatoid Arthritis and Inflammatory Connective Tissue Disease		0.421	0.367	0.371	0.328	0.347	0.264	0.292
MØ5.251	Rheumatoid vasculitis with rheumatoid arthritis of right hip	40	Rheumatoid Arthritis and Inflammatory Connective Tissue Disease		0.421	0.367	0.371	0.328	0.347	0.264	0.292
MØ5.252	Rheumatoid vasculitis with rheumatoid arthritis of left hip	40	Rheumatoid Arthritis and Inflammatory Connective Tissue Disease		0.421	0.367	0.371	0.328	0.347	0.264	0.292
MØ5.259	Rheumatoid vasculitis with rheumatoid arthritis of unspecified hip	40	Rheumatoid Arthritis and Inflammatory Connective Tissue Disease		0.421	0.367	0.371	0.328	0.347	0.264	0.292
MØ5.261	Rheumatoid vasculitis with rheumatoid arthritis of right knee	40	Rheumatoid Arthritis and Inflammatory Connective Tissue Disease		0.421	0.367	0.371	0.328	0.347	0.264	0.292
MØ5.262	Rheumatoid vasculitis with rheumatoid arthritis of left knee	40	Rheumatoid Arthritis and Inflammatory Connective Tissue Disease		0.421	0.367	0.371	0.328	0.347	0.264	0.292
MØ5.269	Rheumatoid vasculitis with rheumatoid arthritis of unspecified knee	40	Rheumatoid Arthritis and Inflammatory Connective Tissue Disease		0.421	0.367	0.371	0.328	0.347	0.264	0.292

ICD-10-CM Code	ICD-10-CM Code Description	V24 CMS-HCC	V24 CMS-HCC Disease Group	V24 CMS-HCC Hierarchies	Community, NonDual, Aged	Community, NonDual, Disabled	Community, FBDual, Aged	Community, FBDual, Disabled	Community, PBDual, Aged	Community, PBDual, Disabled	Institutional
MØ5.271	Rheumatoid vasculitis with rheumatoid arthritis of right ankle and foot	40	Rheumatoid Arthritis and Inflammatory Connective Tissue Disease		0.421	0.367	0.371	0.328	0.347	0.264	0.292
MØ5.272	Rheumatoid vasculitis with rheumatoid arthritis of left ankle and foot	40	Rheumatoid Arthritis and Inflammatory Connective Tissue Disease		0.421	0.367	0.371	0.328	0.347	0.264	0.292
MØ5.279	Rheumatoid vasculitis with rheumatoid arthritis of unspecified ankle and foot	40	Rheumatoid Arthritis and Inflammatory Connective Tissue Disease		0.421	0.367	0.371	0.328	0.347	0.264	0.292
MØ5.29	Rheumatoid vasculitis with rheumatoid arthritis of multiple sites	40	Rheumatoid Arthritis and Inflammatory Connective Tissue Disease		0.421	0.367	0.371	0.328	0.347	0.264	0.292
MØ5.30	Rheumatoid heart disease with rheumatoid arthritis of unspecified site	40	Rheumatoid Arthritis and Inflammatory Connective Tissue Disease		0.421	0.367	0.371	0.328	0.347	0.264	0.292
MØ5.311	Rheumatoid heart disease with rheumatoid arthritis of right shoulder	40	Rheumatoid Arthritis and Inflammatory Connective Tissue Disease		0.421	0.367	0.371	0.328	0.347	0.264	0.292
MØ5.312	Rheumatoid heart disease with rheumatoid arthritis of left shoulder	40	Rheumatoid Arthritis and Inflammatory Connective Tissue Disease		0.421	0.367	0.371	0.328	0.347	0.264	0.292
MØ5.319	Rheumatoid heart disease with rheumatoid arthritis of unspecified shoulder	40	Rheumatoid Arthritis and Inflammatory Connective Tissue Disease		0.421	0.367	0.371	0.328	0.347	0.264	0.292
MØ5.321	Rheumatoid heart disease with rheumatoid arthritis of right elbow	40	Rheumatoid Arthritis and Inflammatory Connective Tissue Disease		0.421	0.367	0.371	0.328	0.347	0.264	0.292
MØ5.322	Rheumatoid heart disease with rheumatoid arthritis of left elbow	40	Rheumatoid Arthritis and Inflammatory Connective Tissue Disease		0.421	0.367	0.371	0.328	0.347	0.264	0.292
MØ5.329	Rheumatoid heart disease with rheumatoid arthritis of unspecified elbow	40	Rheumatoid Arthritis and Inflammatory Connective Tissue Disease		0.421	0.367	0.371	0.328	0.347	0.264	0.292
MØ5.331	Rheumatoid heart disease with rheumatoid arthritis of right wrist	40	Rheumatoid Arthritis and Inflammatory Connective Tissue Disease		0.421	0.367	0.371	0.328	0.347	0.264	0.292
MØ5.332	Rheumatoid heart disease with rheumatoid arthritis of left wrist	40	Rheumatoid Arthritis and Inflammatory Connective Tissue Disease		0.421	0.367	0.371	0.328	0.347	0.264	0.292
MØ5.339	Rheumatoid heart disease with rheumatoid arthritis of unspecified wrist	40	Rheumatoid Arthritis and Inflammatory Connective Tissue Disease		0.421	0.367	0.371	0.328	0.347	0.264	0.292
MØ5.341	Rheumatoid heart disease with rheumatoid arthritis of right hand	40	Rheumatoid Arthritis and Inflammatory Connective Tissue Disease		0.421	0.367	0.371	0.328	0.347	0.264	0.292
MØ5.342	Rheumatoid heart disease with rheumatoid arthritis of left hand	40	Rheumatoid Arthritis and Inflammatory Connective Tissue Disease		0.421	0.367	0.371	0.328	0.347	0.264	0.292
MØ5.349	Rheumatoid heart disease with rheumatoid arthritis of unspecified hand	40	Rheumatoid Arthritis and Inflammatory Connective Tissue Disease		0.421	0.367	0.371	0.328	0.347	0.264	0.292
MØ5.351	Rheumatoid heart disease with rheumatoid arthritis of right hip	40	Rheumatoid Arthritis and Inflammatory Connective Tissue Disease		0.421	0.367	0.371	0.328	0.347	0.264	0.292
MØ5.352	Rheumatoid heart disease with rheumatoid arthritis of left hip	40	Rheumatoid Arthritis and Inflammatory Connective Tissue Disease		0.421	0.367	0.371	0.328	0.347	0.264	0.292
MØ5.359	Rheumatoid heart disease with rheumatoid arthritis of unspecified hip	40	Rheumatoid Arthritis and Inflammatory Connective Tissue Disease		0.421	0.367	0.371	0.328	0.347	0.264	0.292

ICD-10-CM Code	ICD-10-CM Code Description	V24 CMS-HCC	V24 CMS-HCC Disease Group	V24 CMS-HCC Hierarchies	Community, NonDual, Aged	Community, NonDual, Disabled	Community, FBDual, Aged	Community, FBDual, Disabled	Community, PBDual, Aged	Community, PBDual, Disabled	Institutional
M05.361	Rheumatoid heart disease with rheumatoid arthritis of right knee	40	Rheumatoid Arthritis and Inflammatory Connective Tissue Disease		0.421	0.367	0.371	0.328	0.347	0.264	0.292
M05.362	Rheumatoid heart disease with rheumatoid arthritis of left knee	40	Rheumatoid Arthritis and Inflammatory Connective Tissue Disease		0.421	0.367	0.371	0.328	0.347	0.264	0.292
M05.369	Rheumatoid heart disease with rheumatoid arthritis of unspecified knee	40	Rheumatoid Arthritis and Inflammatory Connective Tissue Disease		0.421	0.367	0.371	0.328	0.347	0.264	0.292
M05.371	Rheumatoid heart disease with rheumatoid arthritis of right ankle and foot	40	Rheumatoid Arthritis and Inflammatory Connective Tissue Disease		0.421	0.367	0.371	0.328	0.347	0.264	0.292
M05.372	Rheumatoid heart disease with rheumatoid arthritis of left ankle and foot	40	Rheumatoid Arthritis and Inflammatory Connective Tissue Disease		0.421	0.367	0.371	0.328	0.347	0.264	0.292
M05.379	Rheumatoid heart disease with rheumatoid arthritis of unspecified ankle and foot	40	Rheumatoid Arthritis and Inflammatory Connective Tissue Disease		0.421	0.367	0.371	0.328	0.347	0.264	0.292
M05.39	Rheumatoid heart disease with rheumatoid arthritis of multiple sites	40	Rheumatoid Arthritis and Inflammatory Connective Tissue Disease		0.421	0.367	0.371	0.328	0.347	0.264	0.292
M05.40	Rheumatoid myopathy with rheumatoid arthritis of unspecified site	40	Rheumatoid Arthritis and Inflammatory Connective Tissue Disease		0.421	0.367	0.371	0.328	0.347	0.264	0.292
M05.411	Rheumatoid myopathy with rheumatoid arthritis of right shoulder	40	Rheumatoid Arthritis and Inflammatory Connective Tissue Disease		0.421	0.367	0.371	0.328	0.347	0.264	0.292
M05.412	Rheumatoid myopathy with rheumatoid arthritis of left shoulder	40	Rheumatoid Arthritis and Inflammatory Connective Tissue Disease		0.421	0.367	0.371	0.328	0.347	0.264	0.292
M05.419	Rheumatoid myopathy with rheumatoid arthritis of unspecified shoulder	40	Rheumatoid Arthritis and Inflammatory Connective Tissue Disease		0.421	0.367	0.371	0.328	0.347	0.264	0.292
M05.421	Rheumatoid myopathy with rheumatoid arthritis of right elbow	40	Rheumatoid Arthritis and Inflammatory Connective Tissue Disease		0.421	0.367	0.371	0.328	0.347	0.264	0.292
M05.422	Rheumatoid myopathy with rheumatoid arthritis of left elbow	40	Rheumatoid Arthritis and Inflammatory Connective Tissue Disease		0.421	0.367	0.371	0.328	0.347	0.264	0.292
M05.429	Rheumatoid myopathy with rheumatoid arthritis of unspecified elbow	40	Rheumatoid Arthritis and Inflammatory Connective Tissue Disease		0.421	0.367	0.371	0.328	0.347	0.264	0.292
M05.431	Rheumatoid myopathy with rheumatoid arthritis of right wrist	40	Rheumatoid Arthritis and Inflammatory Connective Tissue Disease		0.421	0.367	0.371	0.328	0.347	0.264	0.292
M05.432	Rheumatoid myopathy with rheumatoid arthritis of left wrist	40	Rheumatoid Arthritis and Inflammatory Connective Tissue Disease		0.421	0.367	0.371	0.328	0.347	0.264	0.292
M05.439	Rheumatoid myopathy with rheumatoid arthritis of unspecified wrist	40	Rheumatoid Arthritis and Inflammatory Connective Tissue Disease		0.421	0.367	0.371	0.328	0.347	0.264	0.292
M05.441	Rheumatoid myopathy with rheumatoid arthritis of right hand	40	Rheumatoid Arthritis and Inflammatory Connective Tissue Disease		0.421	0.367	0.371	0.328	0.347	0.264	0.292
M05.442	Rheumatoid myopathy with rheumatoid arthritis of left hand	40	Rheumatoid Arthritis and Inflammatory Connective Tissue Disease		0.421	0.367	0.371	0.328	0.347	0.264	0.292
M05.449	Rheumatoid myopathy with rheumatoid arthritis of unspecified hand	40	Rheumatoid Arthritis and Inflammatory Connective Tissue Disease		0.421	0.367	0.371	0.328	0.347	0.264	0.292

ICD-10-CM Code	ICD-10-CM Code Description	V24 CMS-HCC	V24 CMS-HCC Disease Group	V24 CMS-HCC Hierarchies	Community, NonDual, Aged	Community, NonDual, Disabled	Community, FBDual, Aged	Community, FBDual, Disabled	Community, PBDual, Aged	Community, PBDual, Disabled	Institutional
M05.451	Rheumatoid myopathy with rheumatoid arthritis of right hip	40	Rheumatoid Arthritis and Inflammatory Connective Tissue Disease		0.421	0.367	0.371	0.328	0.347	0.264	0.292
M05.452	Rheumatoid myopathy with rheumatoid arthritis of left hip	40	Rheumatoid Arthritis and Inflammatory Connective Tissue Disease		0.421	0.367	0.371	0.328	0.347	0.264	0.292
M05.459	Rheumatoid myopathy with rheumatoid arthritis of unspecified hip	40	Rheumatoid Arthritis and Inflammatory Connective Tissue Disease		0.421	0.367	0.371	0.328	0.347	0.264	0.292
M05.461	Rheumatoid myopathy with rheumatoid arthritis of right knee	40	Rheumatoid Arthritis and Inflammatory Connective Tissue Disease		0.421	0.367	0.371	0.328	0.347	0.264	0.292
M05.462	Rheumatoid myopathy with rheumatoid arthritis of left knee	40	Rheumatoid Arthritis and Inflammatory Connective Tissue Disease		0.421	0.367	0.371	0.328	0.347	0.264	0.292
M05.469	Rheumatoid myopathy with rheumatoid arthritis of unspecified knee	40	Rheumatoid Arthritis and Inflammatory Connective Tissue Disease		0.421	0.367	0.371	0.328	0.347	0.264	0.292
M05.471	Rheumatoid myopathy with rheumatoid arthritis of right ankle and foot	40	Rheumatoid Arthritis and Inflammatory Connective Tissue Disease		0.421	0.367	0.371	0.328	0.347	0.264	0.292
M05.472	Rheumatoid myopathy with rheumatoid arthritis of left ankle and foot	40	Rheumatoid Arthritis and Inflammatory Connective Tissue Disease		0.421	0.367	0.371	0.328	0.347	0.264	0.292
M05.479	Rheumatoid myopathy with rheumatoid arthritis of unspecified ankle and foot	40	Rheumatoid Arthritis and Inflammatory Connective Tissue Disease		0.421	0.367	0.371	0.328	0.347	0.264	0.292
M05.49	Rheumatoid myopathy with rheumatoid arthritis of multiple sites	40	Rheumatoid Arthritis and Inflammatory Connective Tissue Disease		0.421	0.367	0.371	0.328	0.347	0.264	0.292
M05.50	Rheumatoid polyneuropathy with rheumatoid arthritis of unspecified site	40	Rheumatoid Arthritis and Inflammatory Connective Tissue Disease		0.421	0.367	0.371	0.328	0.347	0.264	0.292
M05.50	Rheumatoid polyneuropathy with rheumatoid arthritis of unspecified site	75	Myasthenia Gravis/Myoneural Disorders and Guillain-Barre Syndrome/Inflammatory and Toxic Neuropathy		0.472	0.481	0.407	0.404	0.287	0.314	0.332
M05.511	Rheumatoid polyneuropathy with rheumatoid arthritis of right shoulder	40	Rheumatoid Arthritis and Inflammatory Connective Tissue Disease		0.421	0.367	0.371	0.328	0.347	0.264	0.292
M05.511	Rheumatoid polyneuropathy with rheumatoid arthritis of right shoulder	75	Myasthenia Gravis/Myoneural Disorders and Guillain-Barre Syndrome/Inflammatory and Toxic Neuropathy		0.472	0.481	0.407	0.404	0.287	0.314	0.332
M05.512	Rheumatoid polyneuropathy with rheumatoid arthritis of left shoulder	40	Rheumatoid Arthritis and Inflammatory Connective Tissue Disease		0.421	0.367	0.371	0.328	0.347	0.264	0.292
M05.512	Rheumatoid polyneuropathy with rheumatoid arthritis of left shoulder	75	Myasthenia Gravis/Myoneural Disorders and Guillain-Barre Syndrome/Inflammatory and Toxic Neuropathy		0.472	0.481	0.407	0.404	0.287	0.314	0.332
M05.519	Rheumatoid polyneuropathy with rheumatoid arthritis of unspecified shoulder	40	Rheumatoid Arthritis and Inflammatory Connective Tissue Disease		0.421	0.367	0.371	0.328	0.347	0.264	0.292
M05.519	Rheumatoid polyneuropathy with rheumatoid arthritis of unspecified shoulder	75	Myasthenia Gravis/Myoneural Disorders and Guillain-Barre Syndrome/Inflammatory and Toxic Neuropathy		0.472	0.481	0.407	0.404	0.287	0.314	0.332
M05.521	Rheumatoid polyneuropathy with rheumatoid arthritis of right elbow	40	Rheumatoid Arthritis and Inflammatory Connective Tissue Disease		0.421	0.367	0.371	0.328	0.347	0.264	0.292

ICD-10-CM Code	ICD-10-CM Code Description	V24 CMS-HCC	V24 CMS-HCC Disease Group	V24 CMS-HCC Hierarchies	Community, NonDual, Aged	Community, NonDual, Disabled	Community, FBDual, Aged	Community, FBDual, Disabled	Community, PBDual, Aged	Community, PBDual, Disabled	Institutional
M05.521	Rheumatoid polyneuropathy with rheumatoid arthritis of right elbow	75	Myasthenia Gravis/Myoneural Disorders and Guillain-Barre Syndrome/Inflammatory and Toxic Neuropathy		0.472	0.481	0.407	0.404	0.287	0.314	0.332
M05.522	Rheumatoid polyneuropathy with rheumatoid arthritis of left elbow	40	Rheumatoid Arthritis and Inflammatory Connective Tissue Disease		0.421	0.367	0.371	0.328	0.347	0.264	0.292
M05.522	Rheumatoid polyneuropathy with rheumatoid arthritis of left elbow	75	Myasthenia Gravis/Myoneural Disorders and Guillain-Barre Syndrome/Inflammatory and Toxic Neuropathy		0.472	0.481	0.407	0.404	0.287	0.314	0.332
M05.529	Rheumatoid polyneuropathy with rheumatoid arthritis of unspecified elbow	40	Rheumatoid Arthritis and Inflammatory Connective Tissue Disease		0.421	0.367	0.371	0.328	0.347	0.264	0.292
M05.529	Rheumatoid polyneuropathy with rheumatoid arthritis of unspecified elbow	75	Myasthenia Gravis/Myoneural Disorders and Guillain-Barre Syndrome/Inflammatory and Toxic Neuropathy		0.472	0.481	0.407	0.404	0.287	0.314	0.332
M05.531	Rheumatoid polyneuropathy with rheumatoid arthritis of right wrist	40	Rheumatoid Arthritis and Inflammatory Connective Tissue Disease		0.421	0.367	0.371	0.328	0.347	0.264	0.292
M05.531	Rheumatoid polyneuropathy with rheumatoid arthritis of right wrist	75	Myasthenia Gravis/Myoneural Disorders and Guillain-Barre Syndrome/Inflammatory and Toxic Neuropathy		0.472	0.481	0.407	0.404	0.287	0.314	0.332
M05.532	Rheumatoid polyneuropathy with rheumatoid arthritis of left wrist	40	Rheumatoid Arthritis and Inflammatory Connective Tissue Disease		0.421	0.367	0.371	0.328	0.347	0.264	0.292
M05.532	Rheumatoid polyneuropathy with rheumatoid arthritis of left wrist	75	Myasthenia Gravis/Myoneural Disorders and Guillain-Barre Syndrome/Inflammatory and Toxic Neuropathy		0.472	0.481	0.407	0.404	0.287	0.314	0.332
M05.539	Rheumatoid polyneuropathy with rheumatoid arthritis of unspecified wrist	40	Rheumatoid Arthritis and Inflammatory Connective Tissue Disease		0.421	0.367	0.371	0.328	0.347	0.264	0.292
M05.539	Rheumatoid polyneuropathy with rheumatoid arthritis of unspecified wrist	75	Myasthenia Gravis/Myoneural Disorders and Guillain-Barre Syndrome/Inflammatory and Toxic Neuropathy		0.472	0.481	0.407	0.404	0.287	0.314	0.332
M05.541	Rheumatoid polyneuropathy with rheumatoid arthritis of right hand	40	Rheumatoid Arthritis and Inflammatory Connective Tissue Disease		0.421	0.367	0.371	0.328	0.347	0.264	0.292
M05.541	Rheumatoid polyneuropathy with rheumatoid arthritis of right hand	75	Myasthenia Gravis/Myoneural Disorders and Guillain-Barre Syndrome/Inflammatory and Toxic Neuropathy		0.472	0.481	0.407	0.404	0.287	0.314	0.332
M05.542	Rheumatoid polyneuropathy with rheumatoid arthritis of left hand	40	Rheumatoid Arthritis and Inflammatory Connective Tissue Disease		0.421	0.367	0.371	0.328	0.347	0.264	0.292
M05.542	Rheumatoid polyneuropathy with rheumatoid arthritis of left hand	75	Myasthenia Gravis/Myoneural Disorders and Guillain-Barre Syndrome/Inflammatory and Toxic Neuropathy		0.472	0.481	0.407	0.404	0.287	0.314	0.332
M05.549	Rheumatoid polyneuropathy with rheumatoid arthritis of unspecified hand	40	Rheumatoid Arthritis and Inflammatory Connective Tissue Disease		0.421	0.367	0.371	0.328	0.347	0.264	0.292
M05.549	Rheumatoid polyneuropathy with rheumatoid arthritis of unspecified hand	75	Myasthenia Gravis/Myoneural Disorders and Guillain-Barre Syndrome/Inflammatory and Toxic Neuropathy		0.472	0.481	0.407	0.404	0.287	0.314	0.332

ICD-10-CM Code	ICD-10-CM Code Description	V24 CMS-HCC	V24 CMS-HCC Disease Group	V24 CMS-HCC Hierarchies	Community, NonDual, Aged	Community, NonDual, Disabled	Community, FBDual, Aged	Community, FBDual, Disabled	Community, PBDual, Aged	Community, PBDual, Disabled	Institutional
M05.551	Rheumatoid polyneuropathy with rheumatoid arthritis of right hip	40	Rheumatoid Arthritis and Inflammatory Connective Tissue Disease		0.421	0.367	0.371	0.328	0.347	0.264	0.292
M05.551	Rheumatoid polyneuropathy with rheumatoid arthritis of right hip	75	Myasthenia Gravis/Myoneural Disorders and Guillain-Barre Syndrome/Inflammatory and Toxic Neuropathy		0.472	0.481	0.407	0.404	0.287	0.314	0.332
M05.552	Rheumatoid polyneuropathy with rheumatoid arthritis of left hip	40	Rheumatoid Arthritis and Inflammatory Connective Tissue Disease		0.421	0.367	0.371	0.328	0.347	0.264	0.292
M05.552	Rheumatoid polyneuropathy with rheumatoid arthritis of left hip	75	Myasthenia Gravis/Myoneural Disorders and Guillain-Barre Syndrome/Inflammatory and Toxic Neuropathy		0.472	0.481	0.407	0.404	0.287	0.314	0.332
M05.559	Rheumatoid polyneuropathy with rheumatoid arthritis of unspecified hip	40	Rheumatoid Arthritis and Inflammatory Connective Tissue Disease		0.421	0.367	0.371	0.328	0.347	0.264	0.292
M05.559	Rheumatoid polyneuropathy with rheumatoid arthritis of unspecified hip	75	Myasthenia Gravis/Myoneural Disorders and Guillain-Barre Syndrome/Inflammatory and Toxic Neuropathy		0.472	0.481	0.407	0.404	0.287	0.314	0.332
M05.561	Rheumatoid polyneuropathy with rheumatoid arthritis of right knee	40	Rheumatoid Arthritis and Inflammatory Connective Tissue Disease		0.421	0.367	0.371	0.328	0.347	0.264	0.292
M05.561	Rheumatoid polyneuropathy with rheumatoid arthritis of right knee	75	Myasthenia Gravis/Myoneural Disorders and Guillain-Barre Syndrome/Inflammatory and Toxic Neuropathy		0.472	0.481	0.407	0.404	0.287	0.314	0.332
M05.562	Rheumatoid polyneuropathy with rheumatoid arthritis of left knee	40	Rheumatoid Arthritis and Inflammatory Connective Tissue Disease		0.421	0.367	0.371	0.328	0.347	0.264	0.292
M05.562	Rheumatoid polyneuropathy with rheumatoid arthritis of left knee	75	Myasthenia Gravis/Myoneural Disorders and Guillain-Barre Syndrome/Inflammatory and Toxic Neuropathy		0.472	0.481	0.407	0.404	0.287	0.314	0.332
M05.569	Rheumatoid polyneuropathy with rheumatoid arthritis of unspecified knee	40	Rheumatoid Arthritis and Inflammatory Connective Tissue Disease		0.421	0.367	0.371	0.328	0.347	0.264	0.292
M05.569	Rheumatoid polyneuropathy with rheumatoid arthritis of unspecified knee	75	Myasthenia Gravis/Myoneural Disorders and Guillain-Barre Syndrome/Inflammatory and Toxic Neuropathy		0.472	0.481	0.407	0.404	0.287	0.314	0.332
M05.571	Rheumatoid polyneuropathy with rheumatoid arthritis of right ankle and foot	40	Rheumatoid Arthritis and Inflammatory Connective Tissue Disease		0.421	0.367	0.371	0.328	0.347	0.264	0.292
M05.571	Rheumatoid polyneuropathy with rheumatoid arthritis of right ankle and foot	75	Myasthenia Gravis/Myoneural Disorders and Guillain-Barre Syndrome/Inflammatory and Toxic Neuropathy		0.472	0.481	0.407	0.404	0.287	0.314	0.332
M05.572	Rheumatoid polyneuropathy with rheumatoid arthritis of left ankle and foot	40	Rheumatoid Arthritis and Inflammatory Connective Tissue Disease		0.421	0.367	0.371	0.328	0.347	0.264	0.292
M05.572	Rheumatoid polyneuropathy with rheumatoid arthritis of left ankle and foot	75	Myasthenia Gravis/Myoneural Disorders and Guillain-Barre Syndrome/Inflammatory and Toxic Neuropathy		0.472	0.481	0.407	0.404	0.287	0.314	0.332
M05.579	Rheumatoid polyneuropathy with rheumatoid arthritis of unspecified ankle and foot	40	Rheumatoid Arthritis and Inflammatory Connective Tissue Disease		0.421	0.367	0.371	0.328	0.347	0.264	0.292

ICD-10-CM Code	ICD-10-CM Code Description	V24 CMS-HCC	V24 CMS-HCC Disease Group	V24 CMS-HCC Hierarchies	Community, NonDual, Aged	Community, NonDual, Disabled	Community, FBDual, Aged	Community, FBDual, Disabled	Community, PBDual, Aged	Community, PBDual, Disabled	Institutional
M05.579	Rheumatoid polyneuropathy with rheumatoid arthritis of unspecified ankle and foot	75	Myasthenia Gravis/Myoneural Disorders and Guillain-Barre Syndrome/Inflammatory and Toxic Neuropathy		0.472	0.481	0.407	0.404	0.287	0.314	0.332
M05.59	Rheumatoid polyneuropathy with rheumatoid arthritis of multiple sites	40	Rheumatoid Arthritis and Inflammatory Connective Tissue Disease		0.421	0.367	0.371	0.328	0.347	0.264	0.292
M05.59	Rheumatoid polyneuropathy with rheumatoid arthritis of multiple sites	75	Myasthenia Gravis/Myoneural Disorders and Guillain-Barre Syndrome/Inflammatory and Toxic Neuropathy		0.472	0.481	0.407	0.404	0.287	0.314	0.332
M05.60	Rheumatoid arthritis of unspecified site with involvement of other organs and systems	40	Rheumatoid Arthritis and Inflammatory Connective Tissue Disease		0.421	0.367	0.371	0.328	0.347	0.264	0.292
M05.611	Rheumatoid arthritis of right shoulder with involvement of other organs and systems	40	Rheumatoid Arthritis and Inflammatory Connective Tissue Disease		0.421	0.367	0.371	0.328	0.347	0.264	0.292
M05.612	Rheumatoid arthritis of left shoulder with involvement of other organs and systems	40	Rheumatoid Arthritis and Inflammatory Connective Tissue Disease		0.421	0.367	0.371	0.328	0.347	0.264	0.292
M05.619	Rheumatoid arthritis of unspecified shoulder with involvement of other organs and systems	40	Rheumatoid Arthritis and Inflammatory Connective Tissue Disease		0.421	0.367	0.371	0.328	0.347	0.264	0.292
M05.621	Rheumatoid arthritis of right elbow with involvement of other organs and systems	40	Rheumatoid Arthritis and Inflammatory Connective Tissue Disease		0.421	0.367	0.371	0.328	0.347	0.264	0.292
M05.622	Rheumatoid arthritis of left elbow with involvement of other organs and systems	40	Rheumatoid Arthritis and Inflammatory Connective Tissue Disease		0.421	0.367	0.371	0.328	0.347	0.264	0.292
M05.629	Rheumatoid arthritis of unspecified elbow with involvement of other organs and systems	40	Rheumatoid Arthritis and Inflammatory Connective Tissue Disease		0.421	0.367	0.371	0.328	0.347	0.264	0.292
M05.631	Rheumatoid arthritis of right wrist with involvement of other organs and systems	40	Rheumatoid Arthritis and Inflammatory Connective Tissue Disease		0.421	0.367	0.371	0.328	0.347	0.264	0.292
M05.632	Rheumatoid arthritis of left wrist with involvement of other organs and systems	40	Rheumatoid Arthritis and Inflammatory Connective Tissue Disease		0.421	0.367	0.371	0.328	0.347	0.264	0.292
M05.639	Rheumatoid arthritis of unspecified wrist with involvement of other organs and systems	40	Rheumatoid Arthritis and Inflammatory Connective Tissue Disease		0.421	0.367	0.371	0.328	0.347	0.264	0.292
M05.641	Rheumatoid arthritis of right hand with involvement of other organs and systems	40	Rheumatoid Arthritis and Inflammatory Connective Tissue Disease		0.421	0.367	0.371	0.328	0.347	0.264	0.292
M05.642	Rheumatoid arthritis of left hand with involvement of other organs and systems	40	Rheumatoid Arthritis and Inflammatory Connective Tissue Disease		0.421	0.367	0.371	0.328	0.347	0.264	0.292
M05.649	Rheumatoid arthritis of unspecified hand with involvement of other organs and systems	40	Rheumatoid Arthritis and Inflammatory Connective Tissue Disease		0.421	0.367	0.371	0.328	0.347	0.264	0.292
M05.651	Rheumatoid arthritis of right hip with involvement of other organs and systems	40	Rheumatoid Arthritis and Inflammatory Connective Tissue Disease		0.421	0.367	0.371	0.328	0.347	0.264	0.292
M05.652	Rheumatoid arthritis of left hip with involvement of other organs and systems	40	Rheumatoid Arthritis and Inflammatory Connective Tissue Disease		0.421	0.367	0.371	0.328	0.347	0.264	0.292
M05.659	Rheumatoid arthritis of unspecified hip with involvement of other organs and systems	40	Rheumatoid Arthritis and Inflammatory Connective Tissue Disease		0.421	0.367	0.371	0.328	0.347	0.264	0.292
M05.661	Rheumatoid arthritis of right knee with involvement of other organs and systems	40	Rheumatoid Arthritis and Inflammatory Connective Tissue Disease		0.421	0.367	0.371	0.328	0.347	0.264	0.292

ICD-10-CM Code	ICD-10-CM Code Description	V24 CMS-HCC	V24 CMS-HCC Disease Group	V24 CMS-HCC Hierarchies	Community, NonDual, Aged	Community, NonDual, Disabled	Community, FBDual, Aged	Community, FBDual, Disabled	Community, PBDual, Aged	Community, PBDual, Disabled	Institutional
M05.662	Rheumatoid arthritis of left knee with involvement of other organs and systems	40	Rheumatoid Arthritis and Inflammatory Connective Tissue Disease		0.421	0.367	0.371	0.328	0.347	0.264	0.292
M05.669	Rheumatoid arthritis of unspecified knee with involvement of other organs and systems	40	Rheumatoid Arthritis and Inflammatory Connective Tissue Disease		0.421	0.367	0.371	0.328	0.347	0.264	0.292
M05.671	Rheumatoid arthritis of right ankle and foot with involvement of other organs and systems	40	Rheumatoid Arthritis and Inflammatory Connective Tissue Disease		0.421	0.367	0.371	0.328	0.347	0.264	0.292
M05.672	Rheumatoid arthritis of left ankle and foot with involvement of other organs and systems	40	Rheumatoid Arthritis and Inflammatory Connective Tissue Disease		0.421	0.367	0.371	0.328	0.347	0.264	0.292
M05.679	Rheumatoid arthritis of unspecified ankle and foot with involvement of other organs and systems	40	Rheumatoid Arthritis and Inflammatory Connective Tissue Disease		0.421	0.367	0.371	0.328	0.347	0.264	0.292
M05.69	Rheumatoid arthritis of multiple sites with involvement of other organs and systems	40	Rheumatoid Arthritis and Inflammatory Connective Tissue Disease		0.421	0.367	0.371	0.328	0.347	0.264	0.292
M05.70	Rheumatoid arthritis with rheumatoid factor of unspecified site without organ or systems involvement	40	Rheumatoid Arthritis and Inflammatory Connective Tissue Disease		0.421	0.367	0.371	0.328	0.347	0.264	0.292
M05.711	Rheumatoid arthritis with rheumatoid factor of right shoulder without organ or systems involvement	40	Rheumatoid Arthritis and Inflammatory Connective Tissue Disease		0.421	0.367	0.371	0.328	0.347	0.264	0.292
M05.712	Rheumatoid arthritis with rheumatoid factor of left shoulder without organ or systems involvement	40	Rheumatoid Arthritis and Inflammatory Connective Tissue Disease		0.421	0.367	0.371	0.328	0.347	0.264	0.292
M05.719	Rheumatoid arthritis with rheumatoid factor of unspecified shoulder without organ or systems involvement	40	Rheumatoid Arthritis and Inflammatory Connective Tissue Disease		0.421	0.367	0.371	0.328	0.347	0.264	0.292
M05.721	Rheumatoid arthritis with rheumatoid factor of right elbow without organ or systems involvement	40	Rheumatoid Arthritis and Inflammatory Connective Tissue Disease		0.421	0.367	0.371	0.328	0.347	0.264	0.292
M05.722	Rheumatoid arthritis with rheumatoid factor of left elbow without organ or systems involvement	40	Rheumatoid Arthritis and Inflammatory Connective Tissue Disease		0.421	0.367	0.371	0.328	0.347	0.264	0.292
M05.729	Rheumatoid arthritis with rheumatoid factor of unspecified elbow without organ or systems involvement	40	Rheumatoid Arthritis and Inflammatory Connective Tissue Disease		0.421	0.367	0.371	0.328	0.347	0.264	0.292
M05.731	Rheumatoid arthritis with rheumatoid factor of right wrist without organ or systems involvement	40	Rheumatoid Arthritis and Inflammatory Connective Tissue Disease		0.421	0.367	0.371	0.328	0.347	0.264	0.292
M05.732	Rheumatoid arthritis with rheumatoid factor of left wrist without organ or systems involvement	40	Rheumatoid Arthritis and Inflammatory Connective Tissue Disease		0.421	0.367	0.371	0.328	0.347	0.264	0.292
M05.739	Rheumatoid arthritis with rheumatoid factor of unspecified wrist without organ or systems involvement	40	Rheumatoid Arthritis and Inflammatory Connective Tissue Disease		0.421	0.367	0.371	0.328	0.347	0.264	0.292
M05.741	Rheumatoid arthritis with rheumatoid factor of right hand without organ or systems involvement	40	Rheumatoid Arthritis and Inflammatory Connective Tissue Disease		0.421	0.367	0.371	0.328	0.347	0.264	0.292

ICD-10-CM Code	ICD-10-CM Code Description	V24 CMS-HCC	V24 CMS-HCC Disease Group	V24 CMS-HCC Hierarchies	Community, NonDual, Aged	Community, NonDual, Disabled	Community, FBDual, Aged	Community, FBDual, Disabled	Community, PBDual, Aged	Community, PBDual, Disabled	Institutional
M05.742	Rheumatoid arthritis with rheumatoid factor of left hand without organ or systems involvement	40	Rheumatoid Arthritis and Inflammatory Connective Tissue Disease		0.421	0.367	0.371	0.328	0.347	0.264	0.292
M05.749	Rheumatoid arthritis with rheumatoid factor of unspecified hand without organ or systems involvement	40	Rheumatoid Arthritis and Inflammatory Connective Tissue Disease		0.421	0.367	0.371	0.328	0.347	0.264	0.292
M05.751	Rheumatoid arthritis with rheumatoid factor of right hip without organ or systems involvement	40	Rheumatoid Arthritis and Inflammatory Connective Tissue Disease		0.421	0.367	0.371	0.328	0.347	0.264	0.292
M05.752	Rheumatoid arthritis with rheumatoid factor of left hip without organ or systems involvement	40	Rheumatoid Arthritis and Inflammatory Connective Tissue Disease		0.421	0.367	0.371	0.328	0.347	0.264	0.292
M05.759	Rheumatoid arthritis with rheumatoid factor of unspecified hip without organ or systems involvement	40	Rheumatoid Arthritis and Inflammatory Connective Tissue Disease		0.421	0.367	0.371	0.328	0.347	0.264	0.292
M05.761	Rheumatoid arthritis with rheumatoid factor of right knee without organ or systems involvement	40	Rheumatoid Arthritis and Inflammatory Connective Tissue Disease		0.421	0.367	0.371	0.328	0.347	0.264	0.292
M05.762	Rheumatoid arthritis with rheumatoid factor of left knee without organ or systems involvement	40	Rheumatoid Arthritis and Inflammatory Connective Tissue Disease		0.421	0.367	0.371	0.328	0.347	0.264	0.292
M05.769	Rheumatoid arthritis with rheumatoid factor of unspecified knee without organ or systems involvement	40	Rheumatoid Arthritis and Inflammatory Connective Tissue Disease		0.421	0.367	0.371	0.328	0.347	0.264	0.292
M05.771	Rheumatoid arthritis with rheumatoid factor of right ankle and foot without organ or systems involvement	40	Rheumatoid Arthritis and Inflammatory Connective Tissue Disease		0.421	0.367	0.371	0.328	0.347	0.264	0.292
M05.772	Rheumatoid arthritis with rheumatoid factor of left ankle and foot without organ or systems involvement	40	Rheumatoid Arthritis and Inflammatory Connective Tissue Disease		0.421	0.367	0.371	0.328	0.347	0.264	0.292
M05.779	Rheumatoid arthritis with rheumatoid factor of unspecified ankle and foot without organ or systems involvement	40	Rheumatoid Arthritis and Inflammatory Connective Tissue Disease		0.421	0.367	0.371	0.328	0.347	0.264	0.292
M05.79	Rheumatoid arthritis with rheumatoid factor of multiple sites without organ or systems involvement	40	Rheumatoid Arthritis and Inflammatory Connective Tissue Disease		0.421	0.367	0.371	0.328	0.347	0.264	0.292
M05.7A	Rheumatoid arthritis with rheumatoid factor of other specified site without organ or systems involvement	40	Rheumatoid Arthritis and Inflammatory Connective Tissue Disease		0.421	0.367	0.371	0.328	0.347	0.264	0.292
M05.80	Other rheumatoid arthritis with rheumatoid factor of unspecified site	40	Rheumatoid Arthritis and Inflammatory Connective Tissue Disease		0.421	0.367	0.371	0.328	0.347	0.264	0.292
M05.811	Other rheumatoid arthritis with rheumatoid factor of right shoulder	40	Rheumatoid Arthritis and Inflammatory Connective Tissue Disease		0.421	0.367	0.371	0.328	0.347	0.264	0.292
M05.812	Other rheumatoid arthritis with rheumatoid factor of left shoulder	40	Rheumatoid Arthritis and Inflammatory Connective Tissue Disease		0.421	0.367	0.371	0.328	0.347	0.264	0.292
M05.819	Other rheumatoid arthritis with rheumatoid factor of unspecified shoulder	40	Rheumatoid Arthritis and Inflammatory Connective Tissue Disease		0.421	0.367	0.371	0.328	0.347	0.264	0.292

ICD-10-CM Code	ICD-10-CM Code Description	V24 CMS-HCC	V24 CMS-HCC Disease Group	V24 CMS-HCC Hierarchies	Community, NonDual, Aged	Community, NonDual, Disabled	Community, FBDual, Aged	Community, FBDual, Disabled	Community, PBDual, Aged	Community, PBDual, Disabled	Institutional
MØ5.821	Other rheumatoid arthritis with rheumatoid factor of right elbow	40	Rheumatoid Arthritis and Inflammatory Connective Tissue Disease		0.421	0.367	0.371	0.328	0.347	0.264	0.292
MØ5.822	Other rheumatoid arthritis with rheumatoid factor of left elbow	40	Rheumatoid Arthritis and Inflammatory Connective Tissue Disease		0.421	0.367	0.371	0.328	0.347	0.264	0.292
MØ5.829	Other rheumatoid arthritis with rheumatoid factor of unspecified elbow	40	Rheumatoid Arthritis and Inflammatory Connective Tissue Disease		0.421	0.367	0.371	0.328	0.347	0.264	0.292
MØ5.831	Other rheumatoid arthritis with rheumatoid factor of right wrist	40	Rheumatoid Arthritis and Inflammatory Connective Tissue Disease		0.421	0.367	0.371	0.328	0.347	0.264	0.292
MØ5.832	Other rheumatoid arthritis with rheumatoid factor of left wrist	40	Rheumatoid Arthritis and Inflammatory Connective Tissue Disease		0.421	0.367	0.371	0.328	0.347	0.264	0.292
MØ5.839	Other rheumatoid arthritis with rheumatoid factor of unspecified wrist	40	Rheumatoid Arthritis and Inflammatory Connective Tissue Disease		0.421	0.367	0.371	0.328	0.347	0.264	0.292
MØ5.841	Other rheumatoid arthritis with rheumatoid factor of right hand	40	Rheumatoid Arthritis and Inflammatory Connective Tissue Disease		0.421	0.367	0.371	0.328	0.347	0.264	0.292
MØ5.842	Other rheumatoid arthritis with rheumatoid factor of left hand	40	Rheumatoid Arthritis and Inflammatory Connective Tissue Disease		0.421	0.367	0.371	0.328	0.347	0.264	0.292
MØ5.849	Other rheumatoid arthritis with rheumatoid factor of unspecified hand	40	Rheumatoid Arthritis and Inflammatory Connective Tissue Disease		0.421	0.367	0.371	0.328	0.347	0.264	0.292
MØ5.851	Other rheumatoid arthritis with rheumatoid factor of right hip	40	Rheumatoid Arthritis and Inflammatory Connective Tissue Disease		0.421	0.367	0.371	0.328	0.347	0.264	0.292
MØ5.852	Other rheumatoid arthritis with rheumatoid factor of left hip	40	Rheumatoid Arthritis and Inflammatory Connective Tissue Disease		0.421	0.367	0.371	0.328	0.347	0.264	0.292
MØ5.859	Other rheumatoid arthritis with rheumatoid factor of unspecified hip	40	Rheumatoid Arthritis and Inflammatory Connective Tissue Disease		0.421	0.367	0.371	0.328	0.347	0.264	0.292
MØ5.861	Other rheumatoid arthritis with rheumatoid factor of right knee	40	Rheumatoid Arthritis and Inflammatory Connective Tissue Disease		0.421	0.367	0.371	0.328	0.347	0.264	0.292
MØ5.862	Other rheumatoid arthritis with rheumatoid factor of left knee	40	Rheumatoid Arthritis and Inflammatory Connective Tissue Disease		0.421	0.367	0.371	0.328	0.347	0.264	0.292
MØ5.869	Other rheumatoid arthritis with rheumatoid factor of unspecified knee	40	Rheumatoid Arthritis and Inflammatory Connective Tissue Disease		0.421	0.367	0.371	0.328	0.347	0.264	0.292
MØ5.871	Other rheumatoid arthritis with rheumatoid factor of right ankle and foot	40	Rheumatoid Arthritis and Inflammatory Connective Tissue Disease		0.421	0.367	0.371	0.328	0.347	0.264	0.292
MØ5.872	Other rheumatoid arthritis with rheumatoid factor of left ankle and foot	40	Rheumatoid Arthritis and Inflammatory Connective Tissue Disease		0.421	0.367	0.371	0.328	0.347	0.264	0.292
MØ5.879	Other rheumatoid arthritis with rheumatoid factor of unspecified ankle and foot	40	Rheumatoid Arthritis and Inflammatory Connective Tissue Disease		0.421	0.367	0.371	0.328	0.347	0.264	0.292
MØ5.89	Other rheumatoid arthritis with rheumatoid factor of multiple sites	40	Rheumatoid Arthritis and Inflammatory Connective Tissue Disease		0.421	0.367	0.371	0.328	0.347	0.264	0.292
MØ5.8A	Other rheumatoid arthritis with rheumatoid factor of other specified site	40	Rheumatoid Arthritis and Inflammatory Connective Tissue Disease		0.421	0.367	0.371	0.328	0.347	0.264	0.292

ICD-10-CM Code	ICD-10-CM Code Description	V24 CMS-HCC	V24 CMS-HCC Disease Group	V24 CMS-HCC Hierarchies	Community, NonDual, Aged	Community, NonDual, Disabled	Community, FBDual, Aged	Community, FBDual, Disabled	Community, PBDual, Aged	Community, PBDual, Disabled	Institutional
M05.9	Rheumatoid arthritis with rheumatoid factor, unspecified	40	Rheumatoid Arthritis and Inflammatory Connective Tissue Disease		0.421	0.367	0.371	0.328	0.347	0.264	0.292
M06.00	Rheumatoid arthritis without rheumatoid factor, unspecified site	40	Rheumatoid Arthritis and Inflammatory Connective Tissue Disease		0.421	0.367	0.371	0.328	0.347	0.264	0.292
M06.011	Rheumatoid arthritis without rheumatoid factor, right shoulder	40	Rheumatoid Arthritis and Inflammatory Connective Tissue Disease		0.421	0.367	0.371	0.328	0.347	0.264	0.292
M06.012	Rheumatoid arthritis without rheumatoid factor, left shoulder	40	Rheumatoid Arthritis and Inflammatory Connective Tissue Disease		0.421	0.367	0.371	0.328	0.347	0.264	0.292
M06.019	Rheumatoid arthritis without rheumatoid factor, unspecified shoulder	40	Rheumatoid Arthritis and Inflammatory Connective Tissue Disease		0.421	0.367	0.371	0.328	0.347	0.264	0.292
M06.021	Rheumatoid arthritis without rheumatoid factor, right elbow	40	Rheumatoid Arthritis and Inflammatory Connective Tissue Disease		0.421	0.367	0.371	0.328	0.347	0.264	0.292
M06.022	Rheumatoid arthritis without rheumatoid factor, left elbow	40	Rheumatoid Arthritis and Inflammatory Connective Tissue Disease		0.421	0.367	0.371	0.328	0.347	0.264	0.292
M06.029	Rheumatoid arthritis without rheumatoid factor, unspecified elbow	40	Rheumatoid Arthritis and Inflammatory Connective Tissue Disease		0.421	0.367	0.371	0.328	0.347	0.264	0.292
M06.031	Rheumatoid arthritis without rheumatoid factor, right wrist	40	Rheumatoid Arthritis and Inflammatory Connective Tissue Disease		0.421	0.367	0.371	0.328	0.347	0.264	0.292
M06.032	Rheumatoid arthritis without rheumatoid factor, left wrist	40	Rheumatoid Arthritis and Inflammatory Connective Tissue Disease		0.421	0.367	0.371	0.328	0.347	0.264	0.292
M06.039	Rheumatoid arthritis without rheumatoid factor, unspecified wrist	40	Rheumatoid Arthritis and Inflammatory Connective Tissue Disease		0.421	0.367	0.371	0.328	0.347	0.264	0.292
M06.041	Rheumatoid arthritis without rheumatoid factor, right hand	40	Rheumatoid Arthritis and Inflammatory Connective Tissue Disease		0.421	0.367	0.371	0.328	0.347	0.264	0.292
M06.042	Rheumatoid arthritis without rheumatoid factor, left hand	40	Rheumatoid Arthritis and Inflammatory Connective Tissue Disease		0.421	0.367	0.371	0.328	0.347	0.264	0.292
M06.049	Rheumatoid arthritis without rheumatoid factor, unspecified hand	40	Rheumatoid Arthritis and Inflammatory Connective Tissue Disease		0.421	0.367	0.371	0.328	0.347	0.264	0.292
M06.051	Rheumatoid arthritis without rheumatoid factor, right hip	40	Rheumatoid Arthritis and Inflammatory Connective Tissue Disease		0.421	0.367	0.371	0.328	0.347	0.264	0.292
M06.052	Rheumatoid arthritis without rheumatoid factor, left hip	40	Rheumatoid Arthritis and Inflammatory Connective Tissue Disease		0.421	0.367	0.371	0.328	0.347	0.264	0.292
M06.059	Rheumatoid arthritis without rheumatoid factor, unspecified hip	40	Rheumatoid Arthritis and Inflammatory Connective Tissue Disease		0.421	0.367	0.371	0.328	0.347	0.264	0.292
M06.061	Rheumatoid arthritis without rheumatoid factor, right knee	40	Rheumatoid Arthritis and Inflammatory Connective Tissue Disease		0.421	0.367	0.371	0.328	0.347	0.264	0.292
M06.062	Rheumatoid arthritis without rheumatoid factor, left knee	40	Rheumatoid Arthritis and Inflammatory Connective Tissue Disease		0.421	0.367	0.371	0.328	0.347	0.264	0.292
M06.069	Rheumatoid arthritis without rheumatoid factor, unspecified knee	40	Rheumatoid Arthritis and Inflammatory Connective Tissue Disease		0.421	0.367	0.371	0.328	0.347	0.264	0.292

ICD-10-CM Code	ICD-10-CM Code Description	V24 CMS-HCC	V24 CMS-HCC Disease Group	V24 CMS-HCC Hierarchies	Community, NonDual, Aged	Community, NonDual, Disabled	Community, FBDual, Aged	Community, FBDual, Disabled	Community, PBDual, Aged	Community, PBDual, Disabled	Institutional
M06.071	Rheumatoid arthritis without rheumatoid factor, right ankle and foot	40	Rheumatoid Arthritis and Inflammatory Connective Tissue Disease		0.421	0.367	0.371	0.328	0.347	0.264	0.292
M06.072	Rheumatoid arthritis without rheumatoid factor, left ankle and foot	40	Rheumatoid Arthritis and Inflammatory Connective Tissue Disease		0.421	0.367	0.371	0.328	0.347	0.264	0.292
M06.079	Rheumatoid arthritis without rheumatoid factor, unspecified ankle and foot	40	Rheumatoid Arthritis and Inflammatory Connective Tissue Disease		0.421	0.367	0.371	0.328	0.347	0.264	0.292
M06.08	Rheumatoid arthritis without rheumatoid factor, vertebrae	40	Rheumatoid Arthritis and Inflammatory Connective Tissue Disease		0.421	0.367	0.371	0.328	0.347	0.264	0.292
M06.09	Rheumatoid arthritis without rheumatoid factor, multiple sites	40	Rheumatoid Arthritis and Inflammatory Connective Tissue Disease		0.421	0.367	0.371	0.328	0.347	0.264	0.292
M06.0A	Rheumatoid arthritis without rheumatoid factor, other specified site	40	Rheumatoid Arthritis and Inflammatory Connective Tissue Disease		0.421	0.367	0.371	0.328	0.347	0.264	0.292
M06.1	Adult-onset Still's disease	40	Rheumatoid Arthritis and Inflammatory Connective Tissue Disease		0.421	0.367	0.371	0.328	0.347	0.264	0.292
M06.20	Rheumatoid bursitis, unspecified site	40	Rheumatoid Arthritis and Inflammatory Connective Tissue Disease		0.421	0.367	0.371	0.328	0.347	0.264	0.292
M06.211	Rheumatoid bursitis, right shoulder	40	Rheumatoid Arthritis and Inflammatory Connective Tissue Disease		0.421	0.367	0.371	0.328	0.347	0.264	0.292
M06.212	Rheumatoid bursitis, left shoulder	40	Rheumatoid Arthritis and Inflammatory Connective Tissue Disease		0.421	0.367	0.371	0.328	0.347	0.264	0.292
M06.219	Rheumatoid bursitis, unspecified shoulder	40	Rheumatoid Arthritis and Inflammatory Connective Tissue Disease		0.421	0.367	0.371	0.328	0.347	0.264	0.292
M06.221	Rheumatoid bursitis, right elbow	40	Rheumatoid Arthritis and Inflammatory Connective Tissue Disease		0.421	0.367	0.371	0.328	0.347	0.264	0.292
M06.222	Rheumatoid bursitis, left elbow	40	Rheumatoid Arthritis and Inflammatory Connective Tissue Disease		0.421	0.367	0.371	0.328	0.347	0.264	0.292
M06.229	Rheumatoid bursitis, unspecified elbow	40	Rheumatoid Arthritis and Inflammatory Connective Tissue Disease		0.421	0.367	0.371	0.328	0.347	0.264	0.292
M06.231	Rheumatoid bursitis, right wrist	40	Rheumatoid Arthritis and Inflammatory Connective Tissue Disease		0.421	0.367	0.371	0.328	0.347	0.264	0.292
M06.232	Rheumatoid bursitis, left wrist	40	Rheumatoid Arthritis and Inflammatory Connective Tissue Disease		0.421	0.367	0.371	0.328	0.347	0.264	0.292
M06.239	Rheumatoid bursitis, unspecified wrist	40	Rheumatoid Arthritis and Inflammatory Connective Tissue Disease		0.421	0.367	0.371	0.328	0.347	0.264	0.292
M06.241	Rheumatoid bursitis, right hand	40	Rheumatoid Arthritis and Inflammatory Connective Tissue Disease		0.421	0.367	0.371	0.328	0.347	0.264	0.292
M06.242	Rheumatoid bursitis, left hand	40	Rheumatoid Arthritis and Inflammatory Connective Tissue Disease		0.421	0.367	0.371	0.328	0.347	0.264	0.292
M06.249	Rheumatoid bursitis, unspecified hand	40	Rheumatoid Arthritis and Inflammatory Connective Tissue Disease		0.421	0.367	0.371	0.328	0.347	0.264	0.292

ICD-10-CM Code	ICD-10-CM Code Description	V24 CMS-HCC	V24 CMS-HCC Disease Group	V24 CMS-HCC Hierarchies	Community, NonDual, Aged	Community, NonDual, Disabled	Community, FBDual, Aged	Community, FBDual, Disabled	Community, PBDual, Aged	Community, PBDual, Disabled	Institutional
MØ6.251	Rheumatoid bursitis, right hip	40	Rheumatoid Arthritis and Inflammatory Connective Tissue Disease		0.421	0.367	0.371	0.328	0.347	0.264	0.292
MØ6.252	Rheumatoid bursitis, left hip	40	Rheumatoid Arthritis and Inflammatory Connective Tissue Disease		0.421	0.367	0.371	0.328	0.347	0.264	0.292
MØ6.259	Rheumatoid bursitis, unspecified hip	40	Rheumatoid Arthritis and Inflammatory Connective Tissue Disease		0.421	0.367	0.371	0.328	0.347	0.264	0.292
MØ6.261	Rheumatoid bursitis, right knee	40	Rheumatoid Arthritis and Inflammatory Connective Tissue Disease		0.421	0.367	0.371	0.328	0.347	0.264	0.292
MØ6.262	Rheumatoid bursitis, left knee	40	Rheumatoid Arthritis and Inflammatory Connective Tissue Disease		0.421	0.367	0.371	0.328	0.347	0.264	0.292
MØ6.269	Rheumatoid bursitis, unspecified knee	40	Rheumatoid Arthritis and Inflammatory Connective Tissue Disease		0.421	0.367	0.371	0.328	0.347	0.264	0.292
MØ6.271	Rheumatoid bursitis, right ankle and foot	40	Rheumatoid Arthritis and Inflammatory Connective Tissue Disease		0.421	0.367	0.371	0.328	0.347	0.264	0.292
MØ6.272	Rheumatoid bursitis, left ankle and foot	40	Rheumatoid Arthritis and Inflammatory Connective Tissue Disease		0.421	0.367	0.371	0.328	0.347	0.264	0.292
MØ6.279	Rheumatoid bursitis, unspecified ankle and foot	40	Rheumatoid Arthritis and Inflammatory Connective Tissue Disease		0.421	0.367	0.371	0.328	0.347	0.264	0.292
MØ6.28	Rheumatoid bursitis, vertebrae	40	Rheumatoid Arthritis and Inflammatory Connective Tissue Disease		0.421	0.367	0.371	0.328	0.347	0.264	0.292
MØ6.29	Rheumatoid bursitis, multiple sites	40	Rheumatoid Arthritis and Inflammatory Connective Tissue Disease		0.421	0.367	0.371	0.328	0.347	0.264	0.292
MØ6.3Ø	Rheumatoid nodule, unspecified site	40	Rheumatoid Arthritis and Inflammatory Connective Tissue Disease		0.421	0.367	0.371	0.328	0.347	0.264	0.292
MØ6.311	Rheumatoid nodule, right shoulder	40	Rheumatoid Arthritis and Inflammatory Connective Tissue Disease		0.421	0.367	0.371	0.328	0.347	0.264	0.292
MØ6.312	Rheumatoid nodule, left shoulder	40	Rheumatoid Arthritis and Inflammatory Connective Tissue Disease		0.421	0.367	0.371	0.328	0.347	0.264	0.292
MØ6.319	Rheumatoid nodule, unspecified shoulder	40	Rheumatoid Arthritis and Inflammatory Connective Tissue Disease		0.421	0.367	0.371	0.328	0.347	0.264	0.292
MØ6.321	Rheumatoid nodule, right elbow	40	Rheumatoid Arthritis and Inflammatory Connective Tissue Disease		0.421	0.367	0.371	0.328	0.347	0.264	0.292
MØ6.322	Rheumatoid nodule, left elbow	40	Rheumatoid Arthritis and Inflammatory Connective Tissue Disease		0.421	0.367	0.371	0.328	0.347	0.264	0.292
MØ6.329	Rheumatoid nodule, unspecified elbow	40	Rheumatoid Arthritis and Inflammatory Connective Tissue Disease		0.421	0.367	0.371	0.328	0.347	0.264	0.292
MØ6.331	Rheumatoid nodule, right wrist	40	Rheumatoid Arthritis and Inflammatory Connective Tissue Disease		0.421	0.367	0.371	0.328	0.347	0.264	0.292
MØ6.332	Rheumatoid nodule, left wrist	40	Rheumatoid Arthritis and Inflammatory Connective Tissue Disease		0.421	0.367	0.371	0.328	0.347	0.264	0.292

ICD-10-CM Code	ICD-10-CM Code Description	V24 CMS-HCC	V24 CMS-HCC Disease Group	V24 CMS-HCC Hierarchies	Community, NonDual, Aged	Community, NonDual, Disabled	Community, FBDual, Aged	Community, FBDual, Disabled	Community, PBDual, Aged	Community, PBDual, Disabled	Institutional
M06.339	Rheumatoid nodule, unspecified wrist	40	Rheumatoid Arthritis and Inflammatory Connective Tissue Disease		0.421	0.367	0.371	0.328	0.347	0.264	0.292
M06.341	Rheumatoid nodule, right hand	40	Rheumatoid Arthritis and Inflammatory Connective Tissue Disease		0.421	0.367	0.371	0.328	0.347	0.264	0.292
M06.342	Rheumatoid nodule, left hand	40	Rheumatoid Arthritis and Inflammatory Connective Tissue Disease		0.421	0.367	0.371	0.328	0.347	0.264	0.292
M06.349	Rheumatoid nodule, unspecified hand	40	Rheumatoid Arthritis and Inflammatory Connective Tissue Disease		0.421	0.367	0.371	0.328	0.347	0.264	0.292
M06.351	Rheumatoid nodule, right hip	40	Rheumatoid Arthritis and Inflammatory Connective Tissue Disease		0.421	0.367	0.371	0.328	0.347	0.264	0.292
M06.352	Rheumatoid nodule, left hip	40	Rheumatoid Arthritis and Inflammatory Connective Tissue Disease		0.421	0.367	0.371	0.328	0.347	0.264	0.292
M06.359	Rheumatoid nodule, unspecified hip	40	Rheumatoid Arthritis and Inflammatory Connective Tissue Disease		0.421	0.367	0.371	0.328	0.347	0.264	0.292
M06.361	Rheumatoid nodule, right knee	40	Rheumatoid Arthritis and Inflammatory Connective Tissue Disease		0.421	0.367	0.371	0.328	0.347	0.264	0.292
M06.362	Rheumatoid nodule, left knee	40	Rheumatoid Arthritis and Inflammatory Connective Tissue Disease		0.421	0.367	0.371	0.328	0.347	0.264	0.292
M06.369	Rheumatoid nodule, unspecified knee	40	Rheumatoid Arthritis and Inflammatory Connective Tissue Disease		0.421	0.367	0.371	0.328	0.347	0.264	0.292
M06.371	Rheumatoid nodule, right ankle and foot	40	Rheumatoid Arthritis and Inflammatory Connective Tissue Disease		0.421	0.367	0.371	0.328	0.347	0.264	0.292
M06.372	Rheumatoid nodule, left ankle and foot	40	Rheumatoid Arthritis and Inflammatory Connective Tissue Disease		0.421	0.367	0.371	0.328	0.347	0.264	0.292
M06.379	Rheumatoid nodule, unspecified ankle and foot	40	Rheumatoid Arthritis and Inflammatory Connective Tissue Disease		0.421	0.367	0.371	0.328	0.347	0.264	0.292
M06.38	Rheumatoid nodule, vertebrae	40	Rheumatoid Arthritis and Inflammatory Connective Tissue Disease		0.421	0.367	0.371	0.328	0.347	0.264	0.292
M06.39	Rheumatoid nodule, multiple sites	40	Rheumatoid Arthritis and Inflammatory Connective Tissue Disease		0.421	0.367	0.371	0.328	0.347	0.264	0.292
M06.4	Inflammatory polyarthropathy	40	Rheumatoid Arthritis and Inflammatory Connective Tissue Disease		0.421	0.367	0.371	0.328	0.347	0.264	0.292
M06.80	Other specified rheumatoid arthritis, unspecified site	40	Rheumatoid Arthritis and Inflammatory Connective Tissue Disease		0.421	0.367	0.371	0.328	0.347	0.264	0.292
M06.811	Other specified rheumatoid arthritis, right shoulder	40	Rheumatoid Arthritis and Inflammatory Connective Tissue Disease		0.421	0.367	0.371	0.328	0.347	0.264	0.292
M06.812	Other specified rheumatoid arthritis, left shoulder	40	Rheumatoid Arthritis and Inflammatory Connective Tissue Disease		0.421	0.367	0.371	0.328	0.347	0.264	0.292
M06.819	Other specified rheumatoid arthritis, unspecified shoulder	40	Rheumatoid Arthritis and Inflammatory Connective Tissue Disease		0.421	0.367	0.371	0.328	0.347	0.264	0.292

ICD-10-CM Code	ICD-10-CM Code Description	V24 CMS-HCC	V24 CMS-HCC Disease Group	V24 CMS-HCC Hierarchies	Community, NonDual, Aged	Community, NonDual, Disabled	Community, FBDual, Aged	Community, FBDual, Disabled	Community, PBDual, Aged	Community, PBDual, Disabled	Institutional
M06.821	Other specified rheumatoid arthritis, right elbow	40	Rheumatoid Arthritis and Inflammatory Connective Tissue Disease		0.421	0.367	0.371	0.328	0.347	0.264	0.292
M06.822	Other specified rheumatoid arthritis, left elbow	40	Rheumatoid Arthritis and Inflammatory Connective Tissue Disease		0.421	0.367	0.371	0.328	0.347	0.264	0.292
M06.829	Other specified rheumatoid arthritis, unspecified elbow	40	Rheumatoid Arthritis and Inflammatory Connective Tissue Disease		0.421	0.367	0.371	0.328	0.347	0.264	0.292
M06.831	Other specified rheumatoid arthritis, right wrist	40	Rheumatoid Arthritis and Inflammatory Connective Tissue Disease		0.421	0.367	0.371	0.328	0.347	0.264	0.292
M06.832	Other specified rheumatoid arthritis, left wrist	40	Rheumatoid Arthritis and Inflammatory Connective Tissue Disease		0.421	0.367	0.371	0.328	0.347	0.264	0.292
M06.839	Other specified rheumatoid arthritis, unspecified wrist	40	Rheumatoid Arthritis and Inflammatory Connective Tissue Disease		0.421	0.367	0.371	0.328	0.347	0.264	0.292
M06.841	Other specified rheumatoid arthritis, right hand	40	Rheumatoid Arthritis and Inflammatory Connective Tissue Disease		0.421	0.367	0.371	0.328	0.347	0.264	0.292
M06.842	Other specified rheumatoid arthritis, left hand	40	Rheumatoid Arthritis and Inflammatory Connective Tissue Disease		0.421	0.367	0.371	0.328	0.347	0.264	0.292
M06.849	Other specified rheumatoid arthritis, unspecified hand	40	Rheumatoid Arthritis and Inflammatory Connective Tissue Disease		0.421	0.367	0.371	0.328	0.347	0.264	0.292
M06.851	Other specified rheumatoid arthritis, right hip	40	Rheumatoid Arthritis and Inflammatory Connective Tissue Disease		0.421	0.367	0.371	0.328	0.347	0.264	0.292
M06.852	Other specified rheumatoid arthritis, left hip	40	Rheumatoid Arthritis and Inflammatory Connective Tissue Disease		0.421	0.367	0.371	0.328	0.347	0.264	0.292
M06.859	Other specified rheumatoid arthritis, unspecified hip	40	Rheumatoid Arthritis and Inflammatory Connective Tissue Disease		0.421	0.367	0.371	0.328	0.347	0.264	0.292
M06.861	Other specified rheumatoid arthritis, right knee	40	Rheumatoid Arthritis and Inflammatory Connective Tissue Disease		0.421	0.367	0.371	0.328	0.347	0.264	0.292
M06.862	Other specified rheumatoid arthritis, left knee	40	Rheumatoid Arthritis and Inflammatory Connective Tissue Disease		0.421	0.367	0.371	0.328	0.347	0.264	0.292
M06.869	Other specified rheumatoid arthritis, unspecified knee	40	Rheumatoid Arthritis and Inflammatory Connective Tissue Disease		0.421	0.367	0.371	0.328	0.347	0.264	0.292
M06.871	Other specified rheumatoid arthritis, right ankle and foot	40	Rheumatoid Arthritis and Inflammatory Connective Tissue Disease		0.421	0.367	0.371	0.328	0.347	0.264	0.292
M06.872	Other specified rheumatoid arthritis, left ankle and foot	40	Rheumatoid Arthritis and Inflammatory Connective Tissue Disease		0.421	0.367	0.371	0.328	0.347	0.264	0.292
M06.879	Other specified rheumatoid arthritis, unspecified ankle and foot	40	Rheumatoid Arthritis and Inflammatory Connective Tissue Disease		0.421	0.367	0.371	0.328	0.347	0.264	0.292
M06.88	Other specified rheumatoid arthritis, vertebrae	40	Rheumatoid Arthritis and Inflammatory Connective Tissue Disease		0.421	0.367	0.371	0.328	0.347	0.264	0.292
M06.89	Other specified rheumatoid arthritis, multiple sites	40	Rheumatoid Arthritis and Inflammatory Connective Tissue Disease		0.421	0.367	0.371	0.328	0.347	0.264	0.292

ICD-10-CM Code	ICD-10-CM Code Description	V24 CMS-HCC	V24 CMS-HCC Disease Group	V24 CMS-HCC Hierarchies	Community, NonDual, Aged	Community, NonDual, Disabled	Community, FBDual, Aged	Community, FBDual, Disabled	Community, PBDual, Aged	Community, PBDual, Disabled	Institutional
M06.8A	Other specified rheumatoid arthritis, other specified site	40	Rheumatoid Arthritis and Inflammatory Connective Tissue Disease		0.421	0.367	0.371	0.328	0.347	0.264	0.292
M06.9	Rheumatoid arthritis, unspecified	40	Rheumatoid Arthritis and Inflammatory Connective Tissue Disease		0.421	0.367	0.371	0.328	0.347	0.264	0.292
M08.00	Unspecified juvenile rheumatoid arthritis of unspecified site	40	Rheumatoid Arthritis and Inflammatory Connective Tissue Disease		0.421	0.367	0.371	0.328	0.347	0.264	0.292
M08.011	Unspecified juvenile rheumatoid arthritis, right shoulder	40	Rheumatoid Arthritis and Inflammatory Connective Tissue Disease		0.421	0.367	0.371	0.328	0.347	0.264	0.292
M08.012	Unspecified juvenile rheumatoid arthritis, left shoulder	40	Rheumatoid Arthritis and Inflammatory Connective Tissue Disease		0.421	0.367	0.371	0.328	0.347	0.264	0.292
M08.019	Unspecified juvenile rheumatoid arthritis, unspecified shoulder	40	Rheumatoid Arthritis and Inflammatory Connective Tissue Disease		0.421	0.367	0.371	0.328	0.347	0.264	0.292
M08.021	Unspecified juvenile rheumatoid arthritis, right elbow	40	Rheumatoid Arthritis and Inflammatory Connective Tissue Disease		0.421	0.367	0.371	0.328	0.347	0.264	0.292
M08.022	Unspecified juvenile rheumatoid arthritis, left elbow	40	Rheumatoid Arthritis and Inflammatory Connective Tissue Disease		0.421	0.367	0.371	0.328	0.347	0.264	0.292
M08.029	Unspecified juvenile rheumatoid arthritis, unspecified elbow	40	Rheumatoid Arthritis and Inflammatory Connective Tissue Disease		0.421	0.367	0.371	0.328	0.347	0.264	0.292
M08.031	Unspecified juvenile rheumatoid arthritis, right wrist	40	Rheumatoid Arthritis and Inflammatory Connective Tissue Disease		0.421	0.367	0.371	0.328	0.347	0.264	0.292
M08.032	Unspecified juvenile rheumatoid arthritis, left wrist	40	Rheumatoid Arthritis and Inflammatory Connective Tissue Disease		0.421	0.367	0.371	0.328	0.347	0.264	0.292
M08.039	Unspecified juvenile rheumatoid arthritis, unspecified wrist	40	Rheumatoid Arthritis and Inflammatory Connective Tissue Disease		0.421	0.367	0.371	0.328	0.347	0.264	0.292
M08.041	Unspecified juvenile rheumatoid arthritis, right hand	40	Rheumatoid Arthritis and Inflammatory Connective Tissue Disease		0.421	0.367	0.371	0.328	0.347	0.264	0.292
M08.042	Unspecified juvenile rheumatoid arthritis, left hand	40	Rheumatoid Arthritis and Inflammatory Connective Tissue Disease		0.421	0.367	0.371	0.328	0.347	0.264	0.292
M08.049	Unspecified juvenile rheumatoid arthritis, unspecified hand	40	Rheumatoid Arthritis and Inflammatory Connective Tissue Disease		0.421	0.367	0.371	0.328	0.347	0.264	0.292
M08.051	Unspecified juvenile rheumatoid arthritis, right hip	40	Rheumatoid Arthritis and Inflammatory Connective Tissue Disease		0.421	0.367	0.371	0.328	0.347	0.264	0.292
M08.052	Unspecified juvenile rheumatoid arthritis, left hip	40	Rheumatoid Arthritis and Inflammatory Connective Tissue Disease		0.421	0.367	0.371	0.328	0.347	0.264	0.292
M08.059	Unspecified juvenile rheumatoid arthritis, unspecified hip	40	Rheumatoid Arthritis and Inflammatory Connective Tissue Disease		0.421	0.367	0.371	0.328	0.347	0.264	0.292
M08.061	Unspecified juvenile rheumatoid arthritis, right knee	40	Rheumatoid Arthritis and Inflammatory Connective Tissue Disease		0.421	0.367	0.371	0.328	0.347	0.264	0.292
M08.062	Unspecified juvenile rheumatoid arthritis, left knee	40	Rheumatoid Arthritis and Inflammatory Connective Tissue Disease		0.421	0.367	0.371	0.328	0.347	0.264	0.292

ICD-10-CM Code	ICD-10-CM Code Description	V24 CMS-HCC	V24 CMS-HCC Disease Group	V24 CMS-HCC Hierarchies	Community, NonDual, Aged	Community, NonDual, Disabled	Community, FBDual, Aged	Community, FBDual, Disabled	Community, PBDual, Aged	Community, PBDual, Disabled	Institutional
M08.069	Unspecified juvenile rheumatoid arthritis, unspecified knee	40	Rheumatoid Arthritis and Inflammatory Connective Tissue Disease		0.421	0.367	0.371	0.328	0.347	0.264	0.292
M08.071	Unspecified juvenile rheumatoid arthritis, right ankle and foot	40	Rheumatoid Arthritis and Inflammatory Connective Tissue Disease		0.421	0.367	0.371	0.328	0.347	0.264	0.292
M08.072	Unspecified juvenile rheumatoid arthritis, left ankle and foot	40	Rheumatoid Arthritis and Inflammatory Connective Tissue Disease		0.421	0.367	0.371	0.328	0.347	0.264	0.292
M08.079	Unspecified juvenile rheumatoid arthritis, unspecified ankle and foot	40	Rheumatoid Arthritis and Inflammatory Connective Tissue Disease		0.421	0.367	0.371	0.328	0.347	0.264	0.292
M08.08	Unspecified juvenile rheumatoid arthritis, vertebrae	40	Rheumatoid Arthritis and Inflammatory Connective Tissue Disease		0.421	0.367	0.371	0.328	0.347	0.264	0.292
M08.09	Unspecified juvenile rheumatoid arthritis, multiple sites	40	Rheumatoid Arthritis and Inflammatory Connective Tissue Disease		0.421	0.367	0.371	0.328	0.347	0.264	0.292
M08.0A	Unspecified juvenile rheumatoid arthritis, other specified site	40	Rheumatoid Arthritis and Inflammatory Connective Tissue Disease		0.421	0.367	0.371	0.328	0.347	0.264	0.292
M08.1	Juvenile ankylosing spondylitis	40	Rheumatoid Arthritis and Inflammatory Connective Tissue Disease		0.421	0.367	0.371	0.328	0.347	0.264	0.292
M08.20	Juvenile rheumatoid arthritis with systemic onset, unspecified site	40	Rheumatoid Arthritis and Inflammatory Connective Tissue Disease		0.421	0.367	0.371	0.328	0.347	0.264	0.292
M08.211	Juvenile rheumatoid arthritis with systemic onset, right shoulder	40	Rheumatoid Arthritis and Inflammatory Connective Tissue Disease		0.421	0.367	0.371	0.328	0.347	0.264	0.292
M08.212	Juvenile rheumatoid arthritis with systemic onset, left shoulder	40	Rheumatoid Arthritis and Inflammatory Connective Tissue Disease		0.421	0.367	0.371	0.328	0.347	0.264	0.292
M08.219	Juvenile rheumatoid arthritis with systemic onset, unspecified shoulder	40	Rheumatoid Arthritis and Inflammatory Connective Tissue Disease		0.421	0.367	0.371	0.328	0.347	0.264	0.292
M08.221	Juvenile rheumatoid arthritis with systemic onset, right elbow	40	Rheumatoid Arthritis and Inflammatory Connective Tissue Disease		0.421	0.367	0.371	0.328	0.347	0.264	0.292
M08.222	Juvenile rheumatoid arthritis with systemic onset, left elbow	40	Rheumatoid Arthritis and Inflammatory Connective Tissue Disease		0.421	0.367	0.371	0.328	0.347	0.264	0.292
M08.229	Juvenile rheumatoid arthritis with systemic onset, unspecified elbow	40	Rheumatoid Arthritis and Inflammatory Connective Tissue Disease		0.421	0.367	0.371	0.328	0.347	0.264	0.292
M08.231	Juvenile rheumatoid arthritis with systemic onset, right wrist	40	Rheumatoid Arthritis and Inflammatory Connective Tissue Disease		0.421	0.367	0.371	0.328	0.347	0.264	0.292
M08.232	Juvenile rheumatoid arthritis with systemic onset, left wrist	40	Rheumatoid Arthritis and Inflammatory Connective Tissue Disease		0.421	0.367	0.371	0.328	0.347	0.264	0.292
M08.239	Juvenile rheumatoid arthritis with systemic onset, unspecified wrist	40	Rheumatoid Arthritis and Inflammatory Connective Tissue Disease		0.421	0.367	0.371	0.328	0.347	0.264	0.292
M08.241	Juvenile rheumatoid arthritis with systemic onset, right hand	40	Rheumatoid Arthritis and Inflammatory Connective Tissue Disease		0.421	0.367	0.371	0.328	0.347	0.264	0.292
M08.242	Juvenile rheumatoid arthritis with systemic onset, left hand	40	Rheumatoid Arthritis and Inflammatory Connective Tissue Disease		0.421	0.367	0.371	0.328	0.347	0.264	0.292

ICD-10-CM Code	ICD-10-CM Code Description	V24 CMS-HCC	V24 CMS-HCC Disease Group	V24 CMS-HCC Hierarchies	Community, NonDual, Aged	Community, NonDual, Disabled	Community, FBDual, Aged	Community, FBDual, Disabled	Community, PBDual, Aged	Community, PBDual, Disabled	Institutional
M08.249	Juvenile rheumatoid arthritis with systemic onset, unspecified hand	40	Rheumatoid Arthritis and Inflammatory Connective Tissue Disease		0.421	0.367	0.371	0.328	0.347	0.264	0.292
M08.251	Juvenile rheumatoid arthritis with systemic onset, right hip	40	Rheumatoid Arthritis and Inflammatory Connective Tissue Disease		0.421	0.367	0.371	0.328	0.347	0.264	0.292
M08.252	Juvenile rheumatoid arthritis with systemic onset, left hip	40	Rheumatoid Arthritis and Inflammatory Connective Tissue Disease		0.421	0.367	0.371	0.328	0.347	0.264	0.292
M08.259	Juvenile rheumatoid arthritis with systemic onset, unspecified hip	40	Rheumatoid Arthritis and Inflammatory Connective Tissue Disease		0.421	0.367	0.371	0.328	0.347	0.264	0.292
M08.261	Juvenile rheumatoid arthritis with systemic onset, right knee	40	Rheumatoid Arthritis and Inflammatory Connective Tissue Disease		0.421	0.367	0.371	0.328	0.347	0.264	0.292
M08.262	Juvenile rheumatoid arthritis with systemic onset, left knee	40	Rheumatoid Arthritis and Inflammatory Connective Tissue Disease		0.421	0.367	0.371	0.328	0.347	0.264	0.292
M08.269	Juvenile rheumatoid arthritis with systemic onset, unspecified knee	40	Rheumatoid Arthritis and Inflammatory Connective Tissue Disease		0.421	0.367	0.371	0.328	0.347	0.264	0.292
M08.271	Juvenile rheumatoid arthritis with systemic onset, right ankle and foot	40	Rheumatoid Arthritis and Inflammatory Connective Tissue Disease		0.421	0.367	0.371	0.328	0.347	0.264	0.292
M08.272	Juvenile rheumatoid arthritis with systemic onset, left ankle and foot	40	Rheumatoid Arthritis and Inflammatory Connective Tissue Disease		0.421	0.367	0.371	0.328	0.347	0.264	0.292
M08.279	Juvenile rheumatoid arthritis with systemic onset, unspecified ankle and foot	40	Rheumatoid Arthritis and Inflammatory Connective Tissue Disease		0.421	0.367	0.371	0.328	0.347	0.264	0.292
M08.28	Juvenile rheumatoid arthritis with systemic onset, vertebrae	40	Rheumatoid Arthritis and Inflammatory Connective Tissue Disease		0.421	0.367	0.371	0.328	0.347	0.264	0.292
M08.29	Juvenile rheumatoid arthritis with systemic onset, multiple sites	40	Rheumatoid Arthritis and Inflammatory Connective Tissue Disease		0.421	0.367	0.371	0.328	0.347	0.264	0.292
M08.2A	Juvenile rheumatoid arthritis with systemic onset, other specified site	40	Rheumatoid Arthritis and Inflammatory Connective Tissue Disease		0.421	0.367	0.371	0.328	0.347	0.264	0.292
M08.3	Juvenile rheumatoid polyarthritis (seronegative)	40	Rheumatoid Arthritis and Inflammatory Connective Tissue Disease		0.421	0.367	0.371	0.328	0.347	0.264	0.292
M08.40	Pauciarticular juvenile rheumatoid arthritis, unspecified site	40	Rheumatoid Arthritis and Inflammatory Connective Tissue Disease		0.421	0.367	0.371	0.328	0.347	0.264	0.292
M08.411	Pauciarticular juvenile rheumatoid arthritis, right shoulder	40	Rheumatoid Arthritis and Inflammatory Connective Tissue Disease		0.421	0.367	0.371	0.328	0.347	0.264	0.292
M08.412	Pauciarticular juvenile rheumatoid arthritis, left shoulder	40	Rheumatoid Arthritis and Inflammatory Connective Tissue Disease		0.421	0.367	0.371	0.328	0.347	0.264	0.292
M08.419	Pauciarticular juvenile rheumatoid arthritis, unspecified shoulder	40	Rheumatoid Arthritis and Inflammatory Connective Tissue Disease		0.421	0.367	0.371	0.328	0.347	0.264	0.292
M08.421	Pauciarticular juvenile rheumatoid arthritis, right elbow	40	Rheumatoid Arthritis and Inflammatory Connective Tissue Disease		0.421	0.367	0.371	0.328	0.347	0.264	0.292
M08.422	Pauciarticular juvenile rheumatoid arthritis, left elbow	40	Rheumatoid Arthritis and Inflammatory Connective Tissue Disease		0.421	0.367	0.371	0.328	0.347	0.264	0.292

ICD-10-CM Code	ICD-10-CM Code Description	V24 CMS-HCC	V24 CMS-HCC Disease Group	V24 CMS-HCC Hierarchies	Community, NonDual, Aged	Community, NonDual, Disabled	Community, FBDual, Aged	Community, FBDual, Disabled	Community, PBDual, Aged	Community, PBDual, Disabled	Institutional
M08.429	Pauciarticular juvenile rheumatoid arthritis, unspecified elbow	40	Rheumatoid Arthritis and Inflammatory Connective Tissue Disease		0.421	0.367	0.371	0.328	0.347	0.264	0.292
M08.431	Pauciarticular juvenile rheumatoid arthritis, right wrist	40	Rheumatoid Arthritis and Inflammatory Connective Tissue Disease		0.421	0.367	0.371	0.328	0.347	0.264	0.292
M08.432	Pauciarticular juvenile rheumatoid arthritis, left wrist	40	Rheumatoid Arthritis and Inflammatory Connective Tissue Disease		0.421	0.367	0.371	0.328	0.347	0.264	0.292
M08.439	Pauciarticular juvenile rheumatoid arthritis, unspecified wrist	40	Rheumatoid Arthritis and Inflammatory Connective Tissue Disease		0.421	0.367	0.371	0.328	0.347	0.264	0.292
M08.441	Pauciarticular juvenile rheumatoid arthritis, right hand	40	Rheumatoid Arthritis and Inflammatory Connective Tissue Disease		0.421	0.367	0.371	0.328	0.347	0.264	0.292
M08.442	Pauciarticular juvenile rheumatoid arthritis, left hand	40	Rheumatoid Arthritis and Inflammatory Connective Tissue Disease		0.421	0.367	0.371	0.328	0.347	0.264	0.292
M08.449	Pauciarticular juvenile rheumatoid arthritis, unspecified hand	40	Rheumatoid Arthritis and Inflammatory Connective Tissue Disease		0.421	0.367	0.371	0.328	0.347	0.264	0.292
M08.451	Pauciarticular juvenile rheumatoid arthritis, right hip	40	Rheumatoid Arthritis and Inflammatory Connective Tissue Disease		0.421	0.367	0.371	0.328	0.347	0.264	0.292
M08.452	Pauciarticular juvenile rheumatoid arthritis, left hip	40	Rheumatoid Arthritis and Inflammatory Connective Tissue Disease		0.421	0.367	0.371	0.328	0.347	0.264	0.292
M08.459	Pauciarticular juvenile rheumatoid arthritis, unspecified hip	40	Rheumatoid Arthritis and Inflammatory Connective Tissue Disease		0.421	0.367	0.371	0.328	0.347	0.264	0.292
M08.461	Pauciarticular juvenile rheumatoid arthritis, right knee	40	Rheumatoid Arthritis and Inflammatory Connective Tissue Disease		0.421	0.367	0.371	0.328	0.347	0.264	0.292
M08.462	Pauciarticular juvenile rheumatoid arthritis, left knee	40	Rheumatoid Arthritis and Inflammatory Connective Tissue Disease		0.421	0.367	0.371	0.328	0.347	0.264	0.292
M08.469	Pauciarticular juvenile rheumatoid arthritis, unspecified knee	40	Rheumatoid Arthritis and Inflammatory Connective Tissue Disease		0.421	0.367	0.371	0.328	0.347	0.264	0.292
M08.471	Pauciarticular juvenile rheumatoid arthritis, right ankle and foot	40	Rheumatoid Arthritis and Inflammatory Connective Tissue Disease		0.421	0.367	0.371	0.328	0.347	0.264	0.292
M08.472	Pauciarticular juvenile rheumatoid arthritis, left ankle and foot	40	Rheumatoid Arthritis and Inflammatory Connective Tissue Disease		0.421	0.367	0.371	0.328	0.347	0.264	0.292
M08.479	Pauciarticular juvenile rheumatoid arthritis, unspecified ankle and foot	40	Rheumatoid Arthritis and Inflammatory Connective Tissue Disease		0.421	0.367	0.371	0.328	0.347	0.264	0.292
M08.48	Pauciarticular juvenile rheumatoid arthritis, vertebrae	40	Rheumatoid Arthritis and Inflammatory Connective Tissue Disease		0.421	0.367	0.371	0.328	0.347	0.264	0.292
M08.4A	Pauciarticular juvenile rheumatoid arthritis, other specified site	40	Rheumatoid Arthritis and Inflammatory Connective Tissue Disease		0.421	0.367	0.371	0.328	0.347	0.264	0.292
M08.80	Other juvenile arthritis, unspecified site	40	Rheumatoid Arthritis and Inflammatory Connective Tissue Disease		0.421	0.367	0.371	0.328	0.347	0.264	0.292
M08.811	Other juvenile arthritis, right shoulder	40	Rheumatoid Arthritis and Inflammatory Connective Tissue Disease		0.421	0.367	0.371	0.328	0.347	0.264	0.292

ICD-10-CM Code	ICD-10-CM Code Description	V24 CMS-HCC	V24 CMS-HCC Disease Group	V24 CMS-HCC Hierarchies	Community, NonDual, Aged	Community, NonDual, Disabled	Community, FBDual, Aged	Community, FBDual, Disabled	Community, PBDual, Aged	Community, PBDual, Disabled	Institutional
M08.812	Other juvenile arthritis, left shoulder	40	Rheumatoid Arthritis and Inflammatory Connective Tissue Disease		0.421	0.367	0.371	0.328	0.347	0.264	0.292
M08.819	Other juvenile arthritis, unspecified shoulder	40	Rheumatoid Arthritis and Inflammatory Connective Tissue Disease		0.421	0.367	0.371	0.328	0.347	0.264	0.292
M08.821	Other juvenile arthritis, right elbow	40	Rheumatoid Arthritis and Inflammatory Connective Tissue Disease		0.421	0.367	0.371	0.328	0.347	0.264	0.292
M08.822	Other juvenile arthritis, left elbow	40	Rheumatoid Arthritis and Inflammatory Connective Tissue Disease		0.421	0.367	0.371	0.328	0.347	0.264	0.292
M08.829	Other juvenile arthritis, unspecified elbow	40	Rheumatoid Arthritis and Inflammatory Connective Tissue Disease		0.421	0.367	0.371	0.328	0.347	0.264	0.292
M08.831	Other juvenile arthritis, right wrist	40	Rheumatoid Arthritis and Inflammatory Connective Tissue Disease		0.421	0.367	0.371	0.328	0.347	0.264	0.292
M08.832	Other juvenile arthritis, left wrist	40	Rheumatoid Arthritis and Inflammatory Connective Tissue Disease		0.421	0.367	0.371	0.328	0.347	0.264	0.292
M08.839	Other juvenile arthritis, unspecified wrist	40	Rheumatoid Arthritis and Inflammatory Connective Tissue Disease		0.421	0.367	0.371	0.328	0.347	0.264	0.292
M08.841	Other juvenile arthritis, right hand	40	Rheumatoid Arthritis and Inflammatory Connective Tissue Disease		0.421	0.367	0.371	0.328	0.347	0.264	0.292
M08.842	Other juvenile arthritis, left hand	40	Rheumatoid Arthritis and Inflammatory Connective Tissue Disease		0.421	0.367	0.371	0.328	0.347	0.264	0.292
M08.849	Other juvenile arthritis, unspecified hand	40	Rheumatoid Arthritis and Inflammatory Connective Tissue Disease		0.421	0.367	0.371	0.328	0.347	0.264	0.292
M08.851	Other juvenile arthritis, right hip	40	Rheumatoid Arthritis and Inflammatory Connective Tissue Disease		0.421	0.367	0.371	0.328	0.347	0.264	0.292
M08.852	Other juvenile arthritis, left hip	40	Rheumatoid Arthritis and Inflammatory Connective Tissue Disease		0.421	0.367	0.371	0.328	0.347	0.264	0.292
M08.859	Other juvenile arthritis, unspecified hip	40	Rheumatoid Arthritis and Inflammatory Connective Tissue Disease		0.421	0.367	0.371	0.328	0.347	0.264	0.292
M08.861	Other juvenile arthritis, right knee	40	Rheumatoid Arthritis and Inflammatory Connective Tissue Disease		0.421	0.367	0.371	0.328	0.347	0.264	0.292
M08.862	Other juvenile arthritis, left knee	40	Rheumatoid Arthritis and Inflammatory Connective Tissue Disease		0.421	0.367	0.371	0.328	0.347	0.264	0.292
M08.869	Other juvenile arthritis, unspecified knee	40	Rheumatoid Arthritis and Inflammatory Connective Tissue Disease		0.421	0.367	0.371	0.328	0.347	0.264	0.292
M08.871	Other juvenile arthritis, right ankle and foot	40	Rheumatoid Arthritis and Inflammatory Connective Tissue Disease		0.421	0.367	0.371	0.328	0.347	0.264	0.292
M08.872	Other juvenile arthritis, left ankle and foot	40	Rheumatoid Arthritis and Inflammatory Connective Tissue Disease		0.421	0.367	0.371	0.328	0.347	0.264	0.292
M08.879	Other juvenile arthritis, unspecified ankle and foot	40	Rheumatoid Arthritis and Inflammatory Connective Tissue Disease		0.421	0.367	0.371	0.328	0.347	0.264	0.292

ICD-10-CM Code	ICD-10-CM Code Description	V24 CMS-HCC	V24 CMS-HCC Disease Group	V24 CMS-HCC Hierarchies	Community, NonDual, Aged	Community, NonDual, Disabled	Community, FBDual, Aged	Community, FBDual, Disabled	Community, PBDual, Aged	Community, PBDual, Disabled	Institutional
MØ8.88	Other juvenile arthritis, other specified site	40	Rheumatoid Arthritis and Inflammatory Connective Tissue Disease		0.421	0.367	0.371	0.328	0.347	0.264	0.292
MØ8.89	Other juvenile arthritis, multiple sites	40	Rheumatoid Arthritis and Inflammatory Connective Tissue Disease		0.421	0.367	0.371	0.328	0.347	0.264	0.292
MØ8.90	Juvenile arthritis, unspecified, unspecified site	40	Rheumatoid Arthritis and Inflammatory Connective Tissue Disease		0.421	0.367	0.371	0.328	0.347	0.264	0.292
MØ8.911	Juvenile arthritis, unspecified, right shoulder	40	Rheumatoid Arthritis and Inflammatory Connective Tissue Disease		0.421	0.367	0.371	0.328	0.347	0.264	0.292
MØ8.912	Juvenile arthritis, unspecified, left shoulder	40	Rheumatoid Arthritis and Inflammatory Connective Tissue Disease		0.421	0.367	0.371	0.328	0.347	0.264	0.292
MØ8.919	Juvenile arthritis, unspecified, unspecified shoulder	40	Rheumatoid Arthritis and Inflammatory Connective Tissue Disease		0.421	0.367	0.371	0.328	0.347	0.264	0.292
MØ8.921	Juvenile arthritis, unspecified, right elbow	40	Rheumatoid Arthritis and Inflammatory Connective Tissue Disease		0.421	0.367	0.371	0.328	0.347	0.264	0.292
MØ8.922	Juvenile arthritis, unspecified, left elbow	40	Rheumatoid Arthritis and Inflammatory Connective Tissue Disease		0.421	0.367	0.371	0.328	0.347	0.264	0.292
MØ8.929	Juvenile arthritis, unspecified, unspecified elbow	40	Rheumatoid Arthritis and Inflammatory Connective Tissue Disease		0.421	0.367	0.371	0.328	0.347	0.264	0.292
MØ8.931	Juvenile arthritis, unspecified, right wrist	40	Rheumatoid Arthritis and Inflammatory Connective Tissue Disease		0.421	0.367	0.371	0.328	0.347	0.264	0.292
MØ8.932	Juvenile arthritis, unspecified, left wrist	40	Rheumatoid Arthritis and Inflammatory Connective Tissue Disease		0.421	0.367	0.371	0.328	0.347	0.264	0.292
MØ8.939	Juvenile arthritis, unspecified, unspecified wrist	40	Rheumatoid Arthritis and Inflammatory Connective Tissue Disease		0.421	0.367	0.371	0.328	0.347	0.264	0.292
MØ8.941	Juvenile arthritis, unspecified, right hand	40	Rheumatoid Arthritis and Inflammatory Connective Tissue Disease		0.421	0.367	0.371	0.328	0.347	0.264	0.292
MØ8.942	Juvenile arthritis, unspecified, left hand	40	Rheumatoid Arthritis and Inflammatory Connective Tissue Disease		0.421	0.367	0.371	0.328	0.347	0.264	0.292
MØ8.949	Juvenile arthritis, unspecified, unspecified hand	40	Rheumatoid Arthritis and Inflammatory Connective Tissue Disease		0.421	0.367	0.371	0.328	0.347	0.264	0.292
MØ8.951	Juvenile arthritis, unspecified, right hip	40	Rheumatoid Arthritis and Inflammatory Connective Tissue Disease		0.421	0.367	0.371	0.328	0.347	0.264	0.292
MØ8.952	Juvenile arthritis, unspecified, left hip	40	Rheumatoid Arthritis and Inflammatory Connective Tissue Disease		0.421	0.367	0.371	0.328	0.347	0.264	0.292
MØ8.959	Juvenile arthritis, unspecified, unspecified hip	40	Rheumatoid Arthritis and Inflammatory Connective Tissue Disease		0.421	0.367	0.371	0.328	0.347	0.264	0.292
MØ8.961	Juvenile arthritis, unspecified, right knee	40	Rheumatoid Arthritis and Inflammatory Connective Tissue Disease		0.421	0.367	0.371	0.328	0.347	0.264	0.292
MØ8.962	Juvenile arthritis, unspecified, left knee	40	Rheumatoid Arthritis and Inflammatory Connective Tissue Disease		0.421	0.367	0.371	0.328	0.347	0.264	0.292

ICD-10-CM Code	ICD-10-CM Code Description	V24 CMS-HCC	V24 CMS-HCC Disease Group	V24 CMS-HCC Hierarchies	Community, NonDual, Aged	Community, NonDual, Disabled	Community, FBDual, Aged	Community, FBDual, Disabled	Community, PBDual, Aged	Community, PBDual, Disabled	Institutional
M08.969	Juvenile arthritis, unspecified, unspecified knee	40	Rheumatoid Arthritis and Inflammatory Connective Tissue Disease		0.421	0.367	0.371	0.328	0.347	0.264	0.292
M08.971	Juvenile arthritis, unspecified, right ankle and foot	40	Rheumatoid Arthritis and Inflammatory Connective Tissue Disease		0.421	0.367	0.371	0.328	0.347	0.264	0.292
M08.972	Juvenile arthritis, unspecified, left ankle and foot	40	Rheumatoid Arthritis and Inflammatory Connective Tissue Disease		0.421	0.367	0.371	0.328	0.347	0.264	0.292
M08.979	Juvenile arthritis, unspecified, unspecified ankle and foot	40	Rheumatoid Arthritis and Inflammatory Connective Tissue Disease		0.421	0.367	0.371	0.328	0.347	0.264	0.292
M08.98	Juvenile arthritis, unspecified, vertebrae	40	Rheumatoid Arthritis and Inflammatory Connective Tissue Disease		0.421	0.367	0.371	0.328	0.347	0.264	0.292
M08.99	Juvenile arthritis, unspecified, multiple sites	40	Rheumatoid Arthritis and Inflammatory Connective Tissue Disease		0.421	0.367	0.371	0.328	0.347	0.264	0.292
M08.9A	Juvenile arthritis, unspecified, other specified site	40	Rheumatoid Arthritis and Inflammatory Connective Tissue Disease		0.421	0.367	0.371	0.328	0.347	0.264	0.292
M12.00	Chronic postrheumatic arthropathy [Jaccoud], unspecified site	40	Rheumatoid Arthritis and Inflammatory Connective Tissue Disease		0.421	0.367	0.371	0.328	0.347	0.264	0.292
M12.011	Chronic postrheumatic arthropathy [Jaccoud], right shoulder	40	Rheumatoid Arthritis and Inflammatory Connective Tissue Disease		0.421	0.367	0.371	0.328	0.347	0.264	0.292
M12.012	Chronic postrheumatic arthropathy [Jaccoud], left shoulder	40	Rheumatoid Arthritis and Inflammatory Connective Tissue Disease		0.421	0.367	0.371	0.328	0.347	0.264	0.292
M12.019	Chronic postrheumatic arthropathy [Jaccoud], unspecified shoulder	40	Rheumatoid Arthritis and Inflammatory Connective Tissue Disease		0.421	0.367	0.371	0.328	0.347	0.264	0.292
M12.021	Chronic postrheumatic arthropathy [Jaccoud], right elbow	40	Rheumatoid Arthritis and Inflammatory Connective Tissue Disease		0.421	0.367	0.371	0.328	0.347	0.264	0.292
M12.022	Chronic postrheumatic arthropathy [Jaccoud], left elbow	40	Rheumatoid Arthritis and Inflammatory Connective Tissue Disease		0.421	0.367	0.371	0.328	0.347	0.264	0.292
M12.029	Chronic postrheumatic arthropathy [Jaccoud], unspecified elbow	40	Rheumatoid Arthritis and Inflammatory Connective Tissue Disease		0.421	0.367	0.371	0.328	0.347	0.264	0.292
M12.031	Chronic postrheumatic arthropathy [Jaccoud], right wrist	40	Rheumatoid Arthritis and Inflammatory Connective Tissue Disease		0.421	0.367	0.371	0.328	0.347	0.264	0.292
M12.032	Chronic postrheumatic arthropathy [Jaccoud], left wrist	40	Rheumatoid Arthritis and Inflammatory Connective Tissue Disease		0.421	0.367	0.371	0.328	0.347	0.264	0.292
M12.039	Chronic postrheumatic arthropathy [Jaccoud], unspecified wrist	40	Rheumatoid Arthritis and Inflammatory Connective Tissue Disease		0.421	0.367	0.371	0.328	0.347	0.264	0.292
M12.041	Chronic postrheumatic arthropathy [Jaccoud], right hand	40	Rheumatoid Arthritis and Inflammatory Connective Tissue Disease		0.421	0.367	0.371	0.328	0.347	0.264	0.292
M12.042	Chronic postrheumatic arthropathy [Jaccoud], left hand	40	Rheumatoid Arthritis and Inflammatory Connective Tissue Disease		0.421	0.367	0.371	0.328	0.347	0.264	0.292
M12.049	Chronic postrheumatic arthropathy [Jaccoud], unspecified hand	40	Rheumatoid Arthritis and Inflammatory Connective Tissue Disease		0.421	0.367	0.371	0.328	0.347	0.264	0.292

ICD-10-CM Code	ICD-10-CM Code Description	V24 CMS-HCC	V24 CMS-HCC Disease Group	V24 CMS-HCC Hierarchies	Community, NonDual, Aged	Community, NonDual, Disabled	Community, FBDual, Aged	Community, FBDual, Disabled	Community, PBDual, Aged	Community, PBDual, Disabled	Institutional
M12.051	Chronic postrheumatic arthropathy [Jaccoud], right hip	40	Rheumatoid Arthritis and Inflammatory Connective Tissue Disease		0.421	0.367	0.371	0.328	0.347	0.264	0.292
M12.052	Chronic postrheumatic arthropathy [Jaccoud], left hip	40	Rheumatoid Arthritis and Inflammatory Connective Tissue Disease		0.421	0.367	0.371	0.328	0.347	0.264	0.292
M12.059	Chronic postrheumatic arthropathy [Jaccoud], unspecified hip	40	Rheumatoid Arthritis and Inflammatory Connective Tissue Disease		0.421	0.367	0.371	0.328	0.347	0.264	0.292
M12.061	Chronic postrheumatic arthropathy [Jaccoud], right knee	40	Rheumatoid Arthritis and Inflammatory Connective Tissue Disease		0.421	0.367	0.371	0.328	0.347	0.264	0.292
M12.062	Chronic postrheumatic arthropathy [Jaccoud], left knee	40	Rheumatoid Arthritis and Inflammatory Connective Tissue Disease		0.421	0.367	0.371	0.328	0.347	0.264	0.292
M12.069	Chronic postrheumatic arthropathy [Jaccoud], unspecified knee	40	Rheumatoid Arthritis and Inflammatory Connective Tissue Disease		0.421	0.367	0.371	0.328	0.347	0.264	0.292
M12.071	Chronic postrheumatic arthropathy [Jaccoud], right ankle and foot	40	Rheumatoid Arthritis and Inflammatory Connective Tissue Disease		0.421	0.367	0.371	0.328	0.347	0.264	0.292
M12.072	Chronic postrheumatic arthropathy [Jaccoud], left ankle and foot	40	Rheumatoid Arthritis and Inflammatory Connective Tissue Disease		0.421	0.367	0.371	0.328	0.347	0.264	0.292
M12.079	Chronic postrheumatic arthropathy [Jaccoud], unspecified ankle and foot	40	Rheumatoid Arthritis and Inflammatory Connective Tissue Disease		0.421	0.367	0.371	0.328	0.347	0.264	0.292
M12.08	Chronic postrheumatic arthropathy [Jaccoud], other specified site	40	Rheumatoid Arthritis and Inflammatory Connective Tissue Disease		0.421	0.367	0.371	0.328	0.347	0.264	0.292
M12.09	Chronic postrheumatic arthropathy [Jaccoud], multiple sites	40	Rheumatoid Arthritis and Inflammatory Connective Tissue Disease		0.421	0.367	0.371	0.328	0.347	0.264	0.292
M30.0	Polyarteritis nodosa	40	Rheumatoid Arthritis and Inflammatory Connective Tissue Disease		0.421	0.367	0.371	0.328	0.347	0.264	0.292
M30.1	Polyarteritis with lung involvement [Churg-Strauss]	40	Rheumatoid Arthritis and Inflammatory Connective Tissue Disease		0.421	0.367	0.371	0.328	0.347	0.264	0.292
M30.2	Juvenile polyarteritis	40	Rheumatoid Arthritis and Inflammatory Connective Tissue Disease		0.421	0.367	0.371	0.328	0.347	0.264	0.292
M30.3	Mucocutaneous lymph node syndrome [Kawasaki]	40	Rheumatoid Arthritis and Inflammatory Connective Tissue Disease		0.421	0.367	0.371	0.328	0.347	0.264	0.292
M30.8	Other conditions related to polyarteritis nodosa	40	Rheumatoid Arthritis and Inflammatory Connective Tissue Disease		0.421	0.367	0.371	0.328	0.347	0.264	0.292
M31.0	Hypersensitivity angiitis	40	Rheumatoid Arthritis and Inflammatory Connective Tissue Disease		0.421	0.367	0.371	0.328	0.347	0.264	0.292
M31.1	Thrombotic microangiopathy	40	Rheumatoid Arthritis and Inflammatory Connective Tissue Disease		0.421	0.367	0.371	0.328	0.347	0.264	0.292
M31.10	Thrombotic microangiopathy, unspecified	40	Rheumatoid Arthritis and Inflammatory Connective Tissue Disease		0.421	0.367	0.371	0.328	0.347	0.264	0.292
M31.11	Hematopoietic stem cell transplantation-associated thrombotic microangiopathy [HSCT-TMA]	186	Major Organ Transplant or Replacement Status		0.832	0.445	0.728	0.865	0.438	0.613	1.046

ICD-10-CM Code	ICD-10-CM Code Description	V24 CMS-HCC	V24 CMS-HCC Disease Group	V24 CMS-HCC Hierarchies	Community, NonDual, Aged	Community, NonDual, Disabled	Community, FBDual, Aged	Community, FBDual, Disabled	Community, PBDual, Aged	Community, PBDual, Disabled	Institutional
M31.19	Other thrombotic microangiopathy	40	Rheumatoid Arthritis and Inflammatory Connective Tissue Disease		0.421	0.367	0.371	0.328	0.347	0.264	0.292
M31.2	Lethal midline granuloma	40	Rheumatoid Arthritis and Inflammatory Connective Tissue Disease		0.421	0.367	0.371	0.328	0.347	0.264	0.292
M31.30	Wegener's granulomatosis without renal involvement	40	Rheumatoid Arthritis and Inflammatory Connective Tissue Disease		0.421	0.367	0.371	0.328	0.347	0.264	0.292
M31.31	Wegener's granulomatosis with renal involvement	40	Rheumatoid Arthritis and Inflammatory Connective Tissue Disease		0.421	0.367	0.371	0.328	0.347	0.264	0.292
M31.4	Aortic arch syndrome [Takayasu]	40	Rheumatoid Arthritis and Inflammatory Connective Tissue Disease		0.421	0.367	0.371	0.328	0.347	0.264	0.292
M31.5	Giant cell arteritis with polymyalgia rheumatica	40	Rheumatoid Arthritis and Inflammatory Connective Tissue Disease		0.421	0.367	0.371	0.328	0.347	0.264	0.292
M31.6	Other giant cell arteritis	40	Rheumatoid Arthritis and Inflammatory Connective Tissue Disease		0.421	0.367	0.371	0.328	0.347	0.264	0.292
M31.7	Microscopic polyangiitis	40	Rheumatoid Arthritis and Inflammatory Connective Tissue Disease		0.421	0.367	0.371	0.328	0.347	0.264	0.292
M31.8	Other specified necrotizing vasculopathies	108	Vascular Disease		0.288	0.301	0.294	0.267	0.297	0.314	0.093
M31.9	Necrotizing vasculopathy, unspecified	108	Vascular Disease		0.288	0.301	0.294	0.267	0.297	0.314	0.093
M32.0	Drug-induced systemic lupus erythematosus	40	Rheumatoid Arthritis and Inflammatory Connective Tissue Disease		0.421	0.367	0.371	0.328	0.347	0.264	0.292
M32.10	Systemic lupus erythematosus, organ or system involvement unspecified	40	Rheumatoid Arthritis and Inflammatory Connective Tissue Disease		0.421	0.367	0.371	0.328	0.347	0.264	0.292
M32.11	Endocarditis in systemic lupus erythematosus	40	Rheumatoid Arthritis and Inflammatory Connective Tissue Disease		0.421	0.367	0.371	0.328	0.347	0.264	0.292
M32.12	Pericarditis in systemic lupus erythematosus	40	Rheumatoid Arthritis and Inflammatory Connective Tissue Disease		0.421	0.367	0.371	0.328	0.347	0.264	0.292
M32.13	Lung involvement in systemic lupus erythematosus	40	Rheumatoid Arthritis and Inflammatory Connective Tissue Disease		0.421	0.367	0.371	0.328	0.347	0.264	0.292
M32.13	Lung involvement in systemic lupus erythematosus	112	Fibrosis of Lung and Other Chronic Lung Disorders		0.219	0.237	0.161	0.275	0.200	0.229	0.110
M32.14	Glomerular disease in systemic lupus erythematosus	40	Rheumatoid Arthritis and Inflammatory Connective Tissue Disease		0.421	0.367	0.371	0.328	0.347	0.264	0.292
M32.15	Tubulo-interstitial nephropathy in systemic lupus erythematosus	40	Rheumatoid Arthritis and Inflammatory Connective Tissue Disease		0.421	0.367	0.371	0.328	0.347	0.264	0.292
M32.19	Other organ or system involvement in systemic lupus erythematosus	40	Rheumatoid Arthritis and Inflammatory Connective Tissue Disease		0.421	0.367	0.371	0.328	0.347	0.264	0.292
M32.8	Other forms of systemic lupus erythematosus	40	Rheumatoid Arthritis and Inflammatory Connective Tissue Disease		0.421	0.367	0.371	0.328	0.347	0.264	0.292
M32.9	Systemic lupus erythematosus, unspecified	40	Rheumatoid Arthritis and Inflammatory Connective Tissue Disease		0.421	0.367	0.371	0.328	0.347	0.264	0.292

2021 Optum360, LLC

ICD-10-CM Code	ICD-10-CM Code Description	V24 CMS-HCC	V24 CMS-HCC Disease Group	V24 CMS-HCC Hierarchies	Community, NonDual, Aged	Community, NonDual, Disabled	Community, FBDual, Aged	Community, FBDual, Disabled	Community, PBDual, Aged	Community, PBDual, Disabled	Institutional
M33.00	Juvenile dermatomyositis, organ involvement unspecified	40	Rheumatoid Arthritis and Inflammatory Connective Tissue Disease		0.421	0.367	0.371	0.328	0.347	0.264	0.292
M33.01	Juvenile dermatomyositis with respiratory involvement	40	Rheumatoid Arthritis and Inflammatory Connective Tissue Disease		0.421	0.367	0.371	0.328	0.347	0.264	0.292
M33.01	Juvenile dermatomyositis with respiratory involvement	112	Fibrosis of Lung and Other Chronic Lung Disorders		0.219	0.237	0.161	0.275	0.200	0.229	0.110
M33.02	Juvenile dermatomyositis with myopathy	40	Rheumatoid Arthritis and Inflammatory Connective Tissue Disease		0.421	0.367	0.371	0.328	0.347	0.264	0.292
M33.03	Juvenile dermatomyositis without myopathy	40	Rheumatoid Arthritis and Inflammatory Connective Tissue Disease		0.421	0.367	0.371	0.328	0.347	0.264	0.292
M33.09	Juvenile dermatomyositis with other organ involvement	40	Rheumatoid Arthritis and Inflammatory Connective Tissue Disease		0.421	0.367	0.371	0.328	0.347	0.264	0.292
M33.10	Other dermatomyositis, organ involvement unspecified	40	Rheumatoid Arthritis and Inflammatory Connective Tissue Disease		0.421	0.367	0.371	0.328	0.347	0.264	0.292
M33.11	Other dermatomyositis with respiratory involvement	40	Rheumatoid Arthritis and Inflammatory Connective Tissue Disease		0.421	0.367	0.371	0.328	0.347	0.264	0.292
M33.11	Other dermatomyositis with respiratory involvement	112	Fibrosis of Lung and Other Chronic Lung Disorders		0.219	0.237	0.161	0.275	0.200	0.229	0.110
M33.12	Other dermatomyositis with myopathy	40	Rheumatoid Arthritis and Inflammatory Connective Tissue Disease		0.421	0.367	0.371	0.328	0.347	0.264	0.292
M33.13	Other dermatomyositis without myopathy	40	Rheumatoid Arthritis and Inflammatory Connective Tissue Disease		0.421	0.367	0.371	0.328	0.347	0.264	0.292
M33.19	Other dermatomyositis with other organ involvement	40	Rheumatoid Arthritis and Inflammatory Connective Tissue Disease		0.421	0.367	0.371	0.328	0.347	0.264	0.292
M33.20	Polymyositis, organ involvement unspecified	40	Rheumatoid Arthritis and Inflammatory Connective Tissue Disease		0.421	0.367	0.371	0.328	0.347	0.264	0.292
M33.21	Polymyositis with respiratory involvement	40	Rheumatoid Arthritis and Inflammatory Connective Tissue Disease		0.421	0.367	0.371	0.328	0.347	0.264	0.292
M33.21	Polymyositis with respiratory involvement	112	Fibrosis of Lung and Other Chronic Lung Disorders		0.219	0.237	0.161	0.275	0.200	0.229	0.110
M33.22	Polymyositis with myopathy	40	Rheumatoid Arthritis and Inflammatory Connective Tissue Disease		0.421	0.367	0.371	0.328	0.347	0.264	0.292
M33.29	Polymyositis with other organ involvement	40	Rheumatoid Arthritis and Inflammatory Connective Tissue Disease		0.421	0.367	0.371	0.328	0.347	0.264	0.292
M33.90	Dermatopolymyositis, unspecified, organ involvement unspecified	40	Rheumatoid Arthritis and Inflammatory Connective Tissue Disease		0.421	0.367	0.371	0.328	0.347	0.264	0.292
M33.91	Dermatopolymyositis, unspecified with respiratory involvement	40	Rheumatoid Arthritis and Inflammatory Connective Tissue Disease		0.421	0.367	0.371	0.328	0.347	0.264	0.292
M33.91	Dermatopolymyositis, unspecified with respiratory involvement	112	Fibrosis of Lung and Other Chronic Lung Disorders		0.219	0.237	0.161	0.275	0.200	0.229	0.110
M33.92	Dermatopolymyositis, unspecified with myopathy	40	Rheumatoid Arthritis and Inflammatory Connective Tissue Disease		0.421	0.367	0.371	0.328	0.347	0.264	0.292

ICD-10-CM Code	ICD-10-CM Code Description	V24 CMS-HCC	V24 CMS-HCC Disease Group	V24 CMS-HCC Hierarchies	Community, NonDual, Aged	Community, NonDual, Disabled	Community, FBDual, Aged	Community, FBDual, Disabled	Community, PBDual, Aged	Community, PBDual, Disabled	Institutional
M33.93	Dermatopolymyositis, unspecified without myopathy	40	Rheumatoid Arthritis and Inflammatory Connective Tissue Disease		0.421	0.367	0.371	0.328	0.347	0.264	0.292
M33.99	Dermatopolymyositis, unspecified with other organ involvement	40	Rheumatoid Arthritis and Inflammatory Connective Tissue Disease		0.421	0.367	0.371	0.328	0.347	0.264	0.292
M34.0	Progressive systemic sclerosis	40	Rheumatoid Arthritis and Inflammatory Connective Tissue Disease		0.421	0.367	0.371	0.328	0.347	0.264	0.292
M34.1	CR(E)ST syndrome	40	Rheumatoid Arthritis and Inflammatory Connective Tissue Disease		0.421	0.367	0.371	0.328	0.347	0.264	0.292
M34.2	Systemic sclerosis induced by drug and chemical	40	Rheumatoid Arthritis and Inflammatory Connective Tissue Disease		0.421	0.367	0.371	0.328	0.347	0.264	0.292
M34.81	Systemic sclerosis with lung involvement	40	Rheumatoid Arthritis and Inflammatory Connective Tissue Disease		0.421	0.367	0.371	0.328	0.347	0.264	0.292
M34.81	Systemic sclerosis with lung involvement	112	Fibrosis of Lung and Other Chronic Lung Disorders		0.219	0.237	0.161	0.275	0.200	0.229	0.110
M34.82	Systemic sclerosis with myopathy	40	Rheumatoid Arthritis and Inflammatory Connective Tissue Disease		0.421	0.367	0.371	0.328	0.347	0.264	0.292
M34.83	Systemic sclerosis with polyneuropathy	40	Rheumatoid Arthritis and Inflammatory Connective Tissue Disease		0.421	0.367	0.371	0.328	0.347	0.264	0.292
M34.83	Systemic sclerosis with polyneuropathy	75	Myasthenia Gravis/Myoneural Disorders and Guillain-Barre Syndrome/Inflammatory and Toxic Neuropathy		0.472	0.481	0.407	0.404	0.287	0.314	0.332
M34.89	Other systemic sclerosis	40	Rheumatoid Arthritis and Inflammatory Connective Tissue Disease		0.421	0.367	0.371	0.328	0.347	0.264	0.292
M34.9	Systemic sclerosis, unspecified	40	Rheumatoid Arthritis and Inflammatory Connective Tissue Disease		0.421	0.367	0.371	0.328	0.347	0.264	0.292
M35.00	Sjogren syndrome, unspecified	40	Rheumatoid Arthritis and Inflammatory Connective Tissue Disease		0.421	0.367	0.371	0.328	0.347	0.264	0.292
M35.01	Sjogren syndrome with keratoconjunctivitis	40	Rheumatoid Arthritis and Inflammatory Connective Tissue Disease		0.421	0.367	0.371	0.328	0.347	0.264	0.292
M35.02	Sjogren syndrome with lung involvement	40	Rheumatoid Arthritis and Inflammatory Connective Tissue Disease		0.421	0.367	0.371	0.328	0.347	0.264	0.292
M35.02	Sjogren syndrome with lung involvement	112	Fibrosis of Lung and Other Chronic Lung Disorders		0.219	0.237	0.161	0.275	0.200	0.229	0.110
M35.03	Sjogren syndrome with myopathy	40	Rheumatoid Arthritis and Inflammatory Connective Tissue Disease		0.421	0.367	0.371	0.328	0.347	0.264	0.292
M35.04	Sjogren syndrome with tubulo-interstitial nephropathy	40	Rheumatoid Arthritis and Inflammatory Connective Tissue Disease		0.421	0.367	0.371	0.328	0.347	0.264	0.292
M35.05	Sjogren syndrome with inflammatory arthritis	40	Rheumatoid Arthritis and Inflammatory Connective Tissue Disease		0.421	0.367	0.371	0.328	0.347	0.264	0.292
M35.06	Sjogren syndrome with peripheral nervous system involvement	40	Rheumatoid Arthritis and Inflammatory Connective Tissue Disease		0.421	0.367	0.371	0.328	0.347	0.264	0.292

ICD-10-CM Code	ICD-10-CM Code Description	V24 CMS-HCC	V24 CMS-HCC Disease Group	V24 CMS-HCC Hierarchies	Community, NonDual, Aged	Community, NonDual, Disabled	Community, FBDual, Aged	Community, FBDual, Disabled	Community, PBDual, Aged	Community, PBDual, Disabled	Institutional
M35.07	Sjogren syndrome with central nervous system involvement	40	Rheumatoid Arthritis and Inflammatory Connective Tissue Disease		0.421	0.367	0.371	0.328	0.347	0.264	0.292
M35.08	Sjogren syndrome with gastrointestinal involvement	40	Rheumatoid Arthritis and Inflammatory Connective Tissue Disease		0.421	0.367	0.371	0.328	0.347	0.264	0.292
M35.09	Sjogren syndrome with other organ involvement	40	Rheumatoid Arthritis and Inflammatory Connective Tissue Disease		0.421	0.367	0.371	0.328	0.347	0.264	0.292
M35.0A	Sjogren syndrome with glomerular disease	40	Rheumatoid Arthritis and Inflammatory Connective Tissue Disease		0.421	0.367	0.371	0.328	0.347	0.264	0.292
M35.0B	Sjogren syndrome with vasculitis	40	Rheumatoid Arthritis and Inflammatory Connective Tissue Disease		0.421	0.367	0.371	0.328	0.347	0.264	0.292
M35.0C	Sjogren syndrome with dental involvement	40	Rheumatoid Arthritis and Inflammatory Connective Tissue Disease		0.421	0.367	0.371	0.328	0.347	0.264	0.292
M35.1	Other overlap syndromes	40	Rheumatoid Arthritis and Inflammatory Connective Tissue Disease		0.421	0.367	0.371	0.328	0.347	0.264	0.292
M35.2	Behcet's disease	40	Rheumatoid Arthritis and Inflammatory Connective Tissue Disease		0.421	0.367	0.371	0.328	0.347	0.264	0.292
M35.3	Polymyalgia rheumatica	40	Rheumatoid Arthritis and Inflammatory Connective Tissue Disease		0.421	0.367	0.371	0.328	0.347	0.264	0.292
M35.5	Multifocal fibrosclerosis	40	Rheumatoid Arthritis and Inflammatory Connective Tissue Disease		0.421	0.367	0.371	0.328	0.347	0.264	0.292
M35.81	Multisystem inflammatory syndrome	2	Septicemia, Sepsis, Systemic Inflammatory Response Syndrome/ Shock		0.352	0.414	0.453	0.530	0.316	0.297	0.324
M35.89	Other specified systemic involvement of connective tissue	40	Rheumatoid Arthritis and Inflammatory Connective Tissue Disease		0.421	0.367	0.371	0.328	0.347	0.264	0.292
M35.9	Systemic involvement of connective tissue, unspecified	40	Rheumatoid Arthritis and Inflammatory Connective Tissue Disease		0.421	0.367	0.371	0.328	0.347	0.264	0.292
M36.0	Dermato(poly)myositis in neoplastic disease	40	Rheumatoid Arthritis and Inflammatory Connective Tissue Disease		0.421	0.367	0.371	0.328	0.347	0.264	0.292
M36.8	Systemic disorders of connective tissue in other diseases classified elsewhere	40	Rheumatoid Arthritis and Inflammatory Connective Tissue Disease		0.421	0.367	0.371	0.328	0.347	0.264	0.292
M45.0	Ankylosing spondylitis of multiple sites in spine	40	Rheumatoid Arthritis and Inflammatory Connective Tissue Disease		0.421	0.367	0.371	0.328	0.347	0.264	0.292
M45.1	Ankylosing spondylitis of occipito-atlanto-axial region	40	Rheumatoid Arthritis and Inflammatory Connective Tissue Disease		0.421	0.367	0.371	0.328	0.347	0.264	0.292
M45.2	Ankylosing spondylitis of cervical region	40	Rheumatoid Arthritis and Inflammatory Connective Tissue Disease		0.421	0.367	0.371	0.328	0.347	0.264	0.292
M45.3	Ankylosing spondylitis of cervicothoracic region	40	Rheumatoid Arthritis and Inflammatory Connective Tissue Disease		0.421	0.367	0.371	0.328	0.347	0.264	0.292
M45.4	Ankylosing spondylitis of thoracic region	40	Rheumatoid Arthritis and Inflammatory Connective Tissue Disease		0.421	0.367	0.371	0.328	0.347	0.264	0.292

ICD-10-CM Code	ICD-10-CM Code Description	V24 CMS-HCC	V24 CMS-HCC Disease Group	V24 CMS-HCC Hierarchies	Community, NonDual, Aged	Community, NonDual, Disabled	Community, FBDual, Aged	Community, FBDual, Disabled	Community, PBDual, Aged	Community, PBDual, Disabled	Institutional
M45.5	Ankylosing spondylitis of thoracolumbar region	40	Rheumatoid Arthritis and Inflammatory Connective Tissue Disease		0.421	0.367	0.371	0.328	0.347	0.264	0.292
M45.6	Ankylosing spondylitis lumbar region	40	Rheumatoid Arthritis and Inflammatory Connective Tissue Disease		0.421	0.367	0.371	0.328	0.347	0.264	0.292
M45.7	Ankylosing spondylitis of lumbosacral region	40	Rheumatoid Arthritis and Inflammatory Connective Tissue Disease		0.421	0.367	0.371	0.328	0.347	0.264	0.292
M45.8	Ankylosing spondylitis sacral and sacrococcygeal region	40	Rheumatoid Arthritis and Inflammatory Connective Tissue Disease		0.421	0.367	0.371	0.328	0.347	0.264	0.292
M45.9	Ankylosing spondylitis of unspecified sites in spine	40	Rheumatoid Arthritis and Inflammatory Connective Tissue Disease		0.421	0.367	0.371	0.328	0.347	0.264	0.292
M45.A0	Non-radiographic axial spondyloarthritis of unspecified sites in spine	40	Rheumatoid Arthritis and Inflammatory Connective Tissue Disease		0.421	0.367	0.371	0.328	0.347	0.264	0.292
M45.A1	Non-radiographic axial spondyloarthritis of occipito-atlanto-axial region	40	Rheumatoid Arthritis and Inflammatory Connective Tissue Disease		0.421	0.367	0.371	0.328	0.347	0.264	0.292
M45.A2	Non-radiographic axial spondyloarthritis of cervical region	40	Rheumatoid Arthritis and Inflammatory Connective Tissue Disease		0.421	0.367	0.371	0.328	0.347	0.264	0.292
M45.A3	Non-radiographic axial spondyloarthritis of cervicothoracic region	40	Rheumatoid Arthritis and Inflammatory Connective Tissue Disease		0.421	0.367	0.371	0.328	0.347	0.264	0.292
M45.A4	Non-radiographic axial spondyloarthritis of thoracic region	40	Rheumatoid Arthritis and Inflammatory Connective Tissue Disease		0.421	0.367	0.371	0.328	0.347	0.264	0.292
M45.A5	Non-radiographic axial spondyloarthritis of thoracolumbar region	40	Rheumatoid Arthritis and Inflammatory Connective Tissue Disease		0.421	0.367	0.371	0.328	0.347	0.264	0.292
M45.A6	Non-radiographic axial spondyloarthritis of lumbar region	40	Rheumatoid Arthritis and Inflammatory Connective Tissue Disease		0.421	0.367	0.371	0.328	0.347	0.264	0.292
M45.A7	Non-radiographic axial spondyloarthritis of lumbosacral region	40	Rheumatoid Arthritis and Inflammatory Connective Tissue Disease		0.421	0.367	0.371	0.328	0.347	0.264	0.292
M45.A8	Non-radiographic axial spondyloarthritis of sacral and sacrococcygeal region	40	Rheumatoid Arthritis and Inflammatory Connective Tissue Disease		0.421	0.367	0.371	0.328	0.347	0.264	0.292
M45.AB	Non-radiographic axial spondyloarthritis of multiple sites in spine	40	Rheumatoid Arthritis and Inflammatory Connective Tissue Disease		0.421	0.367	0.371	0.328	0.347	0.264	0.292
M46.00	Spinal enthesopathy, site unspecified	40	Rheumatoid Arthritis and Inflammatory Connective Tissue Disease		0.421	0.367	0.371	0.328	0.347	0.264	0.292
M46.01	Spinal enthesopathy, occipito-atlanto-axial region	40	Rheumatoid Arthritis and Inflammatory Connective Tissue Disease		0.421	0.367	0.371	0.328	0.347	0.264	0.292
M46.02	Spinal enthesopathy, cervical region	40	Rheumatoid Arthritis and Inflammatory Connective Tissue Disease		0.421	0.367	0.371	0.328	0.347	0.264	0.292
M46.03	Spinal enthesopathy, cervicothoracic region	40	Rheumatoid Arthritis and Inflammatory Connective Tissue Disease		0.421	0.367	0.371	0.328	0.347	0.264	0.292
M46.04	Spinal enthesopathy, thoracic region	40	Rheumatoid Arthritis and Inflammatory Connective Tissue Disease		0.421	0.367	0.371	0.328	0.347	0.264	0.292

ICD-10-CM Code	ICD-10-CM Code Description	V24 CMS-HCC	V24 CMS-HCC Disease Group	V24 CMS-HCC Hierarchies	Community, NonDual, Aged	Community, NonDual, Disabled	Community, FBDual, Aged	Community, FBDual, Disabled	Community, PBDual, Aged	Community, PBDual, Disabled	Institutional
M46.05	Spinal enthesopathy, thoracolumbar region	40	Rheumatoid Arthritis and Inflammatory Connective Tissue Disease		0.421	0.367	0.371	0.328	0.347	0.264	0.292
M46.06	Spinal enthesopathy, lumbar region	40	Rheumatoid Arthritis and Inflammatory Connective Tissue Disease		0.421	0.367	0.371	0.328	0.347	0.264	0.292
M46.07	Spinal enthesopathy, lumbosacral region	40	Rheumatoid Arthritis and Inflammatory Connective Tissue Disease		0.421	0.367	0.371	0.328	0.347	0.264	0.292
M46.08	Spinal enthesopathy, sacral and sacrococcygeal region	40	Rheumatoid Arthritis and Inflammatory Connective Tissue Disease		0.421	0.367	0.371	0.328	0.347	0.264	0.292
M46.09	Spinal enthesopathy, multiple sites in spine	40	Rheumatoid Arthritis and Inflammatory Connective Tissue Disease		0.421	0.367	0.371	0.328	0.347	0.264	0.292
M46.1	Sacroiliitis, not elsewhere classified	40	Rheumatoid Arthritis and Inflammatory Connective Tissue Disease		0.421	0.367	0.371	0.328	0.347	0.264	0.292
M46.20	Osteomyelitis of vertebra, site unspecified	39	Bone/Joint/Muscle Infections/Necrosis		0.401	0.378	0.558	0.682	0.443	0.435	0.401
M46.21	Osteomyelitis of vertebra, occipito-atlanto-axial region	39	Bone/Joint/Muscle Infections/Necrosis		0.401	0.378	0.558	0.682	0.443	0.435	0.401
M46.22	Osteomyelitis of vertebra, cervical region	39	Bone/Joint/Muscle Infections/Necrosis		0.401	0.378	0.558	0.682	0.443	0.435	0.401
M46.23	Osteomyelitis of vertebra, cervicothoracic region	39	Bone/Joint/Muscle Infections/Necrosis		0.401	0.378	0.558	0.682	0.443	0.435	0.401
M46.24	Osteomyelitis of vertebra, thoracic region	39	Bone/Joint/Muscle Infections/Necrosis		0.401	0.378	0.558	0.682	0.443	0.435	0.401
M46.25	Osteomyelitis of vertebra, thoracolumbar region	39	Bone/Joint/Muscle Infections/Necrosis		0.401	0.378	0.558	0.682	0.443	0.435	0.401
M46.26	Osteomyelitis of vertebra, lumbar region	39	Bone/Joint/Muscle Infections/Necrosis		0.401	0.378	0.558	0.682	0.443	0.435	0.401
M46.27	Osteomyelitis of vertebra, lumbosacral region	39	Bone/Joint/Muscle Infections/Necrosis		0.401	0.378	0.558	0.682	0.443	0.435	0.401
M46.28	Osteomyelitis of vertebra, sacral and sacrococcygeal region	39	Bone/Joint/Muscle Infections/Necrosis		0.401	0.378	0.558	0.682	0.443	0.435	0.401
M46.30	Infection of intervertebral disc (pyogenic), site unspecified	39	Bone/Joint/Muscle Infections/Necrosis		0.401	0.378	0.558	0.682	0.443	0.435	0.401
M46.31	Infection of intervertebral disc (pyogenic), occipito-atlanto-axial region	39	Bone/Joint/Muscle Infections/Necrosis		0.401	0.378	0.558	0.682	0.443	0.435	0.401
M46.32	Infection of intervertebral disc (pyogenic), cervical region	39	Bone/Joint/Muscle Infections/Necrosis		0.401	0.378	0.558	0.682	0.443	0.435	0.401
M46.33	Infection of intervertebral disc (pyogenic), cervicothoracic region	39	Bone/Joint/Muscle Infections/Necrosis		0.401	0.378	0.558	0.682	0.443	0.435	0.401
M46.34	Infection of intervertebral disc (pyogenic), thoracic region	39	Bone/Joint/Muscle Infections/Necrosis		0.401	0.378	0.558	0.682	0.443	0.435	0.401
M46.35	Infection of intervertebral disc (pyogenic), thoracolumbar region	39	Bone/Joint/Muscle Infections/Necrosis		0.401	0.378	0.558	0.682	0.443	0.435	0.401
M46.36	Infection of intervertebral disc (pyogenic), lumbar region	39	Bone/Joint/Muscle Infections/Necrosis		0.401	0.378	0.558	0.682	0.443	0.435	0.401
M46.37	Infection of intervertebral disc (pyogenic), lumbosacral region	39	Bone/Joint/Muscle Infections/Necrosis		0.401	0.378	0.558	0.682	0.443	0.435	0.401
M46.38	Infection of intervertebral disc (pyogenic), sacral and sacrococcygeal region	39	Bone/Joint/Muscle Infections/Necrosis		0.401	0.378	0.558	0.682	0.443	0.435	0.401
M46.39	Infection of intervertebral disc (pyogenic), multiple sites in spine	39	Bone/Joint/Muscle Infections/Necrosis		0.401	0.378	0.558	0.682	0.443	0.435	0.401

ICD-10-CM Code	ICD-10-CM Code Description	V24 CMS-HCC	V24 CMS-HCC Disease Group	V24 CMS-HCC Hierarchies	Community, NonDual, Aged	Community, NonDual, Disabled	Community, FBDual, Aged	Community, FBDual, Disabled	Community, PBDual, Aged	Community, PBDual, Disabled	Institutional
M46.50	Other infective spondylopathies, site unspecified	40	Rheumatoid Arthritis and Inflammatory Connective Tissue Disease		0.421	0.367	0.371	0.328	0.347	0.264	0.292
M46.51	Other infective spondylopathies, occipito-atlanto-axial region	40	Rheumatoid Arthritis and Inflammatory Connective Tissue Disease		0.421	0.367	0.371	0.328	0.347	0.264	0.292
M46.52	Other infective spondylopathies, cervical region	40	Rheumatoid Arthritis and Inflammatory Connective Tissue Disease		0.421	0.367	0.371	0.328	0.347	0.264	0.292
M46.53	Other infective spondylopathies, cervicothoracic region	40	Rheumatoid Arthritis and Inflammatory Connective Tissue Disease		0.421	0.367	0.371	0.328	0.347	0.264	0.292
M46.54	Other infective spondylopathies, thoracic region	40	Rheumatoid Arthritis and Inflammatory Connective Tissue Disease		0.421	0.367	0.371	0.328	0.347	0.264	0.292
M46.55	Other infective spondylopathies, thoracolumbar region	40	Rheumatoid Arthritis and Inflammatory Connective Tissue Disease		0.421	0.367	0.371	0.328	0.347	0.264	0.292
M46.56	Other infective spondylopathies, lumbar region	40	Rheumatoid Arthritis and Inflammatory Connective Tissue Disease		0.421	0.367	0.371	0.328	0.347	0.264	0.292
M46.57	Other infective spondylopathies, lumbosacral region	40	Rheumatoid Arthritis and Inflammatory Connective Tissue Disease		0.421	0.367	0.371	0.328	0.347	0.264	0.292
M46.58	Other infective spondylopathies, sacral and sacrococcygeal region	40	Rheumatoid Arthritis and Inflammatory Connective Tissue Disease		0.421	0.367	0.371	0.328	0.347	0.264	0.292
M46.59	Other infective spondylopathies, multiple sites in spine	40	Rheumatoid Arthritis and Inflammatory Connective Tissue Disease		0.421	0.367	0.371	0.328	0.347	0.264	0.292
M46.80	Other specified inflammatory spondylopathies, site unspecified	40	Rheumatoid Arthritis and Inflammatory Connective Tissue Disease		0.421	0.367	0.371	0.328	0.347	0.264	0.292
M46.81	Other specified inflammatory spondylopathies, occipito-atlanto-axial region	40	Rheumatoid Arthritis and Inflammatory Connective Tissue Disease		0.421	0.367	0.371	0.328	0.347	0.264	0.292
M46.82	Other specified inflammatory spondylopathies, cervical region	40	Rheumatoid Arthritis and Inflammatory Connective Tissue Disease		0.421	0.367	0.371	0.328	0.347	0.264	0.292
M46.83	Other specified inflammatory spondylopathies, cervicothoracic region	40	Rheumatoid Arthritis and Inflammatory Connective Tissue Disease		0.421	0.367	0.371	0.328	0.347	0.264	0.292
M46.84	Other specified inflammatory spondylopathies, thoracic region	40	Rheumatoid Arthritis and Inflammatory Connective Tissue Disease		0.421	0.367	0.371	0.328	0.347	0.264	0.292
M46.85	Other specified inflammatory spondylopathies, thoracolumbar region	40	Rheumatoid Arthritis and Inflammatory Connective Tissue Disease		0.421	0.367	0.371	0.328	0.347	0.264	0.292
M46.86	Other specified inflammatory spondylopathies, lumbar region	40	Rheumatoid Arthritis and Inflammatory Connective Tissue Disease		0.421	0.367	0.371	0.328	0.347	0.264	0.292
M46.87	Other specified inflammatory spondylopathies, lumbosacral region	40	Rheumatoid Arthritis and Inflammatory Connective Tissue Disease		0.421	0.367	0.371	0.328	0.347	0.264	0.292
M46.88	Other specified inflammatory spondylopathies, sacral and sacrococcygeal region	40	Rheumatoid Arthritis and Inflammatory Connective Tissue Disease		0.421	0.367	0.371	0.328	0.347	0.264	0.292
M46.89	Other specified inflammatory spondylopathies, multiple sites in spine	40	Rheumatoid Arthritis and Inflammatory Connective Tissue Disease		0.421	0.367	0.371	0.328	0.347	0.264	0.292

ICD-10-CM Code	ICD-10-CM Code Description	V24 CMS-HCC	V24 CMS-HCC Disease Group	V24 CMS-HCC Hierarchies	Community, NonDual, Aged	Community, NonDual, Disabled	Community, FBDual, Aged	Community, FBDual, Disabled	Community, PBDual, Aged	Community, PBDual, Disabled	Institutional
M46.90	Unspecified inflammatory spondylopathy, site unspecified	40	Rheumatoid Arthritis and Inflammatory Connective Tissue Disease		0.421	0.367	0.371	0.328	0.347	0.264	0.292
M46.91	Unspecified inflammatory spondylopathy, occipito-atlanto-axial region	40	Rheumatoid Arthritis and Inflammatory Connective Tissue Disease		0.421	0.367	0.371	0.328	0.347	0.264	0.292
M46.92	Unspecified inflammatory spondylopathy, cervical region	40	Rheumatoid Arthritis and Inflammatory Connective Tissue Disease		0.421	0.367	0.371	0.328	0.347	0.264	0.292
M46.93	Unspecified inflammatory spondylopathy, cervicothoracic region	40	Rheumatoid Arthritis and Inflammatory Connective Tissue Disease		0.421	0.367	0.371	0.328	0.347	0.264	0.292
M46.94	Unspecified inflammatory spondylopathy, thoracic region	40	Rheumatoid Arthritis and Inflammatory Connective Tissue Disease		0.421	0.367	0.371	0.328	0.347	0.264	0.292
M46.95	Unspecified inflammatory spondylopathy, thoracolumbar region	40	Rheumatoid Arthritis and Inflammatory Connective Tissue Disease		0.421	0.367	0.371	0.328	0.347	0.264	0.292
M46.96	Unspecified inflammatory spondylopathy, lumbar region	40	Rheumatoid Arthritis and Inflammatory Connective Tissue Disease		0.421	0.367	0.371	0.328	0.347	0.264	0.292
M46.97	Unspecified inflammatory spondylopathy, lumbosacral region	40	Rheumatoid Arthritis and Inflammatory Connective Tissue Disease		0.421	0.367	0.371	0.328	0.347	0.264	0.292
M46.98	Unspecified inflammatory spondylopathy, sacral and sacrococcygeal region	40	Rheumatoid Arthritis and Inflammatory Connective Tissue Disease		0.421	0.367	0.371	0.328	0.347	0.264	0.292
M46.99	Unspecified inflammatory spondylopathy, multiple sites in spine	40	Rheumatoid Arthritis and Inflammatory Connective Tissue Disease		0.421	0.367	0.371	0.328	0.347	0.264	0.292
M48.50X A	Collapsed vertebra, not elsewhere classified, site unspecified, initial encounter for fracture	169	Vertebral Fractures without Spinal Cord Injury		0.476	0.369	0.532	0.377	0.512	0.336	0.250
M48.51X A	Collapsed vertebra, not elsewhere classified, occipito-atlanto-axial region, initial encounter for fracture	169	Vertebral Fractures without Spinal Cord Injury		0.476	0.369	0.532	0.377	0.512	0.336	0.250
M48.52X A	Collapsed vertebra, not elsewhere classified, cervical region, initial encounter for fracture	169	Vertebral Fractures without Spinal Cord Injury		0.476	0.369	0.532	0.377	0.512	0.336	0.250
M48.53X A	Collapsed vertebra, not elsewhere classified, cervicothoracic region, initial encounter for fracture	169	Vertebral Fractures without Spinal Cord Injury		0.476	0.369	0.532	0.377	0.512	0.336	0.250
M48.54X A	Collapsed vertebra, not elsewhere classified, thoracic region, initial encounter for fracture	169	Vertebral Fractures without Spinal Cord Injury		0.476	0.369	0.532	0.377	0.512	0.336	0.250
M48.55X A	Collapsed vertebra, not elsewhere classified, thoracolumbar region, initial encounter for fracture	169	Vertebral Fractures without Spinal Cord Injury		0.476	0.369	0.532	0.377	0.512	0.336	0.250
M48.56X A	Collapsed vertebra, not elsewhere classified, lumbar region, initial encounter for fracture	169	Vertebral Fractures without Spinal Cord Injury		0.476	0.369	0.532	0.377	0.512	0.336	0.250
M48.57X A	Collapsed vertebra, not elsewhere classified, lumbosacral region, initial encounter for fracture	169	Vertebral Fractures without Spinal Cord Injury		0.476	0.369	0.532	0.377	0.512	0.336	0.250
M48.58X A	Collapsed vertebra, not elsewhere classified, sacral and sacrococcygeal region, initial encounter for fracture	169	Vertebral Fractures without Spinal Cord Injury		0.476	0.369	0.532	0.377	0.512	0.336	0.250
M48.8X1	Other specified spondylopathies, occipito-atlanto-axial region	40	Rheumatoid Arthritis and Inflammatory Connective Tissue Disease		0.421	0.367	0.371	0.328	0.347	0.264	0.292

ICD-10-CM Code	ICD-10-CM Code Description	V24 CMS-HCC	V24 CMS-HCC Disease Group	V24 CMS-HCC Hierarchies	Community, NonDual, Aged	Community, NonDual, Disabled	Community, FBDual, Aged	Community, FBDual, Disabled	Community, PBDual, Aged	Community, PBDual, Disabled	Institutional
M48.8X2	Other specified spondylopathies, cervical region	40	Rheumatoid Arthritis and Inflammatory Connective Tissue Disease		0.421	0.367	0.371	0.328	0.347	0.264	0.292
M48.8X3	Other specified spondylopathies, cervicothoracic region	40	Rheumatoid Arthritis and Inflammatory Connective Tissue Disease		0.421	0.367	0.371	0.328	0.347	0.264	0.292
M48.8X4	Other specified spondylopathies, thoracic region	40	Rheumatoid Arthritis and Inflammatory Connective Tissue Disease		0.421	0.367	0.371	0.328	0.347	0.264	0.292
M48.8X5	Other specified spondylopathies, thoracolumbar region	40	Rheumatoid Arthritis and Inflammatory Connective Tissue Disease		0.421	0.367	0.371	0.328	0.347	0.264	0.292
M48.8X6	Other specified spondylopathies, lumbar region	40	Rheumatoid Arthritis and Inflammatory Connective Tissue Disease		0.421	0.367	0.371	0.328	0.347	0.264	0.292
M48.8X7	Other specified spondylopathies, lumbosacral region	40	Rheumatoid Arthritis and Inflammatory Connective Tissue Disease		0.421	0.367	0.371	0.328	0.347	0.264	0.292
M48.8X8	Other specified spondylopathies, sacral and sacrococcygeal region	40	Rheumatoid Arthritis and Inflammatory Connective Tissue Disease		0.421	0.367	0.371	0.328	0.347	0.264	0.292
M48.8X9	Other specified spondylopathies, site unspecified	40	Rheumatoid Arthritis and Inflammatory Connective Tissue Disease		0.421	0.367	0.371	0.328	0.347	0.264	0.292
M49.80	Spondylopathy in diseases classified elsewhere, site unspecified	40	Rheumatoid Arthritis and Inflammatory Connective Tissue Disease		0.421	0.367	0.371	0.328	0.347	0.264	0.292
M49.81	Spondylopathy in diseases classified elsewhere, occipito-atlanto-axial region	40	Rheumatoid Arthritis and Inflammatory Connective Tissue Disease		0.421	0.367	0.371	0.328	0.347	0.264	0.292
M49.82	Spondylopathy in diseases classified elsewhere, cervical region	40	Rheumatoid Arthritis and Inflammatory Connective Tissue Disease		0.421	0.367	0.371	0.328	0.347	0.264	0.292
M49.83	Spondylopathy in diseases classified elsewhere, cervicothoracic region	40	Rheumatoid Arthritis and Inflammatory Connective Tissue Disease		0.421	0.367	0.371	0.328	0.347	0.264	0.292
M49.84	Spondylopathy in diseases classified elsewhere, thoracic region	40	Rheumatoid Arthritis and Inflammatory Connective Tissue Disease		0.421	0.367	0.371	0.328	0.347	0.264	0.292
M49.85	Spondylopathy in diseases classified elsewhere, thoracolumbar region	40	Rheumatoid Arthritis and Inflammatory Connective Tissue Disease		0.421	0.367	0.371	0.328	0.347	0.264	0.292
M49.86	Spondylopathy in diseases classified elsewhere, lumbar region	40	Rheumatoid Arthritis and Inflammatory Connective Tissue Disease		0.421	0.367	0.371	0.328	0.347	0.264	0.292
M49.87	Spondylopathy in diseases classified elsewhere, lumbosacral region	40	Rheumatoid Arthritis and Inflammatory Connective Tissue Disease		0.421	0.367	0.371	0.328	0.347	0.264	0.292
M49.88	Spondylopathy in diseases classified elsewhere, sacral and sacrococcygeal region	40	Rheumatoid Arthritis and Inflammatory Connective Tissue Disease		0.421	0.367	0.371	0.328	0.347	0.264	0.292
M49.89	Spondylopathy in diseases classified elsewhere, multiple sites in spine	40	Rheumatoid Arthritis and Inflammatory Connective Tissue Disease		0.421	0.367	0.371	0.328	0.347	0.264	0.292
M72.6	Necrotizing fasciitis	39	Bone/Joint/Muscle Infections/Necrosis		0.401	0.378	0.558	0.682	0.443	0.435	0.401
M80.051A	Age-related osteoporosis with current pathological fracture, right femur, initial encounter for fracture	170	Hip Fracture/Dislocation		0.350	0.394	0.409	0.469	0.354	0.333	—
M80.052A	Age-related osteoporosis with current pathological fracture, left femur, initial encounter for fracture	170	Hip Fracture/Dislocation		0.350	0.394	0.409	0.469	0.354	0.333	—

ICD-10-CM Code	ICD-10-CM Code Description	V24 CMS-HCC	V24 CMS-HCC Disease Group	V24 CMS-HCC Hierarchies	Community, NonDual, Aged	Community, NonDual, Disabled	Community, FBDual, Aged	Community, FBDual, Disabled	Community, PBDual, Aged	Community, PBDual, Disabled	Institutional
M80.059A	Age-related osteoporosis with current pathological fracture, unspecified femur, initial encounter for fracture	170	Hip Fracture/Dislocation		0.350	0.394	0.409	0.469	0.354	0.333	—
M80.08XA	Age-related osteoporosis with current pathological fracture, vertebra(e), initial encounter for fracture	169	Vertebral Fractures without Spinal Cord Injury		0.476	0.369	0.532	0.377	0.512	0.336	0.250
M80.851A	Other osteoporosis with current pathological fracture, right femur, initial encounter for fracture	170	Hip Fracture/Dislocation		0.350	0.394	0.409	0.469	0.354	0.333	—
M80.852A	Other osteoporosis with current pathological fracture, left femur, initial encounter for fracture	170	Hip Fracture/Dislocation		0.350	0.394	0.409	0.469	0.354	0.333	—
M80.859A	Other osteoporosis with current pathological fracture, unspecified femur, initial encounter for fracture	170	Hip Fracture/Dislocation		0.350	0.394	0.409	0.469	0.354	0.333	—
M80.88XA	Other osteoporosis with current pathological fracture, vertebra(e), initial encounter for fracture	169	Vertebral Fractures without Spinal Cord Injury		0.476	0.369	0.532	0.377	0.512	0.336	0.250
M84.451A	Pathological fracture, right femur, initial encounter for fracture	170	Hip Fracture/Dislocation		0.350	0.394	0.409	0.469	0.354	0.333	—
M84.452A	Pathological fracture, left femur, initial encounter for fracture	170	Hip Fracture/Dislocation		0.350	0.394	0.409	0.469	0.354	0.333	—
M84.453A	Pathological fracture, unspecified femur, initial encounter for fracture	170	Hip Fracture/Dislocation		0.350	0.394	0.409	0.469	0.354	0.333	—
M84.459A	Pathological fracture, hip, unspecified, initial encounter for fracture	170	Hip Fracture/Dislocation		0.350	0.394	0.409	0.469	0.354	0.333	—
M84.551A	Pathological fracture in neoplastic disease, right femur, initial encounter for fracture	170	Hip Fracture/Dislocation		0.350	0.394	0.409	0.469	0.354	0.333	—
M84.552A	Pathological fracture in neoplastic disease, left femur, initial encounter for fracture	170	Hip Fracture/Dislocation		0.350	0.394	0.409	0.469	0.354	0.333	—
M84.553A	Pathological fracture in neoplastic disease, unspecified femur, initial encounter for fracture	170	Hip Fracture/Dislocation		0.350	0.394	0.409	0.469	0.354	0.333	—
M84.559A	Pathological fracture in neoplastic disease, hip, unspecified, initial encounter for fracture	170	Hip Fracture/Dislocation		0.350	0.394	0.409	0.469	0.354	0.333	—
M84.651A	Pathological fracture in other disease, right femur, initial encounter for fracture	170	Hip Fracture/Dislocation		0.350	0.394	0.409	0.469	0.354	0.333	—
M84.652A	Pathological fracture in other disease, left femur, initial encounter for fracture	170	Hip Fracture/Dislocation		0.350	0.394	0.409	0.469	0.354	0.333	—
M84.653A	Pathological fracture in other disease, unspecified femur, initial encounter for fracture	170	Hip Fracture/Dislocation		0.350	0.394	0.409	0.469	0.354	0.333	—
M84.659A	Pathological fracture in other disease, hip, unspecified, initial encounter for fracture	170	Hip Fracture/Dislocation		0.350	0.394	0.409	0.469	0.354	0.333	—
M84.754A	Complete transverse atypical femoral fracture, right leg, initial encounter for fracture	170	Hip Fracture/Dislocation		0.350	0.394	0.409	0.469	0.354	0.333	—
M84.755A	Complete transverse atypical femoral fracture, left leg, initial encounter for fracture	170	Hip Fracture/Dislocation		0.350	0.394	0.409	0.469	0.354	0.333	—

ICD-10-CM Code	ICD-10-CM Code Description	V24 CMS-HCC	V24 CMS-HCC Disease Group	V24 CMS-HCC Hierarchies	Community, NonDual, Aged	Community, NonDual, Disabled	Community, FBDual, Aged	Community, FBDual, Disabled	Community, PBDual, Aged	Community, PBDual, Disabled	Institutional
M84.756A	Complete transverse atypical femoral fracture, unspecified leg, initial encounter for fracture	170	Hip Fracture/Dislocation		0.350	0.394	0.409	0.469	0.354	0.333	—
M84.757A	Complete oblique atypical femoral fracture, right leg, initial encounter for fracture	170	Hip Fracture/Dislocation		0.350	0.394	0.409	0.469	0.354	0.333	—
M84.758A	Complete oblique atypical femoral fracture, left leg, initial encounter for fracture	170	Hip Fracture/Dislocation		0.350	0.394	0.409	0.469	0.354	0.333	—
M84.759A	Complete oblique atypical femoral fracture, unspecified leg, initial encounter for fracture	170	Hip Fracture/Dislocation		0.350	0.394	0.409	0.469	0.354	0.333	—
M86.00	Acute hematogenous osteomyelitis, unspecified site	39	Bone/Joint/Muscle Infections/Necrosis		0.401	0.378	0.558	0.682	0.443	0.435	0.401
M86.011	Acute hematogenous osteomyelitis, right shoulder	39	Bone/Joint/Muscle Infections/Necrosis		0.401	0.378	0.558	0.682	0.443	0.435	0.401
M86.012	Acute hematogenous osteomyelitis, left shoulder	39	Bone/Joint/Muscle Infections/Necrosis		0.401	0.378	0.558	0.682	0.443	0.435	0.401
M86.019	Acute hematogenous osteomyelitis, unspecified shoulder	39	Bone/Joint/Muscle Infections/Necrosis		0.401	0.378	0.558	0.682	0.443	0.435	0.401
M86.021	Acute hematogenous osteomyelitis, right humerus	39	Bone/Joint/Muscle Infections/Necrosis		0.401	0.378	0.558	0.682	0.443	0.435	0.401
M86.022	Acute hematogenous osteomyelitis, left humerus	39	Bone/Joint/Muscle Infections/Necrosis		0.401	0.378	0.558	0.682	0.443	0.435	0.401
M86.029	Acute hematogenous osteomyelitis, unspecified humerus	39	Bone/Joint/Muscle Infections/Necrosis		0.401	0.378	0.558	0.682	0.443	0.435	0.401
M86.031	Acute hematogenous osteomyelitis, right radius and ulna	39	Bone/Joint/Muscle Infections/Necrosis		0.401	0.378	0.558	0.682	0.443	0.435	0.401
M86.032	Acute hematogenous osteomyelitis, left radius and ulna	39	Bone/Joint/Muscle Infections/Necrosis		0.401	0.378	0.558	0.682	0.443	0.435	0.401
M86.039	Acute hematogenous osteomyelitis, unspecified radius and ulna	39	Bone/Joint/Muscle Infections/Necrosis		0.401	0.378	0.558	0.682	0.443	0.435	0.401
M86.041	Acute hematogenous osteomyelitis, right hand	39	Bone/Joint/Muscle Infections/Necrosis		0.401	0.378	0.558	0.682	0.443	0.435	0.401
M86.042	Acute hematogenous osteomyelitis, left hand	39	Bone/Joint/Muscle Infections/Necrosis		0.401	0.378	0.558	0.682	0.443	0.435	0.401
M86.049	Acute hematogenous osteomyelitis, unspecified hand	39	Bone/Joint/Muscle Infections/Necrosis		0.401	0.378	0.558	0.682	0.443	0.435	0.401
M86.051	Acute hematogenous osteomyelitis, right femur	39	Bone/Joint/Muscle Infections/Necrosis		0.401	0.378	0.558	0.682	0.443	0.435	0.401
M86.052	Acute hematogenous osteomyelitis, left femur	39	Bone/Joint/Muscle Infections/Necrosis		0.401	0.378	0.558	0.682	0.443	0.435	0.401
M86.059	Acute hematogenous osteomyelitis, unspecified femur	39	Bone/Joint/Muscle Infections/Necrosis		0.401	0.378	0.558	0.682	0.443	0.435	0.401
M86.061	Acute hematogenous osteomyelitis, right tibia and fibula	39	Bone/Joint/Muscle Infections/Necrosis		0.401	0.378	0.558	0.682	0.443	0.435	0.401
M86.062	Acute hematogenous osteomyelitis, left tibia and fibula	39	Bone/Joint/Muscle Infections/Necrosis		0.401	0.378	0.558	0.682	0.443	0.435	0.401
M86.069	Acute hematogenous osteomyelitis, unspecified tibia and fibula	39	Bone/Joint/Muscle Infections/Necrosis		0.401	0.378	0.558	0.682	0.443	0.435	0.401
M86.071	Acute hematogenous osteomyelitis, right ankle and foot	39	Bone/Joint/Muscle Infections/Necrosis		0.401	0.378	0.558	0.682	0.443	0.435	0.401
M86.072	Acute hematogenous osteomyelitis, left ankle and foot	39	Bone/Joint/Muscle Infections/Necrosis		0.401	0.378	0.558	0.682	0.443	0.435	0.401
M86.079	Acute hematogenous osteomyelitis, unspecified ankle and foot	39	Bone/Joint/Muscle Infections/Necrosis		0.401	0.378	0.558	0.682	0.443	0.435	0.401
M86.08	Acute hematogenous osteomyelitis, other sites	39	Bone/Joint/Muscle Infections/Necrosis		0.401	0.378	0.558	0.682	0.443	0.435	0.401

ICD-10-CM Code	ICD-10-CM Code Description	V24 CMS-HCC	V24 CMS-HCC Disease Group	V24 CMS-HCC Hierarchies	Community, NonDual, Aged	Community, NonDual, Disabled	Community, FBDual, Aged	Community, FBDual, Disabled	Community, PBDual, Aged	Community, PBDual, Disabled	Institutional
M86.09	Acute hematogenous osteomyelitis, multiple sites	39	Bone/Joint/Muscle Infections/Necrosis		0.401	0.378	0.558	0.682	0.443	0.435	0.401
M86.10	Other acute osteomyelitis, unspecified site	39	Bone/Joint/Muscle Infections/Necrosis		0.401	0.378	0.558	0.682	0.443	0.435	0.401
M86.111	Other acute osteomyelitis, right shoulder	39	Bone/Joint/Muscle Infections/Necrosis		0.401	0.378	0.558	0.682	0.443	0.435	0.401
M86.112	Other acute osteomyelitis, left shoulder	39	Bone/Joint/Muscle Infections/Necrosis		0.401	0.378	0.558	0.682	0.443	0.435	0.401
M86.119	Other acute osteomyelitis, unspecified shoulder	39	Bone/Joint/Muscle Infections/Necrosis		0.401	0.378	0.558	0.682	0.443	0.435	0.401
M86.121	Other acute osteomyelitis, right humerus	39	Bone/Joint/Muscle Infections/Necrosis		0.401	0.378	0.558	0.682	0.443	0.435	0.401
M86.122	Other acute osteomyelitis, left humerus	39	Bone/Joint/Muscle Infections/Necrosis		0.401	0.378	0.558	0.682	0.443	0.435	0.401
M86.129	Other acute osteomyelitis, unspecified humerus	39	Bone/Joint/Muscle Infections/Necrosis		0.401	0.378	0.558	0.682	0.443	0.435	0.401
M86.131	Other acute osteomyelitis, right radius and ulna	39	Bone/Joint/Muscle Infections/Necrosis		0.401	0.378	0.558	0.682	0.443	0.435	0.401
M86.132	Other acute osteomyelitis, left radius and ulna	39	Bone/Joint/Muscle Infections/Necrosis		0.401	0.378	0.558	0.682	0.443	0.435	0.401
M86.139	Other acute osteomyelitis, unspecified radius and ulna	39	Bone/Joint/Muscle Infections/Necrosis		0.401	0.378	0.558	0.682	0.443	0.435	0.401
M86.141	Other acute osteomyelitis, right hand	39	Bone/Joint/Muscle Infections/Necrosis		0.401	0.378	0.558	0.682	0.443	0.435	0.401
M86.142	Other acute osteomyelitis, left hand	39	Bone/Joint/Muscle Infections/Necrosis		0.401	0.378	0.558	0.682	0.443	0.435	0.401
M86.149	Other acute osteomyelitis, unspecified hand	39	Bone/Joint/Muscle Infections/Necrosis		0.401	0.378	0.558	0.682	0.443	0.435	0.401
M86.151	Other acute osteomyelitis, right femur	39	Bone/Joint/Muscle Infections/Necrosis		0.401	0.378	0.558	0.682	0.443	0.435	0.401
M86.152	Other acute osteomyelitis, left femur	39	Bone/Joint/Muscle Infections/Necrosis		0.401	0.378	0.558	0.682	0.443	0.435	0.401
M86.159	Other acute osteomyelitis, unspecified femur	39	Bone/Joint/Muscle Infections/Necrosis		0.401	0.378	0.558	0.682	0.443	0.435	0.401
M86.161	Other acute osteomyelitis, right tibia and fibula	39	Bone/Joint/Muscle Infections/Necrosis		0.401	0.378	0.558	0.682	0.443	0.435	0.401
M86.162	Other acute osteomyelitis, left tibia and fibula	39	Bone/Joint/Muscle Infections/Necrosis		0.401	0.378	0.558	0.682	0.443	0.435	0.401
M86.169	Other acute osteomyelitis, unspecified tibia and fibula	39	Bone/Joint/Muscle Infections/Necrosis		0.401	0.378	0.558	0.682	0.443	0.435	0.401
M86.171	Other acute osteomyelitis, right ankle and foot	39	Bone/Joint/Muscle Infections/Necrosis		0.401	0.378	0.558	0.682	0.443	0.435	0.401
M86.172	Other acute osteomyelitis, left ankle and foot	39	Bone/Joint/Muscle Infections/Necrosis		0.401	0.378	0.558	0.682	0.443	0.435	0.401
M86.179	Other acute osteomyelitis, unspecified ankle and foot	39	Bone/Joint/Muscle Infections/Necrosis		0.401	0.378	0.558	0.682	0.443	0.435	0.401
M86.18	Other acute osteomyelitis, other site	39	Bone/Joint/Muscle Infections/Necrosis		0.401	0.378	0.558	0.682	0.443	0.435	0.401
M86.19	Other acute osteomyelitis, multiple sites	39	Bone/Joint/Muscle Infections/Necrosis		0.401	0.378	0.558	0.682	0.443	0.435	0.401
M86.20	Subacute osteomyelitis, unspecified site	39	Bone/Joint/Muscle Infections/Necrosis		0.401	0.378	0.558	0.682	0.443	0.435	0.401
M86.211	Subacute osteomyelitis, right shoulder	39	Bone/Joint/Muscle Infections/Necrosis		0.401	0.378	0.558	0.682	0.443	0.435	0.401
M86.212	Subacute osteomyelitis, left shoulder	39	Bone/Joint/Muscle Infections/Necrosis		0.401	0.378	0.558	0.682	0.443	0.435	0.401
M86.219	Subacute osteomyelitis, unspecified shoulder	39	Bone/Joint/Muscle Infections/Necrosis		0.401	0.378	0.558	0.682	0.443	0.435	0.401
M86.221	Subacute osteomyelitis, right humerus	39	Bone/Joint/Muscle Infections/Necrosis		0.401	0.378	0.558	0.682	0.443	0.435	0.401
M86.222	Subacute osteomyelitis, left humerus	39	Bone/Joint/Muscle Infections/Necrosis		0.401	0.378	0.558	0.682	0.443	0.435	0.401
M86.229	Subacute osteomyelitis, unspecified humerus	39	Bone/Joint/Muscle Infections/Necrosis		0.401	0.378	0.558	0.682	0.443	0.435	0.401

ICD-10-CM Code	ICD-10-CM Code Description	V24 CMS-HCC	V24 CMS-HCC Disease Group	V24 CMS-HCC Hierarchies	Community, NonDual, Aged	Community, NonDual, Disabled	Community, FBDual, Aged	Community, FBDual, Disabled	Community, PBDual, Aged	Community, PBDual, Disabled	Institutional
M86.231	Subacute osteomyelitis, right radius and ulna	39	Bone/Joint/Muscle Infections/Necrosis		0.401	0.378	0.558	0.682	0.443	0.435	0.401
M86.232	Subacute osteomyelitis, left radius and ulna	39	Bone/Joint/Muscle Infections/Necrosis		0.401	0.378	0.558	0.682	0.443	0.435	0.401
M86.239	Subacute osteomyelitis, unspecified radius and ulna	39	Bone/Joint/Muscle Infections/Necrosis		0.401	0.378	0.558	0.682	0.443	0.435	0.401
M86.241	Subacute osteomyelitis, right hand	39	Bone/Joint/Muscle Infections/Necrosis		0.401	0.378	0.558	0.682	0.443	0.435	0.401
M86.242	Subacute osteomyelitis, left hand	39	Bone/Joint/Muscle Infections/Necrosis		0.401	0.378	0.558	0.682	0.443	0.435	0.401
M86.249	Subacute osteomyelitis, unspecified hand	39	Bone/Joint/Muscle Infections/Necrosis		0.401	0.378	0.558	0.682	0.443	0.435	0.401
M86.251	Subacute osteomyelitis, right femur	39	Bone/Joint/Muscle Infections/Necrosis		0.401	0.378	0.558	0.682	0.443	0.435	0.401
M86.252	Subacute osteomyelitis, left femur	39	Bone/Joint/Muscle Infections/Necrosis		0.401	0.378	0.558	0.682	0.443	0.435	0.401
M86.259	Subacute osteomyelitis, unspecified femur	39	Bone/Joint/Muscle Infections/Necrosis		0.401	0.378	0.558	0.682	0.443	0.435	0.401
M86.261	Subacute osteomyelitis, right tibia and fibula	39	Bone/Joint/Muscle Infections/Necrosis		0.401	0.378	0.558	0.682	0.443	0.435	0.401
M86.262	Subacute osteomyelitis, left tibia and fibula	39	Bone/Joint/Muscle Infections/Necrosis		0.401	0.378	0.558	0.682	0.443	0.435	0.401
M86.269	Subacute osteomyelitis, unspecified tibia and fibula	39	Bone/Joint/Muscle Infections/Necrosis		0.401	0.378	0.558	0.682	0.443	0.435	0.401
M86.271	Subacute osteomyelitis, right ankle and foot	39	Bone/Joint/Muscle Infections/Necrosis		0.401	0.378	0.558	0.682	0.443	0.435	0.401
M86.272	Subacute osteomyelitis, left ankle and foot	39	Bone/Joint/Muscle Infections/Necrosis		0.401	0.378	0.558	0.682	0.443	0.435	0.401
M86.279	Subacute osteomyelitis, unspecified ankle and foot	39	Bone/Joint/Muscle Infections/Necrosis		0.401	0.378	0.558	0.682	0.443	0.435	0.401
M86.28	Subacute osteomyelitis, other site	39	Bone/Joint/Muscle Infections/Necrosis		0.401	0.378	0.558	0.682	0.443	0.435	0.401
M86.29	Subacute osteomyelitis, multiple sites	39	Bone/Joint/Muscle Infections/Necrosis		0.401	0.378	0.558	0.682	0.443	0.435	0.401
M86.30	Chronic multifocal osteomyelitis, unspecified site	39	Bone/Joint/Muscle Infections/Necrosis		0.401	0.378	0.558	0.682	0.443	0.435	0.401
M86.311	Chronic multifocal osteomyelitis, right shoulder	39	Bone/Joint/Muscle Infections/Necrosis		0.401	0.378	0.558	0.682	0.443	0.435	0.401
M86.312	Chronic multifocal osteomyelitis, left shoulder	39	Bone/Joint/Muscle Infections/Necrosis		0.401	0.378	0.558	0.682	0.443	0.435	0.401
M86.319	Chronic multifocal osteomyelitis, unspecified shoulder	39	Bone/Joint/Muscle Infections/Necrosis		0.401	0.378	0.558	0.682	0.443	0.435	0.401
M86.321	Chronic multifocal osteomyelitis, right humerus	39	Bone/Joint/Muscle Infections/Necrosis		0.401	0.378	0.558	0.682	0.443	0.435	0.401
M86.322	Chronic multifocal osteomyelitis, left humerus	39	Bone/Joint/Muscle Infections/Necrosis		0.401	0.378	0.558	0.682	0.443	0.435	0.401
M86.329	Chronic multifocal osteomyelitis, unspecified humerus	39	Bone/Joint/Muscle Infections/Necrosis		0.401	0.378	0.558	0.682	0.443	0.435	0.401
M86.331	Chronic multifocal osteomyelitis, right radius and ulna	39	Bone/Joint/Muscle Infections/Necrosis		0.401	0.378	0.558	0.682	0.443	0.435	0.401
M86.332	Chronic multifocal osteomyelitis, left radius and ulna	39	Bone/Joint/Muscle Infections/Necrosis		0.401	0.378	0.558	0.682	0.443	0.435	0.401
M86.339	Chronic multifocal osteomyelitis, unspecified radius and ulna	39	Bone/Joint/Muscle Infections/Necrosis		0.401	0.378	0.558	0.682	0.443	0.435	0.401
M86.341	Chronic multifocal osteomyelitis, right hand	39	Bone/Joint/Muscle Infections/Necrosis		0.401	0.378	0.558	0.682	0.443	0.435	0.401
M86.342	Chronic multifocal osteomyelitis, left hand	39	Bone/Joint/Muscle Infections/Necrosis		0.401	0.378	0.558	0.682	0.443	0.435	0.401
M86.349	Chronic multifocal osteomyelitis, unspecified hand	39	Bone/Joint/Muscle Infections/Necrosis		0.401	0.378	0.558	0.682	0.443	0.435	0.401
M86.351	Chronic multifocal osteomyelitis, right femur	39	Bone/Joint/Muscle Infections/Necrosis		0.401	0.378	0.558	0.682	0.443	0.435	0.401
M86.352	Chronic multifocal osteomyelitis, left femur	39	Bone/Joint/Muscle Infections/Necrosis		0.401	0.378	0.558	0.682	0.443	0.435	0.401

ICD-10-CM Code	ICD-10-CM Code Description	V24 CMS-HCC	V24 CMS-HCC Disease Group	V24 CMS-HCC Hierarchies	Community, NonDual, Aged	Community, NonDual, Disabled	Community, FBDual, Aged	Community, FBDual, Disabled	Community, PBDual, Aged	Community, PBDual, Disabled	Institutional
M86.359	Chronic multifocal osteomyelitis, unspecified femur	39	Bone/Joint/Muscle Infections/Necrosis		0.401	0.378	0.558	0.682	0.443	0.435	0.401
M86.361	Chronic multifocal osteomyelitis, right tibia and fibula	39	Bone/Joint/Muscle Infections/Necrosis		0.401	0.378	0.558	0.682	0.443	0.435	0.401
M86.362	Chronic multifocal osteomyelitis, left tibia and fibula	39	Bone/Joint/Muscle Infections/Necrosis		0.401	0.378	0.558	0.682	0.443	0.435	0.401
M86.369	Chronic multifocal osteomyelitis, unspecified tibia and fibula	39	Bone/Joint/Muscle Infections/Necrosis		0.401	0.378	0.558	0.682	0.443	0.435	0.401
M86.371	Chronic multifocal osteomyelitis, right ankle and foot	39	Bone/Joint/Muscle Infections/Necrosis		0.401	0.378	0.558	0.682	0.443	0.435	0.401
M86.372	Chronic multifocal osteomyelitis, left ankle and foot	39	Bone/Joint/Muscle Infections/Necrosis		0.401	0.378	0.558	0.682	0.443	0.435	0.401
M86.379	Chronic multifocal osteomyelitis, unspecified ankle and foot	39	Bone/Joint/Muscle Infections/Necrosis		0.401	0.378	0.558	0.682	0.443	0.435	0.401
M86.38	Chronic multifocal osteomyelitis, other site	39	Bone/Joint/Muscle Infections/Necrosis		0.401	0.378	0.558	0.682	0.443	0.435	0.401
M86.39	Chronic multifocal osteomyelitis, multiple sites	39	Bone/Joint/Muscle Infections/Necrosis		0.401	0.378	0.558	0.682	0.443	0.435	0.401
M86.40	Chronic osteomyelitis with draining sinus, unspecified site	39	Bone/Joint/Muscle Infections/Necrosis		0.401	0.378	0.558	0.682	0.443	0.435	0.401
M86.411	Chronic osteomyelitis with draining sinus, right shoulder	39	Bone/Joint/Muscle Infections/Necrosis		0.401	0.378	0.558	0.682	0.443	0.435	0.401
M86.412	Chronic osteomyelitis with draining sinus, left shoulder	39	Bone/Joint/Muscle Infections/Necrosis		0.401	0.378	0.558	0.682	0.443	0.435	0.401
M86.419	Chronic osteomyelitis with draining sinus, unspecified shoulder	39	Bone/Joint/Muscle Infections/Necrosis		0.401	0.378	0.558	0.682	0.443	0.435	0.401
M86.421	Chronic osteomyelitis with draining sinus, right humerus	39	Bone/Joint/Muscle Infections/Necrosis		0.401	0.378	0.558	0.682	0.443	0.435	0.401
M86.422	Chronic osteomyelitis with draining sinus, left humerus	39	Bone/Joint/Muscle Infections/Necrosis		0.401	0.378	0.558	0.682	0.443	0.435	0.401
M86.429	Chronic osteomyelitis with draining sinus, unspecified humerus	39	Bone/Joint/Muscle Infections/Necrosis		0.401	0.378	0.558	0.682	0.443	0.435	0.401
M86.431	Chronic osteomyelitis with draining sinus, right radius and ulna	39	Bone/Joint/Muscle Infections/Necrosis		0.401	0.378	0.558	0.682	0.443	0.435	0.401
M86.432	Chronic osteomyelitis with draining sinus, left radius and ulna	39	Bone/Joint/Muscle Infections/Necrosis		0.401	0.378	0.558	0.682	0.443	0.435	0.401
M86.439	Chronic osteomyelitis with draining sinus, unspecified radius and ulna	39	Bone/Joint/Muscle Infections/Necrosis		0.401	0.378	0.558	0.682	0.443	0.435	0.401
M86.441	Chronic osteomyelitis with draining sinus, right hand	39	Bone/Joint/Muscle Infections/Necrosis		0.401	0.378	0.558	0.682	0.443	0.435	0.401
M86.442	Chronic osteomyelitis with draining sinus, left hand	39	Bone/Joint/Muscle Infections/Necrosis		0.401	0.378	0.558	0.682	0.443	0.435	0.401
M86.449	Chronic osteomyelitis with draining sinus, unspecified hand	39	Bone/Joint/Muscle Infections/Necrosis		0.401	0.378	0.558	0.682	0.443	0.435	0.401
M86.451	Chronic osteomyelitis with draining sinus, right femur	39	Bone/Joint/Muscle Infections/Necrosis		0.401	0.378	0.558	0.682	0.443	0.435	0.401
M86.452	Chronic osteomyelitis with draining sinus, left femur	39	Bone/Joint/Muscle Infections/Necrosis		0.401	0.378	0.558	0.682	0.443	0.435	0.401
M86.459	Chronic osteomyelitis with draining sinus, unspecified femur	39	Bone/Joint/Muscle Infections/Necrosis		0.401	0.378	0.558	0.682	0.443	0.435	0.401
M86.461	Chronic osteomyelitis with draining sinus, right tibia and fibula	39	Bone/Joint/Muscle Infections/Necrosis		0.401	0.378	0.558	0.682	0.443	0.435	0.401
M86.462	Chronic osteomyelitis with draining sinus, left tibia and fibula	39	Bone/Joint/Muscle Infections/Necrosis		0.401	0.378	0.558	0.682	0.443	0.435	0.401
M86.469	Chronic osteomyelitis with draining sinus, unspecified tibia and fibula	39	Bone/Joint/Muscle Infections/Necrosis		0.401	0.378	0.558	0.682	0.443	0.435	0.401
M86.471	Chronic osteomyelitis with draining sinus, right ankle and foot	39	Bone/Joint/Muscle Infections/Necrosis		0.401	0.378	0.558	0.682	0.443	0.435	0.401

ICD-10-CM Code	ICD-10-CM Code Description	V24 CMS-HCC	V24 CMS-HCC Disease Group	V24 CMS-HCC Hierarchies	Community, NonDual, Aged	Community, NonDual, Disabled	Community, FBDual, Aged	Community, FBDual, Disabled	Community, PBDual, Aged	Community, PBDual, Disabled	Institutional
M86.472	Chronic osteomyelitis with draining sinus, left ankle and foot	39	Bone/Joint/Muscle Infections/Necrosis		0.401	0.378	0.558	0.682	0.443	0.435	0.401
M86.479	Chronic osteomyelitis with draining sinus, unspecified ankle and foot	39	Bone/Joint/Muscle Infections/Necrosis		0.401	0.378	0.558	0.682	0.443	0.435	0.401
M86.48	Chronic osteomyelitis with draining sinus, other site	39	Bone/Joint/Muscle Infections/Necrosis		0.401	0.378	0.558	0.682	0.443	0.435	0.401
M86.49	Chronic osteomyelitis with draining sinus, multiple sites	39	Bone/Joint/Muscle Infections/Necrosis		0.401	0.378	0.558	0.682	0.443	0.435	0.401
M86.50	Other chronic hematogenous osteomyelitis, unspecified site	39	Bone/Joint/Muscle Infections/Necrosis		0.401	0.378	0.558	0.682	0.443	0.435	0.401
M86.511	Other chronic hematogenous osteomyelitis, right shoulder	39	Bone/Joint/Muscle Infections/Necrosis		0.401	0.378	0.558	0.682	0.443	0.435	0.401
M86.512	Other chronic hematogenous osteomyelitis, left shoulder	39	Bone/Joint/Muscle Infections/Necrosis		0.401	0.378	0.558	0.682	0.443	0.435	0.401
M86.519	Other chronic hematogenous osteomyelitis, unspecified shoulder	39	Bone/Joint/Muscle Infections/Necrosis		0.401	0.378	0.558	0.682	0.443	0.435	0.401
M86.521	Other chronic hematogenous osteomyelitis, right humerus	39	Bone/Joint/Muscle Infections/Necrosis		0.401	0.378	0.558	0.682	0.443	0.435	0.401
M86.522	Other chronic hematogenous osteomyelitis, left humerus	39	Bone/Joint/Muscle Infections/Necrosis		0.401	0.378	0.558	0.682	0.443	0.435	0.401
M86.529	Other chronic hematogenous osteomyelitis, unspecified humerus	39	Bone/Joint/Muscle Infections/Necrosis		0.401	0.378	0.558	0.682	0.443	0.435	0.401
M86.531	Other chronic hematogenous osteomyelitis, right radius and ulna	39	Bone/Joint/Muscle Infections/Necrosis		0.401	0.378	0.558	0.682	0.443	0.435	0.401
M86.532	Other chronic hematogenous osteomyelitis, left radius and ulna	39	Bone/Joint/Muscle Infections/Necrosis		0.401	0.378	0.558	0.682	0.443	0.435	0.401
M86.539	Other chronic hematogenous osteomyelitis, unspecified radius and ulna	39	Bone/Joint/Muscle Infections/Necrosis		0.401	0.378	0.558	0.682	0.443	0.435	0.401
M86.541	Other chronic hematogenous osteomyelitis, right hand	39	Bone/Joint/Muscle Infections/Necrosis		0.401	0.378	0.558	0.682	0.443	0.435	0.401
M86.542	Other chronic hematogenous osteomyelitis, left hand	39	Bone/Joint/Muscle Infections/Necrosis		0.401	0.378	0.558	0.682	0.443	0.435	0.401
M86.549	Other chronic hematogenous osteomyelitis, unspecified hand	39	Bone/Joint/Muscle Infections/Necrosis		0.401	0.378	0.558	0.682	0.443	0.435	0.401
M86.551	Other chronic hematogenous osteomyelitis, right femur	39	Bone/Joint/Muscle Infections/Necrosis		0.401	0.378	0.558	0.682	0.443	0.435	0.401
M86.552	Other chronic hematogenous osteomyelitis, left femur	39	Bone/Joint/Muscle Infections/Necrosis		0.401	0.378	0.558	0.682	0.443	0.435	0.401
M86.559	Other chronic hematogenous osteomyelitis, unspecified femur	39	Bone/Joint/Muscle Infections/Necrosis		0.401	0.378	0.558	0.682	0.443	0.435	0.401
M86.561	Other chronic hematogenous osteomyelitis, right tibia and fibula	39	Bone/Joint/Muscle Infections/Necrosis		0.401	0.378	0.558	0.682	0.443	0.435	0.401
M86.562	Other chronic hematogenous osteomyelitis, left tibia and fibula	39	Bone/Joint/Muscle Infections/Necrosis		0.401	0.378	0.558	0.682	0.443	0.435	0.401
M86.569	Other chronic hematogenous osteomyelitis, unspecified tibia and fibula	39	Bone/Joint/Muscle Infections/Necrosis		0.401	0.378	0.558	0.682	0.443	0.435	0.401
M86.571	Other chronic hematogenous osteomyelitis, right ankle and foot	39	Bone/Joint/Muscle Infections/Necrosis		0.401	0.378	0.558	0.682	0.443	0.435	0.401
M86.572	Other chronic hematogenous osteomyelitis, left ankle and foot	39	Bone/Joint/Muscle Infections/Necrosis		0.401	0.378	0.558	0.682	0.443	0.435	0.401
M86.579	Other chronic hematogenous osteomyelitis, unspecified ankle and foot	39	Bone/Joint/Muscle Infections/Necrosis		0.401	0.378	0.558	0.682	0.443	0.435	0.401
M86.58	Other chronic hematogenous osteomyelitis, other site	39	Bone/Joint/Muscle Infections/Necrosis		0.401	0.378	0.558	0.682	0.443	0.435	0.401
M86.59	Other chronic hematogenous osteomyelitis, multiple sites	39	Bone/Joint/Muscle Infections/Necrosis		0.401	0.378	0.558	0.682	0.443	0.435	0.401

ICD-10-CM Code	ICD-10-CM Code Description	V24 CMS-HCC	V24 CMS-HCC Disease Group	V24 CMS-HCC Hierarchies	Community, NonDual, Aged	Community, NonDual, Disabled	Community, FBDual, Aged	Community, FBDual, Disabled	Community, PBDual, Aged	Community, PBDual, Disabled	Institutional
M86.60	Other chronic osteomyelitis, unspecified site	39	Bone/Joint/Muscle Infections/Necrosis		0.401	0.378	0.558	0.682	0.443	0.435	0.401
M86.611	Other chronic osteomyelitis, right shoulder	39	Bone/Joint/Muscle Infections/Necrosis		0.401	0.378	0.558	0.682	0.443	0.435	0.401
M86.612	Other chronic osteomyelitis, left shoulder	39	Bone/Joint/Muscle Infections/Necrosis		0.401	0.378	0.558	0.682	0.443	0.435	0.401
M86.619	Other chronic osteomyelitis, unspecified shoulder	39	Bone/Joint/Muscle Infections/Necrosis		0.401	0.378	0.558	0.682	0.443	0.435	0.401
M86.621	Other chronic osteomyelitis, right humerus	39	Bone/Joint/Muscle Infections/Necrosis		0.401	0.378	0.558	0.682	0.443	0.435	0.401
M86.622	Other chronic osteomyelitis, left humerus	39	Bone/Joint/Muscle Infections/Necrosis		0.401	0.378	0.558	0.682	0.443	0.435	0.401
M86.629	Other chronic osteomyelitis, unspecified humerus	39	Bone/Joint/Muscle Infections/Necrosis		0.401	0.378	0.558	0.682	0.443	0.435	0.401
M86.631	Other chronic osteomyelitis, right radius and ulna	39	Bone/Joint/Muscle Infections/Necrosis		0.401	0.378	0.558	0.682	0.443	0.435	0.401
M86.632	Other chronic osteomyelitis, left radius and ulna	39	Bone/Joint/Muscle Infections/Necrosis		0.401	0.378	0.558	0.682	0.443	0.435	0.401
M86.639	Other chronic osteomyelitis, unspecified radius and ulna	39	Bone/Joint/Muscle Infections/Necrosis		0.401	0.378	0.558	0.682	0.443	0.435	0.401
M86.641	Other chronic osteomyelitis, right hand	39	Bone/Joint/Muscle Infections/Necrosis		0.401	0.378	0.558	0.682	0.443	0.435	0.401
M86.642	Other chronic osteomyelitis, left hand	39	Bone/Joint/Muscle Infections/Necrosis		0.401	0.378	0.558	0.682	0.443	0.435	0.401
M86.649	Other chronic osteomyelitis, unspecified hand	39	Bone/Joint/Muscle Infections/Necrosis		0.401	0.378	0.558	0.682	0.443	0.435	0.401
M86.651	Other chronic osteomyelitis, right thigh	39	Bone/Joint/Muscle Infections/Necrosis		0.401	0.378	0.558	0.682	0.443	0.435	0.401
M86.652	Other chronic osteomyelitis, left thigh	39	Bone/Joint/Muscle Infections/Necrosis		0.401	0.378	0.558	0.682	0.443	0.435	0.401
M86.659	Other chronic osteomyelitis, unspecified thigh	39	Bone/Joint/Muscle Infections/Necrosis		0.401	0.378	0.558	0.682	0.443	0.435	0.401
M86.661	Other chronic osteomyelitis, right tibia and fibula	39	Bone/Joint/Muscle Infections/Necrosis		0.401	0.378	0.558	0.682	0.443	0.435	0.401
M86.662	Other chronic osteomyelitis, left tibia and fibula	39	Bone/Joint/Muscle Infections/Necrosis		0.401	0.378	0.558	0.682	0.443	0.435	0.401
M86.669	Other chronic osteomyelitis, unspecified tibia and fibula	39	Bone/Joint/Muscle Infections/Necrosis		0.401	0.378	0.558	0.682	0.443	0.435	0.401
M86.671	Other chronic osteomyelitis, right ankle and foot	39	Bone/Joint/Muscle Infections/Necrosis		0.401	0.378	0.558	0.682	0.443	0.435	0.401
M86.672	Other chronic osteomyelitis, left ankle and foot	39	Bone/Joint/Muscle Infections/Necrosis		0.401	0.378	0.558	0.682	0.443	0.435	0.401
M86.679	Other chronic osteomyelitis, unspecified ankle and foot	39	Bone/Joint/Muscle Infections/Necrosis		0.401	0.378	0.558	0.682	0.443	0.435	0.401
M86.68	Other chronic osteomyelitis, other site	39	Bone/Joint/Muscle Infections/Necrosis		0.401	0.378	0.558	0.682	0.443	0.435	0.401
M86.69	Other chronic osteomyelitis, multiple sites	39	Bone/Joint/Muscle Infections/Necrosis		0.401	0.378	0.558	0.682	0.443	0.435	0.401
M86.8X0	Other osteomyelitis, multiple sites	39	Bone/Joint/Muscle Infections/Necrosis		0.401	0.378	0.558	0.682	0.443	0.435	0.401
M86.8X1	Other osteomyelitis, shoulder	39	Bone/Joint/Muscle Infections/Necrosis		0.401	0.378	0.558	0.682	0.443	0.435	0.401
M86.8X2	Other osteomyelitis, upper arm	39	Bone/Joint/Muscle Infections/Necrosis		0.401	0.378	0.558	0.682	0.443	0.435	0.401
M86.8X3	Other osteomyelitis, forearm	39	Bone/Joint/Muscle Infections/Necrosis		0.401	0.378	0.558	0.682	0.443	0.435	0.401
M86.8X4	Other osteomyelitis, hand	39	Bone/Joint/Muscle Infections/Necrosis		0.401	0.378	0.558	0.682	0.443	0.435	0.401
M86.8X5	Other osteomyelitis, thigh	39	Bone/Joint/Muscle Infections/Necrosis		0.401	0.378	0.558	0.682	0.443	0.435	0.401
M86.8X6	Other osteomyelitis, lower leg	39	Bone/Joint/Muscle Infections/Necrosis		0.401	0.378	0.558	0.682	0.443	0.435	0.401
M86.8X7	Other osteomyelitis, ankle and foot	39	Bone/Joint/Muscle Infections/Necrosis		0.401	0.378	0.558	0.682	0.443	0.435	0.401
M86.8X8	Other osteomyelitis, other site	39	Bone/Joint/Muscle Infections/Necrosis		0.401	0.378	0.558	0.682	0.443	0.435	0.401
M86.8X9	Other osteomyelitis, unspecified sites	39	Bone/Joint/Muscle Infections/Necrosis		0.401	0.378	0.558	0.682	0.443	0.435	0.401
M86.9	Osteomyelitis, unspecified	39	Bone/Joint/Muscle Infections/Necrosis		0.401	0.378	0.558	0.682	0.443	0.435	0.401

ICD-10-CM Code	ICD-10-CM Code Description	V24 CMS-HCC	V24 CMS-HCC Disease Group	V24 CMS-HCC Hierarchies	Community, NonDual, Aged	Community, NonDual, Disabled	Community, FBDual, Aged	Community, FBDual, Disabled	Community, PBDual, Aged	Community, PBDual, Disabled	Institutional
M87.00	Idiopathic aseptic necrosis of unspecified bone	39	Bone/Joint/Muscle Infections/Necrosis		0.401	0.378	0.558	0.682	0.443	0.435	0.401
M87.011	Idiopathic aseptic necrosis of right shoulder	39	Bone/Joint/Muscle Infections/Necrosis		0.401	0.378	0.558	0.682	0.443	0.435	0.401
M87.012	Idiopathic aseptic necrosis of left shoulder	39	Bone/Joint/Muscle Infections/Necrosis		0.401	0.378	0.558	0.682	0.443	0.435	0.401
M87.019	Idiopathic aseptic necrosis of unspecified shoulder	39	Bone/Joint/Muscle Infections/Necrosis		0.401	0.378	0.558	0.682	0.443	0.435	0.401
M87.021	Idiopathic aseptic necrosis of right humerus	39	Bone/Joint/Muscle Infections/Necrosis		0.401	0.378	0.558	0.682	0.443	0.435	0.401
M87.022	Idiopathic aseptic necrosis of left humerus	39	Bone/Joint/Muscle Infections/Necrosis		0.401	0.378	0.558	0.682	0.443	0.435	0.401
M87.029	Idiopathic aseptic necrosis of unspecified humerus	39	Bone/Joint/Muscle Infections/Necrosis		0.401	0.378	0.558	0.682	0.443	0.435	0.401
M87.031	Idiopathic aseptic necrosis of right radius	39	Bone/Joint/Muscle Infections/Necrosis		0.401	0.378	0.558	0.682	0.443	0.435	0.401
M87.032	Idiopathic aseptic necrosis of left radius	39	Bone/Joint/Muscle Infections/Necrosis		0.401	0.378	0.558	0.682	0.443	0.435	0.401
M87.033	Idiopathic aseptic necrosis of unspecified radius	39	Bone/Joint/Muscle Infections/Necrosis		0.401	0.378	0.558	0.682	0.443	0.435	0.401
M87.034	Idiopathic aseptic necrosis of right ulna	39	Bone/Joint/Muscle Infections/Necrosis		0.401	0.378	0.558	0.682	0.443	0.435	0.401
M87.035	Idiopathic aseptic necrosis of left ulna	39	Bone/Joint/Muscle Infections/Necrosis		0.401	0.378	0.558	0.682	0.443	0.435	0.401
M87.036	Idiopathic aseptic necrosis of unspecified ulna	39	Bone/Joint/Muscle Infections/Necrosis		0.401	0.378	0.558	0.682	0.443	0.435	0.401
M87.037	Idiopathic aseptic necrosis of right carpus	39	Bone/Joint/Muscle Infections/Necrosis		0.401	0.378	0.558	0.682	0.443	0.435	0.401
M87.038	Idiopathic aseptic necrosis of left carpus	39	Bone/Joint/Muscle Infections/Necrosis		0.401	0.378	0.558	0.682	0.443	0.435	0.401
M87.039	Idiopathic aseptic necrosis of unspecified carpus	39	Bone/Joint/Muscle Infections/Necrosis		0.401	0.378	0.558	0.682	0.443	0.435	0.401
M87.041	Idiopathic aseptic necrosis of right hand	39	Bone/Joint/Muscle Infections/Necrosis		0.401	0.378	0.558	0.682	0.443	0.435	0.401
M87.042	Idiopathic aseptic necrosis of left hand	39	Bone/Joint/Muscle Infections/Necrosis		0.401	0.378	0.558	0.682	0.443	0.435	0.401
M87.043	Idiopathic aseptic necrosis of unspecified hand	39	Bone/Joint/Muscle Infections/Necrosis		0.401	0.378	0.558	0.682	0.443	0.435	0.401
M87.044	Idiopathic aseptic necrosis of right finger(s)	39	Bone/Joint/Muscle Infections/Necrosis		0.401	0.378	0.558	0.682	0.443	0.435	0.401
M87.045	Idiopathic aseptic necrosis of left finger(s)	39	Bone/Joint/Muscle Infections/Necrosis		0.401	0.378	0.558	0.682	0.443	0.435	0.401
M87.046	Idiopathic aseptic necrosis of unspecified finger(s)	39	Bone/Joint/Muscle Infections/Necrosis		0.401	0.378	0.558	0.682	0.443	0.435	0.401
M87.050	Idiopathic aseptic necrosis of pelvis	39	Bone/Joint/Muscle Infections/Necrosis		0.401	0.378	0.558	0.682	0.443	0.435	0.401
M87.051	Idiopathic aseptic necrosis of right femur	39	Bone/Joint/Muscle Infections/Necrosis		0.401	0.378	0.558	0.682	0.443	0.435	0.401
M87.052	Idiopathic aseptic necrosis of left femur	39	Bone/Joint/Muscle Infections/Necrosis		0.401	0.378	0.558	0.682	0.443	0.435	0.401
M87.059	Idiopathic aseptic necrosis of unspecified femur	39	Bone/Joint/Muscle Infections/Necrosis		0.401	0.378	0.558	0.682	0.443	0.435	0.401
M87.061	Idiopathic aseptic necrosis of right tibia	39	Bone/Joint/Muscle Infections/Necrosis		0.401	0.378	0.558	0.682	0.443	0.435	0.401
M87.062	Idiopathic aseptic necrosis of left tibia	39	Bone/Joint/Muscle Infections/Necrosis		0.401	0.378	0.558	0.682	0.443	0.435	0.401
M87.063	Idiopathic aseptic necrosis of unspecified tibia	39	Bone/Joint/Muscle Infections/Necrosis		0.401	0.378	0.558	0.682	0.443	0.435	0.401
M87.064	Idiopathic aseptic necrosis of right fibula	39	Bone/Joint/Muscle Infections/Necrosis		0.401	0.378	0.558	0.682	0.443	0.435	0.401

ICD-10-CM Code	ICD-10-CM Code Description	V24 CMS-HCC	V24 CMS-HCC Disease Group	V24 CMS-HCC Hierarchies	Community, NonDual, Aged	Community, NonDual, Disabled	Community, FBDual, Aged	Community, FBDual, Disabled	Community, PBDual, Aged	Community, PBDual, Disabled	Institutional
M87.065	Idiopathic aseptic necrosis of left fibula	39	Bone/Joint/Muscle Infections/Necrosis		0.401	0.378	0.558	0.682	0.443	0.435	0.401
M87.066	Idiopathic aseptic necrosis of unspecified fibula	39	Bone/Joint/Muscle Infections/Necrosis		0.401	0.378	0.558	0.682	0.443	0.435	0.401
M87.071	Idiopathic aseptic necrosis of right ankle	39	Bone/Joint/Muscle Infections/Necrosis		0.401	0.378	0.558	0.682	0.443	0.435	0.401
M87.072	Idiopathic aseptic necrosis of left ankle	39	Bone/Joint/Muscle Infections/Necrosis		0.401	0.378	0.558	0.682	0.443	0.435	0.401
M87.073	Idiopathic aseptic necrosis of unspecified ankle	39	Bone/Joint/Muscle Infections/Necrosis		0.401	0.378	0.558	0.682	0.443	0.435	0.401
M87.074	Idiopathic aseptic necrosis of right foot	39	Bone/Joint/Muscle Infections/Necrosis		0.401	0.378	0.558	0.682	0.443	0.435	0.401
M87.075	Idiopathic aseptic necrosis of left foot	39	Bone/Joint/Muscle Infections/Necrosis		0.401	0.378	0.558	0.682	0.443	0.435	0.401
M87.076	Idiopathic aseptic necrosis of unspecified foot	39	Bone/Joint/Muscle Infections/Necrosis		0.401	0.378	0.558	0.682	0.443	0.435	0.401
M87.077	Idiopathic aseptic necrosis of right toe(s)	39	Bone/Joint/Muscle Infections/Necrosis		0.401	0.378	0.558	0.682	0.443	0.435	0.401
M87.078	Idiopathic aseptic necrosis of left toe(s)	39	Bone/Joint/Muscle Infections/Necrosis		0.401	0.378	0.558	0.682	0.443	0.435	0.401
M87.079	Idiopathic aseptic necrosis of unspecified toe(s)	39	Bone/Joint/Muscle Infections/Necrosis		0.401	0.378	0.558	0.682	0.443	0.435	0.401
M87.08	Idiopathic aseptic necrosis of bone, other site	39	Bone/Joint/Muscle Infections/Necrosis		0.401	0.378	0.558	0.682	0.443	0.435	0.401
M87.09	Idiopathic aseptic necrosis of bone, multiple sites	39	Bone/Joint/Muscle Infections/Necrosis		0.401	0.378	0.558	0.682	0.443	0.435	0.401
M87.10	Osteonecrosis due to drugs, unspecified bone	39	Bone/Joint/Muscle Infections/Necrosis		0.401	0.378	0.558	0.682	0.443	0.435	0.401
M87.111	Osteonecrosis due to drugs, right shoulder	39	Bone/Joint/Muscle Infections/Necrosis		0.401	0.378	0.558	0.682	0.443	0.435	0.401
M87.112	Osteonecrosis due to drugs, left shoulder	39	Bone/Joint/Muscle Infections/Necrosis		0.401	0.378	0.558	0.682	0.443	0.435	0.401
M87.119	Osteonecrosis due to drugs, unspecified shoulder	39	Bone/Joint/Muscle Infections/Necrosis		0.401	0.378	0.558	0.682	0.443	0.435	0.401
M87.121	Osteonecrosis due to drugs, right humerus	39	Bone/Joint/Muscle Infections/Necrosis		0.401	0.378	0.558	0.682	0.443	0.435	0.401
M87.122	Osteonecrosis due to drugs, left humerus	39	Bone/Joint/Muscle Infections/Necrosis		0.401	0.378	0.558	0.682	0.443	0.435	0.401
M87.129	Osteonecrosis due to drugs, unspecified humerus	39	Bone/Joint/Muscle Infections/Necrosis		0.401	0.378	0.558	0.682	0.443	0.435	0.401
M87.131	Osteonecrosis due to drugs of right radius	39	Bone/Joint/Muscle Infections/Necrosis		0.401	0.378	0.558	0.682	0.443	0.435	0.401
M87.132	Osteonecrosis due to drugs of left radius	39	Bone/Joint/Muscle Infections/Necrosis		0.401	0.378	0.558	0.682	0.443	0.435	0.401
M87.133	Osteonecrosis due to drugs of unspecified radius	39	Bone/Joint/Muscle Infections/Necrosis		0.401	0.378	0.558	0.682	0.443	0.435	0.401
M87.134	Osteonecrosis due to drugs of right ulna	39	Bone/Joint/Muscle Infections/Necrosis		0.401	0.378	0.558	0.682	0.443	0.435	0.401
M87.135	Osteonecrosis due to drugs of left ulna	39	Bone/Joint/Muscle Infections/Necrosis		0.401	0.378	0.558	0.682	0.443	0.435	0.401
M87.136	Osteonecrosis due to drugs of unspecified ulna	39	Bone/Joint/Muscle Infections/Necrosis		0.401	0.378	0.558	0.682	0.443	0.435	0.401
M87.137	Osteonecrosis due to drugs of right carpus	39	Bone/Joint/Muscle Infections/Necrosis		0.401	0.378	0.558	0.682	0.443	0.435	0.401
M87.138	Osteonecrosis due to drugs of left carpus	39	Bone/Joint/Muscle Infections/Necrosis		0.401	0.378	0.558	0.682	0.443	0.435	0.401
M87.139	Osteonecrosis due to drugs of unspecified carpus	39	Bone/Joint/Muscle Infections/Necrosis		0.401	0.378	0.558	0.682	0.443	0.435	0.401

ICD-10-CM Code	ICD-10-CM Code Description	V24 CMS-HCC	V24 CMS-HCC Disease Group	V24 CMS-HCC Hierarchies	Community, NonDual, Aged	Community, NonDual, Disabled	Community, FBDual, Aged	Community, FBDual, Disabled	Community, PBDual, Aged	Community, PBDual, Disabled	Institutional
M87.141	Osteonecrosis due to drugs, right hand	39	Bone/Joint/Muscle Infections/Necrosis		0.401	0.378	0.558	0.682	0.443	0.435	0.401
M87.142	Osteonecrosis due to drugs, left hand	39	Bone/Joint/Muscle Infections/Necrosis		0.401	0.378	0.558	0.682	0.443	0.435	0.401
M87.143	Osteonecrosis due to drugs, unspecified hand	39	Bone/Joint/Muscle Infections/Necrosis		0.401	0.378	0.558	0.682	0.443	0.435	0.401
M87.144	Osteonecrosis due to drugs, right finger(s)	39	Bone/Joint/Muscle Infections/Necrosis		0.401	0.378	0.558	0.682	0.443	0.435	0.401
M87.145	Osteonecrosis due to drugs, left finger(s)	39	Bone/Joint/Muscle Infections/Necrosis		0.401	0.378	0.558	0.682	0.443	0.435	0.401
M87.146	Osteonecrosis due to drugs, unspecified finger(s)	39	Bone/Joint/Muscle Infections/Necrosis		0.401	0.378	0.558	0.682	0.443	0.435	0.401
M87.15Ø	Osteonecrosis due to drugs, pelvis	39	Bone/Joint/Muscle Infections/Necrosis		0.401	0.378	0.558	0.682	0.443	0.435	0.401
M87.151	Osteonecrosis due to drugs, right femur	39	Bone/Joint/Muscle Infections/Necrosis		0.401	0.378	0.558	0.682	0.443	0.435	0.401
M87.152	Osteonecrosis due to drugs, left femur	39	Bone/Joint/Muscle Infections/Necrosis		0.401	0.378	0.558	0.682	0.443	0.435	0.401
M87.159	Osteonecrosis due to drugs, unspecified femur	39	Bone/Joint/Muscle Infections/Necrosis		0.401	0.378	0.558	0.682	0.443	0.435	0.401
M87.161	Osteonecrosis due to drugs, right tibia	39	Bone/Joint/Muscle Infections/Necrosis		0.401	0.378	0.558	0.682	0.443	0.435	0.401
M87.162	Osteonecrosis due to drugs, left tibia	39	Bone/Joint/Muscle Infections/Necrosis		0.401	0.378	0.558	0.682	0.443	0.435	0.401
M87.163	Osteonecrosis due to drugs, unspecified tibia	39	Bone/Joint/Muscle Infections/Necrosis		0.401	0.378	0.558	0.682	0.443	0.435	0.401
M87.164	Osteonecrosis due to drugs, right fibula	39	Bone/Joint/Muscle Infections/Necrosis		0.401	0.378	0.558	0.682	0.443	0.435	0.401
M87.165	Osteonecrosis due to drugs, left fibula	39	Bone/Joint/Muscle Infections/Necrosis		0.401	0.378	0.558	0.682	0.443	0.435	0.401
M87.166	Osteonecrosis due to drugs, unspecified fibula	39	Bone/Joint/Muscle Infections/Necrosis		0.401	0.378	0.558	0.682	0.443	0.435	0.401
M87.171	Osteonecrosis due to drugs, right ankle	39	Bone/Joint/Muscle Infections/Necrosis		0.401	0.378	0.558	0.682	0.443	0.435	0.401
M87.172	Osteonecrosis due to drugs, left ankle	39	Bone/Joint/Muscle Infections/Necrosis		0.401	0.378	0.558	0.682	0.443	0.435	0.401
M87.173	Osteonecrosis due to drugs, unspecified ankle	39	Bone/Joint/Muscle Infections/Necrosis		0.401	0.378	0.558	0.682	0.443	0.435	0.401
M87.174	Osteonecrosis due to drugs, right foot	39	Bone/Joint/Muscle Infections/Necrosis		0.401	0.378	0.558	0.682	0.443	0.435	0.401
M87.175	Osteonecrosis due to drugs, left foot	39	Bone/Joint/Muscle Infections/Necrosis		0.401	0.378	0.558	0.682	0.443	0.435	0.401
M87.176	Osteonecrosis due to drugs, unspecified foot	39	Bone/Joint/Muscle Infections/Necrosis		0.401	0.378	0.558	0.682	0.443	0.435	0.401
M87.177	Osteonecrosis due to drugs, right toe(s)	39	Bone/Joint/Muscle Infections/Necrosis		0.401	0.378	0.558	0.682	0.443	0.435	0.401
M87.178	Osteonecrosis due to drugs, left toe(s)	39	Bone/Joint/Muscle Infections/Necrosis		0.401	0.378	0.558	0.682	0.443	0.435	0.401
M87.179	Osteonecrosis due to drugs, unspecified toe(s)	39	Bone/Joint/Muscle Infections/Necrosis		0.401	0.378	0.558	0.682	0.443	0.435	0.401
M87.18Ø	Osteonecrosis due to drugs, jaw	39	Bone/Joint/Muscle Infections/Necrosis		0.401	0.378	0.558	0.682	0.443	0.435	0.401
M87.188	Osteonecrosis due to drugs, other site	39	Bone/Joint/Muscle Infections/Necrosis		0.401	0.378	0.558	0.682	0.443	0.435	0.401
M87.19	Osteonecrosis due to drugs, multiple sites	39	Bone/Joint/Muscle Infections/Necrosis		0.401	0.378	0.558	0.682	0.443	0.435	0.401
M87.2Ø	Osteonecrosis due to previous trauma, unspecified bone	39	Bone/Joint/Muscle Infections/Necrosis		0.401	0.378	0.558	0.682	0.443	0.435	0.401
M87.211	Osteonecrosis due to previous trauma, right shoulder	39	Bone/Joint/Muscle Infections/Necrosis		0.401	0.378	0.558	0.682	0.443	0.435	0.401
M87.212	Osteonecrosis due to previous trauma, left shoulder	39	Bone/Joint/Muscle Infections/Necrosis		0.401	0.378	0.558	0.682	0.443	0.435	0.401
M87.219	Osteonecrosis due to previous trauma, unspecified shoulder	39	Bone/Joint/Muscle Infections/Necrosis		0.401	0.378	0.558	0.682	0.443	0.435	0.401
M87.221	Osteonecrosis due to previous trauma, right humerus	39	Bone/Joint/Muscle Infections/Necrosis		0.401	0.378	0.558	0.682	0.443	0.435	0.401

2021 Optum360, LLC

ICD-10-CM Code	ICD-10-CM Code Description	V24 CMS-HCC	V24 CMS-HCC Disease Group	V24 CMS-HCC Hierarchies	Community, NonDual, Aged	Community, NonDual, Disabled	Community, FBDual, Aged	Community, FBDual, Disabled	Community, PBDual, Aged	Community, PBDual, Disabled	Institutional
M87.222	Osteonecrosis due to previous trauma, left humerus	39	Bone/Joint/Muscle Infections/Necrosis		0.401	0.378	0.558	0.682	0.443	0.435	0.401
M87.229	Osteonecrosis due to previous trauma, unspecified humerus	39	Bone/Joint/Muscle Infections/Necrosis		0.401	0.378	0.558	0.682	0.443	0.435	0.401
M87.231	Osteonecrosis due to previous trauma of right radius	39	Bone/Joint/Muscle Infections/Necrosis		0.401	0.378	0.558	0.682	0.443	0.435	0.401
M87.232	Osteonecrosis due to previous trauma of left radius	39	Bone/Joint/Muscle Infections/Necrosis		0.401	0.378	0.558	0.682	0.443	0.435	0.401
M87.233	Osteonecrosis due to previous trauma of unspecified radius	39	Bone/Joint/Muscle Infections/Necrosis		0.401	0.378	0.558	0.682	0.443	0.435	0.401
M87.234	Osteonecrosis due to previous trauma of right ulna	39	Bone/Joint/Muscle Infections/Necrosis		0.401	0.378	0.558	0.682	0.443	0.435	0.401
M87.235	Osteonecrosis due to previous trauma of left ulna	39	Bone/Joint/Muscle Infections/Necrosis		0.401	0.378	0.558	0.682	0.443	0.435	0.401
M87.236	Osteonecrosis due to previous trauma of unspecified ulna	39	Bone/Joint/Muscle Infections/Necrosis		0.401	0.378	0.558	0.682	0.443	0.435	0.401
M87.237	Osteonecrosis due to previous trauma of right carpus	39	Bone/Joint/Muscle Infections/Necrosis		0.401	0.378	0.558	0.682	0.443	0.435	0.401
M87.238	Osteonecrosis due to previous trauma of left carpus	39	Bone/Joint/Muscle Infections/Necrosis		0.401	0.378	0.558	0.682	0.443	0.435	0.401
M87.239	Osteonecrosis due to previous trauma of unspecified carpus	39	Bone/Joint/Muscle Infections/Necrosis		0.401	0.378	0.558	0.682	0.443	0.435	0.401
M87.241	Osteonecrosis due to previous trauma, right hand	39	Bone/Joint/Muscle Infections/Necrosis		0.401	0.378	0.558	0.682	0.443	0.435	0.401
M87.242	Osteonecrosis due to previous trauma, left hand	39	Bone/Joint/Muscle Infections/Necrosis		0.401	0.378	0.558	0.682	0.443	0.435	0.401
M87.243	Osteonecrosis due to previous trauma, unspecified hand	39	Bone/Joint/Muscle Infections/Necrosis		0.401	0.378	0.558	0.682	0.443	0.435	0.401
M87.244	Osteonecrosis due to previous trauma, right finger(s)	39	Bone/Joint/Muscle Infections/Necrosis		0.401	0.378	0.558	0.682	0.443	0.435	0.401
M87.245	Osteonecrosis due to previous trauma, left finger(s)	39	Bone/Joint/Muscle Infections/Necrosis		0.401	0.378	0.558	0.682	0.443	0.435	0.401
M87.246	Osteonecrosis due to previous trauma, unspecified finger(s)	39	Bone/Joint/Muscle Infections/Necrosis		0.401	0.378	0.558	0.682	0.443	0.435	0.401
M87.250	Osteonecrosis due to previous trauma, pelvis	39	Bone/Joint/Muscle Infections/Necrosis		0.401	0.378	0.558	0.682	0.443	0.435	0.401
M87.251	Osteonecrosis due to previous trauma, right femur	39	Bone/Joint/Muscle Infections/Necrosis		0.401	0.378	0.558	0.682	0.443	0.435	0.401
M87.252	Osteonecrosis due to previous trauma, left femur	39	Bone/Joint/Muscle Infections/Necrosis		0.401	0.378	0.558	0.682	0.443	0.435	0.401
M87.256	Osteonecrosis due to previous trauma, unspecified femur	39	Bone/Joint/Muscle Infections/Necrosis		0.401	0.378	0.558	0.682	0.443	0.435	0.401
M87.261	Osteonecrosis due to previous trauma, right tibia	39	Bone/Joint/Muscle Infections/Necrosis		0.401	0.378	0.558	0.682	0.443	0.435	0.401
M87.262	Osteonecrosis due to previous trauma, left tibia	39	Bone/Joint/Muscle Infections/Necrosis		0.401	0.378	0.558	0.682	0.443	0.435	0.401
M87.263	Osteonecrosis due to previous trauma, unspecified tibia	39	Bone/Joint/Muscle Infections/Necrosis		0.401	0.378	0.558	0.682	0.443	0.435	0.401
M87.264	Osteonecrosis due to previous trauma, right fibula	39	Bone/Joint/Muscle Infections/Necrosis		0.401	0.378	0.558	0.682	0.443	0.435	0.401
M87.265	Osteonecrosis due to previous trauma, left fibula	39	Bone/Joint/Muscle Infections/Necrosis		0.401	0.378	0.558	0.682	0.443	0.435	0.401
M87.266	Osteonecrosis due to previous trauma, unspecified fibula	39	Bone/Joint/Muscle Infections/Necrosis		0.401	0.378	0.558	0.682	0.443	0.435	0.401
M87.271	Osteonecrosis due to previous trauma, right ankle	39	Bone/Joint/Muscle Infections/Necrosis		0.401	0.378	0.558	0.682	0.443	0.435	0.401
M87.272	Osteonecrosis due to previous trauma, left ankle	39	Bone/Joint/Muscle Infections/Necrosis		0.401	0.378	0.558	0.682	0.443	0.435	0.401

ICD-10-CM Code	ICD-10-CM Code Description	V24 CMS-HCC	V24 CMS-HCC Disease Group	V24 CMS-HCC Hierarchies	Community, NonDual, Aged	Community, NonDual, Disabled	Community, FBDual, Aged	Community, FBDual, Disabled	Community, PBDual, Aged	Community, PBDual, Disabled	Institutional
M87.273	Osteonecrosis due to previous trauma, unspecified ankle	39	Bone/Joint/Muscle Infections/Necrosis		0.401	0.378	0.558	0.682	0.443	0.435	0.401
M87.274	Osteonecrosis due to previous trauma, right foot	39	Bone/Joint/Muscle Infections/Necrosis		0.401	0.378	0.558	0.682	0.443	0.435	0.401
M87.275	Osteonecrosis due to previous trauma, left foot	39	Bone/Joint/Muscle Infections/Necrosis		0.401	0.378	0.558	0.682	0.443	0.435	0.401
M87.276	Osteonecrosis due to previous trauma, unspecified foot	39	Bone/Joint/Muscle Infections/Necrosis		0.401	0.378	0.558	0.682	0.443	0.435	0.401
M87.277	Osteonecrosis due to previous trauma, right toe(s)	39	Bone/Joint/Muscle Infections/Necrosis		0.401	0.378	0.558	0.682	0.443	0.435	0.401
M87.278	Osteonecrosis due to previous trauma, left toe(s)	39	Bone/Joint/Muscle Infections/Necrosis		0.401	0.378	0.558	0.682	0.443	0.435	0.401
M87.279	Osteonecrosis due to previous trauma, unspecified toe(s)	39	Bone/Joint/Muscle Infections/Necrosis		0.401	0.378	0.558	0.682	0.443	0.435	0.401
M87.28	Osteonecrosis due to previous trauma, other site	39	Bone/Joint/Muscle Infections/Necrosis		0.401	0.378	0.558	0.682	0.443	0.435	0.401
M87.29	Osteonecrosis due to previous trauma, multiple sites	39	Bone/Joint/Muscle Infections/Necrosis		0.401	0.378	0.558	0.682	0.443	0.435	0.401
M87.30	Other secondary osteonecrosis, unspecified bone	39	Bone/Joint/Muscle Infections/Necrosis		0.401	0.378	0.558	0.682	0.443	0.435	0.401
M87.311	Other secondary osteonecrosis, right shoulder	39	Bone/Joint/Muscle Infections/Necrosis		0.401	0.378	0.558	0.682	0.443	0.435	0.401
M87.312	Other secondary osteonecrosis, left shoulder	39	Bone/Joint/Muscle Infections/Necrosis		0.401	0.378	0.558	0.682	0.443	0.435	0.401
M87.319	Other secondary osteonecrosis, unspecified shoulder	39	Bone/Joint/Muscle Infections/Necrosis		0.401	0.378	0.558	0.682	0.443	0.435	0.401
M87.321	Other secondary osteonecrosis, right humerus	39	Bone/Joint/Muscle Infections/Necrosis		0.401	0.378	0.558	0.682	0.443	0.435	0.401
M87.322	Other secondary osteonecrosis, left humerus	39	Bone/Joint/Muscle Infections/Necrosis		0.401	0.378	0.558	0.682	0.443	0.435	0.401
M87.329	Other secondary osteonecrosis, unspecified humerus	39	Bone/Joint/Muscle Infections/Necrosis		0.401	0.378	0.558	0.682	0.443	0.435	0.401
M87.331	Other secondary osteonecrosis of right radius	39	Bone/Joint/Muscle Infections/Necrosis		0.401	0.378	0.558	0.682	0.443	0.435	0.401
M87.332	Other secondary osteonecrosis of left radius	39	Bone/Joint/Muscle Infections/Necrosis		0.401	0.378	0.558	0.682	0.443	0.435	0.401
M87.333	Other secondary osteonecrosis of unspecified radius	39	Bone/Joint/Muscle Infections/Necrosis		0.401	0.378	0.558	0.682	0.443	0.435	0.401
M87.334	Other secondary osteonecrosis of right ulna	39	Bone/Joint/Muscle Infections/Necrosis		0.401	0.378	0.558	0.682	0.443	0.435	0.401
M87.335	Other secondary osteonecrosis of left ulna	39	Bone/Joint/Muscle Infections/Necrosis		0.401	0.378	0.558	0.682	0.443	0.435	0.401
M87.336	Other secondary osteonecrosis of unspecified ulna	39	Bone/Joint/Muscle Infections/Necrosis		0.401	0.378	0.558	0.682	0.443	0.435	0.401
M87.337	Other secondary osteonecrosis of right carpus	39	Bone/Joint/Muscle Infections/Necrosis		0.401	0.378	0.558	0.682	0.443	0.435	0.401
M87.338	Other secondary osteonecrosis of left carpus	39	Bone/Joint/Muscle Infections/Necrosis		0.401	0.378	0.558	0.682	0.443	0.435	0.401
M87.339	Other secondary osteonecrosis of unspecified carpus	39	Bone/Joint/Muscle Infections/Necrosis		0.401	0.378	0.558	0.682	0.443	0.435	0.401
M87.341	Other secondary osteonecrosis, right hand	39	Bone/Joint/Muscle Infections/Necrosis		0.401	0.378	0.558	0.682	0.443	0.435	0.401
M87.342	Other secondary osteonecrosis, left hand	39	Bone/Joint/Muscle Infections/Necrosis		0.401	0.378	0.558	0.682	0.443	0.435	0.401
M87.343	Other secondary osteonecrosis, unspecified hand	39	Bone/Joint/Muscle Infections/Necrosis		0.401	0.378	0.558	0.682	0.443	0.435	0.401
M87.344	Other secondary osteonecrosis, right finger(s)	39	Bone/Joint/Muscle Infections/Necrosis		0.401	0.378	0.558	0.682	0.443	0.435	0.401

ICD-10-CM Code	ICD-10-CM Code Description	V24 CMS-HCC	V24 CMS-HCC Disease Group	V24 CMS-HCC Hierarchies	Community, NonDual, Aged	Community, NonDual, Disabled	Community, FBDual, Aged	Community, FBDual, Disabled	Community, PBDual, Aged	Community, PBDual, Disabled	Institutional
M87.345	Other secondary osteonecrosis, left finger(s)	39	Bone/Joint/Muscle Infections/Necrosis		0.401	0.378	0.558	0.682	0.443	0.435	0.401
M87.346	Other secondary osteonecrosis, unspecified finger(s)	39	Bone/Joint/Muscle Infections/Necrosis		0.401	0.378	0.558	0.682	0.443	0.435	0.401
M87.350	Other secondary osteonecrosis, pelvis	39	Bone/Joint/Muscle Infections/Necrosis		0.401	0.378	0.558	0.682	0.443	0.435	0.401
M87.351	Other secondary osteonecrosis, right femur	39	Bone/Joint/Muscle Infections/Necrosis		0.401	0.378	0.558	0.682	0.443	0.435	0.401
M87.352	Other secondary osteonecrosis, left femur	39	Bone/Joint/Muscle Infections/Necrosis		0.401	0.378	0.558	0.682	0.443	0.435	0.401
M87.353	Other secondary osteonecrosis, unspecified femur	39	Bone/Joint/Muscle Infections/Necrosis		0.401	0.378	0.558	0.682	0.443	0.435	0.401
M87.361	Other secondary osteonecrosis, right tibia	39	Bone/Joint/Muscle Infections/Necrosis		0.401	0.378	0.558	0.682	0.443	0.435	0.401
M87.362	Other secondary osteonecrosis, left tibia	39	Bone/Joint/Muscle Infections/Necrosis		0.401	0.378	0.558	0.682	0.443	0.435	0.401
M87.363	Other secondary osteonecrosis, unspecified tibia	39	Bone/Joint/Muscle Infections/Necrosis		0.401	0.378	0.558	0.682	0.443	0.435	0.401
M87.364	Other secondary osteonecrosis, right fibula	39	Bone/Joint/Muscle Infections/Necrosis		0.401	0.378	0.558	0.682	0.443	0.435	0.401
M87.365	Other secondary osteonecrosis, left fibula	39	Bone/Joint/Muscle Infections/Necrosis		0.401	0.378	0.558	0.682	0.443	0.435	0.401
M87.366	Other secondary osteonecrosis, unspecified fibula	39	Bone/Joint/Muscle Infections/Necrosis		0.401	0.378	0.558	0.682	0.443	0.435	0.401
M87.371	Other secondary osteonecrosis, right ankle	39	Bone/Joint/Muscle Infections/Necrosis		0.401	0.378	0.558	0.682	0.443	0.435	0.401
M87.372	Other secondary osteonecrosis, left ankle	39	Bone/Joint/Muscle Infections/Necrosis		0.401	0.378	0.558	0.682	0.443	0.435	0.401
M87.373	Other secondary osteonecrosis, unspecified ankle	39	Bone/Joint/Muscle Infections/Necrosis		0.401	0.378	0.558	0.682	0.443	0.435	0.401
M87.374	Other secondary osteonecrosis, right foot	39	Bone/Joint/Muscle Infections/Necrosis		0.401	0.378	0.558	0.682	0.443	0.435	0.401
M87.375	Other secondary osteonecrosis, left foot	39	Bone/Joint/Muscle Infections/Necrosis		0.401	0.378	0.558	0.682	0.443	0.435	0.401
M87.376	Other secondary osteonecrosis, unspecified foot	39	Bone/Joint/Muscle Infections/Necrosis		0.401	0.378	0.558	0.682	0.443	0.435	0.401
M87.377	Other secondary osteonecrosis, right toe(s)	39	Bone/Joint/Muscle Infections/Necrosis		0.401	0.378	0.558	0.682	0.443	0.435	0.401
M87.378	Other secondary osteonecrosis, left toe(s)	39	Bone/Joint/Muscle Infections/Necrosis		0.401	0.378	0.558	0.682	0.443	0.435	0.401
M87.379	Other secondary osteonecrosis, unspecified toe(s)	39	Bone/Joint/Muscle Infections/Necrosis		0.401	0.378	0.558	0.682	0.443	0.435	0.401
M87.38	Other secondary osteonecrosis, other site	39	Bone/Joint/Muscle Infections/Necrosis		0.401	0.378	0.558	0.682	0.443	0.435	0.401
M87.39	Other secondary osteonecrosis, multiple sites	39	Bone/Joint/Muscle Infections/Necrosis		0.401	0.378	0.558	0.682	0.443	0.435	0.401
M87.80	Other osteonecrosis, unspecified bone	39	Bone/Joint/Muscle Infections/Necrosis		0.401	0.378	0.558	0.682	0.443	0.435	0.401
M87.811	Other osteonecrosis, right shoulder	39	Bone/Joint/Muscle Infections/Necrosis		0.401	0.378	0.558	0.682	0.443	0.435	0.401
M87.812	Other osteonecrosis, left shoulder	39	Bone/Joint/Muscle Infections/Necrosis		0.401	0.378	0.558	0.682	0.443	0.435	0.401
M87.819	Other osteonecrosis, unspecified shoulder	39	Bone/Joint/Muscle Infections/Necrosis		0.401	0.378	0.558	0.682	0.443	0.435	0.401
M87.821	Other osteonecrosis, right humerus	39	Bone/Joint/Muscle Infections/Necrosis		0.401	0.378	0.558	0.682	0.443	0.435	0.401
M87.822	Other osteonecrosis, left humerus	39	Bone/Joint/Muscle Infections/Necrosis		0.401	0.378	0.558	0.682	0.443	0.435	0.401
M87.829	Other osteonecrosis, unspecified humerus	39	Bone/Joint/Muscle Infections/Necrosis		0.401	0.378	0.558	0.682	0.443	0.435	0.401
M87.831	Other osteonecrosis of right radius	39	Bone/Joint/Muscle Infections/Necrosis		0.401	0.378	0.558	0.682	0.443	0.435	0.401
M87.832	Other osteonecrosis of left radius	39	Bone/Joint/Muscle Infections/Necrosis		0.401	0.378	0.558	0.682	0.443	0.435	0.401

ICD-10-CM Code	ICD-10-CM Code Description	V24 CMS-HCC	V24 CMS-HCC Disease Group	V24 CMS-HCC Hierarchies	Community, NonDual, Aged	Community, NonDual, Disabled	Community, FBDual, Aged	Community, FBDual, Disabled	Community, PBDual, Aged	Community, PBDual, Disabled	Institutional
M87.833	Other osteonecrosis of unspecified radius	39	Bone/Joint/Muscle Infections/Necrosis		0.401	0.378	0.558	0.682	0.443	0.435	0.401
M87.834	Other osteonecrosis of right ulna	39	Bone/Joint/Muscle Infections/Necrosis		0.401	0.378	0.558	0.682	0.443	0.435	0.401
M87.835	Other osteonecrosis of left ulna	39	Bone/Joint/Muscle Infections/Necrosis		0.401	0.378	0.558	0.682	0.443	0.435	0.401
M87.836	Other osteonecrosis of unspecified ulna	39	Bone/Joint/Muscle Infections/Necrosis		0.401	0.378	0.558	0.682	0.443	0.435	0.401
M87.837	Other osteonecrosis of right carpus	39	Bone/Joint/Muscle Infections/Necrosis		0.401	0.378	0.558	0.682	0.443	0.435	0.401
M87.838	Other osteonecrosis of left carpus	39	Bone/Joint/Muscle Infections/Necrosis		0.401	0.378	0.558	0.682	0.443	0.435	0.401
M87.839	Other osteonecrosis of unspecified carpus	39	Bone/Joint/Muscle Infections/Necrosis		0.401	0.378	0.558	0.682	0.443	0.435	0.401
M87.841	Other osteonecrosis, right hand	39	Bone/Joint/Muscle Infections/Necrosis		0.401	0.378	0.558	0.682	0.443	0.435	0.401
M87.842	Other osteonecrosis, left hand	39	Bone/Joint/Muscle Infections/Necrosis		0.401	0.378	0.558	0.682	0.443	0.435	0.401
M87.843	Other osteonecrosis, unspecified hand	39	Bone/Joint/Muscle Infections/Necrosis		0.401	0.378	0.558	0.682	0.443	0.435	0.401
M87.844	Other osteonecrosis, right finger(s)	39	Bone/Joint/Muscle Infections/Necrosis		0.401	0.378	0.558	0.682	0.443	0.435	0.401
M87.845	Other osteonecrosis, left finger(s)	39	Bone/Joint/Muscle Infections/Necrosis		0.401	0.378	0.558	0.682	0.443	0.435	0.401
M87.849	Other osteonecrosis, unspecified finger(s)	39	Bone/Joint/Muscle Infections/Necrosis		0.401	0.378	0.558	0.682	0.443	0.435	0.401
M87.85Ø	Other osteonecrosis, pelvis	39	Bone/Joint/Muscle Infections/Necrosis		0.401	0.378	0.558	0.682	0.443	0.435	0.401
M87.851	Other osteonecrosis, right femur	39	Bone/Joint/Muscle Infections/Necrosis		0.401	0.378	0.558	0.682	0.443	0.435	0.401
M87.852	Other osteonecrosis, left femur	39	Bone/Joint/Muscle Infections/Necrosis		0.401	0.378	0.558	0.682	0.443	0.435	0.401
M87.859	Other osteonecrosis, unspecified femur	39	Bone/Joint/Muscle Infections/Necrosis		0.401	0.378	0.558	0.682	0.443	0.435	0.401
M87.861	Other osteonecrosis, right tibia	39	Bone/Joint/Muscle Infections/Necrosis		0.401	0.378	0.558	0.682	0.443	0.435	0.401
M87.862	Other osteonecrosis, left tibia	39	Bone/Joint/Muscle Infections/Necrosis		0.401	0.378	0.558	0.682	0.443	0.435	0.401
M87.863	Other osteonecrosis, unspecified tibia	39	Bone/Joint/Muscle Infections/Necrosis		0.401	0.378	0.558	0.682	0.443	0.435	0.401
M87.864	Other osteonecrosis, right fibula	39	Bone/Joint/Muscle Infections/Necrosis		0.401	0.378	0.558	0.682	0.443	0.435	0.401
M87.865	Other osteonecrosis, left fibula	39	Bone/Joint/Muscle Infections/Necrosis		0.401	0.378	0.558	0.682	0.443	0.435	0.401
M87.869	Other osteonecrosis, unspecified fibula	39	Bone/Joint/Muscle Infections/Necrosis		0.401	0.378	0.558	0.682	0.443	0.435	0.401
M87.871	Other osteonecrosis, right ankle	39	Bone/Joint/Muscle Infections/Necrosis		0.401	0.378	0.558	0.682	0.443	0.435	0.401
M87.872	Other osteonecrosis, left ankle	39	Bone/Joint/Muscle Infections/Necrosis		0.401	0.378	0.558	0.682	0.443	0.435	0.401
M87.873	Other osteonecrosis, unspecified ankle	39	Bone/Joint/Muscle Infections/Necrosis		0.401	0.378	0.558	0.682	0.443	0.435	0.401
M87.874	Other osteonecrosis, right foot	39	Bone/Joint/Muscle Infections/Necrosis		0.401	0.378	0.558	0.682	0.443	0.435	0.401
M87.875	Other osteonecrosis, left foot	39	Bone/Joint/Muscle Infections/Necrosis		0.401	0.378	0.558	0.682	0.443	0.435	0.401
M87.876	Other osteonecrosis, unspecified foot	39	Bone/Joint/Muscle Infections/Necrosis		0.401	0.378	0.558	0.682	0.443	0.435	0.401
M87.877	Other osteonecrosis, right toe(s)	39	Bone/Joint/Muscle Infections/Necrosis		0.401	0.378	0.558	0.682	0.443	0.435	0.401
M87.878	Other osteonecrosis, left toe(s)	39	Bone/Joint/Muscle Infections/Necrosis		0.401	0.378	0.558	0.682	0.443	0.435	0.401
M87.879	Other osteonecrosis, unspecified toe(s)	39	Bone/Joint/Muscle Infections/Necrosis		0.401	0.378	0.558	0.682	0.443	0.435	0.401
M87.88	Other osteonecrosis, other site	39	Bone/Joint/Muscle Infections/Necrosis		0.401	0.378	0.558	0.682	0.443	0.435	0.401
M87.89	Other osteonecrosis, multiple sites	39	Bone/Joint/Muscle Infections/Necrosis		0.401	0.378	0.558	0.682	0.443	0.435	0.401
M87.9	Osteonecrosis, unspecified	39	Bone/Joint/Muscle Infections/Necrosis		0.401	0.378	0.558	0.682	0.443	0.435	0.401
M89.6Ø	Osteopathy after poliomyelitis, unspecified site	39	Bone/Joint/Muscle Infections/Necrosis		0.401	0.378	0.558	0.682	0.443	0.435	0.401
M89.611	Osteopathy after poliomyelitis, right shoulder	39	Bone/Joint/Muscle Infections/Necrosis		0.401	0.378	0.558	0.682	0.443	0.435	0.401
M89.612	Osteopathy after poliomyelitis, left shoulder	39	Bone/Joint/Muscle Infections/Necrosis		0.401	0.378	0.558	0.682	0.443	0.435	0.401
M89.619	Osteopathy after poliomyelitis, unspecified shoulder	39	Bone/Joint/Muscle Infections/Necrosis		0.401	0.378	0.558	0.682	0.443	0.435	0.401
M89.621	Osteopathy after poliomyelitis, right upper arm	39	Bone/Joint/Muscle Infections/Necrosis		0.401	0.378	0.558	0.682	0.443	0.435	0.401

ICD-10-CM Code	ICD-10-CM Code Description	V24 CMS-HCC	V24 CMS-HCC Disease Group	V24 CMS-HCC Hierarchies	Community, NonDual, Aged	Community, NonDual, Disabled	Community, FBDual, Aged	Community, FBDual, Disabled	Community, PBDual, Aged	Community, PBDual, Disabled	Institutional
M89.622	Osteopathy after poliomyelitis, left upper arm	39	Bone/Joint/Muscle Infections/Necrosis		0.401	0.378	0.558	0.682	0.443	0.435	0.401
M89.629	Osteopathy after poliomyelitis, unspecified upper arm	39	Bone/Joint/Muscle Infections/Necrosis		0.401	0.378	0.558	0.682	0.443	0.435	0.401
M89.631	Osteopathy after poliomyelitis, right forearm	39	Bone/Joint/Muscle Infections/Necrosis		0.401	0.378	0.558	0.682	0.443	0.435	0.401
M89.632	Osteopathy after poliomyelitis, left forearm	39	Bone/Joint/Muscle Infections/Necrosis		0.401	0.378	0.558	0.682	0.443	0.435	0.401
M89.639	Osteopathy after poliomyelitis, unspecified forearm	39	Bone/Joint/Muscle Infections/Necrosis		0.401	0.378	0.558	0.682	0.443	0.435	0.401
M89.641	Osteopathy after poliomyelitis, right hand	39	Bone/Joint/Muscle Infections/Necrosis		0.401	0.378	0.558	0.682	0.443	0.435	0.401
M89.642	Osteopathy after poliomyelitis, left hand	39	Bone/Joint/Muscle Infections/Necrosis		0.401	0.378	0.558	0.682	0.443	0.435	0.401
M89.649	Osteopathy after poliomyelitis, unspecified hand	39	Bone/Joint/Muscle Infections/Necrosis		0.401	0.378	0.558	0.682	0.443	0.435	0.401
M89.651	Osteopathy after poliomyelitis, right thigh	39	Bone/Joint/Muscle Infections/Necrosis		0.401	0.378	0.558	0.682	0.443	0.435	0.401
M89.652	Osteopathy after poliomyelitis, left thigh	39	Bone/Joint/Muscle Infections/Necrosis		0.401	0.378	0.558	0.682	0.443	0.435	0.401
M89.659	Osteopathy after poliomyelitis, unspecified thigh	39	Bone/Joint/Muscle Infections/Necrosis		0.401	0.378	0.558	0.682	0.443	0.435	0.401
M89.661	Osteopathy after poliomyelitis, right lower leg	39	Bone/Joint/Muscle Infections/Necrosis		0.401	0.378	0.558	0.682	0.443	0.435	0.401
M89.662	Osteopathy after poliomyelitis, left lower leg	39	Bone/Joint/Muscle Infections/Necrosis		0.401	0.378	0.558	0.682	0.443	0.435	0.401
M89.669	Osteopathy after poliomyelitis, unspecified lower leg	39	Bone/Joint/Muscle Infections/Necrosis		0.401	0.378	0.558	0.682	0.443	0.435	0.401
M89.671	Osteopathy after poliomyelitis, right ankle and foot	39	Bone/Joint/Muscle Infections/Necrosis		0.401	0.378	0.558	0.682	0.443	0.435	0.401
M89.672	Osteopathy after poliomyelitis, left ankle and foot	39	Bone/Joint/Muscle Infections/Necrosis		0.401	0.378	0.558	0.682	0.443	0.435	0.401
M89.679	Osteopathy after poliomyelitis, unspecified ankle and foot	39	Bone/Joint/Muscle Infections/Necrosis		0.401	0.378	0.558	0.682	0.443	0.435	0.401
M89.68	Osteopathy after poliomyelitis, other site	39	Bone/Joint/Muscle Infections/Necrosis		0.401	0.378	0.558	0.682	0.443	0.435	0.401
M89.69	Osteopathy after poliomyelitis, multiple sites	39	Bone/Joint/Muscle Infections/Necrosis		0.401	0.378	0.558	0.682	0.443	0.435	0.401
M90.50	Osteonecrosis in diseases classified elsewhere, unspecified site	39	Bone/Joint/Muscle Infections/Necrosis		0.401	0.378	0.558	0.682	0.443	0.435	0.401
M90.511	Osteonecrosis in diseases classified elsewhere, right shoulder	39	Bone/Joint/Muscle Infections/Necrosis		0.401	0.378	0.558	0.682	0.443	0.435	0.401
M90.512	Osteonecrosis in diseases classified elsewhere, left shoulder	39	Bone/Joint/Muscle Infections/Necrosis		0.401	0.378	0.558	0.682	0.443	0.435	0.401
M90.519	Osteonecrosis in diseases classified elsewhere, unspecified shoulder	39	Bone/Joint/Muscle Infections/Necrosis		0.401	0.378	0.558	0.682	0.443	0.435	0.401
M90.521	Osteonecrosis in diseases classified elsewhere, right upper arm	39	Bone/Joint/Muscle Infections/Necrosis		0.401	0.378	0.558	0.682	0.443	0.435	0.401
M90.522	Osteonecrosis in diseases classified elsewhere, left upper arm	39	Bone/Joint/Muscle Infections/Necrosis		0.401	0.378	0.558	0.682	0.443	0.435	0.401
M90.529	Osteonecrosis in diseases classified elsewhere, unspecified upper arm	39	Bone/Joint/Muscle Infections/Necrosis		0.401	0.378	0.558	0.682	0.443	0.435	0.401
M90.531	Osteonecrosis in diseases classified elsewhere, right forearm	39	Bone/Joint/Muscle Infections/Necrosis		0.401	0.378	0.558	0.682	0.443	0.435	0.401
M90.532	Osteonecrosis in diseases classified elsewhere, left forearm	39	Bone/Joint/Muscle Infections/Necrosis		0.401	0.378	0.558	0.682	0.443	0.435	0.401
M90.539	Osteonecrosis in diseases classified elsewhere, unspecified forearm	39	Bone/Joint/Muscle Infections/Necrosis		0.401	0.378	0.558	0.682	0.443	0.435	0.401

ICD-10-CM Code	ICD-10-CM Code Description	V24 CMS-HCC	V24 CMS-HCC Disease Group	V24 CMS-HCC Hierarchies	Community, NonDual, Aged	Community, NonDual, Disabled	Community, FBDual, Aged	Community, FBDual, Disabled	Community, PBDual, Aged	Community, PBDual, Disabled	Institutional
M90.541	Osteonecrosis in diseases classified elsewhere, right hand	39	Bone/Joint/Muscle Infections/Necrosis		0.401	0.378	0.558	0.682	0.443	0.435	0.401
M90.542	Osteonecrosis in diseases classified elsewhere, left hand	39	Bone/Joint/Muscle Infections/Necrosis		0.401	0.378	0.558	0.682	0.443	0.435	0.401
M90.549	Osteonecrosis in diseases classified elsewhere, unspecified hand	39	Bone/Joint/Muscle Infections/Necrosis		0.401	0.378	0.558	0.682	0.443	0.435	0.401
M90.551	Osteonecrosis in diseases classified elsewhere, right thigh	39	Bone/Joint/Muscle Infections/Necrosis		0.401	0.378	0.558	0.682	0.443	0.435	0.401
M90.552	Osteonecrosis in diseases classified elsewhere, left thigh	39	Bone/Joint/Muscle Infections/Necrosis		0.401	0.378	0.558	0.682	0.443	0.435	0.401
M90.559	Osteonecrosis in diseases classified elsewhere, unspecified thigh	39	Bone/Joint/Muscle Infections/Necrosis		0.401	0.378	0.558	0.682	0.443	0.435	0.401
M90.561	Osteonecrosis in diseases classified elsewhere, right lower leg	39	Bone/Joint/Muscle Infections/Necrosis		0.401	0.378	0.558	0.682	0.443	0.435	0.401
M90.562	Osteonecrosis in diseases classified elsewhere, left lower leg	39	Bone/Joint/Muscle Infections/Necrosis		0.401	0.378	0.558	0.682	0.443	0.435	0.401
M90.569	Osteonecrosis in diseases classified elsewhere, unspecified lower leg	39	Bone/Joint/Muscle Infections/Necrosis		0.401	0.378	0.558	0.682	0.443	0.435	0.401
M90.571	Osteonecrosis in diseases classified elsewhere, right ankle and foot	39	Bone/Joint/Muscle Infections/Necrosis		0.401	0.378	0.558	0.682	0.443	0.435	0.401
M90.572	Osteonecrosis in diseases classified elsewhere, left ankle and foot	39	Bone/Joint/Muscle Infections/Necrosis		0.401	0.378	0.558	0.682	0.443	0.435	0.401
M90.579	Osteonecrosis in diseases classified elsewhere, unspecified ankle and foot	39	Bone/Joint/Muscle Infections/Necrosis		0.401	0.378	0.558	0.682	0.443	0.435	0.401
M90.58	Osteonecrosis in diseases classified elsewhere, other site	39	Bone/Joint/Muscle Infections/Necrosis		0.401	0.378	0.558	0.682	0.443	0.435	0.401
M90.59	Osteonecrosis in diseases classified elsewhere, multiple sites	39	Bone/Joint/Muscle Infections/Necrosis		0.401	0.378	0.558	0.682	0.443	0.435	0.401
M96.621	Fracture of humerus following insertion of orthopedic implant, joint prosthesis, or bone plate, right arm	176	Complications of Specified Implanted Device or Graft		0.582	0.911	0.680	0.982	0.520	0.832	0.469
M96.622	Fracture of humerus following insertion of orthopedic implant, joint prosthesis, or bone plate, left arm	176	Complications of Specified Implanted Device or Graft		0.582	0.911	0.680	0.982	0.520	0.832	0.469
M96.629	Fracture of humerus following insertion of orthopedic implant, joint prosthesis, or bone plate, unspecified arm	176	Complications of Specified Implanted Device or Graft		0.582	0.911	0.680	0.982	0.520	0.832	0.469
M96.631	Fracture of radius or ulna following insertion of orthopedic implant, joint prosthesis, or bone plate, right arm	176	Complications of Specified Implanted Device or Graft		0.582	0.911	0.680	0.982	0.520	0.832	0.469
M96.632	Fracture of radius or ulna following insertion of orthopedic implant, joint prosthesis, or bone plate, left arm	176	Complications of Specified Implanted Device or Graft		0.582	0.911	0.680	0.982	0.520	0.832	0.469
M96.639	Fracture of radius or ulna following insertion of orthopedic implant, joint prosthesis, or bone plate, unspecified arm	176	Complications of Specified Implanted Device or Graft		0.582	0.911	0.680	0.982	0.520	0.832	0.469
M96.65	Fracture of pelvis following insertion of orthopedic implant, joint prosthesis, or bone plate	176	Complications of Specified Implanted Device or Graft		0.582	0.911	0.680	0.982	0.520	0.832	0.469
M96.661	Fracture of femur following insertion of orthopedic implant, joint prosthesis, or bone plate, right leg	176	Complications of Specified Implanted Device or Graft		0.582	0.911	0.680	0.982	0.520	0.832	0.469
M96.662	Fracture of femur following insertion of orthopedic implant, joint prosthesis, or bone plate, left leg	176	Complications of Specified Implanted Device or Graft		0.582	0.911	0.680	0.982	0.520	0.832	0.469

ICD-10-CM Code	ICD-10-CM Code Description	V24 CMS-HCC	V24 CMS-HCC Disease Group	V24 CMS-HCC Hierarchies	Community, NonDual, Aged	Community, NonDual, Disabled	Community, FBDual, Aged	Community, FBDual, Disabled	Community, PBDual, Aged	Community, PBDual, Disabled	Institutional
M96.669	Fracture of femur following insertion of orthopedic implant, joint prosthesis, or bone plate, unspecified leg	176	Complications of Specified Implanted Device or Graft		0.582	0.911	0.680	0.982	0.520	0.832	0.469
M96.671	Fracture of tibia or fibula following insertion of orthopedic implant, joint prosthesis, or bone plate, right leg	176	Complications of Specified Implanted Device or Graft		0.582	0.911	0.680	0.982	0.520	0.832	0.469
M96.672	Fracture of tibia or fibula following insertion of orthopedic implant, joint prosthesis, or bone plate, left leg	176	Complications of Specified Implanted Device or Graft		0.582	0.911	0.680	0.982	0.520	0.832	0.469
M96.679	Fracture of tibia or fibula following insertion of orthopedic implant, joint prosthesis, or bone plate, unspecified leg	176	Complications of Specified Implanted Device or Graft		0.582	0.911	0.680	0.982	0.520	0.832	0.469
M96.69	Fracture of other bone following insertion of orthopedic implant, joint prosthesis, or bone plate	176	Complications of Specified Implanted Device or Graft		0.582	0.911	0.680	0.982	0.520	0.832	0.469
M97.01XA	Periprosthetic fracture around internal prosthetic right hip joint, initial encounter	170	Hip Fracture/Dislocation		0.350	0.394	0.409	0.469	0.354	0.333	—
M97.02XA	Periprosthetic fracture around internal prosthetic left hip joint, initial encounter	170	Hip Fracture/Dislocation		0.350	0.394	0.409	0.469	0.354	0.333	—
N17.0	Acute kidney failure with tubular necrosis	135	Acute Renal Failure	136,137, 138	0.435	0.406	0.683	0.594	0.446	0.480	0.468
N17.1	Acute kidney failure with acute cortical necrosis	135	Acute Renal Failure	136,137, 138	0.435	0.406	0.683	0.594	0.446	0.480	0.468
N17.2	Acute kidney failure with medullary necrosis	135	Acute Renal Failure	136,137, 138	0.435	0.406	0.683	0.594	0.446	0.480	0.468
N17.8	Other acute kidney failure	135	Acute Renal Failure	136,137, 138	0.435	0.406	0.683	0.594	0.446	0.480	0.468
N17.9	Acute kidney failure, unspecified	135	Acute Renal Failure	136,137, 138	0.435	0.406	0.683	0.594	0.446	0.480	0.468
N18.30	Chronic kidney disease, stage 3 unspecified	138	Chronic Kidney Disease, Moderate (Stage 3)		0.069	0.021	0.017	—	0.043	—	0.092
N18.31	Chronic kidney disease, stage 3a	138	Chronic Kidney Disease, Moderate (Stage 3)		0.069	0.021	0.017	—	0.043	—	0.092
N18.32	Chronic kidney disease, stage 3b	138	Chronic Kidney Disease, Moderate (Stage 3)		0.069	0.021	0.017	—	0.043	—	0.092
N18.4	Chronic kidney disease, stage 4 (severe)	137	Chronic Kidney Disease, Severe (Stage 4)	138	0.289	0.105	0.260	0.138	0.280	0.039	0.201
N18.5	Chronic kidney disease, stage 5	136	Chronic Kidney Disease, Stage 5	137,138	0.289	0.231	0.260	0.323	0.280	0.261	0.245
N18.6	End stage renal disease	136	Chronic Kidney Disease, Stage 5	137,138	0.289	0.231	0.260	0.323	0.280	0.261	0.245
N25.1	Nephrogenic diabetes insipidus	23	Other Significant Endocrine and Metabolic Disorders		0.194	0.378	0.211	0.299	0.174	0.319	0.379
N25.81	Secondary hyperparathyroidism of renal origin	23	Other Significant Endocrine and Metabolic Disorders		0.194	0.378	0.211	0.299	0.174	0.319	0.379
N28.0	Ischemia and infarction of kidney	107	Vascular Disease with Complications	108	0.383	0.464	0.565	0.653	0.463	0.450	0.299
N99.510	Cystostomy hemorrhage	176	Complications of Specified Implanted Device or Graft		0.582	0.911	0.680	0.982	0.520	0.832	0.469
N99.511	Cystostomy infection	176	Complications of Specified Implanted Device or Graft		0.582	0.911	0.680	0.982	0.520	0.832	0.469
N99.512	Cystostomy malfunction	176	Complications of Specified Implanted Device or Graft		0.582	0.911	0.680	0.982	0.520	0.832	0.469
N99.518	Other cystostomy complication	176	Complications of Specified Implanted Device or Graft		0.582	0.911	0.680	0.982	0.520	0.832	0.469
N99.520	Hemorrhage of incontinent external stoma of urinary tract	176	Complications of Specified Implanted Device or Graft		0.582	0.911	0.680	0.982	0.520	0.832	0.469

ICD-10-CM Code	ICD-10-CM Code Description	V24 CMS-HCC	V24 CMS-HCC Disease Group	V24 CMS-HCC Hierarchies	Community, NonDual, Aged	Community, NonDual, Disabled	Community, FBDual, Aged	Community, FBDual, Disabled	Community, PBDual, Aged	Community, PBDual, Disabled	Institutional
N99.521	Infection of incontinent external stoma of urinary tract	176	Complications of Specified Implanted Device or Graft		0.582	0.911	0.680	0.982	0.520	0.832	0.469
N99.522	Malfunction of incontinent external stoma of urinary tract	176	Complications of Specified Implanted Device or Graft		0.582	0.911	0.680	0.982	0.520	0.832	0.469
N99.523	Herniation of incontinent stoma of urinary tract	176	Complications of Specified Implanted Device or Graft		0.582	0.911	0.680	0.982	0.520	0.832	0.469
N99.524	Stenosis of incontinent stoma of urinary tract	176	Complications of Specified Implanted Device or Graft		0.582	0.911	0.680	0.982	0.520	0.832	0.469
N99.528	Other complication of incontinent external stoma of urinary tract	176	Complications of Specified Implanted Device or Graft		0.582	0.911	0.680	0.982	0.520	0.832	0.469
N99.530	Hemorrhage of continent stoma of urinary tract	176	Complications of Specified Implanted Device or Graft		0.582	0.911	0.680	0.982	0.520	0.832	0.469
N99.531	Infection of continent stoma of urinary tract	176	Complications of Specified Implanted Device or Graft		0.582	0.911	0.680	0.982	0.520	0.832	0.469
N99.532	Malfunction of continent stoma of urinary tract	176	Complications of Specified Implanted Device or Graft		0.582	0.911	0.680	0.982	0.520	0.832	0.469
N99.533	Herniation of continent stoma of urinary tract	176	Complications of Specified Implanted Device or Graft		0.582	0.911	0.680	0.982	0.520	0.832	0.469
N99.534	Stenosis of continent stoma of urinary tract	176	Complications of Specified Implanted Device or Graft		0.582	0.911	0.680	0.982	0.520	0.832	0.469
N99.538	Other complication of continent stoma of urinary tract	176	Complications of Specified Implanted Device or Graft		0.582	0.911	0.680	0.982	0.520	0.832	0.469
P02.70	Newborn affected by fetal inflammatory response syndrome	2	Septicemia, Sepsis, Systemic Inflammatory Response Syndrome/Shock		0.352	0.414	0.453	0.530	0.316	0.297	0.324
P36.0	Sepsis of newborn due to streptococcus, group B	2	Septicemia, Sepsis, Systemic Inflammatory Response Syndrome/Shock		0.352	0.414	0.453	0.530	0.316	0.297	0.324
P36.10	Sepsis of newborn due to unspecified streptococci	2	Septicemia, Sepsis, Systemic Inflammatory Response Syndrome/Shock		0.352	0.414	0.453	0.530	0.316	0.297	0.324
P36.19	Sepsis of newborn due to other streptococci	2	Septicemia, Sepsis, Systemic Inflammatory Response Syndrome/Shock		0.352	0.414	0.453	0.530	0.316	0.297	0.324
P36.2	Sepsis of newborn due to Staphylococcus aureus	2	Septicemia, Sepsis, Systemic Inflammatory Response Syndrome/Shock		0.352	0.414	0.453	0.530	0.316	0.297	0.324
P36.30	Sepsis of newborn due to unspecified staphylococci	2	Septicemia, Sepsis, Systemic Inflammatory Response Syndrome/Shock		0.352	0.414	0.453	0.530	0.316	0.297	0.324
P36.39	Sepsis of newborn due to other staphylococci	2	Septicemia, Sepsis, Systemic Inflammatory Response Syndrome/Shock		0.352	0.414	0.453	0.530	0.316	0.297	0.324
P36.4	Sepsis of newborn due to Escherichia coli	2	Septicemia, Sepsis, Systemic Inflammatory Response Syndrome/Shock		0.352	0.414	0.453	0.530	0.316	0.297	0.324
P36.5	Sepsis of newborn due to anaerobes	2	Septicemia, Sepsis, Systemic Inflammatory Response Syndrome/Shock		0.352	0.414	0.453	0.530	0.316	0.297	0.324
P36.8	Other bacterial sepsis of newborn	2	Septicemia, Sepsis, Systemic Inflammatory Response Syndrome/Shock		0.352	0.414	0.453	0.530	0.316	0.297	0.324
P36.9	Bacterial sepsis of newborn, unspecified	2	Septicemia, Sepsis, Systemic Inflammatory Response Syndrome/Shock		0.352	0.414	0.453	0.530	0.316	0.297	0.324
P91.821	Neonatal cerebral infarction, right side of brain	100	Ischemic or Unspecified Stroke		0.230	0.146	0.380	0.324	0.230	0.163	0.111
P91.822	Neonatal cerebral infarction, left side of brain	100	Ischemic or Unspecified Stroke		0.230	0.146	0.380	0.324	0.230	0.163	0.111
P91.823	Neonatal cerebral infarction, bilateral	100	Ischemic or Unspecified Stroke		0.230	0.146	0.380	0.324	0.230	0.163	0.111

ICD-10-CM Code	ICD-10-CM Code Description	V24 CMS-HCC	V24 CMS-HCC Disease Group	V24 CMS-HCC Hierarchies	Community, NonDual, Aged	Community, NonDual, Disabled	Community, FBDual, Aged	Community, FBDual, Disabled	Community, PBDual, Aged	Community, PBDual, Disabled	Institutional
P91.829	Neonatal cerebral infarction, unspecified side	100	Ischemic or Unspecified Stroke		0.230	0.146	0.380	0.324	0.230	0.163	0.111
Q00.0	Anencephaly	72	Spinal Cord Disorders/Injuries	169	0.481	0.369	0.532	0.377	0.512	0.336	0.289
Q00.1	Craniorachischisis	72	Spinal Cord Disorders/Injuries	169	0.481	0.369	0.532	0.377	0.512	0.336	0.289
Q00.2	Iniencephaly	72	Spinal Cord Disorders/Injuries	169	0.481	0.369	0.532	0.377	0.512	0.336	0.289
Q01.0	Frontal encephalocele	72	Spinal Cord Disorders/Injuries	169	0.481	0.369	0.532	0.377	0.512	0.336	0.289
Q01.1	Nasofrontal encephalocele	72	Spinal Cord Disorders/Injuries	169	0.481	0.369	0.532	0.377	0.512	0.336	0.289
Q01.2	Occipital encephalocele	72	Spinal Cord Disorders/Injuries	169	0.481	0.369	0.532	0.377	0.512	0.336	0.289
Q01.8	Encephalocele of other sites	72	Spinal Cord Disorders/Injuries	169	0.481	0.369	0.532	0.377	0.512	0.336	0.289
Q01.9	Encephalocele, unspecified	72	Spinal Cord Disorders/Injuries	169	0.481	0.369	0.532	0.377	0.512	0.336	0.289
Q02	Microcephaly	72	Spinal Cord Disorders/Injuries	169	0.481	0.369	0.532	0.377	0.512	0.336	0.289
Q03.0	Malformations of aqueduct of Sylvius	72	Spinal Cord Disorders/Injuries	169	0.481	0.369	0.532	0.377	0.512	0.336	0.289
Q03.1	Atresia of foramina of Magendie and Luschka	72	Spinal Cord Disorders/Injuries	169	0.481	0.369	0.532	0.377	0.512	0.336	0.289
Q03.8	Other congenital hydrocephalus	72	Spinal Cord Disorders/Injuries	169	0.481	0.369	0.532	0.377	0.512	0.336	0.289
Q03.9	Congenital hydrocephalus, unspecified	72	Spinal Cord Disorders/Injuries	169	0.481	0.369	0.532	0.377	0.512	0.336	0.289
Q04.0	Congenital malformations of corpus callosum	72	Spinal Cord Disorders/Injuries	169	0.481	0.369	0.532	0.377	0.512	0.336	0.289
Q04.1	Arhinencephaly	72	Spinal Cord Disorders/Injuries	169	0.481	0.369	0.532	0.377	0.512	0.336	0.289
Q04.2	Holoprosencephaly	72	Spinal Cord Disorders/Injuries	169	0.481	0.369	0.532	0.377	0.512	0.336	0.289
Q04.3	Other reduction deformities of brain	72	Spinal Cord Disorders/Injuries	169	0.481	0.369	0.532	0.377	0.512	0.336	0.289
Q04.4	Septo-optic dysplasia of brain	72	Spinal Cord Disorders/Injuries	169	0.481	0.369	0.532	0.377	0.512	0.336	0.289
Q04.5	Megalencephaly	72	Spinal Cord Disorders/Injuries	169	0.481	0.369	0.532	0.377	0.512	0.336	0.289
Q04.6	Congenital cerebral cysts	72	Spinal Cord Disorders/Injuries	169	0.481	0.369	0.532	0.377	0.512	0.336	0.289
Q04.8	Other specified congenital malformations of brain	72	Spinal Cord Disorders/Injuries	169	0.481	0.369	0.532	0.377	0.512	0.336	0.289
Q04.9	Congenital malformation of brain, unspecified	72	Spinal Cord Disorders/Injuries	169	0.481	0.369	0.532	0.377	0.512	0.336	0.289
Q05.0	Cervical spina bifida with hydrocephalus	72	Spinal Cord Disorders/Injuries	169	0.481	0.369	0.532	0.377	0.512	0.336	0.289
Q05.1	Thoracic spina bifida with hydrocephalus	72	Spinal Cord Disorders/Injuries	169	0.481	0.369	0.532	0.377	0.512	0.336	0.289
Q05.2	Lumbar spina bifida with hydrocephalus	72	Spinal Cord Disorders/Injuries	169	0.481	0.369	0.532	0.377	0.512	0.336	0.289
Q05.3	Sacral spina bifida with hydrocephalus	72	Spinal Cord Disorders/Injuries	169	0.481	0.369	0.532	0.377	0.512	0.336	0.289
Q05.4	Unspecified spina bifida with hydrocephalus	72	Spinal Cord Disorders/Injuries	169	0.481	0.369	0.532	0.377	0.512	0.336	0.289
Q05.5	Cervical spina bifida without hydrocephalus	72	Spinal Cord Disorders/Injuries	169	0.481	0.369	0.532	0.377	0.512	0.336	0.289
Q05.6	Thoracic spina bifida without hydrocephalus	72	Spinal Cord Disorders/Injuries	169	0.481	0.369	0.532	0.377	0.512	0.336	0.289
Q05.7	Lumbar spina bifida without hydrocephalus	72	Spinal Cord Disorders/Injuries	169	0.481	0.369	0.532	0.377	0.512	0.336	0.289
Q05.8	Sacral spina bifida without hydrocephalus	72	Spinal Cord Disorders/Injuries	169	0.481	0.369	0.532	0.377	0.512	0.336	0.289
Q05.9	Spina bifida, unspecified	72	Spinal Cord Disorders/Injuries	169	0.481	0.369	0.532	0.377	0.512	0.336	0.289
Q06.0	Amyelia	72	Spinal Cord Disorders/Injuries	169	0.481	0.369	0.532	0.377	0.512	0.336	0.289
Q06.1	Hypoplasia and dysplasia of spinal cord	72	Spinal Cord Disorders/Injuries	169	0.481	0.369	0.532	0.377	0.512	0.336	0.289
Q06.2	Diastematomyelia	72	Spinal Cord Disorders/Injuries	169	0.481	0.369	0.532	0.377	0.512	0.336	0.289
Q06.3	Other congenital cauda equina malformations	72	Spinal Cord Disorders/Injuries	169	0.481	0.369	0.532	0.377	0.512	0.336	0.289
Q06.4	Hydromyelia	72	Spinal Cord Disorders/Injuries	169	0.481	0.369	0.532	0.377	0.512	0.336	0.289

ICD-10-CM Code	ICD-10-CM Code Description	V24 CMS-HCC	V24 CMS-HCC Disease Group	V24 CMS-HCC Hierarchies	Community, NonDual, Aged	Community, NonDual, Disabled	Community, FBDual, Aged	Community, FBDual, Disabled	Community, PBDual, Aged	Community, PBDual, Disabled	Institutional
Q06.8	Other specified congenital malformations of spinal cord	72	Spinal Cord Disorders/Injuries	169	0.481	0.369	0.532	0.377	0.512	0.336	0.289
Q06.9	Congenital malformation of spinal cord, unspecified	72	Spinal Cord Disorders/Injuries	169	0.481	0.369	0.532	0.377	0.512	0.336	0.289
Q07.00	Arnold-Chiari syndrome without spina bifida or hydrocephalus	72	Spinal Cord Disorders/Injuries	169	0.481	0.369	0.532	0.377	0.512	0.336	0.289
Q07.01	Arnold-Chiari syndrome with spina bifida	72	Spinal Cord Disorders/Injuries	169	0.481	0.369	0.532	0.377	0.512	0.336	0.289
Q07.02	Arnold-Chiari syndrome with hydrocephalus	72	Spinal Cord Disorders/Injuries	169	0.481	0.369	0.532	0.377	0.512	0.336	0.289
Q07.03	Arnold-Chiari syndrome with spina bifida and hydrocephalus	72	Spinal Cord Disorders/Injuries	169	0.481	0.369	0.532	0.377	0.512	0.336	0.289
Q07.8	Other specified congenital malformations of nervous system	72	Spinal Cord Disorders/Injuries	169	0.481	0.369	0.532	0.377	0.512	0.336	0.289
Q07.9	Congenital malformation of nervous system, unspecified	72	Spinal Cord Disorders/Injuries	169	0.481	0.369	0.532	0.377	0.512	0.336	0.289
Q85.00	Neurofibromatosis, unspecified	12	Breast, Prostate, and Other Cancers and Tumors		0.150	0.212	0.158	0.212	0.154	0.181	0.210
Q85.01	Neurofibromatosis, type 1	12	Breast, Prostate, and Other Cancers and Tumors		0.150	0.212	0.158	0.212	0.154	0.181	0.210
Q85.02	Neurofibromatosis, type 2	12	Breast, Prostate, and Other Cancers and Tumors		0.150	0.212	0.158	0.212	0.154	0.181	0.210
Q85.03	Schwannomatosis	12	Breast, Prostate, and Other Cancers and Tumors		0.150	0.212	0.158	0.212	0.154	0.181	0.210
Q85.09	Other neurofibromatosis	12	Breast, Prostate, and Other Cancers and Tumors		0.150	0.212	0.158	0.212	0.154	0.181	0.210
Q85.1	Tuberous sclerosis	12	Breast, Prostate, and Other Cancers and Tumors		0.150	0.212	0.158	0.212	0.154	0.181	0.210
Q85.8	Other phakomatoses, not elsewhere classified	12	Breast, Prostate, and Other Cancers and Tumors		0.150	0.212	0.158	0.212	0.154	0.181	0.210
Q85.9	Phakomatosis, unspecified	12	Breast, Prostate, and Other Cancers and Tumors		0.150	0.212	0.158	0.212	0.154	0.181	0.210
R09.2	Respiratory arrest	83	Respiratory Arrest	84	0.354	0.400	0.902	0.531	0.361	0.769	0.511
R40.20	Unspecified coma	80	Coma, Brain Compression/Anoxic Damage		0.486	0.274	0.511	0.105	0.729	0.134	—
R40.2110	Coma scale, eyes open, never, unspecified time	80	Coma, Brain Compression/Anoxic Damage		0.486	0.274	0.511	0.105	0.729	0.134	—
R40.2111	Coma scale, eyes open, never, in the field [EMT or ambulance]	80	Coma, Brain Compression/Anoxic Damage		0.486	0.274	0.511	0.105	0.729	0.134	—
R40.2112	Coma scale, eyes open, never, at arrival to emergency department	80	Coma, Brain Compression/Anoxic Damage		0.486	0.274	0.511	0.105	0.729	0.134	—
R40.2113	Coma scale, eyes open, never, at hospital admission	80	Coma, Brain Compression/Anoxic Damage		0.486	0.274	0.511	0.105	0.729	0.134	—
R40.2114	Coma scale, eyes open, never, 24 hours or more after hospital admission	80	Coma, Brain Compression/Anoxic Damage		0.486	0.274	0.511	0.105	0.729	0.134	—
R40.2120	Coma scale, eyes open, to pain, unspecified time	80	Coma, Brain Compression/Anoxic Damage		0.486	0.274	0.511	0.105	0.729	0.134	—
R40.2121	Coma scale, eyes open, to pain, in the field [EMT or ambulance]	80	Coma, Brain Compression/Anoxic Damage		0.486	0.274	0.511	0.105	0.729	0.134	—
R40.2122	Coma scale, eyes open, to pain, at arrival to emergency department	80	Coma, Brain Compression/Anoxic Damage		0.486	0.274	0.511	0.105	0.729	0.134	—
R40.2123	Coma scale, eyes open, to pain, at hospital admission	80	Coma, Brain Compression/Anoxic Damage		0.486	0.274	0.511	0.105	0.729	0.134	—
R40.2124	Coma scale, eyes open, to pain, 24 hours or more after hospital admission	80	Coma, Brain Compression/Anoxic Damage		0.486	0.274	0.511	0.105	0.729	0.134	—
R40.2210	Coma scale, best verbal response, none, unspecified time	80	Coma, Brain Compression/Anoxic Damage		0.486	0.274	0.511	0.105	0.729	0.134	—

ICD-10-CM Code	ICD-10-CM Code Description	V24 CMS-HCC	V24 CMS-HCC Disease Group	V24 CMS-HCC Hierarchies	Community, NonDual, Aged	Community, NonDual, Disabled	Community, FBDual, Aged	Community, FBDual, Disabled	Community, PBDual, Aged	Community, PBDual, Disabled	Institutional
R40.2211	Coma scale, best verbal response, none, in the field [EMT or ambulance]	80	Coma, Brain Compression/Anoxic Damage		0.486	0.274	0.511	0.105	0.729	0.134	—
R40.2212	Coma scale, best verbal response, none, at arrival to emergency department	80	Coma, Brain Compression/Anoxic Damage		0.486	0.274	0.511	0.105	0.729	0.134	—
R40.2213	Coma scale, best verbal response, none, at hospital admission	80	Coma, Brain Compression/Anoxic Damage		0.486	0.274	0.511	0.105	0.729	0.134	—
R40.2214	Coma scale, best verbal response, none, 24 hours or more after hospital admission	80	Coma, Brain Compression/Anoxic Damage		0.486	0.274	0.511	0.105	0.729	0.134	—
R40.2220	Coma scale, best verbal response, incomprehensible words, unspecified time	80	Coma, Brain Compression/Anoxic Damage		0.486	0.274	0.511	0.105	0.729	0.134	—
R40.2221	Coma scale, best verbal response, incomprehensible words, in the field [EMT or ambulance]	80	Coma, Brain Compression/Anoxic Damage		0.486	0.274	0.511	0.105	0.729	0.134	—
R40.2222	Coma scale, best verbal response, incomprehensible words, at arrival to emergency department	80	Coma, Brain Compression/Anoxic Damage		0.486	0.274	0.511	0.105	0.729	0.134	—
R40.2223	Coma scale, best verbal response, incomprehensible words, at hospital admission	80	Coma, Brain Compression/Anoxic Damage		0.486	0.274	0.511	0.105	0.729	0.134	—
R40.2224	Coma scale, best verbal response, incomprehensible words, 24 hours or more after hospital admission	80	Coma, Brain Compression/Anoxic Damage		0.486	0.274	0.511	0.105	0.729	0.134	—
R40.2310	Coma scale, best motor response, none, unspecified time	80	Coma, Brain Compression/Anoxic Damage		0.486	0.274	0.511	0.105	0.729	0.134	—
R40.2311	Coma scale, best motor response, none, in the field [EMT or ambulance]	80	Coma, Brain Compression/Anoxic Damage		0.486	0.274	0.511	0.105	0.729	0.134	—
R40.2312	Coma scale, best motor response, none, at arrival to emergency department	80	Coma, Brain Compression/Anoxic Damage		0.486	0.274	0.511	0.105	0.729	0.134	—
R40.2313	Coma scale, best motor response, none, at hospital admission	80	Coma, Brain Compression/Anoxic Damage		0.486	0.274	0.511	0.105	0.729	0.134	—
R40.2314	Coma scale, best motor response, none, 24 hours or more after hospital admission	80	Coma, Brain Compression/Anoxic Damage		0.486	0.274	0.511	0.105	0.729	0.134	—
R40.2320	Coma scale, best motor response, extension, unspecified time	80	Coma, Brain Compression/Anoxic Damage		0.486	0.274	0.511	0.105	0.729	0.134	—
R40.2321	Coma scale, best motor response, extension, in the field [EMT or ambulance]	80	Coma, Brain Compression/Anoxic Damage		0.486	0.274	0.511	0.105	0.729	0.134	—
R40.2322	Coma scale, best motor response, extension, at arrival to emergency department	80	Coma, Brain Compression/Anoxic Damage		0.486	0.274	0.511	0.105	0.729	0.134	—
R40.2323	Coma scale, best motor response, extension, at hospital admission	80	Coma, Brain Compression/Anoxic Damage		0.486	0.274	0.511	0.105	0.729	0.134	—
R40.2324	Coma scale, best motor response, extension, 24 hours or more after hospital admission	80	Coma, Brain Compression/Anoxic Damage		0.486	0.274	0.511	0.105	0.729	0.134	—
R40.2340	Coma scale, best motor response, flexion withdrawal, unspecified time	80	Coma, Brain Compression/Anoxic Damage		0.486	0.274	0.511	0.105	0.729	0.134	—
R40.2341	Coma scale, best motor response, flexion withdrawal, in the field [EMT or ambulance]	80	Coma, Brain Compression/Anoxic Damage		0.486	0.274	0.511	0.105	0.729	0.134	—
R40.2342	Coma scale, best motor response, flexion withdrawal, at arrival to emergency department	80	Coma, Brain Compression/Anoxic Damage		0.486	0.274	0.511	0.105	0.729	0.134	—
R40.2343	Coma scale, best motor response, flexion withdrawal, at hospital admission	80	Coma, Brain Compression/Anoxic Damage		0.486	0.274	0.511	0.105	0.729	0.134	—

ICD-10-CM Code	ICD-10-CM Code Description	V24 CMS-HCC	V24 CMS-HCC Disease Group	V24 CMS-HCC Hierarchies	Community, NonDual, Aged	Community, NonDual, Disabled	Community, FBDual, Aged	Community, FBDual, Disabled	Community, PBDual, Aged	Community, PBDual, Disabled	Institutional
R40.2344	Coma scale, best motor response, flexion withdrawal, 24 hours or more after hospital admission	80	Coma, Brain Compression/Anoxic Damage		0.486	0.274	0.511	0.105	0.729	0.134	—
R40.2430	Glasgow coma scale score 3-8, unspecified time	80	Coma, Brain Compression/Anoxic Damage		0.486	0.274	0.511	0.105	0.729	0.134	—
R40.2431	Glasgow coma scale score 3-8, in the field [EMT or ambulance]	80	Coma, Brain Compression/Anoxic Damage		0.486	0.274	0.511	0.105	0.729	0.134	—
R40.2432	Glasgow coma scale score 3-8, at arrival to emergency department	80	Coma, Brain Compression/Anoxic Damage		0.486	0.274	0.511	0.105	0.729	0.134	—
R40.2433	Glasgow coma scale score 3-8, at hospital admission	80	Coma, Brain Compression/Anoxic Damage		0.486	0.274	0.511	0.105	0.729	0.134	—
R40.2434	Glasgow coma scale score 3-8, 24 hours or more after hospital admission	80	Coma, Brain Compression/Anoxic Damage		0.486	0.274	0.511	0.105	0.729	0.134	—
R40.2440	Other coma, without documented Glasgow coma scale score, or with partial score reported, unspecified time	80	Coma, Brain Compression/Anoxic Damage		0.486	0.274	0.511	0.105	0.729	0.134	—
R40.2441	Other coma, without documented Glasgow coma scale score, or with partial score reported, in the field [EMT or ambulance]	80	Coma, Brain Compression/Anoxic Damage		0.486	0.274	0.511	0.105	0.729	0.134	—
R40.2442	Other coma, without documented Glasgow coma scale score, or with partial score reported, at arrival to emergency department	80	Coma, Brain Compression/Anoxic Damage		0.486	0.274	0.511	0.105	0.729	0.134	—
R40.2443	Other coma, without documented Glasgow coma scale score, or with partial score reported, at hospital admission	80	Coma, Brain Compression/Anoxic Damage		0.486	0.274	0.511	0.105	0.729	0.134	—
R40.2444	Other coma, without documented Glasgow coma scale score, or with partial score reported, 24 hours or more after hospital admission	80	Coma, Brain Compression/Anoxic Damage		0.486	0.274	0.511	0.105	0.729	0.134	—
R40.3	Persistent vegetative state	80	Coma, Brain Compression/Anoxic Damage		0.486	0.274	0.511	0.105	0.729	0.134	—
R45.88	Nonsuicidal self-harm	59	Major Depressive, Bipolar, and Paranoid Disorders	60	0.309	0.164	0.299	0.127	0.306	0.109	0.187
R53.2	Functional quadriplegia	70	Quadriplegia	71,72, 103,104, 169	1.242	1.001	1.038	1.000	1.000	1.134	0.549
R56.00	Simple febrile convulsions	79	Seizure Disorders and Convulsions		0.220	0.196	0.237	0.139	0.257	0.169	0.065
R56.01	Complex febrile convulsions	79	Seizure Disorders and Convulsions		0.220	0.196	0.237	0.139	0.257	0.169	0.065
R56.1	Post traumatic seizures	79	Seizure Disorders and Convulsions		0.220	0.196	0.237	0.139	0.257	0.169	0.065
R56.9	Unspecified convulsions	79	Seizure Disorders and Convulsions		0.220	0.196	0.237	0.139	0.257	0.169	0.065
R57.0	Cardiogenic shock	84	Cardio-Respiratory Failure and Shock		0.282	0.385	0.492	0.531	0.361	0.343	0.313
R57.1	Hypovolemic shock	2	Septicemia, Sepsis, Systemic Inflammatory Response Syndrome/Shock		0.352	0.414	0.453	0.530	0.316	0.297	0.324
R57.8	Other shock	2	Septicemia, Sepsis, Systemic Inflammatory Response Syndrome/Shock		0.352	0.414	0.453	0.530	0.316	0.297	0.324
R57.9	Shock, unspecified	84	Cardio-Respiratory Failure and Shock		0.282	0.385	0.492	0.531	0.361	0.343	0.313
R64	Cachexia	21	Protein-Calorie Malnutrition		0.455	0.674	0.693	0.723	0.457	0.679	0.267
R65.10	Systemic inflammatory response syndrome (SIRS) of non-infectious origin without acute organ dysfunction	2	Septicemia, Sepsis, Systemic Inflammatory Response Syndrome/Shock		0.352	0.414	0.453	0.530	0.316	0.297	0.324

ICD-10-CM Code	ICD-10-CM Code Description	V24 CMS-HCC	V24 CMS-HCC Disease Group	V24 CMS-HCC Hierarchies	Community, NonDual, Aged	Community, NonDual, Disabled	Community, FBDual, Aged	Community, FBDual, Disabled	Community, PBDual, Aged	Community, PBDual, Disabled	Institutional
R65.11	Systemic inflammatory response syndrome (SIRS) of non-infectious origin with acute organ dysfunction	2	Septicemia, Sepsis, Systemic Inflammatory Response Syndrome/Shock		0.352	0.414	0.453	0.530	0.316	0.297	0.324
R65.20	Severe sepsis without septic shock	2	Septicemia, Sepsis, Systemic Inflammatory Response Syndrome/Shock		0.352	0.414	0.453	0.530	0.316	0.297	0.324
R65.21	Severe sepsis with septic shock	2	Septicemia, Sepsis, Systemic Inflammatory Response Syndrome/Shock		0.352	0.414	0.453	0.530	0.316	0.297	0.324
S02.0XXA	Fracture of vault of skull, initial encounter for closed fracture	167	Major Head Injury		0.077	—	0.144	0.025	0.034	0.019	—
S02.0XXB	Fracture of vault of skull, initial encounter for open fracture	167	Major Head Injury		0.077	—	0.144	0.025	0.034	0.019	—
S02.0XXS	Fracture of vault of skull, sequela	167	Major Head Injury		0.077	—	0.144	0.025	0.034	0.019	—
S02.101A	Fracture of base of skull, right side, initial encounter for closed fracture	167	Major Head Injury		0.077	—	0.144	0.025	0.034	0.019	—
S02.101B	Fracture of base of skull, right side, initial encounter for open fracture	167	Major Head Injury		0.077	—	0.144	0.025	0.034	0.019	—
S02.101S	Fracture of base of skull, right side, sequela	167	Major Head Injury		0.077	—	0.144	0.025	0.034	0.019	—
S02.102A	Fracture of base of skull, left side, initial encounter for closed fracture	167	Major Head Injury		0.077	—	0.144	0.025	0.034	0.019	—
S02.102B	Fracture of base of skull, left side, initial encounter for open fracture	167	Major Head Injury		0.077	—	0.144	0.025	0.034	0.019	—
S02.102S	Fracture of base of skull, left side, sequela	167	Major Head Injury		0.077	—	0.144	0.025	0.034	0.019	—
S02.109A	Fracture of base of skull, unspecified side, initial encounter for closed fracture	167	Major Head Injury		0.077	—	0.144	0.025	0.034	0.019	—
S02.109B	Fracture of base of skull, unspecified side, initial encounter for open fracture	167	Major Head Injury		0.077	—	0.144	0.025	0.034	0.019	—
S02.109S	Fracture of base of skull, unspecified side, sequela	167	Major Head Injury		0.077	—	0.144	0.025	0.034	0.019	—
S02.110A	Type I occipital condyle fracture, unspecified side, initial encounter for closed fracture	167	Major Head Injury		0.077	—	0.144	0.025	0.034	0.019	—
S02.110B	Type I occipital condyle fracture, unspecified side, initial encounter for open fracture	167	Major Head Injury		0.077	—	0.144	0.025	0.034	0.019	—
S02.110S	Type I occipital condyle fracture, unspecified side, sequela	167	Major Head Injury		0.077	—	0.144	0.025	0.034	0.019	—
S02.111A	Type II occipital condyle fracture, unspecified side, initial encounter for closed fracture	167	Major Head Injury		0.077	—	0.144	0.025	0.034	0.019	—
S02.111B	Type II occipital condyle fracture, unspecified side, initial encounter for open fracture	167	Major Head Injury		0.077	—	0.144	0.025	0.034	0.019	—
S02.111S	Type II occipital condyle fracture, unspecified side, sequela	167	Major Head Injury		0.077	—	0.144	0.025	0.034	0.019	—
S02.112A	Type III occipital condyle fracture, unspecified side, initial encounter for closed fracture	167	Major Head Injury		0.077	—	0.144	0.025	0.034	0.019	—
S02.112B	Type III occipital condyle fracture, unspecified side, initial encounter for open fracture	167	Major Head Injury		0.077	—	0.144	0.025	0.034	0.019	—
S02.112S	Type III occipital condyle fracture, unspecified side, sequela	167	Major Head Injury		0.077	—	0.144	0.025	0.034	0.019	—

ICD-10-CM Code	ICD-10-CM Code Description	V24 CMS-HCC	V24 CMS-HCC Disease Group	V24 CMS-HCC Hierarchies	Community, NonDual, Aged	Community, NonDual, Disabled	Community, FBDual, Aged	Community, FBDual, Disabled	Community, PBDual, Aged	Community, PBDual, Disabled	Institutional
S02.113A	Unspecified occipital condyle fracture, initial encounter for closed fracture	167	Major Head Injury		0.077	—	0.144	0.025	0.034	0.019	—
S02.113B	Unspecified occipital condyle fracture, initial encounter for open fracture	167	Major Head Injury		0.077	—	0.144	0.025	0.034	0.019	—
S02.113S	Unspecified occipital condyle fracture, sequela	167	Major Head Injury		0.077	—	0.144	0.025	0.034	0.019	—
S02.118A	Other fracture of occiput, unspecified side, initial encounter for closed fracture	167	Major Head Injury		0.077	—	0.144	0.025	0.034	0.019	—
S02.118B	Other fracture of occiput, unspecified side, initial encounter for open fracture	167	Major Head Injury		0.077	—	0.144	0.025	0.034	0.019	—
S02.118S	Other fracture of occiput, unspecified side, sequela	167	Major Head Injury		0.077	—	0.144	0.025	0.034	0.019	—
S02.119A	Unspecified fracture of occiput, initial encounter for closed fracture	167	Major Head Injury		0.077	—	0.144	0.025	0.034	0.019	—
S02.119B	Unspecified fracture of occiput, initial encounter for open fracture	167	Major Head Injury		0.077	—	0.144	0.025	0.034	0.019	—
S02.119S	Unspecified fracture of occiput, sequela	167	Major Head Injury		0.077	—	0.144	0.025	0.034	0.019	—
S02.11AA	Type I occipital condyle fracture, right side, initial encounter for closed fracture	167	Major Head Injury		0.077	—	0.144	0.025	0.034	0.019	—
S02.11AB	Type I occipital condyle fracture, right side, initial encounter for open fracture	167	Major Head Injury		0.077	—	0.144	0.025	0.034	0.019	—
S02.11AS	Type I occipital condyle fracture, right side, sequela	167	Major Head Injury		0.077	—	0.144	0.025	0.034	0.019	—
S02.11BA	Type I occipital condyle fracture, left side, initial encounter for closed fracture	167	Major Head Injury		0.077	—	0.144	0.025	0.034	0.019	—
S02.11BB	Type I occipital condyle fracture, left side, initial encounter for open fracture	167	Major Head Injury		0.077	—	0.144	0.025	0.034	0.019	—
S02.11BS	Type I occipital condyle fracture, left side, sequela	167	Major Head Injury		0.077	—	0.144	0.025	0.034	0.019	—
S02.11CA	Type II occipital condyle fracture, right side, initial encounter for closed fracture	167	Major Head Injury		0.077	—	0.144	0.025	0.034	0.019	—
S02.11CB	Type II occipital condyle fracture, right side, initial encounter for open fracture	167	Major Head Injury		0.077	—	0.144	0.025	0.034	0.019	—
S02.11CS	Type II occipital condyle fracture, right side, sequela	167	Major Head Injury		0.077	—	0.144	0.025	0.034	0.019	—
S02.11DA	Type II occipital condyle fracture, left side, initial encounter for closed fracture	167	Major Head Injury		0.077	—	0.144	0.025	0.034	0.019	—
S02.11DB	Type II occipital condyle fracture, left side, initial encounter for open fracture	167	Major Head Injury		0.077	—	0.144	0.025	0.034	0.019	—
S02.11DS	Type II occipital condyle fracture, left side, sequela	167	Major Head Injury		0.077	—	0.144	0.025	0.034	0.019	—
S02.11EA	Type III occipital condyle fracture, right side, initial encounter for closed fracture	167	Major Head Injury		0.077	—	0.144	0.025	0.034	0.019	—
S02.11EB	Type III occipital condyle fracture, right side, initial encounter for open fracture	167	Major Head Injury		0.077	—	0.144	0.025	0.034	0.019	—

2021 Optum360, LLC

ICD-10-CM Code	ICD-10-CM Code Description	V24 CMS-HCC	V24 CMS-HCC Disease Group	V24 CMS-HCC Hierarchies	Community, NonDual, Aged	Community, NonDual, Disabled	Community, FBDual, Aged	Community, FBDual, Disabled	Community, PBDual, Aged	Community, PBDual, Disabled	Institutional
S02.11ES	Type III occipital condyle fracture, right side, sequela	167	Major Head Injury		0.077	—	0.144	0.025	0.034	0.019	—
S02.11FA	Type III occipital condyle fracture, left side, initial encounter for closed fracture	167	Major Head Injury		0.077	—	0.144	0.025	0.034	0.019	—
S02.11FB	Type III occipital condyle fracture, left side, initial encounter for open fracture	167	Major Head Injury		0.077	—	0.144	0.025	0.034	0.019	—
S02.11FS	Type III occipital condyle fracture, left side, sequela	167	Major Head Injury		0.077	—	0.144	0.025	0.034	0.019	—
S02.11GA	Other fracture of occiput, right side, initial encounter for closed fracture	167	Major Head Injury		0.077	—	0.144	0.025	0.034	0.019	—
S02.11GB	Other fracture of occiput, right side, initial encounter for open fracture	167	Major Head Injury		0.077	—	0.144	0.025	0.034	0.019	—
S02.11GS	Other fracture of occiput, right side, sequela	167	Major Head Injury		0.077	—	0.144	0.025	0.034	0.019	—
S02.11HA	Other fracture of occiput, left side, initial encounter for closed fracture	167	Major Head Injury		0.077	—	0.144	0.025	0.034	0.019	—
S02.11HB	Other fracture of occiput, left side, initial encounter for open fracture	167	Major Head Injury		0.077	—	0.144	0.025	0.034	0.019	—
S02.11HS	Other fracture of occiput, left side, sequela	167	Major Head Injury		0.077	—	0.144	0.025	0.034	0.019	—
S02.121A	Fracture of orbital roof, right side, initial encounter for closed fracture	167	Major Head Injury		0.077	—	0.144	0.025	0.034	0.019	—
S02.121B	Fracture of orbital roof, right side, initial encounter for open fracture	167	Major Head Injury		0.077	—	0.144	0.025	0.034	0.019	—
S02.121S	Fracture of orbital roof, right side, sequela	167	Major Head Injury		0.077	—	0.144	0.025	0.034	0.019	—
S02.122A	Fracture of orbital roof, left side, initial encounter for closed fracture	167	Major Head Injury		0.077	—	0.144	0.025	0.034	0.019	—
S02.122B	Fracture of orbital roof, left side, initial encounter for open fracture	167	Major Head Injury		0.077	—	0.144	0.025	0.034	0.019	—
S02.122S	Fracture of orbital roof, left side, sequela	167	Major Head Injury		0.077	—	0.144	0.025	0.034	0.019	—
S02.129A	Fracture of orbital roof, unspecified side, initial encounter for closed fracture	167	Major Head Injury		0.077	—	0.144	0.025	0.034	0.019	—
S02.129B	Fracture of orbital roof, unspecified side, initial encounter for open fracture	167	Major Head Injury		0.077	—	0.144	0.025	0.034	0.019	—
S02.129S	Fracture of orbital roof, unspecified side, sequela	167	Major Head Injury		0.077	—	0.144	0.025	0.034	0.019	—
S02.19XA	Other fracture of base of skull, initial encounter for closed fracture	167	Major Head Injury		0.077	—	0.144	0.025	0.034	0.019	—
S02.19XB	Other fracture of base of skull, initial encounter for open fracture	167	Major Head Injury		0.077	—	0.144	0.025	0.034	0.019	—
S02.19XS	Other fracture of base of skull, sequela	167	Major Head Injury		0.077	—	0.144	0.025	0.034	0.019	—
S02.30XA	Fracture of orbital floor, unspecified side, initial encounter for closed fracture	167	Major Head Injury		0.077	—	0.144	0.025	0.034	0.019	—
S02.30XB	Fracture of orbital floor, unspecified side, initial encounter for open fracture	167	Major Head Injury		0.077	—	0.144	0.025	0.034	0.019	—
S02.30XS	Fracture of orbital floor, unspecified side, sequela	167	Major Head Injury		0.077	—	0.144	0.025	0.034	0.019	—
S02.31XA	Fracture of orbital floor, right side, initial encounter for closed fracture	167	Major Head Injury		0.077	—	0.144	0.025	0.034	0.019	—

ICD-10-CM Code	ICD-10-CM Code Description	V24 CMS-HCC	V24 CMS-HCC Disease Group	V24 CMS-HCC Hierarchies	Community, NonDual, Aged	Community, NonDual, Disabled	Community, FBDual, Aged	Community, FBDual, Disabled	Community, PBDual, Aged	Community, PBDual, Disabled	Institutional
S02.31XB	Fracture of orbital floor, right side, initial encounter for open fracture	167	Major Head Injury		0.077	—	0.144	0.025	0.034	0.019	—
S02.31XS	Fracture of orbital floor, right side, sequela	167	Major Head Injury		0.077	—	0.144	0.025	0.034	0.019	—
S02.32XA	Fracture of orbital floor, left side, initial encounter for closed fracture	167	Major Head Injury		0.077	—	0.144	0.025	0.034	0.019	—
S02.32XB	Fracture of orbital floor, left side, initial encounter for open fracture	167	Major Head Injury		0.077	—	0.144	0.025	0.034	0.019	—
S02.32XS	Fracture of orbital floor, left side, sequela	167	Major Head Injury		0.077	—	0.144	0.025	0.034	0.019	—
S02.400A	Malar fracture, unspecified side, initial encounter for closed fracture	167	Major Head Injury		0.077	—	0.144	0.025	0.034	0.019	—
S02.400B	Malar fracture, unspecified side, initial encounter for open fracture	167	Major Head Injury		0.077	—	0.144	0.025	0.034	0.019	—
S02.400S	Malar fracture, unspecified side, sequela	167	Major Head Injury		0.077	—	0.144	0.025	0.034	0.019	—
S02.401A	Maxillary fracture, unspecified side, initial encounter for closed fracture	167	Major Head Injury		0.077	—	0.144	0.025	0.034	0.019	—
S02.401B	Maxillary fracture, unspecified side, initial encounter for open fracture	167	Major Head Injury		0.077	—	0.144	0.025	0.034	0.019	—
S02.401S	Maxillary fracture, unspecified side, sequela	167	Major Head Injury		0.077	—	0.144	0.025	0.034	0.019	—
S02.402A	Zygomatic fracture, unspecified side, initial encounter for closed fracture	167	Major Head Injury		0.077	—	0.144	0.025	0.034	0.019	—
S02.402B	Zygomatic fracture, unspecified side, initial encounter for open fracture	167	Major Head Injury		0.077	—	0.144	0.025	0.034	0.019	—
S02.402S	Zygomatic fracture, unspecified side, sequela	167	Major Head Injury		0.077	—	0.144	0.025	0.034	0.019	—
S02.40AA	Malar fracture, right side, initial encounter for closed fracture	167	Major Head Injury		0.077	—	0.144	0.025	0.034	0.019	—
S02.40AB	Malar fracture, right side, initial encounter for open fracture	167	Major Head Injury		0.077	—	0.144	0.025	0.034	0.019	—
S02.40AS	Malar fracture, right side, sequela	167	Major Head Injury		0.077	—	0.144	0.025	0.034	0.019	—
S02.40BA	Malar fracture, left side, initial encounter for closed fracture	167	Major Head Injury		0.077	—	0.144	0.025	0.034	0.019	—
S02.40BB	Malar fracture, left side, initial encounter for open fracture	167	Major Head Injury		0.077	—	0.144	0.025	0.034	0.019	—
S02.40BS	Malar fracture, left side, sequela	167	Major Head Injury		0.077	—	0.144	0.025	0.034	0.019	—
S02.40CA	Maxillary fracture, right side, initial encounter for closed fracture	167	Major Head Injury		0.077	—	0.144	0.025	0.034	0.019	—
S02.40CB	Maxillary fracture, right side, initial encounter for open fracture	167	Major Head Injury		0.077	—	0.144	0.025	0.034	0.019	—
S02.40CS	Maxillary fracture, right side, sequela	167	Major Head Injury		0.077	—	0.144	0.025	0.034	0.019	—
S02.40DA	Maxillary fracture, left side, initial encounter for closed fracture	167	Major Head Injury		0.077	—	0.144	0.025	0.034	0.019	—
S02.40DB	Maxillary fracture, left side, initial encounter for open fracture	167	Major Head Injury		0.077	—	0.144	0.025	0.034	0.019	—
S02.40DS	Maxillary fracture, left side, sequela	167	Major Head Injury		0.077	—	0.144	0.025	0.034	0.019	—
S02.40EA	Zygomatic fracture, right side, initial encounter for closed fracture	167	Major Head Injury		0.077	—	0.144	0.025	0.034	0.019	—
S02.40EB	Zygomatic fracture, right side, initial encounter for open fracture	167	Major Head Injury		0.077	—	0.144	0.025	0.034	0.019	—
S02.40ES	Zygomatic fracture, right side, sequela	167	Major Head Injury		0.077	—	0.144	0.025	0.034	0.019	—
S02.40FA	Zygomatic fracture, left side, initial encounter for closed fracture	167	Major Head Injury		0.077	—	0.144	0.025	0.034	0.019	—
S02.40FB	Zygomatic fracture, left side, initial encounter for open fracture	167	Major Head Injury		0.077	—	0.144	0.025	0.034	0.019	—

ICD-10-CM Code	ICD-10-CM Code Description	V24 CMS-HCC	V24 CMS-HCC Disease Group	V24 CMS-HCC Hierarchies	Community, NonDual, Aged	Community, NonDual, Disabled	Community, FBDual, Aged	Community, FBDual, Disabled	Community, PBDual, Aged	Community, PBDual, Disabled	Institutional
S02.40FS	Zygomatic fracture, left side, sequela	167	Major Head Injury		0.077	—	0.144	0.025	0.034	0.019	—
S02.411A	LeFort I fracture, initial encounter for closed fracture	167	Major Head Injury		0.077	—	0.144	0.025	0.034	0.019	—
S02.411B	LeFort I fracture, initial encounter for open fracture	167	Major Head Injury		0.077	—	0.144	0.025	0.034	0.019	—
S02.411S	LeFort I fracture, sequela	167	Major Head Injury		0.077	—	0.144	0.025	0.034	0.019	—
S02.412A	LeFort II fracture, initial encounter for closed fracture	167	Major Head Injury		0.077	—	0.144	0.025	0.034	0.019	—
S02.412B	LeFort II fracture, initial encounter for open fracture	167	Major Head Injury		0.077	—	0.144	0.025	0.034	0.019	—
S02.412S	LeFort II fracture, sequela	167	Major Head Injury		0.077	—	0.144	0.025	0.034	0.019	—
S02.413A	LeFort III fracture, initial encounter for closed fracture	167	Major Head Injury		0.077	—	0.144	0.025	0.034	0.019	—
S02.413B	LeFort III fracture, initial encounter for open fracture	167	Major Head Injury		0.077	—	0.144	0.025	0.034	0.019	—
S02.413S	LeFort III fracture, sequela	167	Major Head Injury		0.077	—	0.144	0.025	0.034	0.019	—
S02.42XA	Fracture of alveolus of maxilla, initial encounter for closed fracture	167	Major Head Injury		0.077	—	0.144	0.025	0.034	0.019	—
S02.42XB	Fracture of alveolus of maxilla, initial encounter for open fracture	167	Major Head Injury		0.077	—	0.144	0.025	0.034	0.019	—
S02.42XS	Fracture of alveolus of maxilla, sequela	167	Major Head Injury		0.077	—	0.144	0.025	0.034	0.019	—
S02.600A	Fracture of unspecified part of body of mandible, unspecified side, initial encounter for closed fracture	167	Major Head Injury		0.077	—	0.144	0.025	0.034	0.019	—
S02.600B	Fracture of unspecified part of body of mandible, unspecified side, initial encounter for open fracture	167	Major Head Injury		0.077	—	0.144	0.025	0.034	0.019	—
S02.600S	Fracture of unspecified part of body of mandible, unspecified side, sequela	167	Major Head Injury		0.077	—	0.144	0.025	0.034	0.019	—
S02.601A	Fracture of unspecified part of body of right mandible, initial encounter for closed fracture	167	Major Head Injury		0.077	—	0.144	0.025	0.034	0.019	—
S02.601B	Fracture of unspecified part of body of right mandible, initial encounter for open fracture	167	Major Head Injury		0.077	—	0.144	0.025	0.034	0.019	—
S02.601S	Fracture of unspecified part of body of right mandible, sequela	167	Major Head Injury		0.077	—	0.144	0.025	0.034	0.019	—
S02.602A	Fracture of unspecified part of body of left mandible, initial encounter for closed fracture	167	Major Head Injury		0.077	—	0.144	0.025	0.034	0.019	—
S02.602B	Fracture of unspecified part of body of left mandible, initial encounter for open fracture	167	Major Head Injury		0.077	—	0.144	0.025	0.034	0.019	—
S02.602S	Fracture of unspecified part of body of left mandible, sequela	167	Major Head Injury		0.077	—	0.144	0.025	0.034	0.019	—
S02.609A	Fracture of mandible, unspecified, initial encounter for closed fracture	167	Major Head Injury		0.077	—	0.144	0.025	0.034	0.019	—
S02.609B	Fracture of mandible, unspecified, initial encounter for open fracture	167	Major Head Injury		0.077	—	0.144	0.025	0.034	0.019	—
S02.609S	Fracture of mandible, unspecified, sequela	167	Major Head Injury		0.077	—	0.144	0.025	0.034	0.019	—
S02.610A	Fracture of condylar process of mandible, unspecified side, initial encounter for closed fracture	167	Major Head Injury		0.077	—	0.144	0.025	0.034	0.019	—
S02.610B	Fracture of condylar process of mandible, unspecified side, initial encounter for open fracture	167	Major Head Injury		0.077	—	0.144	0.025	0.034	0.019	—

ICD-10-CM Code	ICD-10-CM Code Description	V24 CMS-HCC	V24 CMS-HCC Disease Group	V24 CMS-HCC Hierarchies	Community, NonDual, Aged	Community, NonDual, Disabled	Community, FBDual, Aged	Community, FBDual, Disabled	Community, PBDual, Aged	Community, PBDual, Disabled	Institutional
S02.610S	Fracture of condylar process of mandible, unspecified side, sequela	167	Major Head Injury		0.077	—	0.144	0.025	0.034	0.019	—
S02.611A	Fracture of condylar process of right mandible, initial encounter for closed fracture	167	Major Head Injury		0.077	—	0.144	0.025	0.034	0.019	—
S02.611B	Fracture of condylar process of right mandible, initial encounter for open fracture	167	Major Head Injury		0.077	—	0.144	0.025	0.034	0.019	—
S02.611S	Fracture of condylar process of right mandible, sequela	167	Major Head Injury		0.077	—	0.144	0.025	0.034	0.019	—
S02.612A	Fracture of condylar process of left mandible, initial encounter for closed fracture	167	Major Head Injury		0.077	—	0.144	0.025	0.034	0.019	—
S02.612B	Fracture of condylar process of left mandible, initial encounter for open fracture	167	Major Head Injury		0.077	—	0.144	0.025	0.034	0.019	—
S02.612S	Fracture of condylar process of left mandible, sequela	167	Major Head Injury		0.077	—	0.144	0.025	0.034	0.019	—
S02.620A	Fracture of subcondylar process of mandible, unspecified side, initial encounter for closed fracture	167	Major Head Injury		0.077	—	0.144	0.025	0.034	0.019	—
S02.620B	Fracture of subcondylar process of mandible, unspecified side, initial encounter for open fracture	167	Major Head Injury		0.077	—	0.144	0.025	0.034	0.019	—
S02.620S	Fracture of subcondylar process of mandible, unspecified side, sequela	167	Major Head Injury		0.077	—	0.144	0.025	0.034	0.019	—
S02.621A	Fracture of subcondylar process of right mandible, initial encounter for closed fracture	167	Major Head Injury		0.077	—	0.144	0.025	0.034	0.019	—
S02.621B	Fracture of subcondylar process of right mandible, initial encounter for open fracture	167	Major Head Injury		0.077	—	0.144	0.025	0.034	0.019	—
S02.621S	Fracture of subcondylar process of right mandible, sequela	167	Major Head Injury		0.077	—	0.144	0.025	0.034	0.019	—
S02.622A	Fracture of subcondylar process of left mandible, initial encounter for closed fracture	167	Major Head Injury		0.077	—	0.144	0.025	0.034	0.019	—
S02.622B	Fracture of subcondylar process of left mandible, initial encounter for open fracture	167	Major Head Injury		0.077	—	0.144	0.025	0.034	0.019	—
S02.622S	Fracture of subcondylar process of left mandible, sequela	167	Major Head Injury		0.077	—	0.144	0.025	0.034	0.019	—
S02.630A	Fracture of coronoid process of mandible, unspecified side, initial encounter for closed fracture	167	Major Head Injury		0.077	—	0.144	0.025	0.034	0.019	—
S02.630B	Fracture of coronoid process of mandible, unspecified side, initial encounter for open fracture	167	Major Head Injury		0.077	—	0.144	0.025	0.034	0.019	—
S02.630S	Fracture of coronoid process of mandible, unspecified side, sequela	167	Major Head Injury		0.077	—	0.144	0.025	0.034	0.019	—
S02.631A	Fracture of coronoid process of right mandible, initial encounter for closed fracture	167	Major Head Injury		0.077	—	0.144	0.025	0.034	0.019	—
S02.631B	Fracture of coronoid process of right mandible, initial encounter for open fracture	167	Major Head Injury		0.077	—	0.144	0.025	0.034	0.019	—
S02.631S	Fracture of coronoid process of right mandible, sequela	167	Major Head Injury		0.077	—	0.144	0.025	0.034	0.019	—
S02.632A	Fracture of coronoid process of left mandible, initial encounter for closed fracture	167	Major Head Injury		0.077	—	0.144	0.025	0.034	0.019	—

ICD-10-CM Code	ICD-10-CM Code Description	V24 CMS-HCC	V24 CMS-HCC Disease Group	V24 CMS-HCC Hierarchies	Community, NonDual, Aged	Community, NonDual, Disabled	Community, FBDual, Aged	Community, FBDual, Disabled	Community, PBDual, Aged	Community, PBDual, Disabled	Institutional
S02.632B	Fracture of coronoid process of left mandible, initial encounter for open fracture	167	Major Head Injury		0.077	—	0.144	0.025	0.034	0.019	—
S02.632S	Fracture of coronoid process of left mandible, sequela	167	Major Head Injury		0.077	—	0.144	0.025	0.034	0.019	—
S02.640A	Fracture of ramus of mandible, unspecified side, initial encounter for closed fracture	167	Major Head Injury		0.077	—	0.144	0.025	0.034	0.019	—
S02.640B	Fracture of ramus of mandible, unspecified side, initial encounter for open fracture	167	Major Head Injury		0.077	—	0.144	0.025	0.034	0.019	—
S02.640S	Fracture of ramus of mandible, unspecified side, sequela	167	Major Head Injury		0.077	—	0.144	0.025	0.034	0.019	—
S02.641A	Fracture of ramus of right mandible, initial encounter for closed fracture	167	Major Head Injury		0.077	—	0.144	0.025	0.034	0.019	—
S02.641B	Fracture of ramus of right mandible, initial encounter for open fracture	167	Major Head Injury		0.077	—	0.144	0.025	0.034	0.019	—
S02.641S	Fracture of ramus of right mandible, sequela	167	Major Head Injury		0.077	—	0.144	0.025	0.034	0.019	—
S02.642A	Fracture of ramus of left mandible, initial encounter for closed fracture	167	Major Head Injury		0.077	—	0.144	0.025	0.034	0.019	—
S02.642B	Fracture of ramus of left mandible, initial encounter for open fracture	167	Major Head Injury		0.077	—	0.144	0.025	0.034	0.019	—
S02.642S	Fracture of ramus of left mandible, sequela	167	Major Head Injury		0.077	—	0.144	0.025	0.034	0.019	—
S02.650A	Fracture of angle of mandible, unspecified side, initial encounter for closed fracture	167	Major Head Injury		0.077	—	0.144	0.025	0.034	0.019	—
S02.650B	Fracture of angle of mandible, unspecified side, initial encounter for open fracture	167	Major Head Injury		0.077	—	0.144	0.025	0.034	0.019	—
S02.650S	Fracture of angle of mandible, unspecified side, sequela	167	Major Head Injury		0.077	—	0.144	0.025	0.034	0.019	—
S02.651A	Fracture of angle of right mandible, initial encounter for closed fracture	167	Major Head Injury		0.077	—	0.144	0.025	0.034	0.019	—
S02.651B	Fracture of angle of right mandible, initial encounter for open fracture	167	Major Head Injury		0.077	—	0.144	0.025	0.034	0.019	—
S02.651S	Fracture of angle of right mandible, sequela	167	Major Head Injury		0.077	—	0.144	0.025	0.034	0.019	—
S02.652A	Fracture of angle of left mandible, initial encounter for closed fracture	167	Major Head Injury		0.077	—	0.144	0.025	0.034	0.019	—
S02.652B	Fracture of angle of left mandible, initial encounter for open fracture	167	Major Head Injury		0.077	—	0.144	0.025	0.034	0.019	—
S02.652S	Fracture of angle of left mandible, sequela	167	Major Head Injury		0.077	—	0.144	0.025	0.034	0.019	—
S02.66XA	Fracture of symphysis of mandible, initial encounter for closed fracture	167	Major Head Injury		0.077	—	0.144	0.025	0.034	0.019	—
S02.66XB	Fracture of symphysis of mandible, initial encounter for open fracture	167	Major Head Injury		0.077	—	0.144	0.025	0.034	0.019	—
S02.66XS	Fracture of symphysis of mandible, sequela	167	Major Head Injury		0.077	—	0.144	0.025	0.034	0.019	—
S02.670A	Fracture of alveolus of mandible, unspecified side, initial encounter for closed fracture	167	Major Head Injury		0.077	—	0.144	0.025	0.034	0.019	—
S02.670B	Fracture of alveolus of mandible, unspecified side, initial encounter for open fracture	167	Major Head Injury		0.077	—	0.144	0.025	0.034	0.019	—
S02.670S	Fracture of alveolus of mandible, unspecified side, sequela	167	Major Head Injury		0.077	—	0.144	0.025	0.034	0.019	—

ICD-10-CM Code	ICD-10-CM Code Description	V24 CMS-HCC	V24 CMS-HCC Disease Group	V24 CMS-HCC Hierarchies	Community, NonDual, Aged	Community, NonDual, Disabled	Community, FBDual, Aged	Community, FBDual, Disabled	Community, PBDual, Aged	Community, PBDual, Disabled	Institutional
S02.671A	Fracture of alveolus of right mandible, initial encounter for closed fracture	167	Major Head Injury		0.077	—	0.144	0.025	0.034	0.019	—
S02.671B	Fracture of alveolus of right mandible, initial encounter for open fracture	167	Major Head Injury		0.077	—	0.144	0.025	0.034	0.019	—
S02.671S	Fracture of alveolus of right mandible, sequela	167	Major Head Injury		0.077	—	0.144	0.025	0.034	0.019	—
S02.672A	Fracture of alveolus of left mandible, initial encounter for closed fracture	167	Major Head Injury		0.077	—	0.144	0.025	0.034	0.019	—
S02.672B	Fracture of alveolus of left mandible, initial encounter for open fracture	167	Major Head Injury		0.077	—	0.144	0.025	0.034	0.019	—
S02.672S	Fracture of alveolus of left mandible, sequela	167	Major Head Injury		0.077	—	0.144	0.025	0.034	0.019	—
S02.69XA	Fracture of mandible of other specified site, initial encounter for closed fracture	167	Major Head Injury		0.077	—	0.144	0.025	0.034	0.019	—
S02.69XB	Fracture of mandible of other specified site, initial encounter for open fracture	167	Major Head Injury		0.077	—	0.144	0.025	0.034	0.019	—
S02.69XS	Fracture of mandible of other specified site, sequela	167	Major Head Injury		0.077	—	0.144	0.025	0.034	0.019	—
S02.80XA	Fracture of other specified skull and facial bones, unspecified side, initial encounter for closed fracture	167	Major Head Injury		0.077	—	0.144	0.025	0.034	0.019	—
S02.80XB	Fracture of other specified skull and facial bones, unspecified side, initial encounter for open fracture	167	Major Head Injury		0.077	—	0.144	0.025	0.034	0.019	—
S02.80XS	Fracture of other specified skull and facial bones, unspecified side, sequela	167	Major Head Injury		0.077	—	0.144	0.025	0.034	0.019	—
S02.81XA	Fracture of other specified skull and facial bones, right side, initial encounter for closed fracture	167	Major Head Injury		0.077	—	0.144	0.025	0.034	0.019	—
S02.81XB	Fracture of other specified skull and facial bones, right side, initial encounter for open fracture	167	Major Head Injury		0.077	—	0.144	0.025	0.034	0.019	—
S02.81XS	Fracture of other specified skull and facial bones, right side, sequela	167	Major Head Injury		0.077	—	0.144	0.025	0.034	0.019	—
S02.82XA	Fracture of other specified skull and facial bones, left side, initial encounter for closed fracture	167	Major Head Injury		0.077	—	0.144	0.025	0.034	0.019	—
S02.82XB	Fracture of other specified skull and facial bones, left side, initial encounter for open fracture	167	Major Head Injury		0.077	—	0.144	0.025	0.034	0.019	—
S02.82XS	Fracture of other specified skull and facial bones, left side, sequela	167	Major Head Injury		0.077	—	0.144	0.025	0.034	0.019	—
S02.831A	Fracture of medial orbital wall, right side, initial encounter for closed fracture	167	Major Head Injury		0.077	—	0.144	0.025	0.034	0.019	—
S02.831B	Fracture of medial orbital wall, right side, initial encounter for open fracture	167	Major Head Injury		0.077	—	0.144	0.025	0.034	0.019	—
S02.831S	Fracture of medial orbital wall, right side, sequela	167	Major Head Injury		0.077	—	0.144	0.025	0.034	0.019	—
S02.832A	Fracture of medial orbital wall, left side, initial encounter for closed fracture	167	Major Head Injury		0.077	—	0.144	0.025	0.034	0.019	—
S02.832B	Fracture of medial orbital wall, left side, initial encounter for open fracture	167	Major Head Injury		0.077	—	0.144	0.025	0.034	0.019	—

ICD-10-CM Code	ICD-10-CM Code Description	V24 CMS-HCC	V24 CMS-HCC Disease Group	V24 CMS-HCC Hierarchies	Community, NonDual, Aged	Community, NonDual, Disabled	Community, FBDual, Aged	Community, FBDual, Disabled	Community, PBDual, Aged	Community, PBDual, Disabled	Institutional
S02.832S	Fracture of medial orbital wall, left side, sequela	167	Major Head Injury		0.077	—	0.144	0.025	0.034	0.019	—
S02.839A	Fracture of medial orbital wall, unspecified side, initial encounter for closed fracture	167	Major Head Injury		0.077	—	0.144	0.025	0.034	0.019	—
S02.839B	Fracture of medial orbital wall, unspecified side, initial encounter for open fracture	167	Major Head Injury		0.077	—	0.144	0.025	0.034	0.019	—
S02.839S	Fracture of medial orbital wall, unspecified side, sequela	167	Major Head Injury		0.077	—	0.144	0.025	0.034	0.019	—
S02.841A	Fracture of lateral orbital wall, right side, initial encounter for closed fracture	167	Major Head Injury		0.077	—	0.144	0.025	0.034	0.019	—
S02.841B	Fracture of lateral orbital wall, right side, initial encounter for open fracture	167	Major Head Injury		0.077	—	0.144	0.025	0.034	0.019	—
S02.841S	Fracture of lateral orbital wall, right side, sequela	167	Major Head Injury		0.077	—	0.144	0.025	0.034	0.019	—
S02.842A	Fracture of lateral orbital wall, left side, initial encounter for closed fracture	167	Major Head Injury		0.077	—	0.144	0.025	0.034	0.019	—
S02.842B	Fracture of lateral orbital wall, left side, initial encounter for open fracture	167	Major Head Injury		0.077	—	0.144	0.025	0.034	0.019	—
S02.842S	Fracture of lateral orbital wall, left side, sequela	167	Major Head Injury		0.077	—	0.144	0.025	0.034	0.019	—
S02.849A	Fracture of lateral orbital wall, unspecified side, initial encounter for closed fracture	167	Major Head Injury		0.077	—	0.144	0.025	0.034	0.019	—
S02.849B	Fracture of lateral orbital wall, unspecified side, initial encounter for open fracture	167	Major Head Injury		0.077	—	0.144	0.025	0.034	0.019	—
S02.849S	Fracture of lateral orbital wall, unspecified side, sequela	167	Major Head Injury		0.077	—	0.144	0.025	0.034	0.019	—
S02.85XA	Fracture of orbit, unspecified, initial encounter for closed fracture	167	Major Head Injury		0.077	—	0.144	0.025	0.034	0.019	—
S02.85XB	Fracture of orbit, unspecified, initial encounter for open fracture	167	Major Head Injury		0.077	—	0.144	0.025	0.034	0.019	—
S02.85XS	Fracture of orbit, unspecified, sequela	167	Major Head Injury		0.077	—	0.144	0.025	0.034	0.019	—
S02.91XA	Unspecified fracture of skull, initial encounter for closed fracture	167	Major Head Injury		0.077	—	0.144	0.025	0.034	0.019	—
S02.91XB	Unspecified fracture of skull, initial encounter for open fracture	167	Major Head Injury		0.077	—	0.144	0.025	0.034	0.019	—
S02.91XS	Unspecified fracture of skull, sequela	167	Major Head Injury		0.077	—	0.144	0.025	0.034	0.019	—
S02.92XA	Unspecified fracture of facial bones, initial encounter for closed fracture	167	Major Head Injury		0.077	—	0.144	0.025	0.034	0.019	—
S02.92XB	Unspecified fracture of facial bones, initial encounter for open fracture	167	Major Head Injury		0.077	—	0.144	0.025	0.034	0.019	—
S02.92XS	Unspecified fracture of facial bones, sequela	167	Major Head Injury		0.077	—	0.144	0.025	0.034	0.019	—
S06.0X0S	Concussion without loss of consciousness, sequela	167	Major Head Injury		0.077	—	0.144	0.025	0.034	0.019	—
S06.0X1S	Concussion with loss of consciousness of 30 minutes or less, sequela	167	Major Head Injury		0.077	—	0.144	0.025	0.034	0.019	—
S06.0X9S	Concussion with loss of consciousness of unspecified duration, sequela	167	Major Head Injury		0.077	—	0.144	0.025	0.034	0.019	—

ICD-10-CM Code	ICD-10-CM Code Description	V24 CMS-HCC	V24 CMS-HCC Disease Group	V24 CMS-HCC Hierarchies	Community, NonDual, Aged	Community, NonDual, Disabled	Community, FBDual, Aged	Community, FBDual, Disabled	Community, PBDual, Aged	Community, PBDual, Disabled	Institutional
S06.1X0A	Traumatic cerebral edema without loss of consciousness, initial encounter	167	Major Head Injury		0.077	—	0.144	0.025	0.034	0.019	—
S06.1X0S	Traumatic cerebral edema without loss of consciousness, sequela	167	Major Head Injury		0.077	—	0.144	0.025	0.034	0.019	—
S06.1X1A	Traumatic cerebral edema with loss of consciousness of 30 minutes or less, initial encounter	167	Major Head Injury		0.077	—	0.144	0.025	0.034	0.019	—
S06.1X1S	Traumatic cerebral edema with loss of consciousness of 30 minutes or less, sequela	167	Major Head Injury		0.077	—	0.144	0.025	0.034	0.019	—
S06.1X2A	Traumatic cerebral edema with loss of consciousness of 31 minutes to 59 minutes, initial encounter	167	Major Head Injury		0.077	—	0.144	0.025	0.034	0.019	—
S06.1X2S	Traumatic cerebral edema with loss of consciousness of 31 minutes to 59 minutes, sequela	167	Major Head Injury		0.077	—	0.144	0.025	0.034	0.019	—
S06.1X3A	Traumatic cerebral edema with loss of consciousness of 1 hour to 5 hours 59 minutes, initial encounter	166	Severe Head Injury	80,167	0.486	0.274	0.511	0.105	0.729	0.134	—
S06.1X3S	Traumatic cerebral edema with loss of consciousness of 1 hour to 5 hours 59 minutes, sequela	167	Major Head Injury		0.077	—	0.144	0.025	0.034	0.019	—
S06.1X4A	Traumatic cerebral edema with loss of consciousness of 6 hours to 24 hours, initial encounter	166	Severe Head Injury	80,167	0.486	0.274	0.511	0.105	0.729	0.134	—
S06.1X4S	Traumatic cerebral edema with loss of consciousness of 6 hours to 24 hours, sequela	167	Major Head Injury		0.077	—	0.144	0.025	0.034	0.019	—
S06.1X5A	Traumatic cerebral edema with loss of consciousness greater than 24 hours with return to pre-existing conscious level, initial encounter	166	Severe Head Injury	80,167	0.486	0.274	0.511	0.105	0.729	0.134	—
S06.1X5S	Traumatic cerebral edema with loss of consciousness greater than 24 hours with return to pre-existing conscious level, sequela	167	Major Head Injury		0.077	—	0.144	0.025	0.034	0.019	—
S06.1X6A	Traumatic cerebral edema with loss of consciousness greater than 24 hours without return to pre-existing conscious level with patient surviving, initial encounter	166	Severe Head Injury	80,167	0.486	0.274	0.511	0.105	0.729	0.134	—
S06.1X6S	Traumatic cerebral edema with loss of consciousness greater than 24 hours without return to pre-existing conscious level with patient surviving, sequela	167	Major Head Injury		0.077	—	0.144	0.025	0.034	0.019	—
S06.1X9A	Traumatic cerebral edema with loss of consciousness of unspecified duration, initial encounter	167	Major Head Injury		0.077	—	0.144	0.025	0.034	0.019	—
S06.1X9S	Traumatic cerebral edema with loss of consciousness of unspecified duration, sequela	167	Major Head Injury		0.077	—	0.144	0.025	0.034	0.019	—
S06.2X0A	Diffuse traumatic brain injury without loss of consciousness, initial encounter	167	Major Head Injury		0.077	—	0.144	0.025	0.034	0.019	—
S06.2X0S	Diffuse traumatic brain injury without loss of consciousness, sequela	167	Major Head Injury		0.077	—	0.144	0.025	0.034	0.019	—
S06.2X1A	Diffuse traumatic brain injury with loss of consciousness of 30 minutes or less, initial encounter	167	Major Head Injury		0.077	—	0.144	0.025	0.034	0.019	—

ICD-10-CM Code	ICD-10-CM Code Description	V24 CMS-HCC	V24 CMS-HCC Disease Group	V24 CMS-HCC Hierarchies	Community, NonDual, Aged	Community, NonDual, Disabled	Community, FBDual, Aged	Community, FBDual, Disabled	Community, PBDual, Aged	Community, PBDual, Disabled	Institutional
S06.2X1S	Diffuse traumatic brain injury with loss of consciousness of 30 minutes or less, sequela	167	Major Head Injury		0.077	—	0.144	0.025	0.034	0.019	—
S06.2X2A	Diffuse traumatic brain injury with loss of consciousness of 31 minutes to 59 minutes, initial encounter	167	Major Head Injury		0.077	—	0.144	0.025	0.034	0.019	—
S06.2X2S	Diffuse traumatic brain injury with loss of consciousness of 31 minutes to 59 minutes, sequela	167	Major Head Injury		0.077	—	0.144	0.025	0.034	0.019	—
S06.2X3A	Diffuse traumatic brain injury with loss of consciousness of 1 hour to 5 hours 59 minutes, initial encounter	166	Severe Head Injury	80,167	0.486	0.274	0.511	0.105	0.729	0.134	—
S06.2X3S	Diffuse traumatic brain injury with loss of consciousness of 1 hour to 5 hours 59 minutes, sequela	167	Major Head Injury		0.077	—	0.144	0.025	0.034	0.019	—
S06.2X4A	Diffuse traumatic brain injury with loss of consciousness of 6 hours to 24 hours, initial encounter	166	Severe Head Injury	80,167	0.486	0.274	0.511	0.105	0.729	0.134	—
S06.2X4S	Diffuse traumatic brain injury with loss of consciousness of 6 hours to 24 hours, sequela	167	Major Head Injury		0.077	—	0.144	0.025	0.034	0.019	—
S06.2X5A	Diffuse traumatic brain injury with loss of consciousness greater than 24 hours with return to pre-existing conscious levels, initial encounter	166	Severe Head Injury	80,167	0.486	0.274	0.511	0.105	0.729	0.134	—
S06.2X5S	Diffuse traumatic brain injury with loss of consciousness greater than 24 hours with return to pre-existing conscious levels, sequela	167	Major Head Injury		0.077	—	0.144	0.025	0.034	0.019	—
S06.2X6A	Diffuse traumatic brain injury with loss of consciousness greater than 24 hours without return to pre-existing conscious level with patient surviving, initial encounter	166	Severe Head Injury	80,167	0.486	0.274	0.511	0.105	0.729	0.134	—
S06.2X6S	Diffuse traumatic brain injury with loss of consciousness greater than 24 hours without return to pre-existing conscious level with patient surviving, sequela	167	Major Head Injury		0.077	—	0.144	0.025	0.034	0.019	—
S06.2X9A	Diffuse traumatic brain injury with loss of consciousness of unspecified duration, initial encounter	167	Major Head Injury		0.077	—	0.144	0.025	0.034	0.019	—
S06.2X9S	Diffuse traumatic brain injury with loss of consciousness of unspecified duration, sequela	167	Major Head Injury		0.077	—	0.144	0.025	0.034	0.019	—
S06.300A	Unspecified focal traumatic brain injury without loss of consciousness, initial encounter	167	Major Head Injury		0.077	—	0.144	0.025	0.034	0.019	—
S06.300S	Unspecified focal traumatic brain injury without loss of consciousness, sequela	167	Major Head Injury		0.077	—	0.144	0.025	0.034	0.019	—
S06.301A	Unspecified focal traumatic brain injury with loss of consciousness of 30 minutes or less, initial encounter	167	Major Head Injury		0.077	—	0.144	0.025	0.034	0.019	—
S06.301S	Unspecified focal traumatic brain injury with loss of consciousness of 30 minutes or less, sequela	167	Major Head Injury		0.077	—	0.144	0.025	0.034	0.019	—
S06.302A	Unspecified focal traumatic brain injury with loss of consciousness of 31 minutes to 59 minutes, initial encounter	167	Major Head Injury		0.077	—	0.144	0.025	0.034	0.019	—

ICD-10-CM Code	ICD-10-CM Code Description	V24 CMS-HCC	V24 CMS-HCC Disease Group	V24 CMS-HCC Hierarchies	Community, NonDual, Aged	Community, NonDual, Disabled	Community, FBDual, Aged	Community, FBDual, Disabled	Community, PBDual, Aged	Community, PBDual, Disabled	Institutional
S06.302S	Unspecified focal traumatic brain injury with loss of consciousness of 31 minutes to 59 minutes, sequela	167	Major Head Injury		0.077	—	0.144	0.025	0.034	0.019	—
S06.303A	Unspecified focal traumatic brain injury with loss of consciousness of 1 hour to 5 hours 59 minutes, initial encounter	166	Severe Head Injury	80,167	0.486	0.274	0.511	0.105	0.729	0.134	—
S06.303S	Unspecified focal traumatic brain injury with loss of consciousness of 1 hour to 5 hours 59 minutes, sequela	167	Major Head Injury		0.077	—	0.144	0.025	0.034	0.019	—
S06.304A	Unspecified focal traumatic brain injury with loss of consciousness of 6 hours to 24 hours, initial encounter	166	Severe Head Injury	80,167	0.486	0.274	0.511	0.105	0.729	0.134	—
S06.304S	Unspecified focal traumatic brain injury with loss of consciousness of 6 hours to 24 hours, sequela	167	Major Head Injury		0.077	—	0.144	0.025	0.034	0.019	—
S06.305A	Unspecified focal traumatic brain injury with loss of consciousness greater than 24 hours with return to pre-existing conscious level, initial encounter	166	Severe Head Injury	80,167	0.486	0.274	0.511	0.105	0.729	0.134	—
S06.305S	Unspecified focal traumatic brain injury with loss of consciousness greater than 24 hours with return to pre-existing conscious level, sequela	167	Major Head Injury		0.077	—	0.144	0.025	0.034	0.019	—
S06.306A	Unspecified focal traumatic brain injury with loss of consciousness greater than 24 hours without return to pre-existing conscious level with patient surviving, initial encounter	166	Severe Head Injury	80,167	0.486	0.274	0.511	0.105	0.729	0.134	—
S06.306S	Unspecified focal traumatic brain injury with loss of consciousness greater than 24 hours without return to pre-existing conscious level with patient surviving, sequela	167	Major Head Injury		0.077	—	0.144	0.025	0.034	0.019	—
S06.309A	Unspecified focal traumatic brain injury with loss of consciousness of unspecified duration, initial encounter	167	Major Head Injury		0.077	—	0.144	0.025	0.034	0.019	—
S06.309S	Unspecified focal traumatic brain injury with loss of consciousness of unspecified duration, sequela	167	Major Head Injury		0.077	—	0.144	0.025	0.034	0.019	—
S06.310A	Contusion and laceration of right cerebrum without loss of consciousness, initial encounter	167	Major Head Injury		0.077	—	0.144	0.025	0.034	0.019	—
S06.310S	Contusion and laceration of right cerebrum without loss of consciousness, sequela	167	Major Head Injury		0.077	—	0.144	0.025	0.034	0.019	—
S06.311A	Contusion and laceration of right cerebrum with loss of consciousness of 30 minutes or less, initial encounter	167	Major Head Injury		0.077	—	0.144	0.025	0.034	0.019	—
S06.311S	Contusion and laceration of right cerebrum with loss of consciousness of 30 minutes or less, sequela	167	Major Head Injury		0.077	—	0.144	0.025	0.034	0.019	—
S06.312A	Contusion and laceration of right cerebrum with loss of consciousness of 31 minutes to 59 minutes, initial encounter	167	Major Head Injury		0.077	—	0.144	0.025	0.034	0.019	—
S06.312S	Contusion and laceration of right cerebrum with loss of consciousness of 31 minutes to 59 minutes, sequela	167	Major Head Injury		0.077	—	0.144	0.025	0.034	0.019	—

ICD-10-CM Code	ICD-10-CM Code Description	V24 CMS-HCC	V24 CMS-HCC Disease Group	V24 CMS-HCC Hierarchies	Community, NonDual, Aged	Community, NonDual, Disabled	Community, FBDual, Aged	Community, FBDual, Disabled	Community, PBDual, Aged	Community, PBDual, Disabled	Institutional
S06.313A	Contusion and laceration of right cerebrum with loss of consciousness of 1 hour to 5 hours 59 minutes, initial encounter	166	Severe Head Injury	80,167	0.486	0.274	0.511	0.105	0.729	0.134	—
S06.313S	Contusion and laceration of right cerebrum with loss of consciousness of 1 hour to 5 hours 59 minutes, sequela	167	Major Head Injury		0.077	—	0.144	0.025	0.034	0.019	—
S06.314A	Contusion and laceration of right cerebrum with loss of consciousness of 6 hours to 24 hours, initial encounter	166	Severe Head Injury	80,167	0.486	0.274	0.511	0.105	0.729	0.134	—
S06.314S	Contusion and laceration of right cerebrum with loss of consciousness of 6 hours to 24 hours, sequela	167	Major Head Injury		0.077	—	0.144	0.025	0.034	0.019	—
S06.315A	Contusion and laceration of right cerebrum with loss of consciousness greater than 24 hours with return to pre-existing conscious level, initial encounter	166	Severe Head Injury	80,167	0.486	0.274	0.511	0.105	0.729	0.134	—
S06.315S	Contusion and laceration of right cerebrum with loss of consciousness greater than 24 hours with return to pre-existing conscious level, sequela	167	Major Head Injury		0.077	—	0.144	0.025	0.034	0.019	—
S06.316A	Contusion and laceration of right cerebrum with loss of consciousness greater than 24 hours without return to pre-existing conscious level with patient surviving, initial encounter	166	Severe Head Injury	80,167	0.486	0.274	0.511	0.105	0.729	0.134	—
S06.316S	Contusion and laceration of right cerebrum with loss of consciousness greater than 24 hours without return to pre-existing conscious level with patient surviving, sequela	167	Major Head Injury		0.077	—	0.144	0.025	0.034	0.019	—
S06.319A	Contusion and laceration of right cerebrum with loss of consciousness of unspecified duration, initial encounter	167	Major Head Injury		0.077	—	0.144	0.025	0.034	0.019	—
S06.319S	Contusion and laceration of right cerebrum with loss of consciousness of unspecified duration, sequela	167	Major Head Injury		0.077	—	0.144	0.025	0.034	0.019	—
S06.320A	Contusion and laceration of left cerebrum without loss of consciousness, initial encounter	167	Major Head Injury		0.077	—	0.144	0.025	0.034	0.019	—
S06.320S	Contusion and laceration of left cerebrum without loss of consciousness, sequela	167	Major Head Injury		0.077	—	0.144	0.025	0.034	0.019	—
S06.321A	Contusion and laceration of left cerebrum with loss of consciousness of 30 minutes or less, initial encounter	167	Major Head Injury		0.077	—	0.144	0.025	0.034	0.019	—
S06.321S	Contusion and laceration of left cerebrum with loss of consciousness of 30 minutes or less, sequela	167	Major Head Injury		0.077	—	0.144	0.025	0.034	0.019	—
S06.322A	Contusion and laceration of left cerebrum with loss of consciousness of 31 minutes to 59 minutes, initial encounter	167	Major Head Injury		0.077	—	0.144	0.025	0.034	0.019	—
S06.322S	Contusion and laceration of left cerebrum with loss of consciousness of 31 minutes to 59 minutes, sequela	167	Major Head Injury		0.077	—	0.144	0.025	0.034	0.019	—

ICD-10-CM Code	ICD-10-CM Code Description	V24 CMS-HCC	V24 CMS-HCC Disease Group	V24 CMS-HCC Hierarchies	Community, NonDual, Aged	Community, NonDual, Disabled	Community, FBDual, Aged	Community, FBDual, Disabled	Community, PBDual, Aged	Community, PBDual, Disabled	Institutional
S06.323A	Contusion and laceration of left cerebrum with loss of consciousness of 1 hour to 5 hours 59 minutes, initial encounter	166	Severe Head Injury	80,167	0.486	0.274	0.511	0.105	0.729	0.134	—
S06.323S	Contusion and laceration of left cerebrum with loss of consciousness of 1 hour to 5 hours 59 minutes, sequela	167	Major Head Injury		0.077	—	0.144	0.025	0.034	0.019	—
S06.324A	Contusion and laceration of left cerebrum with loss of consciousness of 6 hours to 24 hours, initial encounter	166	Severe Head Injury	80,167	0.486	0.274	0.511	0.105	0.729	0.134	—
S06.324S	Contusion and laceration of left cerebrum with loss of consciousness of 6 hours to 24 hours, sequela	167	Major Head Injury		0.077	—	0.144	0.025	0.034	0.019	—
S06.325A	Contusion and laceration of left cerebrum with loss of consciousness greater than 24 hours with return to pre-existing conscious level, initial encounter	166	Severe Head Injury	80,167	0.486	0.274	0.511	0.105	0.729	0.134	—
S06.325S	Contusion and laceration of left cerebrum with loss of consciousness greater than 24 hours with return to pre-existing conscious level, sequela	167	Major Head Injury		0.077	—	0.144	0.025	0.034	0.019	—
S06.326A	Contusion and laceration of left cerebrum with loss of consciousness greater than 24 hours without return to pre-existing conscious level with patient surviving, initial encounter	166	Severe Head Injury	80,167	0.486	0.274	0.511	0.105	0.729	0.134	—
S06.326S	Contusion and laceration of left cerebrum with loss of consciousness greater than 24 hours without return to pre-existing conscious level with patient surviving, sequela	167	Major Head Injury		0.077	—	0.144	0.025	0.034	0.019	—
S06.329A	Contusion and laceration of left cerebrum with loss of consciousness of unspecified duration, initial encounter	167	Major Head Injury		0.077	—	0.144	0.025	0.034	0.019	—
S06.329S	Contusion and laceration of left cerebrum with loss of consciousness of unspecified duration, sequela	167	Major Head Injury		0.077	—	0.144	0.025	0.034	0.019	—
S06.330A	Contusion and laceration of cerebrum, unspecified, without loss of consciousness, initial encounter	167	Major Head Injury		0.077	—	0.144	0.025	0.034	0.019	—
S06.330S	Contusion and laceration of cerebrum, unspecified, without loss of consciousness, sequela	167	Major Head Injury		0.077	—	0.144	0.025	0.034	0.019	—
S06.331A	Contusion and laceration of cerebrum, unspecified, with loss of consciousness of 30 minutes or less, initial encounter	167	Major Head Injury		0.077	—	0.144	0.025	0.034	0.019	—
S06.331S	Contusion and laceration of cerebrum, unspecified, with loss of consciousness of 30 minutes or less, sequela	167	Major Head Injury		0.077	—	0.144	0.025	0.034	0.019	—
S06.332A	Contusion and laceration of cerebrum, unspecified, with loss of consciousness of 31 minutes to 59 minutes, initial encounter	167	Major Head Injury		0.077	—	0.144	0.025	0.034	0.019	—
S06.332S	Contusion and laceration of cerebrum, unspecified, with loss of consciousness of 31 minutes to 59 minutes, sequela	167	Major Head Injury		0.077	—	0.144	0.025	0.034	0.019	—

2021 Optum360, LLC

ICD-10-CM Code	ICD-10-CM Code Description	V24 CMS-HCC	V24 CMS-HCC Disease Group	V24 CMS-HCC Hierarchies	Community, NonDual, Aged	Community, NonDual, Disabled	Community, FBDual, Aged	Community, FBDual, Disabled	Community, PBDual, Aged	Community, PBDual, Disabled	Institutional
S06.333A	Contusion and laceration of cerebrum, unspecified, with loss of consciousness of 1 hour to 5 hours 59 minutes, initial encounter	166	Severe Head Injury	80,167	0.486	0.274	0.511	0.105	0.729	0.134	—
S06.333S	Contusion and laceration of cerebrum, unspecified, with loss of consciousness of 1 hour to 5 hours 59 minutes, sequela	167	Major Head Injury		0.077	—	0.144	0.025	0.034	0.019	—
S06.334A	Contusion and laceration of cerebrum, unspecified, with loss of consciousness of 6 hours to 24 hours, initial encounter	166	Severe Head Injury	80,167	0.486	0.274	0.511	0.105	0.729	0.134	—
S06.334S	Contusion and laceration of cerebrum, unspecified, with loss of consciousness of 6 hours to 24 hours, sequela	167	Major Head Injury		0.077	—	0.144	0.025	0.034	0.019	—
S06.335A	Contusion and laceration of cerebrum, unspecified, with loss of consciousness greater than 24 hours with return to pre-existing conscious level, initial encounter	166	Severe Head Injury	80,167	0.486	0.274	0.511	0.105	0.729	0.134	—
S06.335S	Contusion and laceration of cerebrum, unspecified, with loss of consciousness greater than 24 hours with return to pre-existing conscious level, sequela	167	Major Head Injury		0.077	—	0.144	0.025	0.034	0.019	—
S06.336A	Contusion and laceration of cerebrum, unspecified, with loss of consciousness greater than 24 hours without return to pre-existing conscious level with patient surviving, initial encounter	166	Severe Head Injury	80,167	0.486	0.274	0.511	0.105	0.729	0.134	—
S06.336S	Contusion and laceration of cerebrum, unspecified, with loss of consciousness greater than 24 hours without return to pre-existing conscious level with patient surviving, sequela	167	Major Head Injury		0.077	—	0.144	0.025	0.034	0.019	—
S06.339A	Contusion and laceration of cerebrum, unspecified, with loss of consciousness of unspecified duration, initial encounter	167	Major Head Injury		0.077	—	0.144	0.025	0.034	0.019	—
S06.339S	Contusion and laceration of cerebrum, unspecified, with loss of consciousness of unspecified duration, sequela	167	Major Head Injury		0.077	—	0.144	0.025	0.034	0.019	—
S06.340A	Traumatic hemorrhage of right cerebrum without loss of consciousness, initial encounter	167	Major Head Injury		0.077	—	0.144	0.025	0.034	0.019	—
S06.340S	Traumatic hemorrhage of right cerebrum without loss of consciousness, sequela	167	Major Head Injury		0.077	—	0.144	0.025	0.034	0.019	—
S06.341A	Traumatic hemorrhage of right cerebrum with loss of consciousness of 30 minutes or less, initial encounter	167	Major Head Injury		0.077	—	0.144	0.025	0.034	0.019	—
S06.341S	Traumatic hemorrhage of right cerebrum with loss of consciousness of 30 minutes or less, sequela	167	Major Head Injury		0.077	—	0.144	0.025	0.034	0.019	—
S06.342A	Traumatic hemorrhage of right cerebrum with loss of consciousness of 31 minutes to 59 minutes, initial encounter	167	Major Head Injury		0.077	—	0.144	0.025	0.034	0.019	—

ICD-10-CM Code	ICD-10-CM Code Description	V24 CMS-HCC	V24 CMS-HCC Disease Group	V24 CMS-HCC Hierarchies	Community, NonDual, Aged	Community, NonDual, Disabled	Community, FBDual, Aged	Community, FBDual, Disabled	Community, PBDual, Aged	Community, PBDual, Disabled	Institutional
SØ6.342S	Traumatic hemorrhage of right cerebrum with loss of consciousness of 31 minutes to 59 minutes, sequela	167	Major Head Injury		0.077	—	0.144	0.025	0.034	0.019	—
SØ6.343A	Traumatic hemorrhage of right cerebrum with loss of consciousness of 1 hours to 5 hours 59 minutes, initial encounter	166	Severe Head Injury	80,167	0.486	0.274	0.511	0.105	0.729	0.134	—
SØ6.343S	Traumatic hemorrhage of right cerebrum with loss of consciousness of 1 hours to 5 hours 59 minutes, sequela	167	Major Head Injury		0.077	—	0.144	0.025	0.034	0.019	—
SØ6.344A	Traumatic hemorrhage of right cerebrum with loss of consciousness of 6 hours to 24 hours, initial encounter	166	Severe Head Injury	80,167	0.486	0.274	0.511	0.105	0.729	0.134	—
SØ6.344S	Traumatic hemorrhage of right cerebrum with loss of consciousness of 6 hours to 24 hours, sequela	167	Major Head Injury		0.077	—	0.144	0.025	0.034	0.019	—
SØ6.345A	Traumatic hemorrhage of right cerebrum with loss of consciousness greater than 24 hours with return to pre-existing conscious level, initial encounter	166	Severe Head Injury	80,167	0.486	0.274	0.511	0.105	0.729	0.134	—
SØ6.345S	Traumatic hemorrhage of right cerebrum with loss of consciousness greater than 24 hours with return to pre-existing conscious level, sequela	167	Major Head Injury		0.077	—	0.144	0.025	0.034	0.019	—
SØ6.346A	Traumatic hemorrhage of right cerebrum with loss of consciousness greater than 24 hours without return to pre-existing conscious level with patient surviving, initial encounter	166	Severe Head Injury	80,167	0.486	0.274	0.511	0.105	0.729	0.134	—
SØ6.346S	Traumatic hemorrhage of right cerebrum with loss of consciousness greater than 24 hours without return to pre-existing conscious level with patient surviving, sequela	167	Major Head Injury		0.077	—	0.144	0.025	0.034	0.019	—
SØ6.349A	Traumatic hemorrhage of right cerebrum with loss of consciousness of unspecified duration, initial encounter	167	Major Head Injury		0.077	—	0.144	0.025	0.034	0.019	—
SØ6.349S	Traumatic hemorrhage of right cerebrum with loss of consciousness of unspecified duration, sequela	167	Major Head Injury		0.077	—	0.144	0.025	0.034	0.019	—
SØ6.35ØA	Traumatic hemorrhage of left cerebrum without loss of consciousness, initial encounter	167	Major Head Injury		0.077	—	0.144	0.025	0.034	0.019	—
SØ6.35ØS	Traumatic hemorrhage of left cerebrum without loss of consciousness, sequela	167	Major Head Injury		0.077	—	0.144	0.025	0.034	0.019	—
SØ6.351A	Traumatic hemorrhage of left cerebrum with loss of consciousness of 30 minutes or less, initial encounter	167	Major Head Injury		0.077	—	0.144	0.025	0.034	0.019	—
SØ6.351S	Traumatic hemorrhage of left cerebrum with loss of consciousness of 30 minutes or less, sequela	167	Major Head Injury		0.077	—	0.144	0.025	0.034	0.019	—
SØ6.352A	Traumatic hemorrhage of left cerebrum with loss of consciousness of 31 minutes to 59 minutes, initial encounter	167	Major Head Injury		0.077	—	0.144	0.025	0.034	0.019	—

ICD-10-CM Code	ICD-10-CM Code Description	V24 CMS-HCC	V24 CMS-HCC Disease Group	V24 CMS-HCC Hierarchies	Community, NonDual, Aged	Community, NonDual, Disabled	Community, FBDual, Aged	Community, FBDual, Disabled	Community, PBDual, Aged	Community, PBDual, Disabled	Institutional
S06.352S	Traumatic hemorrhage of left cerebrum with loss of consciousness of 31 minutes to 59 minutes, sequela	167	Major Head Injury		0.077	—	0.144	0.025	0.034	0.019	—
S06.353A	Traumatic hemorrhage of left cerebrum with loss of consciousness of 1 hours to 5 hours 59 minutes, initial encounter	166	Severe Head Injury	80,167	0.486	0.274	0.511	0.105	0.729	0.134	—
S06.353S	Traumatic hemorrhage of left cerebrum with loss of consciousness of 1 hours to 5 hours 59 minutes, sequela	167	Major Head Injury		0.077	—	0.144	0.025	0.034	0.019	—
S06.354A	Traumatic hemorrhage of left cerebrum with loss of consciousness of 6 hours to 24 hours, initial encounter	166	Severe Head Injury	80,167	0.486	0.274	0.511	0.105	0.729	0.134	—
S06.354S	Traumatic hemorrhage of left cerebrum with loss of consciousness of 6 hours to 24 hours, sequela	167	Major Head Injury		0.077	—	0.144	0.025	0.034	0.019	—
S06.355A	Traumatic hemorrhage of left cerebrum with loss of consciousness greater than 24 hours with return to pre-existing conscious level, initial encounter	166	Severe Head Injury	80,167	0.486	0.274	0.511	0.105	0.729	0.134	—
S06.355S	Traumatic hemorrhage of left cerebrum with loss of consciousness greater than 24 hours with return to pre-existing conscious level, sequela	167	Major Head Injury		0.077	—	0.144	0.025	0.034	0.019	—
S06.356A	Traumatic hemorrhage of left cerebrum with loss of consciousness greater than 24 hours without return to pre-existing conscious level with patient surviving, initial encounter	166	Severe Head Injury	80,167	0.486	0.274	0.511	0.105	0.729	0.134	—
S06.356S	Traumatic hemorrhage of left cerebrum with loss of consciousness greater than 24 hours without return to pre-existing conscious level with patient surviving, sequela	167	Major Head Injury		0.077	—	0.144	0.025	0.034	0.019	—
S06.359A	Traumatic hemorrhage of left cerebrum with loss of consciousness of unspecified duration, initial encounter	167	Major Head Injury		0.077	—	0.144	0.025	0.034	0.019	—
S06.359S	Traumatic hemorrhage of left cerebrum with loss of consciousness of unspecified duration, sequela	167	Major Head Injury		0.077	—	0.144	0.025	0.034	0.019	—
S06.360A	Traumatic hemorrhage of cerebrum, unspecified, without loss of consciousness, initial encounter	167	Major Head Injury		0.077	—	0.144	0.025	0.034	0.019	—
S06.360S	Traumatic hemorrhage of cerebrum, unspecified, without loss of consciousness, sequela	167	Major Head Injury		0.077	—	0.144	0.025	0.034	0.019	—
S06.361A	Traumatic hemorrhage of cerebrum, unspecified, with loss of consciousness of 30 minutes or less, initial encounter	167	Major Head Injury		0.077	—	0.144	0.025	0.034	0.019	—
S06.361S	Traumatic hemorrhage of cerebrum, unspecified, with loss of consciousness of 30 minutes or less, sequela	167	Major Head Injury		0.077	—	0.144	0.025	0.034	0.019	—
S06.362A	Traumatic hemorrhage of cerebrum, unspecified, with loss of consciousness of 31 minutes to 59 minutes, initial encounter	167	Major Head Injury		0.077	—	0.144	0.025	0.034	0.019	—

ICD-10-CM Code	ICD-10-CM Code Description	V24 CMS-HCC	V24 CMS-HCC Disease Group	V24 CMS-HCC Hierarchies	Community, NonDual, Aged	Community, NonDual, Disabled	Community, FBDual, Aged	Community, FBDual, Disabled	Community, PBDual, Aged	Community, PBDual, Disabled	Institutional
S06.362S	Traumatic hemorrhage of cerebrum, unspecified, with loss of consciousness of 31 minutes to 59 minutes, sequela	167	Major Head Injury		0.077	—	0.144	0.025	0.034	0.019	—
S06.363A	Traumatic hemorrhage of cerebrum, unspecified, with loss of consciousness of 1 hours to 5 hours 59 minutes, initial encounter	166	Severe Head Injury	80,167	0.486	0.274	0.511	0.105	0.729	0.134	—
S06.363S	Traumatic hemorrhage of cerebrum, unspecified, with loss of consciousness of 1 hours to 5 hours 59 minutes, sequela	167	Major Head Injury		0.077	—	0.144	0.025	0.034	0.019	—
S06.364A	Traumatic hemorrhage of cerebrum, unspecified, with loss of consciousness of 6 hours to 24 hours, initial encounter	166	Severe Head Injury	80,167	0.486	0.274	0.511	0.105	0.729	0.134	—
S06.364S	Traumatic hemorrhage of cerebrum, unspecified, with loss of consciousness of 6 hours to 24 hours, sequela	167	Major Head Injury		0.077	—	0.144	0.025	0.034	0.019	—
S06.365A	Traumatic hemorrhage of cerebrum, unspecified, with loss of consciousness greater than 24 hours with return to pre-existing conscious level, initial encounter	166	Severe Head Injury	80,167	0.486	0.274	0.511	0.105	0.729	0.134	—
S06.365S	Traumatic hemorrhage of cerebrum, unspecified, with loss of consciousness greater than 24 hours with return to pre-existing conscious level, sequela	167	Major Head Injury		0.077	—	0.144	0.025	0.034	0.019	—
S06.366A	Traumatic hemorrhage of cerebrum, unspecified, with loss of consciousness greater than 24 hours without return to pre-existing conscious level with patient surviving, initial encounter	166	Severe Head Injury	80,167	0.486	0.274	0.511	0.105	0.729	0.134	—
S06.366S	Traumatic hemorrhage of cerebrum, unspecified, with loss of consciousness greater than 24 hours without return to pre-existing conscious level with patient surviving, sequela	167	Major Head Injury		0.077	—	0.144	0.025	0.034	0.019	—
S06.369A	Traumatic hemorrhage of cerebrum, unspecified, with loss of consciousness of unspecified duration, initial encounter	167	Major Head Injury		0.077	—	0.144	0.025	0.034	0.019	—
S06.369S	Traumatic hemorrhage of cerebrum, unspecified, with loss of consciousness of unspecified duration, sequela	167	Major Head Injury		0.077	—	0.144	0.025	0.034	0.019	—
S06.370A	Contusion, laceration, and hemorrhage of cerebellum without loss of consciousness, initial encounter	167	Major Head Injury		0.077	—	0.144	0.025	0.034	0.019	—
S06.370S	Contusion, laceration, and hemorrhage of cerebellum without loss of consciousness, sequela	167	Major Head Injury		0.077	—	0.144	0.025	0.034	0.019	—
S06.371A	Contusion, laceration, and hemorrhage of cerebellum with loss of consciousness of 30 minutes or less, initial encounter	167	Major Head Injury		0.077	—	0.144	0.025	0.034	0.019	—

ICD-10-CM Code	ICD-10-CM Code Description	V24 CMS-HCC	V24 CMS-HCC Disease Group	V24 CMS-HCC Hierarchies	Community, NonDual, Aged	Community, NonDual, Disabled	Community, FBDual, Aged	Community, FBDual, Disabled	Community, PBDual, Aged	Community, PBDual, Disabled	Institutional
S06.371S	Contusion, laceration, and hemorrhage of cerebellum with loss of consciousness of 30 minutes or less, sequela	167	Major Head Injury		0.077	—	0.144	0.025	0.034	0.019	—
S06.372A	Contusion, laceration, and hemorrhage of cerebellum with loss of consciousness of 31 minutes to 59 minutes, initial encounter	167	Major Head Injury		0.077	—	0.144	0.025	0.034	0.019	—
S06.372S	Contusion, laceration, and hemorrhage of cerebellum with loss of consciousness of 31 minutes to 59 minutes, sequela	167	Major Head Injury		0.077	—	0.144	0.025	0.034	0.019	—
S06.373A	Contusion, laceration, and hemorrhage of cerebellum with loss of consciousness of 1 hour to 5 hours 59 minutes, initial encounter	166	Severe Head Injury	80,167	0.486	0.274	0.511	0.105	0.729	0.134	—
S06.373S	Contusion, laceration, and hemorrhage of cerebellum with loss of consciousness of 1 hour to 5 hours 59 minutes, sequela	167	Major Head Injury		0.077	—	0.144	0.025	0.034	0.019	—
S06.374A	Contusion, laceration, and hemorrhage of cerebellum with loss of consciousness of 6 hours to 24 hours, initial encounter	166	Severe Head Injury	80,167	0.486	0.274	0.511	0.105	0.729	0.134	—
S06.374S	Contusion, laceration, and hemorrhage of cerebellum with loss of consciousness of 6 hours to 24 hours, sequela	167	Major Head Injury		0.077	—	0.144	0.025	0.034	0.019	—
S06.375A	Contusion, laceration, and hemorrhage of cerebellum with loss of consciousness greater than 24 hours with return to pre-existing conscious level, initial encounter	166	Severe Head Injury	80,167	0.486	0.274	0.511	0.105	0.729	0.134	—
S06.375S	Contusion, laceration, and hemorrhage of cerebellum with loss of consciousness greater than 24 hours with return to pre-existing conscious level, sequela	167	Major Head Injury		0.077	—	0.144	0.025	0.034	0.019	—
S06.376A	Contusion, laceration, and hemorrhage of cerebellum with loss of consciousness greater than 24 hours without return to pre-existing conscious level with patient surviving, initial encounter	166	Severe Head Injury	80,167	0.486	0.274	0.511	0.105	0.729	0.134	—
S06.376S	Contusion, laceration, and hemorrhage of cerebellum with loss of consciousness greater than 24 hours without return to pre-existing conscious level with patient surviving, sequela	167	Major Head Injury		0.077	—	0.144	0.025	0.034	0.019	—
S06.379A	Contusion, laceration, and hemorrhage of cerebellum with loss of consciousness of unspecified duration, initial encounter	167	Major Head Injury		0.077	—	0.144	0.025	0.034	0.019	—
S06.379S	Contusion, laceration, and hemorrhage of cerebellum with loss of consciousness of unspecified duration, sequela	167	Major Head Injury		0.077	—	0.144	0.025	0.034	0.019	—
S06.380A	Contusion, laceration, and hemorrhage of brainstem without loss of consciousness, initial encounter	167	Major Head Injury		0.077	—	0.144	0.025	0.034	0.019	—

ICD-10-CM Code	ICD-10-CM Code Description	V24 CMS-HCC	V24 CMS-HCC Disease Group	V24 CMS-HCC Hierarchies	Community, NonDual, Aged	Community, NonDual, Disabled	Community, FBDual, Aged	Community, FBDual, Disabled	Community, PBDual, Aged	Community, PBDual, Disabled	Institutional
S06.380S	Contusion, laceration, and hemorrhage of brainstem without loss of consciousness, sequela	167	Major Head Injury		0.077	—	0.144	0.025	0.034	0.019	—
S06.381A	Contusion, laceration, and hemorrhage of brainstem with loss of consciousness of 30 minutes or less, initial encounter	167	Major Head Injury		0.077	—	0.144	0.025	0.034	0.019	—
S06.381S	Contusion, laceration, and hemorrhage of brainstem with loss of consciousness of 30 minutes or less, sequela	167	Major Head Injury		0.077	—	0.144	0.025	0.034	0.019	—
S06.382A	Contusion, laceration, and hemorrhage of brainstem with loss of consciousness of 31 minutes to 59 minutes, initial encounter	167	Major Head Injury		0.077	—	0.144	0.025	0.034	0.019	—
S06.382S	Contusion, laceration, and hemorrhage of brainstem with loss of consciousness of 31 minutes to 59 minutes, sequela	167	Major Head Injury		0.077	—	0.144	0.025	0.034	0.019	—
S06.383A	Contusion, laceration, and hemorrhage of brainstem with loss of consciousness of 1 hour to 5 hours 59 minutes, initial encounter	166	Severe Head Injury	80,167	0.486	0.274	0.511	0.105	0.729	0.134	—
S06.383S	Contusion, laceration, and hemorrhage of brainstem with loss of consciousness of 1 hour to 5 hours 59 minutes, sequela	167	Major Head Injury		0.077	—	0.144	0.025	0.034	0.019	—
S06.384A	Contusion, laceration, and hemorrhage of brainstem with loss of consciousness of 6 hours to 24 hours, initial encounter	166	Severe Head Injury	80,167	0.486	0.274	0.511	0.105	0.729	0.134	—
S06.384S	Contusion, laceration, and hemorrhage of brainstem with loss of consciousness of 6 hours to 24 hours, sequela	167	Major Head Injury		0.077	—	0.144	0.025	0.034	0.019	—
S06.385A	Contusion, laceration, and hemorrhage of brainstem with loss of consciousness greater than 24 hours with return to pre-existing conscious level, initial encounter	166	Severe Head Injury	80,167	0.486	0.274	0.511	0.105	0.729	0.134	—
S06.385S	Contusion, laceration, and hemorrhage of brainstem with loss of consciousness greater than 24 hours with return to pre-existing conscious level, sequela	167	Major Head Injury		0.077	—	0.144	0.025	0.034	0.019	—
S06.386A	Contusion, laceration, and hemorrhage of brainstem with loss of consciousness greater than 24 hours without return to pre-existing conscious level with patient surviving, initial encounter	166	Severe Head Injury	80,167	0.486	0.274	0.511	0.105	0.729	0.134	—
S06.386S	Contusion, laceration, and hemorrhage of brainstem with loss of consciousness greater than 24 hours without return to pre-existing conscious level with patient surviving, sequela	167	Major Head Injury		0.077	—	0.144	0.025	0.034	0.019	—
S06.389A	Contusion, laceration, and hemorrhage of brainstem with loss of consciousness of unspecified duration, initial encounter	167	Major Head Injury		0.077	—	0.144	0.025	0.034	0.019	—

ICD-10-CM Code	ICD-10-CM Code Description	V24 CMS-HCC	V24 CMS-HCC Disease Group	V24 CMS-HCC Hierarchies	Community, NonDual, Aged	Community, NonDual, Disabled	Community, FBDual, Aged	Community, FBDual, Disabled	Community, PBDual, Aged	Community, PBDual, Disabled	Institutional
S06.389S	Contusion, laceration, and hemorrhage of brainstem with loss of consciousness of unspecified duration, sequela	167	Major Head Injury		0.077	—	0.144	0.025	0.034	0.019	—
S06.4X0A	Epidural hemorrhage without loss of consciousness, initial encounter	167	Major Head Injury		0.077	—	0.144	0.025	0.034	0.019	—
S06.4X0S	Epidural hemorrhage without loss of consciousness, sequela	167	Major Head Injury		0.077	—	0.144	0.025	0.034	0.019	—
S06.4X1A	Epidural hemorrhage with loss of consciousness of 30 minutes or less, initial encounter	167	Major Head Injury		0.077	—	0.144	0.025	0.034	0.019	—
S06.4X1S	Epidural hemorrhage with loss of consciousness of 30 minutes or less, sequela	167	Major Head Injury		0.077	—	0.144	0.025	0.034	0.019	—
S06.4X2A	Epidural hemorrhage with loss of consciousness of 31 minutes to 59 minutes, initial encounter	167	Major Head Injury		0.077	—	0.144	0.025	0.034	0.019	—
S06.4X2S	Epidural hemorrhage with loss of consciousness of 31 minutes to 59 minutes, sequela	167	Major Head Injury		0.077	—	0.144	0.025	0.034	0.019	—
S06.4X3A	Epidural hemorrhage with loss of consciousness of 1 hour to 5 hours 59 minutes, initial encounter	166	Severe Head Injury	80,167	0.486	0.274	0.511	0.105	0.729	0.134	—
S06.4X3S	Epidural hemorrhage with loss of consciousness of 1 hour to 5 hours 59 minutes, sequela	167	Major Head Injury		0.077	—	0.144	0.025	0.034	0.019	—
S06.4X4A	Epidural hemorrhage with loss of consciousness of 6 hours to 24 hours, initial encounter	166	Severe Head Injury	80,167	0.486	0.274	0.511	0.105	0.729	0.134	—
S06.4X4S	Epidural hemorrhage with loss of consciousness of 6 hours to 24 hours, sequela	167	Major Head Injury		0.077	—	0.144	0.025	0.034	0.019	—
S06.4X5A	Epidural hemorrhage with loss of consciousness greater than 24 hours with return to pre-existing conscious level, initial encounter	166	Severe Head Injury	80,167	0.486	0.274	0.511	0.105	0.729	0.134	—
S06.4X5S	Epidural hemorrhage with loss of consciousness greater than 24 hours with return to pre-existing conscious level, sequela	167	Major Head Injury		0.077	—	0.144	0.025	0.034	0.019	—
S06.4X6A	Epidural hemorrhage with loss of consciousness greater than 24 hours without return to pre-existing conscious level with patient surviving, initial encounter	166	Severe Head Injury	80,167	0.486	0.274	0.511	0.105	0.729	0.134	—
S06.4X6S	Epidural hemorrhage with loss of consciousness greater than 24 hours without return to pre-existing conscious level with patient surviving, sequela	167	Major Head Injury		0.077	—	0.144	0.025	0.034	0.019	—
S06.4X9A	Epidural hemorrhage with loss of consciousness of unspecified duration, initial encounter	167	Major Head Injury		0.077	—	0.144	0.025	0.034	0.019	—
S06.4X9S	Epidural hemorrhage with loss of consciousness of unspecified duration, sequela	167	Major Head Injury		0.077	—	0.144	0.025	0.034	0.019	—
S06.5X0A	Traumatic subdural hemorrhage without loss of consciousness, initial encounter	167	Major Head Injury		0.077	—	0.144	0.025	0.034	0.019	—
S06.5X0S	Traumatic subdural hemorrhage without loss of consciousness, sequela	167	Major Head Injury		0.077	—	0.144	0.025	0.034	0.019	—

ICD-10-CM Code	ICD-10-CM Code Description	V24 CMS-HCC	V24 CMS-HCC Disease Group	V24 CMS-HCC Hierarchies	Community, NonDual, Aged	Community, NonDual, Disabled	Community, FBDual, Aged	Community, FBDual, Disabled	Community, PBDual, Aged	Community, PBDual, Disabled	Institutional
S06.5X1A	Traumatic subdural hemorrhage with loss of consciousness of 30 minutes or less, initial encounter	167	Major Head Injury		0.077	—	0.144	0.025	0.034	0.019	—
S06.5X1S	Traumatic subdural hemorrhage with loss of consciousness of 30 minutes or less, sequela	167	Major Head Injury		0.077	—	0.144	0.025	0.034	0.019	—
S06.5X2A	Traumatic subdural hemorrhage with loss of consciousness of 31 minutes to 59 minutes, initial encounter	167	Major Head Injury		0.077	—	0.144	0.025	0.034	0.019	—
S06.5X2S	Traumatic subdural hemorrhage with loss of consciousness of 31 minutes to 59 minutes, sequela	167	Major Head Injury		0.077	—	0.144	0.025	0.034	0.019	—
S06.5X3A	Traumatic subdural hemorrhage with loss of consciousness of 1 hour to 5 hours 59 minutes, initial encounter	166	Severe Head Injury	80,167	0.486	0.274	0.511	0.105	0.729	0.134	—
S06.5X3S	Traumatic subdural hemorrhage with loss of consciousness of 1 hour to 5 hours 59 minutes, sequela	167	Major Head Injury		0.077	—	0.144	0.025	0.034	0.019	—
S06.5X4A	Traumatic subdural hemorrhage with loss of consciousness of 6 hours to 24 hours, initial encounter	166	Severe Head Injury	80,167	0.486	0.274	0.511	0.105	0.729	0.134	—
S06.5X4S	Traumatic subdural hemorrhage with loss of consciousness of 6 hours to 24 hours, sequela	167	Major Head Injury		0.077	—	0.144	0.025	0.034	0.019	—
S06.5X5A	Traumatic subdural hemorrhage with loss of consciousness greater than 24 hours with return to pre-existing conscious level, initial encounter	166	Severe Head Injury	80,167	0.486	0.274	0.511	0.105	0.729	0.134	—
S06.5X5S	Traumatic subdural hemorrhage with loss of consciousness greater than 24 hours with return to pre-existing conscious level, sequela	167	Major Head Injury		0.077	—	0.144	0.025	0.034	0.019	—
S06.5X6A	Traumatic subdural hemorrhage with loss of consciousness greater than 24 hours without return to pre-existing conscious level with patient surviving, initial encounter	166	Severe Head Injury	80,167	0.486	0.274	0.511	0.105	0.729	0.134	—
S06.5X6S	Traumatic subdural hemorrhage with loss of consciousness greater than 24 hours without return to pre-existing conscious level with patient surviving, sequela	167	Major Head Injury		0.077	—	0.144	0.025	0.034	0.019	—
S06.5X9A	Traumatic subdural hemorrhage with loss of consciousness of unspecified duration, initial encounter	167	Major Head Injury		0.077	—	0.144	0.025	0.034	0.019	—
S06.5X9S	Traumatic subdural hemorrhage with loss of consciousness of unspecified duration, sequela	167	Major Head Injury		0.077	—	0.144	0.025	0.034	0.019	—
S06.6X0A	Traumatic subarachnoid hemorrhage without loss of consciousness, initial encounter	167	Major Head Injury		0.077	—	0.144	0.025	0.034	0.019	—
S06.6X0S	Traumatic subarachnoid hemorrhage without loss of consciousness, sequela	167	Major Head Injury		0.077	—	0.144	0.025	0.034	0.019	—
S06.6X1A	Traumatic subarachnoid hemorrhage with loss of consciousness of 30 minutes or less, initial encounter	167	Major Head Injury		0.077	—	0.144	0.025	0.034	0.019	—
S06.6X1S	Traumatic subarachnoid hemorrhage with loss of consciousness of 30 minutes or less, sequela	167	Major Head Injury		0.077	—	0.144	0.025	0.034	0.019	—

ICD-10-CM Code	ICD-10-CM Code Description	V24 CMS-HCC	V24 CMS-HCC Disease Group	V24 CMS-HCC Hierarchies	Community, NonDual, Aged	Community, NonDual, Disabled	Community, FBDual, Aged	Community, FBDual, Disabled	Community, PBDual, Aged	Community, PBDual, Disabled	Institutional
S06.6X2A	Traumatic subarachnoid hemorrhage with loss of consciousness of 31 minutes to 59 minutes, initial encounter	167	Major Head Injury		0.077	—	0.144	0.025	0.034	0.019	—
S06.6X2S	Traumatic subarachnoid hemorrhage with loss of consciousness of 31 minutes to 59 minutes, sequela	167	Major Head Injury		0.077	—	0.144	0.025	0.034	0.019	—
S06.6X3A	Traumatic subarachnoid hemorrhage with loss of consciousness of 1 hour to 5 hours 59 minutes, initial encounter	166	Severe Head Injury	80,167	0.486	0.274	0.511	0.105	0.729	0.134	—
S06.6X3S	Traumatic subarachnoid hemorrhage with loss of consciousness of 1 hour to 5 hours 59 minutes, sequela	167	Major Head Injury		0.077	—	0.144	0.025	0.034	0.019	—
S06.6X4A	Traumatic subarachnoid hemorrhage with loss of consciousness of 6 hours to 24 hours, initial encounter	166	Severe Head Injury	80,167	0.486	0.274	0.511	0.105	0.729	0.134	—
S06.6X4S	Traumatic subarachnoid hemorrhage with loss of consciousness of 6 hours to 24 hours, sequela	167	Major Head Injury		0.077	—	0.144	0.025	0.034	0.019	—
S06.6X5A	Traumatic subarachnoid hemorrhage with loss of consciousness greater than 24 hours with return to pre-existing conscious level, initial encounter	166	Severe Head Injury	80,167	0.486	0.274	0.511	0.105	0.729	0.134	—
S06.6X5S	Traumatic subarachnoid hemorrhage with loss of consciousness greater than 24 hours with return to pre-existing conscious level, sequela	167	Major Head Injury		0.077	—	0.144	0.025	0.034	0.019	—
S06.6X6A	Traumatic subarachnoid hemorrhage with loss of consciousness greater than 24 hours without return to pre-existing conscious level with patient surviving, initial encounter	166	Severe Head Injury	80,167	0.486	0.274	0.511	0.105	0.729	0.134	—
S06.6X6S	Traumatic subarachnoid hemorrhage with loss of consciousness greater than 24 hours without return to pre-existing conscious level with patient surviving, sequela	167	Major Head Injury		0.077	—	0.144	0.025	0.034	0.019	—
S06.6X9A	Traumatic subarachnoid hemorrhage with loss of consciousness of unspecified duration, initial encounter	167	Major Head Injury		0.077	—	0.144	0.025	0.034	0.019	—
S06.6X9S	Traumatic subarachnoid hemorrhage with loss of consciousness of unspecified duration, sequela	167	Major Head Injury		0.077	—	0.144	0.025	0.034	0.019	—
S06.810A	Injury of right internal carotid artery, intracranial portion, not elsewhere classified without loss of consciousness, initial encounter	167	Major Head Injury		0.077	—	0.144	0.025	0.034	0.019	—
S06.810S	Injury of right internal carotid artery, intracranial portion, not elsewhere classified without loss of consciousness, sequela	167	Major Head Injury		0.077	—	0.144	0.025	0.034	0.019	—
S06.811A	Injury of right internal carotid artery, intracranial portion, not elsewhere classified with loss of consciousness of 30 minutes or less, initial encounter	167	Major Head Injury		0.077	—	0.144	0.025	0.034	0.019	—
S06.811S	Injury of right internal carotid artery, intracranial portion, not elsewhere classified with loss of consciousness of 30 minutes or less, sequela	167	Major Head Injury		0.077	—	0.144	0.025	0.034	0.019	—

ICD-10-CM Code	ICD-10-CM Code Description	V24 CMS-HCC	V24 CMS-HCC Disease Group	V24 CMS-HCC Hierarchies	Community, NonDual, Aged	Community, NonDual, Disabled	Community, FBDual, Aged	Community, FBDual, Disabled	Community, PBDual, Aged	Community, PBDual, Disabled	Institutional
S06.812A	Injury of right internal carotid artery, intracranial portion, not elsewhere classified with loss of consciousness of 31 minutes to 59 minutes, initial encounter	167	Major Head Injury		0.077	—	0.144	0.025	0.034	0.019	—
S06.812S	Injury of right internal carotid artery, intracranial portion, not elsewhere classified with loss of consciousness of 31 minutes to 59 minutes, sequela	167	Major Head Injury		0.077	—	0.144	0.025	0.034	0.019	—
S06.813A	Injury of right internal carotid artery, intracranial portion, not elsewhere classified with loss of consciousness of 1 hour to 5 hours 59 minutes, initial encounter	166	Severe Head Injury	80,167	0.486	0.274	0.511	0.105	0.729	0.134	—
S06.813S	Injury of right internal carotid artery, intracranial portion, not elsewhere classified with loss of consciousness of 1 hour to 5 hours 59 minutes, sequela	167	Major Head Injury		0.077	—	0.144	0.025	0.034	0.019	—
S06.814A	Injury of right internal carotid artery, intracranial portion, not elsewhere classified with loss of consciousness of 6 hours to 24 hours, initial encounter	166	Severe Head Injury	80,167	0.486	0.274	0.511	0.105	0.729	0.134	—
S06.814S	Injury of right internal carotid artery, intracranial portion, not elsewhere classified with loss of consciousness of 6 hours to 24 hours, sequela	167	Major Head Injury		0.077	—	0.144	0.025	0.034	0.019	—
S06.815A	Injury of right internal carotid artery, intracranial portion, not elsewhere classified with loss of consciousness greater than 24 hours with return to pre-existing conscious level, initial encounter	166	Severe Head Injury	80,167	0.486	0.274	0.511	0.105	0.729	0.134	—
S06.815S	Injury of right internal carotid artery, intracranial portion, not elsewhere classified with loss of consciousness greater than 24 hours with return to pre-existing conscious level, sequela	167	Major Head Injury		0.077	—	0.144	0.025	0.034	0.019	—
S06.816A	Injury of right internal carotid artery, intracranial portion, not elsewhere classified with loss of consciousness greater than 24 hours without return to pre-existing conscious level with patient surviving, initial encounter	166	Severe Head Injury	80,167	0.486	0.274	0.511	0.105	0.729	0.134	—
S06.816S	Injury of right internal carotid artery, intracranial portion, not elsewhere classified with loss of consciousness greater than 24 hours without return to pre-existing conscious level with patient surviving, sequela	167	Major Head Injury		0.077	—	0.144	0.025	0.034	0.019	—
S06.819A	Injury of right internal carotid artery, intracranial portion, not elsewhere classified with loss of consciousness of unspecified duration, initial encounter	167	Major Head Injury		0.077	—	0.144	0.025	0.034	0.019	—
S06.819S	Injury of right internal carotid artery, intracranial portion, not elsewhere classified with loss of consciousness of unspecified duration, sequela	167	Major Head Injury		0.077	—	0.144	0.025	0.034	0.019	—
S06.820A	Injury of left internal carotid artery, intracranial portion, not elsewhere classified without loss of consciousness, initial encounter	167	Major Head Injury		0.077	—	0.144	0.025	0.034	0.019	—

ICD-10-CM Code	ICD-10-CM Code Description	V24 CMS-HCC	V24 CMS-HCC Disease Group	V24 CMS-HCC Hierarchies	Community, NonDual, Aged	Community, NonDual, Disabled	Community, FBDual, Aged	Community, FBDual, Disabled	Community, PBDual, Aged	Community, PBDual, Disabled	Institutional
S06.820S	Injury of left internal carotid artery, intracranial portion, not elsewhere classified without loss of consciousness, sequela	167	Major Head Injury		0.077	—	0.144	0.025	0.034	0.019	—
S06.821A	Injury of left internal carotid artery, intracranial portion, not elsewhere classified with loss of consciousness of 30 minutes or less, initial encounter	167	Major Head Injury		0.077	—	0.144	0.025	0.034	0.019	—
S06.821S	Injury of left internal carotid artery, intracranial portion, not elsewhere classified with loss of consciousness of 30 minutes or less, sequela	167	Major Head Injury		0.077	—	0.144	0.025	0.034	0.019	—
S06.822A	Injury of left internal carotid artery, intracranial portion, not elsewhere classified with loss of consciousness of 31 minutes to 59 minutes, initial encounter	167	Major Head Injury		0.077	—	0.144	0.025	0.034	0.019	—
S06.822S	Injury of left internal carotid artery, intracranial portion, not elsewhere classified with loss of consciousness of 31 minutes to 59 minutes, sequela	167	Major Head Injury		0.077	—	0.144	0.025	0.034	0.019	—
S06.823A	Injury of left internal carotid artery, intracranial portion, not elsewhere classified with loss of consciousness of 1 hour to 5 hours 59 minutes, initial encounter	166	Severe Head Injury	80,167	0.486	0.274	0.511	0.105	0.729	0.134	—
S06.823S	Injury of left internal carotid artery, intracranial portion, not elsewhere classified with loss of consciousness of 1 hour to 5 hours 59 minutes, sequela	167	Major Head Injury		0.077	—	0.144	0.025	0.034	0.019	—
S06.824A	Injury of left internal carotid artery, intracranial portion, not elsewhere classified with loss of consciousness of 6 hours to 24 hours, initial encounter	166	Severe Head Injury	80,167	0.486	0.274	0.511	0.105	0.729	0.134	—
S06.824S	Injury of left internal carotid artery, intracranial portion, not elsewhere classified with loss of consciousness of 6 hours to 24 hours, sequela	167	Major Head Injury		0.077	—	0.144	0.025	0.034	0.019	—
S06.825A	Injury of left internal carotid artery, intracranial portion, not elsewhere classified with loss of consciousness greater than 24 hours with return to pre-existing conscious level, initial encounter	166	Severe Head Injury	80,167	0.486	0.274	0.511	0.105	0.729	0.134	—
S06.825S	Injury of left internal carotid artery, intracranial portion, not elsewhere classified with loss of consciousness greater than 24 hours with return to pre-existing conscious level, sequela	167	Major Head Injury		0.077	—	0.144	0.025	0.034	0.019	—
S06.826A	Injury of left internal carotid artery, intracranial portion, not elsewhere classified with loss of consciousness greater than 24 hours without return to pre-existing conscious level with patient surviving, initial encounter	166	Severe Head Injury	80,167	0.486	0.274	0.511	0.105	0.729	0.134	—
S06.826S	Injury of left internal carotid artery, intracranial portion, not elsewhere classified with loss of consciousness greater than 24 hours without return to pre-existing conscious level with patient surviving, sequela	167	Major Head Injury		0.077	—	0.144	0.025	0.034	0.019	—

ICD-10-CM Code	ICD-10-CM Code Description	V24 CMS-HCC	V24 CMS-HCC Disease Group	V24 CMS-HCC Hierarchies	Community, NonDual, Aged	Community, NonDual, Disabled	Community, FBDual, Aged	Community, FBDual, Disabled	Community, PBDual, Aged	Community, PBDual, Disabled	Institutional
SØ6.829A	Injury of left internal carotid artery, intracranial portion, not elsewhere classified with loss of consciousness of unspecified duration, initial encounter	167	Major Head Injury		0.077	—	0.144	0.025	0.034	0.019	—
SØ6.829S	Injury of left internal carotid artery, intracranial portion, not elsewhere classified with loss of consciousness of unspecified duration, sequela	167	Major Head Injury		0.077	—	0.144	0.025	0.034	0.019	—
SØ6.890A	Other specified intracranial injury without loss of consciousness, initial encounter	167	Major Head Injury		0.077	—	0.144	0.025	0.034	0.019	—
SØ6.890S	Other specified intracranial injury without loss of consciousness, sequela	167	Major Head Injury		0.077	—	0.144	0.025	0.034	0.019	—
SØ6.891A	Other specified intracranial injury with loss of consciousness of 30 minutes or less, initial encounter	167	Major Head Injury		0.077	—	0.144	0.025	0.034	0.019	—
SØ6.891S	Other specified intracranial injury with loss of consciousness of 30 minutes or less, sequela	167	Major Head Injury		0.077	—	0.144	0.025	0.034	0.019	—
SØ6.892A	Other specified intracranial injury with loss of consciousness of 31 minutes to 59 minutes, initial encounter	167	Major Head Injury		0.077	—	0.144	0.025	0.034	0.019	—
SØ6.892S	Other specified intracranial injury with loss of consciousness of 31 minutes to 59 minutes, sequela	167	Major Head Injury		0.077	—	0.144	0.025	0.034	0.019	—
SØ6.893A	Other specified intracranial injury with loss of consciousness of 1 hour to 5 hours 59 minutes, initial encounter	166	Severe Head Injury	80,167	0.486	0.274	0.511	0.105	0.729	0.134	—
SØ6.893S	Other specified intracranial injury with loss of consciousness of 1 hour to 5 hours 59 minutes, sequela	167	Major Head Injury		0.077	—	0.144	0.025	0.034	0.019	—
SØ6.894A	Other specified intracranial injury with loss of consciousness of 6 hours to 24 hours, initial encounter	166	Severe Head Injury	80,167	0.486	0.274	0.511	0.105	0.729	0.134	—
SØ6.894S	Other specified intracranial injury with loss of consciousness of 6 hours to 24 hours, sequela	167	Major Head Injury		0.077	—	0.144	0.025	0.034	0.019	—
SØ6.895A	Other specified intracranial injury with loss of consciousness greater than 24 hours with return to pre-existing conscious level, initial encounter	166	Severe Head Injury	80,167	0.486	0.274	0.511	0.105	0.729	0.134	—
SØ6.895S	Other specified intracranial injury with loss of consciousness greater than 24 hours with return to pre-existing conscious level, sequela	167	Major Head Injury		0.077	—	0.144	0.025	0.034	0.019	—
SØ6.896A	Other specified intracranial injury with loss of consciousness greater than 24 hours without return to pre-existing conscious level with patient surviving, initial encounter	166	Severe Head Injury	80,167	0.486	0.274	0.511	0.105	0.729	0.134	—
SØ6.896S	Other specified intracranial injury with loss of consciousness greater than 24 hours without return to pre-existing conscious level with patient surviving, sequela	167	Major Head Injury		0.077	—	0.144	0.025	0.034	0.019	—

ICD-10-CM Code	ICD-10-CM Code Description	V24 CMS-HCC	V24 CMS-HCC Disease Group	V24 CMS-HCC Hierarchies	Community, NonDual, Aged	Community, NonDual, Disabled	Community, FBDual, Aged	Community, FBDual, Disabled	Community, PBDual, Aged	Community, PBDual, Disabled	Institutional
S06.899A	Other specified intracranial injury with loss of consciousness of unspecified duration, initial encounter	167	Major Head Injury		0.077	—	0.144	0.025	0.034	0.019	—
S06.899S	Other specified intracranial injury with loss of consciousness of unspecified duration, sequela	167	Major Head Injury		0.077	—	0.144	0.025	0.034	0.019	—
S06.9X0A	Unspecified intracranial injury without loss of consciousness, initial encounter	167	Major Head Injury		0.077	—	0.144	0.025	0.034	0.019	—
S06.9X0S	Unspecified intracranial injury without loss of consciousness, sequela	167	Major Head Injury		0.077	—	0.144	0.025	0.034	0.019	—
S06.9X1A	Unspecified intracranial injury with loss of consciousness of 30 minutes or less, initial encounter	167	Major Head Injury		0.077	—	0.144	0.025	0.034	0.019	—
S06.9X1S	Unspecified intracranial injury with loss of consciousness of 30 minutes or less, sequela	167	Major Head Injury		0.077	—	0.144	0.025	0.034	0.019	—
S06.9X2A	Unspecified intracranial injury with loss of consciousness of 31 minutes to 59 minutes, initial encounter	167	Major Head Injury		0.077	—	0.144	0.025	0.034	0.019	—
S06.9X2S	Unspecified intracranial injury with loss of consciousness of 31 minutes to 59 minutes, sequela	167	Major Head Injury		0.077	—	0.144	0.025	0.034	0.019	—
S06.9X3A	Unspecified intracranial injury with loss of consciousness of 1 hour to 5 hours 59 minutes, initial encounter	166	Severe Head Injury	80,167	0.486	0.274	0.511	0.105	0.729	0.134	—
S06.9X3S	Unspecified intracranial injury with loss of consciousness of 1 hour to 5 hours 59 minutes, sequela	167	Major Head Injury		0.077	—	0.144	0.025	0.034	0.019	—
S06.9X4A	Unspecified intracranial injury with loss of consciousness of 6 hours to 24 hours, initial encounter	166	Severe Head Injury	80,167	0.486	0.274	0.511	0.105	0.729	0.134	—
S06.9X4S	Unspecified intracranial injury with loss of consciousness of 6 hours to 24 hours, sequela	167	Major Head Injury		0.077	—	0.144	0.025	0.034	0.019	—
S06.9X5A	Unspecified intracranial injury with loss of consciousness greater than 24 hours with return to pre-existing conscious level, initial encounter	166	Severe Head Injury	80,167	0.486	0.274	0.511	0.105	0.729	0.134	—
S06.9X5S	Unspecified intracranial injury with loss of consciousness greater than 24 hours with return to pre-existing conscious level, sequela	167	Major Head Injury		0.077	—	0.144	0.025	0.034	0.019	—
S06.9X6A	Unspecified intracranial injury with loss of consciousness greater than 24 hours without return to pre-existing conscious level with patient surviving, initial encounter	166	Severe Head Injury	80,167	0.486	0.274	0.511	0.105	0.729	0.134	—
S06.9X6S	Unspecified intracranial injury with loss of consciousness greater than 24 hours without return to pre-existing conscious level with patient surviving, sequela	167	Major Head Injury		0.077	—	0.144	0.025	0.034	0.019	—
S06.9X9A	Unspecified intracranial injury with loss of consciousness of unspecified duration, initial encounter	167	Major Head Injury		0.077	—	0.144	0.025	0.034	0.019	—
S06.9X9S	Unspecified intracranial injury with loss of consciousness of unspecified duration, sequela	167	Major Head Injury		0.077	—	0.144	0.025	0.034	0.019	—

ICD-10-CM Code	ICD-10-CM Code Description	V24 CMS-HCC	V24 CMS-HCC Disease Group	V24 CMS-HCC Hierarchies	Community, NonDual, Aged	Community, NonDual, Disabled	Community, FBDual, Aged	Community, FBDual, Disabled	Community, PBDual, Aged	Community, PBDual, Disabled	Institutional
S06.A0XA	Traumatic brain compression without herniation, initial encounter	167	Major Head Injury		0.077	—	0.144	0.025	0.034	0.019	—
S06.A0XS	Traumatic brain compression without herniation, sequela	167	Major Head Injury		0.077	—	0.144	0.025	0.034	0.019	—
S06.A1XA	Traumatic brain compression with herniation, initial encounter	167	Major Head Injury		0.077	—	0.144	0.025	0.034	0.019	—
S06.A1XS	Traumatic brain compression with herniation, sequela	167	Major Head Injury		0.077	—	0.144	0.025	0.034	0.019	—
S12.000A	Unspecified displaced fracture of first cervical vertebra, initial encounter for closed fracture	169	Vertebral Fractures without Spinal Cord Injury		0.476	0.369	0.532	0.377	0.512	0.336	0.250
S12.000B	Unspecified displaced fracture of first cervical vertebra, initial encounter for open fracture	169	Vertebral Fractures without Spinal Cord Injury		0.476	0.369	0.532	0.377	0.512	0.336	0.250
S12.001A	Unspecified nondisplaced fracture of first cervical vertebra, initial encounter for closed fracture	169	Vertebral Fractures without Spinal Cord Injury		0.476	0.369	0.532	0.377	0.512	0.336	0.250
S12.001B	Unspecified nondisplaced fracture of first cervical vertebra, initial encounter for open fracture	169	Vertebral Fractures without Spinal Cord Injury		0.476	0.369	0.532	0.377	0.512	0.336	0.250
S12.01XA	Stable burst fracture of first cervical vertebra, initial encounter for closed fracture	169	Vertebral Fractures without Spinal Cord Injury		0.476	0.369	0.532	0.377	0.512	0.336	0.250
S12.01XB	Stable burst fracture of first cervical vertebra, initial encounter for open fracture	169	Vertebral Fractures without Spinal Cord Injury		0.476	0.369	0.532	0.377	0.512	0.336	0.250
S12.02XA	Unstable burst fracture of first cervical vertebra, initial encounter for closed fracture	169	Vertebral Fractures without Spinal Cord Injury		0.476	0.369	0.532	0.377	0.512	0.336	0.250
S12.02XB	Unstable burst fracture of first cervical vertebra, initial encounter for open fracture	169	Vertebral Fractures without Spinal Cord Injury		0.476	0.369	0.532	0.377	0.512	0.336	0.250
S12.030A	Displaced posterior arch fracture of first cervical vertebra, initial encounter for closed fracture	169	Vertebral Fractures without Spinal Cord Injury		0.476	0.369	0.532	0.377	0.512	0.336	0.250
S12.030B	Displaced posterior arch fracture of first cervical vertebra, initial encounter for open fracture	169	Vertebral Fractures without Spinal Cord Injury		0.476	0.369	0.532	0.377	0.512	0.336	0.250
S12.031A	Nondisplaced posterior arch fracture of first cervical vertebra, initial encounter for closed fracture	169	Vertebral Fractures without Spinal Cord Injury		0.476	0.369	0.532	0.377	0.512	0.336	0.250
S12.031B	Nondisplaced posterior arch fracture of first cervical vertebra, initial encounter for open fracture	169	Vertebral Fractures without Spinal Cord Injury		0.476	0.369	0.532	0.377	0.512	0.336	0.250
S12.040A	Displaced lateral mass fracture of first cervical vertebra, initial encounter for closed fracture	169	Vertebral Fractures without Spinal Cord Injury		0.476	0.369	0.532	0.377	0.512	0.336	0.250
S12.040B	Displaced lateral mass fracture of first cervical vertebra, initial encounter for open fracture	169	Vertebral Fractures without Spinal Cord Injury		0.476	0.369	0.532	0.377	0.512	0.336	0.250
S12.041A	Nondisplaced lateral mass fracture of first cervical vertebra, initial encounter for closed fracture	169	Vertebral Fractures without Spinal Cord Injury		0.476	0.369	0.532	0.377	0.512	0.336	0.250
S12.041B	Nondisplaced lateral mass fracture of first cervical vertebra, initial encounter for open fracture	169	Vertebral Fractures without Spinal Cord Injury		0.476	0.369	0.532	0.377	0.512	0.336	0.250
S12.090A	Other displaced fracture of first cervical vertebra, initial encounter for closed fracture	169	Vertebral Fractures without Spinal Cord Injury		0.476	0.369	0.532	0.377	0.512	0.336	0.250

ICD-10-CM Code	ICD-10-CM Code Description	V24 CMS-HCC	V24 CMS-HCC Disease Group	V24 CMS-HCC Hierarchies	Community, NonDual, Aged	Community, NonDual, Disabled	Community, FBDual, Aged	Community, FBDual, Disabled	Community, PBDual, Aged	Community, PBDual, Disabled	Institutional
S12.090B	Other displaced fracture of first cervical vertebra, initial encounter for open fracture	169	Vertebral Fractures without Spinal Cord Injury		0.476	0.369	0.532	0.377	0.512	0.336	0.250
S12.091A	Other nondisplaced fracture of first cervical vertebra, initial encounter for closed fracture	169	Vertebral Fractures without Spinal Cord Injury		0.476	0.369	0.532	0.377	0.512	0.336	0.250
S12.091B	Other nondisplaced fracture of first cervical vertebra, initial encounter for open fracture	169	Vertebral Fractures without Spinal Cord Injury		0.476	0.369	0.532	0.377	0.512	0.336	0.250
S12.100A	Unspecified displaced fracture of second cervical vertebra, initial encounter for closed fracture	169	Vertebral Fractures without Spinal Cord Injury		0.476	0.369	0.532	0.377	0.512	0.336	0.250
S12.100B	Unspecified displaced fracture of second cervical vertebra, initial encounter for open fracture	169	Vertebral Fractures without Spinal Cord Injury		0.476	0.369	0.532	0.377	0.512	0.336	0.250
S12.101A	Unspecified nondisplaced fracture of second cervical vertebra, initial encounter for closed fracture	169	Vertebral Fractures without Spinal Cord Injury		0.476	0.369	0.532	0.377	0.512	0.336	0.250
S12.101B	Unspecified nondisplaced fracture of second cervical vertebra, initial encounter for open fracture	169	Vertebral Fractures without Spinal Cord Injury		0.476	0.369	0.532	0.377	0.512	0.336	0.250
S12.110A	Anterior displaced Type II dens fracture, initial encounter for closed fracture	169	Vertebral Fractures without Spinal Cord Injury		0.476	0.369	0.532	0.377	0.512	0.336	0.250
S12.110B	Anterior displaced Type II dens fracture, initial encounter for open fracture	169	Vertebral Fractures without Spinal Cord Injury		0.476	0.369	0.532	0.377	0.512	0.336	0.250
S12.111A	Posterior displaced Type II dens fracture, initial encounter for closed fracture	169	Vertebral Fractures without Spinal Cord Injury		0.476	0.369	0.532	0.377	0.512	0.336	0.250
S12.111B	Posterior displaced Type II dens fracture, initial encounter for open fracture	169	Vertebral Fractures without Spinal Cord Injury		0.476	0.369	0.532	0.377	0.512	0.336	0.250
S12.112A	Nondisplaced Type II dens fracture, initial encounter for closed fracture	169	Vertebral Fractures without Spinal Cord Injury		0.476	0.369	0.532	0.377	0.512	0.336	0.250
S12.112B	Nondisplaced Type II dens fracture, initial encounter for open fracture	169	Vertebral Fractures without Spinal Cord Injury		0.476	0.369	0.532	0.377	0.512	0.336	0.250
S12.120A	Other displaced dens fracture, initial encounter for closed fracture	169	Vertebral Fractures without Spinal Cord Injury		0.476	0.369	0.532	0.377	0.512	0.336	0.250
S12.120B	Other displaced dens fracture, initial encounter for open fracture	169	Vertebral Fractures without Spinal Cord Injury		0.476	0.369	0.532	0.377	0.512	0.336	0.250
S12.121A	Other nondisplaced dens fracture, initial encounter for closed fracture	169	Vertebral Fractures without Spinal Cord Injury		0.476	0.369	0.532	0.377	0.512	0.336	0.250
S12.121B	Other nondisplaced dens fracture, initial encounter for open fracture	169	Vertebral Fractures without Spinal Cord Injury		0.476	0.369	0.532	0.377	0.512	0.336	0.250
S12.130A	Unspecified traumatic displaced spondylolisthesis of second cervical vertebra, initial encounter for closed fracture	169	Vertebral Fractures without Spinal Cord Injury		0.476	0.369	0.532	0.377	0.512	0.336	0.250
S12.130B	Unspecified traumatic displaced spondylolisthesis of second cervical vertebra, initial encounter for open fracture	169	Vertebral Fractures without Spinal Cord Injury		0.476	0.369	0.532	0.377	0.512	0.336	0.250
S12.131A	Unspecified traumatic nondisplaced spondylolisthesis of second cervical vertebra, initial encounter for closed fracture	169	Vertebral Fractures without Spinal Cord Injury		0.476	0.369	0.532	0.377	0.512	0.336	0.250
S12.131B	Unspecified traumatic nondisplaced spondylolisthesis of second cervical vertebra, initial encounter for open fracture	169	Vertebral Fractures without Spinal Cord Injury		0.476	0.369	0.532	0.377	0.512	0.336	0.250

ICD-10-CM Code	ICD-10-CM Code Description	V24 CMS-HCC	V24 CMS-HCC Disease Group	V24 CMS-HCC Hierarchies	Community, NonDual, Aged	Community, NonDual, Disabled	Community, FBDual, Aged	Community, FBDual, Disabled	Community, PBDual, Aged	Community, PBDual, Disabled	Institutional
S12.14XA	Type III traumatic spondylolisthesis of second cervical vertebra, initial encounter for closed fracture	169	Vertebral Fractures without Spinal Cord Injury		0.476	0.369	0.532	0.377	0.512	0.336	0.250
S12.14XB	Type III traumatic spondylolisthesis of second cervical vertebra, initial encounter for open fracture	169	Vertebral Fractures without Spinal Cord Injury		0.476	0.369	0.532	0.377	0.512	0.336	0.250
S12.150A	Other traumatic displaced spondylolisthesis of second cervical vertebra, initial encounter for closed fracture	169	Vertebral Fractures without Spinal Cord Injury		0.476	0.369	0.532	0.377	0.512	0.336	0.250
S12.150B	Other traumatic displaced spondylolisthesis of second cervical vertebra, initial encounter for open fracture	169	Vertebral Fractures without Spinal Cord Injury		0.476	0.369	0.532	0.377	0.512	0.336	0.250
S12.151A	Other traumatic nondisplaced spondylolisthesis of second cervical vertebra, initial encounter for closed fracture	169	Vertebral Fractures without Spinal Cord Injury		0.476	0.369	0.532	0.377	0.512	0.336	0.250
S12.151B	Other traumatic nondisplaced spondylolisthesis of second cervical vertebra, initial encounter for open fracture	169	Vertebral Fractures without Spinal Cord Injury		0.476	0.369	0.532	0.377	0.512	0.336	0.250
S12.190A	Other displaced fracture of second cervical vertebra, initial encounter for closed fracture	169	Vertebral Fractures without Spinal Cord Injury		0.476	0.369	0.532	0.377	0.512	0.336	0.250
S12.190B	Other displaced fracture of second cervical vertebra, initial encounter for open fracture	169	Vertebral Fractures without Spinal Cord Injury		0.476	0.369	0.532	0.377	0.512	0.336	0.250
S12.191A	Other nondisplaced fracture of second cervical vertebra, initial encounter for closed fracture	169	Vertebral Fractures without Spinal Cord Injury		0.476	0.369	0.532	0.377	0.512	0.336	0.250
S12.191B	Other nondisplaced fracture of second cervical vertebra, initial encounter for open fracture	169	Vertebral Fractures without Spinal Cord Injury		0.476	0.369	0.532	0.377	0.512	0.336	0.250
S12.200A	Unspecified displaced fracture of third cervical vertebra, initial encounter for closed fracture	169	Vertebral Fractures without Spinal Cord Injury		0.476	0.369	0.532	0.377	0.512	0.336	0.250
S12.200B	Unspecified displaced fracture of third cervical vertebra, initial encounter for open fracture	169	Vertebral Fractures without Spinal Cord Injury		0.476	0.369	0.532	0.377	0.512	0.336	0.250
S12.201A	Unspecified nondisplaced fracture of third cervical vertebra, initial encounter for closed fracture	169	Vertebral Fractures without Spinal Cord Injury		0.476	0.369	0.532	0.377	0.512	0.336	0.250
S12.201B	Unspecified nondisplaced fracture of third cervical vertebra, initial encounter for open fracture	169	Vertebral Fractures without Spinal Cord Injury		0.476	0.369	0.532	0.377	0.512	0.336	0.250
S12.230A	Unspecified traumatic displaced spondylolisthesis of third cervical vertebra, initial encounter for closed fracture	169	Vertebral Fractures without Spinal Cord Injury		0.476	0.369	0.532	0.377	0.512	0.336	0.250
S12.230B	Unspecified traumatic displaced spondylolisthesis of third cervical vertebra, initial encounter for open fracture	169	Vertebral Fractures without Spinal Cord Injury		0.476	0.369	0.532	0.377	0.512	0.336	0.250
S12.231A	Unspecified traumatic nondisplaced spondylolisthesis of third cervical vertebra, initial encounter for closed fracture	169	Vertebral Fractures without Spinal Cord Injury		0.476	0.369	0.532	0.377	0.512	0.336	0.250
S12.231B	Unspecified traumatic nondisplaced spondylolisthesis of third cervical vertebra, initial encounter for open fracture	169	Vertebral Fractures without Spinal Cord Injury		0.476	0.369	0.532	0.377	0.512	0.336	0.250

ICD-10-CM Code	ICD-10-CM Code Description	V24 CMS-HCC	V24 CMS-HCC Disease Group	V24 CMS-HCC Hierarchies	Community, NonDual, Aged	Community, NonDual, Disabled	Community, FBDual, Aged	Community, FBDual, Disabled	Community, PBDual, Aged	Community, PBDual, Disabled	Institutional
S12.24XA	Type III traumatic spondylolisthesis of third cervical vertebra, initial encounter for closed fracture	169	Vertebral Fractures without Spinal Cord Injury		0.476	0.369	0.532	0.377	0.512	0.336	0.250
S12.24XB	Type III traumatic spondylolisthesis of third cervical vertebra, initial encounter for open fracture	169	Vertebral Fractures without Spinal Cord Injury		0.476	0.369	0.532	0.377	0.512	0.336	0.250
S12.250A	Other traumatic displaced spondylolisthesis of third cervical vertebra, initial encounter for closed fracture	169	Vertebral Fractures without Spinal Cord Injury		0.476	0.369	0.532	0.377	0.512	0.336	0.250
S12.250B	Other traumatic displaced spondylolisthesis of third cervical vertebra, initial encounter for open fracture	169	Vertebral Fractures without Spinal Cord Injury		0.476	0.369	0.532	0.377	0.512	0.336	0.250
S12.251A	Other traumatic nondisplaced spondylolisthesis of third cervical vertebra, initial encounter for closed fracture	169	Vertebral Fractures without Spinal Cord Injury		0.476	0.369	0.532	0.377	0.512	0.336	0.250
S12.251B	Other traumatic nondisplaced spondylolisthesis of third cervical vertebra, initial encounter for open fracture	169	Vertebral Fractures without Spinal Cord Injury		0.476	0.369	0.532	0.377	0.512	0.336	0.250
S12.290A	Other displaced fracture of third cervical vertebra, initial encounter for closed fracture	169	Vertebral Fractures without Spinal Cord Injury		0.476	0.369	0.532	0.377	0.512	0.336	0.250
S12.290B	Other displaced fracture of third cervical vertebra, initial encounter for open fracture	169	Vertebral Fractures without Spinal Cord Injury		0.476	0.369	0.532	0.377	0.512	0.336	0.250
S12.291A	Other nondisplaced fracture of third cervical vertebra, initial encounter for closed fracture	169	Vertebral Fractures without Spinal Cord Injury		0.476	0.369	0.532	0.377	0.512	0.336	0.250
S12.291B	Other nondisplaced fracture of third cervical vertebra, initial encounter for open fracture	169	Vertebral Fractures without Spinal Cord Injury		0.476	0.369	0.532	0.377	0.512	0.336	0.250
S12.300A	Unspecified displaced fracture of fourth cervical vertebra, initial encounter for closed fracture	169	Vertebral Fractures without Spinal Cord Injury		0.476	0.369	0.532	0.377	0.512	0.336	0.250
S12.300B	Unspecified displaced fracture of fourth cervical vertebra, initial encounter for open fracture	169	Vertebral Fractures without Spinal Cord Injury		0.476	0.369	0.532	0.377	0.512	0.336	0.250
S12.301A	Unspecified nondisplaced fracture of fourth cervical vertebra, initial encounter for closed fracture	169	Vertebral Fractures without Spinal Cord Injury		0.476	0.369	0.532	0.377	0.512	0.336	0.250
S12.301B	Unspecified nondisplaced fracture of fourth cervical vertebra, initial encounter for open fracture	169	Vertebral Fractures without Spinal Cord Injury		0.476	0.369	0.532	0.377	0.512	0.336	0.250
S12.330A	Unspecified traumatic displaced spondylolisthesis of fourth cervical vertebra, initial encounter for closed fracture	169	Vertebral Fractures without Spinal Cord Injury		0.476	0.369	0.532	0.377	0.512	0.336	0.250
S12.330B	Unspecified traumatic displaced spondylolisthesis of fourth cervical vertebra, initial encounter for open fracture	169	Vertebral Fractures without Spinal Cord Injury		0.476	0.369	0.532	0.377	0.512	0.336	0.250
S12.331A	Unspecified traumatic nondisplaced spondylolisthesis of fourth cervical vertebra, initial encounter for closed fracture	169	Vertebral Fractures without Spinal Cord Injury		0.476	0.369	0.532	0.377	0.512	0.336	0.250
S12.331B	Unspecified traumatic nondisplaced spondylolisthesis of fourth cervical vertebra, initial encounter for open fracture	169	Vertebral Fractures without Spinal Cord Injury		0.476	0.369	0.532	0.377	0.512	0.336	0.250

ICD-10-CM Code	ICD-10-CM Code Description	V24 CMS-HCC	V24 CMS-HCC Disease Group	V24 CMS-HCC Hierarchies	Community, NonDual, Aged	Community, NonDual, Disabled	Community, FBDual, Aged	Community, FBDual, Disabled	Community, PBDual, Aged	Community, PBDual, Disabled	Institutional
S12.34XA	Type III traumatic spondylolisthesis of fourth cervical vertebra, initial encounter for closed fracture	169	Vertebral Fractures without Spinal Cord Injury		0.476	0.369	0.532	0.377	0.512	0.336	0.250
S12.34XB	Type III traumatic spondylolisthesis of fourth cervical vertebra, initial encounter for open fracture	169	Vertebral Fractures without Spinal Cord Injury		0.476	0.369	0.532	0.377	0.512	0.336	0.250
S12.350A	Other traumatic displaced spondylolisthesis of fourth cervical vertebra, initial encounter for closed fracture	169	Vertebral Fractures without Spinal Cord Injury		0.476	0.369	0.532	0.377	0.512	0.336	0.250
S12.350B	Other traumatic displaced spondylolisthesis of fourth cervical vertebra, initial encounter for open fracture	169	Vertebral Fractures without Spinal Cord Injury		0.476	0.369	0.532	0.377	0.512	0.336	0.250
S12.351A	Other traumatic nondisplaced spondylolisthesis of fourth cervical vertebra, initial encounter for closed fracture	169	Vertebral Fractures without Spinal Cord Injury		0.476	0.369	0.532	0.377	0.512	0.336	0.250
S12.351B	Other traumatic nondisplaced spondylolisthesis of fourth cervical vertebra, initial encounter for open fracture	169	Vertebral Fractures without Spinal Cord Injury		0.476	0.369	0.532	0.377	0.512	0.336	0.250
S12.390A	Other displaced fracture of fourth cervical vertebra, initial encounter for closed fracture	169	Vertebral Fractures without Spinal Cord Injury		0.476	0.369	0.532	0.377	0.512	0.336	0.250
S12.390B	Other displaced fracture of fourth cervical vertebra, initial encounter for open fracture	169	Vertebral Fractures without Spinal Cord Injury		0.476	0.369	0.532	0.377	0.512	0.336	0.250
S12.391A	Other nondisplaced fracture of fourth cervical vertebra, initial encounter for closed fracture	169	Vertebral Fractures without Spinal Cord Injury		0.476	0.369	0.532	0.377	0.512	0.336	0.250
S12.391B	Other nondisplaced fracture of fourth cervical vertebra, initial encounter for open fracture	169	Vertebral Fractures without Spinal Cord Injury		0.476	0.369	0.532	0.377	0.512	0.336	0.250
S12.400A	Unspecified displaced fracture of fifth cervical vertebra, initial encounter for closed fracture	169	Vertebral Fractures without Spinal Cord Injury		0.476	0.369	0.532	0.377	0.512	0.336	0.250
S12.400B	Unspecified displaced fracture of fifth cervical vertebra, initial encounter for open fracture	169	Vertebral Fractures without Spinal Cord Injury		0.476	0.369	0.532	0.377	0.512	0.336	0.250
S12.401A	Unspecified nondisplaced fracture of fifth cervical vertebra, initial encounter for closed fracture	169	Vertebral Fractures without Spinal Cord Injury		0.476	0.369	0.532	0.377	0.512	0.336	0.250
S12.401B	Unspecified nondisplaced fracture of fifth cervical vertebra, initial encounter for open fracture	169	Vertebral Fractures without Spinal Cord Injury		0.476	0.369	0.532	0.377	0.512	0.336	0.250
S12.430A	Unspecified traumatic displaced spondylolisthesis of fifth cervical vertebra, initial encounter for closed fracture	169	Vertebral Fractures without Spinal Cord Injury		0.476	0.369	0.532	0.377	0.512	0.336	0.250
S12.430B	Unspecified traumatic displaced spondylolisthesis of fifth cervical vertebra, initial encounter for open fracture	169	Vertebral Fractures without Spinal Cord Injury		0.476	0.369	0.532	0.377	0.512	0.336	0.250
S12.431A	Unspecified traumatic nondisplaced spondylolisthesis of fifth cervical vertebra, initial encounter for closed fracture	169	Vertebral Fractures without Spinal Cord Injury		0.476	0.369	0.532	0.377	0.512	0.336	0.250
S12.431B	Unspecified traumatic nondisplaced spondylolisthesis of fifth cervical vertebra, initial encounter for open fracture	169	Vertebral Fractures without Spinal Cord Injury		0.476	0.369	0.532	0.377	0.512	0.336	0.250

ICD-10-CM Code	ICD-10-CM Code Description	V24 CMS-HCC	V24 CMS-HCC Disease Group	V24 CMS-HCC Hierarchies	Community, NonDual, Aged	Community, NonDual, Disabled	Community, FBDual, Aged	Community, FBDual, Disabled	Community, PBDual, Aged	Community, PBDual, Disabled	Institutional
S12.44XA	Type III traumatic spondylolisthesis of fifth cervical vertebra, initial encounter for closed fracture	169	Vertebral Fractures without Spinal Cord Injury		0.476	0.369	0.532	0.377	0.512	0.336	0.250
S12.44XB	Type III traumatic spondylolisthesis of fifth cervical vertebra, initial encounter for open fracture	169	Vertebral Fractures without Spinal Cord Injury		0.476	0.369	0.532	0.377	0.512	0.336	0.250
S12.450A	Other traumatic displaced spondylolisthesis of fifth cervical vertebra, initial encounter for closed fracture	169	Vertebral Fractures without Spinal Cord Injury		0.476	0.369	0.532	0.377	0.512	0.336	0.250
S12.450B	Other traumatic displaced spondylolisthesis of fifth cervical vertebra, initial encounter for open fracture	169	Vertebral Fractures without Spinal Cord Injury		0.476	0.369	0.532	0.377	0.512	0.336	0.250
S12.451A	Other traumatic nondisplaced spondylolisthesis of fifth cervical vertebra, initial encounter for closed fracture	169	Vertebral Fractures without Spinal Cord Injury		0.476	0.369	0.532	0.377	0.512	0.336	0.250
S12.451B	Other traumatic nondisplaced spondylolisthesis of fifth cervical vertebra, initial encounter for open fracture	169	Vertebral Fractures without Spinal Cord Injury		0.476	0.369	0.532	0.377	0.512	0.336	0.250
S12.490A	Other displaced fracture of fifth cervical vertebra, initial encounter for closed fracture	169	Vertebral Fractures without Spinal Cord Injury		0.476	0.369	0.532	0.377	0.512	0.336	0.250
S12.490B	Other displaced fracture of fifth cervical vertebra, initial encounter for open fracture	169	Vertebral Fractures without Spinal Cord Injury		0.476	0.369	0.532	0.377	0.512	0.336	0.250
S12.491A	Other nondisplaced fracture of fifth cervical vertebra, initial encounter for closed fracture	169	Vertebral Fractures without Spinal Cord Injury		0.476	0.369	0.532	0.377	0.512	0.336	0.250
S12.491B	Other nondisplaced fracture of fifth cervical vertebra, initial encounter for open fracture	169	Vertebral Fractures without Spinal Cord Injury		0.476	0.369	0.532	0.377	0.512	0.336	0.250
S12.500A	Unspecified displaced fracture of sixth cervical vertebra, initial encounter for closed fracture	169	Vertebral Fractures without Spinal Cord Injury		0.476	0.369	0.532	0.377	0.512	0.336	0.250
S12.500B	Unspecified displaced fracture of sixth cervical vertebra, initial encounter for open fracture	169	Vertebral Fractures without Spinal Cord Injury		0.476	0.369	0.532	0.377	0.512	0.336	0.250
S12.501A	Unspecified nondisplaced fracture of sixth cervical vertebra, initial encounter for closed fracture	169	Vertebral Fractures without Spinal Cord Injury		0.476	0.369	0.532	0.377	0.512	0.336	0.250
S12.501B	Unspecified nondisplaced fracture of sixth cervical vertebra, initial encounter for open fracture	169	Vertebral Fractures without Spinal Cord Injury		0.476	0.369	0.532	0.377	0.512	0.336	0.250
S12.530A	Unspecified traumatic displaced spondylolisthesis of sixth cervical vertebra, initial encounter for closed fracture	169	Vertebral Fractures without Spinal Cord Injury		0.476	0.369	0.532	0.377	0.512	0.336	0.250
S12.530B	Unspecified traumatic displaced spondylolisthesis of sixth cervical vertebra, initial encounter for open fracture	169	Vertebral Fractures without Spinal Cord Injury		0.476	0.369	0.532	0.377	0.512	0.336	0.250
S12.531A	Unspecified traumatic nondisplaced spondylolisthesis of sixth cervical vertebra, initial encounter for closed fracture	169	Vertebral Fractures without Spinal Cord Injury		0.476	0.369	0.532	0.377	0.512	0.336	0.250
S12.531B	Unspecified traumatic nondisplaced spondylolisthesis of sixth cervical vertebra, initial encounter for open fracture	169	Vertebral Fractures without Spinal Cord Injury		0.476	0.369	0.532	0.377	0.512	0.336	0.250

ICD-10-CM Code	ICD-10-CM Code Description	V24 CMS-HCC	V24 CMS-HCC Disease Group	V24 CMS-HCC Hierarchies	Community, NonDual, Aged	Community, NonDual, Disabled	Community, FBDual, Aged	Community, FBDual, Disabled	Community, PBDual, Aged	Community, PBDual, Disabled	Institutional
S12.54XA	Type III traumatic spondylolisthesis of sixth cervical vertebra, initial encounter for closed fracture	169	Vertebral Fractures without Spinal Cord Injury		0.476	0.369	0.532	0.377	0.512	0.336	0.250
S12.54XB	Type III traumatic spondylolisthesis of sixth cervical vertebra, initial encounter for open fracture	169	Vertebral Fractures without Spinal Cord Injury		0.476	0.369	0.532	0.377	0.512	0.336	0.250
S12.550A	Other traumatic displaced spondylolisthesis of sixth cervical vertebra, initial encounter for closed fracture	169	Vertebral Fractures without Spinal Cord Injury		0.476	0.369	0.532	0.377	0.512	0.336	0.250
S12.550B	Other traumatic displaced spondylolisthesis of sixth cervical vertebra, initial encounter for open fracture	169	Vertebral Fractures without Spinal Cord Injury		0.476	0.369	0.532	0.377	0.512	0.336	0.250
S12.551A	Other traumatic nondisplaced spondylolisthesis of sixth cervical vertebra, initial encounter for closed fracture	169	Vertebral Fractures without Spinal Cord Injury		0.476	0.369	0.532	0.377	0.512	0.336	0.250
S12.551B	Other traumatic nondisplaced spondylolisthesis of sixth cervical vertebra, initial encounter for open fracture	169	Vertebral Fractures without Spinal Cord Injury		0.476	0.369	0.532	0.377	0.512	0.336	0.250
S12.590A	Other displaced fracture of sixth cervical vertebra, initial encounter for closed fracture	169	Vertebral Fractures without Spinal Cord Injury		0.476	0.369	0.532	0.377	0.512	0.336	0.250
S12.590B	Other displaced fracture of sixth cervical vertebra, initial encounter for open fracture	169	Vertebral Fractures without Spinal Cord Injury		0.476	0.369	0.532	0.377	0.512	0.336	0.250
S12.591A	Other nondisplaced fracture of sixth cervical vertebra, initial encounter for closed fracture	169	Vertebral Fractures without Spinal Cord Injury		0.476	0.369	0.532	0.377	0.512	0.336	0.250
S12.591B	Other nondisplaced fracture of sixth cervical vertebra, initial encounter for open fracture	169	Vertebral Fractures without Spinal Cord Injury		0.476	0.369	0.532	0.377	0.512	0.336	0.250
S12.600A	Unspecified displaced fracture of seventh cervical vertebra, initial encounter for closed fracture	169	Vertebral Fractures without Spinal Cord Injury		0.476	0.369	0.532	0.377	0.512	0.336	0.250
S12.600B	Unspecified displaced fracture of seventh cervical vertebra, initial encounter for open fracture	169	Vertebral Fractures without Spinal Cord Injury		0.476	0.369	0.532	0.377	0.512	0.336	0.250
S12.601A	Unspecified nondisplaced fracture of seventh cervical vertebra, initial encounter for closed fracture	169	Vertebral Fractures without Spinal Cord Injury		0.476	0.369	0.532	0.377	0.512	0.336	0.250
S12.601B	Unspecified nondisplaced fracture of seventh cervical vertebra, initial encounter for open fracture	169	Vertebral Fractures without Spinal Cord Injury		0.476	0.369	0.532	0.377	0.512	0.336	0.250
S12.630A	Unspecified traumatic displaced spondylolisthesis of seventh cervical vertebra, initial encounter for closed fracture	169	Vertebral Fractures without Spinal Cord Injury		0.476	0.369	0.532	0.377	0.512	0.336	0.250
S12.630B	Unspecified traumatic displaced spondylolisthesis of seventh cervical vertebra, initial encounter for open fracture	169	Vertebral Fractures without Spinal Cord Injury		0.476	0.369	0.532	0.377	0.512	0.336	0.250
S12.631A	Unspecified traumatic nondisplaced spondylolisthesis of seventh cervical vertebra, initial encounter for closed fracture	169	Vertebral Fractures without Spinal Cord Injury		0.476	0.369	0.532	0.377	0.512	0.336	0.250
S12.631B	Unspecified traumatic nondisplaced spondylolisthesis of seventh cervical vertebra, initial encounter for open fracture	169	Vertebral Fractures without Spinal Cord Injury		0.476	0.369	0.532	0.377	0.512	0.336	0.250

ICD-10-CM Code	ICD-10-CM Code Description	V24 CMS-HCC	V24 CMS-HCC Disease Group	V24 CMS-HCC Hierarchies	Community, NonDual, Aged	Community, NonDual, Disabled	Community, FBDual, Aged	Community, FBDual, Disabled	Community, PBDual, Aged	Community, PBDual, Disabled	Institutional
S12.64XA	Type III traumatic spondylolisthesis of seventh cervical vertebra, initial encounter for closed fracture	169	Vertebral Fractures without Spinal Cord Injury		0.476	0.369	0.532	0.377	0.512	0.336	0.250
S12.64XB	Type III traumatic spondylolisthesis of seventh cervical vertebra, initial encounter for open fracture	169	Vertebral Fractures without Spinal Cord Injury		0.476	0.369	0.532	0.377	0.512	0.336	0.250
S12.650A	Other traumatic displaced spondylolisthesis of seventh cervical vertebra, initial encounter for closed fracture	169	Vertebral Fractures without Spinal Cord Injury		0.476	0.369	0.532	0.377	0.512	0.336	0.250
S12.650B	Other traumatic displaced spondylolisthesis of seventh cervical vertebra, initial encounter for open fracture	169	Vertebral Fractures without Spinal Cord Injury		0.476	0.369	0.532	0.377	0.512	0.336	0.250
S12.651A	Other traumatic nondisplaced spondylolisthesis of seventh cervical vertebra, initial encounter for closed fracture	169	Vertebral Fractures without Spinal Cord Injury		0.476	0.369	0.532	0.377	0.512	0.336	0.250
S12.651B	Other traumatic nondisplaced spondylolisthesis of seventh cervical vertebra, initial encounter for open fracture	169	Vertebral Fractures without Spinal Cord Injury		0.476	0.369	0.532	0.377	0.512	0.336	0.250
S12.690A	Other displaced fracture of seventh cervical vertebra, initial encounter for closed fracture	169	Vertebral Fractures without Spinal Cord Injury		0.476	0.369	0.532	0.377	0.512	0.336	0.250
S12.690B	Other displaced fracture of seventh cervical vertebra, initial encounter for open fracture	169	Vertebral Fractures without Spinal Cord Injury		0.476	0.369	0.532	0.377	0.512	0.336	0.250
S12.691A	Other nondisplaced fracture of seventh cervical vertebra, initial encounter for closed fracture	169	Vertebral Fractures without Spinal Cord Injury		0.476	0.369	0.532	0.377	0.512	0.336	0.250
S12.691B	Other nondisplaced fracture of seventh cervical vertebra, initial encounter for open fracture	169	Vertebral Fractures without Spinal Cord Injury		0.476	0.369	0.532	0.377	0.512	0.336	0.250
S12.8XXA	Fracture of other parts of neck, initial encounter	169	Vertebral Fractures without Spinal Cord Injury		0.476	0.369	0.532	0.377	0.512	0.336	0.250
S12.9XXA	Fracture of neck, unspecified, initial encounter	169	Vertebral Fractures without Spinal Cord Injury		0.476	0.369	0.532	0.377	0.512	0.336	0.250
S14.0XXA	Concussion and edema of cervical spinal cord, initial encounter	72	Spinal Cord Disorders/Injuries	169	0.481	0.369	0.532	0.377	0.512	0.336	0.289
S14.0XXD	Concussion and edema of cervical spinal cord, subsequent encounter	72	Spinal Cord Disorders/Injuries	169	0.481	0.369	0.532	0.377	0.512	0.336	0.289
S14.0XXS	Concussion and edema of cervical spinal cord, sequela	72	Spinal Cord Disorders/Injuries	169	0.481	0.369	0.532	0.377	0.512	0.336	0.289
S14.101A	Unspecified injury at C1 level of cervical spinal cord, initial encounter	72	Spinal Cord Disorders/Injuries	169	0.481	0.369	0.532	0.377	0.512	0.336	0.289
S14.101D	Unspecified injury at C1 level of cervical spinal cord, subsequent encounter	72	Spinal Cord Disorders/Injuries	169	0.481	0.369	0.532	0.377	0.512	0.336	0.289
S14.101S	Unspecified injury at C1 level of cervical spinal cord, sequela	72	Spinal Cord Disorders/Injuries	169	0.481	0.369	0.532	0.377	0.512	0.336	0.289
S14.102A	Unspecified injury at C2 level of cervical spinal cord, initial encounter	72	Spinal Cord Disorders/Injuries	169	0.481	0.369	0.532	0.377	0.512	0.336	0.289
S14.102D	Unspecified injury at C2 level of cervical spinal cord, subsequent encounter	72	Spinal Cord Disorders/Injuries	169	0.481	0.369	0.532	0.377	0.512	0.336	0.289
S14.102S	Unspecified injury at C2 level of cervical spinal cord, sequela	72	Spinal Cord Disorders/Injuries	169	0.481	0.369	0.532	0.377	0.512	0.336	0.289
S14.103A	Unspecified injury at C3 level of cervical spinal cord, initial encounter	72	Spinal Cord Disorders/Injuries	169	0.481	0.369	0.532	0.377	0.512	0.336	0.289

ICD-10-CM Code	ICD-10-CM Code Description	V24 CMS-HCC	V24 CMS-HCC Disease Group	V24 CMS-HCC Hierarchies	Community, NonDual, Aged	Community, NonDual, Disabled	Community, FBDual, Aged	Community, FBDual, Disabled	Community, PBDual, Aged	Community, PBDual, Disabled	Institutional
S14.103D	Unspecified injury at C3 level of cervical spinal cord, subsequent encounter	72	Spinal Cord Disorders/Injuries	169	0.481	0.369	0.532	0.377	0.512	0.336	0.289
S14.103S	Unspecified injury at C3 level of cervical spinal cord, sequela	72	Spinal Cord Disorders/Injuries	169	0.481	0.369	0.532	0.377	0.512	0.336	0.289
S14.104A	Unspecified injury at C4 level of cervical spinal cord, initial encounter	72	Spinal Cord Disorders/Injuries	169	0.481	0.369	0.532	0.377	0.512	0.336	0.289
S14.104D	Unspecified injury at C4 level of cervical spinal cord, subsequent encounter	72	Spinal Cord Disorders/Injuries	169	0.481	0.369	0.532	0.377	0.512	0.336	0.289
S14.104S	Unspecified injury at C4 level of cervical spinal cord, sequela	72	Spinal Cord Disorders/Injuries	169	0.481	0.369	0.532	0.377	0.512	0.336	0.289
S14.105A	Unspecified injury at C5 level of cervical spinal cord, initial encounter	72	Spinal Cord Disorders/Injuries	169	0.481	0.369	0.532	0.377	0.512	0.336	0.289
S14.105D	Unspecified injury at C5 level of cervical spinal cord, subsequent encounter	72	Spinal Cord Disorders/Injuries	169	0.481	0.369	0.532	0.377	0.512	0.336	0.289
S14.105S	Unspecified injury at C5 level of cervical spinal cord, sequela	72	Spinal Cord Disorders/Injuries	169	0.481	0.369	0.532	0.377	0.512	0.336	0.289
S14.106A	Unspecified injury at C6 level of cervical spinal cord, initial encounter	72	Spinal Cord Disorders/Injuries	169	0.481	0.369	0.532	0.377	0.512	0.336	0.289
S14.106D	Unspecified injury at C6 level of cervical spinal cord, subsequent encounter	72	Spinal Cord Disorders/Injuries	169	0.481	0.369	0.532	0.377	0.512	0.336	0.289
S14.106S	Unspecified injury at C6 level of cervical spinal cord, sequela	72	Spinal Cord Disorders/Injuries	169	0.481	0.369	0.532	0.377	0.512	0.336	0.289
S14.107A	Unspecified injury at C7 level of cervical spinal cord, initial encounter	72	Spinal Cord Disorders/Injuries	169	0.481	0.369	0.532	0.377	0.512	0.336	0.289
S14.107D	Unspecified injury at C7 level of cervical spinal cord, subsequent encounter	72	Spinal Cord Disorders/Injuries	169	0.481	0.369	0.532	0.377	0.512	0.336	0.289
S14.107S	Unspecified injury at C7 level of cervical spinal cord, sequela	72	Spinal Cord Disorders/Injuries	169	0.481	0.369	0.532	0.377	0.512	0.336	0.289
S14.108A	Unspecified injury at C8 level of cervical spinal cord, initial encounter	72	Spinal Cord Disorders/Injuries	169	0.481	0.369	0.532	0.377	0.512	0.336	0.289
S14.108D	Unspecified injury at C8 level of cervical spinal cord, subsequent encounter	72	Spinal Cord Disorders/Injuries	169	0.481	0.369	0.532	0.377	0.512	0.336	0.289
S14.108S	Unspecified injury at C8 level of cervical spinal cord, sequela	72	Spinal Cord Disorders/Injuries	169	0.481	0.369	0.532	0.377	0.512	0.336	0.289
S14.109A	Unspecified injury at unspecified level of cervical spinal cord, initial encounter	72	Spinal Cord Disorders/Injuries	169	0.481	0.369	0.532	0.377	0.512	0.336	0.289
S14.109D	Unspecified injury at unspecified level of cervical spinal cord, subsequent encounter	72	Spinal Cord Disorders/Injuries	169	0.481	0.369	0.532	0.377	0.512	0.336	0.289
S14.109S	Unspecified injury at unspecified level of cervical spinal cord, sequela	72	Spinal Cord Disorders/Injuries	169	0.481	0.369	0.532	0.377	0.512	0.336	0.289
S14.111A	Complete lesion at C1 level of cervical spinal cord, initial encounter	70	Quadriplegia	71,72, 103,104, 169	1.242	1.001	1.038	1.000	1.000	1.134	0.549
S14.111D	Complete lesion at C1 level of cervical spinal cord, subsequent encounter	70	Quadriplegia	71,72, 103,104, 169	1.242	1.001	1.038	1.000	1.000	1.134	0.549
S14.111S	Complete lesion at C1 level of cervical spinal cord, sequela	70	Quadriplegia	71,72, 103,104, 169	1.242	1.001	1.038	1.000	1.000	1.134	0.549
S14.112A	Complete lesion at C2 level of cervical spinal cord, initial encounter	70	Quadriplegia	71,72, 103,104, 169	1.242	1.001	1.038	1.000	1.000	1.134	0.549

ICD-10-CM Code	ICD-10-CM Code Description	V24 CMS-HCC	V24 CMS-HCC Disease Group	V24 CMS-HCC Hierarchies	Community, NonDual, Aged	Community, NonDual, Disabled	Community, FBDual, Aged	Community, FBDual, Disabled	Community, PBDual, Aged	Community, PBDual, Disabled	Institutional
S14.112D	Complete lesion at C2 level of cervical spinal cord, subsequent encounter	70	Quadriplegia	71,72, 103,104, 169	1.242	1.001	1.038	1.000	1.000	1.134	0.549
S14.112S	Complete lesion at C2 level of cervical spinal cord, sequela	70	Quadriplegia	71,72, 103,104, 169	1.242	1.001	1.038	1.000	1.000	1.134	0.549
S14.113A	Complete lesion at C3 level of cervical spinal cord, initial encounter	70	Quadriplegia	71,72, 103,104, 169	1.242	1.001	1.038	1.000	1.000	1.134	0.549
S14.113D	Complete lesion at C3 level of cervical spinal cord, subsequent encounter	70	Quadriplegia	71,72, 103,104, 169	1.242	1.001	1.038	1.000	1.000	1.134	0.549
S14.113S	Complete lesion at C3 level of cervical spinal cord, sequela	70	Quadriplegia	71,72, 103,104, 169	1.242	1.001	1.038	1.000	1.000	1.134	0.549
S14.114A	Complete lesion at C4 level of cervical spinal cord, initial encounter	70	Quadriplegia	71,72, 103,104, 169	1.242	1.001	1.038	1.000	1.000	1.134	0.549
S14.114D	Complete lesion at C4 level of cervical spinal cord, subsequent encounter	70	Quadriplegia	71,72, 103,104, 169	1.242	1.001	1.038	1.000	1.000	1.134	0.549
S14.114S	Complete lesion at C4 level of cervical spinal cord, sequela	70	Quadriplegia	71,72, 103,104, 169	1.242	1.001	1.038	1.000	1.000	1.134	0.549
S14.115A	Complete lesion at C5 level of cervical spinal cord, initial encounter	70	Quadriplegia	71,72, 103,104, 169	1.242	1.001	1.038	1.000	1.000	1.134	0.549
S14.115D	Complete lesion at C5 level of cervical spinal cord, subsequent encounter	70	Quadriplegia	71,72, 103,104, 169	1.242	1.001	1.038	1.000	1.000	1.134	0.549
S14.115S	Complete lesion at C5 level of cervical spinal cord, sequela	70	Quadriplegia	71,72, 103,104, 169	1.242	1.001	1.038	1.000	1.000	1.134	0.549
S14.116A	Complete lesion at C6 level of cervical spinal cord, initial encounter	70	Quadriplegia	71,72, 103,104, 169	1.242	1.001	1.038	1.000	1.000	1.134	0.549
S14.116D	Complete lesion at C6 level of cervical spinal cord, subsequent encounter	70	Quadriplegia	71,72, 103,104, 169	1.242	1.001	1.038	1.000	1.000	1.134	0.549
S14.116S	Complete lesion at C6 level of cervical spinal cord, sequela	70	Quadriplegia	71,72, 103,104, 169	1.242	1.001	1.038	1.000	1.000	1.134	0.549
S14.117A	Complete lesion at C7 level of cervical spinal cord, initial encounter	70	Quadriplegia	71,72, 103,104, 169	1.242	1.001	1.038	1.000	1.000	1.134	0.549
S14.117D	Complete lesion at C7 level of cervical spinal cord, subsequent encounter	70	Quadriplegia	71,72, 103,104, 169	1.242	1.001	1.038	1.000	1.000	1.134	0.549
S14.117S	Complete lesion at C7 level of cervical spinal cord, sequela	70	Quadriplegia	71,72, 103,104, 169	1.242	1.001	1.038	1.000	1.000	1.134	0.549
S14.118A	Complete lesion at C8 level of cervical spinal cord, initial encounter	70	Quadriplegia	71,72, 103,104, 169	1.242	1.001	1.038	1.000	1.000	1.134	0.549
S14.118D	Complete lesion at C8 level of cervical spinal cord, subsequent encounter	70	Quadriplegia	71,72, 103,104, 169	1.242	1.001	1.038	1.000	1.000	1.134	0.549
S14.118S	Complete lesion at C8 level of cervical spinal cord, sequela	70	Quadriplegia	71,72, 103,104, 169	1.242	1.001	1.038	1.000	1.000	1.134	0.549

ICD-10-CM Code	ICD-10-CM Code Description	V24 CMS-HCC	V24 CMS-HCC Disease Group	V24 CMS-HCC Hierarchies	Community, NonDual, Aged	Community, NonDual, Disabled	Community, FBDual, Aged	Community, FBDual, Disabled	Community, PBDual, Aged	Community, PBDual, Disabled	Institutional
S14.119A	Complete lesion at unspecified level of cervical spinal cord, initial encounter	70	Quadriplegia	71,72, 103,104, 169	1.242	1.001	1.038	1.000	1.000	1.134	0.549
S14.119D	Complete lesion at unspecified level of cervical spinal cord, subsequent encounter	70	Quadriplegia	71,72, 103,104, 169	1.242	1.001	1.038	1.000	1.000	1.134	0.549
S14.119S	Complete lesion at unspecified level of cervical spinal cord, sequela	70	Quadriplegia	71,72, 103,104, 169	1.242	1.001	1.038	1.000	1.000	1.134	0.549
S14.121A	Central cord syndrome at C1 level of cervical spinal cord, initial encounter	72	Spinal Cord Disorders/Injuries	169	0.481	0.369	0.532	0.377	0.512	0.336	0.289
S14.121D	Central cord syndrome at C1 level of cervical spinal cord, subsequent encounter	72	Spinal Cord Disorders/Injuries	169	0.481	0.369	0.532	0.377	0.512	0.336	0.289
S14.121S	Central cord syndrome at C1 level of cervical spinal cord, sequela	72	Spinal Cord Disorders/Injuries	169	0.481	0.369	0.532	0.377	0.512	0.336	0.289
S14.122A	Central cord syndrome at C2 level of cervical spinal cord, initial encounter	72	Spinal Cord Disorders/Injuries	169	0.481	0.369	0.532	0.377	0.512	0.336	0.289
S14.122D	Central cord syndrome at C2 level of cervical spinal cord, subsequent encounter	72	Spinal Cord Disorders/Injuries	169	0.481	0.369	0.532	0.377	0.512	0.336	0.289
S14.122S	Central cord syndrome at C2 level of cervical spinal cord, sequela	72	Spinal Cord Disorders/Injuries	169	0.481	0.369	0.532	0.377	0.512	0.336	0.289
S14.123A	Central cord syndrome at C3 level of cervical spinal cord, initial encounter	72	Spinal Cord Disorders/Injuries	169	0.481	0.369	0.532	0.377	0.512	0.336	0.289
S14.123D	Central cord syndrome at C3 level of cervical spinal cord, subsequent encounter	72	Spinal Cord Disorders/Injuries	169	0.481	0.369	0.532	0.377	0.512	0.336	0.289
S14.123S	Central cord syndrome at C3 level of cervical spinal cord, sequela	72	Spinal Cord Disorders/Injuries	169	0.481	0.369	0.532	0.377	0.512	0.336	0.289
S14.124A	Central cord syndrome at C4 level of cervical spinal cord, initial encounter	72	Spinal Cord Disorders/Injuries	169	0.481	0.369	0.532	0.377	0.512	0.336	0.289
S14.124D	Central cord syndrome at C4 level of cervical spinal cord, subsequent encounter	72	Spinal Cord Disorders/Injuries	169	0.481	0.369	0.532	0.377	0.512	0.336	0.289
S14.124S	Central cord syndrome at C4 level of cervical spinal cord, sequela	72	Spinal Cord Disorders/Injuries	169	0.481	0.369	0.532	0.377	0.512	0.336	0.289
S14.125A	Central cord syndrome at C5 level of cervical spinal cord, initial encounter	72	Spinal Cord Disorders/Injuries	169	0.481	0.369	0.532	0.377	0.512	0.336	0.289
S14.125D	Central cord syndrome at C5 level of cervical spinal cord, subsequent encounter	72	Spinal Cord Disorders/Injuries	169	0.481	0.369	0.532	0.377	0.512	0.336	0.289
S14.125S	Central cord syndrome at C5 level of cervical spinal cord, sequela	72	Spinal Cord Disorders/Injuries	169	0.481	0.369	0.532	0.377	0.512	0.336	0.289
S14.126A	Central cord syndrome at C6 level of cervical spinal cord, initial encounter	72	Spinal Cord Disorders/Injuries	169	0.481	0.369	0.532	0.377	0.512	0.336	0.289
S14.126D	Central cord syndrome at C6 level of cervical spinal cord, subsequent encounter	72	Spinal Cord Disorders/Injuries	169	0.481	0.369	0.532	0.377	0.512	0.336	0.289
S14.126S	Central cord syndrome at C6 level of cervical spinal cord, sequela	72	Spinal Cord Disorders/Injuries	169	0.481	0.369	0.532	0.377	0.512	0.336	0.289
S14.127A	Central cord syndrome at C7 level of cervical spinal cord, initial encounter	72	Spinal Cord Disorders/Injuries	169	0.481	0.369	0.532	0.377	0.512	0.336	0.289
S14.127D	Central cord syndrome at C7 level of cervical spinal cord, subsequent encounter	72	Spinal Cord Disorders/Injuries	169	0.481	0.369	0.532	0.377	0.512	0.336	0.289
S14.127S	Central cord syndrome at C7 level of cervical spinal cord, sequela	72	Spinal Cord Disorders/Injuries	169	0.481	0.369	0.532	0.377	0.512	0.336	0.289
S14.128A	Central cord syndrome at C8 level of cervical spinal cord, initial encounter	72	Spinal Cord Disorders/Injuries	169	0.481	0.369	0.532	0.377	0.512	0.336	0.289

ICD-10-CM Code	ICD-10-CM Code Description	V24 CMS-HCC	V24 CMS-HCC Disease Group	V24 CMS-HCC Hierarchies	Community, NonDual, Aged	Community, NonDual, Disabled	Community, FBDual, Aged	Community, FBDual, Disabled	Community, PBDual, Aged	Community, PBDual, Disabled	Institutional
S14.128D	Central cord syndrome at C8 level of cervical spinal cord, subsequent encounter	72	Spinal Cord Disorders/Injuries	169	0.481	0.369	0.532	0.377	0.512	0.336	0.289
S14.128S	Central cord syndrome at C8 level of cervical spinal cord, sequela	72	Spinal Cord Disorders/Injuries	169	0.481	0.369	0.532	0.377	0.512	0.336	0.289
S14.129A	Central cord syndrome at unspecified level of cervical spinal cord, initial encounter	72	Spinal Cord Disorders/Injuries	169	0.481	0.369	0.532	0.377	0.512	0.336	0.289
S14.129D	Central cord syndrome at unspecified level of cervical spinal cord, subsequent encounter	72	Spinal Cord Disorders/Injuries	169	0.481	0.369	0.532	0.377	0.512	0.336	0.289
S14.129S	Central cord syndrome at unspecified level of cervical spinal cord, sequela	72	Spinal Cord Disorders/Injuries	169	0.481	0.369	0.532	0.377	0.512	0.336	0.289
S14.131A	Anterior cord syndrome at C1 level of cervical spinal cord, initial encounter	72	Spinal Cord Disorders/Injuries	169	0.481	0.369	0.532	0.377	0.512	0.336	0.289
S14.131D	Anterior cord syndrome at C1 level of cervical spinal cord, subsequent encounter	72	Spinal Cord Disorders/Injuries	169	0.481	0.369	0.532	0.377	0.512	0.336	0.289
S14.131S	Anterior cord syndrome at C1 level of cervical spinal cord, sequela	72	Spinal Cord Disorders/Injuries	169	0.481	0.369	0.532	0.377	0.512	0.336	0.289
S14.132A	Anterior cord syndrome at C2 level of cervical spinal cord, initial encounter	72	Spinal Cord Disorders/Injuries	169	0.481	0.369	0.532	0.377	0.512	0.336	0.289
S14.132D	Anterior cord syndrome at C2 level of cervical spinal cord, subsequent encounter	72	Spinal Cord Disorders/Injuries	169	0.481	0.369	0.532	0.377	0.512	0.336	0.289
S14.132S	Anterior cord syndrome at C2 level of cervical spinal cord, sequela	72	Spinal Cord Disorders/Injuries	169	0.481	0.369	0.532	0.377	0.512	0.336	0.289
S14.133A	Anterior cord syndrome at C3 level of cervical spinal cord, initial encounter	72	Spinal Cord Disorders/Injuries	169	0.481	0.369	0.532	0.377	0.512	0.336	0.289
S14.133D	Anterior cord syndrome at C3 level of cervical spinal cord, subsequent encounter	72	Spinal Cord Disorders/Injuries	169	0.481	0.369	0.532	0.377	0.512	0.336	0.289
S14.133S	Anterior cord syndrome at C3 level of cervical spinal cord, sequela	72	Spinal Cord Disorders/Injuries	169	0.481	0.369	0.532	0.377	0.512	0.336	0.289
S14.134A	Anterior cord syndrome at C4 level of cervical spinal cord, initial encounter	72	Spinal Cord Disorders/Injuries	169	0.481	0.369	0.532	0.377	0.512	0.336	0.289
S14.134D	Anterior cord syndrome at C4 level of cervical spinal cord, subsequent encounter	72	Spinal Cord Disorders/Injuries	169	0.481	0.369	0.532	0.377	0.512	0.336	0.289
S14.134S	Anterior cord syndrome at C4 level of cervical spinal cord, sequela	72	Spinal Cord Disorders/Injuries	169	0.481	0.369	0.532	0.377	0.512	0.336	0.289
S14.135A	Anterior cord syndrome at C5 level of cervical spinal cord, initial encounter	72	Spinal Cord Disorders/Injuries	169	0.481	0.369	0.532	0.377	0.512	0.336	0.289
S14.135D	Anterior cord syndrome at C5 level of cervical spinal cord, subsequent encounter	72	Spinal Cord Disorders/Injuries	169	0.481	0.369	0.532	0.377	0.512	0.336	0.289
S14.135S	Anterior cord syndrome at C5 level of cervical spinal cord, sequela	72	Spinal Cord Disorders/Injuries	169	0.481	0.369	0.532	0.377	0.512	0.336	0.289
S14.136A	Anterior cord syndrome at C6 level of cervical spinal cord, initial encounter	72	Spinal Cord Disorders/Injuries	169	0.481	0.369	0.532	0.377	0.512	0.336	0.289
S14.136D	Anterior cord syndrome at C6 level of cervical spinal cord, subsequent encounter	72	Spinal Cord Disorders/Injuries	169	0.481	0.369	0.532	0.377	0.512	0.336	0.289
S14.136S	Anterior cord syndrome at C6 level of cervical spinal cord, sequela	72	Spinal Cord Disorders/Injuries	169	0.481	0.369	0.532	0.377	0.512	0.336	0.289
S14.137A	Anterior cord syndrome at C7 level of cervical spinal cord, initial encounter	72	Spinal Cord Disorders/Injuries	169	0.481	0.369	0.532	0.377	0.512	0.336	0.289
S14.137D	Anterior cord syndrome at C7 level of cervical spinal cord, subsequent encounter	72	Spinal Cord Disorders/Injuries	169	0.481	0.369	0.532	0.377	0.512	0.336	0.289

ICD-10-CM Code	ICD-10-CM Code Description	V24 CMS-HCC	V24 CMS-HCC Disease Group	V24 CMS-HCC Hierarchies	Community, NonDual, Aged	Community, NonDual, Disabled	Community, FBDual, Aged	Community, FBDual, Disabled	Community, PBDual, Aged	Community, PBDual, Disabled	Institutional
S14.137S	Anterior cord syndrome at C7 level of cervical spinal cord, sequela	72	Spinal Cord Disorders/Injuries	169	0.481	0.369	0.532	0.377	0.512	0.336	0.289
S14.138A	Anterior cord syndrome at C8 level of cervical spinal cord, initial encounter	72	Spinal Cord Disorders/Injuries	169	0.481	0.369	0.532	0.377	0.512	0.336	0.289
S14.138D	Anterior cord syndrome at C8 level of cervical spinal cord, subsequent encounter	72	Spinal Cord Disorders/Injuries	169	0.481	0.369	0.532	0.377	0.512	0.336	0.289
S14.138S	Anterior cord syndrome at C8 level of cervical spinal cord, sequela	72	Spinal Cord Disorders/Injuries	169	0.481	0.369	0.532	0.377	0.512	0.336	0.289
S14.139A	Anterior cord syndrome at unspecified level of cervical spinal cord, initial encounter	72	Spinal Cord Disorders/Injuries	169	0.481	0.369	0.532	0.377	0.512	0.336	0.289
S14.139D	Anterior cord syndrome at unspecified level of cervical spinal cord, subsequent encounter	72	Spinal Cord Disorders/Injuries	169	0.481	0.369	0.532	0.377	0.512	0.336	0.289
S14.139S	Anterior cord syndrome at unspecified level of cervical spinal cord, sequela	72	Spinal Cord Disorders/Injuries	169	0.481	0.369	0.532	0.377	0.512	0.336	0.289
S14.141A	Brown-Sequard syndrome at C1 level of cervical spinal cord, initial encounter	72	Spinal Cord Disorders/Injuries	169	0.481	0.369	0.532	0.377	0.512	0.336	0.289
S14.141D	Brown-Sequard syndrome at C1 level of cervical spinal cord, subsequent encounter	72	Spinal Cord Disorders/Injuries	169	0.481	0.369	0.532	0.377	0.512	0.336	0.289
S14.141S	Brown-Sequard syndrome at C1 level of cervical spinal cord, sequela	72	Spinal Cord Disorders/Injuries	169	0.481	0.369	0.532	0.377	0.512	0.336	0.289
S14.142A	Brown-Sequard syndrome at C2 level of cervical spinal cord, initial encounter	72	Spinal Cord Disorders/Injuries	169	0.481	0.369	0.532	0.377	0.512	0.336	0.289
S14.142D	Brown-Sequard syndrome at C2 level of cervical spinal cord, subsequent encounter	72	Spinal Cord Disorders/Injuries	169	0.481	0.369	0.532	0.377	0.512	0.336	0.289
S14.142S	Brown-Sequard syndrome at C2 level of cervical spinal cord, sequela	72	Spinal Cord Disorders/Injuries	169	0.481	0.369	0.532	0.377	0.512	0.336	0.289
S14.143A	Brown-Sequard syndrome at C3 level of cervical spinal cord, initial encounter	72	Spinal Cord Disorders/Injuries	169	0.481	0.369	0.532	0.377	0.512	0.336	0.289
S14.143D	Brown-Sequard syndrome at C3 level of cervical spinal cord, subsequent encounter	72	Spinal Cord Disorders/Injuries	169	0.481	0.369	0.532	0.377	0.512	0.336	0.289
S14.143S	Brown-Sequard syndrome at C3 level of cervical spinal cord, sequela	72	Spinal Cord Disorders/Injuries	169	0.481	0.369	0.532	0.377	0.512	0.336	0.289
S14.144A	Brown-Sequard syndrome at C4 level of cervical spinal cord, initial encounter	72	Spinal Cord Disorders/Injuries	169	0.481	0.369	0.532	0.377	0.512	0.336	0.289
S14.144D	Brown-Sequard syndrome at C4 level of cervical spinal cord, subsequent encounter	72	Spinal Cord Disorders/Injuries	169	0.481	0.369	0.532	0.377	0.512	0.336	0.289
S14.144S	Brown-Sequard syndrome at C4 level of cervical spinal cord, sequela	72	Spinal Cord Disorders/Injuries	169	0.481	0.369	0.532	0.377	0.512	0.336	0.289
S14.145A	Brown-Sequard syndrome at C5 level of cervical spinal cord, initial encounter	72	Spinal Cord Disorders/Injuries	169	0.481	0.369	0.532	0.377	0.512	0.336	0.289
S14.145D	Brown-Sequard syndrome at C5 level of cervical spinal cord, subsequent encounter	72	Spinal Cord Disorders/Injuries	169	0.481	0.369	0.532	0.377	0.512	0.336	0.289
S14.145S	Brown-Sequard syndrome at C5 level of cervical spinal cord, sequela	72	Spinal Cord Disorders/Injuries	169	0.481	0.369	0.532	0.377	0.512	0.336	0.289
S14.146A	Brown-Sequard syndrome at C6 level of cervical spinal cord, initial encounter	72	Spinal Cord Disorders/Injuries	169	0.481	0.369	0.532	0.377	0.512	0.336	0.289

ICD-10-CM Code	ICD-10-CM Code Description	V24 CMS-HCC	V24 CMS-HCC Disease Group	V24 CMS-HCC Hierarchies	Community, NonDual, Aged	Community, NonDual, Disabled	Community, FBDual, Aged	Community, FBDual, Disabled	Community, PBDual, Aged	Community, PBDual, Disabled	Institutional
S14.146D	Brown-Sequard syndrome at C6 level of cervical spinal cord, subsequent encounter	72	Spinal Cord Disorders/Injuries	169	0.481	0.369	0.532	0.377	0.512	0.336	0.289
S14.146S	Brown-Sequard syndrome at C6 level of cervical spinal cord, sequela	72	Spinal Cord Disorders/Injuries	169	0.481	0.369	0.532	0.377	0.512	0.336	0.289
S14.147A	Brown-Sequard syndrome at C7 level of cervical spinal cord, initial encounter	72	Spinal Cord Disorders/Injuries	169	0.481	0.369	0.532	0.377	0.512	0.336	0.289
S14.147D	Brown-Sequard syndrome at C7 level of cervical spinal cord, subsequent encounter	72	Spinal Cord Disorders/Injuries	169	0.481	0.369	0.532	0.377	0.512	0.336	0.289
S14.147S	Brown-Sequard syndrome at C7 level of cervical spinal cord, sequela	72	Spinal Cord Disorders/Injuries	169	0.481	0.369	0.532	0.377	0.512	0.336	0.289
S14.148A	Brown-Sequard syndrome at C8 level of cervical spinal cord, initial encounter	72	Spinal Cord Disorders/Injuries	169	0.481	0.369	0.532	0.377	0.512	0.336	0.289
S14.148D	Brown-Sequard syndrome at C8 level of cervical spinal cord, subsequent encounter	72	Spinal Cord Disorders/Injuries	169	0.481	0.369	0.532	0.377	0.512	0.336	0.289
S14.148S	Brown-Sequard syndrome at C8 level of cervical spinal cord, sequela	72	Spinal Cord Disorders/Injuries	169	0.481	0.369	0.532	0.377	0.512	0.336	0.289
S14.149A	Brown-Sequard syndrome at unspecified level of cervical spinal cord, initial encounter	72	Spinal Cord Disorders/Injuries	169	0.481	0.369	0.532	0.377	0.512	0.336	0.289
S14.149D	Brown-Sequard syndrome at unspecified level of cervical spinal cord, subsequent encounter	72	Spinal Cord Disorders/Injuries	169	0.481	0.369	0.532	0.377	0.512	0.336	0.289
S14.149S	Brown-Sequard syndrome at unspecified level of cervical spinal cord, sequela	72	Spinal Cord Disorders/Injuries	169	0.481	0.369	0.532	0.377	0.512	0.336	0.289
S14.151A	Other incomplete lesion at C1 level of cervical spinal cord, initial encounter	72	Spinal Cord Disorders/Injuries	169	0.481	0.369	0.532	0.377	0.512	0.336	0.289
S14.151D	Other incomplete lesion at C1 level of cervical spinal cord, subsequent encounter	72	Spinal Cord Disorders/Injuries	169	0.481	0.369	0.532	0.377	0.512	0.336	0.289
S14.151S	Other incomplete lesion at C1 level of cervical spinal cord, sequela	72	Spinal Cord Disorders/Injuries	169	0.481	0.369	0.532	0.377	0.512	0.336	0.289
S14.152A	Other incomplete lesion at C2 level of cervical spinal cord, initial encounter	72	Spinal Cord Disorders/Injuries	169	0.481	0.369	0.532	0.377	0.512	0.336	0.289
S14.152D	Other incomplete lesion at C2 level of cervical spinal cord, subsequent encounter	72	Spinal Cord Disorders/Injuries	169	0.481	0.369	0.532	0.377	0.512	0.336	0.289
S14.152S	Other incomplete lesion at C2 level of cervical spinal cord, sequela	72	Spinal Cord Disorders/Injuries	169	0.481	0.369	0.532	0.377	0.512	0.336	0.289
S14.153A	Other incomplete lesion at C3 level of cervical spinal cord, initial encounter	72	Spinal Cord Disorders/Injuries	169	0.481	0.369	0.532	0.377	0.512	0.336	0.289
S14.153D	Other incomplete lesion at C3 level of cervical spinal cord, subsequent encounter	72	Spinal Cord Disorders/Injuries	169	0.481	0.369	0.532	0.377	0.512	0.336	0.289
S14.153S	Other incomplete lesion at C3 level of cervical spinal cord, sequela	72	Spinal Cord Disorders/Injuries	169	0.481	0.369	0.532	0.377	0.512	0.336	0.289
S14.154A	Other incomplete lesion at C4 level of cervical spinal cord, initial encounter	72	Spinal Cord Disorders/Injuries	169	0.481	0.369	0.532	0.377	0.512	0.336	0.289
S14.154D	Other incomplete lesion at C4 level of cervical spinal cord, subsequent encounter	72	Spinal Cord Disorders/Injuries	169	0.481	0.369	0.532	0.377	0.512	0.336	0.289
S14.154S	Other incomplete lesion at C4 level of cervical spinal cord, sequela	72	Spinal Cord Disorders/Injuries	169	0.481	0.369	0.532	0.377	0.512	0.336	0.289
S14.155A	Other incomplete lesion at C5 level of cervical spinal cord, initial encounter	72	Spinal Cord Disorders/Injuries	169	0.481	0.369	0.532	0.377	0.512	0.336	0.289

ICD-10-CM Code	ICD-10-CM Code Description	V24 CMS-HCC	V24 CMS-HCC Disease Group	V24 CMS-HCC Hierarchies	Community, NonDual, Aged	Community, NonDual, Disabled	Community, FBDual, Aged	Community, FBDual, Disabled	Community, PBDual, Aged	Community, PBDual, Disabled	Institutional
S14.155D	Other incomplete lesion at C5 level of cervical spinal cord, subsequent encounter	72	Spinal Cord Disorders/Injuries	169	0.481	0.369	0.532	0.377	0.512	0.336	0.289
S14.155S	Other incomplete lesion at C5 level of cervical spinal cord, sequela	72	Spinal Cord Disorders/Injuries	169	0.481	0.369	0.532	0.377	0.512	0.336	0.289
S14.156A	Other incomplete lesion at C6 level of cervical spinal cord, initial encounter	72	Spinal Cord Disorders/Injuries	169	0.481	0.369	0.532	0.377	0.512	0.336	0.289
S14.156D	Other incomplete lesion at C6 level of cervical spinal cord, subsequent encounter	72	Spinal Cord Disorders/Injuries	169	0.481	0.369	0.532	0.377	0.512	0.336	0.289
S14.156S	Other incomplete lesion at C6 level of cervical spinal cord, sequela	72	Spinal Cord Disorders/Injuries	169	0.481	0.369	0.532	0.377	0.512	0.336	0.289
S14.157A	Other incomplete lesion at C7 level of cervical spinal cord, initial encounter	72	Spinal Cord Disorders/Injuries	169	0.481	0.369	0.532	0.377	0.512	0.336	0.289
S14.157D	Other incomplete lesion at C7 level of cervical spinal cord, subsequent encounter	72	Spinal Cord Disorders/Injuries	169	0.481	0.369	0.532	0.377	0.512	0.336	0.289
S14.157S	Other incomplete lesion at C7 level of cervical spinal cord, sequela	72	Spinal Cord Disorders/Injuries	169	0.481	0.369	0.532	0.377	0.512	0.336	0.289
S14.158A	Other incomplete lesion at C8 level of cervical spinal cord, initial encounter	72	Spinal Cord Disorders/Injuries	169	0.481	0.369	0.532	0.377	0.512	0.336	0.289
S14.158D	Other incomplete lesion at C8 level of cervical spinal cord, subsequent encounter	72	Spinal Cord Disorders/Injuries	169	0.481	0.369	0.532	0.377	0.512	0.336	0.289
S14.158S	Other incomplete lesion at C8 level of cervical spinal cord, sequela	72	Spinal Cord Disorders/Injuries	169	0.481	0.369	0.532	0.377	0.512	0.336	0.289
S14.159A	Other incomplete lesion at unspecified level of cervical spinal cord, initial encounter	72	Spinal Cord Disorders/Injuries	169	0.481	0.369	0.532	0.377	0.512	0.336	0.289
S14.159D	Other incomplete lesion at unspecified level of cervical spinal cord, subsequent encounter	72	Spinal Cord Disorders/Injuries	169	0.481	0.369	0.532	0.377	0.512	0.336	0.289
S14.159S	Other incomplete lesion at unspecified level of cervical spinal cord, sequela	72	Spinal Cord Disorders/Injuries	169	0.481	0.369	0.532	0.377	0.512	0.336	0.289
S22.000A	Wedge compression fracture of unspecified thoracic vertebra, initial encounter for closed fracture	169	Vertebral Fractures without Spinal Cord Injury		0.476	0.369	0.532	0.377	0.512	0.336	0.250
S22.000B	Wedge compression fracture of unspecified thoracic vertebra, initial encounter for open fracture	169	Vertebral Fractures without Spinal Cord Injury		0.476	0.369	0.532	0.377	0.512	0.336	0.250
S22.001A	Stable burst fracture of unspecified thoracic vertebra, initial encounter for closed fracture	169	Vertebral Fractures without Spinal Cord Injury		0.476	0.369	0.532	0.377	0.512	0.336	0.250
S22.001B	Stable burst fracture of unspecified thoracic vertebra, initial encounter for open fracture	169	Vertebral Fractures without Spinal Cord Injury		0.476	0.369	0.532	0.377	0.512	0.336	0.250
S22.002A	Unstable burst fracture of unspecified thoracic vertebra, initial encounter for closed fracture	169	Vertebral Fractures without Spinal Cord Injury		0.476	0.369	0.532	0.377	0.512	0.336	0.250
S22.002B	Unstable burst fracture of unspecified thoracic vertebra, initial encounter for open fracture	169	Vertebral Fractures without Spinal Cord Injury		0.476	0.369	0.532	0.377	0.512	0.336	0.250
S22.008A	Other fracture of unspecified thoracic vertebra, initial encounter for closed fracture	169	Vertebral Fractures without Spinal Cord Injury		0.476	0.369	0.532	0.377	0.512	0.336	0.250
S22.008B	Other fracture of unspecified thoracic vertebra, initial encounter for open fracture	169	Vertebral Fractures without Spinal Cord Injury		0.476	0.369	0.532	0.377	0.512	0.336	0.250

ICD-10-CM Code	ICD-10-CM Code Description	V24 CMS-HCC	V24 CMS-HCC Disease Group	V24 CMS-HCC Hierarchies	Community, NonDual, Aged	Community, NonDual, Disabled	Community, FBDual, Aged	Community, FBDual, Disabled	Community, PBDual, Aged	Community, PBDual, Disabled	Institutional
S22.009A	Unspecified fracture of unspecified thoracic vertebra, initial encounter for closed fracture	169	Vertebral Fractures without Spinal Cord Injury		0.476	0.369	0.532	0.377	0.512	0.336	0.250
S22.009B	Unspecified fracture of unspecified thoracic vertebra, initial encounter for open fracture	169	Vertebral Fractures without Spinal Cord Injury		0.476	0.369	0.532	0.377	0.512	0.336	0.250
S22.010A	Wedge compression fracture of first thoracic vertebra, initial encounter for closed fracture	169	Vertebral Fractures without Spinal Cord Injury		0.476	0.369	0.532	0.377	0.512	0.336	0.250
S22.010B	Wedge compression fracture of first thoracic vertebra, initial encounter for open fracture	169	Vertebral Fractures without Spinal Cord Injury		0.476	0.369	0.532	0.377	0.512	0.336	0.250
S22.011A	Stable burst fracture of first thoracic vertebra, initial encounter for closed fracture	169	Vertebral Fractures without Spinal Cord Injury		0.476	0.369	0.532	0.377	0.512	0.336	0.250
S22.011B	Stable burst fracture of first thoracic vertebra, initial encounter for open fracture	169	Vertebral Fractures without Spinal Cord Injury		0.476	0.369	0.532	0.377	0.512	0.336	0.250
S22.012A	Unstable burst fracture of first thoracic vertebra, initial encounter for closed fracture	169	Vertebral Fractures without Spinal Cord Injury		0.476	0.369	0.532	0.377	0.512	0.336	0.250
S22.012B	Unstable burst fracture of first thoracic vertebra, initial encounter for open fracture	169	Vertebral Fractures without Spinal Cord Injury		0.476	0.369	0.532	0.377	0.512	0.336	0.250
S22.018A	Other fracture of first thoracic vertebra, initial encounter for closed fracture	169	Vertebral Fractures without Spinal Cord Injury		0.476	0.369	0.532	0.377	0.512	0.336	0.250
S22.018B	Other fracture of first thoracic vertebra, initial encounter for open fracture	169	Vertebral Fractures without Spinal Cord Injury		0.476	0.369	0.532	0.377	0.512	0.336	0.250
S22.019A	Unspecified fracture of first thoracic vertebra, initial encounter for closed fracture	169	Vertebral Fractures without Spinal Cord Injury		0.476	0.369	0.532	0.377	0.512	0.336	0.250
S22.019B	Unspecified fracture of first thoracic vertebra, initial encounter for open fracture	169	Vertebral Fractures without Spinal Cord Injury		0.476	0.369	0.532	0.377	0.512	0.336	0.250
S22.020A	Wedge compression fracture of second thoracic vertebra, initial encounter for closed fracture	169	Vertebral Fractures without Spinal Cord Injury		0.476	0.369	0.532	0.377	0.512	0.336	0.250
S22.020B	Wedge compression fracture of second thoracic vertebra, initial encounter for open fracture	169	Vertebral Fractures without Spinal Cord Injury		0.476	0.369	0.532	0.377	0.512	0.336	0.250
S22.021A	Stable burst fracture of second thoracic vertebra, initial encounter for closed fracture	169	Vertebral Fractures without Spinal Cord Injury		0.476	0.369	0.532	0.377	0.512	0.336	0.250
S22.021B	Stable burst fracture of second thoracic vertebra, initial encounter for open fracture	169	Vertebral Fractures without Spinal Cord Injury		0.476	0.369	0.532	0.377	0.512	0.336	0.250
S22.022A	Unstable burst fracture of second thoracic vertebra, initial encounter for closed fracture	169	Vertebral Fractures without Spinal Cord Injury		0.476	0.369	0.532	0.377	0.512	0.336	0.250
S22.022B	Unstable burst fracture of second thoracic vertebra, initial encounter for open fracture	169	Vertebral Fractures without Spinal Cord Injury		0.476	0.369	0.532	0.377	0.512	0.336	0.250
S22.028A	Other fracture of second thoracic vertebra, initial encounter for closed fracture	169	Vertebral Fractures without Spinal Cord Injury		0.476	0.369	0.532	0.377	0.512	0.336	0.250
S22.028B	Other fracture of second thoracic vertebra, initial encounter for open fracture	169	Vertebral Fractures without Spinal Cord Injury		0.476	0.369	0.532	0.377	0.512	0.336	0.250

ICD-10-CM Code	ICD-10-CM Code Description	V24 CMS-HCC	V24 CMS-HCC Disease Group	V24 CMS-HCC Hierarchies	Community, NonDual, Aged	Community, NonDual, Disabled	Community, FBDual, Aged	Community, FBDual, Disabled	Community, PBDual, Aged	Community, PBDual, Disabled	Institutional
S22.029A	Unspecified fracture of second thoracic vertebra, initial encounter for closed fracture	169	Vertebral Fractures without Spinal Cord Injury		0.476	0.369	0.532	0.377	0.512	0.336	0.250
S22.029B	Unspecified fracture of second thoracic vertebra, initial encounter for open fracture	169	Vertebral Fractures without Spinal Cord Injury		0.476	0.369	0.532	0.377	0.512	0.336	0.250
S22.030A	Wedge compression fracture of third thoracic vertebra, initial encounter for closed fracture	169	Vertebral Fractures without Spinal Cord Injury		0.476	0.369	0.532	0.377	0.512	0.336	0.250
S22.030B	Wedge compression fracture of third thoracic vertebra, initial encounter for open fracture	169	Vertebral Fractures without Spinal Cord Injury		0.476	0.369	0.532	0.377	0.512	0.336	0.250
S22.031A	Stable burst fracture of third thoracic vertebra, initial encounter for closed fracture	169	Vertebral Fractures without Spinal Cord Injury		0.476	0.369	0.532	0.377	0.512	0.336	0.250
S22.031B	Stable burst fracture of third thoracic vertebra, initial encounter for open fracture	169	Vertebral Fractures without Spinal Cord Injury		0.476	0.369	0.532	0.377	0.512	0.336	0.250
S22.032A	Unstable burst fracture of third thoracic vertebra, initial encounter for closed fracture	169	Vertebral Fractures without Spinal Cord Injury		0.476	0.369	0.532	0.377	0.512	0.336	0.250
S22.032B	Unstable burst fracture of third thoracic vertebra, initial encounter for open fracture	169	Vertebral Fractures without Spinal Cord Injury		0.476	0.369	0.532	0.377	0.512	0.336	0.250
S22.038A	Other fracture of third thoracic vertebra, initial encounter for closed fracture	169	Vertebral Fractures without Spinal Cord Injury		0.476	0.369	0.532	0.377	0.512	0.336	0.250
S22.038B	Other fracture of third thoracic vertebra, initial encounter for open fracture	169	Vertebral Fractures without Spinal Cord Injury		0.476	0.369	0.532	0.377	0.512	0.336	0.250
S22.039A	Unspecified fracture of third thoracic vertebra, initial encounter for closed fracture	169	Vertebral Fractures without Spinal Cord Injury		0.476	0.369	0.532	0.377	0.512	0.336	0.250
S22.039B	Unspecified fracture of third thoracic vertebra, initial encounter for open fracture	169	Vertebral Fractures without Spinal Cord Injury		0.476	0.369	0.532	0.377	0.512	0.336	0.250
S22.040A	Wedge compression fracture of fourth thoracic vertebra, initial encounter for closed fracture	169	Vertebral Fractures without Spinal Cord Injury		0.476	0.369	0.532	0.377	0.512	0.336	0.250
S22.040B	Wedge compression fracture of fourth thoracic vertebra, initial encounter for open fracture	169	Vertebral Fractures without Spinal Cord Injury		0.476	0.369	0.532	0.377	0.512	0.336	0.250
S22.041A	Stable burst fracture of fourth thoracic vertebra, initial encounter for closed fracture	169	Vertebral Fractures without Spinal Cord Injury		0.476	0.369	0.532	0.377	0.512	0.336	0.250
S22.041B	Stable burst fracture of fourth thoracic vertebra, initial encounter for open fracture	169	Vertebral Fractures without Spinal Cord Injury		0.476	0.369	0.532	0.377	0.512	0.336	0.250
S22.042A	Unstable burst fracture of fourth thoracic vertebra, initial encounter for closed fracture	169	Vertebral Fractures without Spinal Cord Injury		0.476	0.369	0.532	0.377	0.512	0.336	0.250
S22.042B	Unstable burst fracture of fourth thoracic vertebra, initial encounter for open fracture	169	Vertebral Fractures without Spinal Cord Injury		0.476	0.369	0.532	0.377	0.512	0.336	0.250
S22.048A	Other fracture of fourth thoracic vertebra, initial encounter for closed fracture	169	Vertebral Fractures without Spinal Cord Injury		0.476	0.369	0.532	0.377	0.512	0.336	0.250
S22.048B	Other fracture of fourth thoracic vertebra, initial encounter for open fracture	169	Vertebral Fractures without Spinal Cord Injury		0.476	0.369	0.532	0.377	0.512	0.336	0.250

ICD-10-CM Code	ICD-10-CM Code Description	V24 CMS-HCC	V24 CMS-HCC Disease Group	V24 CMS-HCC Hierarchies	Community, NonDual, Aged	Community, NonDual, Disabled	Community, FBDual, Aged	Community, FBDual, Disabled	Community, PBDual, Aged	Community, PBDual, Disabled	Institutional
S22.049A	Unspecified fracture of fourth thoracic vertebra, initial encounter for closed fracture	169	Vertebral Fractures without Spinal Cord Injury		0.476	0.369	0.532	0.377	0.512	0.336	0.250
S22.049B	Unspecified fracture of fourth thoracic vertebra, initial encounter for open fracture	169	Vertebral Fractures without Spinal Cord Injury		0.476	0.369	0.532	0.377	0.512	0.336	0.250
S22.050A	Wedge compression fracture of T5-T6 vertebra, initial encounter for closed fracture	169	Vertebral Fractures without Spinal Cord Injury		0.476	0.369	0.532	0.377	0.512	0.336	0.250
S22.050B	Wedge compression fracture of T5-T6 vertebra, initial encounter for open fracture	169	Vertebral Fractures without Spinal Cord Injury		0.476	0.369	0.532	0.377	0.512	0.336	0.250
S22.051A	Stable burst fracture of T5-T6 vertebra, initial encounter for closed fracture	169	Vertebral Fractures without Spinal Cord Injury		0.476	0.369	0.532	0.377	0.512	0.336	0.250
S22.051B	Stable burst fracture of T5-T6 vertebra, initial encounter for open fracture	169	Vertebral Fractures without Spinal Cord Injury		0.476	0.369	0.532	0.377	0.512	0.336	0.250
S22.052A	Unstable burst fracture of T5-T6 vertebra, initial encounter for closed fracture	169	Vertebral Fractures without Spinal Cord Injury		0.476	0.369	0.532	0.377	0.512	0.336	0.250
S22.052B	Unstable burst fracture of T5-T6 vertebra, initial encounter for open fracture	169	Vertebral Fractures without Spinal Cord Injury		0.476	0.369	0.532	0.377	0.512	0.336	0.250
S22.058A	Other fracture of T5-T6 vertebra, initial encounter for closed fracture	169	Vertebral Fractures without Spinal Cord Injury		0.476	0.369	0.532	0.377	0.512	0.336	0.250
S22.058B	Other fracture of T5-T6 vertebra, initial encounter for open fracture	169	Vertebral Fractures without Spinal Cord Injury		0.476	0.369	0.532	0.377	0.512	0.336	0.250
S22.059A	Unspecified fracture of T5-T6 vertebra, initial encounter for closed fracture	169	Vertebral Fractures without Spinal Cord Injury		0.476	0.369	0.532	0.377	0.512	0.336	0.250
S22.059B	Unspecified fracture of T5-T6 vertebra, initial encounter for open fracture	169	Vertebral Fractures without Spinal Cord Injury		0.476	0.369	0.532	0.377	0.512	0.336	0.250
S22.060A	Wedge compression fracture of T7-T8 vertebra, initial encounter for closed fracture	169	Vertebral Fractures without Spinal Cord Injury		0.476	0.369	0.532	0.377	0.512	0.336	0.250
S22.060B	Wedge compression fracture of T7-T8 vertebra, initial encounter for open fracture	169	Vertebral Fractures without Spinal Cord Injury		0.476	0.369	0.532	0.377	0.512	0.336	0.250
S22.061A	Stable burst fracture of T7-T8 vertebra, initial encounter for closed fracture	169	Vertebral Fractures without Spinal Cord Injury		0.476	0.369	0.532	0.377	0.512	0.336	0.250
S22.061B	Stable burst fracture of T7-T8 vertebra, initial encounter for open fracture	169	Vertebral Fractures without Spinal Cord Injury		0.476	0.369	0.532	0.377	0.512	0.336	0.250
S22.062A	Unstable burst fracture of T7-T8 vertebra, initial encounter for closed fracture	169	Vertebral Fractures without Spinal Cord Injury		0.476	0.369	0.532	0.377	0.512	0.336	0.250
S22.062B	Unstable burst fracture of T7-T8 vertebra, initial encounter for open fracture	169	Vertebral Fractures without Spinal Cord Injury		0.476	0.369	0.532	0.377	0.512	0.336	0.250
S22.068A	Other fracture of T7-T8 thoracic vertebra, initial encounter for closed fracture	169	Vertebral Fractures without Spinal Cord Injury		0.476	0.369	0.532	0.377	0.512	0.336	0.250
S22.068B	Other fracture of T7-T8 thoracic vertebra, initial encounter for open fracture	169	Vertebral Fractures without Spinal Cord Injury		0.476	0.369	0.532	0.377	0.512	0.336	0.250
S22.069A	Unspecified fracture of T7-T8 vertebra, initial encounter for closed fracture	169	Vertebral Fractures without Spinal Cord Injury		0.476	0.369	0.532	0.377	0.512	0.336	0.250

ICD-10-CM Code	ICD-10-CM Code Description	V24 CMS-HCC	V24 CMS-HCC Disease Group	V24 CMS-HCC Hierarchies	Community, NonDual, Aged	Community, NonDual, Disabled	Community, FBDual, Aged	Community, FBDual, Disabled	Community, PBDual, Aged	Community, PBDual, Disabled	Institutional
S22.069B	Unspecified fracture of T7-T8 vertebra, initial encounter for open fracture	169	Vertebral Fractures without Spinal Cord Injury		0.476	0.369	0.532	0.377	0.512	0.336	0.250
S22.070A	Wedge compression fracture of T9-T10 vertebra, initial encounter for closed fracture	169	Vertebral Fractures without Spinal Cord Injury		0.476	0.369	0.532	0.377	0.512	0.336	0.250
S22.070B	Wedge compression fracture of T9-T10 vertebra, initial encounter for open fracture	169	Vertebral Fractures without Spinal Cord Injury		0.476	0.369	0.532	0.377	0.512	0.336	0.250
S22.071A	Stable burst fracture of T9-T10 vertebra, initial encounter for closed fracture	169	Vertebral Fractures without Spinal Cord Injury		0.476	0.369	0.532	0.377	0.512	0.336	0.250
S22.071B	Stable burst fracture of T9-T10 vertebra, initial encounter for open fracture	169	Vertebral Fractures without Spinal Cord Injury		0.476	0.369	0.532	0.377	0.512	0.336	0.250
S22.072A	Unstable burst fracture of T9-T10 vertebra, initial encounter for closed fracture	169	Vertebral Fractures without Spinal Cord Injury		0.476	0.369	0.532	0.377	0.512	0.336	0.250
S22.072B	Unstable burst fracture of T9-T10 vertebra, initial encounter for open fracture	169	Vertebral Fractures without Spinal Cord Injury		0.476	0.369	0.532	0.377	0.512	0.336	0.250
S22.078A	Other fracture of T9-T10 vertebra, initial encounter for closed fracture	169	Vertebral Fractures without Spinal Cord Injury		0.476	0.369	0.532	0.377	0.512	0.336	0.250
S22.078B	Other fracture of T9-T10 vertebra, initial encounter for open fracture	169	Vertebral Fractures without Spinal Cord Injury		0.476	0.369	0.532	0.377	0.512	0.336	0.250
S22.079A	Unspecified fracture of T9-T10 vertebra, initial encounter for closed fracture	169	Vertebral Fractures without Spinal Cord Injury		0.476	0.369	0.532	0.377	0.512	0.336	0.250
S22.079B	Unspecified fracture of T9-T10 vertebra, initial encounter for open fracture	169	Vertebral Fractures without Spinal Cord Injury		0.476	0.369	0.532	0.377	0.512	0.336	0.250
S22.080A	Wedge compression fracture of T11-T12 vertebra, initial encounter for closed fracture	169	Vertebral Fractures without Spinal Cord Injury		0.476	0.369	0.532	0.377	0.512	0.336	0.250
S22.080B	Wedge compression fracture of T11-T12 vertebra, initial encounter for open fracture	169	Vertebral Fractures without Spinal Cord Injury		0.476	0.369	0.532	0.377	0.512	0.336	0.250
S22.081A	Stable burst fracture of T11-T12 vertebra, initial encounter for closed fracture	169	Vertebral Fractures without Spinal Cord Injury		0.476	0.369	0.532	0.377	0.512	0.336	0.250
S22.081B	Stable burst fracture of T11-T12 vertebra, initial encounter for open fracture	169	Vertebral Fractures without Spinal Cord Injury		0.476	0.369	0.532	0.377	0.512	0.336	0.250
S22.082A	Unstable burst fracture of T11-T12 vertebra, initial encounter for closed fracture	169	Vertebral Fractures without Spinal Cord Injury		0.476	0.369	0.532	0.377	0.512	0.336	0.250
S22.082B	Unstable burst fracture of T11-T12 vertebra, initial encounter for open fracture	169	Vertebral Fractures without Spinal Cord Injury		0.476	0.369	0.532	0.377	0.512	0.336	0.250
S22.088A	Other fracture of T11-T12 vertebra, initial encounter for closed fracture	169	Vertebral Fractures without Spinal Cord Injury		0.476	0.369	0.532	0.377	0.512	0.336	0.250
S22.088B	Other fracture of T11-T12 vertebra, initial encounter for open fracture	169	Vertebral Fractures without Spinal Cord Injury		0.476	0.369	0.532	0.377	0.512	0.336	0.250
S22.089A	Unspecified fracture of T11-T12 vertebra, initial encounter for closed fracture	169	Vertebral Fractures without Spinal Cord Injury		0.476	0.369	0.532	0.377	0.512	0.336	0.250
S22.089B	Unspecified fracture of T11-T12 vertebra, initial encounter for open fracture	169	Vertebral Fractures without Spinal Cord Injury		0.476	0.369	0.532	0.377	0.512	0.336	0.250
S24.0XXA	Concussion and edema of thoracic spinal cord, initial encounter	72	Spinal Cord Disorders/Injuries	169	0.481	0.369	0.532	0.377	0.512	0.336	0.289

2021 Optum360, LLC

ICD-10-CM Code	ICD-10-CM Code Description	V24 CMS-HCC	V24 CMS-HCC Disease Group	V24 CMS-HCC Hierarchies	Community, NonDual, Aged	Community, NonDual, Disabled	Community, FBDual, Aged	Community, FBDual, Disabled	Community, PBDual, Aged	Community, PBDual, Disabled	Institutional
S24.0XXD	Concussion and edema of thoracic spinal cord, subsequent encounter	72	Spinal Cord Disorders/Injuries	169	0.481	0.369	0.532	0.377	0.512	0.336	0.289
S24.0XXS	Concussion and edema of thoracic spinal cord, sequela	72	Spinal Cord Disorders/Injuries	169	0.481	0.369	0.532	0.377	0.512	0.336	0.289
S24.101A	Unspecified injury at T1 level of thoracic spinal cord, initial encounter	72	Spinal Cord Disorders/Injuries	169	0.481	0.369	0.532	0.377	0.512	0.336	0.289
S24.101D	Unspecified injury at T1 level of thoracic spinal cord, subsequent encounter	72	Spinal Cord Disorders/Injuries	169	0.481	0.369	0.532	0.377	0.512	0.336	0.289
S24.101S	Unspecified injury at T1 level of thoracic spinal cord, sequela	72	Spinal Cord Disorders/Injuries	169	0.481	0.369	0.532	0.377	0.512	0.336	0.289
S24.102A	Unspecified injury at T2-T6 level of thoracic spinal cord, initial encounter	72	Spinal Cord Disorders/Injuries	169	0.481	0.369	0.532	0.377	0.512	0.336	0.289
S24.102D	Unspecified injury at T2-T6 level of thoracic spinal cord, subsequent encounter	72	Spinal Cord Disorders/Injuries	169	0.481	0.369	0.532	0.377	0.512	0.336	0.289
S24.102S	Unspecified injury at T2-T6 level of thoracic spinal cord, sequela	72	Spinal Cord Disorders/Injuries	169	0.481	0.369	0.532	0.377	0.512	0.336	0.289
S24.103A	Unspecified injury at T7-T10 level of thoracic spinal cord, initial encounter	72	Spinal Cord Disorders/Injuries	169	0.481	0.369	0.532	0.377	0.512	0.336	0.289
S24.103D	Unspecified injury at T7-T10 level of thoracic spinal cord, subsequent encounter	72	Spinal Cord Disorders/Injuries	169	0.481	0.369	0.532	0.377	0.512	0.336	0.289
S24.103S	Unspecified injury at T7-T10 level of thoracic spinal cord, sequela	72	Spinal Cord Disorders/Injuries	169	0.481	0.369	0.532	0.377	0.512	0.336	0.289
S24.104A	Unspecified injury at T11-T12 level of thoracic spinal cord, initial encounter	72	Spinal Cord Disorders/Injuries	169	0.481	0.369	0.532	0.377	0.512	0.336	0.289
S24.104D	Unspecified injury at T11-T12 level of thoracic spinal cord, subsequent encounter	72	Spinal Cord Disorders/Injuries	169	0.481	0.369	0.532	0.377	0.512	0.336	0.289
S24.104S	Unspecified injury at T11-T12 level of thoracic spinal cord, sequela	72	Spinal Cord Disorders/Injuries	169	0.481	0.369	0.532	0.377	0.512	0.336	0.289
S24.109A	Unspecified injury at unspecified level of thoracic spinal cord, initial encounter	72	Spinal Cord Disorders/Injuries	169	0.481	0.369	0.532	0.377	0.512	0.336	0.289
S24.109D	Unspecified injury at unspecified level of thoracic spinal cord, subsequent encounter	72	Spinal Cord Disorders/Injuries	169	0.481	0.369	0.532	0.377	0.512	0.336	0.289
S24.109S	Unspecified injury at unspecified level of thoracic spinal cord, sequela	72	Spinal Cord Disorders/Injuries	169	0.481	0.369	0.532	0.377	0.512	0.336	0.289
S24.111A	Complete lesion at T1 level of thoracic spinal cord, initial encounter	71	Paraplegia	72,104, 169	1.068	0.739	0.921	0.957	1.000	0.933	0.492
S24.111D	Complete lesion at T1 level of thoracic spinal cord, subsequent encounter	71	Paraplegia	72,104, 169	1.068	0.739	0.921	0.957	1.000	0.933	0.492
S24.111S	Complete lesion at T1 level of thoracic spinal cord, sequela	71	Paraplegia	72,104, 169	1.068	0.739	0.921	0.957	1.000	0.933	0.492
S24.112A	Complete lesion at T2-T6 level of thoracic spinal cord, initial encounter	71	Paraplegia	72,104, 169	1.068	0.739	0.921	0.957	1.000	0.933	0.492
S24.112D	Complete lesion at T2-T6 level of thoracic spinal cord, subsequent encounter	71	Paraplegia	72,104, 169	1.068	0.739	0.921	0.957	1.000	0.933	0.492
S24.112S	Complete lesion at T2-T6 level of thoracic spinal cord, sequela	71	Paraplegia	72,104, 169	1.068	0.739	0.921	0.957	1.000	0.933	0.492
S24.113A	Complete lesion at T7-T10 level of thoracic spinal cord, initial encounter	71	Paraplegia	72,104, 169	1.068	0.739	0.921	0.957	1.000	0.933	0.492
S24.113D	Complete lesion at T7-T10 level of thoracic spinal cord, subsequent encounter	71	Paraplegia	72,104, 169	1.068	0.739	0.921	0.957	1.000	0.933	0.492

ICD-10-CM Code	ICD-10-CM Code Description	V24 CMS-HCC	V24 CMS-HCC Disease Group	V24 CMS-HCC Hierarchies	Community, NonDual, Aged	Community, NonDual, Disabled	Community, FBDual, Aged	Community, FBDual, Disabled	Community, PBDual, Aged	Community, PBDual, Disabled	Institutional
S24.113S	Complete lesion at T7-T10 level of thoracic spinal cord, sequela	71	Paraplegia	72,104, 169	1.068	0.739	0.921	0.957	1.000	0.933	0.492
S24.114A	Complete lesion at T11-T12 level of thoracic spinal cord, initial encounter	71	Paraplegia	72,104, 169	1.068	0.739	0.921	0.957	1.000	0.933	0.492
S24.114D	Complete lesion at T11-T12 level of thoracic spinal cord, subsequent encounter	71	Paraplegia	72,104, 169	1.068	0.739	0.921	0.957	1.000	0.933	0.492
S24.114S	Complete lesion at T11-T12 level of thoracic spinal cord, sequela	71	Paraplegia	72,104, 169	1.068	0.739	0.921	0.957	1.000	0.933	0.492
S24.119A	Complete lesion at unspecified level of thoracic spinal cord, initial encounter	71	Paraplegia	72,104, 169	1.068	0.739	0.921	0.957	1.000	0.933	0.492
S24.119D	Complete lesion at unspecified level of thoracic spinal cord, subsequent encounter	71	Paraplegia	72,104, 169	1.068	0.739	0.921	0.957	1.000	0.933	0.492
S24.119S	Complete lesion at unspecified level of thoracic spinal cord, sequela	71	Paraplegia	72,104, 169	1.068	0.739	0.921	0.957	1.000	0.933	0.492
S24.131A	Anterior cord syndrome at T1 level of thoracic spinal cord, initial encounter	72	Spinal Cord Disorders/Injuries	169	0.481	0.369	0.532	0.377	0.512	0.336	0.289
S24.131D	Anterior cord syndrome at T1 level of thoracic spinal cord, subsequent encounter	72	Spinal Cord Disorders/Injuries	169	0.481	0.369	0.532	0.377	0.512	0.336	0.289
S24.131S	Anterior cord syndrome at T1 level of thoracic spinal cord, sequela	72	Spinal Cord Disorders/Injuries	169	0.481	0.369	0.532	0.377	0.512	0.336	0.289
S24.132A	Anterior cord syndrome at T2-T6 level of thoracic spinal cord, initial encounter	72	Spinal Cord Disorders/Injuries	169	0.481	0.369	0.532	0.377	0.512	0.336	0.289
S24.132D	Anterior cord syndrome at T2-T6 level of thoracic spinal cord, subsequent encounter	72	Spinal Cord Disorders/Injuries	169	0.481	0.369	0.532	0.377	0.512	0.336	0.289
S24.132S	Anterior cord syndrome at T2-T6 level of thoracic spinal cord, sequela	72	Spinal Cord Disorders/Injuries	169	0.481	0.369	0.532	0.377	0.512	0.336	0.289
S24.133A	Anterior cord syndrome at T7-T10 level of thoracic spinal cord, initial encounter	72	Spinal Cord Disorders/Injuries	169	0.481	0.369	0.532	0.377	0.512	0.336	0.289
S24.133D	Anterior cord syndrome at T7-T10 level of thoracic spinal cord, subsequent encounter	72	Spinal Cord Disorders/Injuries	169	0.481	0.369	0.532	0.377	0.512	0.336	0.289
S24.133S	Anterior cord syndrome at T7-T10 level of thoracic spinal cord, sequela	72	Spinal Cord Disorders/Injuries	169	0.481	0.369	0.532	0.377	0.512	0.336	0.289
S24.134A	Anterior cord syndrome at T11-T12 level of thoracic spinal cord, initial encounter	72	Spinal Cord Disorders/Injuries	169	0.481	0.369	0.532	0.377	0.512	0.336	0.289
S24.134D	Anterior cord syndrome at T11-T12 level of thoracic spinal cord, subsequent encounter	72	Spinal Cord Disorders/Injuries	169	0.481	0.369	0.532	0.377	0.512	0.336	0.289
S24.134S	Anterior cord syndrome at T11-T12 level of thoracic spinal cord, sequela	72	Spinal Cord Disorders/Injuries	169	0.481	0.369	0.532	0.377	0.512	0.336	0.289
S24.139A	Anterior cord syndrome at unspecified level of thoracic spinal cord, initial encounter	72	Spinal Cord Disorders/Injuries	169	0.481	0.369	0.532	0.377	0.512	0.336	0.289
S24.139D	Anterior cord syndrome at unspecified level of thoracic spinal cord, subsequent encounter	72	Spinal Cord Disorders/Injuries	169	0.481	0.369	0.532	0.377	0.512	0.336	0.289
S24.139S	Anterior cord syndrome at unspecified level of thoracic spinal cord, sequela	72	Spinal Cord Disorders/Injuries	169	0.481	0.369	0.532	0.377	0.512	0.336	0.289
S24.141A	Brown-Sequard syndrome at T1 level of thoracic spinal cord, initial encounter	72	Spinal Cord Disorders/Injuries	169	0.481	0.369	0.532	0.377	0.512	0.336	0.289

ICD-10-CM Code	ICD-10-CM Code Description	V24 CMS-HCC	V24 CMS-HCC Disease Group	V24 CMS-HCC Hierarchies	Community, NonDual, Aged	Community, NonDual, Disabled	Community, FBDual, Aged	Community, FBDual, Disabled	Community, PBDual, Aged	Community, PBDual, Disabled	Institutional
S24.141D	Brown-Sequard syndrome at T1 level of thoracic spinal cord, subsequent encounter	72	Spinal Cord Disorders/Injuries	169	0.481	0.369	0.532	0.377	0.512	0.336	0.289
S24.141S	Brown-Sequard syndrome at T1 level of thoracic spinal cord, sequela	72	Spinal Cord Disorders/Injuries	169	0.481	0.369	0.532	0.377	0.512	0.336	0.289
S24.142A	Brown-Sequard syndrome at T2-T6 level of thoracic spinal cord, initial encounter	72	Spinal Cord Disorders/Injuries	169	0.481	0.369	0.532	0.377	0.512	0.336	0.289
S24.142D	Brown-Sequard syndrome at T2-T6 level of thoracic spinal cord, subsequent encounter	72	Spinal Cord Disorders/Injuries	169	0.481	0.369	0.532	0.377	0.512	0.336	0.289
S24.142S	Brown-Sequard syndrome at T2-T6 level of thoracic spinal cord, sequela	72	Spinal Cord Disorders/Injuries	169	0.481	0.369	0.532	0.377	0.512	0.336	0.289
S24.143A	Brown-Sequard syndrome at T7-T10 level of thoracic spinal cord, initial encounter	72	Spinal Cord Disorders/Injuries	169	0.481	0.369	0.532	0.377	0.512	0.336	0.289
S24.143D	Brown-Sequard syndrome at T7-T10 level of thoracic spinal cord, subsequent encounter	72	Spinal Cord Disorders/Injuries	169	0.481	0.369	0.532	0.377	0.512	0.336	0.289
S24.143S	Brown-Sequard syndrome at T7-T10 level of thoracic spinal cord, sequela	72	Spinal Cord Disorders/Injuries	169	0.481	0.369	0.532	0.377	0.512	0.336	0.289
S24.144A	Brown-Sequard syndrome at T11-T12 level of thoracic spinal cord, initial encounter	72	Spinal Cord Disorders/Injuries	169	0.481	0.369	0.532	0.377	0.512	0.336	0.289
S24.144D	Brown-Sequard syndrome at T11-T12 level of thoracic spinal cord, subsequent encounter	72	Spinal Cord Disorders/Injuries	169	0.481	0.369	0.532	0.377	0.512	0.336	0.289
S24.144S	Brown-Sequard syndrome at T11-T12 level of thoracic spinal cord, sequela	72	Spinal Cord Disorders/Injuries	169	0.481	0.369	0.532	0.377	0.512	0.336	0.289
S24.149A	Brown-Sequard syndrome at unspecified level of thoracic spinal cord, initial encounter	72	Spinal Cord Disorders/Injuries	169	0.481	0.369	0.532	0.377	0.512	0.336	0.289
S24.149D	Brown-Sequard syndrome at unspecified level of thoracic spinal cord, subsequent encounter	72	Spinal Cord Disorders/Injuries	169	0.481	0.369	0.532	0.377	0.512	0.336	0.289
S24.149S	Brown-Sequard syndrome at unspecified level of thoracic spinal cord, sequela	72	Spinal Cord Disorders/Injuries	169	0.481	0.369	0.532	0.377	0.512	0.336	0.289
S24.151A	Other incomplete lesion at T1 level of thoracic spinal cord, initial encounter	72	Spinal Cord Disorders/Injuries	169	0.481	0.369	0.532	0.377	0.512	0.336	0.289
S24.151D	Other incomplete lesion at T1 level of thoracic spinal cord, subsequent encounter	72	Spinal Cord Disorders/Injuries	169	0.481	0.369	0.532	0.377	0.512	0.336	0.289
S24.151S	Other incomplete lesion at T1 level of thoracic spinal cord, sequela	72	Spinal Cord Disorders/Injuries	169	0.481	0.369	0.532	0.377	0.512	0.336	0.289
S24.152A	Other incomplete lesion at T2-T6 level of thoracic spinal cord, initial encounter	72	Spinal Cord Disorders/Injuries	169	0.481	0.369	0.532	0.377	0.512	0.336	0.289
S24.152D	Other incomplete lesion at T2-T6 level of thoracic spinal cord, subsequent encounter	72	Spinal Cord Disorders/Injuries	169	0.481	0.369	0.532	0.377	0.512	0.336	0.289
S24.152S	Other incomplete lesion at T2-T6 level of thoracic spinal cord, sequela	72	Spinal Cord Disorders/Injuries	169	0.481	0.369	0.532	0.377	0.512	0.336	0.289
S24.153A	Other incomplete lesion at T7-T10 level of thoracic spinal cord, initial encounter	72	Spinal Cord Disorders/Injuries	169	0.481	0.369	0.532	0.377	0.512	0.336	0.289
S24.153D	Other incomplete lesion at T7-T10 level of thoracic spinal cord, subsequent encounter	72	Spinal Cord Disorders/Injuries	169	0.481	0.369	0.532	0.377	0.512	0.336	0.289
S24.153S	Other incomplete lesion at T7-T10 level of thoracic spinal cord, sequela	72	Spinal Cord Disorders/Injuries	169	0.481	0.369	0.532	0.377	0.512	0.336	0.289

ICD-10-CM Code	ICD-10-CM Code Description	V24 CMS-HCC	V24 CMS-HCC Disease Group	V24 CMS-HCC Hierarchies	Community, NonDual, Aged	Community, NonDual, Disabled	Community, FBDual, Aged	Community, FBDual, Disabled	Community, PBDual, Aged	Community, PBDual, Disabled	Institutional
S24.154A	Other incomplete lesion at T11-T12 level of thoracic spinal cord, initial encounter	72	Spinal Cord Disorders/Injuries	169	0.481	0.369	0.532	0.377	0.512	0.336	0.289
S24.154D	Other incomplete lesion at T11-T12 level of thoracic spinal cord, subsequent encounter	72	Spinal Cord Disorders/Injuries	169	0.481	0.369	0.532	0.377	0.512	0.336	0.289
S24.154S	Other incomplete lesion at T11-T12 level of thoracic spinal cord, sequela	72	Spinal Cord Disorders/Injuries	169	0.481	0.369	0.532	0.377	0.512	0.336	0.289
S24.159A	Other incomplete lesion at unspecified level of thoracic spinal cord, initial encounter	72	Spinal Cord Disorders/Injuries	169	0.481	0.369	0.532	0.377	0.512	0.336	0.289
S24.159D	Other incomplete lesion at unspecified level of thoracic spinal cord, subsequent encounter	72	Spinal Cord Disorders/Injuries	169	0.481	0.369	0.532	0.377	0.512	0.336	0.289
S24.159S	Other incomplete lesion at unspecified level of thoracic spinal cord, sequela	72	Spinal Cord Disorders/Injuries	169	0.481	0.369	0.532	0.377	0.512	0.336	0.289
S32.000A	Wedge compression fracture of unspecified lumbar vertebra, initial encounter for closed fracture	169	Vertebral Fractures without Spinal Cord Injury		0.476	0.369	0.532	0.377	0.512	0.336	0.250
S32.000B	Wedge compression fracture of unspecified lumbar vertebra, initial encounter for open fracture	169	Vertebral Fractures without Spinal Cord Injury		0.476	0.369	0.532	0.377	0.512	0.336	0.250
S32.001A	Stable burst fracture of unspecified lumbar vertebra, initial encounter for closed fracture	169	Vertebral Fractures without Spinal Cord Injury		0.476	0.369	0.532	0.377	0.512	0.336	0.250
S32.001B	Stable burst fracture of unspecified lumbar vertebra, initial encounter for open fracture	169	Vertebral Fractures without Spinal Cord Injury		0.476	0.369	0.532	0.377	0.512	0.336	0.250
S32.002A	Unstable burst fracture of unspecified lumbar vertebra, initial encounter for closed fracture	169	Vertebral Fractures without Spinal Cord Injury		0.476	0.369	0.532	0.377	0.512	0.336	0.250
S32.002B	Unstable burst fracture of unspecified lumbar vertebra, initial encounter for open fracture	169	Vertebral Fractures without Spinal Cord Injury		0.476	0.369	0.532	0.377	0.512	0.336	0.250
S32.008A	Other fracture of unspecified lumbar vertebra, initial encounter for closed fracture	169	Vertebral Fractures without Spinal Cord Injury		0.476	0.369	0.532	0.377	0.512	0.336	0.250
S32.008B	Other fracture of unspecified lumbar vertebra, initial encounter for open fracture	169	Vertebral Fractures without Spinal Cord Injury		0.476	0.369	0.532	0.377	0.512	0.336	0.250
S32.009A	Unspecified fracture of unspecified lumbar vertebra, initial encounter for closed fracture	169	Vertebral Fractures without Spinal Cord Injury		0.476	0.369	0.532	0.377	0.512	0.336	0.250
S32.009B	Unspecified fracture of unspecified lumbar vertebra, initial encounter for open fracture	169	Vertebral Fractures without Spinal Cord Injury		0.476	0.369	0.532	0.377	0.512	0.336	0.250
S32.010A	Wedge compression fracture of first lumbar vertebra, initial encounter for closed fracture	169	Vertebral Fractures without Spinal Cord Injury		0.476	0.369	0.532	0.377	0.512	0.336	0.250
S32.010B	Wedge compression fracture of first lumbar vertebra, initial encounter for open fracture	169	Vertebral Fractures without Spinal Cord Injury		0.476	0.369	0.532	0.377	0.512	0.336	0.250
S32.011A	Stable burst fracture of first lumbar vertebra, initial encounter for closed fracture	169	Vertebral Fractures without Spinal Cord Injury		0.476	0.369	0.532	0.377	0.512	0.336	0.250
S32.011B	Stable burst fracture of first lumbar vertebra, initial encounter for open fracture	169	Vertebral Fractures without Spinal Cord Injury		0.476	0.369	0.532	0.377	0.512	0.336	0.250

ICD-10-CM Code	ICD-10-CM Code Description	V24 CMS-HCC	V24 CMS-HCC Disease Group	V24 CMS-HCC Hierarchies	Community, NonDual, Aged	Community, NonDual, Disabled	Community, FBDual, Aged	Community, FBDual, Disabled	Community, PBDual, Aged	Community, PBDual, Disabled	Institutional
S32.012A	Unstable burst fracture of first lumbar vertebra, initial encounter for closed fracture	169	Vertebral Fractures without Spinal Cord Injury		0.476	0.369	0.532	0.377	0.512	0.336	0.250
S32.012B	Unstable burst fracture of first lumbar vertebra, initial encounter for open fracture	169	Vertebral Fractures without Spinal Cord Injury		0.476	0.369	0.532	0.377	0.512	0.336	0.250
S32.018A	Other fracture of first lumbar vertebra, initial encounter for closed fracture	169	Vertebral Fractures without Spinal Cord Injury		0.476	0.369	0.532	0.377	0.512	0.336	0.250
S32.018B	Other fracture of first lumbar vertebra, initial encounter for open fracture	169	Vertebral Fractures without Spinal Cord Injury		0.476	0.369	0.532	0.377	0.512	0.336	0.250
S32.019A	Unspecified fracture of first lumbar vertebra, initial encounter for closed fracture	169	Vertebral Fractures without Spinal Cord Injury		0.476	0.369	0.532	0.377	0.512	0.336	0.250
S32.019B	Unspecified fracture of first lumbar vertebra, initial encounter for open fracture	169	Vertebral Fractures without Spinal Cord Injury		0.476	0.369	0.532	0.377	0.512	0.336	0.250
S32.020A	Wedge compression fracture of second lumbar vertebra, initial encounter for closed fracture	169	Vertebral Fractures without Spinal Cord Injury		0.476	0.369	0.532	0.377	0.512	0.336	0.250
S32.020B	Wedge compression fracture of second lumbar vertebra, initial encounter for open fracture	169	Vertebral Fractures without Spinal Cord Injury		0.476	0.369	0.532	0.377	0.512	0.336	0.250
S32.021A	Stable burst fracture of second lumbar vertebra, initial encounter for closed fracture	169	Vertebral Fractures without Spinal Cord Injury		0.476	0.369	0.532	0.377	0.512	0.336	0.250
S32.021B	Stable burst fracture of second lumbar vertebra, initial encounter for open fracture	169	Vertebral Fractures without Spinal Cord Injury		0.476	0.369	0.532	0.377	0.512	0.336	0.250
S32.022A	Unstable burst fracture of second lumbar vertebra, initial encounter for closed fracture	169	Vertebral Fractures without Spinal Cord Injury		0.476	0.369	0.532	0.377	0.512	0.336	0.250
S32.022B	Unstable burst fracture of second lumbar vertebra, initial encounter for open fracture	169	Vertebral Fractures without Spinal Cord Injury		0.476	0.369	0.532	0.377	0.512	0.336	0.250
S32.028A	Other fracture of second lumbar vertebra, initial encounter for closed fracture	169	Vertebral Fractures without Spinal Cord Injury		0.476	0.369	0.532	0.377	0.512	0.336	0.250
S32.028B	Other fracture of second lumbar vertebra, initial encounter for open fracture	169	Vertebral Fractures without Spinal Cord Injury		0.476	0.369	0.532	0.377	0.512	0.336	0.250
S32.029A	Unspecified fracture of second lumbar vertebra, initial encounter for closed fracture	169	Vertebral Fractures without Spinal Cord Injury		0.476	0.369	0.532	0.377	0.512	0.336	0.250
S32.029B	Unspecified fracture of second lumbar vertebra, initial encounter for open fracture	169	Vertebral Fractures without Spinal Cord Injury		0.476	0.369	0.532	0.377	0.512	0.336	0.250
S32.030A	Wedge compression fracture of third lumbar vertebra, initial encounter for closed fracture	169	Vertebral Fractures without Spinal Cord Injury		0.476	0.369	0.532	0.377	0.512	0.336	0.250
S32.030B	Wedge compression fracture of third lumbar vertebra, initial encounter for open fracture	169	Vertebral Fractures without Spinal Cord Injury		0.476	0.369	0.532	0.377	0.512	0.336	0.250
S32.031A	Stable burst fracture of third lumbar vertebra, initial encounter for closed fracture	169	Vertebral Fractures without Spinal Cord Injury		0.476	0.369	0.532	0.377	0.512	0.336	0.250
S32.031B	Stable burst fracture of third lumbar vertebra, initial encounter for open fracture	169	Vertebral Fractures without Spinal Cord Injury		0.476	0.369	0.532	0.377	0.512	0.336	0.250

ICD-10-CM Code	ICD-10-CM Code Description	V24 CMS-HCC	V24 CMS-HCC Disease Group	V24 CMS-HCC Hierarchies	Community, NonDual, Aged	Community, NonDual, Disabled	Community, FBDual, Aged	Community, FBDual, Disabled	Community, PBDual, Aged	Community, PBDual, Disabled	Institutional
S32.032A	Unstable burst fracture of third lumbar vertebra, initial encounter for closed fracture	169	Vertebral Fractures without Spinal Cord Injury		0.476	0.369	0.532	0.377	0.512	0.336	0.250
S32.032B	Unstable burst fracture of third lumbar vertebra, initial encounter for open fracture	169	Vertebral Fractures without Spinal Cord Injury		0.476	0.369	0.532	0.377	0.512	0.336	0.250
S32.038A	Other fracture of third lumbar vertebra, initial encounter for closed fracture	169	Vertebral Fractures without Spinal Cord Injury		0.476	0.369	0.532	0.377	0.512	0.336	0.250
S32.038B	Other fracture of third lumbar vertebra, initial encounter for open fracture	169	Vertebral Fractures without Spinal Cord Injury		0.476	0.369	0.532	0.377	0.512	0.336	0.250
S32.039A	Unspecified fracture of third lumbar vertebra, initial encounter for closed fracture	169	Vertebral Fractures without Spinal Cord Injury		0.476	0.369	0.532	0.377	0.512	0.336	0.250
S32.039B	Unspecified fracture of third lumbar vertebra, initial encounter for open fracture	169	Vertebral Fractures without Spinal Cord Injury		0.476	0.369	0.532	0.377	0.512	0.336	0.250
S32.040A	Wedge compression fracture of fourth lumbar vertebra, initial encounter for closed fracture	169	Vertebral Fractures without Spinal Cord Injury		0.476	0.369	0.532	0.377	0.512	0.336	0.250
S32.040B	Wedge compression fracture of fourth lumbar vertebra, initial encounter for open fracture	169	Vertebral Fractures without Spinal Cord Injury		0.476	0.369	0.532	0.377	0.512	0.336	0.250
S32.041A	Stable burst fracture of fourth lumbar vertebra, initial encounter for closed fracture	169	Vertebral Fractures without Spinal Cord Injury		0.476	0.369	0.532	0.377	0.512	0.336	0.250
S32.041B	Stable burst fracture of fourth lumbar vertebra, initial encounter for open fracture	169	Vertebral Fractures without Spinal Cord Injury		0.476	0.369	0.532	0.377	0.512	0.336	0.250
S32.042A	Unstable burst fracture of fourth lumbar vertebra, initial encounter for closed fracture	169	Vertebral Fractures without Spinal Cord Injury		0.476	0.369	0.532	0.377	0.512	0.336	0.250
S32.042B	Unstable burst fracture of fourth lumbar vertebra, initial encounter for open fracture	169	Vertebral Fractures without Spinal Cord Injury		0.476	0.369	0.532	0.377	0.512	0.336	0.250
S32.048A	Other fracture of fourth lumbar vertebra, initial encounter for closed fracture	169	Vertebral Fractures without Spinal Cord Injury		0.476	0.369	0.532	0.377	0.512	0.336	0.250
S32.048B	Other fracture of fourth lumbar vertebra, initial encounter for open fracture	169	Vertebral Fractures without Spinal Cord Injury		0.476	0.369	0.532	0.377	0.512	0.336	0.250
S32.049A	Unspecified fracture of fourth lumbar vertebra, initial encounter for closed fracture	169	Vertebral Fractures without Spinal Cord Injury		0.476	0.369	0.532	0.377	0.512	0.336	0.250
S32.049B	Unspecified fracture of fourth lumbar vertebra, initial encounter for open fracture	169	Vertebral Fractures without Spinal Cord Injury		0.476	0.369	0.532	0.377	0.512	0.336	0.250
S32.050A	Wedge compression fracture of fifth lumbar vertebra, initial encounter for closed fracture	169	Vertebral Fractures without Spinal Cord Injury		0.476	0.369	0.532	0.377	0.512	0.336	0.250
S32.050B	Wedge compression fracture of fifth lumbar vertebra, initial encounter for open fracture	169	Vertebral Fractures without Spinal Cord Injury		0.476	0.369	0.532	0.377	0.512	0.336	0.250
S32.051A	Stable burst fracture of fifth lumbar vertebra, initial encounter for closed fracture	169	Vertebral Fractures without Spinal Cord Injury		0.476	0.369	0.532	0.377	0.512	0.336	0.250
S32.051B	Stable burst fracture of fifth lumbar vertebra, initial encounter for open fracture	169	Vertebral Fractures without Spinal Cord Injury		0.476	0.369	0.532	0.377	0.512	0.336	0.250

ICD-10-CM Code	ICD-10-CM Code Description	V24 CMS-HCC	V24 CMS-HCC Disease Group	V24 CMS-HCC Hierarchies	Community, NonDual, Aged	Community, NonDual, Disabled	Community, FBDual, Aged	Community, FBDual, Disabled	Community, PBDual, Aged	Community, PBDual, Disabled	Institutional
S32.052A	Unstable burst fracture of fifth lumbar vertebra, initial encounter for closed fracture	169	Vertebral Fractures without Spinal Cord Injury		0.476	0.369	0.532	0.377	0.512	0.336	0.250
S32.052B	Unstable burst fracture of fifth lumbar vertebra, initial encounter for open fracture	169	Vertebral Fractures without Spinal Cord Injury		0.476	0.369	0.532	0.377	0.512	0.336	0.250
S32.058A	Other fracture of fifth lumbar vertebra, initial encounter for closed fracture	169	Vertebral Fractures without Spinal Cord Injury		0.476	0.369	0.532	0.377	0.512	0.336	0.250
S32.058B	Other fracture of fifth lumbar vertebra, initial encounter for open fracture	169	Vertebral Fractures without Spinal Cord Injury		0.476	0.369	0.532	0.377	0.512	0.336	0.250
S32.059A	Unspecified fracture of fifth lumbar vertebra, initial encounter for closed fracture	169	Vertebral Fractures without Spinal Cord Injury		0.476	0.369	0.532	0.377	0.512	0.336	0.250
S32.059B	Unspecified fracture of fifth lumbar vertebra, initial encounter for open fracture	169	Vertebral Fractures without Spinal Cord Injury		0.476	0.369	0.532	0.377	0.512	0.336	0.250
S32.10XA	Unspecified fracture of sacrum, initial encounter for closed fracture	169	Vertebral Fractures without Spinal Cord Injury		0.476	0.369	0.532	0.377	0.512	0.336	0.250
S32.10XB	Unspecified fracture of sacrum, initial encounter for open fracture	169	Vertebral Fractures without Spinal Cord Injury		0.476	0.369	0.532	0.377	0.512	0.336	0.250
S32.110A	Nondisplaced Zone I fracture of sacrum, initial encounter for closed fracture	169	Vertebral Fractures without Spinal Cord Injury		0.476	0.369	0.532	0.377	0.512	0.336	0.250
S32.110B	Nondisplaced Zone I fracture of sacrum, initial encounter for open fracture	169	Vertebral Fractures without Spinal Cord Injury		0.476	0.369	0.532	0.377	0.512	0.336	0.250
S32.111A	Minimally displaced Zone I fracture of sacrum, initial encounter for closed fracture	169	Vertebral Fractures without Spinal Cord Injury		0.476	0.369	0.532	0.377	0.512	0.336	0.250
S32.111B	Minimally displaced Zone I fracture of sacrum, initial encounter for open fracture	169	Vertebral Fractures without Spinal Cord Injury		0.476	0.369	0.532	0.377	0.512	0.336	0.250
S32.112A	Severely displaced Zone I fracture of sacrum, initial encounter for closed fracture	169	Vertebral Fractures without Spinal Cord Injury		0.476	0.369	0.532	0.377	0.512	0.336	0.250
S32.112B	Severely displaced Zone I fracture of sacrum, initial encounter for open fracture	169	Vertebral Fractures without Spinal Cord Injury		0.476	0.369	0.532	0.377	0.512	0.336	0.250
S32.119A	Unspecified Zone I fracture of sacrum, initial encounter for closed fracture	169	Vertebral Fractures without Spinal Cord Injury		0.476	0.369	0.532	0.377	0.512	0.336	0.250
S32.119B	Unspecified Zone I fracture of sacrum, initial encounter for open fracture	169	Vertebral Fractures without Spinal Cord Injury		0.476	0.369	0.532	0.377	0.512	0.336	0.250
S32.120A	Nondisplaced Zone II fracture of sacrum, initial encounter for closed fracture	169	Vertebral Fractures without Spinal Cord Injury		0.476	0.369	0.532	0.377	0.512	0.336	0.250
S32.120B	Nondisplaced Zone II fracture of sacrum, initial encounter for open fracture	169	Vertebral Fractures without Spinal Cord Injury		0.476	0.369	0.532	0.377	0.512	0.336	0.250
S32.121A	Minimally displaced Zone II fracture of sacrum, initial encounter for closed fracture	169	Vertebral Fractures without Spinal Cord Injury		0.476	0.369	0.532	0.377	0.512	0.336	0.250
S32.121B	Minimally displaced Zone II fracture of sacrum, initial encounter for open fracture	169	Vertebral Fractures without Spinal Cord Injury		0.476	0.369	0.532	0.377	0.512	0.336	0.250
S32.122A	Severely displaced Zone II fracture of sacrum, initial encounter for closed fracture	169	Vertebral Fractures without Spinal Cord Injury		0.476	0.369	0.532	0.377	0.512	0.336	0.250

ICD-10-CM Code	ICD-10-CM Code Description	V24 CMS-HCC	V24 CMS-HCC Disease Group	V24 CMS-HCC Hierarchies	Community, NonDual, Aged	Community, NonDual, Disabled	Community, FBDual, Aged	Community, FBDual, Disabled	Community, PBDual, Aged	Community, PBDual, Disabled	Institutional
S32.122B	Severely displaced Zone II fracture of sacrum, initial encounter for open fracture	169	Vertebral Fractures without Spinal Cord Injury		0.476	0.369	0.532	0.377	0.512	0.336	0.250
S32.129A	Unspecified Zone II fracture of sacrum, initial encounter for closed fracture	169	Vertebral Fractures without Spinal Cord Injury		0.476	0.369	0.532	0.377	0.512	0.336	0.250
S32.129B	Unspecified Zone II fracture of sacrum, initial encounter for open fracture	169	Vertebral Fractures without Spinal Cord Injury		0.476	0.369	0.532	0.377	0.512	0.336	0.250
S32.130A	Nondisplaced Zone III fracture of sacrum, initial encounter for closed fracture	169	Vertebral Fractures without Spinal Cord Injury		0.476	0.369	0.532	0.377	0.512	0.336	0.250
S32.130B	Nondisplaced Zone III fracture of sacrum, initial encounter for open fracture	169	Vertebral Fractures without Spinal Cord Injury		0.476	0.369	0.532	0.377	0.512	0.336	0.250
S32.131A	Minimally displaced Zone III fracture of sacrum, initial encounter for closed fracture	169	Vertebral Fractures without Spinal Cord Injury		0.476	0.369	0.532	0.377	0.512	0.336	0.250
S32.131B	Minimally displaced Zone III fracture of sacrum, initial encounter for open fracture	169	Vertebral Fractures without Spinal Cord Injury		0.476	0.369	0.532	0.377	0.512	0.336	0.250
S32.132A	Severely displaced Zone III fracture of sacrum, initial encounter for closed fracture	169	Vertebral Fractures without Spinal Cord Injury		0.476	0.369	0.532	0.377	0.512	0.336	0.250
S32.132B	Severely displaced Zone III fracture of sacrum, initial encounter for open fracture	169	Vertebral Fractures without Spinal Cord Injury		0.476	0.369	0.532	0.377	0.512	0.336	0.250
S32.139A	Unspecified Zone III fracture of sacrum, initial encounter for closed fracture	169	Vertebral Fractures without Spinal Cord Injury		0.476	0.369	0.532	0.377	0.512	0.336	0.250
S32.139B	Unspecified Zone III fracture of sacrum, initial encounter for open fracture	169	Vertebral Fractures without Spinal Cord Injury		0.476	0.369	0.532	0.377	0.512	0.336	0.250
S32.14XA	Type 1 fracture of sacrum, initial encounter for closed fracture	169	Vertebral Fractures without Spinal Cord Injury		0.476	0.369	0.532	0.377	0.512	0.336	0.250
S32.14XB	Type 1 fracture of sacrum, initial encounter for open fracture	169	Vertebral Fractures without Spinal Cord Injury		0.476	0.369	0.532	0.377	0.512	0.336	0.250
S32.15XA	Type 2 fracture of sacrum, initial encounter for closed fracture	169	Vertebral Fractures without Spinal Cord Injury		0.476	0.369	0.532	0.377	0.512	0.336	0.250
S32.15XB	Type 2 fracture of sacrum, initial encounter for open fracture	169	Vertebral Fractures without Spinal Cord Injury		0.476	0.369	0.532	0.377	0.512	0.336	0.250
S32.16XA	Type 3 fracture of sacrum, initial encounter for closed fracture	169	Vertebral Fractures without Spinal Cord Injury		0.476	0.369	0.532	0.377	0.512	0.336	0.250
S32.16XB	Type 3 fracture of sacrum, initial encounter for open fracture	169	Vertebral Fractures without Spinal Cord Injury		0.476	0.369	0.532	0.377	0.512	0.336	0.250
S32.17XA	Type 4 fracture of sacrum, initial encounter for closed fracture	169	Vertebral Fractures without Spinal Cord Injury		0.476	0.369	0.532	0.377	0.512	0.336	0.250
S32.17XB	Type 4 fracture of sacrum, initial encounter for open fracture	169	Vertebral Fractures without Spinal Cord Injury		0.476	0.369	0.532	0.377	0.512	0.336	0.250
S32.19XA	Other fracture of sacrum, initial encounter for closed fracture	169	Vertebral Fractures without Spinal Cord Injury		0.476	0.369	0.532	0.377	0.512	0.336	0.250
S32.19XB	Other fracture of sacrum, initial encounter for open fracture	169	Vertebral Fractures without Spinal Cord Injury		0.476	0.369	0.532	0.377	0.512	0.336	0.250
S32.2XXA	Fracture of coccyx, initial encounter for closed fracture	169	Vertebral Fractures without Spinal Cord Injury		0.476	0.369	0.532	0.377	0.512	0.336	0.250
S32.2XXB	Fracture of coccyx, initial encounter for open fracture	169	Vertebral Fractures without Spinal Cord Injury		0.476	0.369	0.532	0.377	0.512	0.336	0.250
S32.301A	Unspecified fracture of right ilium, initial encounter for closed fracture	170	Hip Fracture/Dislocation		0.350	0.394	0.409	0.469	0.354	0.333	—

ICD-10-CM Code	ICD-10-CM Code Description	V24 CMS-HCC	V24 CMS-HCC Disease Group	V24 CMS-HCC Hierarchies	Community, NonDual, Aged	Community, NonDual, Disabled	Community, FBDual, Aged	Community, FBDual, Disabled	Community, PBDual, Aged	Community, PBDual, Disabled	Institutional
S32.301B	Unspecified fracture of right ilium, initial encounter for open fracture	170	Hip Fracture/Dislocation		0.350	0.394	0.409	0.469	0.354	0.333	—
S32.302A	Unspecified fracture of left ilium, initial encounter for closed fracture	170	Hip Fracture/Dislocation		0.350	0.394	0.409	0.469	0.354	0.333	—
S32.302B	Unspecified fracture of left ilium, initial encounter for open fracture	170	Hip Fracture/Dislocation		0.350	0.394	0.409	0.469	0.354	0.333	—
S32.309A	Unspecified fracture of unspecified ilium, initial encounter for closed fracture	170	Hip Fracture/Dislocation		0.350	0.394	0.409	0.469	0.354	0.333	—
S32.309B	Unspecified fracture of unspecified ilium, initial encounter for open fracture	170	Hip Fracture/Dislocation		0.350	0.394	0.409	0.469	0.354	0.333	—
S32.311A	Displaced avulsion fracture of right ilium, initial encounter for closed fracture	170	Hip Fracture/Dislocation		0.350	0.394	0.409	0.469	0.354	0.333	—
S32.311B	Displaced avulsion fracture of right ilium, initial encounter for open fracture	170	Hip Fracture/Dislocation		0.350	0.394	0.409	0.469	0.354	0.333	—
S32.312A	Displaced avulsion fracture of left ilium, initial encounter for closed fracture	170	Hip Fracture/Dislocation		0.350	0.394	0.409	0.469	0.354	0.333	—
S32.312B	Displaced avulsion fracture of left ilium, initial encounter for open fracture	170	Hip Fracture/Dislocation		0.350	0.394	0.409	0.469	0.354	0.333	—
S32.313A	Displaced avulsion fracture of unspecified ilium, initial encounter for closed fracture	170	Hip Fracture/Dislocation		0.350	0.394	0.409	0.469	0.354	0.333	—
S32.313B	Displaced avulsion fracture of unspecified ilium, initial encounter for open fracture	170	Hip Fracture/Dislocation		0.350	0.394	0.409	0.469	0.354	0.333	—
S32.314A	Nondisplaced avulsion fracture of right ilium, initial encounter for closed fracture	170	Hip Fracture/Dislocation		0.350	0.394	0.409	0.469	0.354	0.333	—
S32.314B	Nondisplaced avulsion fracture of right ilium, initial encounter for open fracture	170	Hip Fracture/Dislocation		0.350	0.394	0.409	0.469	0.354	0.333	—
S32.315A	Nondisplaced avulsion fracture of left ilium, initial encounter for closed fracture	170	Hip Fracture/Dislocation		0.350	0.394	0.409	0.469	0.354	0.333	—
S32.315B	Nondisplaced avulsion fracture of left ilium, initial encounter for open fracture	170	Hip Fracture/Dislocation		0.350	0.394	0.409	0.469	0.354	0.333	—
S32.316A	Nondisplaced avulsion fracture of unspecified ilium, initial encounter for closed fracture	170	Hip Fracture/Dislocation		0.350	0.394	0.409	0.469	0.354	0.333	—
S32.316B	Nondisplaced avulsion fracture of unspecified ilium, initial encounter for open fracture	170	Hip Fracture/Dislocation		0.350	0.394	0.409	0.469	0.354	0.333	—
S32.391A	Other fracture of right ilium, initial encounter for closed fracture	170	Hip Fracture/Dislocation		0.350	0.394	0.409	0.469	0.354	0.333	—
S32.391B	Other fracture of right ilium, initial encounter for open fracture	170	Hip Fracture/Dislocation		0.350	0.394	0.409	0.469	0.354	0.333	—
S32.392A	Other fracture of left ilium, initial encounter for closed fracture	170	Hip Fracture/Dislocation		0.350	0.394	0.409	0.469	0.354	0.333	—
S32.392B	Other fracture of left ilium, initial encounter for open fracture	170	Hip Fracture/Dislocation		0.350	0.394	0.409	0.469	0.354	0.333	—
S32.399A	Other fracture of unspecified ilium, initial encounter for closed fracture	170	Hip Fracture/Dislocation		0.350	0.394	0.409	0.469	0.354	0.333	—
S32.399B	Other fracture of unspecified ilium, initial encounter for open fracture	170	Hip Fracture/Dislocation		0.350	0.394	0.409	0.469	0.354	0.333	—

ICD-10-CM Code	ICD-10-CM Code Description	V24 CMS-HCC	V24 CMS-HCC Disease Group	V24 CMS-HCC Hierarchies	Community, NonDual, Aged	Community, NonDual, Disabled	Community, FBDual, Aged	Community, FBDual, Disabled	Community, PBDual, Aged	Community, PBDual, Disabled	Institutional
S32.401A	Unspecified fracture of right acetabulum, initial encounter for closed fracture	170	Hip Fracture/Dislocation		0.350	0.394	0.409	0.469	0.354	0.333	—
S32.401B	Unspecified fracture of right acetabulum, initial encounter for open fracture	170	Hip Fracture/Dislocation		0.350	0.394	0.409	0.469	0.354	0.333	—
S32.402A	Unspecified fracture of left acetabulum, initial encounter for closed fracture	170	Hip Fracture/Dislocation		0.350	0.394	0.409	0.469	0.354	0.333	—
S32.402B	Unspecified fracture of left acetabulum, initial encounter for open fracture	170	Hip Fracture/Dislocation		0.350	0.394	0.409	0.469	0.354	0.333	—
S32.409A	Unspecified fracture of unspecified acetabulum, initial encounter for closed fracture	170	Hip Fracture/Dislocation		0.350	0.394	0.409	0.469	0.354	0.333	—
S32.409B	Unspecified fracture of unspecified acetabulum, initial encounter for open fracture	170	Hip Fracture/Dislocation		0.350	0.394	0.409	0.469	0.354	0.333	—
S32.411A	Displaced fracture of anterior wall of right acetabulum, initial encounter for closed fracture	170	Hip Fracture/Dislocation		0.350	0.394	0.409	0.469	0.354	0.333	—
S32.411B	Displaced fracture of anterior wall of right acetabulum, initial encounter for open fracture	170	Hip Fracture/Dislocation		0.350	0.394	0.409	0.469	0.354	0.333	—
S32.412A	Displaced fracture of anterior wall of left acetabulum, initial encounter for closed fracture	170	Hip Fracture/Dislocation		0.350	0.394	0.409	0.469	0.354	0.333	—
S32.412B	Displaced fracture of anterior wall of left acetabulum, initial encounter for open fracture	170	Hip Fracture/Dislocation		0.350	0.394	0.409	0.469	0.354	0.333	—
S32.413A	Displaced fracture of anterior wall of unspecified acetabulum, initial encounter for closed fracture	170	Hip Fracture/Dislocation		0.350	0.394	0.409	0.469	0.354	0.333	—
S32.413B	Displaced fracture of anterior wall of unspecified acetabulum, initial encounter for open fracture	170	Hip Fracture/Dislocation		0.350	0.394	0.409	0.469	0.354	0.333	—
S32.414A	Nondisplaced fracture of anterior wall of right acetabulum, initial encounter for closed fracture	170	Hip Fracture/Dislocation		0.350	0.394	0.409	0.469	0.354	0.333	—
S32.414B	Nondisplaced fracture of anterior wall of right acetabulum, initial encounter for open fracture	170	Hip Fracture/Dislocation		0.350	0.394	0.409	0.469	0.354	0.333	—
S32.415A	Nondisplaced fracture of anterior wall of left acetabulum, initial encounter for closed fracture	170	Hip Fracture/Dislocation		0.350	0.394	0.409	0.469	0.354	0.333	—
S32.415B	Nondisplaced fracture of anterior wall of left acetabulum, initial encounter for open fracture	170	Hip Fracture/Dislocation		0.350	0.394	0.409	0.469	0.354	0.333	—
S32.416A	Nondisplaced fracture of anterior wall of unspecified acetabulum, initial encounter for closed fracture	170	Hip Fracture/Dislocation		0.350	0.394	0.409	0.469	0.354	0.333	—
S32.416B	Nondisplaced fracture of anterior wall of unspecified acetabulum, initial encounter for open fracture	170	Hip Fracture/Dislocation		0.350	0.394	0.409	0.469	0.354	0.333	—
S32.421A	Displaced fracture of posterior wall of right acetabulum, initial encounter for closed fracture	170	Hip Fracture/Dislocation		0.350	0.394	0.409	0.469	0.354	0.333	—
S32.421B	Displaced fracture of posterior wall of right acetabulum, initial encounter for open fracture	170	Hip Fracture/Dislocation		0.350	0.394	0.409	0.469	0.354	0.333	—

ICD-10-CM Code	ICD-10-CM Code Description	V24 CMS-HCC	V24 CMS-HCC Disease Group	V24 CMS-HCC Hierarchies	Community, NonDual, Aged	Community, NonDual, Disabled	Community, FBDual, Aged	Community, FBDual, Disabled	Community, PBDual, Aged	Community, PBDual, Disabled	Institutional
S32.422A	Displaced fracture of posterior wall of left acetabulum, initial encounter for closed fracture	170	Hip Fracture/Dislocation		0.350	0.394	0.409	0.469	0.354	0.333	—
S32.422B	Displaced fracture of posterior wall of left acetabulum, initial encounter for open fracture	170	Hip Fracture/Dislocation		0.350	0.394	0.409	0.469	0.354	0.333	—
S32.423A	Displaced fracture of posterior wall of unspecified acetabulum, initial encounter for closed fracture	170	Hip Fracture/Dislocation		0.350	0.394	0.409	0.469	0.354	0.333	—
S32.423B	Displaced fracture of posterior wall of unspecified acetabulum, initial encounter for open fracture	170	Hip Fracture/Dislocation		0.350	0.394	0.409	0.469	0.354	0.333	—
S32.424A	Nondisplaced fracture of posterior wall of right acetabulum, initial encounter for closed fracture	170	Hip Fracture/Dislocation		0.350	0.394	0.409	0.469	0.354	0.333	—
S32.424B	Nondisplaced fracture of posterior wall of right acetabulum, initial encounter for open fracture	170	Hip Fracture/Dislocation		0.350	0.394	0.409	0.469	0.354	0.333	—
S32.425A	Nondisplaced fracture of posterior wall of left acetabulum, initial encounter for closed fracture	170	Hip Fracture/Dislocation		0.350	0.394	0.409	0.469	0.354	0.333	—
S32.425B	Nondisplaced fracture of posterior wall of left acetabulum, initial encounter for open fracture	170	Hip Fracture/Dislocation		0.350	0.394	0.409	0.469	0.354	0.333	—
S32.426A	Nondisplaced fracture of posterior wall of unspecified acetabulum, initial encounter for closed fracture	170	Hip Fracture/Dislocation		0.350	0.394	0.409	0.469	0.354	0.333	—
S32.426B	Nondisplaced fracture of posterior wall of unspecified acetabulum, initial encounter for open fracture	170	Hip Fracture/Dislocation		0.350	0.394	0.409	0.469	0.354	0.333	—
S32.431A	Displaced fracture of anterior column [iliopubic] of right acetabulum, initial encounter for closed fracture	170	Hip Fracture/Dislocation		0.350	0.394	0.409	0.469	0.354	0.333	—
S32.431B	Displaced fracture of anterior column [iliopubic] of right acetabulum, initial encounter for open fracture	170	Hip Fracture/Dislocation		0.350	0.394	0.409	0.469	0.354	0.333	—
S32.432A	Displaced fracture of anterior column [iliopubic] of left acetabulum, initial encounter for closed fracture	170	Hip Fracture/Dislocation		0.350	0.394	0.409	0.469	0.354	0.333	—
S32.432B	Displaced fracture of anterior column [iliopubic] of left acetabulum, initial encounter for open fracture	170	Hip Fracture/Dislocation		0.350	0.394	0.409	0.469	0.354	0.333	—
S32.433A	Displaced fracture of anterior column [iliopubic] of unspecified acetabulum, initial encounter for closed fracture	170	Hip Fracture/Dislocation		0.350	0.394	0.409	0.469	0.354	0.333	—
S32.433B	Displaced fracture of anterior column [iliopubic] of unspecified acetabulum, initial encounter for open fracture	170	Hip Fracture/Dislocation		0.350	0.394	0.409	0.469	0.354	0.333	—
S32.434A	Nondisplaced fracture of anterior column [iliopubic] of right acetabulum, initial encounter for closed fracture	170	Hip Fracture/Dislocation		0.350	0.394	0.409	0.469	0.354	0.333	—
S32.434B	Nondisplaced fracture of anterior column [iliopubic] of right acetabulum, initial encounter for open fracture	170	Hip Fracture/Dislocation		0.350	0.394	0.409	0.469	0.354	0.333	—
S32.435A	Nondisplaced fracture of anterior column [iliopubic] of left acetabulum, initial encounter for closed fracture	170	Hip Fracture/Dislocation		0.350	0.394	0.409	0.469	0.354	0.333	—
S32.435B	Nondisplaced fracture of anterior column [iliopubic] of left acetabulum, initial encounter for open fracture	170	Hip Fracture/Dislocation		0.350	0.394	0.409	0.469	0.354	0.333	—

ICD-10-CM Code	ICD-10-CM Code Description	V24 CMS-HCC	V24 CMS-HCC Disease Group	V24 CMS-HCC Hierarchies	Community, NonDual, Aged	Community, NonDual, Disabled	Community, FBDual, Aged	Community, FBDual, Disabled	Community, PBDual, Aged	Community, PBDual, Disabled	Institutional
S32.436A	Nondisplaced fracture of anterior column [iliopubic] of unspecified acetabulum, initial encounter for closed fracture	170	Hip Fracture/Dislocation		0.350	0.394	0.409	0.469	0.354	0.333	—
S32.436B	Nondisplaced fracture of anterior column [iliopubic] of unspecified acetabulum, initial encounter for open fracture	170	Hip Fracture/Dislocation		0.350	0.394	0.409	0.469	0.354	0.333	—
S32.441A	Displaced fracture of posterior column [ilioischial] of right acetabulum, initial encounter for closed fracture	170	Hip Fracture/Dislocation		0.350	0.394	0.409	0.469	0.354	0.333	—
S32.441B	Displaced fracture of posterior column [ilioischial] of right acetabulum, initial encounter for open fracture	170	Hip Fracture/Dislocation		0.350	0.394	0.409	0.469	0.354	0.333	—
S32.442A	Displaced fracture of posterior column [ilioischial] of left acetabulum, initial encounter for closed fracture	170	Hip Fracture/Dislocation		0.350	0.394	0.409	0.469	0.354	0.333	—
S32.442B	Displaced fracture of posterior column [ilioischial] of left acetabulum, initial encounter for open fracture	170	Hip Fracture/Dislocation		0.350	0.394	0.409	0.469	0.354	0.333	—
S32.443A	Displaced fracture of posterior column [ilioischial] of unspecified acetabulum, initial encounter for closed fracture	170	Hip Fracture/Dislocation		0.350	0.394	0.409	0.469	0.354	0.333	—
S32.443B	Displaced fracture of posterior column [ilioischial] of unspecified acetabulum, initial encounter for open fracture	170	Hip Fracture/Dislocation		0.350	0.394	0.409	0.469	0.354	0.333	—
S32.444A	Nondisplaced fracture of posterior column [ilioischial] of right acetabulum, initial encounter for closed fracture	170	Hip Fracture/Dislocation		0.350	0.394	0.409	0.469	0.354	0.333	—
S32.444B	Nondisplaced fracture of posterior column [ilioischial] of right acetabulum, initial encounter for open fracture	170	Hip Fracture/Dislocation		0.350	0.394	0.409	0.469	0.354	0.333	—
S32.445A	Nondisplaced fracture of posterior column [ilioischial] of left acetabulum, initial encounter for closed fracture	170	Hip Fracture/Dislocation		0.350	0.394	0.409	0.469	0.354	0.333	—
S32.445B	Nondisplaced fracture of posterior column [ilioischial] of left acetabulum, initial encounter for open fracture	170	Hip Fracture/Dislocation		0.350	0.394	0.409	0.469	0.354	0.333	—
S32.446A	Nondisplaced fracture of posterior column [ilioischial] of unspecified acetabulum, initial encounter for closed fracture	170	Hip Fracture/Dislocation		0.350	0.394	0.409	0.469	0.354	0.333	—
S32.446B	Nondisplaced fracture of posterior column [ilioischial] of unspecified acetabulum, initial encounter for open fracture	170	Hip Fracture/Dislocation		0.350	0.394	0.409	0.469	0.354	0.333	—
S32.451A	Displaced transverse fracture of right acetabulum, initial encounter for closed fracture	170	Hip Fracture/Dislocation		0.350	0.394	0.409	0.469	0.354	0.333	—
S32.451B	Displaced transverse fracture of right acetabulum, initial encounter for open fracture	170	Hip Fracture/Dislocation		0.350	0.394	0.409	0.469	0.354	0.333	—

ICD-10-CM Code	ICD-10-CM Code Description	V24 CMS-HCC	V24 CMS-HCC Disease Group	V24 CMS-HCC Hierarchies	Community, NonDual, Aged	Community, NonDual, Disabled	Community, FBDual, Aged	Community, FBDual, Disabled	Community, PBDual, Aged	Community, PBDual, Disabled	Institutional
S32.452A	Displaced transverse fracture of left acetabulum, initial encounter for closed fracture	170	Hip Fracture/Dislocation		0.350	0.394	0.409	0.469	0.354	0.333	—
S32.452B	Displaced transverse fracture of left acetabulum, initial encounter for open fracture	170	Hip Fracture/Dislocation		0.350	0.394	0.409	0.469	0.354	0.333	—
S32.453A	Displaced transverse fracture of unspecified acetabulum, initial encounter for closed fracture	170	Hip Fracture/Dislocation		0.350	0.394	0.409	0.469	0.354	0.333	—
S32.453B	Displaced transverse fracture of unspecified acetabulum, initial encounter for open fracture	170	Hip Fracture/Dislocation		0.350	0.394	0.409	0.469	0.354	0.333	—
S32.454A	Nondisplaced transverse fracture of right acetabulum, initial encounter for closed fracture	170	Hip Fracture/Dislocation		0.350	0.394	0.409	0.469	0.354	0.333	—
S32.454B	Nondisplaced transverse fracture of right acetabulum, initial encounter for open fracture	170	Hip Fracture/Dislocation		0.350	0.394	0.409	0.469	0.354	0.333	—
S32.455A	Nondisplaced transverse fracture of left acetabulum, initial encounter for closed fracture	170	Hip Fracture/Dislocation		0.350	0.394	0.409	0.469	0.354	0.333	—
S32.455B	Nondisplaced transverse fracture of left acetabulum, initial encounter for open fracture	170	Hip Fracture/Dislocation		0.350	0.394	0.409	0.469	0.354	0.333	—
S32.456A	Nondisplaced transverse fracture of unspecified acetabulum, initial encounter for closed fracture	170	Hip Fracture/Dislocation		0.350	0.394	0.409	0.469	0.354	0.333	—
S32.456B	Nondisplaced transverse fracture of unspecified acetabulum, initial encounter for open fracture	170	Hip Fracture/Dislocation		0.350	0.394	0.409	0.469	0.354	0.333	—
S32.461A	Displaced associated transverse-posterior fracture of right acetabulum, initial encounter for closed fracture	170	Hip Fracture/Dislocation		0.350	0.394	0.409	0.469	0.354	0.333	—
S32.461B	Displaced associated transverse-posterior fracture of right acetabulum, initial encounter for open fracture	170	Hip Fracture/Dislocation		0.350	0.394	0.409	0.469	0.354	0.333	—
S32.462A	Displaced associated transverse-posterior fracture of left acetabulum, initial encounter for closed fracture	170	Hip Fracture/Dislocation		0.350	0.394	0.409	0.469	0.354	0.333	—
S32.462B	Displaced associated transverse-posterior fracture of left acetabulum, initial encounter for open fracture	170	Hip Fracture/Dislocation		0.350	0.394	0.409	0.469	0.354	0.333	—
S32.463A	Displaced associated transverse-posterior fracture of unspecified acetabulum, initial encounter for closed fracture	170	Hip Fracture/Dislocation		0.350	0.394	0.409	0.469	0.354	0.333	—
S32.463B	Displaced associated transverse-posterior fracture of unspecified acetabulum, initial encounter for open fracture	170	Hip Fracture/Dislocation		0.350	0.394	0.409	0.469	0.354	0.333	—
S32.464A	Nondisplaced associated transverse-posterior fracture of right acetabulum, initial encounter for closed fracture	170	Hip Fracture/Dislocation		0.350	0.394	0.409	0.469	0.354	0.333	—
S32.464B	Nondisplaced associated transverse-posterior fracture of right acetabulum, initial encounter for open fracture	170	Hip Fracture/Dislocation		0.350	0.394	0.409	0.469	0.354	0.333	—

ICD-10-CM Code	ICD-10-CM Code Description	V24 CMS-HCC	V24 CMS-HCC Disease Group	V24 CMS-HCC Hierarchies	Community, NonDual, Aged	Community, NonDual, Disabled	Community, FBDual, Aged	Community, FBDual, Disabled	Community, PBDual, Aged	Community, PBDual, Disabled	Institutional
S32.465A	Nondisplaced associated transverse-posterior fracture of left acetabulum, initial encounter for closed fracture	170	Hip Fracture/Dislocation		0.350	0.394	0.409	0.469	0.354	0.333	—
S32.465B	Nondisplaced associated transverse-posterior fracture of left acetabulum, initial encounter for open fracture	170	Hip Fracture/Dislocation		0.350	0.394	0.409	0.469	0.354	0.333	—
S32.466A	Nondisplaced associated transverse-posterior fracture of unspecified acetabulum, initial encounter for closed fracture	170	Hip Fracture/Dislocation		0.350	0.394	0.409	0.469	0.354	0.333	—
S32.466B	Nondisplaced associated transverse-posterior fracture of unspecified acetabulum, initial encounter for open fracture	170	Hip Fracture/Dislocation		0.350	0.394	0.409	0.469	0.354	0.333	—
S32.471A	Displaced fracture of medial wall of right acetabulum, initial encounter for closed fracture	170	Hip Fracture/Dislocation		0.350	0.394	0.409	0.469	0.354	0.333	—
S32.471B	Displaced fracture of medial wall of right acetabulum, initial encounter for open fracture	170	Hip Fracture/Dislocation		0.350	0.394	0.409	0.469	0.354	0.333	—
S32.472A	Displaced fracture of medial wall of left acetabulum, initial encounter for closed fracture	170	Hip Fracture/Dislocation		0.350	0.394	0.409	0.469	0.354	0.333	—
S32.472B	Displaced fracture of medial wall of left acetabulum, initial encounter for open fracture	170	Hip Fracture/Dislocation		0.350	0.394	0.409	0.469	0.354	0.333	—
S32.473A	Displaced fracture of medial wall of unspecified acetabulum, initial encounter for closed fracture	170	Hip Fracture/Dislocation		0.350	0.394	0.409	0.469	0.354	0.333	—
S32.473B	Displaced fracture of medial wall of unspecified acetabulum, initial encounter for open fracture	170	Hip Fracture/Dislocation		0.350	0.394	0.409	0.469	0.354	0.333	—
S32.474A	Nondisplaced fracture of medial wall of right acetabulum, initial encounter for closed fracture	170	Hip Fracture/Dislocation		0.350	0.394	0.409	0.469	0.354	0.333	—
S32.474B	Nondisplaced fracture of medial wall of right acetabulum, initial encounter for open fracture	170	Hip Fracture/Dislocation		0.350	0.394	0.409	0.469	0.354	0.333	—
S32.475A	Nondisplaced fracture of medial wall of left acetabulum, initial encounter for closed fracture	170	Hip Fracture/Dislocation		0.350	0.394	0.409	0.469	0.354	0.333	—
S32.475B	Nondisplaced fracture of medial wall of left acetabulum, initial encounter for open fracture	170	Hip Fracture/Dislocation		0.350	0.394	0.409	0.469	0.354	0.333	—
S32.476A	Nondisplaced fracture of medial wall of unspecified acetabulum, initial encounter for closed fracture	170	Hip Fracture/Dislocation		0.350	0.394	0.409	0.469	0.354	0.333	—
S32.476B	Nondisplaced fracture of medial wall of unspecified acetabulum, initial encounter for open fracture	170	Hip Fracture/Dislocation		0.350	0.394	0.409	0.469	0.354	0.333	—
S32.481A	Displaced dome fracture of right acetabulum, initial encounter for closed fracture	170	Hip Fracture/Dislocation		0.350	0.394	0.409	0.469	0.354	0.333	—
S32.481B	Displaced dome fracture of right acetabulum, initial encounter for open fracture	170	Hip Fracture/Dislocation		0.350	0.394	0.409	0.469	0.354	0.333	—
S32.482A	Displaced dome fracture of left acetabulum, initial encounter for closed fracture	170	Hip Fracture/Dislocation		0.350	0.394	0.409	0.469	0.354	0.333	—

2021 Optum360, LLC

ICD-10-CM Code	ICD-10-CM Code Description	V24 CMS-HCC	V24 CMS-HCC Disease Group	V24 CMS-HCC Hierarchies	Community, NonDual, Aged	Community, NonDual, Disabled	Community, FBDual, Aged	Community, FBDual, Disabled	Community, PBDual, Aged	Community, PBDual, Disabled	Institutional
S32.482B	Displaced dome fracture of left acetabulum, initial encounter for open fracture	170	Hip Fracture/Dislocation		0.350	0.394	0.409	0.469	0.354	0.333	—
S32.483A	Displaced dome fracture of unspecified acetabulum, initial encounter for closed fracture	170	Hip Fracture/Dislocation		0.350	0.394	0.409	0.469	0.354	0.333	—
S32.483B	Displaced dome fracture of unspecified acetabulum, initial encounter for open fracture	170	Hip Fracture/Dislocation		0.350	0.394	0.409	0.469	0.354	0.333	—
S32.484A	Nondisplaced dome fracture of right acetabulum, initial encounter for closed fracture	170	Hip Fracture/Dislocation		0.350	0.394	0.409	0.469	0.354	0.333	—
S32.484B	Nondisplaced dome fracture of right acetabulum, initial encounter for open fracture	170	Hip Fracture/Dislocation		0.350	0.394	0.409	0.469	0.354	0.333	—
S32.485A	Nondisplaced dome fracture of left acetabulum, initial encounter for closed fracture	170	Hip Fracture/Dislocation		0.350	0.394	0.409	0.469	0.354	0.333	—
S32.485B	Nondisplaced dome fracture of left acetabulum, initial encounter for open fracture	170	Hip Fracture/Dislocation		0.350	0.394	0.409	0.469	0.354	0.333	—
S32.486A	Nondisplaced dome fracture of unspecified acetabulum, initial encounter for closed fracture	170	Hip Fracture/Dislocation		0.350	0.394	0.409	0.469	0.354	0.333	—
S32.486B	Nondisplaced dome fracture of unspecified acetabulum, initial encounter for open fracture	170	Hip Fracture/Dislocation		0.350	0.394	0.409	0.469	0.354	0.333	—
S32.491A	Other specified fracture of right acetabulum, initial encounter for closed fracture	170	Hip Fracture/Dislocation		0.350	0.394	0.409	0.469	0.354	0.333	—
S32.491B	Other specified fracture of right acetabulum, initial encounter for open fracture	170	Hip Fracture/Dislocation		0.350	0.394	0.409	0.469	0.354	0.333	—
S32.492A	Other specified fracture of left acetabulum, initial encounter for closed fracture	170	Hip Fracture/Dislocation		0.350	0.394	0.409	0.469	0.354	0.333	—
S32.492B	Other specified fracture of left acetabulum, initial encounter for open fracture	170	Hip Fracture/Dislocation		0.350	0.394	0.409	0.469	0.354	0.333	—
S32.499A	Other specified fracture of unspecified acetabulum, initial encounter for closed fracture	170	Hip Fracture/Dislocation		0.350	0.394	0.409	0.469	0.354	0.333	—
S32.499B	Other specified fracture of unspecified acetabulum, initial encounter for open fracture	170	Hip Fracture/Dislocation		0.350	0.394	0.409	0.469	0.354	0.333	—
S32.501A	Unspecified fracture of right pubis, initial encounter for closed fracture	170	Hip Fracture/Dislocation		0.350	0.394	0.409	0.469	0.354	0.333	—
S32.501B	Unspecified fracture of right pubis, initial encounter for open fracture	170	Hip Fracture/Dislocation		0.350	0.394	0.409	0.469	0.354	0.333	—
S32.502A	Unspecified fracture of left pubis, initial encounter for closed fracture	170	Hip Fracture/Dislocation		0.350	0.394	0.409	0.469	0.354	0.333	—
S32.502B	Unspecified fracture of left pubis, initial encounter for open fracture	170	Hip Fracture/Dislocation		0.350	0.394	0.409	0.469	0.354	0.333	—
S32.509A	Unspecified fracture of unspecified pubis, initial encounter for closed fracture	170	Hip Fracture/Dislocation		0.350	0.394	0.409	0.469	0.354	0.333	—
S32.509B	Unspecified fracture of unspecified pubis, initial encounter for open fracture	170	Hip Fracture/Dislocation		0.350	0.394	0.409	0.469	0.354	0.333	—

ICD-10-CM Code	ICD-10-CM Code Description	V24 CMS-HCC	V24 CMS-HCC Disease Group	V24 CMS-HCC Hierarchies	Community, NonDual, Aged	Community, NonDual, Disabled	Community, FBDual, Aged	Community, FBDual, Disabled	Community, PBDual, Aged	Community, PBDual, Disabled	Institutional
S32.511A	Fracture of superior rim of right pubis, initial encounter for closed fracture	170	Hip Fracture/Dislocation		0.350	0.394	0.409	0.469	0.354	0.333	—
S32.511B	Fracture of superior rim of right pubis, initial encounter for open fracture	170	Hip Fracture/Dislocation		0.350	0.394	0.409	0.469	0.354	0.333	—
S32.512A	Fracture of superior rim of left pubis, initial encounter for closed fracture	170	Hip Fracture/Dislocation		0.350	0.394	0.409	0.469	0.354	0.333	—
S32.512B	Fracture of superior rim of left pubis, initial encounter for open fracture	170	Hip Fracture/Dislocation		0.350	0.394	0.409	0.469	0.354	0.333	—
S32.519A	Fracture of superior rim of unspecified pubis, initial encounter for closed fracture	170	Hip Fracture/Dislocation		0.350	0.394	0.409	0.469	0.354	0.333	—
S32.519B	Fracture of superior rim of unspecified pubis, initial encounter for open fracture	170	Hip Fracture/Dislocation		0.350	0.394	0.409	0.469	0.354	0.333	—
S32.591A	Other specified fracture of right pubis, initial encounter for closed fracture	170	Hip Fracture/Dislocation		0.350	0.394	0.409	0.469	0.354	0.333	—
S32.591B	Other specified fracture of right pubis, initial encounter for open fracture	170	Hip Fracture/Dislocation		0.350	0.394	0.409	0.469	0.354	0.333	—
S32.592A	Other specified fracture of left pubis, initial encounter for closed fracture	170	Hip Fracture/Dislocation		0.350	0.394	0.409	0.469	0.354	0.333	—
S32.592B	Other specified fracture of left pubis, initial encounter for open fracture	170	Hip Fracture/Dislocation		0.350	0.394	0.409	0.469	0.354	0.333	—
S32.599A	Other specified fracture of unspecified pubis, initial encounter for closed fracture	170	Hip Fracture/Dislocation		0.350	0.394	0.409	0.469	0.354	0.333	—
S32.599B	Other specified fracture of unspecified pubis, initial encounter for open fracture	170	Hip Fracture/Dislocation		0.350	0.394	0.409	0.469	0.354	0.333	—
S32.601A	Unspecified fracture of right ischium, initial encounter for closed fracture	170	Hip Fracture/Dislocation		0.350	0.394	0.409	0.469	0.354	0.333	—
S32.601B	Unspecified fracture of right ischium, initial encounter for open fracture	170	Hip Fracture/Dislocation		0.350	0.394	0.409	0.469	0.354	0.333	—
S32.602A	Unspecified fracture of left ischium, initial encounter for closed fracture	170	Hip Fracture/Dislocation		0.350	0.394	0.409	0.469	0.354	0.333	—
S32.602B	Unspecified fracture of left ischium, initial encounter for open fracture	170	Hip Fracture/Dislocation		0.350	0.394	0.409	0.469	0.354	0.333	—
S32.609A	Unspecified fracture of unspecified ischium, initial encounter for closed fracture	170	Hip Fracture/Dislocation		0.350	0.394	0.409	0.469	0.354	0.333	—
S32.609B	Unspecified fracture of unspecified ischium, initial encounter for open fracture	170	Hip Fracture/Dislocation		0.350	0.394	0.409	0.469	0.354	0.333	—
S32.611A	Displaced avulsion fracture of right ischium, initial encounter for closed fracture	170	Hip Fracture/Dislocation		0.350	0.394	0.409	0.469	0.354	0.333	—
S32.611B	Displaced avulsion fracture of right ischium, initial encounter for open fracture	170	Hip Fracture/Dislocation		0.350	0.394	0.409	0.469	0.354	0.333	—
S32.612A	Displaced avulsion fracture of left ischium, initial encounter for closed fracture	170	Hip Fracture/Dislocation		0.350	0.394	0.409	0.469	0.354	0.333	—
S32.612B	Displaced avulsion fracture of left ischium, initial encounter for open fracture	170	Hip Fracture/Dislocation		0.350	0.394	0.409	0.469	0.354	0.333	—
S32.613A	Displaced avulsion fracture of unspecified ischium, initial encounter for closed fracture	170	Hip Fracture/Dislocation		0.350	0.394	0.409	0.469	0.354	0.333	—

ICD-10-CM Code	ICD-10-CM Code Description	V24 CMS-HCC	V24 CMS-HCC Disease Group	V24 CMS-HCC Hierarchies	Community, NonDual, Aged	Community, NonDual, Disabled	Community, FBDual, Aged	Community, FBDual, Disabled	Community, PBDual, Aged	Community, PBDual, Disabled	Institutional
S32.613B	Displaced avulsion fracture of unspecified ischium, initial encounter for open fracture	170	Hip Fracture/Dislocation		0.350	0.394	0.409	0.469	0.354	0.333	—
S32.614A	Nondisplaced avulsion fracture of right ischium, initial encounter for closed fracture	170	Hip Fracture/Dislocation		0.350	0.394	0.409	0.469	0.354	0.333	—
S32.614B	Nondisplaced avulsion fracture of right ischium, initial encounter for open fracture	170	Hip Fracture/Dislocation		0.350	0.394	0.409	0.469	0.354	0.333	—
S32.615A	Nondisplaced avulsion fracture of left ischium, initial encounter for closed fracture	170	Hip Fracture/Dislocation		0.350	0.394	0.409	0.469	0.354	0.333	—
S32.615B	Nondisplaced avulsion fracture of left ischium, initial encounter for open fracture	170	Hip Fracture/Dislocation		0.350	0.394	0.409	0.469	0.354	0.333	—
S32.616A	Nondisplaced avulsion fracture of unspecified ischium, initial encounter for closed fracture	170	Hip Fracture/Dislocation		0.350	0.394	0.409	0.469	0.354	0.333	—
S32.616B	Nondisplaced avulsion fracture of unspecified ischium, initial encounter for open fracture	170	Hip Fracture/Dislocation		0.350	0.394	0.409	0.469	0.354	0.333	—
S32.691A	Other specified fracture of right ischium, initial encounter for closed fracture	170	Hip Fracture/Dislocation		0.350	0.394	0.409	0.469	0.354	0.333	—
S32.691B	Other specified fracture of right ischium, initial encounter for open fracture	170	Hip Fracture/Dislocation		0.350	0.394	0.409	0.469	0.354	0.333	—
S32.692A	Other specified fracture of left ischium, initial encounter for closed fracture	170	Hip Fracture/Dislocation		0.350	0.394	0.409	0.469	0.354	0.333	—
S32.692B	Other specified fracture of left ischium, initial encounter for open fracture	170	Hip Fracture/Dislocation		0.350	0.394	0.409	0.469	0.354	0.333	—
S32.699A	Other specified fracture of unspecified ischium, initial encounter for closed fracture	170	Hip Fracture/Dislocation		0.350	0.394	0.409	0.469	0.354	0.333	—
S32.699B	Other specified fracture of unspecified ischium, initial encounter for open fracture	170	Hip Fracture/Dislocation		0.350	0.394	0.409	0.469	0.354	0.333	—
S32.810A	Multiple fractures of pelvis with stable disruption of pelvic ring, initial encounter for closed fracture	170	Hip Fracture/Dislocation		0.350	0.394	0.409	0.469	0.354	0.333	—
S32.810B	Multiple fractures of pelvis with stable disruption of pelvic ring, initial encounter for open fracture	170	Hip Fracture/Dislocation		0.350	0.394	0.409	0.469	0.354	0.333	—
S32.811A	Multiple fractures of pelvis with unstable disruption of pelvic ring, initial encounter for closed fracture	170	Hip Fracture/Dislocation		0.350	0.394	0.409	0.469	0.354	0.333	—
S32.811B	Multiple fractures of pelvis with unstable disruption of pelvic ring, initial encounter for open fracture	170	Hip Fracture/Dislocation		0.350	0.394	0.409	0.469	0.354	0.333	—
S32.82XA	Multiple fractures of pelvis without disruption of pelvic ring, initial encounter for closed fracture	170	Hip Fracture/Dislocation		0.350	0.394	0.409	0.469	0.354	0.333	—
S32.82XB	Multiple fractures of pelvis without disruption of pelvic ring, initial encounter for open fracture	170	Hip Fracture/Dislocation		0.350	0.394	0.409	0.469	0.354	0.333	—
S32.89XA	Fracture of other parts of pelvis, initial encounter for closed fracture	170	Hip Fracture/Dislocation		0.350	0.394	0.409	0.469	0.354	0.333	—
S32.89XB	Fracture of other parts of pelvis, initial encounter for open fracture	170	Hip Fracture/Dislocation		0.350	0.394	0.409	0.469	0.354	0.333	—

ICD-10-CM Code	ICD-10-CM Code Description	V24 CMS-HCC	V24 CMS-HCC Disease Group	V24 CMS-HCC Hierarchies	Community, NonDual, Aged	Community, NonDual, Disabled	Community, FBDual, Aged	Community, FBDual, Disabled	Community, PBDual, Aged	Community, PBDual, Disabled	Institutional
S32.9XXA	Fracture of unspecified parts of lumbosacral spine and pelvis, initial encounter for closed fracture	170	Hip Fracture/Dislocation		0.350	0.394	0.409	0.469	0.354	0.333	—
S32.9XXB	Fracture of unspecified parts of lumbosacral spine and pelvis, initial encounter for open fracture	170	Hip Fracture/Dislocation		0.350	0.394	0.409	0.469	0.354	0.333	—
S34.01XA	Concussion and edema of lumbar spinal cord, initial encounter	72	Spinal Cord Disorders/Injuries	169	0.481	0.369	0.532	0.377	0.512	0.336	0.289
S34.01XD	Concussion and edema of lumbar spinal cord, subsequent encounter	72	Spinal Cord Disorders/Injuries	169	0.481	0.369	0.532	0.377	0.512	0.336	0.289
S34.01XS	Concussion and edema of lumbar spinal cord, sequela	72	Spinal Cord Disorders/Injuries	169	0.481	0.369	0.532	0.377	0.512	0.336	0.289
S34.02XA	Concussion and edema of sacral spinal cord, initial encounter	72	Spinal Cord Disorders/Injuries	169	0.481	0.369	0.532	0.377	0.512	0.336	0.289
S34.02XD	Concussion and edema of sacral spinal cord, subsequent encounter	72	Spinal Cord Disorders/Injuries	169	0.481	0.369	0.532	0.377	0.512	0.336	0.289
S34.02XS	Concussion and edema of sacral spinal cord, sequela	72	Spinal Cord Disorders/Injuries	169	0.481	0.369	0.532	0.377	0.512	0.336	0.289
S34.101A	Unspecified injury to L1 level of lumbar spinal cord, initial encounter	72	Spinal Cord Disorders/Injuries	169	0.481	0.369	0.532	0.377	0.512	0.336	0.289
S34.101D	Unspecified injury to L1 level of lumbar spinal cord, subsequent encounter	72	Spinal Cord Disorders/Injuries	169	0.481	0.369	0.532	0.377	0.512	0.336	0.289
S34.101S	Unspecified injury to L1 level of lumbar spinal cord, sequela	72	Spinal Cord Disorders/Injuries	169	0.481	0.369	0.532	0.377	0.512	0.336	0.289
S34.102A	Unspecified injury to L2 level of lumbar spinal cord, initial encounter	72	Spinal Cord Disorders/Injuries	169	0.481	0.369	0.532	0.377	0.512	0.336	0.289
S34.102D	Unspecified injury to L2 level of lumbar spinal cord, subsequent encounter	72	Spinal Cord Disorders/Injuries	169	0.481	0.369	0.532	0.377	0.512	0.336	0.289
S34.102S	Unspecified injury to L2 level of lumbar spinal cord, sequela	72	Spinal Cord Disorders/Injuries	169	0.481	0.369	0.532	0.377	0.512	0.336	0.289
S34.103A	Unspecified injury to L3 level of lumbar spinal cord, initial encounter	72	Spinal Cord Disorders/Injuries	169	0.481	0.369	0.532	0.377	0.512	0.336	0.289
S34.103D	Unspecified injury to L3 level of lumbar spinal cord, subsequent encounter	72	Spinal Cord Disorders/Injuries	169	0.481	0.369	0.532	0.377	0.512	0.336	0.289
S34.103S	Unspecified injury to L3 level of lumbar spinal cord, sequela	72	Spinal Cord Disorders/Injuries	169	0.481	0.369	0.532	0.377	0.512	0.336	0.289
S34.104A	Unspecified injury to L4 level of lumbar spinal cord, initial encounter	72	Spinal Cord Disorders/Injuries	169	0.481	0.369	0.532	0.377	0.512	0.336	0.289
S34.104D	Unspecified injury to L4 level of lumbar spinal cord, subsequent encounter	72	Spinal Cord Disorders/Injuries	169	0.481	0.369	0.532	0.377	0.512	0.336	0.289
S34.104S	Unspecified injury to L4 level of lumbar spinal cord, sequela	72	Spinal Cord Disorders/Injuries	169	0.481	0.369	0.532	0.377	0.512	0.336	0.289
S34.105A	Unspecified injury to L5 level of lumbar spinal cord, initial encounter	72	Spinal Cord Disorders/Injuries	169	0.481	0.369	0.532	0.377	0.512	0.336	0.289
S34.105D	Unspecified injury to L5 level of lumbar spinal cord, subsequent encounter	72	Spinal Cord Disorders/Injuries	169	0.481	0.369	0.532	0.377	0.512	0.336	0.289
S34.105S	Unspecified injury to L5 level of lumbar spinal cord, sequela	72	Spinal Cord Disorders/Injuries	169	0.481	0.369	0.532	0.377	0.512	0.336	0.289
S34.109A	Unspecified injury to unspecified level of lumbar spinal cord, initial encounter	72	Spinal Cord Disorders/Injuries	169	0.481	0.369	0.532	0.377	0.512	0.336	0.289
S34.109D	Unspecified injury to unspecified level of lumbar spinal cord, subsequent encounter	72	Spinal Cord Disorders/Injuries	169	0.481	0.369	0.532	0.377	0.512	0.336	0.289

ICD-10-CM Code	ICD-10-CM Code Description	V24 CMS-HCC	V24 CMS-HCC Disease Group	V24 CMS-HCC Hierarchies	Community, NonDual, Aged	Community, NonDual, Disabled	Community, FBDual, Aged	Community, FBDual, Disabled	Community, PBDual, Aged	Community, PBDual, Disabled	Institutional
S34.109S	Unspecified injury to unspecified level of lumbar spinal cord, sequela	72	Spinal Cord Disorders/Injuries	169	0.481	0.369	0.532	0.377	0.512	0.336	0.289
S34.111A	Complete lesion of L1 level of lumbar spinal cord, initial encounter	72	Spinal Cord Disorders/Injuries	169	0.481	0.369	0.532	0.377	0.512	0.336	0.289
S34.111D	Complete lesion of L1 level of lumbar spinal cord, subsequent encounter	72	Spinal Cord Disorders/Injuries	169	0.481	0.369	0.532	0.377	0.512	0.336	0.289
S34.111S	Complete lesion of L1 level of lumbar spinal cord, sequela	72	Spinal Cord Disorders/Injuries	169	0.481	0.369	0.532	0.377	0.512	0.336	0.289
S34.112A	Complete lesion of L2 level of lumbar spinal cord, initial encounter	72	Spinal Cord Disorders/Injuries	169	0.481	0.369	0.532	0.377	0.512	0.336	0.289
S34.112D	Complete lesion of L2 level of lumbar spinal cord, subsequent encounter	72	Spinal Cord Disorders/Injuries	169	0.481	0.369	0.532	0.377	0.512	0.336	0.289
S34.112S	Complete lesion of L2 level of lumbar spinal cord, sequela	72	Spinal Cord Disorders/Injuries	169	0.481	0.369	0.532	0.377	0.512	0.336	0.289
S34.113A	Complete lesion of L3 level of lumbar spinal cord, initial encounter	72	Spinal Cord Disorders/Injuries	169	0.481	0.369	0.532	0.377	0.512	0.336	0.289
S34.113D	Complete lesion of L3 level of lumbar spinal cord, subsequent encounter	72	Spinal Cord Disorders/Injuries	169	0.481	0.369	0.532	0.377	0.512	0.336	0.289
S34.113S	Complete lesion of L3 level of lumbar spinal cord, sequela	72	Spinal Cord Disorders/Injuries	169	0.481	0.369	0.532	0.377	0.512	0.336	0.289
S34.114A	Complete lesion of L4 level of lumbar spinal cord, initial encounter	72	Spinal Cord Disorders/Injuries	169	0.481	0.369	0.532	0.377	0.512	0.336	0.289
S34.114D	Complete lesion of L4 level of lumbar spinal cord, subsequent encounter	72	Spinal Cord Disorders/Injuries	169	0.481	0.369	0.532	0.377	0.512	0.336	0.289
S34.114S	Complete lesion of L4 level of lumbar spinal cord, sequela	72	Spinal Cord Disorders/Injuries	169	0.481	0.369	0.532	0.377	0.512	0.336	0.289
S34.115A	Complete lesion of L5 level of lumbar spinal cord, initial encounter	72	Spinal Cord Disorders/Injuries	169	0.481	0.369	0.532	0.377	0.512	0.336	0.289
S34.115D	Complete lesion of L5 level of lumbar spinal cord, subsequent encounter	72	Spinal Cord Disorders/Injuries	169	0.481	0.369	0.532	0.377	0.512	0.336	0.289
S34.115S	Complete lesion of L5 level of lumbar spinal cord, sequela	72	Spinal Cord Disorders/Injuries	169	0.481	0.369	0.532	0.377	0.512	0.336	0.289
S34.119A	Complete lesion of unspecified level of lumbar spinal cord, initial encounter	72	Spinal Cord Disorders/Injuries	169	0.481	0.369	0.532	0.377	0.512	0.336	0.289
S34.119D	Complete lesion of unspecified level of lumbar spinal cord, subsequent encounter	72	Spinal Cord Disorders/Injuries	169	0.481	0.369	0.532	0.377	0.512	0.336	0.289
S34.119S	Complete lesion of unspecified level of lumbar spinal cord, sequela	72	Spinal Cord Disorders/Injuries	169	0.481	0.369	0.532	0.377	0.512	0.336	0.289
S34.121A	Incomplete lesion of L1 level of lumbar spinal cord, initial encounter	72	Spinal Cord Disorders/Injuries	169	0.481	0.369	0.532	0.377	0.512	0.336	0.289
S34.121D	Incomplete lesion of L1 level of lumbar spinal cord, subsequent encounter	72	Spinal Cord Disorders/Injuries	169	0.481	0.369	0.532	0.377	0.512	0.336	0.289
S34.121S	Incomplete lesion of L1 level of lumbar spinal cord, sequela	72	Spinal Cord Disorders/Injuries	169	0.481	0.369	0.532	0.377	0.512	0.336	0.289
S34.122A	Incomplete lesion of L2 level of lumbar spinal cord, initial encounter	72	Spinal Cord Disorders/Injuries	169	0.481	0.369	0.532	0.377	0.512	0.336	0.289
S34.122D	Incomplete lesion of L2 level of lumbar spinal cord, subsequent encounter	72	Spinal Cord Disorders/Injuries	169	0.481	0.369	0.532	0.377	0.512	0.336	0.289
S34.122S	Incomplete lesion of L2 level of lumbar spinal cord, sequela	72	Spinal Cord Disorders/Injuries	169	0.481	0.369	0.532	0.377	0.512	0.336	0.289
S34.123A	Incomplete lesion of L3 level of lumbar spinal cord, initial encounter	72	Spinal Cord Disorders/Injuries	169	0.481	0.369	0.532	0.377	0.512	0.336	0.289
S34.123D	Incomplete lesion of L3 level of lumbar spinal cord, subsequent encounter	72	Spinal Cord Disorders/Injuries	169	0.481	0.369	0.532	0.377	0.512	0.336	0.289

ICD-10-CM Code	ICD-10-CM Code Description	V24 CMS-HCC	V24 CMS-HCC Disease Group	V24 CMS-HCC Hierarchies	Community, NonDual, Aged	Community, NonDual, Disabled	Community, FBDual, Aged	Community, FBDual, Disabled	Community, PBDual, Aged	Community, PBDual, Disabled	Institutional
S34.123S	Incomplete lesion of L3 level of lumbar spinal cord, sequela	72	Spinal Cord Disorders/Injuries	169	0.481	0.369	0.532	0.377	0.512	0.336	0.289
S34.124A	Incomplete lesion of L4 level of lumbar spinal cord, initial encounter	72	Spinal Cord Disorders/Injuries	169	0.481	0.369	0.532	0.377	0.512	0.336	0.289
S34.124D	Incomplete lesion of L4 level of lumbar spinal cord, subsequent encounter	72	Spinal Cord Disorders/Injuries	169	0.481	0.369	0.532	0.377	0.512	0.336	0.289
S34.124S	Incomplete lesion of L4 level of lumbar spinal cord, sequela	72	Spinal Cord Disorders/Injuries	169	0.481	0.369	0.532	0.377	0.512	0.336	0.289
S34.125A	Incomplete lesion of L5 level of lumbar spinal cord, initial encounter	72	Spinal Cord Disorders/Injuries	169	0.481	0.369	0.532	0.377	0.512	0.336	0.289
S34.125D	Incomplete lesion of L5 level of lumbar spinal cord, subsequent encounter	72	Spinal Cord Disorders/Injuries	169	0.481	0.369	0.532	0.377	0.512	0.336	0.289
S34.125S	Incomplete lesion of L5 level of lumbar spinal cord, sequela	72	Spinal Cord Disorders/Injuries	169	0.481	0.369	0.532	0.377	0.512	0.336	0.289
S34.129A	Incomplete lesion of unspecified level of lumbar spinal cord, initial encounter	72	Spinal Cord Disorders/Injuries	169	0.481	0.369	0.532	0.377	0.512	0.336	0.289
S34.129D	Incomplete lesion of unspecified level of lumbar spinal cord, subsequent encounter	72	Spinal Cord Disorders/Injuries	169	0.481	0.369	0.532	0.377	0.512	0.336	0.289
S34.129S	Incomplete lesion of unspecified level of lumbar spinal cord, sequela	72	Spinal Cord Disorders/Injuries	169	0.481	0.369	0.532	0.377	0.512	0.336	0.289
S34.131A	Complete lesion of sacral spinal cord, initial encounter	72	Spinal Cord Disorders/Injuries	169	0.481	0.369	0.532	0.377	0.512	0.336	0.289
S34.131D	Complete lesion of sacral spinal cord, subsequent encounter	72	Spinal Cord Disorders/Injuries	169	0.481	0.369	0.532	0.377	0.512	0.336	0.289
S34.131S	Complete lesion of sacral spinal cord, sequela	72	Spinal Cord Disorders/Injuries	169	0.481	0.369	0.532	0.377	0.512	0.336	0.289
S34.132A	Incomplete lesion of sacral spinal cord, initial encounter	72	Spinal Cord Disorders/Injuries	169	0.481	0.369	0.532	0.377	0.512	0.336	0.289
S34.132D	Incomplete lesion of sacral spinal cord, subsequent encounter	72	Spinal Cord Disorders/Injuries	169	0.481	0.369	0.532	0.377	0.512	0.336	0.289
S34.132S	Incomplete lesion of sacral spinal cord, sequela	72	Spinal Cord Disorders/Injuries	169	0.481	0.369	0.532	0.377	0.512	0.336	0.289
S34.139A	Unspecified injury to sacral spinal cord, initial encounter	72	Spinal Cord Disorders/Injuries	169	0.481	0.369	0.532	0.377	0.512	0.336	0.289
S34.139D	Unspecified injury to sacral spinal cord, subsequent encounter	72	Spinal Cord Disorders/Injuries	169	0.481	0.369	0.532	0.377	0.512	0.336	0.289
S34.139S	Unspecified injury to sacral spinal cord, sequela	72	Spinal Cord Disorders/Injuries	169	0.481	0.369	0.532	0.377	0.512	0.336	0.289
S34.3XXA	Injury of cauda equina, initial encounter	72	Spinal Cord Disorders/Injuries	169	0.481	0.369	0.532	0.377	0.512	0.336	0.289
S48.011A	Complete traumatic amputation at right shoulder joint, initial encounter	173	Traumatic Amputations and Complications		0.208	0.172	0.221	0.525	0.176	0.180	0.092
S48.011S	Complete traumatic amputation at right shoulder joint, sequela	189	Amputation Status, Lower Limb/ Amputation Complications		0.519	0.437	0.795	0.934	0.697	0.626	0.357
S48.012A	Complete traumatic amputation at left shoulder joint, initial encounter	173	Traumatic Amputations and Complications		0.208	0.172	0.221	0.525	0.176	0.180	0.092
S48.012S	Complete traumatic amputation at left shoulder joint, sequela	189	Amputation Status, Lower Limb/ Amputation Complications		0.519	0.437	0.795	0.934	0.697	0.626	0.357
S48.019A	Complete traumatic amputation at unspecified shoulder joint, initial encounter	173	Traumatic Amputations and Complications		0.208	0.172	0.221	0.525	0.176	0.180	0.092
S48.019S	Complete traumatic amputation at unspecified shoulder joint, sequela	189	Amputation Status, Lower Limb/ Amputation Complications		0.519	0.437	0.795	0.934	0.697	0.626	0.357
S48.021A	Partial traumatic amputation at right shoulder joint, initial encounter	173	Traumatic Amputations and Complications		0.208	0.172	0.221	0.525	0.176	0.180	0.092

ICD-10-CM Code	ICD-10-CM Code Description	V24 CMS-HCC	V24 CMS-HCC Disease Group	V24 CMS-HCC Hierarchies	Community, NonDual, Aged	Community, NonDual, Disabled	Community, FBDual, Aged	Community, FBDual, Disabled	Community, PBDual, Aged	Community, PBDual, Disabled	Institutional
S48.021S	Partial traumatic amputation at right shoulder joint, sequela	189	Amputation Status, Lower Limb/ Amputation Complications		0.519	0.437	0.795	0.934	0.697	0.626	0.357
S48.022A	Partial traumatic amputation at left shoulder joint, initial encounter	173	Traumatic Amputations and Complications		0.208	0.172	0.221	0.525	0.176	0.180	0.092
S48.022S	Partial traumatic amputation at left shoulder joint, sequela	189	Amputation Status, Lower Limb/ Amputation Complications		0.519	0.437	0.795	0.934	0.697	0.626	0.357
S48.029A	Partial traumatic amputation at unspecified shoulder joint, initial encounter	173	Traumatic Amputations and Complications		0.208	0.172	0.221	0.525	0.176	0.180	0.092
S48.029S	Partial traumatic amputation at unspecified shoulder joint, sequela	189	Amputation Status, Lower Limb/ Amputation Complications		0.519	0.437	0.795	0.934	0.697	0.626	0.357
S48.111A	Complete traumatic amputation at level between right shoulder and elbow, initial encounter	173	Traumatic Amputations and Complications		0.208	0.172	0.221	0.525	0.176	0.180	0.092
S48.111S	Complete traumatic amputation at level between right shoulder and elbow, sequela	189	Amputation Status, Lower Limb/ Amputation Complications		0.519	0.437	0.795	0.934	0.697	0.626	0.357
S48.112A	Complete traumatic amputation at level between left shoulder and elbow, initial encounter	173	Traumatic Amputations and Complications		0.208	0.172	0.221	0.525	0.176	0.180	0.092
S48.112S	Complete traumatic amputation at level between left shoulder and elbow, sequela	189	Amputation Status, Lower Limb/ Amputation Complications		0.519	0.437	0.795	0.934	0.697	0.626	0.357
S48.119A	Complete traumatic amputation at level between unspecified shoulder and elbow, initial encounter	173	Traumatic Amputations and Complications		0.208	0.172	0.221	0.525	0.176	0.180	0.092
S48.119S	Complete traumatic amputation at level between unspecified shoulder and elbow, sequela	189	Amputation Status, Lower Limb/ Amputation Complications		0.519	0.437	0.795	0.934	0.697	0.626	0.357
S48.121A	Partial traumatic amputation at level between right shoulder and elbow, initial encounter	173	Traumatic Amputations and Complications		0.208	0.172	0.221	0.525	0.176	0.180	0.092
S48.121S	Partial traumatic amputation at level between right shoulder and elbow, sequela	189	Amputation Status, Lower Limb/ Amputation Complications		0.519	0.437	0.795	0.934	0.697	0.626	0.357
S48.122A	Partial traumatic amputation at level between left shoulder and elbow, initial encounter	173	Traumatic Amputations and Complications		0.208	0.172	0.221	0.525	0.176	0.180	0.092
S48.122S	Partial traumatic amputation at level between left shoulder and elbow, sequela	189	Amputation Status, Lower Limb/ Amputation Complications		0.519	0.437	0.795	0.934	0.697	0.626	0.357
S48.129A	Partial traumatic amputation at level between unspecified shoulder and elbow, initial encounter	173	Traumatic Amputations and Complications		0.208	0.172	0.221	0.525	0.176	0.180	0.092
S48.129S	Partial traumatic amputation at level between unspecified shoulder and elbow, sequela	189	Amputation Status, Lower Limb/ Amputation Complications		0.519	0.437	0.795	0.934	0.697	0.626	0.357
S48.911A	Complete traumatic amputation of right shoulder and upper arm, level unspecified, initial encounter	173	Traumatic Amputations and Complications		0.208	0.172	0.221	0.525	0.176	0.180	0.092
S48.911S	Complete traumatic amputation of right shoulder and upper arm, level unspecified, sequela	189	Amputation Status, Lower Limb/ Amputation Complications		0.519	0.437	0.795	0.934	0.697	0.626	0.357
S48.912A	Complete traumatic amputation of left shoulder and upper arm, level unspecified, initial encounter	173	Traumatic Amputations and Complications		0.208	0.172	0.221	0.525	0.176	0.180	0.092
S48.912S	Complete traumatic amputation of left shoulder and upper arm, level unspecified, sequela	189	Amputation Status, Lower Limb/ Amputation Complications		0.519	0.437	0.795	0.934	0.697	0.626	0.357

ICD-10-CM Code	ICD-10-CM Code Description	V24 CMS-HCC	V24 CMS-HCC Disease Group	V24 CMS-HCC Hierarchies	Community, NonDual, Aged	Community, NonDual, Disabled	Community, FBDual, Aged	Community, FBDual, Disabled	Community, PBDual, Aged	Community, PBDual, Disabled	Institutional
S48.919A	Complete traumatic amputation of unspecified shoulder and upper arm, level unspecified, initial encounter	173	Traumatic Amputations and Complications		0.208	0.172	0.221	0.525	0.176	0.180	0.092
S48.919S	Complete traumatic amputation of unspecified shoulder and upper arm, level unspecified, sequela	189	Amputation Status, Lower Limb/ Amputation Complications		0.519	0.437	0.795	0.934	0.697	0.626	0.357
S48.921A	Partial traumatic amputation of right shoulder and upper arm, level unspecified, initial encounter	173	Traumatic Amputations and Complications		0.208	0.172	0.221	0.525	0.176	0.180	0.092
S48.921S	Partial traumatic amputation of right shoulder and upper arm, level unspecified, sequela	189	Amputation Status, Lower Limb/ Amputation Complications		0.519	0.437	0.795	0.934	0.697	0.626	0.357
S48.922A	Partial traumatic amputation of left shoulder and upper arm, level unspecified, initial encounter	173	Traumatic Amputations and Complications		0.208	0.172	0.221	0.525	0.176	0.180	0.092
S48.922S	Partial traumatic amputation of left shoulder and upper arm, level unspecified, sequela	189	Amputation Status, Lower Limb/ Amputation Complications		0.519	0.437	0.795	0.934	0.697	0.626	0.357
S48.929A	Partial traumatic amputation of unspecified shoulder and upper arm, level unspecified, initial encounter	173	Traumatic Amputations and Complications		0.208	0.172	0.221	0.525	0.176	0.180	0.092
S48.929S	Partial traumatic amputation of unspecified shoulder and upper arm, level unspecified, sequela	189	Amputation Status, Lower Limb/ Amputation Complications		0.519	0.437	0.795	0.934	0.697	0.626	0.357
S58.011A	Complete traumatic amputation at elbow level, right arm, initial encounter	173	Traumatic Amputations and Complications		0.208	0.172	0.221	0.525	0.176	0.180	0.092
S58.011S	Complete traumatic amputation at elbow level, right arm, sequela	189	Amputation Status, Lower Limb/ Amputation Complications		0.519	0.437	0.795	0.934	0.697	0.626	0.357
S58.012A	Complete traumatic amputation at elbow level, left arm, initial encounter	173	Traumatic Amputations and Complications		0.208	0.172	0.221	0.525	0.176	0.180	0.092
S58.012S	Complete traumatic amputation at elbow level, left arm, sequela	189	Amputation Status, Lower Limb/ Amputation Complications		0.519	0.437	0.795	0.934	0.697	0.626	0.357
S58.019A	Complete traumatic amputation at elbow level, unspecified arm, initial encounter	173	Traumatic Amputations and Complications		0.208	0.172	0.221	0.525	0.176	0.180	0.092
S58.019S	Complete traumatic amputation at elbow level, unspecified arm, sequela	189	Amputation Status, Lower Limb/ Amputation Complications		0.519	0.437	0.795	0.934	0.697	0.626	0.357
S58.021A	Partial traumatic amputation at elbow level, right arm, initial encounter	173	Traumatic Amputations and Complications		0.208	0.172	0.221	0.525	0.176	0.180	0.092
S58.021S	Partial traumatic amputation at elbow level, right arm, sequela	189	Amputation Status, Lower Limb/ Amputation Complications		0.519	0.437	0.795	0.934	0.697	0.626	0.357
S58.022A	Partial traumatic amputation at elbow level, left arm, initial encounter	173	Traumatic Amputations and Complications		0.208	0.172	0.221	0.525	0.176	0.180	0.092
S58.022S	Partial traumatic amputation at elbow level, left arm, sequela	189	Amputation Status, Lower Limb/ Amputation Complications		0.519	0.437	0.795	0.934	0.697	0.626	0.357
S58.029A	Partial traumatic amputation at elbow level, unspecified arm, initial encounter	173	Traumatic Amputations and Complications		0.208	0.172	0.221	0.525	0.176	0.180	0.092
S58.029S	Partial traumatic amputation at elbow level, unspecified arm, sequela	189	Amputation Status, Lower Limb/ Amputation Complications		0.519	0.437	0.795	0.934	0.697	0.626	0.357
S58.111A	Complete traumatic amputation at level between elbow and wrist, right arm, initial encounter	173	Traumatic Amputations and Complications		0.208	0.172	0.221	0.525	0.176	0.180	0.092
S58.111S	Complete traumatic amputation at level between elbow and wrist, right arm, sequela	189	Amputation Status, Lower Limb/ Amputation Complications		0.519	0.437	0.795	0.934	0.697	0.626	0.357
S58.112A	Complete traumatic amputation at level between elbow and wrist, left arm, initial encounter	173	Traumatic Amputations and Complications		0.208	0.172	0.221	0.525	0.176	0.180	0.092

ICD-10-CM Code	ICD-10-CM Code Description	V24 CMS-HCC	V24 CMS-HCC Disease Group	V24 CMS-HCC Hierarchies	Community, NonDual, Aged	Community, NonDual, Disabled	Community, FBDual, Aged	Community, FBDual, Disabled	Community, PBDual, Aged	Community, PBDual, Disabled	Institutional
S58.112S	Complete traumatic amputation at level between elbow and wrist, left arm, sequela	189	Amputation Status, Lower Limb/ Amputation Complications		0.519	0.437	0.795	0.934	0.697	0.626	0.357
S58.119A	Complete traumatic amputation at level between elbow and wrist, unspecified arm, initial encounter	173	Traumatic Amputations and Complications		0.208	0.172	0.221	0.525	0.176	0.180	0.092
S58.119S	Complete traumatic amputation at level between elbow and wrist, unspecified arm, sequela	189	Amputation Status, Lower Limb/ Amputation Complications		0.519	0.437	0.795	0.934	0.697	0.626	0.357
S58.121A	Partial traumatic amputation at level between elbow and wrist, right arm, initial encounter	173	Traumatic Amputations and Complications		0.208	0.172	0.221	0.525	0.176	0.180	0.092
S58.121S	Partial traumatic amputation at level between elbow and wrist, right arm, sequela	189	Amputation Status, Lower Limb/ Amputation Complications		0.519	0.437	0.795	0.934	0.697	0.626	0.357
S58.122A	Partial traumatic amputation at level between elbow and wrist, left arm, initial encounter	173	Traumatic Amputations and Complications		0.208	0.172	0.221	0.525	0.176	0.180	0.092
S58.122S	Partial traumatic amputation at level between elbow and wrist, left arm, sequela	189	Amputation Status, Lower Limb/ Amputation Complications		0.519	0.437	0.795	0.934	0.697	0.626	0.357
S58.129A	Partial traumatic amputation at level between elbow and wrist, unspecified arm, initial encounter	173	Traumatic Amputations and Complications		0.208	0.172	0.221	0.525	0.176	0.180	0.092
S58.129S	Partial traumatic amputation at level between elbow and wrist, unspecified arm, sequela	189	Amputation Status, Lower Limb/ Amputation Complications		0.519	0.437	0.795	0.934	0.697	0.626	0.357
S58.911A	Complete traumatic amputation of right forearm, level unspecified, initial encounter	173	Traumatic Amputations and Complications		0.208	0.172	0.221	0.525	0.176	0.180	0.092
S58.911S	Complete traumatic amputation of right forearm, level unspecified, sequela	189	Amputation Status, Lower Limb/ Amputation Complications		0.519	0.437	0.795	0.934	0.697	0.626	0.357
S58.912A	Complete traumatic amputation of left forearm, level unspecified, initial encounter	173	Traumatic Amputations and Complications		0.208	0.172	0.221	0.525	0.176	0.180	0.092
S58.912S	Complete traumatic amputation of left forearm, level unspecified, sequela	189	Amputation Status, Lower Limb/ Amputation Complications		0.519	0.437	0.795	0.934	0.697	0.626	0.357
S58.919A	Complete traumatic amputation of unspecified forearm, level unspecified, initial encounter	173	Traumatic Amputations and Complications		0.208	0.172	0.221	0.525	0.176	0.180	0.092
S58.919S	Complete traumatic amputation of unspecified forearm, level unspecified, sequela	189	Amputation Status, Lower Limb/ Amputation Complications		0.519	0.437	0.795	0.934	0.697	0.626	0.357
S58.921A	Partial traumatic amputation of right forearm, level unspecified, initial encounter	173	Traumatic Amputations and Complications		0.208	0.172	0.221	0.525	0.176	0.180	0.092
S58.921S	Partial traumatic amputation of right forearm, level unspecified, sequela	189	Amputation Status, Lower Limb/ Amputation Complications		0.519	0.437	0.795	0.934	0.697	0.626	0.357
S58.922A	Partial traumatic amputation of left forearm, level unspecified, initial encounter	173	Traumatic Amputations and Complications		0.208	0.172	0.221	0.525	0.176	0.180	0.092
S58.922S	Partial traumatic amputation of left forearm, level unspecified, sequela	189	Amputation Status, Lower Limb/ Amputation Complications		0.519	0.437	0.795	0.934	0.697	0.626	0.357
S58.929A	Partial traumatic amputation of unspecified forearm, level unspecified, initial encounter	173	Traumatic Amputations and Complications		0.208	0.172	0.221	0.525	0.176	0.180	0.092
S58.929S	Partial traumatic amputation of unspecified forearm, level unspecified, sequela	189	Amputation Status, Lower Limb/ Amputation Complications		0.519	0.437	0.795	0.934	0.697	0.626	0.357

ICD-10-CM Code	ICD-10-CM Code Description	V24 CMS-HCC	V24 CMS-HCC Disease Group	V24 CMS-HCC Hierarchies	Community, NonDual, Aged	Community, NonDual, Disabled	Community, FBDual, Aged	Community, FBDual, Disabled	Community, PBDual, Aged	Community, PBDual, Disabled	Institutional
S68.011S	Complete traumatic metacarpophalangeal amputation of right thumb, sequela	189	Amputation Status, Lower Limb/ Amputation Complications		0.519	0.437	0.795	0.934	0.697	0.626	0.357
S68.012S	Complete traumatic metacarpophalangeal amputation of left thumb, sequela	189	Amputation Status, Lower Limb/ Amputation Complications		0.519	0.437	0.795	0.934	0.697	0.626	0.357
S68.019S	Complete traumatic metacarpophalangeal amputation of unspecified thumb, sequela	189	Amputation Status, Lower Limb/ Amputation Complications		0.519	0.437	0.795	0.934	0.697	0.626	0.357
S68.021S	Partial traumatic metacarpophalangeal amputation of right thumb, sequela	189	Amputation Status, Lower Limb/ Amputation Complications		0.519	0.437	0.795	0.934	0.697	0.626	0.357
S68.022S	Partial traumatic metacarpophalangeal amputation of left thumb, sequela	189	Amputation Status, Lower Limb/ Amputation Complications		0.519	0.437	0.795	0.934	0.697	0.626	0.357
S68.029S	Partial traumatic metacarpophalangeal amputation of unspecified thumb, sequela	189	Amputation Status, Lower Limb/ Amputation Complications		0.519	0.437	0.795	0.934	0.697	0.626	0.357
S68.110S	Complete traumatic metacarpophalangeal amputation of right index finger, sequela	189	Amputation Status, Lower Limb/ Amputation Complications		0.519	0.437	0.795	0.934	0.697	0.626	0.357
S68.111S	Complete traumatic metacarpophalangeal amputation of left index finger, sequela	189	Amputation Status, Lower Limb/ Amputation Complications		0.519	0.437	0.795	0.934	0.697	0.626	0.357
S68.112S	Complete traumatic metacarpophalangeal amputation of right middle finger, sequela	189	Amputation Status, Lower Limb/ Amputation Complications		0.519	0.437	0.795	0.934	0.697	0.626	0.357
S68.113S	Complete traumatic metacarpophalangeal amputation of left middle finger, sequela	189	Amputation Status, Lower Limb/ Amputation Complications		0.519	0.437	0.795	0.934	0.697	0.626	0.357
S68.114S	Complete traumatic metacarpophalangeal amputation of right ring finger, sequela	189	Amputation Status, Lower Limb/ Amputation Complications		0.519	0.437	0.795	0.934	0.697	0.626	0.357
S68.115S	Complete traumatic metacarpophalangeal amputation of left ring finger, sequela	189	Amputation Status, Lower Limb/ Amputation Complications		0.519	0.437	0.795	0.934	0.697	0.626	0.357
S68.116S	Complete traumatic metacarpophalangeal amputation of right little finger, sequela	189	Amputation Status, Lower Limb/ Amputation Complications		0.519	0.437	0.795	0.934	0.697	0.626	0.357
S68.117S	Complete traumatic metacarpophalangeal amputation of left little finger, sequela	189	Amputation Status, Lower Limb/ Amputation Complications		0.519	0.437	0.795	0.934	0.697	0.626	0.357
S68.118S	Complete traumatic metacarpophalangeal amputation of other finger, sequela	189	Amputation Status, Lower Limb/ Amputation Complications		0.519	0.437	0.795	0.934	0.697	0.626	0.357
S68.119S	Complete traumatic metacarpophalangeal amputation of unspecified finger, sequela	189	Amputation Status, Lower Limb/ Amputation Complications		0.519	0.437	0.795	0.934	0.697	0.626	0.357
S68.120S	Partial traumatic metacarpophalangeal amputation of right index finger, sequela	189	Amputation Status, Lower Limb/ Amputation Complications		0.519	0.437	0.795	0.934	0.697	0.626	0.357
S68.121S	Partial traumatic metacarpophalangeal amputation of left index finger, sequela	189	Amputation Status, Lower Limb/ Amputation Complications		0.519	0.437	0.795	0.934	0.697	0.626	0.357
S68.122S	Partial traumatic metacarpophalangeal amputation of right middle finger, sequela	189	Amputation Status, Lower Limb/ Amputation Complications		0.519	0.437	0.795	0.934	0.697	0.626	0.357
S68.123S	Partial traumatic metacarpophalangeal amputation of left middle finger, sequela	189	Amputation Status, Lower Limb/ Amputation Complications		0.519	0.437	0.795	0.934	0.697	0.626	0.357

ICD-10-CM Code	ICD-10-CM Code Description	V24 CMS-HCC	V24 CMS-HCC Disease Group	V24 CMS-HCC Hierarchies	Community, NonDual, Aged	Community, NonDual, Disabled	Community, FBDual, Aged	Community, FBDual, Disabled	Community, PBDual, Aged	Community, PBDual, Disabled	Institutional
S68.124S	Partial traumatic metacarpophalangeal amputation of right ring finger, sequela	189	Amputation Status, Lower Limb/ Amputation Complications		0.519	0.437	0.795	0.934	0.697	0.626	0.357
S68.125S	Partial traumatic metacarpophalangeal amputation of left ring finger, sequela	189	Amputation Status, Lower Limb/ Amputation Complications		0.519	0.437	0.795	0.934	0.697	0.626	0.357
S68.126S	Partial traumatic metacarpophalangeal amputation of right little finger, sequela	189	Amputation Status, Lower Limb/ Amputation Complications		0.519	0.437	0.795	0.934	0.697	0.626	0.357
S68.127S	Partial traumatic metacarpophalangeal amputation of left little finger, sequela	189	Amputation Status, Lower Limb/ Amputation Complications		0.519	0.437	0.795	0.934	0.697	0.626	0.357
S68.128S	Partial traumatic metacarpophalangeal amputation of other finger, sequela	189	Amputation Status, Lower Limb/ Amputation Complications		0.519	0.437	0.795	0.934	0.697	0.626	0.357
S68.129S	Partial traumatic metacarpophalangeal amputation of unspecified finger, sequela	189	Amputation Status, Lower Limb/ Amputation Complications		0.519	0.437	0.795	0.934	0.697	0.626	0.357
S68.411A	Complete traumatic amputation of right hand at wrist level, initial encounter	173	Traumatic Amputations and Complications		0.208	0.172	0.221	0.525	0.176	0.180	0.092
S68.411S	Complete traumatic amputation of right hand at wrist level, sequela	189	Amputation Status, Lower Limb/ Amputation Complications		0.519	0.437	0.795	0.934	0.697	0.626	0.357
S68.412A	Complete traumatic amputation of left hand at wrist level, initial encounter	173	Traumatic Amputations and Complications		0.208	0.172	0.221	0.525	0.176	0.180	0.092
S68.412S	Complete traumatic amputation of left hand at wrist level, sequela	189	Amputation Status, Lower Limb/ Amputation Complications		0.519	0.437	0.795	0.934	0.697	0.626	0.357
S68.419A	Complete traumatic amputation of unspecified hand at wrist level, initial encounter	173	Traumatic Amputations and Complications		0.208	0.172	0.221	0.525	0.176	0.180	0.092
S68.419S	Complete traumatic amputation of unspecified hand at wrist level, sequela	189	Amputation Status, Lower Limb/ Amputation Complications		0.519	0.437	0.795	0.934	0.697	0.626	0.357
S68.421A	Partial traumatic amputation of right hand at wrist level, initial encounter	173	Traumatic Amputations and Complications		0.208	0.172	0.221	0.525	0.176	0.180	0.092
S68.421S	Partial traumatic amputation of right hand at wrist level, sequela	189	Amputation Status, Lower Limb/ Amputation Complications		0.519	0.437	0.795	0.934	0.697	0.626	0.357
S68.422A	Partial traumatic amputation of left hand at wrist level, initial encounter	173	Traumatic Amputations and Complications		0.208	0.172	0.221	0.525	0.176	0.180	0.092
S68.422S	Partial traumatic amputation of left hand at wrist level, sequela	189	Amputation Status, Lower Limb/ Amputation Complications		0.519	0.437	0.795	0.934	0.697	0.626	0.357
S68.429A	Partial traumatic amputation of unspecified hand at wrist level, initial encounter	173	Traumatic Amputations and Complications		0.208	0.172	0.221	0.525	0.176	0.180	0.092
S68.429S	Partial traumatic amputation of unspecified hand at wrist level, sequela	189	Amputation Status, Lower Limb/ Amputation Complications		0.519	0.437	0.795	0.934	0.697	0.626	0.357
S68.511S	Complete traumatic transphalangeal amputation of right thumb, sequela	189	Amputation Status, Lower Limb/ Amputation Complications		0.519	0.437	0.795	0.934	0.697	0.626	0.357
S68.512S	Complete traumatic transphalangeal amputation of left thumb, sequela	189	Amputation Status, Lower Limb/ Amputation Complications		0.519	0.437	0.795	0.934	0.697	0.626	0.357
S68.519S	Complete traumatic transphalangeal amputation of unspecified thumb, sequela	189	Amputation Status, Lower Limb/ Amputation Complications		0.519	0.437	0.795	0.934	0.697	0.626	0.357
S68.521S	Partial traumatic transphalangeal amputation of right thumb, sequela	189	Amputation Status, Lower Limb/ Amputation Complications		0.519	0.437	0.795	0.934	0.697	0.626	0.357
S68.522S	Partial traumatic transphalangeal amputation of left thumb, sequela	189	Amputation Status, Lower Limb/ Amputation Complications		0.519	0.437	0.795	0.934	0.697	0.626	0.357

ICD-10-CM Code	ICD-10-CM Code Description	V24 CMS-HCC	V24 CMS-HCC Disease Group	V24 CMS-HCC Hierarchies	Community, NonDual, Aged	Community, NonDual, Disabled	Community, FBDual, Aged	Community, FBDual, Disabled	Community, PBDual, Aged	Community, PBDual, Disabled	Institutional
S68.529S	Partial traumatic transphalangeal amputation of unspecified thumb, sequela	189	Amputation Status, Lower Limb/ Amputation Complications		0.519	0.437	0.795	0.934	0.697	0.626	0.357
S68.610S	Complete traumatic transphalangeal amputation of right index finger, sequela	189	Amputation Status, Lower Limb/ Amputation Complications		0.519	0.437	0.795	0.934	0.697	0.626	0.357
S68.611S	Complete traumatic transphalangeal amputation of left index finger, sequela	189	Amputation Status, Lower Limb/ Amputation Complications		0.519	0.437	0.795	0.934	0.697	0.626	0.357
S68.612S	Complete traumatic transphalangeal amputation of right middle finger, sequela	189	Amputation Status, Lower Limb/ Amputation Complications		0.519	0.437	0.795	0.934	0.697	0.626	0.357
S68.613S	Complete traumatic transphalangeal amputation of left middle finger, sequela	189	Amputation Status, Lower Limb/ Amputation Complications		0.519	0.437	0.795	0.934	0.697	0.626	0.357
S68.614S	Complete traumatic transphalangeal amputation of right ring finger, sequela	189	Amputation Status, Lower Limb/ Amputation Complications		0.519	0.437	0.795	0.934	0.697	0.626	0.357
S68.615S	Complete traumatic transphalangeal amputation of left ring finger, sequela	189	Amputation Status, Lower Limb/ Amputation Complications		0.519	0.437	0.795	0.934	0.697	0.626	0.357
S68.616S	Complete traumatic transphalangeal amputation of right little finger, sequela	189	Amputation Status, Lower Limb/ Amputation Complications		0.519	0.437	0.795	0.934	0.697	0.626	0.357
S68.617S	Complete traumatic transphalangeal amputation of left little finger, sequela	189	Amputation Status, Lower Limb/ Amputation Complications		0.519	0.437	0.795	0.934	0.697	0.626	0.357
S68.618S	Complete traumatic transphalangeal amputation of other finger, sequela	189	Amputation Status, Lower Limb/ Amputation Complications		0.519	0.437	0.795	0.934	0.697	0.626	0.357
S68.619S	Complete traumatic transphalangeal amputation of unspecified finger, sequela	189	Amputation Status, Lower Limb/ Amputation Complications		0.519	0.437	0.795	0.934	0.697	0.626	0.357
S68.620S	Partial traumatic transphalangeal amputation of right index finger, sequela	189	Amputation Status, Lower Limb/ Amputation Complications		0.519	0.437	0.795	0.934	0.697	0.626	0.357
S68.621S	Partial traumatic transphalangeal amputation of left index finger, sequela	189	Amputation Status, Lower Limb/ Amputation Complications		0.519	0.437	0.795	0.934	0.697	0.626	0.357
S68.622S	Partial traumatic transphalangeal amputation of right middle finger, sequela	189	Amputation Status, Lower Limb/ Amputation Complications		0.519	0.437	0.795	0.934	0.697	0.626	0.357
S68.623S	Partial traumatic transphalangeal amputation of left middle finger, sequela	189	Amputation Status, Lower Limb/ Amputation Complications		0.519	0.437	0.795	0.934	0.697	0.626	0.357
S68.624S	Partial traumatic transphalangeal amputation of right ring finger, sequela	189	Amputation Status, Lower Limb/ Amputation Complications		0.519	0.437	0.795	0.934	0.697	0.626	0.357
S68.625S	Partial traumatic transphalangeal amputation of left ring finger, sequela	189	Amputation Status, Lower Limb/ Amputation Complications		0.519	0.437	0.795	0.934	0.697	0.626	0.357
S68.626S	Partial traumatic transphalangeal amputation of right little finger, sequela	189	Amputation Status, Lower Limb/ Amputation Complications		0.519	0.437	0.795	0.934	0.697	0.626	0.357
S68.627S	Partial traumatic transphalangeal amputation of left little finger, sequela	189	Amputation Status, Lower Limb/ Amputation Complications		0.519	0.437	0.795	0.934	0.697	0.626	0.357
S68.628S	Partial traumatic transphalangeal amputation of other finger, sequela	189	Amputation Status, Lower Limb/ Amputation Complications		0.519	0.437	0.795	0.934	0.697	0.626	0.357
S68.629S	Partial traumatic transphalangeal amputation of unspecified finger, sequela	189	Amputation Status, Lower Limb/ Amputation Complications		0.519	0.437	0.795	0.934	0.697	0.626	0.357

ICD-10-CM Code	ICD-10-CM Code Description	V24 CMS-HCC	V24 CMS-HCC Disease Group	V24 CMS-HCC Hierarchies	Community, NonDual, Aged	Community, NonDual, Disabled	Community, FBDual, Aged	Community, FBDual, Disabled	Community, PBDual, Aged	Community, PBDual, Disabled	Institutional
S68.711A	Complete traumatic transmetacarpal amputation of right hand, initial encounter	173	Traumatic Amputations and Complications		0.208	0.172	0.221	0.525	0.176	0.180	0.092
S68.711S	Complete traumatic transmetacarpal amputation of right hand, sequela	189	Amputation Status, Lower Limb/ Amputation Complications		0.519	0.437	0.795	0.934	0.697	0.626	0.357
S68.712A	Complete traumatic transmetacarpal amputation of left hand, initial encounter	173	Traumatic Amputations and Complications		0.208	0.172	0.221	0.525	0.176	0.180	0.092
S68.712S	Complete traumatic transmetacarpal amputation of left hand, sequela	189	Amputation Status, Lower Limb/ Amputation Complications		0.519	0.437	0.795	0.934	0.697	0.626	0.357
S68.719A	Complete traumatic transmetacarpal amputation of unspecified hand, initial encounter	173	Traumatic Amputations and Complications		0.208	0.172	0.221	0.525	0.176	0.180	0.092
S68.719S	Complete traumatic transmetacarpal amputation of unspecified hand, sequela	189	Amputation Status, Lower Limb/ Amputation Complications		0.519	0.437	0.795	0.934	0.697	0.626	0.357
S68.721A	Partial traumatic transmetacarpal amputation of right hand, initial encounter	173	Traumatic Amputations and Complications		0.208	0.172	0.221	0.525	0.176	0.180	0.092
S68.721S	Partial traumatic transmetacarpal amputation of right hand, sequela	189	Amputation Status, Lower Limb/ Amputation Complications		0.519	0.437	0.795	0.934	0.697	0.626	0.357
S68.722A	Partial traumatic transmetacarpal amputation of left hand, initial encounter	173	Traumatic Amputations and Complications		0.208	0.172	0.221	0.525	0.176	0.180	0.092
S68.722S	Partial traumatic transmetacarpal amputation of left hand, sequela	189	Amputation Status, Lower Limb/ Amputation Complications		0.519	0.437	0.795	0.934	0.697	0.626	0.357
S68.729A	Partial traumatic transmetacarpal amputation of unspecified hand, initial encounter	173	Traumatic Amputations and Complications		0.208	0.172	0.221	0.525	0.176	0.180	0.092
S68.729S	Partial traumatic transmetacarpal amputation of unspecified hand, sequela	189	Amputation Status, Lower Limb/ Amputation Complications		0.519	0.437	0.795	0.934	0.697	0.626	0.357
S72.001A	Fracture of unspecified part of neck of right femur, initial encounter for closed fracture	170	Hip Fracture/Dislocation		0.350	0.394	0.409	0.469	0.354	0.333	—
S72.001B	Fracture of unspecified part of neck of right femur, initial encounter for open fracture type I or II	170	Hip Fracture/Dislocation		0.350	0.394	0.409	0.469	0.354	0.333	—
S72.001C	Fracture of unspecified part of neck of right femur, initial encounter for open fracture type IIIA, IIIB, or IIIC	170	Hip Fracture/Dislocation		0.350	0.394	0.409	0.469	0.354	0.333	—
S72.002A	Fracture of unspecified part of neck of left femur, initial encounter for closed fracture	170	Hip Fracture/Dislocation		0.350	0.394	0.409	0.469	0.354	0.333	—
S72.002B	Fracture of unspecified part of neck of left femur, initial encounter for open fracture type I or II	170	Hip Fracture/Dislocation		0.350	0.394	0.409	0.469	0.354	0.333	—
S72.002C	Fracture of unspecified part of neck of left femur, initial encounter for open fracture type IIIA, IIIB, or IIIC	170	Hip Fracture/Dislocation		0.350	0.394	0.409	0.469	0.354	0.333	—
S72.009A	Fracture of unspecified part of neck of unspecified femur, initial encounter for closed fracture	170	Hip Fracture/Dislocation		0.350	0.394	0.409	0.469	0.354	0.333	—
S72.009B	Fracture of unspecified part of neck of unspecified femur, initial encounter for open fracture type I or II	170	Hip Fracture/Dislocation		0.350	0.394	0.409	0.469	0.354	0.333	—
S72.009C	Fracture of unspecified part of neck of unspecified femur, initial encounter for open fracture type IIIA, IIIB, or IIIC	170	Hip Fracture/Dislocation		0.350	0.394	0.409	0.469	0.354	0.333	—

ICD-10-CM Code	ICD-10-CM Code Description	V24 CMS-HCC	V24 CMS-HCC Disease Group	V24 CMS-HCC Hierarchies	Community, NonDual, Aged	Community, NonDual, Disabled	Community, FBDual, Aged	Community, FBDual, Disabled	Community, PBDual, Aged	Community, PBDual, Disabled	Institutional
S72.011A	Unspecified intracapsular fracture of right femur, initial encounter for closed fracture	170	Hip Fracture/Dislocation		0.350	0.394	0.409	0.469	0.354	0.333	—
S72.011B	Unspecified intracapsular fracture of right femur, initial encounter for open fracture type I or II	170	Hip Fracture/Dislocation		0.350	0.394	0.409	0.469	0.354	0.333	—
S72.011C	Unspecified intracapsular fracture of right femur, initial encounter for open fracture type IIIA, IIIB, or IIIC	170	Hip Fracture/Dislocation		0.350	0.394	0.409	0.469	0.354	0.333	—
S72.012A	Unspecified intracapsular fracture of left femur, initial encounter for closed fracture	170	Hip Fracture/Dislocation		0.350	0.394	0.409	0.469	0.354	0.333	—
S72.012B	Unspecified intracapsular fracture of left femur, initial encounter for open fracture type I or II	170	Hip Fracture/Dislocation		0.350	0.394	0.409	0.469	0.354	0.333	—
S72.012C	Unspecified intracapsular fracture of left femur, initial encounter for open fracture type IIIA, IIIB, or IIIC	170	Hip Fracture/Dislocation		0.350	0.394	0.409	0.469	0.354	0.333	—
S72.019A	Unspecified intracapsular fracture of unspecified femur, initial encounter for closed fracture	170	Hip Fracture/Dislocation		0.350	0.394	0.409	0.469	0.354	0.333	—
S72.019B	Unspecified intracapsular fracture of unspecified femur, initial encounter for open fracture type I or II	170	Hip Fracture/Dislocation		0.350	0.394	0.409	0.469	0.354	0.333	—
S72.019C	Unspecified intracapsular fracture of unspecified femur, initial encounter for open fracture type IIIA, IIIB, or IIIC	170	Hip Fracture/Dislocation		0.350	0.394	0.409	0.469	0.354	0.333	—
S72.021A	Displaced fracture of epiphysis (separation) (upper) of right femur, initial encounter for closed fracture	170	Hip Fracture/Dislocation		0.350	0.394	0.409	0.469	0.354	0.333	—
S72.021B	Displaced fracture of epiphysis (separation) (upper) of right femur, initial encounter for open fracture type I or II	170	Hip Fracture/Dislocation		0.350	0.394	0.409	0.469	0.354	0.333	—
S72.021C	Displaced fracture of epiphysis (separation) (upper) of right femur, initial encounter for open fracture type IIIA, IIIB, or IIIC	170	Hip Fracture/Dislocation		0.350	0.394	0.409	0.469	0.354	0.333	—
S72.022A	Displaced fracture of epiphysis (separation) (upper) of left femur, initial encounter for closed fracture	170	Hip Fracture/Dislocation		0.350	0.394	0.409	0.469	0.354	0.333	—
S72.022B	Displaced fracture of epiphysis (separation) (upper) of left femur, initial encounter for open fracture type I or II	170	Hip Fracture/Dislocation		0.350	0.394	0.409	0.469	0.354	0.333	—
S72.022C	Displaced fracture of epiphysis (separation) (upper) of left femur, initial encounter for open fracture type IIIB, or IIIC	170	Hip Fracture/Dislocation		0.350	0.394	0.409	0.469	0.354	0.333	—
S72.023A	Displaced fracture of epiphysis (separation) (upper) of unspecified femur, initial encounter for closed fracture	170	Hip Fracture/Dislocation		0.350	0.394	0.409	0.469	0.354	0.333	—
S72.023B	Displaced fracture of epiphysis (separation) (upper) of unspecified femur, initial encounter for open fracture type I or II	170	Hip Fracture/Dislocation		0.350	0.394	0.409	0.469	0.354	0.333	—
S72.023C	Displaced fracture of epiphysis (separation) (upper) of unspecified femur, initial encounter for open fracture type IIIA, IIIB, or IIIC	170	Hip Fracture/Dislocation		0.350	0.394	0.409	0.469	0.354	0.333	—

ICD-10-CM Code	ICD-10-CM Code Description	V24 CMS-HCC	V24 CMS-HCC Disease Group	V24 CMS-HCC Hierarchies	Community, NonDual, Aged	Community, NonDual, Disabled	Community, FBDual, Aged	Community, FBDual, Disabled	Community, PBDual, Aged	Community, PBDual, Disabled	Institutional
S72.024A	Nondisplaced fracture of epiphysis (separation) (upper) of right femur, initial encounter for closed fracture	170	Hip Fracture/Dislocation		0.350	0.394	0.409	0.469	0.354	0.333	—
S72.024B	Nondisplaced fracture of epiphysis (separation) (upper) of right femur, initial encounter for open fracture type I or II	170	Hip Fracture/Dislocation		0.350	0.394	0.409	0.469	0.354	0.333	—
S72.024C	Nondisplaced fracture of epiphysis (separation) (upper) of right femur, initial encounter for open fracture type IIIA, IIIB, or IIIC	170	Hip Fracture/Dislocation		0.350	0.394	0.409	0.469	0.354	0.333	—
S72.025A	Nondisplaced fracture of epiphysis (separation) (upper) of left femur, initial encounter for closed fracture	170	Hip Fracture/Dislocation		0.350	0.394	0.409	0.469	0.354	0.333	—
S72.025B	Nondisplaced fracture of epiphysis (separation) (upper) of left femur, initial encounter for open fracture type I or II	170	Hip Fracture/Dislocation		0.350	0.394	0.409	0.469	0.354	0.333	—
S72.025C	Nondisplaced fracture of epiphysis (separation) (upper) of left femur, initial encounter for open fracture type IIIA, IIIB, or IIIC	170	Hip Fracture/Dislocation		0.350	0.394	0.409	0.469	0.354	0.333	—
S72.026A	Nondisplaced fracture of epiphysis (separation) (upper) of unspecified femur, initial encounter for closed fracture	170	Hip Fracture/Dislocation		0.350	0.394	0.409	0.469	0.354	0.333	—
S72.026B	Nondisplaced fracture of epiphysis (separation) (upper) of unspecified femur, initial encounter for open fracture type I or II	170	Hip Fracture/Dislocation		0.350	0.394	0.409	0.469	0.354	0.333	—
S72.026C	Nondisplaced fracture of epiphysis (separation) (upper) of unspecified femur, initial encounter for open fracture type IIIA, IIIB, or IIIC	170	Hip Fracture/Dislocation		0.350	0.394	0.409	0.469	0.354	0.333	—
S72.031A	Displaced midcervical fracture of right femur, initial encounter for closed fracture	170	Hip Fracture/Dislocation		0.350	0.394	0.409	0.469	0.354	0.333	—
S72.031B	Displaced midcervical fracture of right femur, initial encounter for open fracture type I or II	170	Hip Fracture/Dislocation		0.350	0.394	0.409	0.469	0.354	0.333	—
S72.031C	Displaced midcervical fracture of right femur, initial encounter for open fracture type IIIA, IIIB, or IIIC	170	Hip Fracture/Dislocation		0.350	0.394	0.409	0.469	0.354	0.333	—
S72.032A	Displaced midcervical fracture of left femur, initial encounter for closed fracture	170	Hip Fracture/Dislocation		0.350	0.394	0.409	0.469	0.354	0.333	—
S72.032B	Displaced midcervical fracture of left femur, initial encounter for open fracture type I or II	170	Hip Fracture/Dislocation		0.350	0.394	0.409	0.469	0.354	0.333	—
S72.032C	Displaced midcervical fracture of left femur, initial encounter for open fracture type IIIA, IIIB, or IIIC	170	Hip Fracture/Dislocation		0.350	0.394	0.409	0.469	0.354	0.333	—
S72.033A	Displaced midcervical fracture of unspecified femur, initial encounter for closed fracture	170	Hip Fracture/Dislocation		0.350	0.394	0.409	0.469	0.354	0.333	—
S72.033B	Displaced midcervical fracture of unspecified femur, initial encounter for open fracture type I or II	170	Hip Fracture/Dislocation		0.350	0.394	0.409	0.469	0.354	0.333	—
S72.033C	Displaced midcervical fracture of unspecified femur, initial encounter for open fracture type IIIA, IIIB, or IIIC	170	Hip Fracture/Dislocation		0.350	0.394	0.409	0.469	0.354	0.333	—

ICD-10-CM Code	ICD-10-CM Code Description	V24 CMS-HCC	V24 CMS-HCC Disease Group	V24 CMS-HCC Hierarchies	Community, NonDual, Aged	Community, NonDual, Disabled	Community, FBDual, Aged	Community, FBDual, Disabled	Community, PBDual, Aged	Community, PBDual, Disabled	Institutional
S72.034A	Nondisplaced midcervical fracture of right femur, initial encounter for closed fracture	170	Hip Fracture/Dislocation		0.350	0.394	0.409	0.469	0.354	0.333	—
S72.034B	Nondisplaced midcervical fracture of right femur, initial encounter for open fracture type I or II	170	Hip Fracture/Dislocation		0.350	0.394	0.409	0.469	0.354	0.333	—
S72.034C	Nondisplaced midcervical fracture of right femur, initial encounter for open fracture type IIIA, IIIB, or IIIC	170	Hip Fracture/Dislocation		0.350	0.394	0.409	0.469	0.354	0.333	—
S72.035A	Nondisplaced midcervical fracture of left femur, initial encounter for closed fracture	170	Hip Fracture/Dislocation		0.350	0.394	0.409	0.469	0.354	0.333	—
S72.035B	Nondisplaced midcervical fracture of left femur, initial encounter for open fracture type I or II	170	Hip Fracture/Dislocation		0.350	0.394	0.409	0.469	0.354	0.333	—
S72.035C	Nondisplaced midcervical fracture of left femur, initial encounter for open fracture type IIIA, IIIB, or IIIC	170	Hip Fracture/Dislocation		0.350	0.394	0.409	0.469	0.354	0.333	—
S72.036A	Nondisplaced midcervical fracture of unspecified femur, initial encounter for closed fracture	170	Hip Fracture/Dislocation		0.350	0.394	0.409	0.469	0.354	0.333	—
S72.036B	Nondisplaced midcervical fracture of unspecified femur, initial encounter for open fracture type I or II	170	Hip Fracture/Dislocation		0.350	0.394	0.409	0.469	0.354	0.333	—
S72.036C	Nondisplaced midcervical fracture of unspecified femur, initial encounter for open fracture type IIIA, IIIB, or IIIC	170	Hip Fracture/Dislocation		0.350	0.394	0.409	0.469	0.354	0.333	—
S72.041A	Displaced fracture of base of neck of right femur, initial encounter for closed fracture	170	Hip Fracture/Dislocation		0.350	0.394	0.409	0.469	0.354	0.333	—
S72.041B	Displaced fracture of base of neck of right femur, initial encounter for open fracture type I or II	170	Hip Fracture/Dislocation		0.350	0.394	0.409	0.469	0.354	0.333	—
S72.041C	Displaced fracture of base of neck of right femur, initial encounter for open fracture type IIIA, IIIB, or IIIC	170	Hip Fracture/Dislocation		0.350	0.394	0.409	0.469	0.354	0.333	—
S72.042A	Displaced fracture of base of neck of left femur, initial encounter for closed fracture	170	Hip Fracture/Dislocation		0.350	0.394	0.409	0.469	0.354	0.333	—
S72.042B	Displaced fracture of base of neck of left femur, initial encounter for open fracture type I or II	170	Hip Fracture/Dislocation		0.350	0.394	0.409	0.469	0.354	0.333	—
S72.042C	Displaced fracture of base of neck of left femur, initial encounter for open fracture type IIIA, IIIB, or IIIC	170	Hip Fracture/Dislocation		0.350	0.394	0.409	0.469	0.354	0.333	—
S72.043A	Displaced fracture of base of neck of unspecified femur, initial encounter for closed fracture	170	Hip Fracture/Dislocation		0.350	0.394	0.409	0.469	0.354	0.333	—
S72.043B	Displaced fracture of base of neck of unspecified femur, initial encounter for open fracture type I or II	170	Hip Fracture/Dislocation		0.350	0.394	0.409	0.469	0.354	0.333	—
S72.043C	Displaced fracture of base of neck of unspecified femur, initial encounter for open fracture type IIIA, IIIB, or IIIC	170	Hip Fracture/Dislocation		0.350	0.394	0.409	0.469	0.354	0.333	—
S72.044A	Nondisplaced fracture of base of neck of right femur, initial encounter for closed fracture	170	Hip Fracture/Dislocation		0.350	0.394	0.409	0.469	0.354	0.333	—
S72.044B	Nondisplaced fracture of base of neck of right femur, initial encounter for open fracture type I or II	170	Hip Fracture/Dislocation		0.350	0.394	0.409	0.469	0.354	0.333	—

ICD-10-CM Code	ICD-10-CM Code Description	V24 CMS-HCC	V24 CMS-HCC Disease Group	V24 CMS-HCC Hierarchies	Community, NonDual, Aged	Community, NonDual, Disabled	Community, FBDual, Aged	Community, FBDual, Disabled	Community, PBDual, Aged	Community, PBDual, Disabled	Institutional
S72.044C	Nondisplaced fracture of base of neck of right femur, initial encounter for open fracture type IIIA, IIIB, or IIIC	170	Hip Fracture/Dislocation		0.350	0.394	0.409	0.469	0.354	0.333	—
S72.045A	Nondisplaced fracture of base of neck of left femur, initial encounter for closed fracture	170	Hip Fracture/Dislocation		0.350	0.394	0.409	0.469	0.354	0.333	—
S72.045B	Nondisplaced fracture of base of neck of left femur, initial encounter for open fracture type I or II	170	Hip Fracture/Dislocation		0.350	0.394	0.409	0.469	0.354	0.333	—
S72.045C	Nondisplaced fracture of base of neck of left femur, initial encounter for open fracture type IIIA, IIIB, or IIIC	170	Hip Fracture/Dislocation		0.350	0.394	0.409	0.469	0.354	0.333	—
S72.046A	Nondisplaced fracture of base of neck of unspecified femur, initial encounter for closed fracture	170	Hip Fracture/Dislocation		0.350	0.394	0.409	0.469	0.354	0.333	—
S72.046B	Nondisplaced fracture of base of neck of unspecified femur, initial encounter for open fracture type I or II	170	Hip Fracture/Dislocation		0.350	0.394	0.409	0.469	0.354	0.333	—
S72.046C	Nondisplaced fracture of base of neck of unspecified femur, initial encounter for open fracture type IIIA, IIIB, or IIIC	170	Hip Fracture/Dislocation		0.350	0.394	0.409	0.469	0.354	0.333	—
S72.051A	Unspecified fracture of head of right femur, initial encounter for closed fracture	170	Hip Fracture/Dislocation		0.350	0.394	0.409	0.469	0.354	0.333	—
S72.051B	Unspecified fracture of head of right femur, initial encounter for open fracture type I or II	170	Hip Fracture/Dislocation		0.350	0.394	0.409	0.469	0.354	0.333	—
S72.051C	Unspecified fracture of head of right femur, initial encounter for open fracture type IIIA, IIIB, or IIIC	170	Hip Fracture/Dislocation		0.350	0.394	0.409	0.469	0.354	0.333	—
S72.052A	Unspecified fracture of head of left femur, initial encounter for closed fracture	170	Hip Fracture/Dislocation		0.350	0.394	0.409	0.469	0.354	0.333	—
S72.052B	Unspecified fracture of head of left femur, initial encounter for open fracture type I or II	170	Hip Fracture/Dislocation		0.350	0.394	0.409	0.469	0.354	0.333	—
S72.052C	Unspecified fracture of head of left femur, initial encounter for open fracture type IIIA, IIIB, or IIIC	170	Hip Fracture/Dislocation		0.350	0.394	0.409	0.469	0.354	0.333	—
S72.059A	Unspecified fracture of head of unspecified femur, initial encounter for closed fracture	170	Hip Fracture/Dislocation		0.350	0.394	0.409	0.469	0.354	0.333	—
S72.059B	Unspecified fracture of head of unspecified femur, initial encounter for open fracture type I or II	170	Hip Fracture/Dislocation		0.350	0.394	0.409	0.469	0.354	0.333	—
S72.059C	Unspecified fracture of head of unspecified femur, initial encounter for open fracture type IIIA, IIIB, or IIIC	170	Hip Fracture/Dislocation		0.350	0.394	0.409	0.469	0.354	0.333	—
S72.061A	Displaced articular fracture of head of right femur, initial encounter for closed fracture	170	Hip Fracture/Dislocation		0.350	0.394	0.409	0.469	0.354	0.333	—
S72.061B	Displaced articular fracture of head of right femur, initial encounter for open fracture type I or II	170	Hip Fracture/Dislocation		0.350	0.394	0.409	0.469	0.354	0.333	—
S72.061C	Displaced articular fracture of head of right femur, initial encounter for open fracture type IIIA, IIIB, or IIIC	170	Hip Fracture/Dislocation		0.350	0.394	0.409	0.469	0.354	0.333	—
S72.062A	Displaced articular fracture of head of left femur, initial encounter for closed fracture	170	Hip Fracture/Dislocation		0.350	0.394	0.409	0.469	0.354	0.333	—

ICD-10-CM Code	ICD-10-CM Code Description	V24 CMS-HCC	V24 CMS-HCC Disease Group	V24 CMS-HCC Hierarchies	Community, NonDual, Aged	Community, NonDual, Disabled	Community, FBDual, Aged	Community, FBDual, Disabled	Community, PBDual, Aged	Community, PBDual, Disabled	Institutional
S72.062B	Displaced articular fracture of head of left femur, initial encounter for open fracture type I or II	170	Hip Fracture/Dislocation		0.350	0.394	0.409	0.469	0.354	0.333	—
S72.062C	Displaced articular fracture of head of left femur, initial encounter for open fracture type IIIA, IIIB, or IIIC	170	Hip Fracture/Dislocation		0.350	0.394	0.409	0.469	0.354	0.333	—
S72.063A	Displaced articular fracture of head of unspecified femur, initial encounter for closed fracture	170	Hip Fracture/Dislocation		0.350	0.394	0.409	0.469	0.354	0.333	—
S72.063B	Displaced articular fracture of head of unspecified femur, initial encounter for open fracture type I or II	170	Hip Fracture/Dislocation		0.350	0.394	0.409	0.469	0.354	0.333	—
S72.063C	Displaced articular fracture of head of unspecified femur, initial encounter for open fracture type IIIA, IIIB, or IIIC	170	Hip Fracture/Dislocation		0.350	0.394	0.409	0.469	0.354	0.333	—
S72.064A	Nondisplaced articular fracture of head of right femur, initial encounter for closed fracture	170	Hip Fracture/Dislocation		0.350	0.394	0.409	0.469	0.354	0.333	—
S72.064B	Nondisplaced articular fracture of head of right femur, initial encounter for open fracture type I or II	170	Hip Fracture/Dislocation		0.350	0.394	0.409	0.469	0.354	0.333	—
S72.064C	Nondisplaced articular fracture of head of right femur, initial encounter for open fracture type IIIA, IIIB, or IIIC	170	Hip Fracture/Dislocation		0.350	0.394	0.409	0.469	0.354	0.333	—
S72.065A	Nondisplaced articular fracture of head of left femur, initial encounter for closed fracture	170	Hip Fracture/Dislocation		0.350	0.394	0.409	0.469	0.354	0.333	—
S72.065B	Nondisplaced articular fracture of head of left femur, initial encounter for open fracture type I or II	170	Hip Fracture/Dislocation		0.350	0.394	0.409	0.469	0.354	0.333	—
S72.065C	Nondisplaced articular fracture of head of left femur, initial encounter for open fracture type IIIA, IIIB, or IIIC	170	Hip Fracture/Dislocation		0.350	0.394	0.409	0.469	0.354	0.333	—
S72.066A	Nondisplaced articular fracture of head of unspecified femur, initial encounter for closed fracture	170	Hip Fracture/Dislocation		0.350	0.394	0.409	0.469	0.354	0.333	—
S72.066B	Nondisplaced articular fracture of head of unspecified femur, initial encounter for open fracture type I or II	170	Hip Fracture/Dislocation		0.350	0.394	0.409	0.469	0.354	0.333	—
S72.066C	Nondisplaced articular fracture of head of unspecified femur, initial encounter for open fracture type IIIA, IIIB, or IIIC	170	Hip Fracture/Dislocation		0.350	0.394	0.409	0.469	0.354	0.333	—
S72.091A	Other fracture of head and neck of right femur, initial encounter for closed fracture	170	Hip Fracture/Dislocation		0.350	0.394	0.409	0.469	0.354	0.333	—
S72.091B	Other fracture of head and neck of right femur, initial encounter for open fracture type I or II	170	Hip Fracture/Dislocation		0.350	0.394	0.409	0.469	0.354	0.333	—
S72.091C	Other fracture of head and neck of right femur, initial encounter for open fracture type IIIA, IIIB, or IIIC	170	Hip Fracture/Dislocation		0.350	0.394	0.409	0.469	0.354	0.333	—
S72.092A	Other fracture of head and neck of left femur, initial encounter for closed fracture	170	Hip Fracture/Dislocation		0.350	0.394	0.409	0.469	0.354	0.333	—
S72.092B	Other fracture of head and neck of left femur, initial encounter for open fracture type I or II	170	Hip Fracture/Dislocation		0.350	0.394	0.409	0.469	0.354	0.333	—
S72.092C	Other fracture of head and neck of left femur, initial encounter for open fracture type IIIA, IIIB, or IIIC	170	Hip Fracture/Dislocation		0.350	0.394	0.409	0.469	0.354	0.333	—

ICD-10-CM Code	ICD-10-CM Code Description	V24 CMS-HCC	V24 CMS-HCC Disease Group	V24 CMS-HCC Hierarchies	Community, NonDual, Aged	Community, NonDual, Disabled	Community, FBDual, Aged	Community, FBDual, Disabled	Community, PBDual, Aged	Community, PBDual, Disabled	Institutional
S72.099A	Other fracture of head and neck of unspecified femur, initial encounter for closed fracture	170	Hip Fracture/Dislocation		0.350	0.394	0.409	0.469	0.354	0.333	—
S72.099B	Other fracture of head and neck of unspecified femur, initial encounter for open fracture type I or II	170	Hip Fracture/Dislocation		0.350	0.394	0.409	0.469	0.354	0.333	—
S72.099C	Other fracture of head and neck of unspecified femur, initial encounter for open fracture type IIIA, IIIB, or IIIC	170	Hip Fracture/Dislocation		0.350	0.394	0.409	0.469	0.354	0.333	—
S72.101A	Unspecified trochanteric fracture of right femur, initial encounter for closed fracture	170	Hip Fracture/Dislocation		0.350	0.394	0.409	0.469	0.354	0.333	—
S72.101B	Unspecified trochanteric fracture of right femur, initial encounter for open fracture type I or II	170	Hip Fracture/Dislocation		0.350	0.394	0.409	0.469	0.354	0.333	—
S72.101C	Unspecified trochanteric fracture of right femur, initial encounter for open fracture type IIIA, IIIB, or IIIC	170	Hip Fracture/Dislocation		0.350	0.394	0.409	0.469	0.354	0.333	—
S72.102A	Unspecified trochanteric fracture of left femur, initial encounter for closed fracture	170	Hip Fracture/Dislocation		0.350	0.394	0.409	0.469	0.354	0.333	—
S72.102B	Unspecified trochanteric fracture of left femur, initial encounter for open fracture type I or II	170	Hip Fracture/Dislocation		0.350	0.394	0.409	0.469	0.354	0.333	—
S72.102C	Unspecified trochanteric fracture of left femur, initial encounter for open fracture type IIIA, IIIB, or IIIC	170	Hip Fracture/Dislocation		0.350	0.394	0.409	0.469	0.354	0.333	—
S72.109A	Unspecified trochanteric fracture of unspecified femur, initial encounter for closed fracture	170	Hip Fracture/Dislocation		0.350	0.394	0.409	0.469	0.354	0.333	—
S72.109B	Unspecified trochanteric fracture of unspecified femur, initial encounter for open fracture type I or II	170	Hip Fracture/Dislocation		0.350	0.394	0.409	0.469	0.354	0.333	—
S72.109C	Unspecified trochanteric fracture of unspecified femur, initial encounter for open fracture type IIIA, IIIB, or IIIC	170	Hip Fracture/Dislocation		0.350	0.394	0.409	0.469	0.354	0.333	—
S72.111A	Displaced fracture of greater trochanter of right femur, initial encounter for closed fracture	170	Hip Fracture/Dislocation		0.350	0.394	0.409	0.469	0.354	0.333	—
S72.111B	Displaced fracture of greater trochanter of right femur, initial encounter for open fracture type I or II	170	Hip Fracture/Dislocation		0.350	0.394	0.409	0.469	0.354	0.333	—
S72.111C	Displaced fracture of greater trochanter of right femur, initial encounter for open fracture type IIIA, IIIB, or IIIC	170	Hip Fracture/Dislocation		0.350	0.394	0.409	0.469	0.354	0.333	—
S72.112A	Displaced fracture of greater trochanter of left femur, initial encounter for closed fracture	170	Hip Fracture/Dislocation		0.350	0.394	0.409	0.469	0.354	0.333	—
S72.112B	Displaced fracture of greater trochanter of left femur, initial encounter for open fracture type I or II	170	Hip Fracture/Dislocation		0.350	0.394	0.409	0.469	0.354	0.333	—
S72.112C	Displaced fracture of greater trochanter of left femur, initial encounter for open fracture type IIIA, IIIB, or IIIC	170	Hip Fracture/Dislocation		0.350	0.394	0.409	0.469	0.354	0.333	—
S72.113A	Displaced fracture of greater trochanter of unspecified femur, initial encounter for closed fracture	170	Hip Fracture/Dislocation		0.350	0.394	0.409	0.469	0.354	0.333	—

ICD-10-CM Code	ICD-10-CM Code Description	V24 CMS-HCC	V24 CMS-HCC Disease Group	V24 CMS-HCC Hierarchies	Community, NonDual, Aged	Community, NonDual, Disabled	Community, FBDual, Aged	Community, FBDual, Disabled	Community, PBDual, Aged	Community, PBDual, Disabled	Institutional
S72.113B	Displaced fracture of greater trochanter of unspecified femur, initial encounter for open fracture type I or II	170	Hip Fracture/Dislocation		0.350	0.394	0.409	0.469	0.354	0.333	—
S72.113C	Displaced fracture of greater trochanter of unspecified femur, initial encounter for open fracture type IIIA, IIIB, or IIIC	170	Hip Fracture/Dislocation		0.350	0.394	0.409	0.469	0.354	0.333	—
S72.114A	Nondisplaced fracture of greater trochanter of right femur, initial encounter for closed fracture	170	Hip Fracture/Dislocation		0.350	0.394	0.409	0.469	0.354	0.333	—
S72.114B	Nondisplaced fracture of greater trochanter of right femur, initial encounter for open fracture type I or II	170	Hip Fracture/Dislocation		0.350	0.394	0.409	0.469	0.354	0.333	—
S72.114C	Nondisplaced fracture of greater trochanter of right femur, initial encounter for open fracture type IIIA, IIIB, or IIIC	170	Hip Fracture/Dislocation		0.350	0.394	0.409	0.469	0.354	0.333	—
S72.115A	Nondisplaced fracture of greater trochanter of left femur, initial encounter for closed fracture	170	Hip Fracture/Dislocation		0.350	0.394	0.409	0.469	0.354	0.333	—
S72.115B	Nondisplaced fracture of greater trochanter of left femur, initial encounter for open fracture type I or II	170	Hip Fracture/Dislocation		0.350	0.394	0.409	0.469	0.354	0.333	—
S72.115C	Nondisplaced fracture of greater trochanter of left femur, initial encounter for open fracture type IIIA, IIIB, or IIIC	170	Hip Fracture/Dislocation		0.350	0.394	0.409	0.469	0.354	0.333	—
S72.116A	Nondisplaced fracture of greater trochanter of unspecified femur, initial encounter for closed fracture	170	Hip Fracture/Dislocation		0.350	0.394	0.409	0.469	0.354	0.333	—
S72.116B	Nondisplaced fracture of greater trochanter of unspecified femur, initial encounter for open fracture type I or II	170	Hip Fracture/Dislocation		0.350	0.394	0.409	0.469	0.354	0.333	—
S72.116C	Nondisplaced fracture of greater trochanter of unspecified femur, initial encounter for open fracture type IIIA, IIIB, or IIIC	170	Hip Fracture/Dislocation		0.350	0.394	0.409	0.469	0.354	0.333	—
S72.121A	Displaced fracture of lesser trochanter of right femur, initial encounter for closed fracture	170	Hip Fracture/Dislocation		0.350	0.394	0.409	0.469	0.354	0.333	—
S72.121B	Displaced fracture of lesser trochanter of right femur, initial encounter for open fracture type I or II	170	Hip Fracture/Dislocation		0.350	0.394	0.409	0.469	0.354	0.333	—
S72.121C	Displaced fracture of lesser trochanter of right femur, initial encounter for open fracture type IIIA, IIIB, or IIIC	170	Hip Fracture/Dislocation		0.350	0.394	0.409	0.469	0.354	0.333	—
S72.122A	Displaced fracture of lesser trochanter of left femur, initial encounter for closed fracture	170	Hip Fracture/Dislocation		0.350	0.394	0.409	0.469	0.354	0.333	—
S72.122B	Displaced fracture of lesser trochanter of left femur, initial encounter for open fracture type I or II	170	Hip Fracture/Dislocation		0.350	0.394	0.409	0.469	0.354	0.333	—
S72.122C	Displaced fracture of lesser trochanter of left femur, initial encounter for open fracture type IIIA, IIIB, or IIIC	170	Hip Fracture/Dislocation		0.350	0.394	0.409	0.469	0.354	0.333	—

ICD-10-CM Code	ICD-10-CM Code Description	V24 CMS-HCC	V24 CMS-HCC Disease Group	V24 CMS-HCC Hierarchies	Community, NonDual, Aged	Community, NonDual, Disabled	Community, FBDual, Aged	Community, FBDual, Disabled	Community, PBDual, Aged	Community, PBDual, Disabled	Institutional
S72.123A	Displaced fracture of lesser trochanter of unspecified femur, initial encounter for closed fracture	170	Hip Fracture/Dislocation		0.350	0.394	0.409	0.469	0.354	0.333	—
S72.123B	Displaced fracture of lesser trochanter of unspecified femur, initial encounter for open fracture type I or II	170	Hip Fracture/Dislocation		0.350	0.394	0.409	0.469	0.354	0.333	—
S72.123C	Displaced fracture of lesser trochanter of unspecified femur, initial encounter for open fracture type IIIA, IIIB, or IIIC	170	Hip Fracture/Dislocation		0.350	0.394	0.409	0.469	0.354	0.333	—
S72.124A	Nondisplaced fracture of lesser trochanter of right femur, initial encounter for closed fracture	170	Hip Fracture/Dislocation		0.350	0.394	0.409	0.469	0.354	0.333	—
S72.124B	Nondisplaced fracture of lesser trochanter of right femur, initial encounter for open fracture type I or II	170	Hip Fracture/Dislocation		0.350	0.394	0.409	0.469	0.354	0.333	—
S72.124C	Nondisplaced fracture of lesser trochanter of right femur, initial encounter for open fracture type IIIA, IIIB, or IIIC	170	Hip Fracture/Dislocation		0.350	0.394	0.409	0.469	0.354	0.333	—
S72.125A	Nondisplaced fracture of lesser trochanter of left femur, initial encounter for closed fracture	170	Hip Fracture/Dislocation		0.350	0.394	0.409	0.469	0.354	0.333	—
S72.125B	Nondisplaced fracture of lesser trochanter of left femur, initial encounter for open fracture type I or II	170	Hip Fracture/Dislocation		0.350	0.394	0.409	0.469	0.354	0.333	—
S72.125C	Nondisplaced fracture of lesser trochanter of left femur, initial encounter for open fracture type IIIA, IIIB, or IIIC	170	Hip Fracture/Dislocation		0.350	0.394	0.409	0.469	0.354	0.333	—
S72.126A	Nondisplaced fracture of lesser trochanter of unspecified femur, initial encounter for closed fracture	170	Hip Fracture/Dislocation		0.350	0.394	0.409	0.469	0.354	0.333	—
S72.126B	Nondisplaced fracture of lesser trochanter of unspecified femur, initial encounter for open fracture type I or II	170	Hip Fracture/Dislocation		0.350	0.394	0.409	0.469	0.354	0.333	—
S72.126C	Nondisplaced fracture of lesser trochanter of unspecified femur, initial encounter for open fracture type IIIA, IIIB, or IIIC	170	Hip Fracture/Dislocation		0.350	0.394	0.409	0.469	0.354	0.333	—
S72.131A	Displaced apophyseal fracture of right femur, initial encounter for closed fracture	170	Hip Fracture/Dislocation		0.350	0.394	0.409	0.469	0.354	0.333	—
S72.131B	Displaced apophyseal fracture of right femur, initial encounter for open fracture type I or II	170	Hip Fracture/Dislocation		0.350	0.394	0.409	0.469	0.354	0.333	—
S72.131C	Displaced apophyseal fracture of right femur, initial encounter for open fracture type IIIA, IIIB, or IIIC	170	Hip Fracture/Dislocation		0.350	0.394	0.409	0.469	0.354	0.333	—
S72.132A	Displaced apophyseal fracture of left femur, initial encounter for closed fracture	170	Hip Fracture/Dislocation		0.350	0.394	0.409	0.469	0.354	0.333	—
S72.132B	Displaced apophyseal fracture of left femur, initial encounter for open fracture type I or II	170	Hip Fracture/Dislocation		0.350	0.394	0.409	0.469	0.354	0.333	—
S72.132C	Displaced apophyseal fracture of left femur, initial encounter for open fracture type IIIA, IIIB, or IIIC	170	Hip Fracture/Dislocation		0.350	0.394	0.409	0.469	0.354	0.333	—

ICD-10-CM Code	ICD-10-CM Code Description	V24 CMS-HCC	V24 CMS-HCC Disease Group	V24 CMS-HCC Hierarchies	Community, NonDual, Aged	Community, NonDual, Disabled	Community, FBDual, Aged	Community, FBDual, Disabled	Community, PBDual, Aged	Community, PBDual, Disabled	Institutional
S72.133A	Displaced apophyseal fracture of unspecified femur, initial encounter for closed fracture	170	Hip Fracture/Dislocation		0.350	0.394	0.409	0.469	0.354	0.333	—
S72.133B	Displaced apophyseal fracture of unspecified femur, initial encounter for open fracture type I or II	170	Hip Fracture/Dislocation		0.350	0.394	0.409	0.469	0.354	0.333	—
S72.133C	Displaced apophyseal fracture of unspecified femur, initial encounter for open fracture type IIIA, IIIB, or IIIC	170	Hip Fracture/Dislocation		0.350	0.394	0.409	0.469	0.354	0.333	—
S72.134A	Nondisplaced apophyseal fracture of right femur, initial encounter for closed fracture	170	Hip Fracture/Dislocation		0.350	0.394	0.409	0.469	0.354	0.333	—
S72.134B	Nondisplaced apophyseal fracture of right femur, initial encounter for open fracture type I or II	170	Hip Fracture/Dislocation		0.350	0.394	0.409	0.469	0.354	0.333	—
S72.134C	Nondisplaced apophyseal fracture of right femur, initial encounter for open fracture type IIIA, IIIB, or IIIC	170	Hip Fracture/Dislocation		0.350	0.394	0.409	0.469	0.354	0.333	—
S72.135A	Nondisplaced apophyseal fracture of left femur, initial encounter for closed fracture	170	Hip Fracture/Dislocation		0.350	0.394	0.409	0.469	0.354	0.333	—
S72.135B	Nondisplaced apophyseal fracture of left femur, initial encounter for open fracture type I or II	170	Hip Fracture/Dislocation		0.350	0.394	0.409	0.469	0.354	0.333	—
S72.135C	Nondisplaced apophyseal fracture of left femur, initial encounter for open fracture type IIIA, IIIB, or IIIC	170	Hip Fracture/Dislocation		0.350	0.394	0.409	0.469	0.354	0.333	—
S72.136A	Nondisplaced apophyseal fracture of unspecified femur, initial encounter for closed fracture	170	Hip Fracture/Dislocation		0.350	0.394	0.409	0.469	0.354	0.333	—
S72.136B	Nondisplaced apophyseal fracture of unspecified femur, initial encounter for open fracture type I or II	170	Hip Fracture/Dislocation		0.350	0.394	0.409	0.469	0.354	0.333	—
S72.136C	Nondisplaced apophyseal fracture of unspecified femur, initial encounter for open fracture type IIIA, IIIB, or IIIC	170	Hip Fracture/Dislocation		0.350	0.394	0.409	0.469	0.354	0.333	—
S72.141A	Displaced intertrochanteric fracture of right femur, initial encounter for closed fracture	170	Hip Fracture/Dislocation		0.350	0.394	0.409	0.469	0.354	0.333	—
S72.141B	Displaced intertrochanteric fracture of right femur, initial encounter for open fracture type I or II	170	Hip Fracture/Dislocation		0.350	0.394	0.409	0.469	0.354	0.333	—
S72.141C	Displaced intertrochanteric fracture of right femur, initial encounter for open fracture type IIIA, IIIB, or IIIC	170	Hip Fracture/Dislocation		0.350	0.394	0.409	0.469	0.354	0.333	—
S72.142A	Displaced intertrochanteric fracture of left femur, initial encounter for closed fracture	170	Hip Fracture/Dislocation		0.350	0.394	0.409	0.469	0.354	0.333	—
S72.142B	Displaced intertrochanteric fracture of left femur, initial encounter for open fracture type I or II	170	Hip Fracture/Dislocation		0.350	0.394	0.409	0.469	0.354	0.333	—
S72.142C	Displaced intertrochanteric fracture of left femur, initial encounter for open fracture type IIIA, IIIB, or IIIC	170	Hip Fracture/Dislocation		0.350	0.394	0.409	0.469	0.354	0.333	—
S72.143A	Displaced intertrochanteric fracture of unspecified femur, initial encounter for closed fracture	170	Hip Fracture/Dislocation		0.350	0.394	0.409	0.469	0.354	0.333	—
S72.143B	Displaced intertrochanteric fracture of unspecified femur, initial encounter for open fracture type I or II	170	Hip Fracture/Dislocation		0.350	0.394	0.409	0.469	0.354	0.333	—

ICD-10-CM Code	ICD-10-CM Code Description	V24 CMS-HCC	V24 CMS-HCC Disease Group	V24 CMS-HCC Hierarchies	Community, NonDual, Aged	Community, NonDual, Disabled	Community, FBDual, Aged	Community, FBDual, Disabled	Community, PBDual, Aged	Community, PBDual, Disabled	Institutional
S72.143C	Displaced intertrochanteric fracture of unspecified femur, initial encounter for open fracture type IIIA, IIIB, or IIIC	170	Hip Fracture/Dislocation		0.350	0.394	0.409	0.469	0.354	0.333	—
S72.144A	Nondisplaced intertrochanteric fracture of right femur, initial encounter for closed fracture	170	Hip Fracture/Dislocation		0.350	0.394	0.409	0.469	0.354	0.333	—
S72.144B	Nondisplaced intertrochanteric fracture of right femur, initial encounter for open fracture type I or II	170	Hip Fracture/Dislocation		0.350	0.394	0.409	0.469	0.354	0.333	—
S72.144C	Nondisplaced intertrochanteric fracture of right femur, initial encounter for open fracture type IIIA, IIIB, or IIIC	170	Hip Fracture/Dislocation		0.350	0.394	0.409	0.469	0.354	0.333	—
S72.145A	Nondisplaced intertrochanteric fracture of left femur, initial encounter for closed fracture	170	Hip Fracture/Dislocation		0.350	0.394	0.409	0.469	0.354	0.333	—
S72.145B	Nondisplaced intertrochanteric fracture of left femur, initial encounter for open fracture type I or II	170	Hip Fracture/Dislocation		0.350	0.394	0.409	0.469	0.354	0.333	—
S72.145C	Nondisplaced intertrochanteric fracture of left femur, initial encounter for open fracture type IIIA, IIIB, or IIIC	170	Hip Fracture/Dislocation		0.350	0.394	0.409	0.469	0.354	0.333	—
S72.146A	Nondisplaced intertrochanteric fracture of unspecified femur, initial encounter for closed fracture	170	Hip Fracture/Dislocation		0.350	0.394	0.409	0.469	0.354	0.333	—
S72.146B	Nondisplaced intertrochanteric fracture of unspecified femur, initial encounter for open fracture type I or II	170	Hip Fracture/Dislocation		0.350	0.394	0.409	0.469	0.354	0.333	—
S72.146C	Nondisplaced intertrochanteric fracture of unspecified femur, initial encounter for open fracture type IIIA, IIIB, or IIIC	170	Hip Fracture/Dislocation		0.350	0.394	0.409	0.469	0.354	0.333	—
S72.21XA	Displaced subtrochanteric fracture of right femur, initial encounter for closed fracture	170	Hip Fracture/Dislocation		0.350	0.394	0.409	0.469	0.354	0.333	—
S72.21XB	Displaced subtrochanteric fracture of right femur, initial encounter for open fracture type I or II	170	Hip Fracture/Dislocation		0.350	0.394	0.409	0.469	0.354	0.333	—
S72.21XC	Displaced subtrochanteric fracture of right femur, initial encounter for open fracture type IIIA, IIIB, or IIIC	170	Hip Fracture/Dislocation		0.350	0.394	0.409	0.469	0.354	0.333	—
S72.22XA	Displaced subtrochanteric fracture of left femur, initial encounter for closed fracture	170	Hip Fracture/Dislocation		0.350	0.394	0.409	0.469	0.354	0.333	—
S72.22XB	Displaced subtrochanteric fracture of left femur, initial encounter for open fracture type I or II	170	Hip Fracture/Dislocation		0.350	0.394	0.409	0.469	0.354	0.333	—
S72.22XC	Displaced subtrochanteric fracture of left femur, initial encounter for open fracture type IIIA, IIIB, or IIIC	170	Hip Fracture/Dislocation		0.350	0.394	0.409	0.469	0.354	0.333	—
S72.23XA	Displaced subtrochanteric fracture of unspecified femur, initial encounter for closed fracture	170	Hip Fracture/Dislocation		0.350	0.394	0.409	0.469	0.354	0.333	—
S72.23XB	Displaced subtrochanteric fracture of unspecified femur, initial encounter for open fracture type I or II	170	Hip Fracture/Dislocation		0.350	0.394	0.409	0.469	0.354	0.333	—

ICD-10-CM Code	ICD-10-CM Code Description	V24 CMS-HCC	V24 CMS-HCC Disease Group	V24 CMS-HCC Hierarchies	Community, NonDual, Aged	Community, NonDual, Disabled	Community, FBDual, Aged	Community, FBDual, Disabled	Community, PBDual, Aged	Community, PBDual, Disabled	Institutional
S72.23XC	Displaced subtrochanteric fracture of unspecified femur, initial encounter for open fracture type IIIA, IIIB, or IIIC	170	Hip Fracture/Dislocation		0.350	0.394	0.409	0.469	0.354	0.333	—
S72.24XA	Nondisplaced subtrochanteric fracture of right femur, initial encounter for closed fracture	170	Hip Fracture/Dislocation		0.350	0.394	0.409	0.469	0.354	0.333	—
S72.24XB	Nondisplaced subtrochanteric fracture of right femur, initial encounter for open fracture type I or II	170	Hip Fracture/Dislocation		0.350	0.394	0.409	0.469	0.354	0.333	—
S72.24XC	Nondisplaced subtrochanteric fracture of right femur, initial encounter for open fracture type IIIA, IIIB, or IIIC	170	Hip Fracture/Dislocation		0.350	0.394	0.409	0.469	0.354	0.333	—
S72.25XA	Nondisplaced subtrochanteric fracture of left femur, initial encounter for closed fracture	170	Hip Fracture/Dislocation		0.350	0.394	0.409	0.469	0.354	0.333	—
S72.25XB	Nondisplaced subtrochanteric fracture of left femur, initial encounter for open fracture type I or II	170	Hip Fracture/Dislocation		0.350	0.394	0.409	0.469	0.354	0.333	—
S72.25XC	Nondisplaced subtrochanteric fracture of left femur, initial encounter for open fracture type IIIA, IIIB, or IIIC	170	Hip Fracture/Dislocation		0.350	0.394	0.409	0.469	0.354	0.333	—
S72.26XA	Nondisplaced subtrochanteric fracture of unspecified femur, initial encounter for closed fracture	170	Hip Fracture/Dislocation		0.350	0.394	0.409	0.469	0.354	0.333	—
S72.26XB	Nondisplaced subtrochanteric fracture of unspecified femur, initial encounter for open fracture type I or II	170	Hip Fracture/Dislocation		0.350	0.394	0.409	0.469	0.354	0.333	—
S72.26XC	Nondisplaced subtrochanteric fracture of unspecified femur, initial encounter for open fracture type IIIA, IIIB, or IIIC	170	Hip Fracture/Dislocation		0.350	0.394	0.409	0.469	0.354	0.333	—
S72.301A	Unspecified fracture of shaft of right femur, initial encounter for closed fracture	170	Hip Fracture/Dislocation		0.350	0.394	0.409	0.469	0.354	0.333	—
S72.301B	Unspecified fracture of shaft of right femur, initial encounter for open fracture type I or II	170	Hip Fracture/Dislocation		0.350	0.394	0.409	0.469	0.354	0.333	—
S72.301C	Unspecified fracture of shaft of right femur, initial encounter for open fracture type IIIA, IIIB, or IIIC	170	Hip Fracture/Dislocation		0.350	0.394	0.409	0.469	0.354	0.333	—
S72.302A	Unspecified fracture of shaft of left femur, initial encounter for closed fracture	170	Hip Fracture/Dislocation		0.350	0.394	0.409	0.469	0.354	0.333	—
S72.302B	Unspecified fracture of shaft of left femur, initial encounter for open fracture type I or II	170	Hip Fracture/Dislocation		0.350	0.394	0.409	0.469	0.354	0.333	—
S72.302C	Unspecified fracture of shaft of left femur, initial encounter for open fracture type IIIA, IIIB, or IIIC	170	Hip Fracture/Dislocation		0.350	0.394	0.409	0.469	0.354	0.333	—
S72.309A	Unspecified fracture of shaft of unspecified femur, initial encounter for closed fracture	170	Hip Fracture/Dislocation		0.350	0.394	0.409	0.469	0.354	0.333	—
S72.309B	Unspecified fracture of shaft of unspecified femur, initial encounter for open fracture type I or II	170	Hip Fracture/Dislocation		0.350	0.394	0.409	0.469	0.354	0.333	—

ICD-10-CM Code	ICD-10-CM Code Description	V24 CMS-HCC	V24 CMS-HCC Disease Group	V24 CMS-HCC Hierarchies	Community, NonDual, Aged	Community, NonDual, Disabled	Community, FBDual, Aged	Community, FBDual, Disabled	Community, PBDual, Aged	Community, PBDual, Disabled	Institutional
S72.309C	Unspecified fracture of shaft of unspecified femur, initial encounter for open fracture type IIIA, IIIB, or IIIC	170	Hip Fracture/Dislocation		0.350	0.394	0.409	0.469	0.354	0.333	—
S72.321A	Displaced transverse fracture of shaft of right femur, initial encounter for closed fracture	170	Hip Fracture/Dislocation		0.350	0.394	0.409	0.469	0.354	0.333	—
S72.321B	Displaced transverse fracture of shaft of right femur, initial encounter for open fracture type I or II	170	Hip Fracture/Dislocation		0.350	0.394	0.409	0.469	0.354	0.333	—
S72.321C	Displaced transverse fracture of shaft of right femur, initial encounter for open fracture type IIIA, IIIB, or IIIC	170	Hip Fracture/Dislocation		0.350	0.394	0.409	0.469	0.354	0.333	—
S72.322A	Displaced transverse fracture of shaft of left femur, initial encounter for closed fracture	170	Hip Fracture/Dislocation		0.350	0.394	0.409	0.469	0.354	0.333	—
S72.322B	Displaced transverse fracture of shaft of left femur, initial encounter for open fracture type I or II	170	Hip Fracture/Dislocation		0.350	0.394	0.409	0.469	0.354	0.333	—
S72.322C	Displaced transverse fracture of shaft of left femur, initial encounter for open fracture type IIIA, IIIB, or IIIC	170	Hip Fracture/Dislocation		0.350	0.394	0.409	0.469	0.354	0.333	—
S72.323A	Displaced transverse fracture of shaft of unspecified femur, initial encounter for closed fracture	170	Hip Fracture/Dislocation		0.350	0.394	0.409	0.469	0.354	0.333	—
S72.323B	Displaced transverse fracture of shaft of unspecified femur, initial encounter for open fracture type I or II	170	Hip Fracture/Dislocation		0.350	0.394	0.409	0.469	0.354	0.333	—
S72.323C	Displaced transverse fracture of shaft of unspecified femur, initial encounter for open fracture type IIIA, IIIB, or IIIC	170	Hip Fracture/Dislocation		0.350	0.394	0.409	0.469	0.354	0.333	—
S72.324A	Nondisplaced transverse fracture of shaft of right femur, initial encounter for closed fracture	170	Hip Fracture/Dislocation		0.350	0.394	0.409	0.469	0.354	0.333	—
S72.324B	Nondisplaced transverse fracture of shaft of right femur, initial encounter for open fracture type I or II	170	Hip Fracture/Dislocation		0.350	0.394	0.409	0.469	0.354	0.333	—
S72.324C	Nondisplaced transverse fracture of shaft of right femur, initial encounter for open fracture type IIIA, IIIB, or IIIC	170	Hip Fracture/Dislocation		0.350	0.394	0.409	0.469	0.354	0.333	—
S72.325A	Nondisplaced transverse fracture of shaft of left femur, initial encounter for closed fracture	170	Hip Fracture/Dislocation		0.350	0.394	0.409	0.469	0.354	0.333	—
S72.325B	Nondisplaced transverse fracture of shaft of left femur, initial encounter for open fracture type I or II	170	Hip Fracture/Dislocation		0.350	0.394	0.409	0.469	0.354	0.333	—
S72.325C	Nondisplaced transverse fracture of shaft of left femur, initial encounter for open fracture type IIIA, IIIB, or IIIC	170	Hip Fracture/Dislocation		0.350	0.394	0.409	0.469	0.354	0.333	—
S72.326A	Nondisplaced transverse fracture of shaft of unspecified femur, initial encounter for closed fracture	170	Hip Fracture/Dislocation		0.350	0.394	0.409	0.469	0.354	0.333	—
S72.326B	Nondisplaced transverse fracture of shaft of unspecified femur, initial encounter for open fracture type I or II	170	Hip Fracture/Dislocation		0.350	0.394	0.409	0.469	0.354	0.333	—
S72.326C	Nondisplaced transverse fracture of shaft of unspecified femur, initial encounter for open fracture type IIIA, IIIB, or IIIC	170	Hip Fracture/Dislocation		0.350	0.394	0.409	0.469	0.354	0.333	—

ICD-10-CM Code	ICD-10-CM Code Description	V24 CMS-HCC	V24 CMS-HCC Disease Group	V24 CMS-HCC Hierarchies	Community, NonDual, Aged	Community, NonDual, Disabled	Community, FBDual, Aged	Community, FBDual, Disabled	Community, PBDual, Aged	Community, PBDual, Disabled	Institutional
S72.331A	Displaced oblique fracture of shaft of right femur, initial encounter for closed fracture	170	Hip Fracture/Dislocation		0.350	0.394	0.409	0.469	0.354	0.333	—
S72.331B	Displaced oblique fracture of shaft of right femur, initial encounter for open fracture type I or II	170	Hip Fracture/Dislocation		0.350	0.394	0.409	0.469	0.354	0.333	—
S72.331C	Displaced oblique fracture of shaft of right femur, initial encounter for open fracture type IIIA, IIIB, or IIIC	170	Hip Fracture/Dislocation		0.350	0.394	0.409	0.469	0.354	0.333	—
S72.332A	Displaced oblique fracture of shaft of left femur, initial encounter for closed fracture	170	Hip Fracture/Dislocation		0.350	0.394	0.409	0.469	0.354	0.333	—
S72.332B	Displaced oblique fracture of shaft of left femur, initial encounter for open fracture type I or II	170	Hip Fracture/Dislocation		0.350	0.394	0.409	0.469	0.354	0.333	—
S72.332C	Displaced oblique fracture of shaft of left femur, initial encounter for open fracture type IIIA, IIIB, or IIIC	170	Hip Fracture/Dislocation		0.350	0.394	0.409	0.469	0.354	0.333	—
S72.333A	Displaced oblique fracture of shaft of unspecified femur, initial encounter for closed fracture	170	Hip Fracture/Dislocation		0.350	0.394	0.409	0.469	0.354	0.333	—
S72.333B	Displaced oblique fracture of shaft of unspecified femur, initial encounter for open fracture type I or II	170	Hip Fracture/Dislocation		0.350	0.394	0.409	0.469	0.354	0.333	—
S72.333C	Displaced oblique fracture of shaft of unspecified femur, initial encounter for open fracture type IIIA, IIIB, or IIIC	170	Hip Fracture/Dislocation		0.350	0.394	0.409	0.469	0.354	0.333	—
S72.334A	Nondisplaced oblique fracture of shaft of right femur, initial encounter for closed fracture	170	Hip Fracture/Dislocation		0.350	0.394	0.409	0.469	0.354	0.333	—
S72.334B	Nondisplaced oblique fracture of shaft of right femur, initial encounter for open fracture type I or II	170	Hip Fracture/Dislocation		0.350	0.394	0.409	0.469	0.354	0.333	—
S72.334C	Nondisplaced oblique fracture of shaft of right femur, initial encounter for open fracture type IIIA, IIIB, or IIIC	170	Hip Fracture/Dislocation		0.350	0.394	0.409	0.469	0.354	0.333	—
S72.335A	Nondisplaced oblique fracture of shaft of left femur, initial encounter for closed fracture	170	Hip Fracture/Dislocation		0.350	0.394	0.409	0.469	0.354	0.333	—
S72.335B	Nondisplaced oblique fracture of shaft of left femur, initial encounter for open fracture type I or II	170	Hip Fracture/Dislocation		0.350	0.394	0.409	0.469	0.354	0.333	—
S72.335C	Nondisplaced oblique fracture of shaft of left femur, initial encounter for open fracture type IIIA, IIIB, or IIIC	170	Hip Fracture/Dislocation		0.350	0.394	0.409	0.469	0.354	0.333	—
S72.336A	Nondisplaced oblique fracture of shaft of unspecified femur, initial encounter for closed fracture	170	Hip Fracture/Dislocation		0.350	0.394	0.409	0.469	0.354	0.333	—
S72.336B	Nondisplaced oblique fracture of shaft of unspecified femur, initial encounter for open fracture type I or II	170	Hip Fracture/Dislocation		0.350	0.394	0.409	0.469	0.354	0.333	—
S72.336C	Nondisplaced oblique fracture of shaft of unspecified femur, initial encounter for open fracture type IIIA, IIIB, or IIIC	170	Hip Fracture/Dislocation		0.350	0.394	0.409	0.469	0.354	0.333	—
S72.341A	Displaced spiral fracture of shaft of right femur, initial encounter for closed fracture	170	Hip Fracture/Dislocation		0.350	0.394	0.409	0.469	0.354	0.333	—
S72.341B	Displaced spiral fracture of shaft of right femur, initial encounter for open fracture type I or II	170	Hip Fracture/Dislocation		0.350	0.394	0.409	0.469	0.354	0.333	—

ICD-10-CM Code	ICD-10-CM Code Description	V24 CMS-HCC	V24 CMS-HCC Disease Group	V24 CMS-HCC Hierarchies	Community, NonDual, Aged	Community, NonDual, Disabled	Community, FBDual, Aged	Community, FBDual, Disabled	Community, PBDual, Aged	Community, PBDual, Disabled	Institutional
S72.341C	Displaced spiral fracture of shaft of right femur, initial encounter for open fracture type IIIA, IIIB, or IIIC	170	Hip Fracture/Dislocation		0.350	0.394	0.409	0.469	0.354	0.333	—
S72.342A	Displaced spiral fracture of shaft of left femur, initial encounter for closed fracture	170	Hip Fracture/Dislocation		0.350	0.394	0.409	0.469	0.354	0.333	—
S72.342B	Displaced spiral fracture of shaft of left femur, initial encounter for open fracture type I or II	170	Hip Fracture/Dislocation		0.350	0.394	0.409	0.469	0.354	0.333	—
S72.342C	Displaced spiral fracture of shaft of left femur, initial encounter for open fracture type IIIA, IIIB, or IIIC	170	Hip Fracture/Dislocation		0.350	0.394	0.409	0.469	0.354	0.333	—
S72.343A	Displaced spiral fracture of shaft of unspecified femur, initial encounter for closed fracture	170	Hip Fracture/Dislocation		0.350	0.394	0.409	0.469	0.354	0.333	—
S72.343B	Displaced spiral fracture of shaft of unspecified femur, initial encounter for open fracture type I or II	170	Hip Fracture/Dislocation		0.350	0.394	0.409	0.469	0.354	0.333	—
S72.343C	Displaced spiral fracture of shaft of unspecified femur, initial encounter for open fracture type IIIA, IIIB, or IIIC	170	Hip Fracture/Dislocation		0.350	0.394	0.409	0.469	0.354	0.333	—
S72.344A	Nondisplaced spiral fracture of shaft of right femur, initial encounter for closed fracture	170	Hip Fracture/Dislocation		0.350	0.394	0.409	0.469	0.354	0.333	—
S72.344B	Nondisplaced spiral fracture of shaft of right femur, initial encounter for open fracture type I or II	170	Hip Fracture/Dislocation		0.350	0.394	0.409	0.469	0.354	0.333	—
S72.344C	Nondisplaced spiral fracture of shaft of right femur, initial encounter for open fracture type IIIA, IIIB, or IIIC	170	Hip Fracture/Dislocation		0.350	0.394	0.409	0.469	0.354	0.333	—
S72.345A	Nondisplaced spiral fracture of shaft of left femur, initial encounter for closed fracture	170	Hip Fracture/Dislocation		0.350	0.394	0.409	0.469	0.354	0.333	—
S72.345B	Nondisplaced spiral fracture of shaft of left femur, initial encounter for open fracture type I or II	170	Hip Fracture/Dislocation		0.350	0.394	0.409	0.469	0.354	0.333	—
S72.345C	Nondisplaced spiral fracture of shaft of left femur, initial encounter for open fracture type IIIA, IIIB, or IIIC	170	Hip Fracture/Dislocation		0.350	0.394	0.409	0.469	0.354	0.333	—
S72.346A	Nondisplaced spiral fracture of shaft of unspecified femur, initial encounter for closed fracture	170	Hip Fracture/Dislocation		0.350	0.394	0.409	0.469	0.354	0.333	—
S72.346B	Nondisplaced spiral fracture of shaft of unspecified femur, initial encounter for open fracture type I or II	170	Hip Fracture/Dislocation		0.350	0.394	0.409	0.469	0.354	0.333	—
S72.346C	Nondisplaced spiral fracture of shaft of unspecified femur, initial encounter for open fracture type IIIA, IIIB, or IIIC	170	Hip Fracture/Dislocation		0.350	0.394	0.409	0.469	0.354	0.333	—
S72.351A	Displaced comminuted fracture of shaft of right femur, initial encounter for closed fracture	170	Hip Fracture/Dislocation		0.350	0.394	0.409	0.469	0.354	0.333	—
S72.351B	Displaced comminuted fracture of shaft of right femur, initial encounter for open fracture type I or II	170	Hip Fracture/Dislocation		0.350	0.394	0.409	0.469	0.354	0.333	—
S72.351C	Displaced comminuted fracture of shaft of right femur, initial encounter for open fracture type IIIA, IIIB, or IIIC	170	Hip Fracture/Dislocation		0.350	0.394	0.409	0.469	0.354	0.333	—
S72.352A	Displaced comminuted fracture of shaft of left femur, initial encounter for closed fracture	170	Hip Fracture/Dislocation		0.350	0.394	0.409	0.469	0.354	0.333	—

ICD-10-CM Code	ICD-10-CM Code Description	V24 CMS-HCC	V24 CMS-HCC Disease Group	V24 CMS-HCC Hierarchies	Community, NonDual, Aged	Community, NonDual, Disabled	Community, FBDual, Aged	Community, FBDual, Disabled	Community, PBDual, Aged	Community, PBDual, Disabled	Institutional
S72.352B	Displaced comminuted fracture of shaft of left femur, initial encounter for open fracture type I or II	170	Hip Fracture/Dislocation		0.350	0.394	0.409	0.469	0.354	0.333	—
S72.352C	Displaced comminuted fracture of shaft of left femur, initial encounter for open fracture type IIIA, IIIB, or IIIC	170	Hip Fracture/Dislocation		0.350	0.394	0.409	0.469	0.354	0.333	—
S72.353A	Displaced comminuted fracture of shaft of unspecified femur, initial encounter for closed fracture	170	Hip Fracture/Dislocation		0.350	0.394	0.409	0.469	0.354	0.333	—
S72.353B	Displaced comminuted fracture of shaft of unspecified femur, initial encounter for open fracture type I or II	170	Hip Fracture/Dislocation		0.350	0.394	0.409	0.469	0.354	0.333	—
S72.353C	Displaced comminuted fracture of shaft of unspecified femur, initial encounter for open fracture type IIIA, IIIB, or IIIC	170	Hip Fracture/Dislocation		0.350	0.394	0.409	0.469	0.354	0.333	—
S72.354A	Nondisplaced comminuted fracture of shaft of right femur, initial encounter for closed fracture	170	Hip Fracture/Dislocation		0.350	0.394	0.409	0.469	0.354	0.333	—
S72.354B	Nondisplaced comminuted fracture of shaft of right femur, initial encounter for open fracture type I or II	170	Hip Fracture/Dislocation		0.350	0.394	0.409	0.469	0.354	0.333	—
S72.354C	Nondisplaced comminuted fracture of shaft of right femur, initial encounter for open fracture type IIIA, IIIB, or IIIC	170	Hip Fracture/Dislocation		0.350	0.394	0.409	0.469	0.354	0.333	—
S72.355A	Nondisplaced comminuted fracture of shaft of left femur, initial encounter for closed fracture	170	Hip Fracture/Dislocation		0.350	0.394	0.409	0.469	0.354	0.333	—
S72.355B	Nondisplaced comminuted fracture of shaft of left femur, initial encounter for open fracture type I or II	170	Hip Fracture/Dislocation		0.350	0.394	0.409	0.469	0.354	0.333	—
S72.355C	Nondisplaced comminuted fracture of shaft of left femur, initial encounter for open fracture type IIIA, IIIB, or IIIC	170	Hip Fracture/Dislocation		0.350	0.394	0.409	0.469	0.354	0.333	—
S72.356A	Nondisplaced comminuted fracture of shaft of unspecified femur, initial encounter for closed fracture	170	Hip Fracture/Dislocation		0.350	0.394	0.409	0.469	0.354	0.333	—
S72.356B	Nondisplaced comminuted fracture of shaft of unspecified femur, initial encounter for open fracture type I or II	170	Hip Fracture/Dislocation		0.350	0.394	0.409	0.469	0.354	0.333	—
S72.356C	Nondisplaced comminuted fracture of shaft of unspecified femur, initial encounter for open fracture type IIIA, IIIB, or IIIC	170	Hip Fracture/Dislocation		0.350	0.394	0.409	0.469	0.354	0.333	—
S72.361A	Displaced segmental fracture of shaft of right femur, initial encounter for closed fracture	170	Hip Fracture/Dislocation		0.350	0.394	0.409	0.469	0.354	0.333	—
S72.361B	Displaced segmental fracture of shaft of right femur, initial encounter for open fracture type I or II	170	Hip Fracture/Dislocation		0.350	0.394	0.409	0.469	0.354	0.333	—
S72.361C	Displaced segmental fracture of shaft of right femur, initial encounter for open fracture type IIIA, IIIB, or IIIC	170	Hip Fracture/Dislocation		0.350	0.394	0.409	0.469	0.354	0.333	—
S72.362A	Displaced segmental fracture of shaft of left femur, initial encounter for closed fracture	170	Hip Fracture/Dislocation		0.350	0.394	0.409	0.469	0.354	0.333	—

ICD-10-CM Code	ICD-10-CM Code Description	V24 CMS-HCC	V24 CMS-HCC Disease Group	V24 CMS-HCC Hierarchies	Community, NonDual, Aged	Community, NonDual, Disabled	Community, FBDual, Aged	Community, FBDual, Disabled	Community, PBDual, Aged	Community, PBDual, Disabled	Institutional
S72.362B	Displaced segmental fracture of shaft of left femur, initial encounter for open fracture type I or II	170	Hip Fracture/Dislocation		0.350	0.394	0.409	0.469	0.354	0.333	—
S72.362C	Displaced segmental fracture of shaft of left femur, initial encounter for open fracture type IIIA, IIIB, or IIIC	170	Hip Fracture/Dislocation		0.350	0.394	0.409	0.469	0.354	0.333	—
S72.363A	Displaced segmental fracture of shaft of unspecified femur, initial encounter for closed fracture	170	Hip Fracture/Dislocation		0.350	0.394	0.409	0.469	0.354	0.333	—
S72.363B	Displaced segmental fracture of shaft of unspecified femur, initial encounter for open fracture type I or II	170	Hip Fracture/Dislocation		0.350	0.394	0.409	0.469	0.354	0.333	—
S72.363C	Displaced segmental fracture of shaft of unspecified femur, initial encounter for open fracture type IIIA, IIIB, or IIIC	170	Hip Fracture/Dislocation		0.350	0.394	0.409	0.469	0.354	0.333	—
S72.364A	Nondisplaced segmental fracture of shaft of right femur, initial encounter for closed fracture	170	Hip Fracture/Dislocation		0.350	0.394	0.409	0.469	0.354	0.333	—
S72.364B	Nondisplaced segmental fracture of shaft of right femur, initial encounter for open fracture type I or II	170	Hip Fracture/Dislocation		0.350	0.394	0.409	0.469	0.354	0.333	—
S72.364C	Nondisplaced segmental fracture of shaft of right femur, initial encounter for open fracture type IIIA, IIIB, or IIIC	170	Hip Fracture/Dislocation		0.350	0.394	0.409	0.469	0.354	0.333	—
S72.365A	Nondisplaced segmental fracture of shaft of left femur, initial encounter for closed fracture	170	Hip Fracture/Dislocation		0.350	0.394	0.409	0.469	0.354	0.333	—
S72.365B	Nondisplaced segmental fracture of shaft of left femur, initial encounter for open fracture type I or II	170	Hip Fracture/Dislocation		0.350	0.394	0.409	0.469	0.354	0.333	—
S72.365C	Nondisplaced segmental fracture of shaft of left femur, initial encounter for open fracture type IIIA, IIIB, or IIIC	170	Hip Fracture/Dislocation		0.350	0.394	0.409	0.469	0.354	0.333	—
S72.366A	Nondisplaced segmental fracture of shaft of unspecified femur, initial encounter for closed fracture	170	Hip Fracture/Dislocation		0.350	0.394	0.409	0.469	0.354	0.333	—
S72.366B	Nondisplaced segmental fracture of shaft of unspecified femur, initial encounter for open fracture type I or II	170	Hip Fracture/Dislocation		0.350	0.394	0.409	0.469	0.354	0.333	—
S72.366C	Nondisplaced segmental fracture of shaft of unspecified femur, initial encounter for open fracture type IIIA, IIIB, or IIIC	170	Hip Fracture/Dislocation		0.350	0.394	0.409	0.469	0.354	0.333	—
S72.391A	Other fracture of shaft of right femur, initial encounter for closed fracture	170	Hip Fracture/Dislocation		0.350	0.394	0.409	0.469	0.354	0.333	—
S72.391B	Other fracture of shaft of right femur, initial encounter for open fracture type I or II	170	Hip Fracture/Dislocation		0.350	0.394	0.409	0.469	0.354	0.333	—
S72.391C	Other fracture of shaft of right femur, initial encounter for open fracture type IIIA, IIIB, or IIIC	170	Hip Fracture/Dislocation		0.350	0.394	0.409	0.469	0.354	0.333	—
S72.392A	Other fracture of shaft of left femur, initial encounter for closed fracture	170	Hip Fracture/Dislocation		0.350	0.394	0.409	0.469	0.354	0.333	—
S72.392B	Other fracture of shaft of left femur, initial encounter for open fracture type I or II	170	Hip Fracture/Dislocation		0.350	0.394	0.409	0.469	0.354	0.333	—
S72.392C	Other fracture of shaft of left femur, initial encounter for open fracture type IIIA, IIIB, or IIIC	170	Hip Fracture/Dislocation		0.350	0.394	0.409	0.469	0.354	0.333	—

ICD-10-CM Code	ICD-10-CM Code Description	V24 CMS-HCC	V24 CMS-HCC Disease Group	V24 CMS-HCC Hierarchies	Community, NonDual, Aged	Community, NonDual, Disabled	Community, FBDual, Aged	Community, FBDual, Disabled	Community, PBDual, Aged	Community, PBDual, Disabled	Institutional
S72.399A	Other fracture of shaft of unspecified femur, initial encounter for closed fracture	170	Hip Fracture/Dislocation		0.350	0.394	0.409	0.469	0.354	0.333	—
S72.399B	Other fracture of shaft of unspecified femur, initial encounter for open fracture type I or II	170	Hip Fracture/Dislocation		0.350	0.394	0.409	0.469	0.354	0.333	—
S72.399C	Other fracture of shaft of unspecified femur, initial encounter for open fracture type IIIA, IIIB, or IIIC	170	Hip Fracture/Dislocation		0.350	0.394	0.409	0.469	0.354	0.333	—
S72.401A	Unspecified fracture of lower end of right femur, initial encounter for closed fracture	170	Hip Fracture/Dislocation		0.350	0.394	0.409	0.469	0.354	0.333	—
S72.401B	Unspecified fracture of lower end of right femur, initial encounter for open fracture type I or II	170	Hip Fracture/Dislocation		0.350	0.394	0.409	0.469	0.354	0.333	—
S72.401C	Unspecified fracture of lower end of right femur, initial encounter for open fracture type IIIA, IIIB, or IIIC	170	Hip Fracture/Dislocation		0.350	0.394	0.409	0.469	0.354	0.333	—
S72.402A	Unspecified fracture of lower end of left femur, initial encounter for closed fracture	170	Hip Fracture/Dislocation		0.350	0.394	0.409	0.469	0.354	0.333	—
S72.402B	Unspecified fracture of lower end of left femur, initial encounter for open fracture type I or II	170	Hip Fracture/Dislocation		0.350	0.394	0.409	0.469	0.354	0.333	—
S72.402C	Unspecified fracture of lower end of left femur, initial encounter for open fracture type IIIA, IIIB, or IIIC	170	Hip Fracture/Dislocation		0.350	0.394	0.409	0.469	0.354	0.333	—
S72.409A	Unspecified fracture of lower end of unspecified femur, initial encounter for closed fracture	170	Hip Fracture/Dislocation		0.350	0.394	0.409	0.469	0.354	0.333	—
S72.409B	Unspecified fracture of lower end of unspecified femur, initial encounter for open fracture type I or II	170	Hip Fracture/Dislocation		0.350	0.394	0.409	0.469	0.354	0.333	—
S72.409C	Unspecified fracture of lower end of unspecified femur, initial encounter for open fracture type IIIA, IIIB, or IIIC	170	Hip Fracture/Dislocation		0.350	0.394	0.409	0.469	0.354	0.333	—
S72.411A	Displaced unspecified condyle fracture of lower end of right femur, initial encounter for closed fracture	170	Hip Fracture/Dislocation		0.350	0.394	0.409	0.469	0.354	0.333	—
S72.411B	Displaced unspecified condyle fracture of lower end of right femur, initial encounter for open fracture type I or II	170	Hip Fracture/Dislocation		0.350	0.394	0.409	0.469	0.354	0.333	—
S72.411C	Displaced unspecified condyle fracture of lower end of right femur, initial encounter for open fracture type IIIA, IIIB, or IIIC	170	Hip Fracture/Dislocation		0.350	0.394	0.409	0.469	0.354	0.333	—
S72.412A	Displaced unspecified condyle fracture of lower end of left femur, initial encounter for closed fracture	170	Hip Fracture/Dislocation		0.350	0.394	0.409	0.469	0.354	0.333	—
S72.412B	Displaced unspecified condyle fracture of lower end of left femur, initial encounter for open fracture type I or II	170	Hip Fracture/Dislocation		0.350	0.394	0.409	0.469	0.354	0.333	—
S72.412C	Displaced unspecified condyle fracture of lower end of left femur, initial encounter for open fracture type IIIA, IIIB, or IIIC	170	Hip Fracture/Dislocation		0.350	0.394	0.409	0.469	0.354	0.333	—
S72.413A	Displaced unspecified condyle fracture of lower end of unspecified femur, initial encounter for closed fracture	170	Hip Fracture/Dislocation		0.350	0.394	0.409	0.469	0.354	0.333	—

ICD-10-CM Code	ICD-10-CM Code Description	V24 CMS-HCC	V24 CMS-HCC Disease Group	V24 CMS-HCC Hierarchies	Community, NonDual, Aged	Community, NonDual, Disabled	Community, FBDual, Aged	Community, FBDual, Disabled	Community, PBDual, Aged	Community, PBDual, Disabled	Institutional
S72.413B	Displaced unspecified condyle fracture of lower end of unspecified femur, initial encounter for open fracture type I or II	170	Hip Fracture/Dislocation		0.350	0.394	0.409	0.469	0.354	0.333	—
S72.413C	Displaced unspecified condyle fracture of lower end of unspecified femur, initial encounter for open fracture type IIIA, IIIB, or IIIC	170	Hip Fracture/Dislocation		0.350	0.394	0.409	0.469	0.354	0.333	—
S72.414A	Nondisplaced unspecified condyle fracture of lower end of right femur, initial encounter for closed fracture	170	Hip Fracture/Dislocation		0.350	0.394	0.409	0.469	0.354	0.333	—
S72.414B	Nondisplaced unspecified condyle fracture of lower end of right femur, initial encounter for open fracture type I or II	170	Hip Fracture/Dislocation		0.350	0.394	0.409	0.469	0.354	0.333	—
S72.414C	Nondisplaced unspecified condyle fracture of lower end of right femur, initial encounter for open fracture type IIIA, IIIB, or IIIC	170	Hip Fracture/Dislocation		0.350	0.394	0.409	0.469	0.354	0.333	—
S72.415A	Nondisplaced unspecified condyle fracture of lower end of left femur, initial encounter for closed fracture	170	Hip Fracture/Dislocation		0.350	0.394	0.409	0.469	0.354	0.333	—
S72.415B	Nondisplaced unspecified condyle fracture of lower end of left femur, initial encounter for open fracture type I or II	170	Hip Fracture/Dislocation		0.350	0.394	0.409	0.469	0.354	0.333	—
S72.415C	Nondisplaced unspecified condyle fracture of lower end of left femur, initial encounter for open fracture type IIIA, IIIB, or IIIC	170	Hip Fracture/Dislocation		0.350	0.394	0.409	0.469	0.354	0.333	—
S72.416A	Nondisplaced unspecified condyle fracture of lower end of unspecified femur, initial encounter for closed fracture	170	Hip Fracture/Dislocation		0.350	0.394	0.409	0.469	0.354	0.333	—
S72.416B	Nondisplaced unspecified condyle fracture of lower end of unspecified femur, initial encounter for open fracture type I or II	170	Hip Fracture/Dislocation		0.350	0.394	0.409	0.469	0.354	0.333	—
S72.416C	Nondisplaced unspecified condyle fracture of lower end of unspecified femur, initial encounter for open fracture type IIIA, IIIB, or IIIC	170	Hip Fracture/Dislocation		0.350	0.394	0.409	0.469	0.354	0.333	—
S72.421A	Displaced fracture of lateral condyle of right femur, initial encounter for closed fracture	170	Hip Fracture/Dislocation		0.350	0.394	0.409	0.469	0.354	0.333	—
S72.421B	Displaced fracture of lateral condyle of right femur, initial encounter for open fracture type I or II	170	Hip Fracture/Dislocation		0.350	0.394	0.409	0.469	0.354	0.333	—
S72.421C	Displaced fracture of lateral condyle of right femur, initial encounter for open fracture type IIIA, IIIB, or IIIC	170	Hip Fracture/Dislocation		0.350	0.394	0.409	0.469	0.354	0.333	—
S72.422A	Displaced fracture of lateral condyle of left femur, initial encounter for closed fracture	170	Hip Fracture/Dislocation		0.350	0.394	0.409	0.469	0.354	0.333	—
S72.422B	Displaced fracture of lateral condyle of left femur, initial encounter for open fracture type I or II	170	Hip Fracture/Dislocation		0.350	0.394	0.409	0.469	0.354	0.333	—
S72.422C	Displaced fracture of lateral condyle of left femur, initial encounter for open fracture type IIIA, IIIB, or IIIC	170	Hip Fracture/Dislocation		0.350	0.394	0.409	0.469	0.354	0.333	—

ICD-10-CM Code	ICD-10-CM Code Description	V24 CMS-HCC	V24 CMS-HCC Disease Group	V24 CMS-HCC Hierarchies	Community, NonDual, Aged	Community, NonDual, Disabled	Community, FBDual, Aged	Community, FBDual, Disabled	Community, PBDual, Aged	Community, PBDual, Disabled	Institutional
S72.423A	Displaced fracture of lateral condyle of unspecified femur, initial encounter for closed fracture	170	Hip Fracture/Dislocation		0.350	0.394	0.409	0.469	0.354	0.333	—
S72.423B	Displaced fracture of lateral condyle of unspecified femur, initial encounter for open fracture type I or II	170	Hip Fracture/Dislocation		0.350	0.394	0.409	0.469	0.354	0.333	—
S72.423C	Displaced fracture of lateral condyle of unspecified femur, initial encounter for open fracture type IIIA, IIIB, or IIIC	170	Hip Fracture/Dislocation		0.350	0.394	0.409	0.469	0.354	0.333	—
S72.424A	Nondisplaced fracture of lateral condyle of right femur, initial encounter for closed fracture	170	Hip Fracture/Dislocation		0.350	0.394	0.409	0.469	0.354	0.333	—
S72.424B	Nondisplaced fracture of lateral condyle of right femur, initial encounter for open fracture type I or II	170	Hip Fracture/Dislocation		0.350	0.394	0.409	0.469	0.354	0.333	—
S72.424C	Nondisplaced fracture of lateral condyle of right femur, initial encounter for open fracture type IIIA, IIIB, or IIIC	170	Hip Fracture/Dislocation		0.350	0.394	0.409	0.469	0.354	0.333	—
S72.425A	Nondisplaced fracture of lateral condyle of left femur, initial encounter for closed fracture	170	Hip Fracture/Dislocation		0.350	0.394	0.409	0.469	0.354	0.333	—
S72.425B	Nondisplaced fracture of lateral condyle of left femur, initial encounter for open fracture type I or II	170	Hip Fracture/Dislocation		0.350	0.394	0.409	0.469	0.354	0.333	—
S72.425C	Nondisplaced fracture of lateral condyle of left femur, initial encounter for open fracture type IIIA, IIIB, or IIIC	170	Hip Fracture/Dislocation		0.350	0.394	0.409	0.469	0.354	0.333	—
S72.426A	Nondisplaced fracture of lateral condyle of unspecified femur, initial encounter for closed fracture	170	Hip Fracture/Dislocation		0.350	0.394	0.409	0.469	0.354	0.333	—
S72.426B	Nondisplaced fracture of lateral condyle of unspecified femur, initial encounter for open fracture type I or II	170	Hip Fracture/Dislocation		0.350	0.394	0.409	0.469	0.354	0.333	—
S72.426C	Nondisplaced fracture of lateral condyle of unspecified femur, initial encounter for open fracture type IIIA, IIIB, or IIIC	170	Hip Fracture/Dislocation		0.350	0.394	0.409	0.469	0.354	0.333	—
S72.431A	Displaced fracture of medial condyle of right femur, initial encounter for closed fracture	170	Hip Fracture/Dislocation		0.350	0.394	0.409	0.469	0.354	0.333	—
S72.431B	Displaced fracture of medial condyle of right femur, initial encounter for open fracture type I or II	170	Hip Fracture/Dislocation		0.350	0.394	0.409	0.469	0.354	0.333	—
S72.431C	Displaced fracture of medial condyle of right femur, initial encounter for open fracture type IIIA, IIIB, or IIIC	170	Hip Fracture/Dislocation		0.350	0.394	0.409	0.469	0.354	0.333	—
S72.432A	Displaced fracture of medial condyle of left femur, initial encounter for closed fracture	170	Hip Fracture/Dislocation		0.350	0.394	0.409	0.469	0.354	0.333	—
S72.432B	Displaced fracture of medial condyle of left femur, initial encounter for open fracture type I or II	170	Hip Fracture/Dislocation		0.350	0.394	0.409	0.469	0.354	0.333	—
S72.432C	Displaced fracture of medial condyle of left femur, initial encounter for open fracture type IIIA, IIIB, or IIIC	170	Hip Fracture/Dislocation		0.350	0.394	0.409	0.469	0.354	0.333	—

ICD-10-CM Code	ICD-10-CM Code Description	V24 CMS-HCC	V24 CMS-HCC Disease Group	V24 CMS-HCC Hierarchies	Community, NonDual, Aged	Community, NonDual, Disabled	Community, FBDual, Aged	Community, FBDual, Disabled	Community, PBDual, Aged	Community, PBDual, Disabled	Institutional
S72.433A	Displaced fracture of medial condyle of unspecified femur, initial encounter for closed fracture	170	Hip Fracture/Dislocation		0.350	0.394	0.409	0.469	0.354	0.333	—
S72.433B	Displaced fracture of medial condyle of unspecified femur, initial encounter for open fracture type I or II	170	Hip Fracture/Dislocation		0.350	0.394	0.409	0.469	0.354	0.333	—
S72.433C	Displaced fracture of medial condyle of unspecified femur, initial encounter for open fracture type IIIA, IIIB, or IIIC	170	Hip Fracture/Dislocation		0.350	0.394	0.409	0.469	0.354	0.333	—
S72.434A	Nondisplaced fracture of medial condyle of right femur, initial encounter for closed fracture	170	Hip Fracture/Dislocation		0.350	0.394	0.409	0.469	0.354	0.333	—
S72.434B	Nondisplaced fracture of medial condyle of right femur, initial encounter for open fracture type I or II	170	Hip Fracture/Dislocation		0.350	0.394	0.409	0.469	0.354	0.333	—
S72.434C	Nondisplaced fracture of medial condyle of right femur, initial encounter for open fracture type IIIA, IIIB, or IIIC	170	Hip Fracture/Dislocation		0.350	0.394	0.409	0.469	0.354	0.333	—
S72.435A	Nondisplaced fracture of medial condyle of left femur, initial encounter for closed fracture	170	Hip Fracture/Dislocation		0.350	0.394	0.409	0.469	0.354	0.333	—
S72.435B	Nondisplaced fracture of medial condyle of left femur, initial encounter for open fracture type I or II	170	Hip Fracture/Dislocation		0.350	0.394	0.409	0.469	0.354	0.333	—
S72.435C	Nondisplaced fracture of medial condyle of left femur, initial encounter for open fracture type IIIA, IIIB, or IIIC	170	Hip Fracture/Dislocation		0.350	0.394	0.409	0.469	0.354	0.333	—
S72.436A	Nondisplaced fracture of medial condyle of unspecified femur, initial encounter for closed fracture	170	Hip Fracture/Dislocation		0.350	0.394	0.409	0.469	0.354	0.333	—
S72.436B	Nondisplaced fracture of medial condyle of unspecified femur, initial encounter for open fracture type I or II	170	Hip Fracture/Dislocation		0.350	0.394	0.409	0.469	0.354	0.333	—
S72.436C	Nondisplaced fracture of medial condyle of unspecified femur, initial encounter for open fracture type IIIA, IIIB, or IIIC	170	Hip Fracture/Dislocation		0.350	0.394	0.409	0.469	0.354	0.333	—
S72.441A	Displaced fracture of lower epiphysis (separation) of right femur, initial encounter for closed fracture	170	Hip Fracture/Dislocation		0.350	0.394	0.409	0.469	0.354	0.333	—
S72.441B	Displaced fracture of lower epiphysis (separation) of right femur, initial encounter for open fracture type I or II	170	Hip Fracture/Dislocation		0.350	0.394	0.409	0.469	0.354	0.333	—
S72.441C	Displaced fracture of lower epiphysis (separation) of right femur, initial encounter for open fracture type IIIA, IIIB, or IIIC	170	Hip Fracture/Dislocation		0.350	0.394	0.409	0.469	0.354	0.333	—
S72.442A	Displaced fracture of lower epiphysis (separation) of left femur, initial encounter for closed fracture	170	Hip Fracture/Dislocation		0.350	0.394	0.409	0.469	0.354	0.333	—
S72.442B	Displaced fracture of lower epiphysis (separation) of left femur, initial encounter for open fracture type I or II	170	Hip Fracture/Dislocation		0.350	0.394	0.409	0.469	0.354	0.333	—

ICD-10-CM Code	ICD-10-CM Code Description	V24 CMS-HCC	V24 CMS-HCC Disease Group	V24 CMS-HCC Hierarchies	Community, NonDual, Aged	Community, NonDual, Disabled	Community, FBDual, Aged	Community, FBDual, Disabled	Community, PBDual, Aged	Community, PBDual, Disabled	Institutional
S72.442C	Displaced fracture of lower epiphysis (separation) of left femur, initial encounter for open fracture type IIIA, IIIB, or IIIC	170	Hip Fracture/Dislocation		0.350	0.394	0.409	0.469	0.354	0.333	—
S72.443A	Displaced fracture of lower epiphysis (separation) of unspecified femur, initial encounter for closed fracture	170	Hip Fracture/Dislocation		0.350	0.394	0.409	0.469	0.354	0.333	—
S72.443B	Displaced fracture of lower epiphysis (separation) of unspecified femur, initial encounter for open fracture type I or II	170	Hip Fracture/Dislocation		0.350	0.394	0.409	0.469	0.354	0.333	—
S72.443C	Displaced fracture of lower epiphysis (separation) of unspecified femur, initial encounter for open fracture type IIIA, IIIB, or IIIC	170	Hip Fracture/Dislocation		0.350	0.394	0.409	0.469	0.354	0.333	—
S72.444A	Nondisplaced fracture of lower epiphysis (separation) of right femur, initial encounter for closed fracture	170	Hip Fracture/Dislocation		0.350	0.394	0.409	0.469	0.354	0.333	—
S72.444B	Nondisplaced fracture of lower epiphysis (separation) of right femur, initial encounter for open fracture type I or II	170	Hip Fracture/Dislocation		0.350	0.394	0.409	0.469	0.354	0.333	—
S72.444C	Nondisplaced fracture of lower epiphysis (separation) of right femur, initial encounter for open fracture type IIIA, IIIB, or IIIC	170	Hip Fracture/Dislocation		0.350	0.394	0.409	0.469	0.354	0.333	—
S72.445A	Nondisplaced fracture of lower epiphysis (separation) of left femur, initial encounter for closed fracture	170	Hip Fracture/Dislocation		0.350	0.394	0.409	0.469	0.354	0.333	—
S72.445B	Nondisplaced fracture of lower epiphysis (separation) of left femur, initial encounter for open fracture type I or II	170	Hip Fracture/Dislocation		0.350	0.394	0.409	0.469	0.354	0.333	—
S72.445C	Nondisplaced fracture of lower epiphysis (separation) of left femur, initial encounter for open fracture type IIIA, IIIB, or IIIC	170	Hip Fracture/Dislocation		0.350	0.394	0.409	0.469	0.354	0.333	—
S72.446A	Nondisplaced fracture of lower epiphysis (separation) of unspecified femur, initial encounter for closed fracture	170	Hip Fracture/Dislocation		0.350	0.394	0.409	0.469	0.354	0.333	—
S72.446B	Nondisplaced fracture of lower epiphysis (separation) of unspecified femur, initial encounter for open fracture type I or II	170	Hip Fracture/Dislocation		0.350	0.394	0.409	0.469	0.354	0.333	—
S72.446C	Nondisplaced fracture of lower epiphysis (separation) of unspecified femur, initial encounter for open fracture type IIIA, IIIB, or IIIC	170	Hip Fracture/Dislocation		0.350	0.394	0.409	0.469	0.354	0.333	—
S72.451A	Displaced supracondylar fracture without intracondylar extension of lower end of right femur, initial encounter for closed fracture	170	Hip Fracture/Dislocation		0.350	0.394	0.409	0.469	0.354	0.333	—
S72.451B	Displaced supracondylar fracture without intracondylar extension of lower end of right femur, initial encounter for open fracture type I or II	170	Hip Fracture/Dislocation		0.350	0.394	0.409	0.469	0.354	0.333	—
S72.451C	Displaced supracondylar fracture without intracondylar extension of lower end of right femur, initial encounter for open fracture type IIIA, IIIB, or IIIC	170	Hip Fracture/Dislocation		0.350	0.394	0.409	0.469	0.354	0.333	—

2021 Optum360, LLC

ICD-10-CM Code	ICD-10-CM Code Description	V24 CMS-HCC	V24 CMS-HCC Disease Group	V24 CMS-HCC Hierarchies	Community, NonDual, Aged	Community, NonDual, Disabled	Community, FBDual, Aged	Community, FBDual, Disabled	Community, PBDual, Aged	Community, PBDual, Disabled	Institutional
S72.452A	Displaced supracondylar fracture without intracondylar extension of lower end of left femur, initial encounter for closed fracture	170	Hip Fracture/Dislocation		0.350	0.394	0.409	0.469	0.354	0.333	—
S72.452B	Displaced supracondylar fracture without intracondylar extension of lower end of left femur, initial encounter for open fracture type I or II	170	Hip Fracture/Dislocation		0.350	0.394	0.409	0.469	0.354	0.333	—
S72.452C	Displaced supracondylar fracture without intracondylar extension of lower end of left femur, initial encounter for open fracture type IIIA, IIIB, or IIIC	170	Hip Fracture/Dislocation		0.350	0.394	0.409	0.469	0.354	0.333	—
S72.453A	Displaced supracondylar fracture without intracondylar extension of lower end of unspecified femur, initial encounter for closed fracture	170	Hip Fracture/Dislocation		0.350	0.394	0.409	0.469	0.354	0.333	—
S72.453B	Displaced supracondylar fracture without intracondylar extension of lower end of unspecified femur, initial encounter for open fracture type I or II	170	Hip Fracture/Dislocation		0.350	0.394	0.409	0.469	0.354	0.333	—
S72.453C	Displaced supracondylar fracture without intracondylar extension of lower end of unspecified femur, initial encounter for open fracture type IIIA, IIIB, or IIIC	170	Hip Fracture/Dislocation		0.350	0.394	0.409	0.469	0.354	0.333	—
S72.454A	Nondisplaced supracondylar fracture without intracondylar extension of lower end of right femur, initial encounter for closed fracture	170	Hip Fracture/Dislocation		0.350	0.394	0.409	0.469	0.354	0.333	—
S72.454B	Nondisplaced supracondylar fracture without intracondylar extension of lower end of right femur, initial encounter for open fracture type I or II	170	Hip Fracture/Dislocation		0.350	0.394	0.409	0.469	0.354	0.333	—
S72.454C	Nondisplaced supracondylar fracture without intracondylar extension of lower end of right femur, initial encounter for open fracture type IIIA, IIIB, or IIIC	170	Hip Fracture/Dislocation		0.350	0.394	0.409	0.469	0.354	0.333	—
S72.455A	Nondisplaced supracondylar fracture without intracondylar extension of lower end of left femur, initial encounter for closed fracture	170	Hip Fracture/Dislocation		0.350	0.394	0.409	0.469	0.354	0.333	—
S72.455B	Nondisplaced supracondylar fracture without intracondylar extension of lower end of left femur, initial encounter for open fracture type I or II	170	Hip Fracture/Dislocation		0.350	0.394	0.409	0.469	0.354	0.333	—
S72.455C	Nondisplaced supracondylar fracture without intracondylar extension of lower end of left femur, initial encounter for open fracture type IIIA, IIIB, or IIIC	170	Hip Fracture/Dislocation		0.350	0.394	0.409	0.469	0.354	0.333	—
S72.456A	Nondisplaced supracondylar fracture without intracondylar extension of lower end of unspecified femur, initial encounter for closed fracture	170	Hip Fracture/Dislocation		0.350	0.394	0.409	0.469	0.354	0.333	—

ICD-10-CM Code	ICD-10-CM Code Description	V24 CMS-HCC	V24 CMS-HCC Disease Group	V24 CMS-HCC Hierarchies	Community, NonDual, Aged	Community, NonDual, Disabled	Community, FBDual, Aged	Community, FBDual, Disabled	Community, PBDual, Aged	Community, PBDual, Disabled	Institutional
S72.456B	Nondisplaced supracondylar fracture without intracondylar extension of lower end of unspecified femur, initial encounter for open fracture type I or II	170	Hip Fracture/Dislocation		0.350	0.394	0.409	0.469	0.354	0.333	—
S72.456C	Nondisplaced supracondylar fracture without intracondylar extension of lower end of unspecified femur, initial encounter for open fracture type IIIA, IIIB, or IIIC	170	Hip Fracture/Dislocation		0.350	0.394	0.409	0.469	0.354	0.333	—
S72.461A	Displaced supracondylar fracture with intracondylar extension of lower end of right femur, initial encounter for closed fracture	170	Hip Fracture/Dislocation		0.350	0.394	0.409	0.469	0.354	0.333	—
S72.461B	Displaced supracondylar fracture with intracondylar extension of lower end of right femur, initial encounter for open fracture type I or II	170	Hip Fracture/Dislocation		0.350	0.394	0.409	0.469	0.354	0.333	—
S72.461C	Displaced supracondylar fracture with intracondylar extension of lower end of right femur, initial encounter for open fracture type IIIA, IIIB, or IIIC	170	Hip Fracture/Dislocation		0.350	0.394	0.409	0.469	0.354	0.333	—
S72.462A	Displaced supracondylar fracture with intracondylar extension of lower end of left femur, initial encounter for closed fracture	170	Hip Fracture/Dislocation		0.350	0.394	0.409	0.469	0.354	0.333	—
S72.462B	Displaced supracondylar fracture with intracondylar extension of lower end of left femur, initial encounter for open fracture type I or II	170	Hip Fracture/Dislocation		0.350	0.394	0.409	0.469	0.354	0.333	—
S72.462C	Displaced supracondylar fracture with intracondylar extension of lower end of left femur, initial encounter for open fracture type IIIA, IIIB, or IIIC	170	Hip Fracture/Dislocation		0.350	0.394	0.409	0.469	0.354	0.333	—
S72.463A	Displaced supracondylar fracture with intracondylar extension of lower end of unspecified femur, initial encounter for closed fracture	170	Hip Fracture/Dislocation		0.350	0.394	0.409	0.469	0.354	0.333	—
S72.463B	Displaced supracondylar fracture with intracondylar extension of lower end of unspecified femur, initial encounter for open fracture type I or II	170	Hip Fracture/Dislocation		0.350	0.394	0.409	0.469	0.354	0.333	—
S72.463C	Displaced supracondylar fracture with intracondylar extension of lower end of unspecified femur, initial encounter for open fracture type IIIA, IIIB, or IIIC	170	Hip Fracture/Dislocation		0.350	0.394	0.409	0.469	0.354	0.333	—
S72.464A	Nondisplaced supracondylar fracture with intracondylar extension of lower end of right femur, initial encounter for closed fracture	170	Hip Fracture/Dislocation		0.350	0.394	0.409	0.469	0.354	0.333	—
S72.464B	Nondisplaced supracondylar fracture with intracondylar extension of lower end of right femur, initial encounter for open fracture type I or II	170	Hip Fracture/Dislocation		0.350	0.394	0.409	0.469	0.354	0.333	—
S72.464C	Nondisplaced supracondylar fracture with intracondylar extension of lower end of right femur, initial encounter for open fracture type IIIA, IIIB, or IIIC	170	Hip Fracture/Dislocation		0.350	0.394	0.409	0.469	0.354	0.333	—

ICD-10-CM Code	ICD-10-CM Code Description	V24 CMS-HCC	V24 CMS-HCC Disease Group	V24 CMS-HCC Hierarchies	Community, NonDual, Aged	Community, NonDual, Disabled	Community, FBDual, Aged	Community, FBDual, Disabled	Community, PBDual, Aged	Community, PBDual, Disabled	Institutional
S72.465A	Nondisplaced supracondylar fracture with intracondylar extension of lower end of left femur, initial encounter for closed fracture	170	Hip Fracture/Dislocation		0.350	0.394	0.409	0.469	0.354	0.333	—
S72.465B	Nondisplaced supracondylar fracture with intracondylar extension of lower end of left femur, initial encounter for open fracture type I or II	170	Hip Fracture/Dislocation		0.350	0.394	0.409	0.469	0.354	0.333	—
S72.465C	Nondisplaced supracondylar fracture with intracondylar extension of lower end of left femur, initial encounter for open fracture type IIIA, IIIB, or IIIC	170	Hip Fracture/Dislocation		0.350	0.394	0.409	0.469	0.354	0.333	—
S72.466A	Nondisplaced supracondylar fracture with intracondylar extension of lower end of unspecified femur, initial encounter for closed fracture	170	Hip Fracture/Dislocation		0.350	0.394	0.409	0.469	0.354	0.333	—
S72.466B	Nondisplaced supracondylar fracture with intracondylar extension of lower end of unspecified femur, initial encounter for open fracture type I or II	170	Hip Fracture/Dislocation		0.350	0.394	0.409	0.469	0.354	0.333	—
S72.466C	Nondisplaced supracondylar fracture with intracondylar extension of lower end of unspecified femur, initial encounter for open fracture type IIIA, IIIB, or IIIC	170	Hip Fracture/Dislocation		0.350	0.394	0.409	0.469	0.354	0.333	—
S72.471A	Torus fracture of lower end of right femur, initial encounter for closed fracture	170	Hip Fracture/Dislocation		0.350	0.394	0.409	0.469	0.354	0.333	—
S72.472A	Torus fracture of lower end of left femur, initial encounter for closed fracture	170	Hip Fracture/Dislocation		0.350	0.394	0.409	0.469	0.354	0.333	—
S72.479A	Torus fracture of lower end of unspecified femur, initial encounter for closed fracture	170	Hip Fracture/Dislocation		0.350	0.394	0.409	0.469	0.354	0.333	—
S72.491A	Other fracture of lower end of right femur, initial encounter for closed fracture	170	Hip Fracture/Dislocation		0.350	0.394	0.409	0.469	0.354	0.333	—
S72.491B	Other fracture of lower end of right femur, initial encounter for open fracture type I or II	170	Hip Fracture/Dislocation		0.350	0.394	0.409	0.469	0.354	0.333	—
S72.491C	Other fracture of lower end of right femur, initial encounter for open fracture type IIIA, IIIB, or IIIC	170	Hip Fracture/Dislocation		0.350	0.394	0.409	0.469	0.354	0.333	—
S72.492A	Other fracture of lower end of left femur, initial encounter for closed fracture	170	Hip Fracture/Dislocation		0.350	0.394	0.409	0.469	0.354	0.333	—
S72.492B	Other fracture of lower end of left femur, initial encounter for open fracture type I or II	170	Hip Fracture/Dislocation		0.350	0.394	0.409	0.469	0.354	0.333	—
S72.492C	Other fracture of lower end of left femur, initial encounter for open fracture type IIIA, IIIB, or IIIC	170	Hip Fracture/Dislocation		0.350	0.394	0.409	0.469	0.354	0.333	—
S72.499A	Other fracture of lower end of unspecified femur, initial encounter for closed fracture	170	Hip Fracture/Dislocation		0.350	0.394	0.409	0.469	0.354	0.333	—
S72.499B	Other fracture of lower end of unspecified femur, initial encounter for open fracture type I or II	170	Hip Fracture/Dislocation		0.350	0.394	0.409	0.469	0.354	0.333	—
S72.499C	Other fracture of lower end of unspecified femur, initial encounter for open fracture type IIIA, IIIB, or IIIC	170	Hip Fracture/Dislocation		0.350	0.394	0.409	0.469	0.354	0.333	—

ICD-10-CM Code	ICD-10-CM Code Description	V24 CMS-HCC	V24 CMS-HCC Disease Group	V24 CMS-HCC Hierarchies	Community, NonDual, Aged	Community, NonDual, Disabled	Community, FBDual, Aged	Community, FBDual, Disabled	Community, PBDual, Aged	Community, PBDual, Disabled	Institutional
S72.8X1A	Other fracture of right femur, initial encounter for closed fracture	170	Hip Fracture/Dislocation		0.350	0.394	0.409	0.469	0.354	0.333	—
S72.8X1B	Other fracture of right femur, initial encounter for open fracture type I or II	170	Hip Fracture/Dislocation		0.350	0.394	0.409	0.469	0.354	0.333	—
S72.8X1C	Other fracture of right femur, initial encounter for open fracture type IIIA, IIIB, or IIIC	170	Hip Fracture/Dislocation		0.350	0.394	0.409	0.469	0.354	0.333	—
S72.8X2A	Other fracture of left femur, initial encounter for closed fracture	170	Hip Fracture/Dislocation		0.350	0.394	0.409	0.469	0.354	0.333	—
S72.8X2B	Other fracture of left femur, initial encounter for open fracture type I or II	170	Hip Fracture/Dislocation		0.350	0.394	0.409	0.469	0.354	0.333	—
S72.8X2C	Other fracture of left femur, initial encounter for open fracture type IIIA, IIIB, or IIIC	170	Hip Fracture/Dislocation		0.350	0.394	0.409	0.469	0.354	0.333	—
S72.8X9A	Other fracture of unspecified femur, initial encounter for closed fracture	170	Hip Fracture/Dislocation		0.350	0.394	0.409	0.469	0.354	0.333	—
S72.8X9B	Other fracture of unspecified femur, initial encounter for open fracture type I or II	170	Hip Fracture/Dislocation		0.350	0.394	0.409	0.469	0.354	0.333	—
S72.8X9C	Other fracture of unspecified femur, initial encounter for open fracture type IIIA, IIIB, or IIIC	170	Hip Fracture/Dislocation		0.350	0.394	0.409	0.469	0.354	0.333	—
S72.90XA	Unspecified fracture of unspecified femur, initial encounter for closed fracture	170	Hip Fracture/Dislocation		0.350	0.394	0.409	0.469	0.354	0.333	—
S72.90XB	Unspecified fracture of unspecified femur, initial encounter for open fracture type I or II	170	Hip Fracture/Dislocation		0.350	0.394	0.409	0.469	0.354	0.333	—
S72.90XC	Unspecified fracture of unspecified femur, initial encounter for open fracture type IIIA, IIIB, or IIIC	170	Hip Fracture/Dislocation		0.350	0.394	0.409	0.469	0.354	0.333	—
S72.91XA	Unspecified fracture of right femur, initial encounter for closed fracture	170	Hip Fracture/Dislocation		0.350	0.394	0.409	0.469	0.354	0.333	—
S72.91XB	Unspecified fracture of right femur, initial encounter for open fracture type I or II	170	Hip Fracture/Dislocation		0.350	0.394	0.409	0.469	0.354	0.333	—
S72.91XC	Unspecified fracture of right femur, initial encounter for open fracture type IIIA, IIIB, or IIIC	170	Hip Fracture/Dislocation		0.350	0.394	0.409	0.469	0.354	0.333	—
S72.92XA	Unspecified fracture of left femur, initial encounter for closed fracture	170	Hip Fracture/Dislocation		0.350	0.394	0.409	0.469	0.354	0.333	—
S72.92XB	Unspecified fracture of left femur, initial encounter for open fracture type I or II	170	Hip Fracture/Dislocation		0.350	0.394	0.409	0.469	0.354	0.333	—
S72.92XC	Unspecified fracture of left femur, initial encounter for open fracture type IIIA, IIIB, or IIIC	170	Hip Fracture/Dislocation		0.350	0.394	0.409	0.469	0.354	0.333	—
S73.001A	Unspecified subluxation of right hip, initial encounter	170	Hip Fracture/Dislocation		0.350	0.394	0.409	0.469	0.354	0.333	—
S73.002A	Unspecified subluxation of left hip, initial encounter	170	Hip Fracture/Dislocation		0.350	0.394	0.409	0.469	0.354	0.333	—
S73.003A	Unspecified subluxation of unspecified hip, initial encounter	170	Hip Fracture/Dislocation		0.350	0.394	0.409	0.469	0.354	0.333	—
S73.004A	Unspecified dislocation of right hip, initial encounter	170	Hip Fracture/Dislocation		0.350	0.394	0.409	0.469	0.354	0.333	—
S73.005A	Unspecified dislocation of left hip, initial encounter	170	Hip Fracture/Dislocation		0.350	0.394	0.409	0.469	0.354	0.333	—

ICD-10-CM Code	ICD-10-CM Code Description	V24 CMS-HCC	V24 CMS-HCC Disease Group	V24 CMS-HCC Hierarchies	Community, NonDual, Aged	Community, NonDual, Disabled	Community, FBDual, Aged	Community, FBDual, Disabled	Community, PBDual, Aged	Community, PBDual, Disabled	Institutional
S73.006A	Unspecified dislocation of unspecified hip, initial encounter	170	Hip Fracture/Dislocation		0.350	0.394	0.409	0.469	0.354	0.333	—
S73.011A	Posterior subluxation of right hip, initial encounter	170	Hip Fracture/Dislocation		0.350	0.394	0.409	0.469	0.354	0.333	—
S73.012A	Posterior subluxation of left hip, initial encounter	170	Hip Fracture/Dislocation		0.350	0.394	0.409	0.469	0.354	0.333	—
S73.013A	Posterior subluxation of unspecified hip, initial encounter	170	Hip Fracture/Dislocation		0.350	0.394	0.409	0.469	0.354	0.333	—
S73.014A	Posterior dislocation of right hip, initial encounter	170	Hip Fracture/Dislocation		0.350	0.394	0.409	0.469	0.354	0.333	—
S73.015A	Posterior dislocation of left hip, initial encounter	170	Hip Fracture/Dislocation		0.350	0.394	0.409	0.469	0.354	0.333	—
S73.016A	Posterior dislocation of unspecified hip, initial encounter	170	Hip Fracture/Dislocation		0.350	0.394	0.409	0.469	0.354	0.333	—
S73.021A	Obturator subluxation of right hip, initial encounter	170	Hip Fracture/Dislocation		0.350	0.394	0.409	0.469	0.354	0.333	—
S73.022A	Obturator subluxation of left hip, initial encounter	170	Hip Fracture/Dislocation		0.350	0.394	0.409	0.469	0.354	0.333	—
S73.023A	Obturator subluxation of unspecified hip, initial encounter	170	Hip Fracture/Dislocation		0.350	0.394	0.409	0.469	0.354	0.333	—
S73.024A	Obturator dislocation of right hip, initial encounter	170	Hip Fracture/Dislocation		0.350	0.394	0.409	0.469	0.354	0.333	—
S73.025A	Obturator dislocation of left hip, initial encounter	170	Hip Fracture/Dislocation		0.350	0.394	0.409	0.469	0.354	0.333	—
S73.026A	Obturator dislocation of unspecified hip, initial encounter	170	Hip Fracture/Dislocation		0.350	0.394	0.409	0.469	0.354	0.333	—
S73.031A	Other anterior subluxation of right hip, initial encounter	170	Hip Fracture/Dislocation		0.350	0.394	0.409	0.469	0.354	0.333	—
S73.032A	Other anterior subluxation of left hip, initial encounter	170	Hip Fracture/Dislocation		0.350	0.394	0.409	0.469	0.354	0.333	—
S73.033A	Other anterior subluxation of unspecified hip, initial encounter	170	Hip Fracture/Dislocation		0.350	0.394	0.409	0.469	0.354	0.333	—
S73.034A	Other anterior dislocation of right hip, initial encounter	170	Hip Fracture/Dislocation		0.350	0.394	0.409	0.469	0.354	0.333	—
S73.035A	Other anterior dislocation of left hip, initial encounter	170	Hip Fracture/Dislocation		0.350	0.394	0.409	0.469	0.354	0.333	—
S73.036A	Other anterior dislocation of unspecified hip, initial encounter	170	Hip Fracture/Dislocation		0.350	0.394	0.409	0.469	0.354	0.333	—
S73.041A	Central subluxation of right hip, initial encounter	170	Hip Fracture/Dislocation		0.350	0.394	0.409	0.469	0.354	0.333	—
S73.042A	Central subluxation of left hip, initial encounter	170	Hip Fracture/Dislocation		0.350	0.394	0.409	0.469	0.354	0.333	—
S73.043A	Central subluxation of unspecified hip, initial encounter	170	Hip Fracture/Dislocation		0.350	0.394	0.409	0.469	0.354	0.333	—
S73.044A	Central dislocation of right hip, initial encounter	170	Hip Fracture/Dislocation		0.350	0.394	0.409	0.469	0.354	0.333	—
S73.045A	Central dislocation of left hip, initial encounter	170	Hip Fracture/Dislocation		0.350	0.394	0.409	0.469	0.354	0.333	—
S73.046A	Central dislocation of unspecified hip, initial encounter	170	Hip Fracture/Dislocation		0.350	0.394	0.409	0.469	0.354	0.333	—
S78.011A	Complete traumatic amputation at right hip joint, initial encounter	173	Traumatic Amputations and Complications		0.208	0.172	0.221	0.525	0.176	0.180	0.092
S78.011D	Complete traumatic amputation at right hip joint, subsequent encounter	189	Amputation Status, Lower Limb/Amputation Complications		0.519	0.437	0.795	0.934	0.697	0.626	0.357
S78.011S	Complete traumatic amputation at right hip joint, sequela	189	Amputation Status, Lower Limb/Amputation Complications		0.519	0.437	0.795	0.934	0.697	0.626	0.357
S78.012A	Complete traumatic amputation at left hip joint, initial encounter	173	Traumatic Amputations and Complications		0.208	0.172	0.221	0.525	0.176	0.180	0.092

ICD-10-CM Code	ICD-10-CM Code Description	V24 CMS-HCC	V24 CMS-HCC Disease Group	V24 CMS-HCC Hierarchies	Community, NonDual, Aged	Community, NonDual, Disabled	Community, FBDual, Aged	Community, FBDual, Disabled	Community, PBDual, Aged	Community, PBDual, Disabled	Institutional
S78.012D	Complete traumatic amputation at left hip joint, subsequent encounter	189	Amputation Status, Lower Limb/ Amputation Complications		0.519	0.437	0.795	0.934	0.697	0.626	0.357
S78.012S	Complete traumatic amputation at left hip joint, sequela	189	Amputation Status, Lower Limb/ Amputation Complications		0.519	0.437	0.795	0.934	0.697	0.626	0.357
S78.019A	Complete traumatic amputation at unspecified hip joint, initial encounter	173	Traumatic Amputations and Complications		0.208	0.172	0.221	0.525	0.176	0.180	0.092
S78.019D	Complete traumatic amputation at unspecified hip joint, subsequent encounter	189	Amputation Status, Lower Limb/ Amputation Complications		0.519	0.437	0.795	0.934	0.697	0.626	0.357
S78.019S	Complete traumatic amputation at unspecified hip joint, sequela	189	Amputation Status, Lower Limb/ Amputation Complications		0.519	0.437	0.795	0.934	0.697	0.626	0.357
S78.021A	Partial traumatic amputation at right hip joint, initial encounter	173	Traumatic Amputations and Complications		0.208	0.172	0.221	0.525	0.176	0.180	0.092
S78.021D	Partial traumatic amputation at right hip joint, subsequent encounter	189	Amputation Status, Lower Limb/ Amputation Complications		0.519	0.437	0.795	0.934	0.697	0.626	0.357
S78.021S	Partial traumatic amputation at right hip joint, sequela	189	Amputation Status, Lower Limb/ Amputation Complications		0.519	0.437	0.795	0.934	0.697	0.626	0.357
S78.022A	Partial traumatic amputation at left hip joint, initial encounter	173	Traumatic Amputations and Complications		0.208	0.172	0.221	0.525	0.176	0.180	0.092
S78.022D	Partial traumatic amputation at left hip joint, subsequent encounter	189	Amputation Status, Lower Limb/ Amputation Complications		0.519	0.437	0.795	0.934	0.697	0.626	0.357
S78.022S	Partial traumatic amputation at left hip joint, sequela	189	Amputation Status, Lower Limb/ Amputation Complications		0.519	0.437	0.795	0.934	0.697	0.626	0.357
S78.029A	Partial traumatic amputation at unspecified hip joint, initial encounter	173	Traumatic Amputations and Complications		0.208	0.172	0.221	0.525	0.176	0.180	0.092
S78.029D	Partial traumatic amputation at unspecified hip joint, subsequent encounter	189	Amputation Status, Lower Limb/ Amputation Complications		0.519	0.437	0.795	0.934	0.697	0.626	0.357
S78.029S	Partial traumatic amputation at unspecified hip joint, sequela	189	Amputation Status, Lower Limb/ Amputation Complications		0.519	0.437	0.795	0.934	0.697	0.626	0.357
S78.111A	Complete traumatic amputation at level between right hip and knee, initial encounter	173	Traumatic Amputations and Complications		0.208	0.172	0.221	0.525	0.176	0.180	0.092
S78.111D	Complete traumatic amputation at level between right hip and knee, subsequent encounter	189	Amputation Status, Lower Limb/ Amputation Complications		0.519	0.437	0.795	0.934	0.697	0.626	0.357
S78.111S	Complete traumatic amputation at level between right hip and knee, sequela	189	Amputation Status, Lower Limb/ Amputation Complications		0.519	0.437	0.795	0.934	0.697	0.626	0.357
S78.112A	Complete traumatic amputation at level between left hip and knee, initial encounter	173	Traumatic Amputations and Complications		0.208	0.172	0.221	0.525	0.176	0.180	0.092
S78.112D	Complete traumatic amputation at level between left hip and knee, subsequent encounter	189	Amputation Status, Lower Limb/ Amputation Complications		0.519	0.437	0.795	0.934	0.697	0.626	0.357
S78.112S	Complete traumatic amputation at level between left hip and knee, sequela	189	Amputation Status, Lower Limb/ Amputation Complications		0.519	0.437	0.795	0.934	0.697	0.626	0.357
S78.119A	Complete traumatic amputation at level between unspecified hip and knee, initial encounter	173	Traumatic Amputations and Complications		0.208	0.172	0.221	0.525	0.176	0.180	0.092
S78.119D	Complete traumatic amputation at level between unspecified hip and knee, subsequent encounter	189	Amputation Status, Lower Limb/ Amputation Complications		0.519	0.437	0.795	0.934	0.697	0.626	0.357
S78.119S	Complete traumatic amputation at level between unspecified hip and knee, sequela	189	Amputation Status, Lower Limb/ Amputation Complications		0.519	0.437	0.795	0.934	0.697	0.626	0.357

ICD-10-CM Code	ICD-10-CM Code Description	V24 CMS-HCC	V24 CMS-HCC Disease Group	V24 CMS-HCC Hierarchies	Community, NonDual, Aged	Community, NonDual, Disabled	Community, FBDual, Aged	Community, FBDual, Disabled	Community, PBDual, Aged	Community, PBDual, Disabled	Institutional
S78.121A	Partial traumatic amputation at level between right hip and knee, initial encounter	173	Traumatic Amputations and Complications		0.208	0.172	0.221	0.525	0.176	0.180	0.092
S78.121D	Partial traumatic amputation at level between right hip and knee, subsequent encounter	189	Amputation Status, Lower Limb/ Amputation Complications		0.519	0.437	0.795	0.934	0.697	0.626	0.357
S78.121S	Partial traumatic amputation at level between right hip and knee, sequela	189	Amputation Status, Lower Limb/ Amputation Complications		0.519	0.437	0.795	0.934	0.697	0.626	0.357
S78.122A	Partial traumatic amputation at level between left hip and knee, initial encounter	173	Traumatic Amputations and Complications		0.208	0.172	0.221	0.525	0.176	0.180	0.092
S78.122D	Partial traumatic amputation at level between left hip and knee, subsequent encounter	189	Amputation Status, Lower Limb/ Amputation Complications		0.519	0.437	0.795	0.934	0.697	0.626	0.357
S78.122S	Partial traumatic amputation at level between left hip and knee, sequela	189	Amputation Status, Lower Limb/ Amputation Complications		0.519	0.437	0.795	0.934	0.697	0.626	0.357
S78.129A	Partial traumatic amputation at level between unspecified hip and knee, initial encounter	173	Traumatic Amputations and Complications		0.208	0.172	0.221	0.525	0.176	0.180	0.092
S78.129D	Partial traumatic amputation at level between unspecified hip and knee, subsequent encounter	189	Amputation Status, Lower Limb/ Amputation Complications		0.519	0.437	0.795	0.934	0.697	0.626	0.357
S78.129S	Partial traumatic amputation at level between unspecified hip and knee, sequela	189	Amputation Status, Lower Limb/ Amputation Complications		0.519	0.437	0.795	0.934	0.697	0.626	0.357
S78.911A	Complete traumatic amputation of right hip and thigh, level unspecified, initial encounter	173	Traumatic Amputations and Complications		0.208	0.172	0.221	0.525	0.176	0.180	0.092
S78.911D	Complete traumatic amputation of right hip and thigh, level unspecified, subsequent encounter	189	Amputation Status, Lower Limb/ Amputation Complications		0.519	0.437	0.795	0.934	0.697	0.626	0.357
S78.911S	Complete traumatic amputation of right hip and thigh, level unspecified, sequela	189	Amputation Status, Lower Limb/ Amputation Complications		0.519	0.437	0.795	0.934	0.697	0.626	0.357
S78.912A	Complete traumatic amputation of left hip and thigh, level unspecified, initial encounter	173	Traumatic Amputations and Complications		0.208	0.172	0.221	0.525	0.176	0.180	0.092
S78.912D	Complete traumatic amputation of left hip and thigh, level unspecified, subsequent encounter	189	Amputation Status, Lower Limb/ Amputation Complications		0.519	0.437	0.795	0.934	0.697	0.626	0.357
S78.912S	Complete traumatic amputation of left hip and thigh, level unspecified, sequela	189	Amputation Status, Lower Limb/ Amputation Complications		0.519	0.437	0.795	0.934	0.697	0.626	0.357
S78.919A	Complete traumatic amputation of unspecified hip and thigh, level unspecified, initial encounter	173	Traumatic Amputations and Complications		0.208	0.172	0.221	0.525	0.176	0.180	0.092
S78.919D	Complete traumatic amputation of unspecified hip and thigh, level unspecified, subsequent encounter	189	Amputation Status, Lower Limb/ Amputation Complications		0.519	0.437	0.795	0.934	0.697	0.626	0.357
S78.919S	Complete traumatic amputation of unspecified hip and thigh, level unspecified, sequela	189	Amputation Status, Lower Limb/ Amputation Complications		0.519	0.437	0.795	0.934	0.697	0.626	0.357
S78.921A	Partial traumatic amputation of right hip and thigh, level unspecified, initial encounter	173	Traumatic Amputations and Complications		0.208	0.172	0.221	0.525	0.176	0.180	0.092
S78.921D	Partial traumatic amputation of right hip and thigh, level unspecified, subsequent encounter	189	Amputation Status, Lower Limb/ Amputation Complications		0.519	0.437	0.795	0.934	0.697	0.626	0.357
S78.921S	Partial traumatic amputation of right hip and thigh, level unspecified, sequela	189	Amputation Status, Lower Limb/ Amputation Complications		0.519	0.437	0.795	0.934	0.697	0.626	0.357

ICD-10-CM Code	ICD-10-CM Code Description	V24 CMS-HCC	V24 CMS-HCC Disease Group	V24 CMS-HCC Hierarchies	Community, NonDual, Aged	Community, NonDual, Disabled	Community, FBDual, Aged	Community, FBDual, Disabled	Community, PBDual, Aged	Community, PBDual, Disabled	Institutional
S78.922A	Partial traumatic amputation of left hip and thigh, level unspecified, initial encounter	173	Traumatic Amputations and Complications		0.208	0.172	0.221	0.525	0.176	0.180	0.092
S78.922D	Partial traumatic amputation of left hip and thigh, level unspecified, subsequent encounter	189	Amputation Status, Lower Limb/ Amputation Complications		0.519	0.437	0.795	0.934	0.697	0.626	0.357
S78.922S	Partial traumatic amputation of left hip and thigh, level unspecified, sequela	189	Amputation Status, Lower Limb/ Amputation Complications		0.519	0.437	0.795	0.934	0.697	0.626	0.357
S78.929A	Partial traumatic amputation of unspecified hip and thigh, level unspecified, initial encounter	173	Traumatic Amputations and Complications		0.208	0.172	0.221	0.525	0.176	0.180	0.092
S78.929D	Partial traumatic amputation of unspecified hip and thigh, level unspecified, subsequent encounter	189	Amputation Status, Lower Limb/ Amputation Complications		0.519	0.437	0.795	0.934	0.697	0.626	0.357
S78.929S	Partial traumatic amputation of unspecified hip and thigh, level unspecified, sequela	189	Amputation Status, Lower Limb/ Amputation Complications		0.519	0.437	0.795	0.934	0.697	0.626	0.357
S79.001A	Unspecified physeal fracture of upper end of right femur, initial encounter for closed fracture	170	Hip Fracture/Dislocation		0.350	0.394	0.409	0.469	0.354	0.333	—
S79.002A	Unspecified physeal fracture of upper end of left femur, initial encounter for closed fracture	170	Hip Fracture/Dislocation		0.350	0.394	0.409	0.469	0.354	0.333	—
S79.009A	Unspecified physeal fracture of upper end of unspecified femur, initial encounter for closed fracture	170	Hip Fracture/Dislocation		0.350	0.394	0.409	0.469	0.354	0.333	—
S79.011A	Salter-Harris Type I physeal fracture of upper end of right femur, initial encounter for closed fracture	170	Hip Fracture/Dislocation		0.350	0.394	0.409	0.469	0.354	0.333	—
S79.012A	Salter-Harris Type I physeal fracture of upper end of left femur, initial encounter for closed fracture	170	Hip Fracture/Dislocation		0.350	0.394	0.409	0.469	0.354	0.333	—
S79.019A	Salter-Harris Type I physeal fracture of upper end of unspecified femur, initial encounter for closed fracture	170	Hip Fracture/Dislocation		0.350	0.394	0.409	0.469	0.354	0.333	—
S79.091A	Other physeal fracture of upper end of right femur, initial encounter for closed fracture	170	Hip Fracture/Dislocation		0.350	0.394	0.409	0.469	0.354	0.333	—
S79.092A	Other physeal fracture of upper end of left femur, initial encounter for closed fracture	170	Hip Fracture/Dislocation		0.350	0.394	0.409	0.469	0.354	0.333	—
S79.099A	Other physeal fracture of upper end of unspecified femur, initial encounter for closed fracture	170	Hip Fracture/Dislocation		0.350	0.394	0.409	0.469	0.354	0.333	—
S79.101A	Unspecified physeal fracture of lower end of right femur, initial encounter for closed fracture	170	Hip Fracture/Dislocation		0.350	0.394	0.409	0.469	0.354	0.333	—
S79.102A	Unspecified physeal fracture of lower end of left femur, initial encounter for closed fracture	170	Hip Fracture/Dislocation		0.350	0.394	0.409	0.469	0.354	0.333	—
S79.109A	Unspecified physeal fracture of lower end of unspecified femur, initial encounter for closed fracture	170	Hip Fracture/Dislocation		0.350	0.394	0.409	0.469	0.354	0.333	—
S79.111A	Salter-Harris Type I physeal fracture of lower end of right femur, initial encounter for closed fracture	170	Hip Fracture/Dislocation		0.350	0.394	0.409	0.469	0.354	0.333	—
S79.112A	Salter-Harris Type I physeal fracture of lower end of left femur, initial encounter for closed fracture	170	Hip Fracture/Dislocation		0.350	0.394	0.409	0.469	0.354	0.333	—

ICD-10-CM Code	ICD-10-CM Code Description	V24 CMS-HCC	V24 CMS-HCC Disease Group	V24 CMS-HCC Hierarchies	Community, NonDual, Aged	Community, NonDual, Disabled	Community, FBDual, Aged	Community, FBDual, Disabled	Community, PBDual, Aged	Community, PBDual, Disabled	Institutional
S79.119A	Salter-Harris Type I physeal fracture of lower end of unspecified femur, initial encounter for closed fracture	170	Hip Fracture/Dislocation		0.350	0.394	0.409	0.469	0.354	0.333	—
S79.121A	Salter-Harris Type II physeal fracture of lower end of right femur, initial encounter for closed fracture	170	Hip Fracture/Dislocation		0.350	0.394	0.409	0.469	0.354	0.333	—
S79.122A	Salter-Harris Type II physeal fracture of lower end of left femur, initial encounter for closed fracture	170	Hip Fracture/Dislocation		0.350	0.394	0.409	0.469	0.354	0.333	—
S79.129A	Salter-Harris Type II physeal fracture of lower end of unspecified femur, initial encounter for closed fracture	170	Hip Fracture/Dislocation		0.350	0.394	0.409	0.469	0.354	0.333	—
S79.131A	Salter-Harris Type III physeal fracture of lower end of right femur, initial encounter for closed fracture	170	Hip Fracture/Dislocation		0.350	0.394	0.409	0.469	0.354	0.333	—
S79.132A	Salter-Harris Type III physeal fracture of lower end of left femur, initial encounter for closed fracture	170	Hip Fracture/Dislocation		0.350	0.394	0.409	0.469	0.354	0.333	—
S79.139A	Salter-Harris Type III physeal fracture of lower end of unspecified femur, initial encounter for closed fracture	170	Hip Fracture/Dislocation		0.350	0.394	0.409	0.469	0.354	0.333	—
S79.141A	Salter-Harris Type IV physeal fracture of lower end of right femur, initial encounter for closed fracture	170	Hip Fracture/Dislocation		0.350	0.394	0.409	0.469	0.354	0.333	—
S79.142A	Salter-Harris Type IV physeal fracture of lower end of left femur, initial encounter for closed fracture	170	Hip Fracture/Dislocation		0.350	0.394	0.409	0.469	0.354	0.333	—
S79.149A	Salter-Harris Type IV physeal fracture of lower end of unspecified femur, initial encounter for closed fracture	170	Hip Fracture/Dislocation		0.350	0.394	0.409	0.469	0.354	0.333	—
S79.191A	Other physeal fracture of lower end of right femur, initial encounter for closed fracture	170	Hip Fracture/Dislocation		0.350	0.394	0.409	0.469	0.354	0.333	—
S79.192A	Other physeal fracture of lower end of left femur, initial encounter for closed fracture	170	Hip Fracture/Dislocation		0.350	0.394	0.409	0.469	0.354	0.333	—
S79.199A	Other physeal fracture of lower end of unspecified femur, initial encounter for closed fracture	170	Hip Fracture/Dislocation		0.350	0.394	0.409	0.469	0.354	0.333	—
S88.011A	Complete traumatic amputation at knee level, right lower leg, initial encounter	173	Traumatic Amputations and Complications		0.208	0.172	0.221	0.525	0.176	0.180	0.092
S88.011D	Complete traumatic amputation at knee level, right lower leg, subsequent encounter	189	Amputation Status, Lower Limb/Amputation Complications		0.519	0.437	0.795	0.934	0.697	0.626	0.357
S88.011S	Complete traumatic amputation at knee level, right lower leg, sequela	189	Amputation Status, Lower Limb/Amputation Complications		0.519	0.437	0.795	0.934	0.697	0.626	0.357
S88.012A	Complete traumatic amputation at knee level, left lower leg, initial encounter	173	Traumatic Amputations and Complications		0.208	0.172	0.221	0.525	0.176	0.180	0.092
S88.012D	Complete traumatic amputation at knee level, left lower leg, subsequent encounter	189	Amputation Status, Lower Limb/Amputation Complications		0.519	0.437	0.795	0.934	0.697	0.626	0.357
S88.012S	Complete traumatic amputation at knee level, left lower leg, sequela	189	Amputation Status, Lower Limb/Amputation Complications		0.519	0.437	0.795	0.934	0.697	0.626	0.357
S88.019A	Complete traumatic amputation at knee level, unspecified lower leg, initial encounter	173	Traumatic Amputations and Complications		0.208	0.172	0.221	0.525	0.176	0.180	0.092
S88.019D	Complete traumatic amputation at knee level, unspecified lower leg, subsequent encounter	189	Amputation Status, Lower Limb/Amputation Complications		0.519	0.437	0.795	0.934	0.697	0.626	0.357

ICD-10-CM Code	ICD-10-CM Code Description	V24 CMS-HCC	V24 CMS-HCC Disease Group	V24 CMS-HCC Hierarchies	Community, NonDual, Aged	Community, NonDual, Disabled	Community, FBDual, Aged	Community, FBDual, Disabled	Community, PBDual, Aged	Community, PBDual, Disabled	Institutional
S88.019S	Complete traumatic amputation at knee level, unspecified lower leg, sequela	189	Amputation Status, Lower Limb/ Amputation Complications		0.519	0.437	0.795	0.934	0.697	0.626	0.357
S88.021A	Partial traumatic amputation at knee level, right lower leg, initial encounter	173	Traumatic Amputations and Complications		0.208	0.172	0.221	0.525	0.176	0.180	0.092
S88.021D	Partial traumatic amputation at knee level, right lower leg, subsequent encounter	189	Amputation Status, Lower Limb/ Amputation Complications		0.519	0.437	0.795	0.934	0.697	0.626	0.357
S88.021S	Partial traumatic amputation at knee level, right lower leg, sequela	189	Amputation Status, Lower Limb/ Amputation Complications		0.519	0.437	0.795	0.934	0.697	0.626	0.357
S88.022A	Partial traumatic amputation at knee level, left lower leg, initial encounter	173	Traumatic Amputations and Complications		0.208	0.172	0.221	0.525	0.176	0.180	0.092
S88.022D	Partial traumatic amputation at knee level, left lower leg, subsequent encounter	189	Amputation Status, Lower Limb/ Amputation Complications		0.519	0.437	0.795	0.934	0.697	0.626	0.357
S88.022S	Partial traumatic amputation at knee level, left lower leg, sequela	189	Amputation Status, Lower Limb/ Amputation Complications		0.519	0.437	0.795	0.934	0.697	0.626	0.357
S88.029A	Partial traumatic amputation at knee level, unspecified lower leg, initial encounter	173	Traumatic Amputations and Complications		0.208	0.172	0.221	0.525	0.176	0.180	0.092
S88.029D	Partial traumatic amputation at knee level, unspecified lower leg, subsequent encounter	189	Amputation Status, Lower Limb/ Amputation Complications		0.519	0.437	0.795	0.934	0.697	0.626	0.357
S88.029S	Partial traumatic amputation at knee level, unspecified lower leg, sequela	189	Amputation Status, Lower Limb/ Amputation Complications		0.519	0.437	0.795	0.934	0.697	0.626	0.357
S88.111A	Complete traumatic amputation at level between knee and ankle, right lower leg, initial encounter	173	Traumatic Amputations and Complications		0.208	0.172	0.221	0.525	0.176	0.180	0.092
S88.111D	Complete traumatic amputation at level between knee and ankle, right lower leg, subsequent encounter	189	Amputation Status, Lower Limb/ Amputation Complications		0.519	0.437	0.795	0.934	0.697	0.626	0.357
S88.111S	Complete traumatic amputation at level between knee and ankle, right lower leg, sequela	189	Amputation Status, Lower Limb/ Amputation Complications		0.519	0.437	0.795	0.934	0.697	0.626	0.357
S88.112A	Complete traumatic amputation at level between knee and ankle, left lower leg, initial encounter	173	Traumatic Amputations and Complications		0.208	0.172	0.221	0.525	0.176	0.180	0.092
S88.112D	Complete traumatic amputation at level between knee and ankle, left lower leg, subsequent encounter	189	Amputation Status, Lower Limb/ Amputation Complications		0.519	0.437	0.795	0.934	0.697	0.626	0.357
S88.112S	Complete traumatic amputation at level between knee and ankle, left lower leg, sequela	189	Amputation Status, Lower Limb/ Amputation Complications		0.519	0.437	0.795	0.934	0.697	0.626	0.357
S88.119A	Complete traumatic amputation at level between knee and ankle, unspecified lower leg, initial encounter	173	Traumatic Amputations and Complications		0.208	0.172	0.221	0.525	0.176	0.180	0.092
S88.119D	Complete traumatic amputation at level between knee and ankle, unspecified lower leg, subsequent encounter	189	Amputation Status, Lower Limb/ Amputation Complications		0.519	0.437	0.795	0.934	0.697	0.626	0.357
S88.119S	Complete traumatic amputation at level between knee and ankle, unspecified lower leg, sequela	189	Amputation Status, Lower Limb/ Amputation Complications		0.519	0.437	0.795	0.934	0.697	0.626	0.357
S88.121A	Partial traumatic amputation at level between knee and ankle, right lower leg, initial encounter	173	Traumatic Amputations and Complications		0.208	0.172	0.221	0.525	0.176	0.180	0.092
S88.121D	Partial traumatic amputation at level between knee and ankle, right lower leg, subsequent encounter	189	Amputation Status, Lower Limb/ Amputation Complications		0.519	0.437	0.795	0.934	0.697	0.626	0.357

ICD-10-CM Code	ICD-10-CM Code Description	V24 CMS-HCC	V24 CMS-HCC Disease Group	V24 CMS-HCC Hierarchies	Community, NonDual, Aged	Community, NonDual, Disabled	Community, FBDual, Aged	Community, FBDual, Disabled	Community, PBDual, Aged	Community, PBDual, Disabled	Institutional
S88.121S	Partial traumatic amputation at level between knee and ankle, right lower leg, sequela	189	Amputation Status, Lower Limb/ Amputation Complications		0.519	0.437	0.795	0.934	0.697	0.626	0.357
S88.122A	Partial traumatic amputation at level between knee and ankle, left lower leg, initial encounter	173	Traumatic Amputations and Complications		0.208	0.172	0.221	0.525	0.176	0.180	0.092
S88.122D	Partial traumatic amputation at level between knee and ankle, left lower leg, subsequent encounter	189	Amputation Status, Lower Limb/ Amputation Complications		0.519	0.437	0.795	0.934	0.697	0.626	0.357
S88.122S	Partial traumatic amputation at level between knee and ankle, left lower leg, sequela	189	Amputation Status, Lower Limb/ Amputation Complications		0.519	0.437	0.795	0.934	0.697	0.626	0.357
S88.129A	Partial traumatic amputation at level between knee and ankle, unspecified lower leg, initial encounter	173	Traumatic Amputations and Complications		0.208	0.172	0.221	0.525	0.176	0.180	0.092
S88.129D	Partial traumatic amputation at level between knee and ankle, unspecified lower leg, subsequent encounter	189	Amputation Status, Lower Limb/ Amputation Complications		0.519	0.437	0.795	0.934	0.697	0.626	0.357
S88.129S	Partial traumatic amputation at level between knee and ankle, unspecified lower leg, sequela	189	Amputation Status, Lower Limb/ Amputation Complications		0.519	0.437	0.795	0.934	0.697	0.626	0.357
S88.911A	Complete traumatic amputation of right lower leg, level unspecified, initial encounter	173	Traumatic Amputations and Complications		0.208	0.172	0.221	0.525	0.176	0.180	0.092
S88.911D	Complete traumatic amputation of right lower leg, level unspecified, subsequent encounter	189	Amputation Status, Lower Limb/ Amputation Complications		0.519	0.437	0.795	0.934	0.697	0.626	0.357
S88.911S	Complete traumatic amputation of right lower leg, level unspecified, sequela	189	Amputation Status, Lower Limb/ Amputation Complications		0.519	0.437	0.795	0.934	0.697	0.626	0.357
S88.912A	Complete traumatic amputation of left lower leg, level unspecified, initial encounter	173	Traumatic Amputations and Complications		0.208	0.172	0.221	0.525	0.176	0.180	0.092
S88.912D	Complete traumatic amputation of left lower leg, level unspecified, subsequent encounter	189	Amputation Status, Lower Limb/ Amputation Complications		0.519	0.437	0.795	0.934	0.697	0.626	0.357
S88.912S	Complete traumatic amputation of left lower leg, level unspecified, sequela	189	Amputation Status, Lower Limb/ Amputation Complications		0.519	0.437	0.795	0.934	0.697	0.626	0.357
S88.919A	Complete traumatic amputation of unspecified lower leg, level unspecified, initial encounter	173	Traumatic Amputations and Complications		0.208	0.172	0.221	0.525	0.176	0.180	0.092
S88.919D	Complete traumatic amputation of unspecified lower leg, level unspecified, subsequent encounter	189	Amputation Status, Lower Limb/ Amputation Complications		0.519	0.437	0.795	0.934	0.697	0.626	0.357
S88.919S	Complete traumatic amputation of unspecified lower leg, level unspecified, sequela	189	Amputation Status, Lower Limb/ Amputation Complications		0.519	0.437	0.795	0.934	0.697	0.626	0.357
S88.921A	Partial traumatic amputation of right lower leg, level unspecified, initial encounter	173	Traumatic Amputations and Complications		0.208	0.172	0.221	0.525	0.176	0.180	0.092
S88.921D	Partial traumatic amputation of right lower leg, level unspecified, subsequent encounter	189	Amputation Status, Lower Limb/ Amputation Complications		0.519	0.437	0.795	0.934	0.697	0.626	0.357
S88.921S	Partial traumatic amputation of right lower leg, level unspecified, sequela	189	Amputation Status, Lower Limb/ Amputation Complications		0.519	0.437	0.795	0.934	0.697	0.626	0.357
S88.922A	Partial traumatic amputation of left lower leg, level unspecified, initial encounter	173	Traumatic Amputations and Complications		0.208	0.172	0.221	0.525	0.176	0.180	0.092

ICD-10-CM Code	ICD-10-CM Code Description	V24 CMS-HCC	V24 CMS-HCC Disease Group	V24 CMS-HCC Hierarchies	Community, NonDual, Aged	Community, NonDual, Disabled	Community, FBDual, Aged	Community, FBDual, Disabled	Community, PBDual, Aged	Community, PBDual, Disabled	Institutional
S88.922D	Partial traumatic amputation of left lower leg, level unspecified, subsequent encounter	189	Amputation Status, Lower Limb/ Amputation Complications		0.519	0.437	0.795	0.934	0.697	0.626	0.357
S88.922S	Partial traumatic amputation of left lower leg, level unspecified, sequela	189	Amputation Status, Lower Limb/ Amputation Complications		0.519	0.437	0.795	0.934	0.697	0.626	0.357
S88.929A	Partial traumatic amputation of unspecified lower leg, level unspecified, initial encounter	173	Traumatic Amputations and Complications		0.208	0.172	0.221	0.525	0.176	0.180	0.092
S88.929D	Partial traumatic amputation of unspecified lower leg, level unspecified, subsequent encounter	189	Amputation Status, Lower Limb/ Amputation Complications		0.519	0.437	0.795	0.934	0.697	0.626	0.357
S88.929S	Partial traumatic amputation of unspecified lower leg, level unspecified, sequela	189	Amputation Status, Lower Limb/ Amputation Complications		0.519	0.437	0.795	0.934	0.697	0.626	0.357
S98.011A	Complete traumatic amputation of right foot at ankle level, initial encounter	173	Traumatic Amputations and Complications		0.208	0.172	0.221	0.525	0.176	0.180	0.092
S98.011D	Complete traumatic amputation of right foot at ankle level, subsequent encounter	189	Amputation Status, Lower Limb/ Amputation Complications		0.519	0.437	0.795	0.934	0.697	0.626	0.357
S98.011S	Complete traumatic amputation of right foot at ankle level, sequela	189	Amputation Status, Lower Limb/ Amputation Complications		0.519	0.437	0.795	0.934	0.697	0.626	0.357
S98.012A	Complete traumatic amputation of left foot at ankle level, initial encounter	173	Traumatic Amputations and Complications		0.208	0.172	0.221	0.525	0.176	0.180	0.092
S98.012D	Complete traumatic amputation of left foot at ankle level, subsequent encounter	189	Amputation Status, Lower Limb/ Amputation Complications		0.519	0.437	0.795	0.934	0.697	0.626	0.357
S98.012S	Complete traumatic amputation of left foot at ankle level, sequela	189	Amputation Status, Lower Limb/ Amputation Complications		0.519	0.437	0.795	0.934	0.697	0.626	0.357
S98.019A	Complete traumatic amputation of unspecified foot at ankle level, initial encounter	173	Traumatic Amputations and Complications		0.208	0.172	0.221	0.525	0.176	0.180	0.092
S98.019D	Complete traumatic amputation of unspecified foot at ankle level, subsequent encounter	189	Amputation Status, Lower Limb/ Amputation Complications		0.519	0.437	0.795	0.934	0.697	0.626	0.357
S98.019S	Complete traumatic amputation of unspecified foot at ankle level, sequela	189	Amputation Status, Lower Limb/ Amputation Complications		0.519	0.437	0.795	0.934	0.697	0.626	0.357
S98.021A	Partial traumatic amputation of right foot at ankle level, initial encounter	173	Traumatic Amputations and Complications		0.208	0.172	0.221	0.525	0.176	0.180	0.092
S98.021D	Partial traumatic amputation of right foot at ankle level, subsequent encounter	189	Amputation Status, Lower Limb/ Amputation Complications		0.519	0.437	0.795	0.934	0.697	0.626	0.357
S98.021S	Partial traumatic amputation of right foot at ankle level, sequela	189	Amputation Status, Lower Limb/ Amputation Complications		0.519	0.437	0.795	0.934	0.697	0.626	0.357
S98.022A	Partial traumatic amputation of left foot at ankle level, initial encounter	173	Traumatic Amputations and Complications		0.208	0.172	0.221	0.525	0.176	0.180	0.092
S98.022D	Partial traumatic amputation of left foot at ankle level, subsequent encounter	189	Amputation Status, Lower Limb/ Amputation Complications		0.519	0.437	0.795	0.934	0.697	0.626	0.357
S98.022S	Partial traumatic amputation of left foot at ankle level, sequela	189	Amputation Status, Lower Limb/ Amputation Complications		0.519	0.437	0.795	0.934	0.697	0.626	0.357
S98.029A	Partial traumatic amputation of unspecified foot at ankle level, initial encounter	173	Traumatic Amputations and Complications		0.208	0.172	0.221	0.525	0.176	0.180	0.092
S98.029D	Partial traumatic amputation of unspecified foot at ankle level, subsequent encounter	189	Amputation Status, Lower Limb/ Amputation Complications		0.519	0.437	0.795	0.934	0.697	0.626	0.357

ICD-10-CM Code	ICD-10-CM Code Description	V24 CMS-HCC	V24 CMS-HCC Disease Group	V24 CMS-HCC Hierarchies	Community, NonDual, Aged	Community, NonDual, Disabled	Community, FBDual, Aged	Community, FBDual, Disabled	Community, PBDual, Aged	Community, PBDual, Disabled	Institutional
S98.029S	Partial traumatic amputation of unspecified foot at ankle level, sequela	189	Amputation Status, Lower Limb/ Amputation Complications		0.519	0.437	0.795	0.934	0.697	0.626	0.357
S98.111A	Complete traumatic amputation of right great toe, initial encounter	173	Traumatic Amputations and Complications		0.208	0.172	0.221	0.525	0.176	0.180	0.092
S98.111D	Complete traumatic amputation of right great toe, subsequent encounter	189	Amputation Status, Lower Limb/ Amputation Complications		0.519	0.437	0.795	0.934	0.697	0.626	0.357
S98.111S	Complete traumatic amputation of right great toe, sequela	189	Amputation Status, Lower Limb/ Amputation Complications		0.519	0.437	0.795	0.934	0.697	0.626	0.357
S98.112A	Complete traumatic amputation of left great toe, initial encounter	173	Traumatic Amputations and Complications		0.208	0.172	0.221	0.525	0.176	0.180	0.092
S98.112D	Complete traumatic amputation of left great toe, subsequent encounter	189	Amputation Status, Lower Limb/ Amputation Complications		0.519	0.437	0.795	0.934	0.697	0.626	0.357
S98.112S	Complete traumatic amputation of left great toe, sequela	189	Amputation Status, Lower Limb/ Amputation Complications		0.519	0.437	0.795	0.934	0.697	0.626	0.357
S98.119A	Complete traumatic amputation of unspecified great toe, initial encounter	173	Traumatic Amputations and Complications		0.208	0.172	0.221	0.525	0.176	0.180	0.092
S98.119D	Complete traumatic amputation of unspecified great toe, subsequent encounter	189	Amputation Status, Lower Limb/ Amputation Complications		0.519	0.437	0.795	0.934	0.697	0.626	0.357
S98.119S	Complete traumatic amputation of unspecified great toe, sequela	189	Amputation Status, Lower Limb/ Amputation Complications		0.519	0.437	0.795	0.934	0.697	0.626	0.357
S98.121A	Partial traumatic amputation of right great toe, initial encounter	173	Traumatic Amputations and Complications		0.208	0.172	0.221	0.525	0.176	0.180	0.092
S98.121D	Partial traumatic amputation of right great toe, subsequent encounter	189	Amputation Status, Lower Limb/ Amputation Complications		0.519	0.437	0.795	0.934	0.697	0.626	0.357
S98.121S	Partial traumatic amputation of right great toe, sequela	189	Amputation Status, Lower Limb/ Amputation Complications		0.519	0.437	0.795	0.934	0.697	0.626	0.357
S98.122A	Partial traumatic amputation of left great toe, initial encounter	173	Traumatic Amputations and Complications		0.208	0.172	0.221	0.525	0.176	0.180	0.092
S98.122D	Partial traumatic amputation of left great toe, subsequent encounter	189	Amputation Status, Lower Limb/ Amputation Complications		0.519	0.437	0.795	0.934	0.697	0.626	0.357
S98.122S	Partial traumatic amputation of left great toe, sequela	189	Amputation Status, Lower Limb/ Amputation Complications		0.519	0.437	0.795	0.934	0.697	0.626	0.357
S98.129A	Partial traumatic amputation of unspecified great toe, initial encounter	173	Traumatic Amputations and Complications		0.208	0.172	0.221	0.525	0.176	0.180	0.092
S98.129D	Partial traumatic amputation of unspecified great toe, subsequent encounter	189	Amputation Status, Lower Limb/ Amputation Complications		0.519	0.437	0.795	0.934	0.697	0.626	0.357
S98.129S	Partial traumatic amputation of unspecified great toe, sequela	189	Amputation Status, Lower Limb/ Amputation Complications		0.519	0.437	0.795	0.934	0.697	0.626	0.357
S98.131A	Complete traumatic amputation of one right lesser toe, initial encounter	173	Traumatic Amputations and Complications		0.208	0.172	0.221	0.525	0.176	0.180	0.092
S98.131D	Complete traumatic amputation of one right lesser toe, subsequent encounter	189	Amputation Status, Lower Limb/ Amputation Complications		0.519	0.437	0.795	0.934	0.697	0.626	0.357
S98.131S	Complete traumatic amputation of one right lesser toe, sequela	189	Amputation Status, Lower Limb/ Amputation Complications		0.519	0.437	0.795	0.934	0.697	0.626	0.357
S98.132A	Complete traumatic amputation of one left lesser toe, initial encounter	173	Traumatic Amputations and Complications		0.208	0.172	0.221	0.525	0.176	0.180	0.092
S98.132D	Complete traumatic amputation of one left lesser toe, subsequent encounter	189	Amputation Status, Lower Limb/ Amputation Complications		0.519	0.437	0.795	0.934	0.697	0.626	0.357
S98.132S	Complete traumatic amputation of one left lesser toe, sequela	189	Amputation Status, Lower Limb/ Amputation Complications		0.519	0.437	0.795	0.934	0.697	0.626	0.357

ICD-10-CM Code	ICD-10-CM Code Description	V24 CMS-HCC	V24 CMS-HCC Disease Group	V24 CMS-HCC Hierarchies	Community, NonDual, Aged	Community, NonDual, Disabled	Community, FBDual, Aged	Community, FBDual, Disabled	Community, PBDual, Aged	Community, PBDual, Disabled	Institutional
S98.139A	Complete traumatic amputation of one unspecified lesser toe, initial encounter	173	Traumatic Amputations and Complications		0.208	0.172	0.221	0.525	0.176	0.180	0.092
S98.139D	Complete traumatic amputation of one unspecified lesser toe, subsequent encounter	189	Amputation Status, Lower Limb/ Amputation Complications		0.519	0.437	0.795	0.934	0.697	0.626	0.357
S98.139S	Complete traumatic amputation of one unspecified lesser toe, sequela	189	Amputation Status, Lower Limb/ Amputation Complications		0.519	0.437	0.795	0.934	0.697	0.626	0.357
S98.141A	Partial traumatic amputation of one right lesser toe, initial encounter	173	Traumatic Amputations and Complications		0.208	0.172	0.221	0.525	0.176	0.180	0.092
S98.141D	Partial traumatic amputation of one right lesser toe, subsequent encounter	189	Amputation Status, Lower Limb/ Amputation Complications		0.519	0.437	0.795	0.934	0.697	0.626	0.357
S98.141S	Partial traumatic amputation of one right lesser toe, sequela	189	Amputation Status, Lower Limb/ Amputation Complications		0.519	0.437	0.795	0.934	0.697	0.626	0.357
S98.142A	Partial traumatic amputation of one left lesser toe, initial encounter	173	Traumatic Amputations and Complications		0.208	0.172	0.221	0.525	0.176	0.180	0.092
S98.142D	Partial traumatic amputation of one left lesser toe, subsequent encounter	189	Amputation Status, Lower Limb/ Amputation Complications		0.519	0.437	0.795	0.934	0.697	0.626	0.357
S98.142S	Partial traumatic amputation of one left lesser toe, sequela	189	Amputation Status, Lower Limb/ Amputation Complications		0.519	0.437	0.795	0.934	0.697	0.626	0.357
S98.149A	Partial traumatic amputation of one unspecified lesser toe, initial encounter	173	Traumatic Amputations and Complications		0.208	0.172	0.221	0.525	0.176	0.180	0.092
S98.149D	Partial traumatic amputation of one unspecified lesser toe, subsequent encounter	189	Amputation Status, Lower Limb/ Amputation Complications		0.519	0.437	0.795	0.934	0.697	0.626	0.357
S98.149S	Partial traumatic amputation of one unspecified lesser toe, sequela	189	Amputation Status, Lower Limb/ Amputation Complications		0.519	0.437	0.795	0.934	0.697	0.626	0.357
S98.211A	Complete traumatic amputation of two or more right lesser toes, initial encounter	173	Traumatic Amputations and Complications		0.208	0.172	0.221	0.525	0.176	0.180	0.092
S98.211D	Complete traumatic amputation of two or more right lesser toes, subsequent encounter	189	Amputation Status, Lower Limb/ Amputation Complications		0.519	0.437	0.795	0.934	0.697	0.626	0.357
S98.211S	Complete traumatic amputation of two or more right lesser toes, sequela	189	Amputation Status, Lower Limb/ Amputation Complications		0.519	0.437	0.795	0.934	0.697	0.626	0.357
S98.212A	Complete traumatic amputation of two or more left lesser toes, initial encounter	173	Traumatic Amputations and Complications		0.208	0.172	0.221	0.525	0.176	0.180	0.092
S98.212D	Complete traumatic amputation of two or more left lesser toes, subsequent encounter	189	Amputation Status, Lower Limb/ Amputation Complications		0.519	0.437	0.795	0.934	0.697	0.626	0.357
S98.212S	Complete traumatic amputation of two or more left lesser toes, sequela	189	Amputation Status, Lower Limb/ Amputation Complications		0.519	0.437	0.795	0.934	0.697	0.626	0.357
S98.219A	Complete traumatic amputation of two or more unspecified lesser toes, initial encounter	173	Traumatic Amputations and Complications		0.208	0.172	0.221	0.525	0.176	0.180	0.092
S98.219D	Complete traumatic amputation of two or more unspecified lesser toes, subsequent encounter	189	Amputation Status, Lower Limb/ Amputation Complications		0.519	0.437	0.795	0.934	0.697	0.626	0.357
S98.219S	Complete traumatic amputation of two or more unspecified lesser toes, sequela	189	Amputation Status, Lower Limb/ Amputation Complications		0.519	0.437	0.795	0.934	0.697	0.626	0.357
S98.221A	Partial traumatic amputation of two or more right lesser toes, initial encounter	173	Traumatic Amputations and Complications		0.208	0.172	0.221	0.525	0.176	0.180	0.092
S98.221D	Partial traumatic amputation of two or more right lesser toes, subsequent encounter	189	Amputation Status, Lower Limb/ Amputation Complications		0.519	0.437	0.795	0.934	0.697	0.626	0.357

ICD-10-CM Code	ICD-10-CM Code Description	V24 CMS-HCC	V24 CMS-HCC Disease Group	V24 CMS-HCC Hierarchies	Community, NonDual, Aged	Community, NonDual, Disabled	Community, FBDual, Aged	Community, FBDual, Disabled	Community, PBDual, Aged	Community, PBDual, Disabled	Institutional
S98.221S	Partial traumatic amputation of two or more right lesser toes, sequela	189	Amputation Status, Lower Limb/ Amputation Complications		0.519	0.437	0.795	0.934	0.697	0.626	0.357
S98.222A	Partial traumatic amputation of two or more left lesser toes, initial encounter	173	Traumatic Amputations and Complications		0.208	0.172	0.221	0.525	0.176	0.180	0.092
S98.222D	Partial traumatic amputation of two or more left lesser toes, subsequent encounter	189	Amputation Status, Lower Limb/ Amputation Complications		0.519	0.437	0.795	0.934	0.697	0.626	0.357
S98.222S	Partial traumatic amputation of two or more left lesser toes, sequela	189	Amputation Status, Lower Limb/ Amputation Complications		0.519	0.437	0.795	0.934	0.697	0.626	0.357
S98.229A	Partial traumatic amputation of two or more unspecified lesser toes, initial encounter	173	Traumatic Amputations and Complications		0.208	0.172	0.221	0.525	0.176	0.180	0.092
S98.229D	Partial traumatic amputation of two or more unspecified lesser toes, subsequent encounter	189	Amputation Status, Lower Limb/ Amputation Complications		0.519	0.437	0.795	0.934	0.697	0.626	0.357
S98.229S	Partial traumatic amputation of two or more unspecified lesser toes, sequela	189	Amputation Status, Lower Limb/ Amputation Complications		0.519	0.437	0.795	0.934	0.697	0.626	0.357
S98.311A	Complete traumatic amputation of right midfoot, initial encounter	173	Traumatic Amputations and Complications		0.208	0.172	0.221	0.525	0.176	0.180	0.092
S98.311D	Complete traumatic amputation of right midfoot, subsequent encounter	189	Amputation Status, Lower Limb/ Amputation Complications		0.519	0.437	0.795	0.934	0.697	0.626	0.357
S98.311S	Complete traumatic amputation of right midfoot, sequela	189	Amputation Status, Lower Limb/ Amputation Complications		0.519	0.437	0.795	0.934	0.697	0.626	0.357
S98.312A	Complete traumatic amputation of left midfoot, initial encounter	173	Traumatic Amputations and Complications		0.208	0.172	0.221	0.525	0.176	0.180	0.092
S98.312D	Complete traumatic amputation of left midfoot, subsequent encounter	189	Amputation Status, Lower Limb/ Amputation Complications		0.519	0.437	0.795	0.934	0.697	0.626	0.357
S98.312S	Complete traumatic amputation of left midfoot, sequela	189	Amputation Status, Lower Limb/ Amputation Complications		0.519	0.437	0.795	0.934	0.697	0.626	0.357
S98.319A	Complete traumatic amputation of unspecified midfoot, initial encounter	173	Traumatic Amputations and Complications		0.208	0.172	0.221	0.525	0.176	0.180	0.092
S98.319D	Complete traumatic amputation of unspecified midfoot, subsequent encounter	189	Amputation Status, Lower Limb/ Amputation Complications		0.519	0.437	0.795	0.934	0.697	0.626	0.357
S98.319S	Complete traumatic amputation of unspecified midfoot, sequela	189	Amputation Status, Lower Limb/ Amputation Complications		0.519	0.437	0.795	0.934	0.697	0.626	0.357
S98.321A	Partial traumatic amputation of right midfoot, initial encounter	173	Traumatic Amputations and Complications		0.208	0.172	0.221	0.525	0.176	0.180	0.092
S98.321D	Partial traumatic amputation of right midfoot, subsequent encounter	189	Amputation Status, Lower Limb/ Amputation Complications		0.519	0.437	0.795	0.934	0.697	0.626	0.357
S98.321S	Partial traumatic amputation of right midfoot, sequela	189	Amputation Status, Lower Limb/ Amputation Complications		0.519	0.437	0.795	0.934	0.697	0.626	0.357
S98.322A	Partial traumatic amputation of left midfoot, initial encounter	173	Traumatic Amputations and Complications		0.208	0.172	0.221	0.525	0.176	0.180	0.092
S98.322D	Partial traumatic amputation of left midfoot, subsequent encounter	189	Amputation Status, Lower Limb/ Amputation Complications		0.519	0.437	0.795	0.934	0.697	0.626	0.357
S98.322S	Partial traumatic amputation of left midfoot, sequela	189	Amputation Status, Lower Limb/ Amputation Complications		0.519	0.437	0.795	0.934	0.697	0.626	0.357
S98.329A	Partial traumatic amputation of unspecified midfoot, initial encounter	173	Traumatic Amputations and Complications		0.208	0.172	0.221	0.525	0.176	0.180	0.092
S98.329D	Partial traumatic amputation of unspecified midfoot, subsequent encounter	189	Amputation Status, Lower Limb/ Amputation Complications		0.519	0.437	0.795	0.934	0.697	0.626	0.357
S98.329S	Partial traumatic amputation of unspecified midfoot, sequela	189	Amputation Status, Lower Limb/ Amputation Complications		0.519	0.437	0.795	0.934	0.697	0.626	0.357
S98.911A	Complete traumatic amputation of right foot, level unspecified, initial encounter	173	Traumatic Amputations and Complications		0.208	0.172	0.221	0.525	0.176	0.180	0.092

ICD-10-CM Code	ICD-10-CM Code Description	V24 CMS-HCC	V24 CMS-HCC Disease Group	V24 CMS-HCC Hierarchies	Community, NonDual, Aged	Community, NonDual, Disabled	Community, FBDual, Aged	Community, FBDual, Disabled	Community, PBDual, Aged	Community, PBDual, Disabled	Institutional
S98.911D	Complete traumatic amputation of right foot, level unspecified, subsequent encounter	189	Amputation Status, Lower Limb/ Amputation Complications		0.519	0.437	0.795	0.934	0.697	0.626	0.357
S98.911S	Complete traumatic amputation of right foot, level unspecified, sequela	189	Amputation Status, Lower Limb/ Amputation Complications		0.519	0.437	0.795	0.934	0.697	0.626	0.357
S98.912A	Complete traumatic amputation of left foot, level unspecified, initial encounter	173	Traumatic Amputations and Complications		0.208	0.172	0.221	0.525	0.176	0.180	0.092
S98.912D	Complete traumatic amputation of left foot, level unspecified, subsequent encounter	189	Amputation Status, Lower Limb/ Amputation Complications		0.519	0.437	0.795	0.934	0.697	0.626	0.357
S98.912S	Complete traumatic amputation of left foot, level unspecified, sequela	189	Amputation Status, Lower Limb/ Amputation Complications		0.519	0.437	0.795	0.934	0.697	0.626	0.357
S98.919A	Complete traumatic amputation of unspecified foot, level unspecified, initial encounter	173	Traumatic Amputations and Complications		0.208	0.172	0.221	0.525	0.176	0.180	0.092
S98.919D	Complete traumatic amputation of unspecified foot, level unspecified, subsequent encounter	189	Amputation Status, Lower Limb/ Amputation Complications		0.519	0.437	0.795	0.934	0.697	0.626	0.357
S98.919S	Complete traumatic amputation of unspecified foot, level unspecified, sequela	189	Amputation Status, Lower Limb/ Amputation Complications		0.519	0.437	0.795	0.934	0.697	0.626	0.357
S98.921A	Partial traumatic amputation of right foot, level unspecified, initial encounter	173	Traumatic Amputations and Complications		0.208	0.172	0.221	0.525	0.176	0.180	0.092
S98.921D	Partial traumatic amputation of right foot, level unspecified, subsequent encounter	189	Amputation Status, Lower Limb/ Amputation Complications		0.519	0.437	0.795	0.934	0.697	0.626	0.357
S98.921S	Partial traumatic amputation of right foot, level unspecified, sequela	189	Amputation Status, Lower Limb/ Amputation Complications		0.519	0.437	0.795	0.934	0.697	0.626	0.357
S98.922A	Partial traumatic amputation of left foot, level unspecified, initial encounter	173	Traumatic Amputations and Complications		0.208	0.172	0.221	0.525	0.176	0.180	0.092
S98.922D	Partial traumatic amputation of left foot, level unspecified, subsequent encounter	189	Amputation Status, Lower Limb/ Amputation Complications		0.519	0.437	0.795	0.934	0.697	0.626	0.357
S98.922S	Partial traumatic amputation of left foot, level unspecified, sequela	189	Amputation Status, Lower Limb/ Amputation Complications		0.519	0.437	0.795	0.934	0.697	0.626	0.357
S98.929A	Partial traumatic amputation of unspecified foot, level unspecified, initial encounter	173	Traumatic Amputations and Complications		0.208	0.172	0.221	0.525	0.176	0.180	0.092
S98.929D	Partial traumatic amputation of unspecified foot, level unspecified, subsequent encounter	189	Amputation Status, Lower Limb/ Amputation Complications		0.519	0.437	0.795	0.934	0.697	0.626	0.357
S98.929S	Partial traumatic amputation of unspecified foot, level unspecified, sequela	189	Amputation Status, Lower Limb/ Amputation Complications		0.519	0.437	0.795	0.934	0.697	0.626	0.357
T14.91XA	Suicide attempt, initial encounter	59	Major Depressive, Bipolar, and Paranoid Disorders	60	0.309	0.164	0.299	0.127	0.306	0.109	0.187
T14.91XD	Suicide attempt, subsequent encounter	59	Major Depressive, Bipolar, and Paranoid Disorders	60	0.309	0.164	0.299	0.127	0.306	0.109	0.187
T14.91XS	Suicide attempt, sequela	59	Major Depressive, Bipolar, and Paranoid Disorders	60	0.309	0.164	0.299	0.127	0.306	0.109	0.187
T31.11	Burns involving 10-19% of body surface with 10-19% third degree burns	162	Severe Skin Burn or Condition		0.224	0.506	0.162	0.308	—	0.324	—
T31.21	Burns involving 20-29% of body surface with 10-19% third degree burns	162	Severe Skin Burn or Condition		0.224	0.506	0.162	0.308	—	0.324	—

ICD-10-CM Code	ICD-10-CM Code Description	V24 CMS-HCC	V24 CMS-HCC Disease Group	V24 CMS-HCC Hierarchies	Community, NonDual, Aged	Community, NonDual, Disabled	Community, FBDual, Aged	Community, FBDual, Disabled	Community, PBDual, Aged	Community, PBDual, Disabled	Institutional
T31.22	Burns involving 20-29% of body surface with 20-29% third degree burns	162	Severe Skin Burn or Condition		0.224	0.506	0.162	0.308	—	0.324	—
T31.31	Burns involving 30-39% of body surface with 10-19% third degree burns	162	Severe Skin Burn or Condition		0.224	0.506	0.162	0.308	—	0.324	—
T31.32	Burns involving 30-39% of body surface with 20-29% third degree burns	162	Severe Skin Burn or Condition		0.224	0.506	0.162	0.308	—	0.324	—
T31.33	Burns involving 30-39% of body surface with 30-39% third degree burns	162	Severe Skin Burn or Condition		0.224	0.506	0.162	0.308	—	0.324	—
T31.41	Burns involving 40-49% of body surface with 10-19% third degree burns	162	Severe Skin Burn or Condition		0.224	0.506	0.162	0.308	—	0.324	—
T31.42	Burns involving 40-49% of body surface with 20-29% third degree burns	162	Severe Skin Burn or Condition		0.224	0.506	0.162	0.308	—	0.324	—
T31.43	Burns involving 40-49% of body surface with 30-39% third degree burns	162	Severe Skin Burn or Condition		0.224	0.506	0.162	0.308	—	0.324	—
T31.44	Burns involving 40-49% of body surface with 40-49% third degree burns	162	Severe Skin Burn or Condition		0.224	0.506	0.162	0.308	—	0.324	—
T31.51	Burns involving 50-59% of body surface with 10-19% third degree burns	162	Severe Skin Burn or Condition		0.224	0.506	0.162	0.308	—	0.324	—
T31.52	Burns involving 50-59% of body surface with 20-29% third degree burns	162	Severe Skin Burn or Condition		0.224	0.506	0.162	0.308	—	0.324	—
T31.53	Burns involving 50-59% of body surface with 30-39% third degree burns	162	Severe Skin Burn or Condition		0.224	0.506	0.162	0.308	—	0.324	—
T31.54	Burns involving 50-59% of body surface with 40-49% third degree burns	162	Severe Skin Burn or Condition		0.224	0.506	0.162	0.308	—	0.324	—
T31.55	Burns involving 50-59% of body surface with 50-59% third degree burns	162	Severe Skin Burn or Condition		0.224	0.506	0.162	0.308	—	0.324	—
T31.61	Burns involving 60-69% of body surface with 10-19% third degree burns	162	Severe Skin Burn or Condition		0.224	0.506	0.162	0.308	—	0.324	—
T31.62	Burns involving 60-69% of body surface with 20-29% third degree burns	162	Severe Skin Burn or Condition		0.224	0.506	0.162	0.308	—	0.324	—
T31.63	Burns involving 60-69% of body surface with 30-39% third degree burns	162	Severe Skin Burn or Condition		0.224	0.506	0.162	0.308	—	0.324	—
T31.64	Burns involving 60-69% of body surface with 40-49% third degree burns	162	Severe Skin Burn or Condition		0.224	0.506	0.162	0.308	—	0.324	—
T31.65	Burns involving 60-69% of body surface with 50-59% third degree burns	162	Severe Skin Burn or Condition		0.224	0.506	0.162	0.308	—	0.324	—
T31.66	Burns involving 60-69% of body surface with 60-69% third degree burns	162	Severe Skin Burn or Condition		0.224	0.506	0.162	0.308	—	0.324	—
T31.71	Burns involving 70-79% of body surface with 10-19% third degree burns	162	Severe Skin Burn or Condition		0.224	0.506	0.162	0.308	—	0.324	—

ICD-10-CM Code	ICD-10-CM Code Description	V24 CMS-HCC	V24 CMS-HCC Disease Group	V24 CMS-HCC Hierarchies	Community, NonDual, Aged	Community, NonDual, Disabled	Community, FBDual, Aged	Community, FBDual, Disabled	Community, PBDual, Aged	Community, PBDual, Disabled	Institutional
T31.72	Burns involving 70-79% of body surface with 20-29% third degree burns	162	Severe Skin Burn or Condition		0.224	0.506	0.162	0.308	—	0.324	—
T31.73	Burns involving 70-79% of body surface with 30-39% third degree burns	162	Severe Skin Burn or Condition		0.224	0.506	0.162	0.308	—	0.324	—
T31.74	Burns involving 70-79% of body surface with 40-49% third degree burns	162	Severe Skin Burn or Condition		0.224	0.506	0.162	0.308	—	0.324	—
T31.75	Burns involving 70-79% of body surface with 50-59% third degree burns	162	Severe Skin Burn or Condition		0.224	0.506	0.162	0.308	—	0.324	—
T31.76	Burns involving 70-79% of body surface with 60-69% third degree burns	162	Severe Skin Burn or Condition		0.224	0.506	0.162	0.308	—	0.324	—
T31.77	Burns involving 70-79% of body surface with 70-79% third degree burns	162	Severe Skin Burn or Condition		0.224	0.506	0.162	0.308	—	0.324	—
T31.81	Burns involving 80-89% of body surface with 10-19% third degree burns	162	Severe Skin Burn or Condition		0.224	0.506	0.162	0.308	—	0.324	—
T31.82	Burns involving 80-89% of body surface with 20-29% third degree burns	162	Severe Skin Burn or Condition		0.224	0.506	0.162	0.308	—	0.324	—
T31.83	Burns involving 80-89% of body surface with 30-39% third degree burns	162	Severe Skin Burn or Condition		0.224	0.506	0.162	0.308	—	0.324	—
T31.84	Burns involving 80-89% of body surface with 40-49% third degree burns	162	Severe Skin Burn or Condition		0.224	0.506	0.162	0.308	—	0.324	—
T31.85	Burns involving 80-89% of body surface with 50-59% third degree burns	162	Severe Skin Burn or Condition		0.224	0.506	0.162	0.308	—	0.324	—
T31.86	Burns involving 80-89% of body surface with 60-69% third degree burns	162	Severe Skin Burn or Condition		0.224	0.506	0.162	0.308	—	0.324	—
T31.87	Burns involving 80-89% of body surface with 70-79% third degree burns	162	Severe Skin Burn or Condition		0.224	0.506	0.162	0.308	—	0.324	—
T31.88	Burns involving 80-89% of body surface with 80-89% third degree burns	162	Severe Skin Burn or Condition		0.224	0.506	0.162	0.308	—	0.324	—
T31.91	Burns involving 90% or more of body surface with 10-19% third degree burns	162	Severe Skin Burn or Condition		0.224	0.506	0.162	0.308	—	0.324	—
T31.92	Burns involving 90% or more of body surface with 20-29% third degree burns	162	Severe Skin Burn or Condition		0.224	0.506	0.162	0.308	—	0.324	—
T31.93	Burns involving 90% or more of body surface with 30-39% third degree burns	162	Severe Skin Burn or Condition		0.224	0.506	0.162	0.308	—	0.324	—
T31.94	Burns involving 90% or more of body surface with 40-49% third degree burns	162	Severe Skin Burn or Condition		0.224	0.506	0.162	0.308	—	0.324	—
T31.95	Burns involving 90% or more of body surface with 50-59% third degree burns	162	Severe Skin Burn or Condition		0.224	0.506	0.162	0.308	—	0.324	—
T31.96	Burns involving 90% or more of body surface with 60-69% third degree burns	162	Severe Skin Burn or Condition		0.224	0.506	0.162	0.308	—	0.324	—

ICD-10-CM Code	ICD-10-CM Code Description	V24 CMS-HCC	V24 CMS-HCC Disease Group	V24 CMS-HCC Hierarchies	Community, NonDual, Aged	Community, NonDual, Disabled	Community, FBDual, Aged	Community, FBDual, Disabled	Community, PBDual, Aged	Community, PBDual, Disabled	Institutional
T31.97	Burns involving 90% or more of body surface with 70-79% third degree burns	162	Severe Skin Burn or Condition		0.224	0.506	0.162	0.308	—	0.324	—
T31.98	Burns involving 90% or more of body surface with 80-89% third degree burns	162	Severe Skin Burn or Condition		0.224	0.506	0.162	0.308	—	0.324	—
T31.99	Burns involving 90% or more of body surface with 90% or more third degree burns	162	Severe Skin Burn or Condition		0.224	0.506	0.162	0.308	—	0.324	—
T32.11	Corrosions involving 10-19% of body surface with 10-19% third degree corrosion	162	Severe Skin Burn or Condition		0.224	0.506	0.162	0.308	—	0.324	—
T32.21	Corrosions involving 20-29% of body surface with 10-19% third degree corrosion	162	Severe Skin Burn or Condition		0.224	0.506	0.162	0.308	—	0.324	—
T32.22	Corrosions involving 20-29% of body surface with 20-29% third degree corrosion	162	Severe Skin Burn or Condition		0.224	0.506	0.162	0.308	—	0.324	—
T32.31	Corrosions involving 30-39% of body surface with 10-19% third degree corrosion	162	Severe Skin Burn or Condition		0.224	0.506	0.162	0.308	—	0.324	—
T32.32	Corrosions involving 30-39% of body surface with 20-29% third degree corrosion	162	Severe Skin Burn or Condition		0.224	0.506	0.162	0.308	—	0.324	—
T32.33	Corrosions involving 30-39% of body surface with 30-39% third degree corrosion	162	Severe Skin Burn or Condition		0.224	0.506	0.162	0.308	—	0.324	—
T32.41	Corrosions involving 40-49% of body surface with 10-19% third degree corrosion	162	Severe Skin Burn or Condition		0.224	0.506	0.162	0.308	—	0.324	—
T32.42	Corrosions involving 40-49% of body surface with 20-29% third degree corrosion	162	Severe Skin Burn or Condition		0.224	0.506	0.162	0.308	—	0.324	—
T32.43	Corrosions involving 40-49% of body surface with 30-39% third degree corrosion	162	Severe Skin Burn or Condition		0.224	0.506	0.162	0.308	—	0.324	—
T32.44	Corrosions involving 40-49% of body surface with 40-49% third degree corrosion	162	Severe Skin Burn or Condition		0.224	0.506	0.162	0.308	—	0.324	—
T32.51	Corrosions involving 50-59% of body surface with 10-19% third degree corrosion	162	Severe Skin Burn or Condition		0.224	0.506	0.162	0.308	—	0.324	—
T32.52	Corrosions involving 50-59% of body surface with 20-29% third degree corrosion	162	Severe Skin Burn or Condition		0.224	0.506	0.162	0.308	—	0.324	—
T32.53	Corrosions involving 50-59% of body surface with 30-39% third degree corrosion	162	Severe Skin Burn or Condition		0.224	0.506	0.162	0.308	—	0.324	—
T32.54	Corrosions involving 50-59% of body surface with 40-49% third degree corrosion	162	Severe Skin Burn or Condition		0.224	0.506	0.162	0.308	—	0.324	—
T32.55	Corrosions involving 50-59% of body surface with 50-59% third degree corrosion	162	Severe Skin Burn or Condition		0.224	0.506	0.162	0.308	—	0.324	—
T32.61	Corrosions involving 60-69% of body surface with 10-19% third degree corrosion	162	Severe Skin Burn or Condition		0.224	0.506	0.162	0.308	—	0.324	—
T32.62	Corrosions involving 60-69% of body surface with 20-29% third degree corrosion	162	Severe Skin Burn or Condition		0.224	0.506	0.162	0.308	—	0.324	—

ICD-10-CM Code	ICD-10-CM Code Description	V24 CMS-HCC	V24 CMS-HCC Disease Group	V24 CMS-HCC Hierarchies	Community, NonDual, Aged	Community, NonDual, Disabled	Community, FBDual, Aged	Community, FBDual, Disabled	Community, PBDual, Aged	Community, PBDual, Disabled	Institutional
T32.63	Corrosions involving 60-69% of body surface with 30-39% third degree corrosion	162	Severe Skin Burn or Condition		0.224	0.506	0.162	0.308	—	0.324	—
T32.64	Corrosions involving 60-69% of body surface with 40-49% third degree corrosion	162	Severe Skin Burn or Condition		0.224	0.506	0.162	0.308	—	0.324	—
T32.65	Corrosions involving 60-69% of body surface with 50-59% third degree corrosion	162	Severe Skin Burn or Condition		0.224	0.506	0.162	0.308	—	0.324	—
T32.66	Corrosions involving 60-69% of body surface with 60-69% third degree corrosion	162	Severe Skin Burn or Condition		0.224	0.506	0.162	0.308	—	0.324	—
T32.71	Corrosions involving 70-79% of body surface with 10-19% third degree corrosion	162	Severe Skin Burn or Condition		0.224	0.506	0.162	0.308	—	0.324	—
T32.72	Corrosions involving 70-79% of body surface with 20-29% third degree corrosion	162	Severe Skin Burn or Condition		0.224	0.506	0.162	0.308	—	0.324	—
T32.73	Corrosions involving 70-79% of body surface with 30-39% third degree corrosion	162	Severe Skin Burn or Condition		0.224	0.506	0.162	0.308	—	0.324	—
T32.74	Corrosions involving 70-79% of body surface with 40-49% third degree corrosion	162	Severe Skin Burn or Condition		0.224	0.506	0.162	0.308	—	0.324	—
T32.75	Corrosions involving 70-79% of body surface with 50-59% third degree corrosion	162	Severe Skin Burn or Condition		0.224	0.506	0.162	0.308	—	0.324	—
T32.76	Corrosions involving 70-79% of body surface with 60-69% third degree corrosion	162	Severe Skin Burn or Condition		0.224	0.506	0.162	0.308	—	0.324	—
T32.77	Corrosions involving 70-79% of body surface with 70-79% third degree corrosion	162	Severe Skin Burn or Condition		0.224	0.506	0.162	0.308	—	0.324	—
T32.81	Corrosions involving 80-89% of body surface with 10-19% third degree corrosion	162	Severe Skin Burn or Condition		0.224	0.506	0.162	0.308	—	0.324	—
T32.82	Corrosions involving 80-89% of body surface with 20-29% third degree corrosion	162	Severe Skin Burn or Condition		0.224	0.506	0.162	0.308	—	0.324	—
T32.83	Corrosions involving 80-89% of body surface with 30-39% third degree corrosion	162	Severe Skin Burn or Condition		0.224	0.506	0.162	0.308	—	0.324	—
T32.84	Corrosions involving 80-89% of body surface with 40-49% third degree corrosion	162	Severe Skin Burn or Condition		0.224	0.506	0.162	0.308	—	0.324	—
T32.85	Corrosions involving 80-89% of body surface with 50-59% third degree corrosion	162	Severe Skin Burn or Condition		0.224	0.506	0.162	0.308	—	0.324	—
T32.86	Corrosions involving 80-89% of body surface with 60-69% third degree corrosion	162	Severe Skin Burn or Condition		0.224	0.506	0.162	0.308	—	0.324	—
T32.87	Corrosions involving 80-89% of body surface with 70-79% third degree corrosion	162	Severe Skin Burn or Condition		0.224	0.506	0.162	0.308	—	0.324	—
T32.88	Corrosions involving 80-89% of body surface with 80-89% third degree corrosion	162	Severe Skin Burn or Condition		0.224	0.506	0.162	0.308	—	0.324	—
T32.91	Corrosions involving 90% or more of body surface with 10-19% third degree corrosion	162	Severe Skin Burn or Condition		0.224	0.506	0.162	0.308	—	0.324	—

ICD-10-CM Code	ICD-10-CM Code Description	V24 CMS-HCC	V24 CMS-HCC Disease Group	V24 CMS-HCC Hierarchies	Community, NonDual, Aged	Community, NonDual, Disabled	Community, FBDual, Aged	Community, FBDual, Disabled	Community, PBDual, Aged	Community, PBDual, Disabled	Institutional
T32.92	Corrosions involving 90% or more of body surface with 20-29% third degree corrosion	162	Severe Skin Burn or Condition		0.224	0.506	0.162	0.308	—	0.324	—
T32.93	Corrosions involving 90% or more of body surface with 30-39% third degree corrosion	162	Severe Skin Burn or Condition		0.224	0.506	0.162	0.308	—	0.324	—
T32.94	Corrosions involving 90% or more of body surface with 40-49% third degree corrosion	162	Severe Skin Burn or Condition		0.224	0.506	0.162	0.308	—	0.324	—
T32.95	Corrosions involving 90% or more of body surface with 50-59% third degree corrosion	162	Severe Skin Burn or Condition		0.224	0.506	0.162	0.308	—	0.324	—
T32.96	Corrosions involving 90% or more of body surface with 60-69% third degree corrosion	162	Severe Skin Burn or Condition		0.224	0.506	0.162	0.308	—	0.324	—
T32.97	Corrosions involving 90% or more of body surface with 70-79% third degree corrosion	162	Severe Skin Burn or Condition		0.224	0.506	0.162	0.308	—	0.324	—
T32.98	Corrosions involving 90% or more of body surface with 80-89% third degree corrosion	162	Severe Skin Burn or Condition		0.224	0.506	0.162	0.308	—	0.324	—
T32.99	Corrosions involving 90% or more of body surface with 90% or more third degree corrosion	162	Severe Skin Burn or Condition		0.224	0.506	0.162	0.308	—	0.324	—
T36.0X2A	Poisoning by penicillins, intentional self-harm, initial encounter	59	Major Depressive, Bipolar, and Paranoid Disorders	60	0.309	0.164	0.299	0.127	0.306	0.109	0.187
T36.0X2S	Poisoning by penicillins, intentional self-harm, sequela	59	Major Depressive, Bipolar, and Paranoid Disorders	60	0.309	0.164	0.299	0.127	0.306	0.109	0.187
T36.1X2A	Poisoning by cephalosporins and other beta-lactam antibiotics, intentional self-harm, initial encounter	59	Major Depressive, Bipolar, and Paranoid Disorders	60	0.309	0.164	0.299	0.127	0.306	0.109	0.187
T36.1X2S	Poisoning by cephalosporins and other beta-lactam antibiotics, intentional self-harm, sequela	59	Major Depressive, Bipolar, and Paranoid Disorders	60	0.309	0.164	0.299	0.127	0.306	0.109	0.187
T36.2X2A	Poisoning by chloramphenicol group, intentional self-harm, initial encounter	59	Major Depressive, Bipolar, and Paranoid Disorders	60	0.309	0.164	0.299	0.127	0.306	0.109	0.187
T36.2X2S	Poisoning by chloramphenicol group, intentional self-harm, sequela	59	Major Depressive, Bipolar, and Paranoid Disorders	60	0.309	0.164	0.299	0.127	0.306	0.109	0.187
T36.3X2A	Poisoning by macrolides, intentional self-harm, initial encounter	59	Major Depressive, Bipolar, and Paranoid Disorders	60	0.309	0.164	0.299	0.127	0.306	0.109	0.187
T36.3X2S	Poisoning by macrolides, intentional self-harm, sequela	59	Major Depressive, Bipolar, and Paranoid Disorders	60	0.309	0.164	0.299	0.127	0.306	0.109	0.187
T36.4X2A	Poisoning by tetracyclines, intentional self-harm, initial encounter	59	Major Depressive, Bipolar, and Paranoid Disorders	60	0.309	0.164	0.299	0.127	0.306	0.109	0.187
T36.4X2S	Poisoning by tetracyclines, intentional self-harm, sequela	59	Major Depressive, Bipolar, and Paranoid Disorders	60	0.309	0.164	0.299	0.127	0.306	0.109	0.187
T36.5X2A	Poisoning by aminoglycosides, intentional self-harm, initial encounter	59	Major Depressive, Bipolar, and Paranoid Disorders	60	0.309	0.164	0.299	0.127	0.306	0.109	0.187
T36.5X2S	Poisoning by aminoglycosides, intentional self-harm, sequela	59	Major Depressive, Bipolar, and Paranoid Disorders	60	0.309	0.164	0.299	0.127	0.306	0.109	0.187
T36.6X2A	Poisoning by rifampicins, intentional self-harm, initial encounter	59	Major Depressive, Bipolar, and Paranoid Disorders	60	0.309	0.164	0.299	0.127	0.306	0.109	0.187
T36.6X2S	Poisoning by rifampicins, intentional self-harm, sequela	59	Major Depressive, Bipolar, and Paranoid Disorders	60	0.309	0.164	0.299	0.127	0.306	0.109	0.187
T36.7X2A	Poisoning by antifungal antibiotics, systemically used, intentional self-harm, initial encounter	59	Major Depressive, Bipolar, and Paranoid Disorders	60	0.309	0.164	0.299	0.127	0.306	0.109	0.187

ICD-10-CM Code	ICD-10-CM Code Description	V24 CMS-HCC	V24 CMS-HCC Disease Group	V24 CMS-HCC Hierarchies	Community, NonDual, Aged	Community, NonDual, Disabled	Community, FBDual, Aged	Community, FBDual, Disabled	Community, PBDual, Aged	Community, PBDual, Disabled	Institutional
T36.7X2S	Poisoning by antifungal antibiotics, systemically used, intentional self-harm, sequela	59	Major Depressive, Bipolar, and Paranoid Disorders	60	0.309	0.164	0.299	0.127	0.306	0.109	0.187
T36.8X2A	Poisoning by other systemic antibiotics, intentional self-harm, initial encounter	59	Major Depressive, Bipolar, and Paranoid Disorders	60	0.309	0.164	0.299	0.127	0.306	0.109	0.187
T36.8X2S	Poisoning by other systemic antibiotics, intentional self-harm, sequela	59	Major Depressive, Bipolar, and Paranoid Disorders	60	0.309	0.164	0.299	0.127	0.306	0.109	0.187
T36.92XA	Poisoning by unspecified systemic antibiotic, intentional self-harm, initial encounter	59	Major Depressive, Bipolar, and Paranoid Disorders	60	0.309	0.164	0.299	0.127	0.306	0.109	0.187
T36.92XS	Poisoning by unspecified systemic antibiotic, intentional self-harm, sequela	59	Major Depressive, Bipolar, and Paranoid Disorders	60	0.309	0.164	0.299	0.127	0.306	0.109	0.187
T37.0X2A	Poisoning by sulfonamides, intentional self-harm, initial encounter	59	Major Depressive, Bipolar, and Paranoid Disorders	60	0.309	0.164	0.299	0.127	0.306	0.109	0.187
T37.0X2S	Poisoning by sulfonamides, intentional self-harm, sequela	59	Major Depressive, Bipolar, and Paranoid Disorders	60	0.309	0.164	0.299	0.127	0.306	0.109	0.187
T37.1X2A	Poisoning by antimycobacterial drugs, intentional self-harm, initial encounter	59	Major Depressive, Bipolar, and Paranoid Disorders	60	0.309	0.164	0.299	0.127	0.306	0.109	0.187
T37.1X2S	Poisoning by antimycobacterial drugs, intentional self-harm, sequela	59	Major Depressive, Bipolar, and Paranoid Disorders	60	0.309	0.164	0.299	0.127	0.306	0.109	0.187
T37.2X2A	Poisoning by antimalarials and drugs acting on other blood protozoa, intentional self-harm, initial encounter	59	Major Depressive, Bipolar, and Paranoid Disorders	60	0.309	0.164	0.299	0.127	0.306	0.109	0.187
T37.2X2S	Poisoning by antimalarials and drugs acting on other blood protozoa, intentional self-harm, sequela	59	Major Depressive, Bipolar, and Paranoid Disorders	60	0.309	0.164	0.299	0.127	0.306	0.109	0.187
T37.3X2A	Poisoning by other antiprotozoal drugs, intentional self-harm, initial encounter	59	Major Depressive, Bipolar, and Paranoid Disorders	60	0.309	0.164	0.299	0.127	0.306	0.109	0.187
T37.3X2S	Poisoning by other antiprotozoal drugs, intentional self-harm, sequela	59	Major Depressive, Bipolar, and Paranoid Disorders	60	0.309	0.164	0.299	0.127	0.306	0.109	0.187
T37.4X2A	Poisoning by anthelminthics, intentional self-harm, initial encounter	59	Major Depressive, Bipolar, and Paranoid Disorders	60	0.309	0.164	0.299	0.127	0.306	0.109	0.187
T37.4X2S	Poisoning by anthelminthics, intentional self-harm, sequela	59	Major Depressive, Bipolar, and Paranoid Disorders	60	0.309	0.164	0.299	0.127	0.306	0.109	0.187
T37.5X2A	Poisoning by antiviral drugs, intentional self-harm, initial encounter	59	Major Depressive, Bipolar, and Paranoid Disorders	60	0.309	0.164	0.299	0.127	0.306	0.109	0.187
T37.5X2S	Poisoning by antiviral drugs, intentional self-harm, sequela	59	Major Depressive, Bipolar, and Paranoid Disorders	60	0.309	0.164	0.299	0.127	0.306	0.109	0.187
T37.8X2A	Poisoning by other specified systemic anti-infectives and antiparasitics, intentional self-harm, initial encounter	59	Major Depressive, Bipolar, and Paranoid Disorders	60	0.309	0.164	0.299	0.127	0.306	0.109	0.187
T37.8X2S	Poisoning by other specified systemic anti-infectives and antiparasitics, intentional self-harm, sequela	59	Major Depressive, Bipolar, and Paranoid Disorders	60	0.309	0.164	0.299	0.127	0.306	0.109	0.187
T37.92XA	Poisoning by unspecified systemic anti-infective and antiparasitics, intentional self-harm, initial encounter	59	Major Depressive, Bipolar, and Paranoid Disorders	60	0.309	0.164	0.299	0.127	0.306	0.109	0.187
T37.92XS	Poisoning by unspecified systemic anti-infective and antiparasitics, intentional self-harm, sequela	59	Major Depressive, Bipolar, and Paranoid Disorders	60	0.309	0.164	0.299	0.127	0.306	0.109	0.187

ICD-10-CM Code	ICD-10-CM Code Description	V24 CMS-HCC	V24 CMS-HCC Disease Group	V24 CMS-HCC Hierarchies	Community, NonDual, Aged	Community, NonDual, Disabled	Community, FBDual, Aged	Community, FBDual, Disabled	Community, PBDual, Aged	Community, PBDual, Disabled	Institutional
T38.0X2A	Poisoning by glucocorticoids and synthetic analogues, intentional self-harm, initial encounter	59	Major Depressive, Bipolar, and Paranoid Disorders	60	0.309	0.164	0.299	0.127	0.306	0.109	0.187
T38.0X2S	Poisoning by glucocorticoids and synthetic analogues, intentional self-harm, sequela	59	Major Depressive, Bipolar, and Paranoid Disorders	60	0.309	0.164	0.299	0.127	0.306	0.109	0.187
T38.1X2A	Poisoning by thyroid hormones and substitutes, intentional self-harm, initial encounter	59	Major Depressive, Bipolar, and Paranoid Disorders	60	0.309	0.164	0.299	0.127	0.306	0.109	0.187
T38.1X2S	Poisoning by thyroid hormones and substitutes, intentional self-harm, sequela	59	Major Depressive, Bipolar, and Paranoid Disorders	60	0.309	0.164	0.299	0.127	0.306	0.109	0.187
T38.2X2A	Poisoning by antithyroid drugs, intentional self-harm, initial encounter	59	Major Depressive, Bipolar, and Paranoid Disorders	60	0.309	0.164	0.299	0.127	0.306	0.109	0.187
T38.2X2S	Poisoning by antithyroid drugs, intentional self-harm, sequela	59	Major Depressive, Bipolar, and Paranoid Disorders	60	0.309	0.164	0.299	0.127	0.306	0.109	0.187
T38.3X2A	Poisoning by insulin and oral hypoglycemic [antidiabetic] drugs, intentional self-harm, initial encounter	59	Major Depressive, Bipolar, and Paranoid Disorders	60	0.309	0.164	0.299	0.127	0.306	0.109	0.187
T38.3X2S	Poisoning by insulin and oral hypoglycemic [antidiabetic] drugs, intentional self-harm, sequela	59	Major Depressive, Bipolar, and Paranoid Disorders	60	0.309	0.164	0.299	0.127	0.306	0.109	0.187
T38.4X2A	Poisoning by oral contraceptives, intentional self-harm, initial encounter	59	Major Depressive, Bipolar, and Paranoid Disorders	60	0.309	0.164	0.299	0.127	0.306	0.109	0.187
T38.4X2S	Poisoning by oral contraceptives, intentional self-harm, sequela	59	Major Depressive, Bipolar, and Paranoid Disorders	60	0.309	0.164	0.299	0.127	0.306	0.109	0.187
T38.5X2A	Poisoning by other estrogens and progestogens, intentional self-harm, initial encounter	59	Major Depressive, Bipolar, and Paranoid Disorders	60	0.309	0.164	0.299	0.127	0.306	0.109	0.187
T38.5X2S	Poisoning by other estrogens and progestogens, intentional self-harm, sequela	59	Major Depressive, Bipolar, and Paranoid Disorders	60	0.309	0.164	0.299	0.127	0.306	0.109	0.187
T38.6X2A	Poisoning by antigonadotrophins, antiestrogens, antiandrogens, not elsewhere classified, intentional self-harm, initial encounter	59	Major Depressive, Bipolar, and Paranoid Disorders	60	0.309	0.164	0.299	0.127	0.306	0.109	0.187
T38.6X2S	Poisoning by antigonadotrophins, antiestrogens, antiandrogens, not elsewhere classified, intentional self-harm, sequela	59	Major Depressive, Bipolar, and Paranoid Disorders	60	0.309	0.164	0.299	0.127	0.306	0.109	0.187
T38.7X2A	Poisoning by androgens and anabolic congeners, intentional self-harm, initial encounter	59	Major Depressive, Bipolar, and Paranoid Disorders	60	0.309	0.164	0.299	0.127	0.306	0.109	0.187
T38.7X2S	Poisoning by androgens and anabolic congeners, intentional self-harm, sequela	59	Major Depressive, Bipolar, and Paranoid Disorders	60	0.309	0.164	0.299	0.127	0.306	0.109	0.187
T38.802A	Poisoning by unspecified hormones and synthetic substitutes, intentional self-harm, initial encounter	59	Major Depressive, Bipolar, and Paranoid Disorders	60	0.309	0.164	0.299	0.127	0.306	0.109	0.187
T38.802S	Poisoning by unspecified hormones and synthetic substitutes, intentional self-harm, sequela	59	Major Depressive, Bipolar, and Paranoid Disorders	60	0.309	0.164	0.299	0.127	0.306	0.109	0.187
T38.812A	Poisoning by anterior pituitary [adenohypophyseal] hormones, intentional self-harm, initial encounter	59	Major Depressive, Bipolar, and Paranoid Disorders	60	0.309	0.164	0.299	0.127	0.306	0.109	0.187
T38.812S	Poisoning by anterior pituitary [adenohypophyseal] hormones, intentional self-harm, sequela	59	Major Depressive, Bipolar, and Paranoid Disorders	60	0.309	0.164	0.299	0.127	0.306	0.109	0.187

ICD-10-CM Code	ICD-10-CM Code Description	V24 CMS-HCC	V24 CMS-HCC Disease Group	V24 CMS-HCC Hierarchies	Community, NonDual, Aged	Community, NonDual, Disabled	Community, FBDual, Aged	Community, FBDual, Disabled	Community, PBDual, Aged	Community, PBDual, Disabled	Institutional
T38.892A	Poisoning by other hormones and synthetic substitutes, intentional self-harm, initial encounter	59	Major Depressive, Bipolar, and Paranoid Disorders	60	0.309	0.164	0.299	0.127	0.306	0.109	0.187
T38.892S	Poisoning by other hormones and synthetic substitutes, intentional self-harm, sequela	59	Major Depressive, Bipolar, and Paranoid Disorders	60	0.309	0.164	0.299	0.127	0.306	0.109	0.187
T38.902A	Poisoning by unspecified hormone antagonists, intentional self-harm, initial encounter	59	Major Depressive, Bipolar, and Paranoid Disorders	60	0.309	0.164	0.299	0.127	0.306	0.109	0.187
T38.902S	Poisoning by unspecified hormone antagonists, intentional self-harm, sequela	59	Major Depressive, Bipolar, and Paranoid Disorders	60	0.309	0.164	0.299	0.127	0.306	0.109	0.187
T38.992A	Poisoning by other hormone antagonists, intentional self-harm, initial encounter	59	Major Depressive, Bipolar, and Paranoid Disorders	60	0.309	0.164	0.299	0.127	0.306	0.109	0.187
T38.992S	Poisoning by other hormone antagonists, intentional self-harm, sequela	59	Major Depressive, Bipolar, and Paranoid Disorders	60	0.309	0.164	0.299	0.127	0.306	0.109	0.187
T39.012A	Poisoning by aspirin, intentional self-harm, initial encounter	59	Major Depressive, Bipolar, and Paranoid Disorders	60	0.309	0.164	0.299	0.127	0.306	0.109	0.187
T39.012S	Poisoning by aspirin, intentional self-harm, sequela	59	Major Depressive, Bipolar, and Paranoid Disorders	60	0.309	0.164	0.299	0.127	0.306	0.109	0.187
T39.092A	Poisoning by salicylates, intentional self-harm, initial encounter	59	Major Depressive, Bipolar, and Paranoid Disorders	60	0.309	0.164	0.299	0.127	0.306	0.109	0.187
T39.092S	Poisoning by salicylates, intentional self-harm, sequela	59	Major Depressive, Bipolar, and Paranoid Disorders	60	0.309	0.164	0.299	0.127	0.306	0.109	0.187
T39.1X2A	Poisoning by 4-Aminophenol derivatives, intentional self-harm, initial encounter	59	Major Depressive, Bipolar, and Paranoid Disorders	60	0.309	0.164	0.299	0.127	0.306	0.109	0.187
T39.1X2S	Poisoning by 4-Aminophenol derivatives, intentional self-harm, sequela	59	Major Depressive, Bipolar, and Paranoid Disorders	60	0.309	0.164	0.299	0.127	0.306	0.109	0.187
T39.2X2A	Poisoning by pyrazolone derivatives, intentional self-harm, initial encounter	59	Major Depressive, Bipolar, and Paranoid Disorders	60	0.309	0.164	0.299	0.127	0.306	0.109	0.187
T39.2X2S	Poisoning by pyrazolone derivatives, intentional self-harm, sequela	59	Major Depressive, Bipolar, and Paranoid Disorders	60	0.309	0.164	0.299	0.127	0.306	0.109	0.187
T39.312A	Poisoning by propionic acid derivatives, intentional self-harm, initial encounter	59	Major Depressive, Bipolar, and Paranoid Disorders	60	0.309	0.164	0.299	0.127	0.306	0.109	0.187
T39.312S	Poisoning by propionic acid derivatives, intentional self-harm, sequela	59	Major Depressive, Bipolar, and Paranoid Disorders	60	0.309	0.164	0.299	0.127	0.306	0.109	0.187
T39.392A	Poisoning by other nonsteroidal anti-inflammatory drugs [NSAID], intentional self-harm, initial encounter	59	Major Depressive, Bipolar, and Paranoid Disorders	60	0.309	0.164	0.299	0.127	0.306	0.109	0.187
T39.392S	Poisoning by other nonsteroidal anti-inflammatory drugs [NSAID], intentional self-harm, sequela	59	Major Depressive, Bipolar, and Paranoid Disorders	60	0.309	0.164	0.299	0.127	0.306	0.109	0.187
T39.4X2A	Poisoning by antirheumatics, not elsewhere classified, intentional self-harm, initial encounter	59	Major Depressive, Bipolar, and Paranoid Disorders	60	0.309	0.164	0.299	0.127	0.306	0.109	0.187
T39.4X2S	Poisoning by antirheumatics, not elsewhere classified, intentional self-harm, sequela	59	Major Depressive, Bipolar, and Paranoid Disorders	60	0.309	0.164	0.299	0.127	0.306	0.109	0.187
T39.8X2A	Poisoning by other nonopioid analgesics and antipyretics, not elsewhere classified, intentional self-harm, initial encounter	59	Major Depressive, Bipolar, and Paranoid Disorders	60	0.309	0.164	0.299	0.127	0.306	0.109	0.187

ICD-10-CM Code	ICD-10-CM Code Description	V24 CMS-HCC	V24 CMS-HCC Disease Group	V24 CMS-HCC Hierarchies	Community, NonDual, Aged	Community, NonDual, Disabled	Community, FBDual, Aged	Community, FBDual, Disabled	Community, PBDual, Aged	Community, PBDual, Disabled	Institutional
T39.8X2S	Poisoning by other nonopioid analgesics and antipyretics, not elsewhere classified, intentional self-harm, sequela	59	Major Depressive, Bipolar, and Paranoid Disorders	60	0.309	0.164	0.299	0.127	0.306	0.109	0.187
T39.92XA	Poisoning by unspecified nonopioid analgesic, antipyretic and antirheumatic, intentional self-harm, initial encounter	59	Major Depressive, Bipolar, and Paranoid Disorders	60	0.309	0.164	0.299	0.127	0.306	0.109	0.187
T39.92XS	Poisoning by unspecified nonopioid analgesic, antipyretic and antirheumatic, intentional self-harm, sequela	59	Major Depressive, Bipolar, and Paranoid Disorders	60	0.309	0.164	0.299	0.127	0.306	0.109	0.187
T40.0X1A	Poisoning by opium, accidental (unintentional), initial encounter	55	Substance Use Disorder, Moderate/Severe, or Substance Use with Complications	56	0.329	0.279	0.538	0.356	0.372	0.275	0.178
T40.0X2A	Poisoning by opium, intentional self-harm, initial encounter	59	Major Depressive, Bipolar, and Paranoid Disorders	60	0.309	0.164	0.299	0.127	0.306	0.109	0.187
T40.0X2S	Poisoning by opium, intentional self-harm, sequela	59	Major Depressive, Bipolar, and Paranoid Disorders	60	0.309	0.164	0.299	0.127	0.306	0.109	0.187
T40.0X4A	Poisoning by opium, undetermined, initial encounter	55	Substance Use Disorder, Moderate/Severe, or Substance Use with Complications	56	0.329	0.279	0.538	0.356	0.372	0.275	0.178
T40.1X1A	Poisoning by heroin, accidental (unintentional), initial encounter	55	Substance Use Disorder, Moderate/Severe, or Substance Use with Complications	56	0.329	0.279	0.538	0.356	0.372	0.275	0.178
T40.1X2A	Poisoning by heroin, intentional self-harm, initial encounter	59	Major Depressive, Bipolar, and Paranoid Disorders	60	0.309	0.164	0.299	0.127	0.306	0.109	0.187
T40.1X2S	Poisoning by heroin, intentional self-harm, sequela	59	Major Depressive, Bipolar, and Paranoid Disorders	60	0.309	0.164	0.299	0.127	0.306	0.109	0.187
T40.1X4A	Poisoning by heroin, undetermined, initial encounter	55	Substance Use Disorder, Moderate/Severe, or Substance Use with Complications	56	0.329	0.279	0.538	0.356	0.372	0.275	0.178
T40.2X1A	Poisoning by other opioids, accidental (unintentional), initial encounter	55	Substance Use Disorder, Moderate/Severe, or Substance Use with Complications	56	0.329	0.279	0.538	0.356	0.372	0.275	0.178
T40.2X2A	Poisoning by other opioids, intentional self-harm, initial encounter	59	Major Depressive, Bipolar, and Paranoid Disorders	60	0.309	0.164	0.299	0.127	0.306	0.109	0.187
T40.2X2S	Poisoning by other opioids, intentional self-harm, sequela	59	Major Depressive, Bipolar, and Paranoid Disorders	60	0.309	0.164	0.299	0.127	0.306	0.109	0.187
T40.2X4A	Poisoning by other opioids, undetermined, initial encounter	55	Substance Use Disorder, Moderate/Severe, or Substance Use with Complications	56	0.329	0.279	0.538	0.356	0.372	0.275	0.178
T40.3X1A	Poisoning by methadone, accidental (unintentional), initial encounter	55	Substance Use Disorder, Moderate/Severe, or Substance Use with Complications	56	0.329	0.279	0.538	0.356	0.372	0.275	0.178
T40.3X2A	Poisoning by methadone, intentional self-harm, initial encounter	59	Major Depressive, Bipolar, and Paranoid Disorders	60	0.309	0.164	0.299	0.127	0.306	0.109	0.187
T40.3X2S	Poisoning by methadone, intentional self-harm, sequela	59	Major Depressive, Bipolar, and Paranoid Disorders	60	0.309	0.164	0.299	0.127	0.306	0.109	0.187
T40.3X4A	Poisoning by methadone, undetermined, initial encounter	55	Substance Use Disorder, Moderate/Severe, or Substance Use with Complications	56	0.329	0.279	0.538	0.356	0.372	0.275	0.178
T40.411A	Poisoning by fentanyl or fentanyl analogs, accidental (unintentional), initial encounter	55	Substance Use Disorder, Moderate/Severe, or Substance Use with Complications	56	0.329	0.279	0.538	0.356	0.372	0.275	0.178
T40.412A	Poisoning by fentanyl or fentanyl analogs, intentional self-harm, initial encounter	59	Major Depressive, Bipolar, and Paranoid Disorders	60	0.309	0.164	0.299	0.127	0.306	0.109	0.187

ICD-10-CM Code	ICD-10-CM Code Description	V24 CMS-HCC	V24 CMS-HCC Disease Group	V24 CMS-HCC Hierarchies	Community, NonDual, Aged	Community, NonDual, Disabled	Community, FBDual, Aged	Community, FBDual, Disabled	Community, PBDual, Aged	Community, PBDual, Disabled	Institutional
T40.412S	Poisoning by fentanyl or fentanyl analogs, intentional self-harm, sequela	59	Major Depressive, Bipolar, and Paranoid Disorders	60	0.309	0.164	0.299	0.127	0.306	0.109	0.187
T40.414A	Poisoning by fentanyl or fentanyl analogs, undetermined, initial encounter	55	Substance Use Disorder, Moderate/ Severe, or Substance Use with Complications	56	0.329	0.279	0.538	0.356	0.372	0.275	0.178
T40.421A	Poisoning by tramadol, accidental (unintentional), initial encounter	55	Substance Use Disorder, Moderate/ Severe, or Substance Use with Complications	56	0.329	0.279	0.538	0.356	0.372	0.275	0.178
T40.422A	Poisoning by tramadol, intentional self-harm, initial encounter	59	Major Depressive, Bipolar, and Paranoid Disorders	60	0.309	0.164	0.299	0.127	0.306	0.109	0.187
T40.422S	Poisoning by tramadol, intentional self-harm, sequela	59	Major Depressive, Bipolar, and Paranoid Disorders	60	0.309	0.164	0.299	0.127	0.306	0.109	0.187
T40.424A	Poisoning by tramadol, undetermined, initial encounter	55	Substance Use Disorder, Moderate/ Severe, or Substance Use with Complications	56	0.329	0.279	0.538	0.356	0.372	0.275	0.178
T40.491A	Poisoning by other synthetic narcotics, accidental (unintentional), initial encounter	55	Substance Use Disorder, Moderate/ Severe, or Substance Use with Complications	56	0.329	0.279	0.538	0.356	0.372	0.275	0.178
T40.492A	Poisoning by other synthetic narcotics, intentional self-harm, initial encounter	59	Major Depressive, Bipolar, and Paranoid Disorders	60	0.309	0.164	0.299	0.127	0.306	0.109	0.187
T40.492S	Poisoning by other synthetic narcotics, intentional self-harm, sequela	59	Major Depressive, Bipolar, and Paranoid Disorders	60	0.309	0.164	0.299	0.127	0.306	0.109	0.187
T40.494A	Poisoning by other synthetic narcotics, undetermined, initial encounter	55	Substance Use Disorder, Moderate/ Severe, or Substance Use with Complications	56	0.329	0.279	0.538	0.356	0.372	0.275	0.178
T40.5X1A	Poisoning by cocaine, accidental (unintentional), initial encounter	55	Substance Use Disorder, Moderate/ Severe, or Substance Use with Complications	56	0.329	0.279	0.538	0.356	0.372	0.275	0.178
T40.5X2A	Poisoning by cocaine, intentional self-harm, initial encounter	59	Major Depressive, Bipolar, and Paranoid Disorders	60	0.309	0.164	0.299	0.127	0.306	0.109	0.187
T40.5X2S	Poisoning by cocaine, intentional self-harm, sequela	59	Major Depressive, Bipolar, and Paranoid Disorders	60	0.309	0.164	0.299	0.127	0.306	0.109	0.187
T40.5X4A	Poisoning by cocaine, undetermined, initial encounter	55	Substance Use Disorder, Moderate/ Severe, or Substance Use with Complications	56	0.329	0.279	0.538	0.356	0.372	0.275	0.178
T40.601A	Poisoning by unspecified narcotics, accidental (unintentional), initial encounter	55	Substance Use Disorder, Moderate/ Severe, or Substance Use with Complications	56	0.329	0.279	0.538	0.356	0.372	0.275	0.178
T40.602A	Poisoning by unspecified narcotics, intentional self-harm, initial encounter	59	Major Depressive, Bipolar, and Paranoid Disorders	60	0.309	0.164	0.299	0.127	0.306	0.109	0.187
T40.602S	Poisoning by unspecified narcotics, intentional self-harm, sequela	59	Major Depressive, Bipolar, and Paranoid Disorders	60	0.309	0.164	0.299	0.127	0.306	0.109	0.187
T40.604A	Poisoning by unspecified narcotics, undetermined, initial encounter	55	Substance Use Disorder, Moderate/ Severe, or Substance Use with Complications	56	0.329	0.279	0.538	0.356	0.372	0.275	0.178
T40.691A	Poisoning by other narcotics, accidental (unintentional), initial encounter	55	Substance Use Disorder, Moderate/ Severe, or Substance Use with Complications	56	0.329	0.279	0.538	0.356	0.372	0.275	0.178
T40.692A	Poisoning by other narcotics, intentional self-harm, initial encounter	59	Major Depressive, Bipolar, and Paranoid Disorders	60	0.309	0.164	0.299	0.127	0.306	0.109	0.187
T40.692S	Poisoning by other narcotics, intentional self-harm, sequela	59	Major Depressive, Bipolar, and Paranoid Disorders	60	0.309	0.164	0.299	0.127	0.306	0.109	0.187
T40.694A	Poisoning by other narcotics, undetermined, initial encounter	55	Substance Use Disorder, Moderate/ Severe, or Substance Use with Complications	56	0.329	0.279	0.538	0.356	0.372	0.275	0.178

ICD-10-CM Code	ICD-10-CM Code Description	V24 CMS-HCC	V24 CMS-HCC Disease Group	V24 CMS-HCC Hierarchies	Community, NonDual, Aged	Community, NonDual, Disabled	Community, FBDual, Aged	Community, FBDual, Disabled	Community, PBDual, Aged	Community, PBDual, Disabled	Institutional
T40.712A	Poisoning by cannabis, intentional self-harm, initial encounter	59	Major Depressive, Bipolar, and Paranoid Disorders	60	0.309	0.164	0.299	0.127	0.306	0.109	0.187
T40.712S	Poisoning by cannabis, intentional self-harm, sequela	59	Major Depressive, Bipolar, and Paranoid Disorders	60	0.309	0.164	0.299	0.127	0.306	0.109	0.187
T40.722A	Poisoning by synthetic cannabinoids, intentional self-harm, initial encounter	59	Major Depressive, Bipolar, and Paranoid Disorders	60	0.309	0.164	0.299	0.127	0.306	0.109	0.187
T40.722S	Poisoning by synthetic cannabinoids, intentional self-harm, sequela	59	Major Depressive, Bipolar, and Paranoid Disorders	60	0.309	0.164	0.299	0.127	0.306	0.109	0.187
T40.7X2A	Poisoning by cannabis (derivatives), intentional self-harm, initial encounter	59	Major Depressive, Bipolar, and Paranoid Disorders	60	0.309	0.164	0.299	0.127	0.306	0.109	0.187
T40.7X2S	Poisoning by cannabis (derivatives), intentional self-harm, sequela	59	Major Depressive, Bipolar, and Paranoid Disorders	60	0.309	0.164	0.299	0.127	0.306	0.109	0.187
T40.8X1A	Poisoning by lysergide [LSD], accidental (unintentional), initial encounter	55	Substance Use Disorder, Moderate/Severe, or Substance Use with Complications	56	0.329	0.279	0.538	0.356	0.372	0.275	0.178
T40.8X2A	Poisoning by lysergide [LSD], intentional self-harm, initial encounter	59	Major Depressive, Bipolar, and Paranoid Disorders	60	0.309	0.164	0.299	0.127	0.306	0.109	0.187
T40.8X2S	Poisoning by lysergide [LSD], intentional self-harm, sequela	59	Major Depressive, Bipolar, and Paranoid Disorders	60	0.309	0.164	0.299	0.127	0.306	0.109	0.187
T40.8X4A	Poisoning by lysergide [LSD], undetermined, initial encounter	55	Substance Use Disorder, Moderate/Severe, or Substance Use with Complications	56	0.329	0.279	0.538	0.356	0.372	0.275	0.178
T40.901A	Poisoning by unspecified psychodysleptics [hallucinogens], accidental (unintentional), initial encounter	55	Substance Use Disorder, Moderate/Severe, or Substance Use with Complications	56	0.329	0.279	0.538	0.356	0.372	0.275	0.178
T40.902A	Poisoning by unspecified psychodysleptics [hallucinogens], intentional self-harm, initial encounter	59	Major Depressive, Bipolar, and Paranoid Disorders	60	0.309	0.164	0.299	0.127	0.306	0.109	0.187
T40.902S	Poisoning by unspecified psychodysleptics [hallucinogens], intentional self-harm, sequela	59	Major Depressive, Bipolar, and Paranoid Disorders	60	0.309	0.164	0.299	0.127	0.306	0.109	0.187
T40.904A	Poisoning by unspecified psychodysleptics [hallucinogens], undetermined, initial encounter	55	Substance Use Disorder, Moderate/Severe, or Substance Use with Complications	56	0.329	0.279	0.538	0.356	0.372	0.275	0.178
T40.991A	Poisoning by other psychodysleptics [hallucinogens], accidental (unintentional), initial encounter	55	Substance Use Disorder, Moderate/Severe, or Substance Use with Complications	56	0.329	0.279	0.538	0.356	0.372	0.275	0.178
T40.992A	Poisoning by other psychodysleptics [hallucinogens], intentional self-harm, initial encounter	59	Major Depressive, Bipolar, and Paranoid Disorders	60	0.309	0.164	0.299	0.127	0.306	0.109	0.187
T40.992S	Poisoning by other psychodysleptics [hallucinogens], intentional self-harm, sequela	59	Major Depressive, Bipolar, and Paranoid Disorders	60	0.309	0.164	0.299	0.127	0.306	0.109	0.187
T40.994A	Poisoning by other psychodysleptics [hallucinogens], undetermined, initial encounter	55	Substance Use Disorder, Moderate/Severe, or Substance Use with Complications	56	0.329	0.279	0.538	0.356	0.372	0.275	0.178
T41.0X2A	Poisoning by inhaled anesthetics, intentional self-harm, initial encounter	59	Major Depressive, Bipolar, and Paranoid Disorders	60	0.309	0.164	0.299	0.127	0.306	0.109	0.187
T41.0X2S	Poisoning by inhaled anesthetics, intentional self-harm, sequela	59	Major Depressive, Bipolar, and Paranoid Disorders	60	0.309	0.164	0.299	0.127	0.306	0.109	0.187
T41.1X2A	Poisoning by intravenous anesthetics, intentional self-harm, initial encounter	59	Major Depressive, Bipolar, and Paranoid Disorders	60	0.309	0.164	0.299	0.127	0.306	0.109	0.187

ICD-10-CM Code	ICD-10-CM Code Description	V24 CMS-HCC	V24 CMS-HCC Disease Group	V24 CMS-HCC Hierarchies	Community, NonDual, Aged	Community, NonDual, Disabled	Community, FBDual, Aged	Community, FBDual, Disabled	Community, PBDual, Aged	Community, PBDual, Disabled	Institutional
T41.1X2S	Poisoning by intravenous anesthetics, intentional self-harm, sequela	59	Major Depressive, Bipolar, and Paranoid Disorders	60	0.309	0.164	0.299	0.127	0.306	0.109	0.187
T41.202A	Poisoning by unspecified general anesthetics, intentional self-harm, initial encounter	59	Major Depressive, Bipolar, and Paranoid Disorders	60	0.309	0.164	0.299	0.127	0.306	0.109	0.187
T41.202S	Poisoning by unspecified general anesthetics, intentional self-harm, sequela	59	Major Depressive, Bipolar, and Paranoid Disorders	60	0.309	0.164	0.299	0.127	0.306	0.109	0.187
T41.292A	Poisoning by other general anesthetics, intentional self-harm, initial encounter	59	Major Depressive, Bipolar, and Paranoid Disorders	60	0.309	0.164	0.299	0.127	0.306	0.109	0.187
T41.292S	Poisoning by other general anesthetics, intentional self-harm, sequela	59	Major Depressive, Bipolar, and Paranoid Disorders	60	0.309	0.164	0.299	0.127	0.306	0.109	0.187
T41.3X2A	Poisoning by local anesthetics, intentional self-harm, initial encounter	59	Major Depressive, Bipolar, and Paranoid Disorders	60	0.309	0.164	0.299	0.127	0.306	0.109	0.187
T41.3X2S	Poisoning by local anesthetics, intentional self-harm, sequela	59	Major Depressive, Bipolar, and Paranoid Disorders	60	0.309	0.164	0.299	0.127	0.306	0.109	0.187
T41.42XA	Poisoning by unspecified anesthetic, intentional self-harm, initial encounter	59	Major Depressive, Bipolar, and Paranoid Disorders	60	0.309	0.164	0.299	0.127	0.306	0.109	0.187
T41.42XS	Poisoning by unspecified anesthetic, intentional self-harm, sequela	59	Major Depressive, Bipolar, and Paranoid Disorders	60	0.309	0.164	0.299	0.127	0.306	0.109	0.187
T41.5X2A	Poisoning by therapeutic gases, intentional self-harm, initial encounter	59	Major Depressive, Bipolar, and Paranoid Disorders	60	0.309	0.164	0.299	0.127	0.306	0.109	0.187
T41.5X2S	Poisoning by therapeutic gases, intentional self-harm, sequela	59	Major Depressive, Bipolar, and Paranoid Disorders	60	0.309	0.164	0.299	0.127	0.306	0.109	0.187
T42.0X2A	Poisoning by hydantoin derivatives, intentional self-harm, initial encounter	59	Major Depressive, Bipolar, and Paranoid Disorders	60	0.309	0.164	0.299	0.127	0.306	0.109	0.187
T42.0X2S	Poisoning by hydantoin derivatives, intentional self-harm, sequela	59	Major Depressive, Bipolar, and Paranoid Disorders	60	0.309	0.164	0.299	0.127	0.306	0.109	0.187
T42.1X2A	Poisoning by iminostilbenes, intentional self-harm, initial encounter	59	Major Depressive, Bipolar, and Paranoid Disorders	60	0.309	0.164	0.299	0.127	0.306	0.109	0.187
T42.1X2S	Poisoning by iminostilbenes, intentional self-harm, sequela	59	Major Depressive, Bipolar, and Paranoid Disorders	60	0.309	0.164	0.299	0.127	0.306	0.109	0.187
T42.2X2A	Poisoning by succinimides and oxazolidinediones, intentional self-harm, initial encounter	59	Major Depressive, Bipolar, and Paranoid Disorders	60	0.309	0.164	0.299	0.127	0.306	0.109	0.187
T42.2X2S	Poisoning by succinimides and oxazolidinediones, intentional self-harm, sequela	59	Major Depressive, Bipolar, and Paranoid Disorders	60	0.309	0.164	0.299	0.127	0.306	0.109	0.187
T42.3X2A	Poisoning by barbiturates, intentional self-harm, initial encounter	59	Major Depressive, Bipolar, and Paranoid Disorders	60	0.309	0.164	0.299	0.127	0.306	0.109	0.187
T42.3X2S	Poisoning by barbiturates, intentional self-harm, sequela	59	Major Depressive, Bipolar, and Paranoid Disorders	60	0.309	0.164	0.299	0.127	0.306	0.109	0.187
T42.4X2A	Poisoning by benzodiazepines, intentional self-harm, initial encounter	59	Major Depressive, Bipolar, and Paranoid Disorders	60	0.309	0.164	0.299	0.127	0.306	0.109	0.187
T42.4X2S	Poisoning by benzodiazepines, intentional self-harm, sequela	59	Major Depressive, Bipolar, and Paranoid Disorders	60	0.309	0.164	0.299	0.127	0.306	0.109	0.187
T42.5X2A	Poisoning by mixed antiepileptics, intentional self-harm, initial encounter	59	Major Depressive, Bipolar, and Paranoid Disorders	60	0.309	0.164	0.299	0.127	0.306	0.109	0.187
T42.5X2S	Poisoning by mixed antiepileptics, intentional self-harm, sequela	59	Major Depressive, Bipolar, and Paranoid Disorders	60	0.309	0.164	0.299	0.127	0.306	0.109	0.187

ICD-10-CM Code	ICD-10-CM Code Description	V24 CMS-HCC	V24 CMS-HCC Disease Group	V24 CMS-HCC Hierarchies	Community, NonDual, Aged	Community, NonDual, Disabled	Community, FBDual, Aged	Community, FBDual, Disabled	Community, PBDual, Aged	Community, PBDual, Disabled	Institutional
T42.6X2A	Poisoning by other antiepileptic and sedative-hypnotic drugs, intentional self-harm, initial encounter	59	Major Depressive, Bipolar, and Paranoid Disorders	60	0.309	0.164	0.299	0.127	0.306	0.109	0.187
T42.6X2S	Poisoning by other antiepileptic and sedative-hypnotic drugs, intentional self-harm, sequela	59	Major Depressive, Bipolar, and Paranoid Disorders	60	0.309	0.164	0.299	0.127	0.306	0.109	0.187
T42.72XA	Poisoning by unspecified antiepileptic and sedative-hypnotic drugs, intentional self-harm, initial encounter	59	Major Depressive, Bipolar, and Paranoid Disorders	60	0.309	0.164	0.299	0.127	0.306	0.109	0.187
T42.72XS	Poisoning by unspecified antiepileptic and sedative-hypnotic drugs, intentional self-harm, sequela	59	Major Depressive, Bipolar, and Paranoid Disorders	60	0.309	0.164	0.299	0.127	0.306	0.109	0.187
T42.8X2A	Poisoning by antiparkinsonism drugs and other central muscle-tone depressants, intentional self-harm, initial encounter	59	Major Depressive, Bipolar, and Paranoid Disorders	60	0.309	0.164	0.299	0.127	0.306	0.109	0.187
T42.8X2S	Poisoning by antiparkinsonism drugs and other central muscle-tone depressants, intentional self-harm, sequela	59	Major Depressive, Bipolar, and Paranoid Disorders	60	0.309	0.164	0.299	0.127	0.306	0.109	0.187
T43.012A	Poisoning by tricyclic antidepressants, intentional self-harm, initial encounter	59	Major Depressive, Bipolar, and Paranoid Disorders	60	0.309	0.164	0.299	0.127	0.306	0.109	0.187
T43.012S	Poisoning by tricyclic antidepressants, intentional self-harm, sequela	59	Major Depressive, Bipolar, and Paranoid Disorders	60	0.309	0.164	0.299	0.127	0.306	0.109	0.187
T43.022A	Poisoning by tetracyclic antidepressants, intentional self-harm, initial encounter	59	Major Depressive, Bipolar, and Paranoid Disorders	60	0.309	0.164	0.299	0.127	0.306	0.109	0.187
T43.022S	Poisoning by tetracyclic antidepressants, intentional self-harm, sequela	59	Major Depressive, Bipolar, and Paranoid Disorders	60	0.309	0.164	0.299	0.127	0.306	0.109	0.187
T43.1X2A	Poisoning by monoamine-oxidase-inhibitor antidepressants, intentional self-harm, initial encounter	59	Major Depressive, Bipolar, and Paranoid Disorders	60	0.309	0.164	0.299	0.127	0.306	0.109	0.187
T43.1X2S	Poisoning by monoamine-oxidase-inhibitor antidepressants, intentional self-harm, sequela	59	Major Depressive, Bipolar, and Paranoid Disorders	60	0.309	0.164	0.299	0.127	0.306	0.109	0.187
T43.202A	Poisoning by unspecified antidepressants, intentional self-harm, initial encounter	59	Major Depressive, Bipolar, and Paranoid Disorders	60	0.309	0.164	0.299	0.127	0.306	0.109	0.187
T43.202S	Poisoning by unspecified antidepressants, intentional self-harm, sequela	59	Major Depressive, Bipolar, and Paranoid Disorders	60	0.309	0.164	0.299	0.127	0.306	0.109	0.187
T43.212A	Poisoning by selective serotonin and norepinephrine reuptake inhibitors, intentional self-harm, initial encounter	59	Major Depressive, Bipolar, and Paranoid Disorders	60	0.309	0.164	0.299	0.127	0.306	0.109	0.187
T43.212S	Poisoning by selective serotonin and norepinephrine reuptake inhibitors, intentional self-harm, sequela	59	Major Depressive, Bipolar, and Paranoid Disorders	60	0.309	0.164	0.299	0.127	0.306	0.109	0.187
T43.222A	Poisoning by selective serotonin reuptake inhibitors, intentional self-harm, initial encounter	59	Major Depressive, Bipolar, and Paranoid Disorders	60	0.309	0.164	0.299	0.127	0.306	0.109	0.187
T43.222S	Poisoning by selective serotonin reuptake inhibitors, intentional self-harm, sequela	59	Major Depressive, Bipolar, and Paranoid Disorders	60	0.309	0.164	0.299	0.127	0.306	0.109	0.187

ICD-10-CM Code	ICD-10-CM Code Description	V24 CMS-HCC	V24 CMS-HCC Disease Group	V24 CMS-HCC Hierarchies	Community, NonDual, Aged	Community, NonDual, Disabled	Community, FBDual, Aged	Community, FBDual, Disabled	Community, PBDual, Aged	Community, PBDual, Disabled	Institutional
T43.292A	Poisoning by other antidepressants, intentional self-harm, initial encounter	59	Major Depressive, Bipolar, and Paranoid Disorders	60	0.309	0.164	0.299	0.127	0.306	0.109	0.187
T43.292S	Poisoning by other antidepressants, intentional self-harm, sequela	59	Major Depressive, Bipolar, and Paranoid Disorders	60	0.309	0.164	0.299	0.127	0.306	0.109	0.187
T43.3X2A	Poisoning by phenothiazine antipsychotics and neuroleptics, intentional self-harm, initial encounter	59	Major Depressive, Bipolar, and Paranoid Disorders	60	0.309	0.164	0.299	0.127	0.306	0.109	0.187
T43.3X2S	Poisoning by phenothiazine antipsychotics and neuroleptics, intentional self-harm, sequela	59	Major Depressive, Bipolar, and Paranoid Disorders	60	0.309	0.164	0.299	0.127	0.306	0.109	0.187
T43.4X2A	Poisoning by butyrophenone and thiothixene neuroleptics, intentional self-harm, initial encounter	59	Major Depressive, Bipolar, and Paranoid Disorders	60	0.309	0.164	0.299	0.127	0.306	0.109	0.187
T43.4X2S	Poisoning by butyrophenone and thiothixene neuroleptics, intentional self-harm, sequela	59	Major Depressive, Bipolar, and Paranoid Disorders	60	0.309	0.164	0.299	0.127	0.306	0.109	0.187
T43.502A	Poisoning by unspecified antipsychotics and neuroleptics, intentional self-harm, initial encounter	59*	Major Depressive, Bipolar, and Paranoid Disorders	60	0.309	0.164	0.299	0.127	0.306	0.109	0.187
T43.502S	Poisoning by unspecified antipsychotics and neuroleptics, intentional self-harm, sequela	59	Major Depressive, Bipolar, and Paranoid Disorders	60	0.309	0.164	0.299	0.127	0.306	0.109	0.187
T43.592A	Poisoning by other antipsychotics and neuroleptics, intentional self-harm, initial encounter	59	Major Depressive, Bipolar, and Paranoid Disorders	60	0.309	0.164	0.299	0.127	0.306	0.109	0.187
T43.592S	Poisoning by other antipsychotics and neuroleptics, intentional self-harm, sequela	59	Major Depressive, Bipolar, and Paranoid Disorders	60	0.309	0.164	0.299	0.127	0.306	0.109	0.187
T43.601A	Poisoning by unspecified psychostimulants, accidental (unintentional), initial encounter	55	Substance Use Disorder, Moderate/Severe, or Substance Use with Complications	56	0.329	0.279	0.538	0.356	0.372	0.275	0.178
T43.602A	Poisoning by unspecified psychostimulants, intentional self-harm, initial encounter	59	Major Depressive, Bipolar, and Paranoid Disorders	60	0.309	0.164	0.299	0.127	0.306	0.109	0.187
T43.602S	Poisoning by unspecified psychostimulants, intentional self-harm, sequela	59	Major Depressive, Bipolar, and Paranoid Disorders	60	0.309	0.164	0.299	0.127	0.306	0.109	0.187
T43.604A	Poisoning by unspecified psychostimulants, undetermined, initial encounter	55	Substance Use Disorder, Moderate/Severe, or Substance Use with Complications	56	0.329	0.279	0.538	0.356	0.372	0.275	0.178
T43.611A	Poisoning by caffeine, accidental (unintentional), initial encounter	55	Substance Use Disorder, Moderate/Severe, or Substance Use with Complications	56	0.329	0.279	0.538	0.356	0.372	0.275	0.178
T43.612A	Poisoning by caffeine, intentional self-harm, initial encounter	59	Major Depressive, Bipolar, and Paranoid Disorders	60	0.309	0.164	0.299	0.127	0.306	0.109	0.187
T43.612S	Poisoning by caffeine, intentional self-harm, sequela	59	Major Depressive, Bipolar, and Paranoid Disorders	60	0.309	0.164	0.299	0.127	0.306	0.109	0.187
T43.614A	Poisoning by caffeine, undetermined, initial encounter	55	Substance Use Disorder, Moderate/Severe, or Substance Use with Complications	56	0.329	0.279	0.538	0.356	0.372	0.275	0.178
T43.621A	Poisoning by amphetamines, accidental (unintentional), initial encounter	55	Substance Use Disorder, Moderate/Severe, or Substance Use with Complications	56	0.329	0.279	0.538	0.356	0.372	0.275	0.178
T43.622A	Poisoning by amphetamines, intentional self-harm, initial encounter	59	Major Depressive, Bipolar, and Paranoid Disorders	60	0.309	0.164	0.299	0.127	0.306	0.109	0.187
T43.622S	Poisoning by amphetamines, intentional self-harm, sequela	59	Major Depressive, Bipolar, and Paranoid Disorders	60	0.309	0.164	0.299	0.127	0.306	0.109	0.187

ICD-10-CM Code	ICD-10-CM Code Description	V24 CMS-HCC	V24 CMS-HCC Disease Group	V24 CMS-HCC Hierarchies	Community, NonDual, Aged	Community, NonDual, Disabled	Community, FBDual, Aged	Community, FBDual, Disabled	Community, PBDual, Aged	Community, PBDual, Disabled	Institutional
T43.624A	Poisoning by amphetamines, undetermined, initial encounter	55	Substance Use Disorder, Moderate/Severe, or Substance Use with Complications	56	0.329	0.279	0.538	0.356	0.372	0.275	0.178
T43.631A	Poisoning by methylphenidate, accidental (unintentional), initial encounter	55	Substance Use Disorder, Moderate/Severe, or Substance Use with Complications	56	0.329	0.279	0.538	0.356	0.372	0.275	0.178
T43.632A	Poisoning by methylphenidate, intentional self-harm, initial encounter	59	Major Depressive, Bipolar, and Paranoid Disorders	60	0.309	0.164	0.299	0.127	0.306	0.109	0.187
T43.632S	Poisoning by methylphenidate, intentional self-harm, sequela	59	Major Depressive, Bipolar, and Paranoid Disorders	60	0.309	0.164	0.299	0.127	0.306	0.109	0.187
T43.634A	Poisoning by methylphenidate, undetermined, initial encounter	55	Substance Use Disorder, Moderate/Severe, or Substance Use with Complications	56	0.329	0.279	0.538	0.356	0.372	0.275	0.178
T43.641A	Poisoning by ecstasy, accidental (unintentional), initial encounter	55	Substance Use Disorder, Moderate/Severe, or Substance Use with Complications	56	0.329	0.279	0.538	0.356	0.372	0.275	0.178
T43.642A	Poisoning by ecstasy, intentional self-harm, initial encounter	59	Major Depressive, Bipolar, and Paranoid Disorders	60	0.309	0.164	0.299	0.127	0.306	0.109	0.187
T43.642S	Poisoning by ecstasy, intentional self-harm, sequela	59	Major Depressive, Bipolar, and Paranoid Disorders	60	0.309	0.164	0.299	0.127	0.306	0.109	0.187
T43.644A	Poisoning by ecstasy, undetermined, initial encounter	55	Substance Use Disorder, Moderate/Severe, or Substance Use with Complications	56	0.329	0.279	0.538	0.356	0.372	0.275	0.178
T43.691A	Poisoning by other psychostimulants, accidental (unintentional), initial encounter	55	Substance Use Disorder, Moderate/Severe, or Substance Use with Complications	56	0.329	0.279	0.538	0.356	0.372	0.275	0.178
T43.692A	Poisoning by other psychostimulants, intentional self-harm, initial encounter	59	Major Depressive, Bipolar, and Paranoid Disorders	60	0.309	0.164	0.299	0.127	0.306	0.109	0.187
T43.692S	Poisoning by other psychostimulants, intentional self-harm, sequela	59	Major Depressive, Bipolar, and Paranoid Disorders	60	0.309	0.164	0.299	0.127	0.306	0.109	0.187
T43.694A	Poisoning by other psychostimulants, undetermined, initial encounter	55	Substance Use Disorder, Moderate/Severe, or Substance Use with Complications	56	0.329	0.279	0.538	0.356	0.372	0.275	0.178
T43.8X2A	Poisoning by other psychotropic drugs, intentional self-harm, initial encounter	59	Major Depressive, Bipolar, and Paranoid Disorders	60	0.309	0.164	0.299	0.127	0.306	0.109	0.187
T43.8X2S	Poisoning by other psychotropic drugs, intentional self-harm, sequela	59	Major Depressive, Bipolar, and Paranoid Disorders	60	0.309	0.164	0.299	0.127	0.306	0.109	0.187
T43.92XA	Poisoning by unspecified psychotropic drug, intentional self-harm, initial encounter	59	Major Depressive, Bipolar, and Paranoid Disorders	60	0.309	0.164	0.299	0.127	0.306	0.109	0.187
T43.92XS	Poisoning by unspecified psychotropic drug, intentional self-harm, sequela	59	Major Depressive, Bipolar, and Paranoid Disorders	60	0.309	0.164	0.299	0.127	0.306	0.109	0.187
T44.0X2A	Poisoning by anticholinesterase agents, intentional self-harm, initial encounter	59	Major Depressive, Bipolar, and Paranoid Disorders	60	0.309	0.164	0.299	0.127	0.306	0.109	0.187
T44.0X2S	Poisoning by anticholinesterase agents, intentional self-harm, sequela	59	Major Depressive, Bipolar, and Paranoid Disorders	60	0.309	0.164	0.299	0.127	0.306	0.109	0.187
T44.1X2A	Poisoning by other parasympathomimetics [cholinergics], intentional self-harm, initial encounter	59	Major Depressive, Bipolar, and Paranoid Disorders	60	0.309	0.164	0.299	0.127	0.306	0.109	0.187
T44.1X2S	Poisoning by other parasympathomimetics [cholinergics], intentional self-harm, sequela	59	Major Depressive, Bipolar, and Paranoid Disorders	60	0.309	0.164	0.299	0.127	0.306	0.109	0.187

ICD-10-CM Code	ICD-10-CM Code Description	V24 CMS-HCC	V24 CMS-HCC Disease Group	V24 CMS-HCC Hierarchies	Community, NonDual, Aged	Community, NonDual, Disabled	Community, FBDual, Aged	Community, FBDual, Disabled	Community, PBDual, Aged	Community, PBDual, Disabled	Institutional
T44.2X2A	Poisoning by ganglionic blocking drugs, intentional self-harm, initial encounter	59	Major Depressive, Bipolar, and Paranoid Disorders	60	0.309	0.164	0.299	0.127	0.306	0.109	0.187
T44.2X2S	Poisoning by ganglionic blocking drugs, intentional self-harm, sequela	59	Major Depressive, Bipolar, and Paranoid Disorders	60	0.309	0.164	0.299	0.127	0.306	0.109	0.187
T44.3X2A	Poisoning by other parasympatholytics [anticholinergics and antimuscarinics] and spasmolytics, intentional self-harm, initial encounter	59	Major Depressive, Bipolar, and Paranoid Disorders	60	0.309	0.164	0.299	0.127	0.306	0.109	0.187
T44.3X2S	Poisoning by other parasympatholytics [anticholinergics and antimuscarinics] and spasmolytics, intentional self-harm, sequela	59	Major Depressive, Bipolar, and Paranoid Disorders	60	0.309	0.164	0.299	0.127	0.306	0.109	0.187
T44.4X2A	Poisoning by predominantly alpha-adrenoreceptor agonists, intentional self-harm, initial encounter	59	Major Depressive, Bipolar, and Paranoid Disorders	60	0.309	0.164	0.299	0.127	0.306	0.109	0.187
T44.4X2S	Poisoning by predominantly alpha-adrenoreceptor agonists, intentional self-harm, sequela	59	Major Depressive, Bipolar, and Paranoid Disorders	60	0.309	0.164	0.299	0.127	0.306	0.109	0.187
T44.5X2A	Poisoning by predominantly beta-adrenoreceptor agonists, intentional self-harm, initial encounter	59	Major Depressive, Bipolar, and Paranoid Disorders	60	0.309	0.164	0.299	0.127	0.306	0.109	0.187
T44.5X2S	Poisoning by predominantly beta-adrenoreceptor agonists, intentional self-harm, sequela	59	Major Depressive, Bipolar, and Paranoid Disorders	60	0.309	0.164	0.299	0.127	0.306	0.109	0.187
T44.6X2A	Poisoning by alpha-adrenoreceptor antagonists, intentional self-harm, initial encounter	59	Major Depressive, Bipolar, and Paranoid Disorders	60	0.309	0.164	0.299	0.127	0.306	0.109	0.187
T44.6X2S	Poisoning by alpha-adrenoreceptor antagonists, intentional self-harm, sequela	59	Major Depressive, Bipolar, and Paranoid Disorders	60	0.309	0.164	0.299	0.127	0.306	0.109	0.187
T44.7X2A	Poisoning by beta-adrenoreceptor antagonists, intentional self-harm, initial encounter	59	Major Depressive, Bipolar, and Paranoid Disorders	60	0.309	0.164	0.299	0.127	0.306	0.109	0.187
T44.7X2S	Poisoning by beta-adrenoreceptor antagonists, intentional self-harm, sequela	59	Major Depressive, Bipolar, and Paranoid Disorders	60	0.309	0.164	0.299	0.127	0.306	0.109	0.187
T44.8X2A	Poisoning by centrally-acting and adrenergic-neuron-blocking agents, intentional self-harm, initial encounter	59	Major Depressive, Bipolar, and Paranoid Disorders	60	0.309	0.164	0.299	0.127	0.306	0.109	0.187
T44.8X2S	Poisoning by centrally-acting and adrenergic-neuron-blocking agents, intentional self-harm, sequela	59	Major Depressive, Bipolar, and Paranoid Disorders	60	0.309	0.164	0.299	0.127	0.306	0.109	0.187
T44.902A	Poisoning by unspecified drugs primarily affecting the autonomic nervous system, intentional self-harm, initial encounter	59	Major Depressive, Bipolar, and Paranoid Disorders	60	0.309	0.164	0.299	0.127	0.306	0.109	0.187
T44.902S	Poisoning by unspecified drugs primarily affecting the autonomic nervous system, intentional self-harm, sequela	59	Major Depressive, Bipolar, and Paranoid Disorders	60	0.309	0.164	0.299	0.127	0.306	0.109	0.187
T44.992A	Poisoning by other drug primarily affecting the autonomic nervous system, intentional self-harm, initial encounter	59	Major Depressive, Bipolar, and Paranoid Disorders	60	0.309	0.164	0.299	0.127	0.306	0.109	0.187

ICD-10-CM Code	ICD-10-CM Code Description	V24 CMS-HCC	V24 CMS-HCC Disease Group	V24 CMS-HCC Hierarchies	Community, NonDual, Aged	Community, NonDual, Disabled	Community, FBDual, Aged	Community, FBDual, Disabled	Community, PBDual, Aged	Community, PBDual, Disabled	Institutional
T44.992S	Poisoning by other drug primarily affecting the autonomic nervous system, intentional self-harm, sequela	59	Major Depressive, Bipolar, and Paranoid Disorders	60	0.309	0.164	0.299	0.127	0.306	0.109	0.187
T45.0X2A	Poisoning by antiallergic and antiemetic drugs, intentional self-harm, initial encounter	59	Major Depressive, Bipolar, and Paranoid Disorders	60	0.309	0.164	0.299	0.127	0.306	0.109	0.187
T45.0X2S	Poisoning by antiallergic and antiemetic drugs, intentional self-harm, sequela	59	Major Depressive, Bipolar, and Paranoid Disorders	60	0.309	0.164	0.299	0.127	0.306	0.109	0.187
T45.1X2A	Poisoning by antineoplastic and immunosuppressive drugs, intentional self-harm, initial encounter	59	Major Depressive, Bipolar, and Paranoid Disorders	60	0.309	0.164	0.299	0.127	0.306	0.109	0.187
T45.1X2S	Poisoning by antineoplastic and immunosuppressive drugs, intentional self-harm, sequela	59	Major Depressive, Bipolar, and Paranoid Disorders	60	0.309	0.164	0.299	0.127	0.306	0.109	0.187
T45.2X2A	Poisoning by vitamins, intentional self-harm, initial encounter	59	Major Depressive, Bipolar, and Paranoid Disorders	60	0.309	0.164	0.299	0.127	0.306	0.109	0.187
T45.2X2S	Poisoning by vitamins, intentional self-harm, sequela	59	Major Depressive, Bipolar, and Paranoid Disorders	60	0.309	0.164	0.299	0.127	0.306	0.109	0.187
T45.3X2A	Poisoning by enzymes, intentional self-harm, initial encounter	59	Major Depressive, Bipolar, and Paranoid Disorders	60	0.309	0.164	0.299	0.127	0.306	0.109	0.187
T45.3X2S	Poisoning by enzymes, intentional self-harm, sequela	59	Major Depressive, Bipolar, and Paranoid Disorders	60	0.309	0.164	0.299	0.127	0.306	0.109	0.187
T45.4X2A	Poisoning by iron and its compounds, intentional self-harm, initial encounter	59	Major Depressive, Bipolar, and Paranoid Disorders	60	0.309	0.164	0.299	0.127	0.306	0.109	0.187
T45.4X2S	Poisoning by iron and its compounds, intentional self-harm, sequela	59	Major Depressive, Bipolar, and Paranoid Disorders	60	0.309	0.164	0.299	0.127	0.306	0.109	0.187
T45.512A	Poisoning by anticoagulants, intentional self-harm, initial encounter	59	Major Depressive, Bipolar, and Paranoid Disorders	60	0.309	0.164	0.299	0.127	0.306	0.109	0.187
T45.512S	Poisoning by anticoagulants, intentional self-harm, sequela	59	Major Depressive, Bipolar, and Paranoid Disorders	60	0.309	0.164	0.299	0.127	0.306	0.109	0.187
T45.522A	Poisoning by antithrombotic drugs, intentional self-harm, initial encounter	59	Major Depressive, Bipolar, and Paranoid Disorders	60	0.309	0.164	0.299	0.127	0.306	0.109	0.187
T45.522S	Poisoning by antithrombotic drugs, intentional self-harm, sequela	59	Major Depressive, Bipolar, and Paranoid Disorders	60	0.309	0.164	0.299	0.127	0.306	0.109	0.187
T45.602A	Poisoning by unspecified fibrinolysis-affecting drugs, intentional self-harm, initial encounter	59	Major Depressive, Bipolar, and Paranoid Disorders	60	0.309	0.164	0.299	0.127	0.306	0.109	0.187
T45.602S	Poisoning by unspecified fibrinolysis-affecting drugs, intentional self-harm, sequela	59	Major Depressive, Bipolar, and Paranoid Disorders	60	0.309	0.164	0.299	0.127	0.306	0.109	0.187
T45.612A	Poisoning by thrombolytic drug, intentional self-harm, initial encounter	59	Major Depressive, Bipolar, and Paranoid Disorders	60	0.309	0.164	0.299	0.127	0.306	0.109	0.187
T45.612S	Poisoning by thrombolytic drug, intentional self-harm, sequela	59	Major Depressive, Bipolar, and Paranoid Disorders	60	0.309	0.164	0.299	0.127	0.306	0.109	0.187
T45.622A	Poisoning by hemostatic drug, intentional self-harm, initial encounter	59	Major Depressive, Bipolar, and Paranoid Disorders	60	0.309	0.164	0.299	0.127	0.306	0.109	0.187
T45.622S	Poisoning by hemostatic drug, intentional self-harm, sequela	59	Major Depressive, Bipolar, and Paranoid Disorders	60	0.309	0.164	0.299	0.127	0.306	0.109	0.187
T45.692A	Poisoning by other fibrinolysis-affecting drugs, intentional self-harm, initial encounter	59	Major Depressive, Bipolar, and Paranoid Disorders	60	0.309	0.164	0.299	0.127	0.306	0.109	0.187

ICD-10-CM Code	ICD-10-CM Code Description	V24 CMS-HCC	V24 CMS-HCC Disease Group	V24 CMS-HCC Hierarchies	Community, NonDual, Aged	Community, NonDual, Disabled	Community, FBDual, Aged	Community, FBDual, Disabled	Community, PBDual, Aged	Community, PBDual, Disabled	Institutional
T45.692S	Poisoning by other fibrinolysis-affecting drugs, intentional self-harm, sequela	59	Major Depressive, Bipolar, and Paranoid Disorders	60	0.309	0.164	0.299	0.127	0.306	0.109	0.187
T45.7X2A	Poisoning by anticoagulant antagonists, vitamin K and other coagulants, intentional self-harm, initial encounter	59	Major Depressive, Bipolar, and Paranoid Disorders	60	0.309	0.164	0.299	0.127	0.306	0.109	0.187
T45.7X2S	Poisoning by anticoagulant antagonists, vitamin K and other coagulants, intentional self-harm, sequela	59	Major Depressive, Bipolar, and Paranoid Disorders	60	0.309	0.164	0.299	0.127	0.306	0.109	0.187
T45.8X2A	Poisoning by other primarily systemic and hematological agents, intentional self-harm, initial encounter	59	Major Depressive, Bipolar, and Paranoid Disorders	60	0.309	0.164	0.299	0.127	0.306	0.109	0.187
T45.8X2S	Poisoning by other primarily systemic and hematological agents, intentional self-harm, sequela	59	Major Depressive, Bipolar, and Paranoid Disorders	60	0.309	0.164	0.299	0.127	0.306	0.109	0.187
T45.92XA	Poisoning by unspecified primarily systemic and hematological agent, intentional self-harm, initial encounter	59	Major Depressive, Bipolar, and Paranoid Disorders	60	0.309	0.164	0.299	0.127	0.306	0.109	0.187
T45.92XS	Poisoning by unspecified primarily systemic and hematological agent, intentional self-harm, sequela	59	Major Depressive, Bipolar, and Paranoid Disorders	60	0.309	0.164	0.299	0.127	0.306	0.109	0.187
T46.0X2A	Poisoning by cardiac-stimulant glycosides and drugs of similar action, intentional self-harm, initial encounter	59	Major Depressive, Bipolar, and Paranoid Disorders	60	0.309	0.164	0.299	0.127	0.306	0.109	0.187
T46.0X2S	Poisoning by cardiac-stimulant glycosides and drugs of similar action, intentional self-harm, sequela	59	Major Depressive, Bipolar, and Paranoid Disorders	60	0.309	0.164	0.299	0.127	0.306	0.109	0.187
T46.1X2A	Poisoning by calcium-channel blockers, intentional self-harm, initial encounter	59	Major Depressive, Bipolar, and Paranoid Disorders	60	0.309	0.164	0.299	0.127	0.306	0.109	0.187
T46.1X2S	Poisoning by calcium-channel blockers, intentional self-harm, sequela	59	Major Depressive, Bipolar, and Paranoid Disorders	60	0.309	0.164	0.299	0.127	0.306	0.109	0.187
T46.2X2A	Poisoning by other antidysrhythmic drugs, intentional self-harm, initial encounter	59	Major Depressive, Bipolar, and Paranoid Disorders	60	0.309	0.164	0.299	0.127	0.306	0.109	0.187
T46.2X2S	Poisoning by other antidysrhythmic drugs, intentional self-harm, sequela	59	Major Depressive, Bipolar, and Paranoid Disorders	60	0.309	0.164	0.299	0.127	0.306	0.109	0.187
T46.3X2A	Poisoning by coronary vasodilators, intentional self-harm, initial encounter	59	Major Depressive, Bipolar, and Paranoid Disorders	60	0.309	0.164	0.299	0.127	0.306	0.109	0.187
T46.3X2S	Poisoning by coronary vasodilators, intentional self-harm, sequela	59	Major Depressive, Bipolar, and Paranoid Disorders	60	0.309	0.164	0.299	0.127	0.306	0.109	0.187
T46.4X2A	Poisoning by angiotensin-converting-enzyme inhibitors, intentional self-harm, initial encounter	59	Major Depressive, Bipolar, and Paranoid Disorders	60	0.309	0.164	0.299	0.127	0.306	0.109	0.187
T46.4X2S	Poisoning by angiotensin-converting-enzyme inhibitors, intentional self-harm, sequela	59	Major Depressive, Bipolar, and Paranoid Disorders	60	0.309	0.164	0.299	0.127	0.306	0.109	0.187
T46.5X2A	Poisoning by other antihypertensive drugs, intentional self-harm, initial encounter	59	Major Depressive, Bipolar, and Paranoid Disorders	60	0.309	0.164	0.299	0.127	0.306	0.109	0.187
T46.5X2S	Poisoning by other antihypertensive drugs, intentional self-harm, sequela	59	Major Depressive, Bipolar, and Paranoid Disorders	60	0.309	0.164	0.299	0.127	0.306	0.109	0.187

                                                                              2021 Optum360, LLC

ICD-10-CM Code	ICD-10-CM Code Description	V24 CMS-HCC	V24 CMS-HCC Disease Group	V24 CMS-HCC Hierarchies	Community, NonDual, Aged	Community, NonDual, Disabled	Community, FBDual, Aged	Community, FBDual, Disabled	Community, PBDual, Aged	Community, PBDual, Disabled	Institutional
T46.6X2A	Poisoning by antihyperlipidemic and antiarteriosclerotic drugs, intentional self-harm, initial encounter	59	Major Depressive, Bipolar, and Paranoid Disorders	60	0.309	0.164	0.299	0.127	0.306	0.109	0.187
T46.6X2S	Poisoning by antihyperlipidemic and antiarteriosclerotic drugs, intentional self-harm, sequela	59	Major Depressive, Bipolar, and Paranoid Disorders	60	0.309	0.164	0.299	0.127	0.306	0.109	0.187
T46.7X2A	Poisoning by peripheral vasodilators, intentional self-harm, initial encounter	59	Major Depressive, Bipolar, and Paranoid Disorders	60	0.309	0.164	0.299	0.127	0.306	0.109	0.187
T46.7X2S	Poisoning by peripheral vasodilators, intentional self-harm, sequela	59	Major Depressive, Bipolar, and Paranoid Disorders	60	0.309	0.164	0.299	0.127	0.306	0.109	0.187
T46.8X2A	Poisoning by antivaricose drugs, including sclerosing agents, intentional self-harm, initial encounter	59	Major Depressive, Bipolar, and Paranoid Disorders	60	0.309	0.164	0.299	0.127	0.306	0.109	0.187
T46.8X2S	Poisoning by antivaricose drugs, including sclerosing agents, intentional self-harm, sequela	59	Major Depressive, Bipolar, and Paranoid Disorders	60	0.309	0.164	0.299	0.127	0.306	0.109	0.187
T46.902A	Poisoning by unspecified agents primarily affecting the cardiovascular system, intentional self-harm, initial encounter	59	Major Depressive, Bipolar, and Paranoid Disorders	60	0.309	0.164	0.299	0.127	0.306	0.109	0.187
T46.902S	Poisoning by unspecified agents primarily affecting the cardiovascular system, intentional self-harm, sequela	59	Major Depressive, Bipolar, and Paranoid Disorders	60	0.309	0.164	0.299	0.127	0.306	0.109	0.187
T46.992A	Poisoning by other agents primarily affecting the cardiovascular system, intentional self-harm, initial encounter	59	Major Depressive, Bipolar, and Paranoid Disorders	60	0.309	0.164	0.299	0.127	0.306	0.109	0.187
T46.992S	Poisoning by other agents primarily affecting the cardiovascular system, intentional self-harm, sequela	59	Major Depressive, Bipolar, and Paranoid Disorders	60	0.309	0.164	0.299	0.127	0.306	0.109	0.187
T47.0X2A	Poisoning by histamine H2-receptor blockers, intentional self-harm, initial encounter	59	Major Depressive, Bipolar, and Paranoid Disorders	60	0.309	0.164	0.299	0.127	0.306	0.109	0.187
T47.0X2S	Poisoning by histamine H2-receptor blockers, intentional self-harm, sequela	59	Major Depressive, Bipolar, and Paranoid Disorders	60	0.309	0.164	0.299	0.127	0.306	0.109	0.187
T47.1X2A	Poisoning by other antacids and anti-gastric-secretion drugs, intentional self-harm, initial encounter	59	Major Depressive, Bipolar, and Paranoid Disorders	60	0.309	0.164	0.299	0.127	0.306	0.109	0.187
T47.1X2S	Poisoning by other antacids and anti-gastric-secretion drugs, intentional self-harm, sequela	59	Major Depressive, Bipolar, and Paranoid Disorders	60	0.309	0.164	0.299	0.127	0.306	0.109	0.187
T47.2X2A	Poisoning by stimulant laxatives, intentional self-harm, initial encounter	59	Major Depressive, Bipolar, and Paranoid Disorders	60	0.309	0.164	0.299	0.127	0.306	0.109	0.187
T47.2X2S	Poisoning by stimulant laxatives, intentional self-harm, sequela	59	Major Depressive, Bipolar, and Paranoid Disorders	60	0.309	0.164	0.299	0.127	0.306	0.109	0.187
T47.3X2A	Poisoning by saline and osmotic laxatives, intentional self-harm, initial encounter	59	Major Depressive, Bipolar, and Paranoid Disorders	60	0.309	0.164	0.299	0.127	0.306	0.109	0.187
T47.3X2S	Poisoning by saline and osmotic laxatives, intentional self-harm, sequela	59	Major Depressive, Bipolar, and Paranoid Disorders	60	0.309	0.164	0.299	0.127	0.306	0.109	0.187
T47.4X2A	Poisoning by other laxatives, intentional self-harm, initial encounter	59	Major Depressive, Bipolar, and Paranoid Disorders	60	0.309	0.164	0.299	0.127	0.306	0.109	0.187
T47.4X2S	Poisoning by other laxatives, intentional self-harm, sequela	59	Major Depressive, Bipolar, and Paranoid Disorders	60	0.309	0.164	0.299	0.127	0.306	0.109	0.187

ICD-10-CM Code	ICD-10-CM Code Description	V24 CMS-HCC	V24 CMS-HCC Disease Group	V24 CMS-HCC Hierarchies	Community, NonDual, Aged	Community, NonDual, Disabled	Community, FBDual, Aged	Community, FBDual, Disabled	Community, PBDual, Aged	Community, PBDual, Disabled	Institutional
T47.5X2A	Poisoning by digestants, intentional self-harm, initial encounter	59	Major Depressive, Bipolar, and Paranoid Disorders	60	0.309	0.164	0.299	0.127	0.306	0.109	0.187
T47.5X2S	Poisoning by digestants, intentional self-harm, sequela	59	Major Depressive, Bipolar, and Paranoid Disorders	60	0.309	0.164	0.299	0.127	0.306	0.109	0.187
T47.6X2A	Poisoning by antidiarrheal drugs, intentional self-harm, initial encounter	59	Major Depressive, Bipolar, and Paranoid Disorders	60	0.309	0.164	0.299	0.127	0.306	0.109	0.187
T47.6X2S	Poisoning by antidiarrheal drugs, intentional self-harm, sequela	59	Major Depressive, Bipolar, and Paranoid Disorders	60	0.309	0.164	0.299	0.127	0.306	0.109	0.187
T47.7X2A	Poisoning by emetics, intentional self-harm, initial encounter	59	Major Depressive, Bipolar, and Paranoid Disorders	60	0.309	0.164	0.299	0.127	0.306	0.109	0.187
T47.7X2S	Poisoning by emetics, intentional self-harm, sequela	59	Major Depressive, Bipolar, and Paranoid Disorders	60	0.309	0.164	0.299	0.127	0.306	0.109	0.187
T47.8X2A	Poisoning by other agents primarily affecting gastrointestinal system, intentional self-harm, initial encounter	59	Major Depressive, Bipolar, and Paranoid Disorders	60	0.309	0.164	0.299	0.127	0.306	0.109	0.187
T47.8X2S	Poisoning by other agents primarily affecting gastrointestinal system, intentional self-harm, sequela	59	Major Depressive, Bipolar, and Paranoid Disorders	60	0.309	0.164	0.299	0.127	0.306	0.109	0.187
T47.92XA	Poisoning by unspecified agents primarily affecting the gastrointestinal system, intentional self-harm, initial encounter	59	Major Depressive, Bipolar, and Paranoid Disorders	60	0.309	0.164	0.299	0.127	0.306	0.109	0.187
T47.92XS	Poisoning by unspecified agents primarily affecting the gastrointestinal system, intentional self-harm, sequela	59	Major Depressive, Bipolar, and Paranoid Disorders	60	0.309	0.164	0.299	0.127	0.306	0.109	0.187
T48.0X2A	Poisoning by oxytocic drugs, intentional self-harm, initial encounter	59	Major Depressive, Bipolar, and Paranoid Disorders	60	0.309	0.164	0.299	0.127	0.306	0.109	0.187
T48.0X2S	Poisoning by oxytocic drugs, intentional self-harm, sequela	59	Major Depressive, Bipolar, and Paranoid Disorders	60	0.309	0.164	0.299	0.127	0.306	0.109	0.187
T48.1X2A	Poisoning by skeletal muscle relaxants [neuromuscular blocking agents], intentional self-harm, initial encounter	59	Major Depressive, Bipolar, and Paranoid Disorders	60	0.309	0.164	0.299	0.127	0.306	0.109	0.187
T48.1X2S	Poisoning by skeletal muscle relaxants [neuromuscular blocking agents], intentional self-harm, sequela	59	Major Depressive, Bipolar, and Paranoid Disorders	60	0.309	0.164	0.299	0.127	0.306	0.109	0.187
T48.202A	Poisoning by unspecified drugs acting on muscles, intentional self-harm, initial encounter	59	Major Depressive, Bipolar, and Paranoid Disorders	60	0.309	0.164	0.299	0.127	0.306	0.109	0.187
T48.202S	Poisoning by unspecified drugs acting on muscles, intentional self-harm, sequela	59	Major Depressive, Bipolar, and Paranoid Disorders	60	0.309	0.164	0.299	0.127	0.306	0.109	0.187
T48.292A	Poisoning by other drugs acting on muscles, intentional self-harm, initial encounter	59	Major Depressive, Bipolar, and Paranoid Disorders	60	0.309	0.164	0.299	0.127	0.306	0.109	0.187
T48.292S	Poisoning by other drugs acting on muscles, intentional self-harm, sequela	59	Major Depressive, Bipolar, and Paranoid Disorders	60	0.309	0.164	0.299	0.127	0.306	0.109	0.187
T48.3X2A	Poisoning by antitussives, intentional self-harm, initial encounter	59	Major Depressive, Bipolar, and Paranoid Disorders	60	0.309	0.164	0.299	0.127	0.306	0.109	0.187
T48.3X2S	Poisoning by antitussives, intentional self-harm, sequela	59	Major Depressive, Bipolar, and Paranoid Disorders	60	0.309	0.164	0.299	0.127	0.306	0.109	0.187
T48.4X2A	Poisoning by expectorants, intentional self-harm, initial encounter	59	Major Depressive, Bipolar, and Paranoid Disorders	60	0.309	0.164	0.299	0.127	0.306	0.109	0.187

ICD-10-CM Code	ICD-10-CM Code Description	V24 CMS-HCC	V24 CMS-HCC Disease Group	V24 CMS-HCC Hierarchies	Community, NonDual, Aged	Community, NonDual, Disabled	Community, FBDual, Aged	Community, FBDual, Disabled	Community, PBDual, Aged	Community, PBDual, Disabled	Institutional
T48.4X2S	Poisoning by expectorants, intentional self-harm, sequela	59	Major Depressive, Bipolar, and Paranoid Disorders	60	0.309	0.164	0.299	0.127	0.306	0.109	0.187
T48.5X2A	Poisoning by other anti-common-cold drugs, intentional self-harm, initial encounter	59	Major Depressive, Bipolar, and Paranoid Disorders	60	0.309	0.164	0.299	0.127	0.306	0.109	0.187
T48.5X2S	Poisoning by other anti-common-cold drugs, intentional self-harm, sequela	59	Major Depressive, Bipolar, and Paranoid Disorders	60	0.309	0.164	0.299	0.127	0.306	0.109	0.187
T48.6X2A	Poisoning by antiasthmatics, intentional self-harm, initial encounter	59	Major Depressive, Bipolar, and Paranoid Disorders	60	0.309	0.164	0.299	0.127	0.306	0.109	0.187
T48.6X2S	Poisoning by antiasthmatics, intentional self-harm, sequela	59	Major Depressive, Bipolar, and Paranoid Disorders	60	0.309	0.164	0.299	0.127	0.306	0.109	0.187
T48.902A	Poisoning by unspecified agents primarily acting on the respiratory system, intentional self-harm, initial encounter	59	Major Depressive, Bipolar, and Paranoid Disorders	60	0.309	0.164	0.299	0.127	0.306	0.109	0.187
T48.902S	Poisoning by unspecified agents primarily acting on the respiratory system, intentional self-harm, sequela	59	Major Depressive, Bipolar, and Paranoid Disorders	60	0.309	0.164	0.299	0.127	0.306	0.109	0.187
T48.992A	Poisoning by other agents primarily acting on the respiratory system, intentional self-harm, initial encounter	59	Major Depressive, Bipolar, and Paranoid Disorders	60	0.309	0.164	0.299	0.127	0.306	0.109	0.187
T48.992S	Poisoning by other agents primarily acting on the respiratory system, intentional self-harm, sequela	59	Major Depressive, Bipolar, and Paranoid Disorders	60	0.309	0.164	0.299	0.127	0.306	0.109	0.187
T49.0X2A	Poisoning by local antifungal, anti-infective and anti-inflammatory drugs, intentional self-harm, initial encounter	59	Major Depressive, Bipolar, and Paranoid Disorders	60	0.309	0.164	0.299	0.127	0.306	0.109	0.187
T49.0X2S	Poisoning by local antifungal, anti-infective and anti-inflammatory drugs, intentional self-harm, sequela	59	Major Depressive, Bipolar, and Paranoid Disorders	60	0.309	0.164	0.299	0.127	0.306	0.109	0.187
T49.1X2A	Poisoning by antipruritics, intentional self-harm, initial encounter	59	Major Depressive, Bipolar, and Paranoid Disorders	60	0.309	0.164	0.299	0.127	0.306	0.109	0.187
T49.1X2S	Poisoning by antipruritics, intentional self-harm, sequela	59	Major Depressive, Bipolar, and Paranoid Disorders	60	0.309	0.164	0.299	0.127	0.306	0.109	0.187
T49.2X2A	Poisoning by local astringents and local detergents, intentional self-harm, initial encounter	59	Major Depressive, Bipolar, and Paranoid Disorders	60	0.309	0.164	0.299	0.127	0.306	0.109	0.187
T49.2X2S	Poisoning by local astringents and local detergents, intentional self-harm, sequela	59	Major Depressive, Bipolar, and Paranoid Disorders	60	0.309	0.164	0.299	0.127	0.306	0.109	0.187
T49.3X2A	Poisoning by emollients, demulcents and protectants, intentional self-harm, initial encounter	59	Major Depressive, Bipolar, and Paranoid Disorders	60	0.309	0.164	0.299	0.127	0.306	0.109	0.187
T49.3X2S	Poisoning by emollients, demulcents and protectants, intentional self-harm, sequela	59	Major Depressive, Bipolar, and Paranoid Disorders	60	0.309	0.164	0.299	0.127	0.306	0.109	0.187
T49.4X2A	Poisoning by keratolytics, keratoplastics, and other hair treatment drugs and preparations, intentional self-harm, initial encounter	59	Major Depressive, Bipolar, and Paranoid Disorders	60	0.309	0.164	0.299	0.127	0.306	0.109	0.187
T49.4X2S	Poisoning by keratolytics, keratoplastics, and other hair treatment drugs and preparations, intentional self-harm, sequela	59	Major Depressive, Bipolar, and Paranoid Disorders	60	0.309	0.164	0.299	0.127	0.306	0.109	0.187

ICD-10-CM Code	ICD-10-CM Code Description	V24 CMS-HCC	V24 CMS-HCC Disease Group	V24 CMS-HCC Hierarchies	Community, NonDual, Aged	Community, NonDual, Disabled	Community, FBDual, Aged	Community, FBDual, Disabled	Community, PBDual, Aged	Community, PBDual, Disabled	Institutional
T49.5X2A	Poisoning by ophthalmological drugs and preparations, intentional self-harm, initial encounter	59	Major Depressive, Bipolar, and Paranoid Disorders	60	0.309	0.164	0.299	0.127	0.306	0.109	0.187
T49.5X2S	Poisoning by ophthalmological drugs and preparations, intentional self-harm, sequela	59	Major Depressive, Bipolar, and Paranoid Disorders	60	0.309	0.164	0.299	0.127	0.306	0.109	0.187
T49.6X2A	Poisoning by otorhinolaryngological drugs and preparations, intentional self-harm, initial encounter	59	Major Depressive, Bipolar, and Paranoid Disorders	60	0.309	0.164	0.299	0.127	0.306	0.109	0.187
T49.6X2S	Poisoning by otorhinolaryngological drugs and preparations, intentional self-harm, sequela	59	Major Depressive, Bipolar, and Paranoid Disorders	60	0.309	0.164	0.299	0.127	0.306	0.109	0.187
T49.7X2A	Poisoning by dental drugs, topically applied, intentional self-harm, initial encounter	59	Major Depressive, Bipolar, and Paranoid Disorders	60	0.309	0.164	0.299	0.127	0.306	0.109	0.187
T49.7X2S	Poisoning by dental drugs, topically applied, intentional self-harm, sequela	59	Major Depressive, Bipolar, and Paranoid Disorders	60	0.309	0.164	0.299	0.127	0.306	0.109	0.187
T49.8X2A	Poisoning by other topical agents, intentional self-harm, initial encounter	59	Major Depressive, Bipolar, and Paranoid Disorders	60	0.309	0.164	0.299	0.127	0.306	0.109	0.187
T49.8X2S	Poisoning by other topical agents, intentional self-harm, sequela	59	Major Depressive, Bipolar, and Paranoid Disorders	60	0.309	0.164	0.299	0.127	0.306	0.109	0.187
T49.92XA	Poisoning by unspecified topical agent, intentional self-harm, initial encounter	59	Major Depressive, Bipolar, and Paranoid Disorders	60	0.309	0.164	0.299	0.127	0.306	0.109	0.187
T49.92XS	Poisoning by unspecified topical agent, intentional self-harm, sequela	59	Major Depressive, Bipolar, and Paranoid Disorders	60	0.309	0.164	0.299	0.127	0.306	0.109	0.187
T50.0X2A	Poisoning by mineralocorticoids and their antagonists, intentional self-harm, initial encounter	59	Major Depressive, Bipolar, and Paranoid Disorders	60	0.309	0.164	0.299	0.127	0.306	0.109	0.187
T50.0X2S	Poisoning by mineralocorticoids and their antagonists, intentional self-harm, sequela	59	Major Depressive, Bipolar, and Paranoid Disorders	60	0.309	0.164	0.299	0.127	0.306	0.109	0.187
T50.1X2A	Poisoning by loop [high-ceiling] diuretics, intentional self-harm, initial encounter	59	Major Depressive, Bipolar, and Paranoid Disorders	60	0.309	0.164	0.299	0.127	0.306	0.109	0.187
T50.1X2S	Poisoning by loop [high-ceiling] diuretics, intentional self-harm, sequela	59	Major Depressive, Bipolar, and Paranoid Disorders	60	0.309	0.164	0.299	0.127	0.306	0.109	0.187
T50.2X2A	Poisoning by carbonic-anhydrase inhibitors, benzothiadiazides and other diuretics, intentional self-harm, initial encounter	59	Major Depressive, Bipolar, and Paranoid Disorders	60	0.309	0.164	0.299	0.127	0.306	0.109	0.187
T50.2X2S	Poisoning by carbonic-anhydrase inhibitors, benzothiadiazides and other diuretics, intentional self-harm, sequela	59	Major Depressive, Bipolar, and Paranoid Disorders	60	0.309	0.164	0.299	0.127	0.306	0.109	0.187
T50.3X2A	Poisoning by electrolytic, caloric and water-balance agents, intentional self-harm, initial encounter	59	Major Depressive, Bipolar, and Paranoid Disorders	60	0.309	0.164	0.299	0.127	0.306	0.109	0.187
T50.3X2S	Poisoning by electrolytic, caloric and water-balance agents, intentional self-harm, sequela	59	Major Depressive, Bipolar, and Paranoid Disorders	60	0.309	0.164	0.299	0.127	0.306	0.109	0.187
T50.4X2A	Poisoning by drugs affecting uric acid metabolism, intentional self-harm, initial encounter	59	Major Depressive, Bipolar, and Paranoid Disorders	60	0.309	0.164	0.299	0.127	0.306	0.109	0.187
T50.4X2S	Poisoning by drugs affecting uric acid metabolism, intentional self-harm, sequela	59	Major Depressive, Bipolar, and Paranoid Disorders	60	0.309	0.164	0.299	0.127	0.306	0.109	0.187

ICD-10-CM Code	ICD-10-CM Code Description	V24 CMS-HCC	V24 CMS-HCC Disease Group	V24 CMS-HCC Hierarchies	Community, NonDual, Aged	Community, NonDual, Disabled	Community, FBDual, Aged	Community, FBDual, Disabled	Community, PBDual, Aged	Community, PBDual, Disabled	Institutional
T50.5X2A	Poisoning by appetite depressants, intentional self-harm, initial encounter	59	Major Depressive, Bipolar, and Paranoid Disorders	60	0.309	0.164	0.299	0.127	0.306	0.109	0.187
T50.5X2S	Poisoning by appetite depressants, intentional self-harm, sequela	59	Major Depressive, Bipolar, and Paranoid Disorders	60	0.309	0.164	0.299	0.127	0.306	0.109	0.187
T50.6X2A	Poisoning by antidotes and chelating agents, intentional self-harm, initial encounter	59	Major Depressive, Bipolar, and Paranoid Disorders	60	0.309	0.164	0.299	0.127	0.306	0.109	0.187
T50.6X2S	Poisoning by antidotes and chelating agents, intentional self-harm, sequela	59	Major Depressive, Bipolar, and Paranoid Disorders	60	0.309	0.164	0.299	0.127	0.306	0.109	0.187
T50.7X2A	Poisoning by analeptics and opioid receptor antagonists, intentional self-harm, initial encounter	59	Major Depressive, Bipolar, and Paranoid Disorders	60	0.309	0.164	0.299	0.127	0.306	0.109	0.187
T50.7X2S	Poisoning by analeptics and opioid receptor antagonists, intentional self-harm, sequela	59	Major Depressive, Bipolar, and Paranoid Disorders	60	0.309	0.164	0.299	0.127	0.306	0.109	0.187
T50.8X2A	Poisoning by diagnostic agents, intentional self-harm, initial encounter	59	Major Depressive, Bipolar, and Paranoid Disorders	60	0.309	0.164	0.299	0.127	0.306	0.109	0.187
T50.8X2S	Poisoning by diagnostic agents, intentional self-harm, sequela	59	Major Depressive, Bipolar, and Paranoid Disorders	60	0.309	0.164	0.299	0.127	0.306	0.109	0.187
T50.902A	Poisoning by unspecified drugs, medicaments and biological substances, intentional self-harm, initial encounter	59	Major Depressive, Bipolar, and Paranoid Disorders	60	0.309	0.164	0.299	0.127	0.306	0.109	0.187
T50.902S	Poisoning by unspecified drugs, medicaments and biological substances, intentional self-harm, sequela	59	Major Depressive, Bipolar, and Paranoid Disorders	60	0.309	0.164	0.299	0.127	0.306	0.109	0.187
T50.912A	Poisoning by multiple unspecified drugs, medicaments and biological substances, intentional self-harm, initial encounter	59	Major Depressive, Bipolar, and Paranoid Disorders	60	0.309	0.164	0.299	0.127	0.306	0.109	0.187
T50.912S	Poisoning by multiple unspecified drugs, medicaments and biological substances, intentional self-harm, sequela	59	Major Depressive, Bipolar, and Paranoid Disorders	60	0.309	0.164	0.299	0.127	0.306	0.109	0.187
T50.992A	Poisoning by other drugs, medicaments and biological substances, intentional self-harm, initial encounter	59	Major Depressive, Bipolar, and Paranoid Disorders	60	0.309	0.164	0.299	0.127	0.306	0.109	0.187
T50.992S	Poisoning by other drugs, medicaments and biological substances, intentional self-harm, sequela	59	Major Depressive, Bipolar, and Paranoid Disorders	60	0.309	0.164	0.299	0.127	0.306	0.109	0.187
T50.A12A	Poisoning by pertussis vaccine, including combinations with a pertussis component, intentional self-harm, initial encounter	59	Major Depressive, Bipolar, and Paranoid Disorders	60	0.309	0.164	0.299	0.127	0.306	0.109	0.187
T50.A12S	Poisoning by pertussis vaccine, including combinations with a pertussis component, intentional self-harm, sequela	59	Major Depressive, Bipolar, and Paranoid Disorders	60	0.309	0.164	0.299	0.127	0.306	0.109	0.187
T50.A22A	Poisoning by mixed bacterial vaccines without a pertussis component, intentional self-harm, initial encounter	59	Major Depressive, Bipolar, and Paranoid Disorders	60	0.309	0.164	0.299	0.127	0.306	0.109	0.187
T50.A22S	Poisoning by mixed bacterial vaccines without a pertussis component, intentional self-harm, sequela	59	Major Depressive, Bipolar, and Paranoid Disorders	60	0.309	0.164	0.299	0.127	0.306	0.109	0.187

ICD-10-CM Code	ICD-10-CM Code Description	V24 CMS-HCC	V24 CMS-HCC Disease Group	V24 CMS-HCC Hierarchies	Community, NonDual, Aged	Community, NonDual, Disabled	Community, FBDual, Aged	Community, FBDual, Disabled	Community, PBDual, Aged	Community, PBDual, Disabled	Institutional
T50.A92A	Poisoning by other bacterial vaccines, intentional self-harm, initial encounter	59	Major Depressive, Bipolar, and Paranoid Disorders	60	0.309	0.164	0.299	0.127	0.306	0.109	0.187
T50.A92S	Poisoning by other bacterial vaccines, intentional self-harm, sequela	59	Major Depressive, Bipolar, and Paranoid Disorders	60	0.309	0.164	0.299	0.127	0.306	0.109	0.187
T50.B12A	Poisoning by smallpox vaccines, intentional self-harm, initial encounter	59	Major Depressive, Bipolar, and Paranoid Disorders	60	0.309	0.164	0.299	0.127	0.306	0.109	0.187
T50.B12S	Poisoning by smallpox vaccines, intentional self-harm, sequela	59	Major Depressive, Bipolar, and Paranoid Disorders	60	0.309	0.164	0.299	0.127	0.306	0.109	0.187
T50.B92A	Poisoning by other viral vaccines, intentional self-harm, initial encounter	59	Major Depressive, Bipolar, and Paranoid Disorders	60	0.309	0.164	0.299	0.127	0.306	0.109	0.187
T50.B92S	Poisoning by other viral vaccines, intentional self-harm, sequela	59	Major Depressive, Bipolar, and Paranoid Disorders	60	0.309	0.164	0.299	0.127	0.306	0.109	0.187
T50.Z12A	Poisoning by immunoglobulin, intentional self-harm, initial encounter	59	Major Depressive, Bipolar, and Paranoid Disorders	60	0.309	0.164	0.299	0.127	0.306	0.109	0.187
T50.Z12S	Poisoning by immunoglobulin, intentional self-harm, sequela	59	Major Depressive, Bipolar, and Paranoid Disorders	60	0.309	0.164	0.299	0.127	0.306	0.109	0.187
T50.Z92A	Poisoning by other vaccines and biological substances, intentional self-harm, initial encounter	59	Major Depressive, Bipolar, and Paranoid Disorders	60	0.309	0.164	0.299	0.127	0.306	0.109	0.187
T50.Z92S	Poisoning by other vaccines and biological substances, intentional self-harm, sequela	59	Major Depressive, Bipolar, and Paranoid Disorders	60	0.309	0.164	0.299	0.127	0.306	0.109	0.187
T51.0X1A	Toxic effect of ethanol, accidental (unintentional), initial encounter	55	Substance Use Disorder, Moderate/Severe, or Substance Use with Complications	56	0.329	0.279	0.538	0.356	0.372	0.275	0.178
T51.0X2A	Toxic effect of ethanol, intentional self-harm, initial encounter	59	Major Depressive, Bipolar, and Paranoid Disorders	60	0.309	0.164	0.299	0.127	0.306	0.109	0.187
T51.0X2S	Toxic effect of ethanol, intentional self-harm, sequela	59	Major Depressive, Bipolar, and Paranoid Disorders	60	0.309	0.164	0.299	0.127	0.306	0.109	0.187
T51.0X4A	Toxic effect of ethanol, undetermined, initial encounter	55	Substance Use Disorder, Moderate/Severe, or Substance Use with Complications	56	0.329	0.279	0.538	0.356	0.372	0.275	0.178
T51.1X2A	Toxic effect of methanol, intentional self-harm, initial encounter	59	Major Depressive, Bipolar, and Paranoid Disorders	60	0.309	0.164	0.299	0.127	0.306	0.109	0.187
T51.1X2S	Toxic effect of methanol, intentional self-harm, sequela	59	Major Depressive, Bipolar, and Paranoid Disorders	60	0.309	0.164	0.299	0.127	0.306	0.109	0.187
T51.2X2A	Toxic effect of 2-Propanol, intentional self-harm, initial encounter	59	Major Depressive, Bipolar, and Paranoid Disorders	60	0.309	0.164	0.299	0.127	0.306	0.109	0.187
T51.2X2S	Toxic effect of 2-Propanol, intentional self-harm, sequela	59	Major Depressive, Bipolar, and Paranoid Disorders	60	0.309	0.164	0.299	0.127	0.306	0.109	0.187
T51.3X2A	Toxic effect of fusel oil, intentional self-harm, initial encounter	59	Major Depressive, Bipolar, and Paranoid Disorders	60	0.309	0.164	0.299	0.127	0.306	0.109	0.187
T51.3X2S	Toxic effect of fusel oil, intentional self-harm, sequela	59	Major Depressive, Bipolar, and Paranoid Disorders	60	0.309	0.164	0.299	0.127	0.306	0.109	0.187
T51.8X2A	Toxic effect of other alcohols, intentional self-harm, initial encounter	59	Major Depressive, Bipolar, and Paranoid Disorders	60	0.309	0.164	0.299	0.127	0.306	0.109	0.187
T51.8X2S	Toxic effect of other alcohols, intentional self-harm, sequela	59	Major Depressive, Bipolar, and Paranoid Disorders	60	0.309	0.164	0.299	0.127	0.306	0.109	0.187
T51.92XA	Toxic effect of unspecified alcohol, intentional self-harm, initial encounter	59	Major Depressive, Bipolar, and Paranoid Disorders	60	0.309	0.164	0.299	0.127	0.306	0.109	0.187
T51.92XS	Toxic effect of unspecified alcohol, intentional self-harm, sequela	59	Major Depressive, Bipolar, and Paranoid Disorders	60	0.309	0.164	0.299	0.127	0.306	0.109	0.187

ICD-10-CM Code	ICD-10-CM Code Description	V24 CMS-HCC	V24 CMS-HCC Disease Group	V24 CMS-HCC Hierarchies	Community, NonDual, Aged	Community, NonDual, Disabled	Community, FBDual, Aged	Community, FBDual, Disabled	Community, PBDual, Aged	Community, PBDual, Disabled	Institutional
T52.0X2A	Toxic effect of petroleum products, intentional self-harm, initial encounter	59	Major Depressive, Bipolar, and Paranoid Disorders	60	0.309	0.164	0.299	0.127	0.306	0.109	0.187
T52.0X2S	Toxic effect of petroleum products, intentional self-harm, sequela	59	Major Depressive, Bipolar, and Paranoid Disorders	60	0.309	0.164	0.299	0.127	0.306	0.109	0.187
T52.1X2A	Toxic effect of benzene, intentional self-harm, initial encounter	59	Major Depressive, Bipolar, and Paranoid Disorders	60	0.309	0.164	0.299	0.127	0.306	0.109	0.187
T52.1X2S	Toxic effect of benzene, intentional self-harm, sequela	59	Major Depressive, Bipolar, and Paranoid Disorders	60	0.309	0.164	0.299	0.127	0.306	0.109	0.187
T52.2X2A	Toxic effect of homologues of benzene, intentional self-harm, initial encounter	59	Major Depressive, Bipolar, and Paranoid Disorders	60	0.309	0.164	0.299	0.127	0.306	0.109	0.187
T52.2X2S	Toxic effect of homologues of benzene, intentional self-harm, sequela	59	Major Depressive, Bipolar, and Paranoid Disorders	60	0.309	0.164	0.299	0.127	0.306	0.109	0.187
T52.3X2A	Toxic effect of glycols, intentional self-harm, initial encounter	59	Major Depressive, Bipolar, and Paranoid Disorders	60	0.309	0.164	0.299	0.127	0.306	0.109	0.187
T52.3X2S	Toxic effect of glycols, intentional self-harm, sequela	59	Major Depressive, Bipolar, and Paranoid Disorders	60	0.309	0.164	0.299	0.127	0.306	0.109	0.187
T52.4X2A	Toxic effect of ketones, intentional self-harm, initial encounter	59	Major Depressive, Bipolar, and Paranoid Disorders	60	0.309	0.164	0.299	0.127	0.306	0.109	0.187
T52.4X2S	Toxic effect of ketones, intentional self-harm, sequela	59	Major Depressive, Bipolar, and Paranoid Disorders	60	0.309	0.164	0.299	0.127	0.306	0.109	0.187
T52.8X2A	Toxic effect of other organic solvents, intentional self-harm, initial encounter	59	Major Depressive, Bipolar, and Paranoid Disorders	60	0.309	0.164	0.299	0.127	0.306	0.109	0.187
T52.8X2S	Toxic effect of other organic solvents, intentional self-harm, sequela	59	Major Depressive, Bipolar, and Paranoid Disorders	60	0.309	0.164	0.299	0.127	0.306	0.109	0.187
T52.92XA	Toxic effect of unspecified organic solvent, intentional self-harm, initial encounter	59	Major Depressive, Bipolar, and Paranoid Disorders	60	0.309	0.164	0.299	0.127	0.306	0.109	0.187
T52.92XS	Toxic effect of unspecified organic solvent, intentional self-harm, sequela	59	Major Depressive, Bipolar, and Paranoid Disorders	60	0.309	0.164	0.299	0.127	0.306	0.109	0.187
T53.0X2A	Toxic effect of carbon tetrachloride, intentional self-harm, initial encounter	59	Major Depressive, Bipolar, and Paranoid Disorders	60	0.309	0.164	0.299	0.127	0.306	0.109	0.187
T53.0X2S	Toxic effect of carbon tetrachloride, intentional self-harm, sequela	59	Major Depressive, Bipolar, and Paranoid Disorders	60	0.309	0.164	0.299	0.127	0.306	0.109	0.187
T53.1X2A	Toxic effect of chloroform, intentional self-harm, initial encounter	59	Major Depressive, Bipolar, and Paranoid Disorders	60	0.309	0.164	0.299	0.127	0.306	0.109	0.187
T53.1X2S	Toxic effect of chloroform, intentional self-harm, sequela	59	Major Depressive, Bipolar, and Paranoid Disorders	60	0.309	0.164	0.299	0.127	0.306	0.109	0.187
T53.2X2A	Toxic effect of trichloroethylene, intentional self-harm, initial encounter	59	Major Depressive, Bipolar, and Paranoid Disorders	60	0.309	0.164	0.299	0.127	0.306	0.109	0.187
T53.2X2S	Toxic effect of trichloroethylene, intentional self-harm, sequela	59	Major Depressive, Bipolar, and Paranoid Disorders	60	0.309	0.164	0.299	0.127	0.306	0.109	0.187
T53.3X2A	Toxic effect of tetrachloroethylene, intentional self-harm, initial encounter	59	Major Depressive, Bipolar, and Paranoid Disorders	60	0.309	0.164	0.299	0.127	0.306	0.109	0.187
T53.3X2S	Toxic effect of tetrachloroethylene, intentional self-harm, sequela	59	Major Depressive, Bipolar, and Paranoid Disorders	60	0.309	0.164	0.299	0.127	0.306	0.109	0.187
T53.4X2A	Toxic effect of dichloromethane, intentional self-harm, initial encounter	59	Major Depressive, Bipolar, and Paranoid Disorders	60	0.309	0.164	0.299	0.127	0.306	0.109	0.187
T53.4X2S	Toxic effect of dichloromethane, intentional self-harm, sequela	59	Major Depressive, Bipolar, and Paranoid Disorders	60	0.309	0.164	0.299	0.127	0.306	0.109	0.187

ICD-10-CM Code	ICD-10-CM Code Description	V24 CMS-HCC	V24 CMS-HCC Disease Group	V24 CMS-HCC Hierarchies	Community, NonDual, Aged	Community, NonDual, Disabled	Community, FBDual, Aged	Community, FBDual, Disabled	Community, PBDual, Aged	Community, PBDual, Disabled	Institutional
T53.5X2A	Toxic effect of chlorofluorocarbons, intentional self-harm, initial encounter	59	Major Depressive, Bipolar, and Paranoid Disorders	60	0.309	0.164	0.299	0.127	0.306	0.109	0.187
T53.5X2S	Toxic effect of chlorofluorocarbons, intentional self-harm, sequela	59	Major Depressive, Bipolar, and Paranoid Disorders	60	0.309	0.164	0.299	0.127	0.306	0.109	0.187
T53.6X2A	Toxic effect of other halogen derivatives of aliphatic hydrocarbons, intentional self-harm, initial encounter	59	Major Depressive, Bipolar, and Paranoid Disorders	60	0.309	0.164	0.299	0.127	0.306	0.109	0.187
T53.6X2S	Toxic effect of other halogen derivatives of aliphatic hydrocarbons, intentional self-harm, sequela	59	Major Depressive, Bipolar, and Paranoid Disorders	60	0.309	0.164	0.299	0.127	0.306	0.109	0.187
T53.7X2A	Toxic effect of other halogen derivatives of aromatic hydrocarbons, intentional self-harm, initial encounter	59	Major Depressive, Bipolar, and Paranoid Disorders	60	0.309	0.164	0.299	0.127	0.306	0.109	0.187
T53.7X2S	Toxic effect of other halogen derivatives of aromatic hydrocarbons, intentional self-harm, sequela	59	Major Depressive, Bipolar, and Paranoid Disorders	60	0.309	0.164	0.299	0.127	0.306	0.109	0.187
T53.92XA	Toxic effect of unspecified halogen derivatives of aliphatic and aromatic hydrocarbons, intentional self-harm, initial encounter	59	Major Depressive, Bipolar, and Paranoid Disorders	60	0.309	0.164	0.299	0.127	0.306	0.109	0.187
T53.92XS	Toxic effect of unspecified halogen derivatives of aliphatic and aromatic hydrocarbons, intentional self-harm, sequela	59	Major Depressive, Bipolar, and Paranoid Disorders	60	0.309	0.164	0.299	0.127	0.306	0.109	0.187
T54.0X2A	Toxic effect of phenol and phenol homologues, intentional self-harm, initial encounter	59	Major Depressive, Bipolar, and Paranoid Disorders	60	0.309	0.164	0.299	0.127	0.306	0.109	0.187
T54.0X2S	Toxic effect of phenol and phenol homologues, intentional self-harm, sequela	59	Major Depressive, Bipolar, and Paranoid Disorders	60	0.309	0.164	0.299	0.127	0.306	0.109	0.187
T54.1X2A	Toxic effect of other corrosive organic compounds, intentional self-harm, initial encounter	59	Major Depressive, Bipolar, and Paranoid Disorders	60	0.309	0.164	0.299	0.127	0.306	0.109	0.187
T54.1X2S	Toxic effect of other corrosive organic compounds, intentional self-harm, sequela	59	Major Depressive, Bipolar, and Paranoid Disorders	60	0.309	0.164	0.299	0.127	0.306	0.109	0.187
T54.2X2A	Toxic effect of corrosive acids and acid-like substances, intentional self-harm, initial encounter	59	Major Depressive, Bipolar, and Paranoid Disorders	60	0.309	0.164	0.299	0.127	0.306	0.109	0.187
T54.2X2S	Toxic effect of corrosive acids and acid-like substances, intentional self-harm, sequela	59	Major Depressive, Bipolar, and Paranoid Disorders	60	0.309	0.164	0.299	0.127	0.306	0.109	0.187
T54.3X2A	Toxic effect of corrosive alkalis and alkali-like substances, intentional self-harm, initial encounter	59	Major Depressive, Bipolar, and Paranoid Disorders	60	0.309	0.164	0.299	0.127	0.306	0.109	0.187
T54.3X2S	Toxic effect of corrosive alkalis and alkali-like substances, intentional self-harm, sequela	59	Major Depressive, Bipolar, and Paranoid Disorders	60	0.309	0.164	0.299	0.127	0.306	0.109	0.187
T54.92XA	Toxic effect of unspecified corrosive substance, intentional self-harm, initial encounter	59	Major Depressive, Bipolar, and Paranoid Disorders	60	0.309	0.164	0.299	0.127	0.306	0.109	0.187
T54.92XS	Toxic effect of unspecified corrosive substance, intentional self-harm, sequela	59	Major Depressive, Bipolar, and Paranoid Disorders	60	0.309	0.164	0.299	0.127	0.306	0.109	0.187
T55.0X2A	Toxic effect of soaps, intentional self-harm, initial encounter	59	Major Depressive, Bipolar, and Paranoid Disorders	60	0.309	0.164	0.299	0.127	0.306	0.109	0.187
T55.0X2S	Toxic effect of soaps, intentional self-harm, sequela	59	Major Depressive, Bipolar, and Paranoid Disorders	60	0.309	0.164	0.299	0.127	0.306	0.109	0.187

ICD-10-CM Code	ICD-10-CM Code Description	V24 CMS-HCC	V24 CMS-HCC Disease Group	V24 CMS-HCC Hierarchies	Community, NonDual, Aged	Community, NonDual, Disabled	Community, FBDual, Aged	Community, FBDual, Disabled	Community, PBDual, Aged	Community, PBDual, Disabled	Institutional
T55.1X2A	Toxic effect of detergents, intentional self-harm, initial encounter	59	Major Depressive, Bipolar, and Paranoid Disorders	60	0.309	0.164	0.299	0.127	0.306	0.109	0.187
T55.1X2S	Toxic effect of detergents, intentional self-harm, sequela	59	Major Depressive, Bipolar, and Paranoid Disorders	60	0.309	0.164	0.299	0.127	0.306	0.109	0.187
T56.0X2A	Toxic effect of lead and its compounds, intentional self-harm, initial encounter	59	Major Depressive, Bipolar, and Paranoid Disorders	60	0.309	0.164	0.299	0.127	0.306	0.109	0.187
T56.0X2S	Toxic effect of lead and its compounds, intentional self-harm, sequela	59	Major Depressive, Bipolar, and Paranoid Disorders	60	0.309	0.164	0.299	0.127	0.306	0.109	0.187
T56.1X2A	Toxic effect of mercury and its compounds, intentional self-harm, initial encounter	59	Major Depressive, Bipolar, and Paranoid Disorders	60	0.309	0.164	0.299	0.127	0.306	0.109	0.187
T56.1X2S	Toxic effect of mercury and its compounds, intentional self-harm, sequela	59	Major Depressive, Bipolar, and Paranoid Disorders	60	0.309	0.164	0.299	0.127	0.306	0.109	0.187
T56.2X2A	Toxic effect of chromium and its compounds, intentional self-harm, initial encounter	59	Major Depressive, Bipolar, and Paranoid Disorders	60	0.309	0.164	0.299	0.127	0.306	0.109	0.187
T56.2X2S	Toxic effect of chromium and its compounds, intentional self-harm, sequela	59	Major Depressive, Bipolar, and Paranoid Disorders	60	0.309	0.164	0.299	0.127	0.306	0.109	0.187
T56.3X2A	Toxic effect of cadmium and its compounds, intentional self-harm, initial encounter	59	Major Depressive, Bipolar, and Paranoid Disorders	60	0.309	0.164	0.299	0.127	0.306	0.109	0.187
T56.3X2S	Toxic effect of cadmium and its compounds, intentional self-harm, sequela	59	Major Depressive, Bipolar, and Paranoid Disorders	60	0.309	0.164	0.299	0.127	0.306	0.109	0.187
T56.4X2A	Toxic effect of copper and its compounds, intentional self-harm, initial encounter	59	Major Depressive, Bipolar, and Paranoid Disorders	60	0.309	0.164	0.299	0.127	0.306	0.109	0.187
T56.4X2S	Toxic effect of copper and its compounds, intentional self-harm, sequela	59	Major Depressive, Bipolar, and Paranoid Disorders	60	0.309	0.164	0.299	0.127	0.306	0.109	0.187
T56.5X2A	Toxic effect of zinc and its compounds, intentional self-harm, initial encounter	59	Major Depressive, Bipolar, and Paranoid Disorders	60	0.309	0.164	0.299	0.127	0.306	0.109	0.187
T56.5X2S	Toxic effect of zinc and its compounds, intentional self-harm, sequela	59	Major Depressive, Bipolar, and Paranoid Disorders	60	0.309	0.164	0.299	0.127	0.306	0.109	0.187
T56.6X2A	Toxic effect of tin and its compounds, intentional self-harm, initial encounter	59	Major Depressive, Bipolar, and Paranoid Disorders	60	0.309	0.164	0.299	0.127	0.306	0.109	0.187
T56.6X2S	Toxic effect of tin and its compounds, intentional self-harm, sequela	59	Major Depressive, Bipolar, and Paranoid Disorders	60	0.309	0.164	0.299	0.127	0.306	0.109	0.187
T56.7X2A	Toxic effect of beryllium and its compounds, intentional self-harm, initial encounter	59	Major Depressive, Bipolar, and Paranoid Disorders	60	0.309	0.164	0.299	0.127	0.306	0.109	0.187
T56.7X2S	Toxic effect of beryllium and its compounds, intentional self-harm, sequela	59	Major Depressive, Bipolar, and Paranoid Disorders	60	0.309	0.164	0.299	0.127	0.306	0.109	0.187
T56.812A	Toxic effect of thallium, intentional self-harm, initial encounter	59	Major Depressive, Bipolar, and Paranoid Disorders	60	0.309	0.164	0.299	0.127	0.306	0.109	0.187
T56.812S	Toxic effect of thallium, intentional self-harm, sequela	59	Major Depressive, Bipolar, and Paranoid Disorders	60	0.309	0.164	0.299	0.127	0.306	0.109	0.187
T56.892A	Toxic effect of other metals, intentional self-harm, initial encounter	59	Major Depressive, Bipolar, and Paranoid Disorders	60	0.309	0.164	0.299	0.127	0.306	0.109	0.187
T56.892S	Toxic effect of other metals, intentional self-harm, sequela	59	Major Depressive, Bipolar, and Paranoid Disorders	60	0.309	0.164	0.299	0.127	0.306	0.109	0.187

ICD-10-CM Code	ICD-10-CM Code Description	V24 CMS-HCC	V24 CMS-HCC Disease Group	V24 CMS-HCC Hierarchies	Community, NonDual, Aged	Community, NonDual, Disabled	Community, FBDual, Aged	Community, FBDual, Disabled	Community, PBDual, Aged	Community, PBDual, Disabled	Institutional
T56.92XA	Toxic effect of unspecified metal, intentional self-harm, initial encounter	59	Major Depressive, Bipolar, and Paranoid Disorders	60	0.309	0.164	0.299	0.127	0.306	0.109	0.187
T56.92XS	Toxic effect of unspecified metal, intentional self-harm, sequela	59	Major Depressive, Bipolar, and Paranoid Disorders	60	0.309	0.164	0.299	0.127	0.306	0.109	0.187
T57.0X2A	Toxic effect of arsenic and its compounds, intentional self-harm, initial encounter	59	Major Depressive, Bipolar, and Paranoid Disorders	60	0.309	0.164	0.299	0.127	0.306	0.109	0.187
T57.0X2S	Toxic effect of arsenic and its compounds, intentional self-harm, sequela	59	Major Depressive, Bipolar, and Paranoid Disorders	60	0.309	0.164	0.299	0.127	0.306	0.109	0.187
T57.1X2A	Toxic effect of phosphorus and its compounds, intentional self-harm, initial encounter	59	Major Depressive, Bipolar, and Paranoid Disorders	60	0.309	0.164	0.299	0.127	0.306	0.109	0.187
T57.1X2S	Toxic effect of phosphorus and its compounds, intentional self-harm, sequela	59	Major Depressive, Bipolar, and Paranoid Disorders	60	0.309	0.164	0.299	0.127	0.306	0.109	0.187
T57.2X2A	Toxic effect of manganese and its compounds, intentional self-harm, initial encounter	59	Major Depressive, Bipolar, and Paranoid Disorders	60	0.309	0.164	0.299	0.127	0.306	0.109	0.187
T57.2X2S	Toxic effect of manganese and its compounds, intentional self-harm, sequela	59	Major Depressive, Bipolar, and Paranoid Disorders	60	0.309	0.164	0.299	0.127	0.306	0.109	0.187
T57.3X2A	Toxic effect of hydrogen cyanide, intentional self-harm, initial encounter	59	Major Depressive, Bipolar, and Paranoid Disorders	60	0.309	0.164	0.299	0.127	0.306	0.109	0.187
T57.3X2S	Toxic effect of hydrogen cyanide, intentional self-harm, sequela	59	Major Depressive, Bipolar, and Paranoid Disorders	60	0.309	0.164	0.299	0.127	0.306	0.109	0.187
T57.8X2A	Toxic effect of other specified inorganic substances, intentional self-harm, initial encounter	59	Major Depressive, Bipolar, and Paranoid Disorders	60	0.309	0.164	0.299	0.127	0.306	0.109	0.187
T57.8X2S	Toxic effect of other specified inorganic substances, intentional self-harm, sequela	59	Major Depressive, Bipolar, and Paranoid Disorders	60	0.309	0.164	0.299	0.127	0.306	0.109	0.187
T57.92XA	Toxic effect of unspecified inorganic substance, intentional self-harm, initial encounter	59	Major Depressive, Bipolar, and Paranoid Disorders	60	0.309	0.164	0.299	0.127	0.306	0.109	0.187
T57.92XS	Toxic effect of unspecified inorganic substance, intentional self-harm, sequela	59	Major Depressive, Bipolar, and Paranoid Disorders	60	0.309	0.164	0.299	0.127	0.306	0.109	0.187
T58.02XA	Toxic effect of carbon monoxide from motor vehicle exhaust, intentional self-harm, initial encounter	59	Major Depressive, Bipolar, and Paranoid Disorders	60	0.309	0.164	0.299	0.127	0.306	0.109	0.187
T58.02XS	Toxic effect of carbon monoxide from motor vehicle exhaust, intentional self-harm, sequela	59	Major Depressive, Bipolar, and Paranoid Disorders	60	0.309	0.164	0.299	0.127	0.306	0.109	0.187
T58.12XA	Toxic effect of carbon monoxide from utility gas, intentional self-harm, initial encounter	59	Major Depressive, Bipolar, and Paranoid Disorders	60	0.309	0.164	0.299	0.127	0.306	0.109	0.187
T58.12XS	Toxic effect of carbon monoxide from utility gas, intentional self-harm, sequela	59	Major Depressive, Bipolar, and Paranoid Disorders	60	0.309	0.164	0.299	0.127	0.306	0.109	0.187
T58.2X2A	Toxic effect of carbon monoxide from incomplete combustion of other domestic fuels, intentional self-harm, initial encounter	59	Major Depressive, Bipolar, and Paranoid Disorders	60	0.309	0.164	0.299	0.127	0.306	0.109	0.187
T58.2X2S	Toxic effect of carbon monoxide from incomplete combustion of other domestic fuels, intentional self-harm, sequela	59	Major Depressive, Bipolar, and Paranoid Disorders	60	0.309	0.164	0.299	0.127	0.306	0.109	0.187

ICD-10-CM Code	ICD-10-CM Code Description	V24 CMS-HCC	V24 CMS-HCC Disease Group	V24 CMS-HCC Hierarchies	Community, NonDual, Aged	Community, NonDual, Disabled	Community, FBDual, Aged	Community, FBDual, Disabled	Community, PBDual, Aged	Community, PBDual, Disabled	Institutional
T58.8X2A	Toxic effect of carbon monoxide from other source, intentional self-harm, initial encounter	59	Major Depressive, Bipolar, and Paranoid Disorders	60	0.309	0.164	0.299	0.127	0.306	0.109	0.187
T58.8X2S	Toxic effect of carbon monoxide from other source, intentional self-harm, sequela	59	Major Depressive, Bipolar, and Paranoid Disorders	60	0.309	0.164	0.299	0.127	0.306	0.109	0.187
T58.92XA	Toxic effect of carbon monoxide from unspecified source, intentional self-harm, initial encounter	59	Major Depressive, Bipolar, and Paranoid Disorders	60	0.309	0.164	0.299	0.127	0.306	0.109	0.187
T58.92XS	Toxic effect of carbon monoxide from unspecified source, intentional self-harm, sequela	59	Major Depressive, Bipolar, and Paranoid Disorders	60	0.309	0.164	0.299	0.127	0.306	0.109	0.187
T59.0X2A	Toxic effect of nitrogen oxides, intentional self-harm, initial encounter	59	Major Depressive, Bipolar, and Paranoid Disorders	60	0.309	0.164	0.299	0.127	0.306	0.109	0.187
T59.0X2S	Toxic effect of nitrogen oxides, intentional self-harm, sequela	59	Major Depressive, Bipolar, and Paranoid Disorders	60	0.309	0.164	0.299	0.127	0.306	0.109	0.187
T59.1X2A	Toxic effect of sulfur dioxide, intentional self-harm, initial encounter	59	Major Depressive, Bipolar, and Paranoid Disorders	60	0.309	0.164	0.299	0.127	0.306	0.109	0.187
T59.1X2S	Toxic effect of sulfur dioxide, intentional self-harm, sequela	59	Major Depressive, Bipolar, and Paranoid Disorders	60	0.309	0.164	0.299	0.127	0.306	0.109	0.187
T59.2X2A	Toxic effect of formaldehyde, intentional self-harm, initial encounter	59	Major Depressive, Bipolar, and Paranoid Disorders	60	0.309	0.164	0.299	0.127	0.306	0.109	0.187
T59.2X2S	Toxic effect of formaldehyde, intentional self-harm, sequela	59	Major Depressive, Bipolar, and Paranoid Disorders	60	0.309	0.164	0.299	0.127	0.306	0.109	0.187
T59.3X2A	Toxic effect of lacrimogenic gas, intentional self-harm, initial encounter	59	Major Depressive, Bipolar, and Paranoid Disorders	60	0.309	0.164	0.299	0.127	0.306	0.109	0.187
T59.3X2S	Toxic effect of lacrimogenic gas, intentional self-harm, sequela	59	Major Depressive, Bipolar, and Paranoid Disorders	60	0.309	0.164	0.299	0.127	0.306	0.109	0.187
T59.4X2A	Toxic effect of chlorine gas, intentional self-harm, initial encounter	59	Major Depressive, Bipolar, and Paranoid Disorders	60	0.309	0.164	0.299	0.127	0.306	0.109	0.187
T59.4X2S	Toxic effect of chlorine gas, intentional self-harm, sequela	59	Major Depressive, Bipolar, and Paranoid Disorders	60	0.309	0.164	0.299	0.127	0.306	0.109	0.187
T59.5X2A	Toxic effect of fluorine gas and hydrogen fluoride, intentional self-harm, initial encounter	59	Major Depressive, Bipolar, and Paranoid Disorders	60	0.309	0.164	0.299	0.127	0.306	0.109	0.187
T59.5X2S	Toxic effect of fluorine gas and hydrogen fluoride, intentional self-harm, sequela	59	Major Depressive, Bipolar, and Paranoid Disorders	60	0.309	0.164	0.299	0.127	0.306	0.109	0.187
T59.6X2A	Toxic effect of hydrogen sulfide, intentional self-harm, initial encounter	59	Major Depressive, Bipolar, and Paranoid Disorders	60	0.309	0.164	0.299	0.127	0.306	0.109	0.187
T59.6X2S	Toxic effect of hydrogen sulfide, intentional self-harm, sequela	59	Major Depressive, Bipolar, and Paranoid Disorders	60	0.309	0.164	0.299	0.127	0.306	0.109	0.187
T59.7X2A	Toxic effect of carbon dioxide, intentional self-harm, initial encounter	59	Major Depressive, Bipolar, and Paranoid Disorders	60	0.309	0.164	0.299	0.127	0.306	0.109	0.187
T59.7X2S	Toxic effect of carbon dioxide, intentional self-harm, sequela	59	Major Depressive, Bipolar, and Paranoid Disorders	60	0.309	0.164	0.299	0.127	0.306	0.109	0.187
T59.812A	Toxic effect of smoke, intentional self-harm, initial encounter	59	Major Depressive, Bipolar, and Paranoid Disorders	60	0.309	0.164	0.299	0.127	0.306	0.109	0.187
T59.812S	Toxic effect of smoke, intentional self-harm, sequela	59	Major Depressive, Bipolar, and Paranoid Disorders	60	0.309	0.164	0.299	0.127	0.306	0.109	0.187
T59.892A	Toxic effect of other specified gases, fumes and vapors, intentional self-harm, initial encounter	59	Major Depressive, Bipolar, and Paranoid Disorders	60	0.309	0.164	0.299	0.127	0.306	0.109	0.187

ICD-10-CM Code	ICD-10-CM Code Description	V24 CMS-HCC	V24 CMS-HCC Disease Group	V24 CMS-HCC Hierarchies	Community, NonDual, Aged	Community, NonDual, Disabled	Community, FBDual, Aged	Community, FBDual, Disabled	Community, PBDual, Aged	Community, PBDual, Disabled	Institutional
T59.892S	Toxic effect of other specified gases, fumes and vapors, intentional self-harm, sequela	59	Major Depressive, Bipolar, and Paranoid Disorders	60	0.309	0.164	0.299	0.127	0.306	0.109	0.187
T59.92XA	Toxic effect of unspecified gases, fumes and vapors, intentional self-harm, initial encounter	59	Major Depressive, Bipolar, and Paranoid Disorders	60	0.309	0.164	0.299	0.127	0.306	0.109	0.187
T59.92XS	Toxic effect of unspecified gases, fumes and vapors, intentional self-harm, sequela	59	Major Depressive, Bipolar, and Paranoid Disorders	60	0.309	0.164	0.299	0.127	0.306	0.109	0.187
T60.0X2A	Toxic effect of organophosphate and carbamate insecticides, intentional self-harm, initial encounter	59	Major Depressive, Bipolar, and Paranoid Disorders	60	0.309	0.164	0.299	0.127	0.306	0.109	0.187
T60.0X2S	Toxic effect of organophosphate and carbamate insecticides, intentional self-harm, sequela	59	Major Depressive, Bipolar, and Paranoid Disorders	60	0.309	0.164	0.299	0.127	0.306	0.109	0.187
T60.1X2A	Toxic effect of halogenated insecticides, intentional self-harm, initial encounter	59	Major Depressive, Bipolar, and Paranoid Disorders	60	0.309	0.164	0.299	0.127	0.306	0.109	0.187
T60.1X2S	Toxic effect of halogenated insecticides, intentional self-harm, sequela	59	Major Depressive, Bipolar, and Paranoid Disorders	60	0.309	0.164	0.299	0.127	0.306	0.109	0.187
T60.2X2A	Toxic effect of other insecticides, intentional self-harm, initial encounter	59	Major Depressive, Bipolar, and Paranoid Disorders	60	0.309	0.164	0.299	0.127	0.306	0.109	0.187
T60.2X2S	Toxic effect of other insecticides, intentional self-harm, sequela	59	Major Depressive, Bipolar, and Paranoid Disorders	60	0.309	0.164	0.299	0.127	0.306	0.109	0.187
T60.3X2A	Toxic effect of herbicides and fungicides, intentional self-harm, initial encounter	59	Major Depressive, Bipolar, and Paranoid Disorders	60	0.309	0.164	0.299	0.127	0.306	0.109	0.187
T60.3X2S	Toxic effect of herbicides and fungicides, intentional self-harm, sequela	59	Major Depressive, Bipolar, and Paranoid Disorders	60	0.309	0.164	0.299	0.127	0.306	0.109	0.187
T60.4X2A	Toxic effect of rodenticides, intentional self-harm, initial encounter	59	Major Depressive, Bipolar, and Paranoid Disorders	60	0.309	0.164	0.299	0.127	0.306	0.109	0.187
T60.4X2S	Toxic effect of rodenticides, intentional self-harm, sequela	59	Major Depressive, Bipolar, and Paranoid Disorders	60	0.309	0.164	0.299	0.127	0.306	0.109	0.187
T60.8X2A	Toxic effect of other pesticides, intentional self-harm, initial encounter	59	Major Depressive, Bipolar, and Paranoid Disorders	60	0.309	0.164	0.299	0.127	0.306	0.109	0.187
T60.8X2S	Toxic effect of other pesticides, intentional self-harm, sequela	59	Major Depressive, Bipolar, and Paranoid Disorders	60	0.309	0.164	0.299	0.127	0.306	0.109	0.187
T60.92XA	Toxic effect of unspecified pesticide, intentional self-harm, initial encounter	59	Major Depressive, Bipolar, and Paranoid Disorders	60	0.309	0.164	0.299	0.127	0.306	0.109	0.187
T60.92XS	Toxic effect of unspecified pesticide, intentional self-harm, sequela	59	Major Depressive, Bipolar, and Paranoid Disorders	60	0.309	0.164	0.299	0.127	0.306	0.109	0.187
T61.02XA	Ciguatera fish poisoning, intentional self-harm, initial encounter	59	Major Depressive, Bipolar, and Paranoid Disorders	60	0.309	0.164	0.299	0.127	0.306	0.109	0.187
T61.02XS	Ciguatera fish poisoning, intentional self-harm, sequela	59	Major Depressive, Bipolar, and Paranoid Disorders	60	0.309	0.164	0.299	0.127	0.306	0.109	0.187
T61.12XA	Scombroid fish poisoning, intentional self-harm, initial encounter	59	Major Depressive, Bipolar, and Paranoid Disorders	60	0.309	0.164	0.299	0.127	0.306	0.109	0.187
T61.12XS	Scombroid fish poisoning, intentional self-harm, sequela	59	Major Depressive, Bipolar, and Paranoid Disorders	60	0.309	0.164	0.299	0.127	0.306	0.109	0.187
T61.772A	Other fish poisoning, intentional self-harm, initial encounter	59	Major Depressive, Bipolar, and Paranoid Disorders	60	0.309	0.164	0.299	0.127	0.306	0.109	0.187
T61.772S	Other fish poisoning, intentional self-harm, sequela	59	Major Depressive, Bipolar, and Paranoid Disorders	60	0.309	0.164	0.299	0.127	0.306	0.109	0.187

ICD-10-CM Code	ICD-10-CM Code Description	V24 CMS-HCC	V24 CMS-HCC Disease Group	V24 CMS-HCC Hierarchies	Community, NonDual, Aged	Community, NonDual, Disabled	Community, FBDual, Aged	Community, FBDual, Disabled	Community, PBDual, Aged	Community, PBDual, Disabled	Institutional
T61.782A	Other shellfish poisoning, intentional self-harm, initial encounter	59	Major Depressive, Bipolar, and Paranoid Disorders	60	0.309	0.164	0.299	0.127	0.306	0.109	0.187
T61.782S	Other shellfish poisoning, intentional self-harm, sequela	59	Major Depressive, Bipolar, and Paranoid Disorders	60	0.309	0.164	0.299	0.127	0.306	0.109	0.187
T61.8X2A	Toxic effect of other seafood, intentional self-harm, initial encounter	59	Major Depressive, Bipolar, and Paranoid Disorders	60	0.309	0.164	0.299	0.127	0.306	0.109	0.187
T61.8X2S	Toxic effect of other seafood, intentional self-harm, sequela	59	Major Depressive, Bipolar, and Paranoid Disorders	60	0.309	0.164	0.299	0.127	0.306	0.109	0.187
T61.92XA	Toxic effect of unspecified seafood, intentional self-harm, initial encounter	59	Major Depressive, Bipolar, and Paranoid Disorders	60	0.309	0.164	0.299	0.127	0.306	0.109	0.187
T61.92XS	Toxic effect of unspecified seafood, intentional self-harm, sequela	59	Major Depressive, Bipolar, and Paranoid Disorders	60	0.309	0.164	0.299	0.127	0.306	0.109	0.187
T62.0X2A	Toxic effect of ingested mushrooms, intentional self-harm, initial encounter	59	Major Depressive, Bipolar, and Paranoid Disorders	60	0.309	0.164	0.299	0.127	0.306	0.109	0.187
T62.0X2S	Toxic effect of ingested mushrooms, intentional self-harm, sequela	59	Major Depressive, Bipolar, and Paranoid Disorders	60	0.309	0.164	0.299	0.127	0.306	0.109	0.187
T62.1X2A	Toxic effect of ingested berries, intentional self-harm, initial encounter	59	Major Depressive, Bipolar, and Paranoid Disorders	60	0.309	0.164	0.299	0.127	0.306	0.109	0.187
T62.1X2S	Toxic effect of ingested berries, intentional self-harm, sequela	59	Major Depressive, Bipolar, and Paranoid Disorders	60	0.309	0.164	0.299	0.127	0.306	0.109	0.187
T62.2X2A	Toxic effect of other ingested (parts of) plant(s), intentional self-harm, initial encounter	59	Major Depressive, Bipolar, and Paranoid Disorders	60	0.309	0.164	0.299	0.127	0.306	0.109	0.187
T62.2X2S	Toxic effect of other ingested (parts of) plant(s), intentional self-harm, sequela	59	Major Depressive, Bipolar, and Paranoid Disorders	60	0.309	0.164	0.299	0.127	0.306	0.109	0.187
T62.8X2A	Toxic effect of other specified noxious substances eaten as food, intentional self-harm, initial encounter	59	Major Depressive, Bipolar, and Paranoid Disorders	60	0.309	0.164	0.299	0.127	0.306	0.109	0.187
T62.8X2S	Toxic effect of other specified noxious substances eaten as food, intentional self-harm, sequela	59	Major Depressive, Bipolar, and Paranoid Disorders	60	0.309	0.164	0.299	0.127	0.306	0.109	0.187
T62.92XA	Toxic effect of unspecified noxious substance eaten as food, intentional self-harm, initial encounter	59	Major Depressive, Bipolar, and Paranoid Disorders	60	0.309	0.164	0.299	0.127	0.306	0.109	0.187
T62.92XS	Toxic effect of unspecified noxious substance eaten as food, intentional self-harm, sequela	59	Major Depressive, Bipolar, and Paranoid Disorders	60	0.309	0.164	0.299	0.127	0.306	0.109	0.187
T63.002A	Toxic effect of unspecified snake venom, intentional self-harm, initial encounter	59	Major Depressive, Bipolar, and Paranoid Disorders	60	0.309	0.164	0.299	0.127	0.306	0.109	0.187
T63.002S	Toxic effect of unspecified snake venom, intentional self-harm, sequela	59	Major Depressive, Bipolar, and Paranoid Disorders	60	0.309	0.164	0.299	0.127	0.306	0.109	0.187
T63.012A	Toxic effect of rattlesnake venom, intentional self-harm, initial encounter	59	Major Depressive, Bipolar, and Paranoid Disorders	60	0.309	0.164	0.299	0.127	0.306	0.109	0.187
T63.012S	Toxic effect of rattlesnake venom, intentional self-harm, sequela	59	Major Depressive, Bipolar, and Paranoid Disorders	60	0.309	0.164	0.299	0.127	0.306	0.109	0.187
T63.022A	Toxic effect of coral snake venom, intentional self-harm, initial encounter	59	Major Depressive, Bipolar, and Paranoid Disorders	60	0.309	0.164	0.299	0.127	0.306	0.109	0.187
T63.022S	Toxic effect of coral snake venom, intentional self-harm, sequela	59	Major Depressive, Bipolar, and Paranoid Disorders	60	0.309	0.164	0.299	0.127	0.306	0.109	0.187
T63.032A	Toxic effect of taipan venom, intentional self-harm, initial encounter	59	Major Depressive, Bipolar, and Paranoid Disorders	60	0.309	0.164	0.299	0.127	0.306	0.109	0.187

ICD-10-CM Code	ICD-10-CM Code Description	V24 CMS-HCC	V24 CMS-HCC Disease Group	V24 CMS-HCC Hierarchies	Community, NonDual, Aged	Community, NonDual, Disabled	Community, FBDual, Aged	Community, FBDual, Disabled	Community, PBDual, Aged	Community, PBDual, Disabled	Institutional
T63.032S	Toxic effect of taipan venom, intentional self-harm, sequela	59	Major Depressive, Bipolar, and Paranoid Disorders	60	0.309	0.164	0.299	0.127	0.306	0.109	0.187
T63.042A	Toxic effect of cobra venom, intentional self-harm, initial encounter	59	Major Depressive, Bipolar, and Paranoid Disorders	60	0.309	0.164	0.299	0.127	0.306	0.109	0.187
T63.042S	Toxic effect of cobra venom, intentional self-harm, sequela	59	Major Depressive, Bipolar, and Paranoid Disorders	60	0.309	0.164	0.299	0.127	0.306	0.109	0.187
T63.062A	Toxic effect of venom of other North and South American snake, intentional self-harm, initial encounter	59	Major Depressive, Bipolar, and Paranoid Disorders	60	0.309	0.164	0.299	0.127	0.306	0.109	0.187
T63.062S	Toxic effect of venom of other North and South American snake, intentional self-harm, sequela	59	Major Depressive, Bipolar, and Paranoid Disorders	60	0.309	0.164	0.299	0.127	0.306	0.109	0.187
T63.072A	Toxic effect of venom of other Australian snake, intentional self-harm, initial encounter	59	Major Depressive, Bipolar, and Paranoid Disorders	60	0.309	0.164	0.299	0.127	0.306	0.109	0.187
T63.072S	Toxic effect of venom of other Australian snake, intentional self-harm, sequela	59	Major Depressive, Bipolar, and Paranoid Disorders	60	0.309	0.164	0.299	0.127	0.306	0.109	0.187
T63.082A	Toxic effect of venom of other African and Asian snake, intentional self-harm, initial encounter	59	Major Depressive, Bipolar, and Paranoid Disorders	60	0.309	0.164	0.299	0.127	0.306	0.109	0.187
T63.082S	Toxic effect of venom of other African and Asian snake, intentional self-harm, sequela	59	Major Depressive, Bipolar, and Paranoid Disorders	60	0.309	0.164	0.299	0.127	0.306	0.109	0.187
T63.092A	Toxic effect of venom of other snake, intentional self-harm, initial encounter	59	Major Depressive, Bipolar, and Paranoid Disorders	60	0.309	0.164	0.299	0.127	0.306	0.109	0.187
T63.092S	Toxic effect of venom of other snake, intentional self-harm, sequela	59	Major Depressive, Bipolar, and Paranoid Disorders	60	0.309	0.164	0.299	0.127	0.306	0.109	0.187
T63.112A	Toxic effect of venom of gila monster, intentional self-harm, initial encounter	59	Major Depressive, Bipolar, and Paranoid Disorders	60	0.309	0.164	0.299	0.127	0.306	0.109	0.187
T63.112S	Toxic effect of venom of gila monster, intentional self-harm, sequela	59	Major Depressive, Bipolar, and Paranoid Disorders	60	0.309	0.164	0.299	0.127	0.306	0.109	0.187
T63.122A	Toxic effect of venom of other venomous lizard, intentional self-harm, initial encounter	59	Major Depressive, Bipolar, and Paranoid Disorders	60	0.309	0.164	0.299	0.127	0.306	0.109	0.187
T63.122S	Toxic effect of venom of other venomous lizard, intentional self-harm, sequela	59	Major Depressive, Bipolar, and Paranoid Disorders	60	0.309	0.164	0.299	0.127	0.306	0.109	0.187
T63.192A	Toxic effect of venom of other reptiles, intentional self-harm, initial encounter	59	Major Depressive, Bipolar, and Paranoid Disorders	60	0.309	0.164	0.299	0.127	0.306	0.109	0.187
T63.192S	Toxic effect of venom of other reptiles, intentional self-harm, sequela	59	Major Depressive, Bipolar, and Paranoid Disorders	60	0.309	0.164	0.299	0.127	0.306	0.109	0.187
T63.2X2A	Toxic effect of venom of scorpion, intentional self-harm, initial encounter	59	Major Depressive, Bipolar, and Paranoid Disorders	60	0.309	0.164	0.299	0.127	0.306	0.109	0.187
T63.2X2S	Toxic effect of venom of scorpion, intentional self-harm, sequela	59	Major Depressive, Bipolar, and Paranoid Disorders	60	0.309	0.164	0.299	0.127	0.306	0.109	0.187
T63.302A	Toxic effect of unspecified spider venom, intentional self-harm, initial encounter	59	Major Depressive, Bipolar, and Paranoid Disorders	60	0.309	0.164	0.299	0.127	0.306	0.109	0.187
T63.302S	Toxic effect of unspecified spider venom, intentional self-harm, sequela	59	Major Depressive, Bipolar, and Paranoid Disorders	60	0.309	0.164	0.299	0.127	0.306	0.109	0.187

ICD-10-CM Code	ICD-10-CM Code Description	V24 CMS-HCC	V24 CMS-HCC Disease Group	V24 CMS-HCC Hierarchies	Community, NonDual, Aged	Community, NonDual, Disabled	Community, FBDual, Aged	Community, FBDual, Disabled	Community, PBDual, Aged	Community, PBDual, Disabled	Institutional
T63.312A	Toxic effect of venom of black widow spider, intentional self-harm, initial encounter	59	Major Depressive, Bipolar, and Paranoid Disorders	60	0.309	0.164	0.299	0.127	0.306	0.109	0.187
T63.312S	Toxic effect of venom of black widow spider, intentional self-harm, sequela	59	Major Depressive, Bipolar, and Paranoid Disorders	60	0.309	0.164	0.299	0.127	0.306	0.109	0.187
T63.322A	Toxic effect of venom of tarantula, intentional self-harm, initial encounter	59	Major Depressive, Bipolar, and Paranoid Disorders	60	0.309	0.164	0.299	0.127	0.306	0.109	0.187
T63.322S	Toxic effect of venom of tarantula, intentional self-harm, sequela	59	Major Depressive, Bipolar, and Paranoid Disorders	60	0.309	0.164	0.299	0.127	0.306	0.109	0.187
T63.332A	Toxic effect of venom of brown recluse spider, intentional self-harm, initial encounter	59	Major Depressive, Bipolar, and Paranoid Disorders	60	0.309	0.164	0.299	0.127	0.306	0.109	0.187
T63.332S	Toxic effect of venom of brown recluse spider, intentional self-harm, sequela	59	Major Depressive, Bipolar, and Paranoid Disorders	60	0.309	0.164	0.299	0.127	0.306	0.109	0.187
T63.392A	Toxic effect of venom of other spider, intentional self-harm, initial encounter	59	Major Depressive, Bipolar, and Paranoid Disorders	60	0.309	0.164	0.299	0.127	0.306	0.109	0.187
T63.392S	Toxic effect of venom of other spider, intentional self-harm, sequela	59	Major Depressive, Bipolar, and Paranoid Disorders	60	0.309	0.164	0.299	0.127	0.306	0.109	0.187
T63.412A	Toxic effect of venom of centipedes and venomous millipedes, intentional self-harm, initial encounter	59	Major Depressive, Bipolar, and Paranoid Disorders	60	0.309	0.164	0.299	0.127	0.306	0.109	0.187
T63.412S	Toxic effect of venom of centipedes and venomous millipedes, intentional self-harm, sequela	59	Major Depressive, Bipolar, and Paranoid Disorders	60	0.309	0.164	0.299	0.127	0.306	0.109	0.187
T63.422A	Toxic effect of venom of ants, intentional self-harm, initial encounter	59	Major Depressive, Bipolar, and Paranoid Disorders	60	0.309	0.164	0.299	0.127	0.306	0.109	0.187
T63.422S	Toxic effect of venom of ants, intentional self-harm, sequela	59	Major Depressive, Bipolar, and Paranoid Disorders	60	0.309	0.164	0.299	0.127	0.306	0.109	0.187
T63.432A	Toxic effect of venom of caterpillars, intentional self-harm, initial encounter	59	Major Depressive, Bipolar, and Paranoid Disorders	60	0.309	0.164	0.299	0.127	0.306	0.109	0.187
T63.432S	Toxic effect of venom of caterpillars, intentional self-harm, sequela	59	Major Depressive, Bipolar, and Paranoid Disorders	60	0.309	0.164	0.299	0.127	0.306	0.109	0.187
T63.442A	Toxic effect of venom of bees, intentional self-harm, initial encounter	59	Major Depressive, Bipolar, and Paranoid Disorders	60	0.309	0.164	0.299	0.127	0.306	0.109	0.187
T63.442S	Toxic effect of venom of bees, intentional self-harm, sequela	59	Major Depressive, Bipolar, and Paranoid Disorders	60	0.309	0.164	0.299	0.127	0.306	0.109	0.187
T63.452A	Toxic effect of venom of hornets, intentional self-harm, initial encounter	59	Major Depressive, Bipolar, and Paranoid Disorders	60	0.309	0.164	0.299	0.127	0.306	0.109	0.187
T63.452S	Toxic effect of venom of hornets, intentional self-harm, sequela	59	Major Depressive, Bipolar, and Paranoid Disorders	60	0.309	0.164	0.299	0.127	0.306	0.109	0.187
T63.462A	Toxic effect of venom of wasps, intentional self-harm, initial encounter	59	Major Depressive, Bipolar, and Paranoid Disorders	60	0.309	0.164	0.299	0.127	0.306	0.109	0.187
T63.462S	Toxic effect of venom of wasps, intentional self-harm, sequela	59	Major Depressive, Bipolar, and Paranoid Disorders	60	0.309	0.164	0.299	0.127	0.306	0.109	0.187
T63.482A	Toxic effect of venom of other arthropod, intentional self-harm, initial encounter	59	Major Depressive, Bipolar, and Paranoid Disorders	60	0.309	0.164	0.299	0.127	0.306	0.109	0.187
T63.482S	Toxic effect of venom of other arthropod, intentional self-harm, sequela	59	Major Depressive, Bipolar, and Paranoid Disorders	60	0.309	0.164	0.299	0.127	0.306	0.109	0.187

ICD-10-CM Code	ICD-10-CM Code Description	V24 CMS-HCC	V24 CMS-HCC Disease Group	V24 CMS-HCC Hierarchies	Community, NonDual, Aged	Community, NonDual, Disabled	Community, FBDual, Aged	Community, FBDual, Disabled	Community, PBDual, Aged	Community, PBDual, Disabled	Institutional
T63.512A	Toxic effect of contact with stingray, intentional self-harm, initial encounter	59	Major Depressive, Bipolar, and Paranoid Disorders	60	0.309	0.164	0.299	0.127	0.306	0.109	0.187
T63.512S	Toxic effect of contact with stingray, intentional self-harm, sequela	59	Major Depressive, Bipolar, and Paranoid Disorders	60	0.309	0.164	0.299	0.127	0.306	0.109	0.187
T63.592A	Toxic effect of contact with other venomous fish, intentional self-harm, initial encounter	59	Major Depressive, Bipolar, and Paranoid Disorders	60	0.309	0.164	0.299	0.127	0.306	0.109	0.187
T63.592S	Toxic effect of contact with other venomous fish, intentional self-harm, sequela	59	Major Depressive, Bipolar, and Paranoid Disorders	60	0.309	0.164	0.299	0.127	0.306	0.109	0.187
T63.612A	Toxic effect of contact with Portuguese Man-o-war, intentional self-harm, initial encounter	59	Major Depressive, Bipolar, and Paranoid Disorders	60	0.309	0.164	0.299	0.127	0.306	0.109	0.187
T63.612S	Toxic effect of contact with Portuguese Man-o-war, intentional self-harm, sequela	59	Major Depressive, Bipolar, and Paranoid Disorders	60	0.309	0.164	0.299	0.127	0.306	0.109	0.187
T63.622A	Toxic effect of contact with other jellyfish, intentional self-harm, initial encounter	59	Major Depressive, Bipolar, and Paranoid Disorders	60	0.309	0.164	0.299	0.127	0.306	0.109	0.187
T63.622S	Toxic effect of contact with other jellyfish, intentional self-harm, sequela	59	Major Depressive, Bipolar, and Paranoid Disorders	60	0.309	0.164	0.299	0.127	0.306	0.109	0.187
T63.632A	Toxic effect of contact with sea anemone, intentional self-harm, initial encounter	59	Major Depressive, Bipolar, and Paranoid Disorders	60	0.309	0.164	0.299	0.127	0.306	0.109	0.187
T63.632S	Toxic effect of contact with sea anemone, intentional self-harm, sequela	59	Major Depressive, Bipolar, and Paranoid Disorders	60	0.309	0.164	0.299	0.127	0.306	0.109	0.187
T63.692A	Toxic effect of contact with other venomous marine animals, intentional self-harm, initial encounter	59	Major Depressive, Bipolar, and Paranoid Disorders	60	0.309	0.164	0.299	0.127	0.306	0.109	0.187
T63.692S	Toxic effect of contact with other venomous marine animals, intentional self-harm, sequela	59	Major Depressive, Bipolar, and Paranoid Disorders	60	0.309	0.164	0.299	0.127	0.306	0.109	0.187
T63.712A	Toxic effect of contact with venomous marine plant, intentional self-harm, initial encounter	59	Major Depressive, Bipolar, and Paranoid Disorders	60	0.309	0.164	0.299	0.127	0.306	0.109	0.187
T63.712S	Toxic effect of contact with venomous marine plant, intentional self-harm, sequela	59	Major Depressive, Bipolar, and Paranoid Disorders	60	0.309	0.164	0.299	0.127	0.306	0.109	0.187
T63.792A	Toxic effect of contact with other venomous plant, intentional self-harm, initial encounter	59	Major Depressive, Bipolar, and Paranoid Disorders	60	0.309	0.164	0.299	0.127	0.306	0.109	0.187
T63.792S	Toxic effect of contact with other venomous plant, intentional self-harm, sequela	59	Major Depressive, Bipolar, and Paranoid Disorders	60	0.309	0.164	0.299	0.127	0.306	0.109	0.187
T63.812A	Toxic effect of contact with venomous frog, intentional self-harm, initial encounter	59	Major Depressive, Bipolar, and Paranoid Disorders	60	0.309	0.164	0.299	0.127	0.306	0.109	0.187
T63.812S	Toxic effect of contact with venomous frog, intentional self-harm, sequela	59	Major Depressive, Bipolar, and Paranoid Disorders	60	0.309	0.164	0.299	0.127	0.306	0.109	0.187
T63.822A	Toxic effect of contact with venomous toad, intentional self-harm, initial encounter	59	Major Depressive, Bipolar, and Paranoid Disorders	60	0.309	0.164	0.299	0.127	0.306	0.109	0.187
T63.822S	Toxic effect of contact with venomous toad, intentional self-harm, sequela	59	Major Depressive, Bipolar, and Paranoid Disorders	60	0.309	0.164	0.299	0.127	0.306	0.109	0.187

ICD-10-CM Code	ICD-10-CM Code Description	V24 CMS-HCC	V24 CMS-HCC Disease Group	V24 CMS-HCC Hierarchies	Community, NonDual, Aged	Community, NonDual, Disabled	Community, FBDual, Aged	Community, FBDual, Disabled	Community, PBDual, Aged	Community, PBDual, Disabled	Institutional
T63.832A	Toxic effect of contact with other venomous amphibian, intentional self-harm, initial encounter	59	Major Depressive, Bipolar, and Paranoid Disorders	60	0.309	0.164	0.299	0.127	0.306	0.109	0.187
T63.832S	Toxic effect of contact with other venomous amphibian, intentional self-harm, sequela	59	Major Depressive, Bipolar, and Paranoid Disorders	60	0.309	0.164	0.299	0.127	0.306	0.109	0.187
T63.892A	Toxic effect of contact with other venomous animals, intentional self-harm, initial encounter	59	Major Depressive, Bipolar, and Paranoid Disorders	60	0.309	0.164	0.299	0.127	0.306	0.109	0.187
T63.892S	Toxic effect of contact with other venomous animals, intentional self-harm, sequela	59	Major Depressive, Bipolar, and Paranoid Disorders	60	0.309	0.164	0.299	0.127	0.306	0.109	0.187
T63.92XA	Toxic effect of contact with unspecified venomous animal, intentional self-harm, initial encounter	59	Major Depressive, Bipolar, and Paranoid Disorders	60	0.309	0.164	0.299	0.127	0.306	0.109	0.187
T63.92XS	Toxic effect of contact with unspecified venomous animal, intentional self-harm, sequela	59	Major Depressive, Bipolar, and Paranoid Disorders	60	0.309	0.164	0.299	0.127	0.306	0.109	0.187
T64.02XA	Toxic effect of aflatoxin, intentional self-harm, initial encounter	59	Major Depressive, Bipolar, and Paranoid Disorders	60	0.309	0.164	0.299	0.127	0.306	0.109	0.187
T64.02XS	Toxic effect of aflatoxin, intentional self-harm, sequela	59	Major Depressive, Bipolar, and Paranoid Disorders	60	0.309	0.164	0.299	0.127	0.306	0.109	0.187
T64.82XA	Toxic effect of other mycotoxin food contaminants, intentional self-harm, initial encounter	59	Major Depressive, Bipolar, and Paranoid Disorders	60	0.309	0.164	0.299	0.127	0.306	0.109	0.187
T64.82XS	Toxic effect of other mycotoxin food contaminants, intentional self-harm, sequela	59	Major Depressive, Bipolar, and Paranoid Disorders	60	0.309	0.164	0.299	0.127	0.306	0.109	0.187
T65.0X2A	Toxic effect of cyanides, intentional self-harm, initial encounter	59	Major Depressive, Bipolar, and Paranoid Disorders	60	0.309	0.164	0.299	0.127	0.306	0.109	0.187
T65.0X2S	Toxic effect of cyanides, intentional self-harm, sequela	59	Major Depressive, Bipolar, and Paranoid Disorders	60	0.309	0.164	0.299	0.127	0.306	0.109	0.187
T65.1X2A	Toxic effect of strychnine and its salts, intentional self-harm, initial encounter	59	Major Depressive, Bipolar, and Paranoid Disorders	60	0.309	0.164	0.299	0.127	0.306	0.109	0.187
T65.1X2S	Toxic effect of strychnine and its salts, intentional self-harm, sequela	59	Major Depressive, Bipolar, and Paranoid Disorders	60	0.309	0.164	0.299	0.127	0.306	0.109	0.187
T65.212A	Toxic effect of chewing tobacco, intentional self-harm, initial encounter	59	Major Depressive, Bipolar, and Paranoid Disorders	60	0.309	0.164	0.299	0.127	0.306	0.109	0.187
T65.212S	Toxic effect of chewing tobacco, intentional self-harm, sequela	59	Major Depressive, Bipolar, and Paranoid Disorders	60	0.309	0.164	0.299	0.127	0.306	0.109	0.187
T65.222A	Toxic effect of tobacco cigarettes, intentional self-harm, initial encounter	59	Major Depressive, Bipolar, and Paranoid Disorders	60	0.309	0.164	0.299	0.127	0.306	0.109	0.187
T65.222S	Toxic effect of tobacco cigarettes, intentional self-harm, sequela	59	Major Depressive, Bipolar, and Paranoid Disorders	60	0.309	0.164	0.299	0.127	0.306	0.109	0.187
T65.292A	Toxic effect of other tobacco and nicotine, intentional self-harm, initial encounter	59	Major Depressive, Bipolar, and Paranoid Disorders	60	0.309	0.164	0.299	0.127	0.306	0.109	0.187
T65.292S	Toxic effect of other tobacco and nicotine, intentional self-harm, sequela	59	Major Depressive, Bipolar, and Paranoid Disorders	60	0.309	0.164	0.299	0.127	0.306	0.109	0.187
T65.3X2A	Toxic effect of nitroderivatives and aminoderivatives of benzene and its homologues, intentional self-harm, initial encounter	59	Major Depressive, Bipolar, and Paranoid Disorders	60	0.309	0.164	0.299	0.127	0.306	0.109	0.187

ICD-10-CM Code	ICD-10-CM Code Description	V24 CMS-HCC	V24 CMS-HCC Disease Group	V24 CMS-HCC Hierarchies	Community, NonDual, Aged	Community, NonDual, Disabled	Community, FBDual, Aged	Community, FBDual, Disabled	Community, PBDual, Aged	Community, PBDual, Disabled	Institutional
T65.3X2S	Toxic effect of nitroderivatives and aminoderivatives of benzene and its homologues, intentional self-harm, sequela	59	Major Depressive, Bipolar, and Paranoid Disorders	60	0.309	0.164	0.299	0.127	0.306	0.109	0.187
T65.4X2A	Toxic effect of carbon disulfide, intentional self-harm, initial encounter	59	Major Depressive, Bipolar, and Paranoid Disorders	60	0.309	0.164	0.299	0.127	0.306	0.109	0.187
T65.4X2S	Toxic effect of carbon disulfide, intentional self-harm, sequela	59	Major Depressive, Bipolar, and Paranoid Disorders	60	0.309	0.164	0.299	0.127	0.306	0.109	0.187
T65.5X2A	Toxic effect of nitroglycerin and other nitric acids and esters, intentional self-harm, initial encounter	59	Major Depressive, Bipolar, and Paranoid Disorders	60	0.309	0.164	0.299	0.127	0.306	0.109	0.187
T65.5X2S	Toxic effect of nitroglycerin and other nitric acids and esters, intentional self-harm, sequela	59	Major Depressive, Bipolar, and Paranoid Disorders	60	0.309	0.164	0.299	0.127	0.306	0.109	0.187
T65.6X2A	Toxic effect of paints and dyes, not elsewhere classified, intentional self-harm, initial encounter	59	Major Depressive, Bipolar, and Paranoid Disorders	60	0.309	0.164	0.299	0.127	0.306	0.109	0.187
T65.6X2S	Toxic effect of paints and dyes, not elsewhere classified, intentional self-harm, sequela	59	Major Depressive, Bipolar, and Paranoid Disorders	60	0.309	0.164	0.299	0.127	0.306	0.109	0.187
T65.812A	Toxic effect of latex, intentional self-harm, initial encounter	59	Major Depressive, Bipolar, and Paranoid Disorders	60	0.309	0.164	0.299	0.127	0.306	0.109	0.187
T65.812S	Toxic effect of latex, intentional self-harm, sequela	59	Major Depressive, Bipolar, and Paranoid Disorders	60	0.309	0.164	0.299	0.127	0.306	0.109	0.187
T65.822A	Toxic effect of harmful algae and algae toxins, intentional self-harm, initial encounter	59	Major Depressive, Bipolar, and Paranoid Disorders	60	0.309	0.164	0.299	0.127	0.306	0.109	0.187
T65.822S	Toxic effect of harmful algae and algae toxins, intentional self-harm, sequela	59	Major Depressive, Bipolar, and Paranoid Disorders	60	0.309	0.164	0.299	0.127	0.306	0.109	0.187
T65.832A	Toxic effect of fiberglass, intentional self-harm, initial encounter	59	Major Depressive, Bipolar, and Paranoid Disorders	60	0.309	0.164	0.299	0.127	0.306	0.109	0.187
T65.832S	Toxic effect of fiberglass, intentional self-harm, sequela	59	Major Depressive, Bipolar, and Paranoid Disorders	60	0.309	0.164	0.299	0.127	0.306	0.109	0.187
T65.892A	Toxic effect of other specified substances, intentional self-harm, initial encounter	59	Major Depressive, Bipolar, and Paranoid Disorders	60	0.309	0.164	0.299	0.127	0.306	0.109	0.187
T65.892S	Toxic effect of other specified substances, intentional self-harm, sequela	59	Major Depressive, Bipolar, and Paranoid Disorders	60	0.309	0.164	0.299	0.127	0.306	0.109	0.187
T65.92XA	Toxic effect of unspecified substance, intentional self-harm, initial encounter	59	Major Depressive, Bipolar, and Paranoid Disorders	60	0.309	0.164	0.299	0.127	0.306	0.109	0.187
T65.92XS	Toxic effect of unspecified substance, intentional self-harm, sequela	59	Major Depressive, Bipolar, and Paranoid Disorders	60	0.309	0.164	0.299	0.127	0.306	0.109	0.187
T71.112A	Asphyxiation due to smothering under pillow, intentional self-harm, initial encounter	59	Major Depressive, Bipolar, and Paranoid Disorders	60	0.309	0.164	0.299	0.127	0.306	0.109	0.187
T71.112S	Asphyxiation due to smothering under pillow, intentional self-harm, sequela	59	Major Depressive, Bipolar, and Paranoid Disorders	60	0.309	0.164	0.299	0.127	0.306	0.109	0.187
T71.122A	Asphyxiation due to plastic bag, intentional self-harm, initial encounter	59	Major Depressive, Bipolar, and Paranoid Disorders	60	0.309	0.164	0.299	0.127	0.306	0.109	0.187
T71.122S	Asphyxiation due to plastic bag, intentional self-harm, sequela	59	Major Depressive, Bipolar, and Paranoid Disorders	60	0.309	0.164	0.299	0.127	0.306	0.109	0.187
T71.132A	Asphyxiation due to being trapped in bed linens, intentional self-harm, initial encounter	59	Major Depressive, Bipolar, and Paranoid Disorders	60	0.309	0.164	0.299	0.127	0.306	0.109	0.187

ICD-10-CM Code	ICD-10-CM Code Description	V24 CMS-HCC	V24 CMS-HCC Disease Group	V24 CMS-HCC Hierarchies	Community, NonDual, Aged	Community, NonDual, Disabled	Community, FBDual, Aged	Community, FBDual, Disabled	Community, PBDual, Aged	Community, PBDual, Disabled	Institutional
T71.132S	Asphyxiation due to being trapped in bed linens, intentional self-harm, sequela	59	Major Depressive, Bipolar, and Paranoid Disorders	60	0.309	0.164	0.299	0.127	0.306	0.109	0.187
T71.152A	Asphyxiation due to smothering in furniture, intentional self-harm, initial encounter	59	Major Depressive, Bipolar, and Paranoid Disorders	60	0.309	0.164	0.299	0.127	0.306	0.109	0.187
T71.152S	Asphyxiation due to smothering in furniture, intentional self-harm, sequela	59	Major Depressive, Bipolar, and Paranoid Disorders	60	0.309	0.164	0.299	0.127	0.306	0.109	0.187
T71.162A	Asphyxiation due to hanging, intentional self-harm, initial encounter	59	Major Depressive, Bipolar, and Paranoid Disorders	60	0.309	0.164	0.299	0.127	0.306	0.109	0.187
T71.162S	Asphyxiation due to hanging, intentional self-harm, sequela	59	Major Depressive, Bipolar, and Paranoid Disorders	60	0.309	0.164	0.299	0.127	0.306	0.109	0.187
T71.192A	Asphyxiation due to mechanical threat to breathing due to other causes, intentional self-harm, initial encounter	59	Major Depressive, Bipolar, and Paranoid Disorders	60	0.309	0.164	0.299	0.127	0.306	0.109	0.187
T71.192S	Asphyxiation due to mechanical threat to breathing due to other causes, intentional self-harm, sequela	59	Major Depressive, Bipolar, and Paranoid Disorders	60	0.309	0.164	0.299	0.127	0.306	0.109	0.187
T71.222A	Asphyxiation due to being trapped in a car trunk, intentional self-harm, initial encounter	59	Major Depressive, Bipolar, and Paranoid Disorders	60	0.309	0.164	0.299	0.127	0.306	0.109	0.187
T71.222S	Asphyxiation due to being trapped in a car trunk, intentional self-harm, sequela	59	Major Depressive, Bipolar, and Paranoid Disorders	60	0.309	0.164	0.299	0.127	0.306	0.109	0.187
T71.232A	Asphyxiation due to being trapped in a (discarded) refrigerator, intentional self-harm, initial encounter	59	Major Depressive, Bipolar, and Paranoid Disorders	60	0.309	0.164	0.299	0.127	0.306	0.109	0.187
T71.232S	Asphyxiation due to being trapped in a (discarded) refrigerator, intentional self-harm, sequela	59	Major Depressive, Bipolar, and Paranoid Disorders	60	0.309	0.164	0.299	0.127	0.306	0.109	0.187
T79.0XXA	Air embolism (traumatic), initial encounter	173	Traumatic Amputations and Complications		0.208	0.172	0.221	0.525	0.176	0.180	0.092
T79.1XXA	Fat embolism (traumatic), initial encounter	173	Traumatic Amputations and Complications		0.208	0.172	0.221	0.525	0.176	0.180	0.092
T79.2XXA	Traumatic secondary and recurrent hemorrhage and seroma, initial encounter	173	Traumatic Amputations and Complications		0.208	0.172	0.221	0.525	0.176	0.180	0.092
T79.4XXA	Traumatic shock, initial encounter	173	Traumatic Amputations and Complications		0.208	0.172	0.221	0.525	0.176	0.180	0.092
T79.5XXA	Traumatic anuria, initial encounter	173	Traumatic Amputations and Complications		0.208	0.172	0.221	0.525	0.176	0.180	0.092
T79.6XXA	Traumatic ischemia of muscle, initial encounter	173	Traumatic Amputations and Complications		0.208	0.172	0.221	0.525	0.176	0.180	0.092
T79.7XXA	Traumatic subcutaneous emphysema, initial encounter	173	Traumatic Amputations and Complications		0.208	0.172	0.221	0.525	0.176	0.180	0.092
T79.8XXA	Other early complications of trauma, initial encounter	173	Traumatic Amputations and Complications		0.208	0.172	0.221	0.525	0.176	0.180	0.092
T79.9XXA	Unspecified early complication of trauma, initial encounter	173	Traumatic Amputations and Complications		0.208	0.172	0.221	0.525	0.176	0.180	0.092
T79.A0XA	Compartment syndrome, unspecified, initial encounter	173	Traumatic Amputations and Complications		0.208	0.172	0.221	0.525	0.176	0.180	0.092
T79.A11A	Traumatic compartment syndrome of right upper extremity, initial encounter	173	Traumatic Amputations and Complications		0.208	0.172	0.221	0.525	0.176	0.180	0.092
T79.A12A	Traumatic compartment syndrome of left upper extremity, initial encounter	173	Traumatic Amputations and Complications		0.208	0.172	0.221	0.525	0.176	0.180	0.092

ICD-10-CM Code	ICD-10-CM Code Description	V24 CMS-HCC	V24 CMS-HCC Disease Group	V24 CMS-HCC Hierarchies	Community, NonDual, Aged	Community, NonDual, Disabled	Community, FBDual, Aged	Community, FBDual, Disabled	Community, PBDual, Aged	Community, PBDual, Disabled	Institutional
T79.A19A	Traumatic compartment syndrome of unspecified upper extremity, initial encounter	173	Traumatic Amputations and Complications		0.208	0.172	0.221	0.525	0.176	0.180	0.092
T79.A21A	Traumatic compartment syndrome of right lower extremity, initial encounter	173	Traumatic Amputations and Complications		0.208	0.172	0.221	0.525	0.176	0.180	0.092
T79.A22A	Traumatic compartment syndrome of left lower extremity, initial encounter	173	Traumatic Amputations and Complications		0.208	0.172	0.221	0.525	0.176	0.180	0.092
T79.A29A	Traumatic compartment syndrome of unspecified lower extremity, initial encounter	173	Traumatic Amputations and Complications		0.208	0.172	0.221	0.525	0.176	0.180	0.092
T79.A3XA	Traumatic compartment syndrome of abdomen, initial encounter	173	Traumatic Amputations and Complications		0.208	0.172	0.221	0.525	0.176	0.180	0.092
T79.A9XA	Traumatic compartment syndrome of other sites, initial encounter	173	Traumatic Amputations and Complications		0.208	0.172	0.221	0.525	0.176	0.180	0.092
T81.11XA	Postprocedural cardiogenic shock, initial encounter	84	Cardio-Respiratory Failure and Shock		0.282	0.385	0.492	0.531	0.361	0.343	0.313
T81.12XA	Postprocedural septic shock, initial encounter	2	Septicemia, Sepsis, Systemic Inflammatory Response Syndrome/ Shock		0.352	0.414	0.453	0.530	0.316	0.297	0.324
T81.44XA	Sepsis following a procedure, initial encounter	2	Septicemia, Sepsis, Systemic Inflammatory Response Syndrome/ Shock		0.352	0.414	0.453	0.530	0.316	0.297	0.324
T81.502A	Unspecified complication of foreign body accidentally left in body following kidney dialysis, initial encounter	134	Dialysis Status	135,136, 137,138	0.435	0.406	0.683	0.594	0.446	0.480	0.468
T81.502D	Unspecified complication of foreign body accidentally left in body following kidney dialysis, subsequent encounter	134	Dialysis Status	135,136, 137,138	0.435	0.406	0.683	0.594	0.446	0.480	0.468
T81.502S	Unspecified complication of foreign body accidentally left in body following kidney dialysis, sequela	134	Dialysis Status	135,136, 137,138	0.435	0.406	0.683	0.594	0.446	0.480	0.468
T81.512A	Adhesions due to foreign body accidentally left in body following kidney dialysis, initial encounter	134	Dialysis Status	135,136, 137,138	0.435	0.406	0.683	0.594	0.446	0.480	0.468
T81.512D	Adhesions due to foreign body accidentally left in body following kidney dialysis, subsequent encounter	134	Dialysis Status	135,136, 137,138	0.435	0.406	0.683	0.594	0.446	0.480	0.468
T81.512S	Adhesions due to foreign body accidentally left in body following kidney dialysis, sequela	134	Dialysis Status	135,136, 137,138	0.435	0.406	0.683	0.594	0.446	0.480	0.468
T81.522A	Obstruction due to foreign body accidentally left in body following kidney dialysis, initial encounter	134	Dialysis Status	135,136, 137,138	0.435	0.406	0.683	0.594	0.446	0.480	0.468
T81.522D	Obstruction due to foreign body accidentally left in body following kidney dialysis, subsequent encounter	134	Dialysis Status	135,136, 137,138	0.435	0.406	0.683	0.594	0.446	0.480	0.468
T81.522S	Obstruction due to foreign body accidentally left in body following kidney dialysis, sequela	134	Dialysis Status	135,136, 137,138	0.435	0.406	0.683	0.594	0.446	0.480	0.468
T81.532A	Perforation due to foreign body accidentally left in body following kidney dialysis, initial encounter	134	Dialysis Status	135,136, 137,138	0.435	0.406	0.683	0.594	0.446	0.480	0.468
T81.532D	Perforation due to foreign body accidentally left in body following kidney dialysis, subsequent encounter	134	Dialysis Status	135,136, 137,138	0.435	0.406	0.683	0.594	0.446	0.480	0.468

ICD-10-CM Code	ICD-10-CM Code Description	V24 CMS-HCC	V24 CMS-HCC Disease Group	V24 CMS-HCC Hierarchies	Community, NonDual, Aged	Community, NonDual, Disabled	Community, FBDual, Aged	Community, FBDual, Disabled	Community, PBDual, Aged	Community, PBDual, Disabled	Institutional
T81.532S	Perforation due to foreign body accidentally left in body following kidney dialysis, sequela	134	Dialysis Status	135,136, 137,138	0.435	0.406	0.683	0.594	0.446	0.480	0.468
T81.592A	Other complications of foreign body accidentally left in body following kidney dialysis, initial encounter	134	Dialysis Status	135,136, 137,138	0.435	0.406	0.683	0.594	0.446	0.480	0.468
T81.592D	Other complications of foreign body accidentally left in body following kidney dialysis, subsequent encounter	134	Dialysis Status	135,136, 137,138	0.435	0.406	0.683	0.594	0.446	0.480	0.468
T81.592S	Other complications of foreign body accidentally left in body following kidney dialysis, sequela	134	Dialysis Status	135,136, 137,138	0.435	0.406	0.683	0.594	0.446	0.480	0.468
T82.310A	Breakdown (mechanical) of aortic (bifurcation) graft (replacement), initial encounter	176	Complications of Specified Implanted Device or Graft		0.582	0.911	0.680	0.982	0.520	0.832	0.469
T82.311A	Breakdown (mechanical) of carotid arterial graft (bypass), initial encounter	176	Complications of Specified Implanted Device or Graft		0.582	0.911	0.680	0.982	0.520	0.832	0.469
T82.312A	Breakdown (mechanical) of femoral arterial graft (bypass), initial encounter	176	Complications of Specified Implanted Device or Graft		0.582	0.911	0.680	0.982	0.520	0.832	0.469
T82.318A	Breakdown (mechanical) of other vascular grafts, initial encounter	176	Complications of Specified Implanted Device or Graft		0.582	0.911	0.680	0.982	0.520	0.832	0.469
T82.319A	Breakdown (mechanical) of unspecified vascular grafts, initial encounter	176	Complications of Specified Implanted Device or Graft		0.582	0.911	0.680	0.982	0.520	0.832	0.469
T82.320A	Displacement of aortic (bifurcation) graft (replacement), initial encounter	176	Complications of Specified Implanted Device or Graft		0.582	0.911	0.680	0.982	0.520	0.832	0.469
T82.321A	Displacement of carotid arterial graft (bypass), initial encounter	176	Complications of Specified Implanted Device or Graft		0.582	0.911	0.680	0.982	0.520	0.832	0.469
T82.322A	Displacement of femoral arterial graft (bypass), initial encounter	176	Complications of Specified Implanted Device or Graft		0.582	0.911	0.680	0.982	0.520	0.832	0.469
T82.328A	Displacement of other vascular grafts, initial encounter	176	Complications of Specified Implanted Device or Graft		0.582	0.911	0.680	0.982	0.520	0.832	0.469
T82.329A	Displacement of unspecified vascular grafts, initial encounter	176	Complications of Specified Implanted Device or Graft		0.582	0.911	0.680	0.982	0.520	0.832	0.469
T82.330A	Leakage of aortic (bifurcation) graft (replacement), initial encounter	176	Complications of Specified Implanted Device or Graft		0.582	0.911	0.680	0.982	0.520	0.832	0.469
T82.331A	Leakage of carotid arterial graft (bypass), initial encounter	176	Complications of Specified Implanted Device or Graft		0.582	0.911	0.680	0.982	0.520	0.832	0.469
T82.332A	Leakage of femoral arterial graft (bypass), initial encounter	176	Complications of Specified Implanted Device or Graft		0.582	0.911	0.680	0.982	0.520	0.832	0.469
T82.338A	Leakage of other vascular grafts, initial encounter	176	Complications of Specified Implanted Device or Graft		0.582	0.911	0.680	0.982	0.520	0.832	0.469
T82.339A	Leakage of unspecified vascular graft, initial encounter	176	Complications of Specified Implanted Device or Graft		0.582	0.911	0.680	0.982	0.520	0.832	0.469
T82.390A	Other mechanical complication of aortic (bifurcation) graft (replacement), initial encounter	176	Complications of Specified Implanted Device or Graft		0.582	0.911	0.680	0.982	0.520	0.832	0.469
T82.391A	Other mechanical complication of carotid arterial graft (bypass), initial encounter	176	Complications of Specified Implanted Device or Graft		0.582	0.911	0.680	0.982	0.520	0.832	0.469
T82.392A	Other mechanical complication of femoral arterial graft (bypass), initial encounter	176	Complications of Specified Implanted Device or Graft		0.582	0.911	0.680	0.982	0.520	0.832	0.469
T82.398A	Other mechanical complication of other vascular grafts, initial encounter	176	Complications of Specified Implanted Device or Graft		0.582	0.911	0.680	0.982	0.520	0.832	0.469

ICD-10-CM Code	ICD-10-CM Code Description	V24 CMS-HCC	V24 CMS-HCC Disease Group	V24 CMS-HCC Hierarchies	Community, NonDual, Aged	Community, NonDual, Disabled	Community, FBDual, Aged	Community, FBDual, Disabled	Community, PBDual, Aged	Community, PBDual, Disabled	Institutional
T82.399A	Other mechanical complication of unspecified vascular grafts, initial encounter	176	Complications of Specified Implanted Device or Graft		0.582	0.911	0.680	0.982	0.520	0.832	0.469
T82.41XA	Breakdown (mechanical) of vascular dialysis catheter, initial encounter	134	Dialysis Status	135,136, 137,138	0.435	0.406	0.683	0.594	0.446	0.480	0.468
T82.41XD	Breakdown (mechanical) of vascular dialysis catheter, subsequent encounter	134	Dialysis Status	135,136, 137,138	0.435	0.406	0.683	0.594	0.446	0.480	0.468
T82.41XS	Breakdown (mechanical) of vascular dialysis catheter, sequela	134	Dialysis Status	135,136, 137,138	0.435	0.406	0.683	0.594	0.446	0.480	0.468
T82.42XA	Displacement of vascular dialysis catheter, initial encounter	134	Dialysis Status	135,136, 137,138	0.435	0.406	0.683	0.594	0.446	0.480	0.468
T82.42XD	Displacement of vascular dialysis catheter, subsequent encounter	134	Dialysis Status	135,136, 137,138	0.435	0.406	0.683	0.594	0.446	0.480	0.468
T82.42XS	Displacement of vascular dialysis catheter, sequela	134	Dialysis Status	135,136, 137,138	0.435	0.406	0.683	0.594	0.446	0.480	0.468
T82.43XA	Leakage of vascular dialysis catheter, initial encounter	134	Dialysis Status	135,136, 137,138	0.435	0.406	0.683	0.594	0.446	0.480	0.468
T82.43XD	Leakage of vascular dialysis catheter, subsequent encounter	134	Dialysis Status	135,136, 137,138	0.435	0.406	0.683	0.594	0.446	0.480	0.468
T82.43XS	Leakage of vascular dialysis catheter, sequela	134	Dialysis Status	135,136, 137,138	0.435	0.406	0.683	0.594	0.446	0.480	0.468
T82.49XA	Other complication of vascular dialysis catheter, initial encounter	134	Dialysis Status	135,136, 137,138	0.435	0.406	0.683	0.594	0.446	0.480	0.468
T82.49XD	Other complication of vascular dialysis catheter, subsequent encounter	134	Dialysis Status	135,136, 137,138	0.435	0.406	0.683	0.594	0.446	0.480	0.468
T82.49XS	Other complication of vascular dialysis catheter, sequela	134	Dialysis Status	135,136, 137,138	0.435	0.406	0.683	0.594	0.446	0.480	0.468
T82.510A	Breakdown (mechanical) of surgically created arteriovenous fistula, initial encounter	176	Complications of Specified Implanted Device or Graft		0.582	0.911	0.680	0.982	0.520	0.832	0.469
T82.511A	Breakdown (mechanical) of surgically created arteriovenous shunt, initial encounter	176	Complications of Specified Implanted Device or Graft		0.582	0.911	0.680	0.982	0.520	0.832	0.469
T82.513A	Breakdown (mechanical) of balloon (counterpulsation) device, initial encounter	176	Complications of Specified Implanted Device or Graft		0.582	0.911	0.680	0.982	0.520	0.832	0.469
T82.514A	Breakdown (mechanical) of infusion catheter, initial encounter	176	Complications of Specified Implanted Device or Graft		0.582	0.911	0.680	0.982	0.520	0.832	0.469
T82.515A	Breakdown (mechanical) of umbrella device, initial encounter	176	Complications of Specified Implanted Device or Graft		0.582	0.911	0.680	0.982	0.520	0.832	0.469
T82.518A	Breakdown (mechanical) of other cardiac and vascular devices and implants, initial encounter	176	Complications of Specified Implanted Device or Graft		0.582	0.911	0.680	0.982	0.520	0.832	0.469
T82.520A	Displacement of surgically created arteriovenous fistula, initial encounter	176	Complications of Specified Implanted Device or Graft		0.582	0.911	0.680	0.982	0.520	0.832	0.469
T82.521A	Displacement of surgically created arteriovenous shunt, initial encounter	176	Complications of Specified Implanted Device or Graft		0.582	0.911	0.680	0.982	0.520	0.832	0.469
T82.523A	Displacement of balloon (counterpulsation) device, initial encounter	176	Complications of Specified Implanted Device or Graft		0.582	0.911	0.680	0.982	0.520	0.832	0.469
T82.524A	Displacement of infusion catheter, initial encounter	176	Complications of Specified Implanted Device or Graft		0.582	0.911	0.680	0.982	0.520	0.832	0.469
T82.525A	Displacement of umbrella device, initial encounter	176	Complications of Specified Implanted Device or Graft		0.582	0.911	0.680	0.982	0.520	0.832	0.469
T82.528A	Displacement of other cardiac and vascular devices and implants, initial encounter	176	Complications of Specified Implanted Device or Graft		0.582	0.911	0.680	0.982	0.520	0.832	0.469

ICD-10-CM Code	ICD-10-CM Code Description	V24 CMS-HCC	V24 CMS-HCC Disease Group	V24 CMS-HCC Hierarchies	Community, NonDual, Aged	Community, NonDual, Disabled	Community, FBDual, Aged	Community, FBDual, Disabled	Community, PBDual, Aged	Community, PBDual, Disabled	Institutional
T82.530A	Leakage of surgically created arteriovenous fistula, initial encounter	176	Complications of Specified Implanted Device or Graft		0.582	0.911	0.680	0.982	0.520	0.832	0.469
T82.531A	Leakage of surgically created arteriovenous shunt, initial encounter	176	Complications of Specified Implanted Device or Graft		0.582	0.911	0.680	0.982	0.520	0.832	0.469
T82.533A	Leakage of balloon (counterpulsation) device, initial encounter	176	Complications of Specified Implanted Device or Graft		0.582	0.911	0.680	0.982	0.520	0.832	0.469
T82.534A	Leakage of infusion catheter, initial encounter	176	Complications of Specified Implanted Device or Graft		0.582	0.911	0.680	0.982	0.520	0.832	0.469
T82.535A	Leakage of umbrella device, initial encounter	176	Complications of Specified Implanted Device or Graft		0.582	0.911	0.680	0.982	0.520	0.832	0.469
T82.538A	Leakage of other cardiac and vascular devices and implants, initial encounter	176	Complications of Specified Implanted Device or Graft		0.582	0.911	0.680	0.982	0.520	0.832	0.469
T82.590A	Other mechanical complication of surgically created arteriovenous fistula, initial encounter	176	Complications of Specified Implanted Device or Graft		0.582	0.911	0.680	0.982	0.520	0.832	0.469
T82.591A	Other mechanical complication of surgically created arteriovenous shunt, initial encounter	176	Complications of Specified Implanted Device or Graft		0.582	0.911	0.680	0.982	0.520	0.832	0.469
T82.593A	Other mechanical complication of balloon (counterpulsation) device, initial encounter	176	Complications of Specified Implanted Device or Graft		0.582	0.911	0.680	0.982	0.520	0.832	0.469
T82.594A	Other mechanical complication of infusion catheter, initial encounter	176	Complications of Specified Implanted Device or Graft		0.582	0.911	0.680	0.982	0.520	0.832	0.469
T82.595A	Other mechanical complication of umbrella device, initial encounter	176	Complications of Specified Implanted Device or Graft		0.582	0.911	0.680	0.982	0.520	0.832	0.469
T82.598A	Other mechanical complication of other cardiac and vascular devices and implants, initial encounter	176	Complications of Specified Implanted Device or Graft		0.582	0.911	0.680	0.982	0.520	0.832	0.469
T82.6XXA	Infection and inflammatory reaction due to cardiac valve prosthesis, initial encounter	176	Complications of Specified Implanted Device or Graft		0.582	0.911	0.680	0.982	0.520	0.832	0.469
T82.7XXA	Infection and inflammatory reaction due to other cardiac and vascular devices, implants and grafts, initial encounter	176	Complications of Specified Implanted Device or Graft		0.582	0.911	0.680	0.982	0.520	0.832	0.469
T82.818A	Embolism due to vascular prosthetic devices, implants and grafts, initial encounter	176	Complications of Specified Implanted Device or Graft		0.582	0.911	0.680	0.982	0.520	0.832	0.469
T82.828A	Fibrosis due to vascular prosthetic devices, implants and grafts, initial encounter	176	Complications of Specified Implanted Device or Graft		0.582	0.911	0.680	0.982	0.520	0.832	0.469
T82.838A	Hemorrhage due to vascular prosthetic devices, implants and grafts, initial encounter	176	Complications of Specified Implanted Device or Graft		0.582	0.911	0.680	0.982	0.520	0.832	0.469
T82.848A	Pain due to vascular prosthetic devices, implants and grafts, initial encounter	176	Complications of Specified Implanted Device or Graft		0.582	0.911	0.680	0.982	0.520	0.832	0.469
T82.856A	Stenosis of peripheral vascular stent, initial encounter	176	Complications of Specified Implanted Device or Graft		0.582	0.911	0.680	0.982	0.520	0.832	0.469
T82.858A	Stenosis of other vascular prosthetic devices, implants and grafts, initial encounter	176	Complications of Specified Implanted Device or Graft		0.582	0.911	0.680	0.982	0.520	0.832	0.469
T82.868A	Thrombosis due to vascular prosthetic devices, implants and grafts, initial encounter	176	Complications of Specified Implanted Device or Graft		0.582	0.911	0.680	0.982	0.520	0.832	0.469
T82.898A	Other specified complication of vascular prosthetic devices, implants and grafts, initial encounter	176	Complications of Specified Implanted Device or Graft		0.582	0.911	0.680	0.982	0.520	0.832	0.469

ICD-10-CM Code	ICD-10-CM Code Description	V24 CMS-HCC	V24 CMS-HCC Disease Group	V24 CMS-HCC Hierarchies	Community, NonDual, Aged	Community, NonDual, Disabled	Community, FBDual, Aged	Community, FBDual, Disabled	Community, PBDual, Aged	Community, PBDual, Disabled	Institutional
T83.010A	Breakdown (mechanical) of cystostomy catheter, initial encounter	176	Complications of Specified Implanted Device or Graft		0.582	0.911	0.680	0.982	0.520	0.832	0.469
T83.011A	Breakdown (mechanical) of indwelling urethral catheter, initial encounter	176	Complications of Specified Implanted Device or Graft		0.582	0.911	0.680	0.982	0.520	0.832	0.469
T83.012A	Breakdown (mechanical) of nephrostomy catheter, initial encounter	176	Complications of Specified Implanted Device or Graft		0.582	0.911	0.680	0.982	0.520	0.832	0.469
T83.018A	Breakdown (mechanical) of other urinary catheter, initial encounter	176	Complications of Specified Implanted Device or Graft		0.582	0.911	0.680	0.982	0.520	0.832	0.469
T83.020A	Displacement of cystostomy catheter, initial encounter	176	Complications of Specified Implanted Device or Graft		0.582	0.911	0.680	0.982	0.520	0.832	0.469
T83.021A	Displacement of indwelling urethral catheter, initial encounter	176	Complications of Specified Implanted Device or Graft		0.582	0.911	0.680	0.982	0.520	0.832	0.469
T83.022A	Displacement of nephrostomy catheter, initial encounter	176	Complications of Specified Implanted Device or Graft		0.582	0.911	0.680	0.982	0.520	0.832	0.469
T83.028A	Displacement of other urinary catheter, initial encounter	176	Complications of Specified Implanted Device or Graft		0.582	0.911	0.680	0.982	0.520	0.832	0.469
T83.030A	Leakage of cystostomy catheter, initial encounter	176	Complications of Specified Implanted Device or Graft		0.582	0.911	0.680	0.982	0.520	0.832	0.469
T83.031A	Leakage of indwelling urethral catheter, initial encounter	176	Complications of Specified Implanted Device or Graft		0.582	0.911	0.680	0.982	0.520	0.832	0.469
T83.032A	Leakage of nephrostomy catheter, initial encounter	176	Complications of Specified Implanted Device or Graft		0.582	0.911	0.680	0.982	0.520	0.832	0.469
T83.038A	Leakage of other urinary catheter, initial encounter	176	Complications of Specified Implanted Device or Graft		0.582	0.911	0.680	0.982	0.520	0.832	0.469
T83.090A	Other mechanical complication of cystostomy catheter, initial encounter	176	Complications of Specified Implanted Device or Graft		0.582	0.911	0.680	0.982	0.520	0.832	0.469
T83.091A	Other mechanical complication of indwelling urethral catheter, initial encounter	176	Complications of Specified Implanted Device or Graft		0.582	0.911	0.680	0.982	0.520	0.832	0.469
T83.092A	Other mechanical complication of nephrostomy catheter, initial encounter	176	Complications of Specified Implanted Device or Graft		0.582	0.911	0.680	0.982	0.520	0.832	0.469
T83.098A	Other mechanical complication of other urinary catheter, initial encounter	176	Complications of Specified Implanted Device or Graft		0.582	0.911	0.680	0.982	0.520	0.832	0.469
T83.110A	Breakdown (mechanical) of urinary electronic stimulator device, initial encounter	176	Complications of Specified Implanted Device or Graft		0.582	0.911	0.680	0.982	0.520	0.832	0.469
T83.111A	Breakdown (mechanical) of implanted urinary sphincter, initial encounter	176	Complications of Specified Implanted Device or Graft		0.582	0.911	0.680	0.982	0.520	0.832	0.469
T83.112A	Breakdown (mechanical) of indwelling ureteral stent, initial encounter	176	Complications of Specified Implanted Device or Graft		0.582	0.911	0.680	0.982	0.520	0.832	0.469
T83.113A	Breakdown (mechanical) of other urinary stents, initial encounter	176	Complications of Specified Implanted Device or Graft		0.582	0.911	0.680	0.982	0.520	0.832	0.469
T83.118A	Breakdown (mechanical) of other urinary devices and implants, initial encounter	176	Complications of Specified Implanted Device or Graft		0.582	0.911	0.680	0.982	0.520	0.832	0.469
T83.120A	Displacement of urinary electronic stimulator device, initial encounter	176	Complications of Specified Implanted Device or Graft		0.582	0.911	0.680	0.982	0.520	0.832	0.469
T83.121A	Displacement of implanted urinary sphincter, initial encounter	176	Complications of Specified Implanted Device or Graft		0.582	0.911	0.680	0.982	0.520	0.832	0.469
T83.122A	Displacement of indwelling ureteral stent, initial encounter	176	Complications of Specified Implanted Device or Graft		0.582	0.911	0.680	0.982	0.520	0.832	0.469

ICD-10-CM Code	ICD-10-CM Code Description	V24 CMS-HCC	V24 CMS-HCC Disease Group	V24 CMS-HCC Hierarchies	Community, NonDual, Aged	Community, NonDual, Disabled	Community, FBDual, Aged	Community, FBDual, Disabled	Community, PBDual, Aged	Community, PBDual, Disabled	Institutional
T83.123A	Displacement of other urinary stents, initial encounter	176	Complications of Specified Implanted Device or Graft		0.582	0.911	0.680	0.982	0.520	0.832	0.469
T83.128A	Displacement of other urinary devices and implants, initial encounter	176	Complications of Specified Implanted Device or Graft		0.582	0.911	0.680	0.982	0.520	0.832	0.469
T83.190A	Other mechanical complication of urinary electronic stimulator device, initial encounter	176	Complications of Specified Implanted Device or Graft		0.582	0.911	0.680	0.982	0.520	0.832	0.469
T83.191A	Other mechanical complication of implanted urinary sphincter, initial encounter	176	Complications of Specified Implanted Device or Graft		0.582	0.911	0.680	0.982	0.520	0.832	0.469
T83.192A	Other mechanical complication of indwelling ureteral stent, initial encounter	176	Complications of Specified Implanted Device or Graft		0.582	0.911	0.680	0.982	0.520	0.832	0.469
T83.193A	Other mechanical complication of other urinary stent, initial encounter	176	Complications of Specified Implanted Device or Graft		0.582	0.911	0.680	0.982	0.520	0.832	0.469
T83.198A	Other mechanical complication of other urinary devices and implants, initial encounter	176	Complications of Specified Implanted Device or Graft		0.582	0.911	0.680	0.982	0.520	0.832	0.469
T83.21XA	Breakdown (mechanical) of graft of urinary organ, initial encounter	176	Complications of Specified Implanted Device or Graft		0.582	0.911	0.680	0.982	0.520	0.832	0.469
T83.22XA	Displacement of graft of urinary organ, initial encounter	176	Complications of Specified Implanted Device or Graft		0.582	0.911	0.680	0.982	0.520	0.832	0.469
T83.23XA	Leakage of graft of urinary organ, initial encounter	176	Complications of Specified Implanted Device or Graft		0.582	0.911	0.680	0.982	0.520	0.832	0.469
T83.24XA	Erosion of graft of urinary organ, initial encounter	176	Complications of Specified Implanted Device or Graft		0.582	0.911	0.680	0.982	0.520	0.832	0.469
T83.25XA	Exposure of graft of urinary organ, initial encounter	176	Complications of Specified Implanted Device or Graft		0.582	0.911	0.680	0.982	0.520	0.832	0.469
T83.29XA	Other mechanical complication of graft of urinary organ, initial encounter	176	Complications of Specified Implanted Device or Graft		0.582	0.911	0.680	0.982	0.520	0.832	0.469
T83.410A	Breakdown (mechanical) of implanted penile prosthesis, initial encounter	176	Complications of Specified Implanted Device or Graft		0.582	0.911	0.680	0.982	0.520	0.832	0.469
T83.411A	Breakdown (mechanical) of implanted testicular prosthesis, initial encounter	176	Complications of Specified Implanted Device or Graft		0.582	0.911	0.680	0.982	0.520	0.832	0.469
T83.418A	Breakdown (mechanical) of other prosthetic devices, implants and grafts of genital tract, initial encounter	176	Complications of Specified Implanted Device or Graft		0.582	0.911	0.680	0.982	0.520	0.832	0.469
T83.420A	Displacement of implanted penile prosthesis, initial encounter	176	Complications of Specified Implanted Device or Graft		0.582	0.911	0.680	0.982	0.520	0.832	0.469
T83.421A	Displacement of implanted testicular prosthesis, initial encounter	176	Complications of Specified Implanted Device or Graft		0.582	0.911	0.680	0.982	0.520	0.832	0.469
T83.428A	Displacement of other prosthetic devices, implants and grafts of genital tract, initial encounter	176	Complications of Specified Implanted Device or Graft		0.582	0.911	0.680	0.982	0.520	0.832	0.469
T83.490A	Other mechanical complication of implanted penile prosthesis, initial encounter	176	Complications of Specified Implanted Device or Graft		0.582	0.911	0.680	0.982	0.520	0.832	0.469
T83.491A	Other mechanical complication of implanted testicular prosthesis, initial encounter	176	Complications of Specified Implanted Device or Graft		0.582	0.911	0.680	0.982	0.520	0.832	0.469
T83.498A	Other mechanical complication of other prosthetic devices, implants and grafts of genital tract, initial encounter	176	Complications of Specified Implanted Device or Graft		0.582	0.911	0.680	0.982	0.520	0.832	0.469

ICD-10-CM Code	ICD-10-CM Code Description	V24 CMS-HCC	V24 CMS-HCC Disease Group	V24 CMS-HCC Hierarchies	Community, NonDual, Aged	Community, NonDual, Disabled	Community, FBDual, Aged	Community, FBDual, Disabled	Community, PBDual, Aged	Community, PBDual, Disabled	Institutional
T83.510A	Infection and inflammatory reaction due to cystostomy catheter, initial encounter	176	Complications of Specified Implanted Device or Graft		0.582	0.911	0.680	0.982	0.520	0.832	0.469
T83.511A	Infection and inflammatory reaction due to indwelling urethral catheter, initial encounter	176	Complications of Specified Implanted Device or Graft		0.582	0.911	0.680	0.982	0.520	0.832	0.469
T83.512A	Infection and inflammatory reaction due to nephrostomy catheter, initial encounter	176	Complications of Specified Implanted Device or Graft		0.582	0.911	0.680	0.982	0.520	0.832	0.469
T83.518A	Infection and inflammatory reaction due to other urinary catheter, initial encounter	176	Complications of Specified Implanted Device or Graft		0.582	0.911	0.680	0.982	0.520	0.832	0.469
T83.590A	Infection and inflammatory reaction due to implanted urinary neurostimulation device, initial encounter	176	Complications of Specified Implanted Device or Graft		0.582	0.911	0.680	0.982	0.520	0.832	0.469
T83.591A	Infection and inflammatory reaction due to implanted urinary sphincter, initial encounter	176	Complications of Specified Implanted Device or Graft		0.582	0.911	0.680	0.982	0.520	0.832	0.469
T83.592A	Infection and inflammatory reaction due to indwelling ureteral stent, initial encounter	176	Complications of Specified Implanted Device or Graft		0.582	0.911	0.680	0.982	0.520	0.832	0.469
T83.593A	Infection and inflammatory reaction due to other urinary stents, initial encounter	176	Complications of Specified Implanted Device or Graft		0.582	0.911	0.680	0.982	0.520	0.832	0.469
T83.598A	Infection and inflammatory reaction due to other prosthetic device, implant and graft in urinary system, initial encounter	176	Complications of Specified Implanted Device or Graft		0.582	0.911	0.680	0.982	0.520	0.832	0.469
T83.61XA	Infection and inflammatory reaction due to implanted penile prosthesis, initial encounter	176	Complications of Specified Implanted Device or Graft		0.582	0.911	0.680	0.982	0.520	0.832	0.469
T83.62XA	Infection and inflammatory reaction due to implanted testicular prosthesis, initial encounter	176	Complications of Specified Implanted Device or Graft		0.582	0.911	0.680	0.982	0.520	0.832	0.469
T83.69XA	Infection and inflammatory reaction due to other prosthetic device, implant and graft in genital tract, initial encounter	176	Complications of Specified Implanted Device or Graft		0.582	0.911	0.680	0.982	0.520	0.832	0.469
T83.711A	Erosion of implanted vaginal mesh to surrounding organ or tissue, initial encounter	176	Complications of Specified Implanted Device or Graft		0.582	0.911	0.680	0.982	0.520	0.832	0.469
T83.712A	Erosion of implanted urethral mesh to surrounding organ or tissue, initial encounter	176	Complications of Specified Implanted Device or Graft		0.582	0.911	0.680	0.982	0.520	0.832	0.469
T83.713A	Erosion of implanted urethral bulking agent to surrounding organ or tissue, initial encounter	176	Complications of Specified Implanted Device or Graft		0.582	0.911	0.680	0.982	0.520	0.832	0.469
T83.714A	Erosion of implanted ureteral bulking agent to surrounding organ or tissue, initial encounter	176	Complications of Specified Implanted Device or Graft		0.582	0.911	0.680	0.982	0.520	0.832	0.469
T83.718A	Erosion of other implanted mesh to organ or tissue, initial encounter	176	Complications of Specified Implanted Device or Graft		0.582	0.911	0.680	0.982	0.520	0.832	0.469
T83.719A	Erosion of other prosthetic materials to surrounding organ or tissue, initial encounter	176	Complications of Specified Implanted Device or Graft		0.582	0.911	0.680	0.982	0.520	0.832	0.469
T83.721A	Exposure of implanted vaginal mesh into vagina, initial encounter	176	Complications of Specified Implanted Device or Graft		0.582	0.911	0.680	0.982	0.520	0.832	0.469
T83.722A	Exposure of implanted urethral mesh into urethra, initial encounter	176	Complications of Specified Implanted Device or Graft		0.582	0.911	0.680	0.982	0.520	0.832	0.469

ICD-10-CM Code	ICD-10-CM Code Description	V24 CMS-HCC	V24 CMS-HCC Disease Group	V24 CMS-HCC Hierarchies	Community, NonDual, Aged	Community, NonDual, Disabled	Community, FBDual, Aged	Community, FBDual, Disabled	Community, PBDual, Aged	Community, PBDual, Disabled	Institutional
X71.9XXA	Intentional self-harm by drowning and submersion, unspecified, initial encounter	59	Major Depressive, Bipolar, and Paranoid Disorders	60	0.309	0.164	0.299	0.127	0.306	0.109	0.187
X71.9XXD	Intentional self-harm by drowning and submersion, unspecified, subsequent encounter	59	Major Depressive, Bipolar, and Paranoid Disorders	60	0.309	0.164	0.299	0.127	0.306	0.109	0.187
X71.9XXS	Intentional self-harm by drowning and submersion, unspecified, sequela	59	Major Depressive, Bipolar, and Paranoid Disorders	60	0.309	0.164	0.299	0.127	0.306	0.109	0.187
X72.XXXA	Intentional self-harm by handgun discharge, initial encounter	59	Major Depressive, Bipolar, and Paranoid Disorders	60	0.309	0.164	0.299	0.127	0.306	0.109	0.187
X72.XXXD	Intentional self-harm by handgun discharge, subsequent encounter	59	Major Depressive, Bipolar, and Paranoid Disorders	60	0.309	0.164	0.299	0.127	0.306	0.109	0.187
X72.XXXS	Intentional self-harm by handgun discharge, sequela	59	Major Depressive, Bipolar, and Paranoid Disorders	60	0.309	0.164	0.299	0.127	0.306	0.109	0.187
X73.0XXA	Intentional self-harm by shotgun discharge, initial encounter	59	Major Depressive, Bipolar, and Paranoid Disorders	60	0.309	0.164	0.299	0.127	0.306	0.109	0.187
X73.0XXD	Intentional self-harm by shotgun discharge, subsequent encounter	59	Major Depressive, Bipolar, and Paranoid Disorders	60	0.309	0.164	0.299	0.127	0.306	0.109	0.187
X73.0XXS	Intentional self-harm by shotgun discharge, sequela	59	Major Depressive, Bipolar, and Paranoid Disorders	60	0.309	0.164	0.299	0.127	0.306	0.109	0.187
X73.1XXA	Intentional self-harm by hunting rifle discharge, initial encounter	59	Major Depressive, Bipolar, and Paranoid Disorders	60	0.309	0.164	0.299	0.127	0.306	0.109	0.187
X73.1XXD	Intentional self-harm by hunting rifle discharge, subsequent encounter	59	Major Depressive, Bipolar, and Paranoid Disorders	60	0.309	0.164	0.299	0.127	0.306	0.109	0.187
X73.1XXS	Intentional self-harm by hunting rifle discharge, sequela	59	Major Depressive, Bipolar, and Paranoid Disorders	60	0.309	0.164	0.299	0.127	0.306	0.109	0.187
X73.2XXA	Intentional self-harm by machine gun discharge, initial encounter	59	Major Depressive, Bipolar, and Paranoid Disorders	60	0.309	0.164	0.299	0.127	0.306	0.109	0.187
X73.2XXD	Intentional self-harm by machine gun discharge, subsequent encounter	59	Major Depressive, Bipolar, and Paranoid Disorders	60	0.309	0.164	0.299	0.127	0.306	0.109	0.187
X73.2XXS	Intentional self-harm by machine gun discharge, sequela	59	Major Depressive, Bipolar, and Paranoid Disorders	60	0.309	0.164	0.299	0.127	0.306	0.109	0.187
X73.8XXA	Intentional self-harm by other larger firearm discharge, initial encounter	59	Major Depressive, Bipolar, and Paranoid Disorders	60	0.309	0.164	0.299	0.127	0.306	0.109	0.187
X73.8XXD	Intentional self-harm by other larger firearm discharge, subsequent encounter	59	Major Depressive, Bipolar, and Paranoid Disorders	60	0.309	0.164	0.299	0.127	0.306	0.109	0.187
X73.8XXS	Intentional self-harm by other larger firearm discharge, sequela	59	Major Depressive, Bipolar, and Paranoid Disorders	60	0.309	0.164	0.299	0.127	0.306	0.109	0.187
X73.9XXA	Intentional self-harm by unspecified larger firearm discharge, initial encounter	59	Major Depressive, Bipolar, and Paranoid Disorders	60	0.309	0.164	0.299	0.127	0.306	0.109	0.187
X73.9XXD	Intentional self-harm by unspecified larger firearm discharge, subsequent encounter	59	Major Depressive, Bipolar, and Paranoid Disorders	60	0.309	0.164	0.299	0.127	0.306	0.109	0.187
X73.9XXS	Intentional self-harm by unspecified larger firearm discharge, sequela	59	Major Depressive, Bipolar, and Paranoid Disorders	60	0.309	0.164	0.299	0.127	0.306	0.109	0.187
X74.01XA	Intentional self-harm by airgun, initial encounter	59	Major Depressive, Bipolar, and Paranoid Disorders	60	0.309	0.164	0.299	0.127	0.306	0.109	0.187
X74.01XD	Intentional self-harm by airgun, subsequent encounter	59	Major Depressive, Bipolar, and Paranoid Disorders	60	0.309	0.164	0.299	0.127	0.306	0.109	0.187
X74.01XS	Intentional self-harm by airgun, sequela	59	Major Depressive, Bipolar, and Paranoid Disorders	60	0.309	0.164	0.299	0.127	0.306	0.109	0.187
X74.02XA	Intentional self-harm by paintball gun, initial encounter	59	Major Depressive, Bipolar, and Paranoid Disorders	60	0.309	0.164	0.299	0.127	0.306	0.109	0.187
X74.02XD	Intentional self-harm by paintball gun, subsequent encounter	59	Major Depressive, Bipolar, and Paranoid Disorders	60	0.309	0.164	0.299	0.127	0.306	0.109	0.187
X74.02XS	Intentional self-harm by paintball gun, sequela	59	Major Depressive, Bipolar, and Paranoid Disorders	60	0.309	0.164	0.299	0.127	0.306	0.109	0.187

ICD-10-CM Code	ICD-10-CM Code Description	V24 CMS-HCC	V24 CMS-HCC Disease Group	V24 CMS-HCC Hierarchies	Community, NonDual, Aged	Community, NonDual, Disabled	Community, FBDual, Aged	Community, FBDual, Disabled	Community, PBDual, Aged	Community, PBDual, Disabled	Institutional
X74.Ø9XA	Intentional self-harm by other gas, air or spring-operated gun, initial encounter	59	Major Depressive, Bipolar, and Paranoid Disorders	60	0.309	0.164	0.299	0.127	0.306	0.109	0.187
X74.Ø9XD	Intentional self-harm by other gas, air or spring-operated gun, subsequent encounter	59	Major Depressive, Bipolar, and Paranoid Disorders	60	0.309	0.164	0.299	0.127	0.306	0.109	0.187
X74.Ø9XS	Intentional self-harm by other gas, air or spring-operated gun, sequela	59	Major Depressive, Bipolar, and Paranoid Disorders	60	0.309	0.164	0.299	0.127	0.306	0.109	0.187
X74.8XXA	Intentional self-harm by other firearm discharge, initial encounter	59	Major Depressive, Bipolar, and Paranoid Disorders	60	0.309	0.164	0.299	0.127	0.306	0.109	0.187
X74.8XXD	Intentional self-harm by other firearm discharge, subsequent encounter	59	Major Depressive, Bipolar, and Paranoid Disorders	60	0.309	0.164	0.299	0.127	0.306	0.109	0.187
X74.8XXS	Intentional self-harm by other firearm discharge, sequela	59	Major Depressive, Bipolar, and Paranoid Disorders	60	0.309	0.164	0.299	0.127	0.306	0.109	0.187
X74.9XXA	Intentional self-harm by unspecified firearm discharge, initial encounter	59	Major Depressive, Bipolar, and Paranoid Disorders	60	0.309	0.164	0.299	0.127	0.306	0.109	0.187
X74.9XXD	Intentional self-harm by unspecified firearm discharge, subsequent encounter	59	Major Depressive, Bipolar, and Paranoid Disorders	60	0.309	0.164	0.299	0.127	0.306	0.109	0.187
X74.9XXS	Intentional self-harm by unspecified firearm discharge, sequela	59	Major Depressive, Bipolar, and Paranoid Disorders	60	0.309	0.164	0.299	0.127	0.306	0.109	0.187
X75.XXXA	Intentional self-harm by explosive material, initial encounter	59	Major Depressive, Bipolar, and Paranoid Disorders	60	0.309	0.164	0.299	0.127	0.306	0.109	0.187
X75.XXXD	Intentional self-harm by explosive material, subsequent encounter	59	Major Depressive, Bipolar, and Paranoid Disorders	60	0.309	0.164	0.299	0.127	0.306	0.109	0.187
X75.XXXS	Intentional self-harm by explosive material, sequela	59	Major Depressive, Bipolar, and Paranoid Disorders	60	0.309	0.164	0.299	0.127	0.306	0.109	0.187
X76.XXXA	Intentional self-harm by smoke, fire and flames, initial encounter	59	Major Depressive, Bipolar, and Paranoid Disorders	60	0.309	0.164	0.299	0.127	0.306	0.109	0.187
X76.XXXD	Intentional self-harm by smoke, fire and flames, subsequent encounter	59	Major Depressive, Bipolar, and Paranoid Disorders	60	0.309	0.164	0.299	0.127	0.306	0.109	0.187
X76.XXXS	Intentional self-harm by smoke, fire and flames, sequela	59	Major Depressive, Bipolar, and Paranoid Disorders	60	0.309	0.164	0.299	0.127	0.306	0.109	0.187
X77.ØXXA	Intentional self-harm by steam or hot vapors, initial encounter	59	Major Depressive, Bipolar, and Paranoid Disorders	60	0.309	0.164	0.299	0.127	0.306	0.109	0.187
X77.ØXXD	Intentional self-harm by steam or hot vapors, subsequent encounter	59	Major Depressive, Bipolar, and Paranoid Disorders	60	0.309	0.164	0.299	0.127	0.306	0.109	0.187
X77.ØXXS	Intentional self-harm by steam or hot vapors, sequela	59	Major Depressive, Bipolar, and Paranoid Disorders	60	0.309	0.164	0.299	0.127	0.306	0.109	0.187
X77.1XXA	Intentional self-harm by hot tap water, initial encounter	59	Major Depressive, Bipolar, and Paranoid Disorders	60	0.309	0.164	0.299	0.127	0.306	0.109	0.187
X77.1XXD	Intentional self-harm by hot tap water, subsequent encounter	59	Major Depressive, Bipolar, and Paranoid Disorders	60	0.309	0.164	0.299	0.127	0.306	0.109	0.187
X77.1XXS	Intentional self-harm by hot tap water, sequela	59	Major Depressive, Bipolar, and Paranoid Disorders	60	0.309	0.164	0.299	0.127	0.306	0.109	0.187
X77.2XXA	Intentional self-harm by other hot fluids, initial encounter	59	Major Depressive, Bipolar, and Paranoid Disorders	60	0.309	0.164	0.299	0.127	0.306	0.109	0.187
X77.2XXD	Intentional self-harm by other hot fluids, subsequent encounter	59	Major Depressive, Bipolar, and Paranoid Disorders	60	0.309	0.164	0.299	0.127	0.306	0.109	0.187
X77.2XXS	Intentional self-harm by other hot fluids, sequela	59	Major Depressive, Bipolar, and Paranoid Disorders	60	0.309	0.164	0.299	0.127	0.306	0.109	0.187
X77.3XXA	Intentional self-harm by hot household appliances, initial encounter	59	Major Depressive, Bipolar, and Paranoid Disorders	60	0.309	0.164	0.299	0.127	0.306	0.109	0.187
X77.3XXD	Intentional self-harm by hot household appliances, subsequent encounter	59	Major Depressive, Bipolar, and Paranoid Disorders	60	0.309	0.164	0.299	0.127	0.306	0.109	0.187
X77.3XXS	Intentional self-harm by hot household appliances, sequela	59	Major Depressive, Bipolar, and Paranoid Disorders	60	0.309	0.164	0.299	0.127	0.306	0.109	0.187

ICD-10-CM Code	ICD-10-CM Code Description	V24 CMS-HCC	V24 CMS-HCC Disease Group	V24 CMS-HCC Hierarchies	Community, NonDual, Aged	Community, NonDual, Disabled	Community, FBDual, Aged	Community, FBDual, Disabled	Community, PBDual, Aged	Community, PBDual, Disabled	Institutional
X77.8XXA	Intentional self-harm by other hot objects, initial encounter	59	Major Depressive, Bipolar, and Paranoid Disorders	60	0.309	0.164	0.299	0.127	0.306	0.109	0.187
X77.8XXD	Intentional self-harm by other hot objects, subsequent encounter	59	Major Depressive, Bipolar, and Paranoid Disorders	60	0.309	0.164	0.299	0.127	0.306	0.109	0.187
X77.8XXS	Intentional self-harm by other hot objects, sequela	59	Major Depressive, Bipolar, and Paranoid Disorders	60	0.309	0.164	0.299	0.127	0.306	0.109	0.187
X77.9XXA	Intentional self-harm by unspecified hot objects, initial encounter	59	Major Depressive, Bipolar, and Paranoid Disorders	60	0.309	0.164	0.299	0.127	0.306	0.109	0.187
X77.9XXD	Intentional self-harm by unspecified hot objects, subsequent encounter	59	Major Depressive, Bipolar, and Paranoid Disorders	60	0.309	0.164	0.299	0.127	0.306	0.109	0.187
X77.9XXS	Intentional self-harm by unspecified hot objects, sequela	59	Major Depressive, Bipolar, and Paranoid Disorders	60	0.309	0.164	0.299	0.127	0.306	0.109	0.187
X78.0XXA	Intentional self-harm by sharp glass, initial encounter	59	Major Depressive, Bipolar, and Paranoid Disorders	60	0.309	0.164	0.299	0.127	0.306	0.109	0.187
X78.0XXD	Intentional self-harm by sharp glass, subsequent encounter	59	Major Depressive, Bipolar, and Paranoid Disorders	60	0.309	0.164	0.299	0.127	0.306	0.109	0.187
X78.0XXS	Intentional self-harm by sharp glass, sequela	59	Major Depressive, Bipolar, and Paranoid Disorders	60	0.309	0.164	0.299	0.127	0.306	0.109	0.187
X78.1XXA	Intentional self-harm by knife, initial encounter	59	Major Depressive, Bipolar, and Paranoid Disorders	60	0.309	0.164	0.299	0.127	0.306	0.109	0.187
X78.1XXD	Intentional self-harm by knife, subsequent encounter	59	Major Depressive, Bipolar, and Paranoid Disorders	60	0.309	0.164	0.299	0.127	0.306	0.109	0.187
X78.1XXS	Intentional self-harm by knife, sequela	59	Major Depressive, Bipolar, and Paranoid Disorders	60	0.309	0.164	0.299	0.127	0.306	0.109	0.187
X78.2XXA	Intentional self-harm by sword or dagger, initial encounter	59	Major Depressive, Bipolar, and Paranoid Disorders	60	0.309	0.164	0.299	0.127	0.306	0.109	0.187
X78.2XXD	Intentional self-harm by sword or dagger, subsequent encounter	59	Major Depressive, Bipolar, and Paranoid Disorders	60	0.309	0.164	0.299	0.127	0.306	0.109	0.187
X78.2XXS	Intentional self-harm by sword or dagger, sequela	59	Major Depressive, Bipolar, and Paranoid Disorders	60	0.309	0.164	0.299	0.127	0.306	0.109	0.187
X78.8XXA	Intentional self-harm by other sharp object, initial encounter	59	Major Depressive, Bipolar, and Paranoid Disorders	60	0.309	0.164	0.299	0.127	0.306	0.109	0.187
X78.8XXD	Intentional self-harm by other sharp object, subsequent encounter	59	Major Depressive, Bipolar, and Paranoid Disorders	60	0.309	0.164	0.299	0.127	0.306	0.109	0.187
X78.8XXS	Intentional self-harm by other sharp object, sequela	59	Major Depressive, Bipolar, and Paranoid Disorders	60	0.309	0.164	0.299	0.127	0.306	0.109	0.187
X78.9XXA	Intentional self-harm by unspecified sharp object, initial encounter	59	Major Depressive, Bipolar, and Paranoid Disorders	60	0.309	0.164	0.299	0.127	0.306	0.109	0.187
X78.9XXD	Intentional self-harm by unspecified sharp object, subsequent encounter	59	Major Depressive, Bipolar, and Paranoid Disorders	60	0.309	0.164	0.299	0.127	0.306	0.109	0.187
X78.9XXS	Intentional self-harm by unspecified sharp object, sequela	59	Major Depressive, Bipolar, and Paranoid Disorders	60	0.309	0.164	0.299	0.127	0.306	0.109	0.187
X79.XXXA	Intentional self-harm by blunt object, initial encounter	59	Major Depressive, Bipolar, and Paranoid Disorders	60	0.309	0.164	0.299	0.127	0.306	0.109	0.187
X79.XXXD	Intentional self-harm by blunt object, subsequent encounter	59	Major Depressive, Bipolar, and Paranoid Disorders	60	0.309	0.164	0.299	0.127	0.306	0.109	0.187
X79.XXXS	Intentional self-harm by blunt object, sequela	59	Major Depressive, Bipolar, and Paranoid Disorders	60	0.309	0.164	0.299	0.127	0.306	0.109	0.187
X80.XXXA	Intentional self-harm by jumping from a high place, initial encounter	59	Major Depressive, Bipolar, and Paranoid Disorders	60	0.309	0.164	0.299	0.127	0.306	0.109	0.187
X80.XXXD	Intentional self-harm by jumping from a high place, subsequent encounter	59	Major Depressive, Bipolar, and Paranoid Disorders	60	0.309	0.164	0.299	0.127	0.306	0.109	0.187
X80.XXXS	Intentional self-harm by jumping from a high place, sequela	59	Major Depressive, Bipolar, and Paranoid Disorders	60	0.309	0.164	0.299	0.127	0.306	0.109	0.187
X81.0XXA	Intentional self-harm by jumping or lying in front of motor vehicle, initial encounter	59	Major Depressive, Bipolar, and Paranoid Disorders	60	0.309	0.164	0.299	0.127	0.306	0.109	0.187

ICD-10-CM Code	ICD-10-CM Code Description	V24 CMS-HCC	V24 CMS-HCC Disease Group	V24 CMS-HCC Hierarchies	Community, NonDual, Aged	Community, NonDual, Disabled	Community, FBDual, Aged	Community, FBDual, Disabled	Community, PBDual, Aged	Community, PBDual, Disabled	Institutional
X81.0XXD	Intentional self-harm by jumping or lying in front of motor vehicle, subsequent encounter	59	Major Depressive, Bipolar, and Paranoid Disorders	60	0.309	0.164	0.299	0.127	0.306	0.109	0.187
X81.0XXS	Intentional self-harm by jumping or lying in front of motor vehicle, sequela	59	Major Depressive, Bipolar, and Paranoid Disorders	60	0.309	0.164	0.299	0.127	0.306	0.109	0.187
X81.1XXA	Intentional self-harm by jumping or lying in front of (subway) train, initial encounter	59	Major Depressive, Bipolar, and Paranoid Disorders	60	0.309	0.164	0.299	0.127	0.306	0.109	0.187
X81.1XXD	Intentional self-harm by jumping or lying in front of (subway) train, subsequent encounter	59	Major Depressive, Bipolar, and Paranoid Disorders	60	0.309	0.164	0.299	0.127	0.306	0.109	0.187
X81.1XXS	Intentional self-harm by jumping or lying in front of (subway) train, sequela	59	Major Depressive, Bipolar, and Paranoid Disorders	60	0.309	0.164	0.299	0.127	0.306	0.109	0.187
X81.8XXA	Intentional self-harm by jumping or lying in front of other moving object, initial encounter	59	Major Depressive, Bipolar, and Paranoid Disorders	60	0.309	0.164	0.299	0.127	0.306	0.109	0.187
X81.8XXD	Intentional self-harm by jumping or lying in front of other moving object, subsequent encounter	59	Major Depressive, Bipolar, and Paranoid Disorders	60	0.309	0.164	0.299	0.127	0.306	0.109	0.187
X81.8XXS	Intentional self-harm by jumping or lying in front of other moving object, sequela	59	Major Depressive, Bipolar, and Paranoid Disorders	60	0.309	0.164	0.299	0.127	0.306	0.109	0.187
X82.0XXA	Intentional collision of motor vehicle with other motor vehicle, initial encounter	59	Major Depressive, Bipolar, and Paranoid Disorders	60	0.309	0.164	0.299	0.127	0.306	0.109	0.187
X82.0XXD	Intentional collision of motor vehicle with other motor vehicle, subsequent encounter	59	Major Depressive, Bipolar, and Paranoid Disorders	60	0.309	0.164	0.299	0.127	0.306	0.109	0.187
X82.0XXS	Intentional collision of motor vehicle with other motor vehicle, sequela	59	Major Depressive, Bipolar, and Paranoid Disorders	60	0.309	0.164	0.299	0.127	0.306	0.109	0.187
X82.1XXA	Intentional collision of motor vehicle with train, initial encounter	59	Major Depressive, Bipolar, and Paranoid Disorders	60	0.309	0.164	0.299	0.127	0.306	0.109	0.187
X82.1XXD	Intentional collision of motor vehicle with train, subsequent encounter	59	Major Depressive, Bipolar, and Paranoid Disorders	60	0.309	0.164	0.299	0.127	0.306	0.109	0.187
X82.1XXS	Intentional collision of motor vehicle with train, sequela	59	Major Depressive, Bipolar, and Paranoid Disorders	60	0.309	0.164	0.299	0.127	0.306	0.109	0.187
X82.2XXA	Intentional collision of motor vehicle with tree, initial encounter	59	Major Depressive, Bipolar, and Paranoid Disorders	60	0.309	0.164	0.299	0.127	0.306	0.109	0.187
X82.2XXD	Intentional collision of motor vehicle with tree, subsequent encounter	59	Major Depressive, Bipolar, and Paranoid Disorders	60	0.309	0.164	0.299	0.127	0.306	0.109	0.187
X82.2XXS	Intentional collision of motor vehicle with tree, sequela	59	Major Depressive, Bipolar, and Paranoid Disorders	60	0.309	0.164	0.299	0.127	0.306	0.109	0.187
X82.8XXA	Other intentional self-harm by crashing of motor vehicle, initial encounter	59	Major Depressive, Bipolar, and Paranoid Disorders	60	0.309	0.164	0.299	0.127	0.306	0.109	0.187
X82.8XXD	Other intentional self-harm by crashing of motor vehicle, subsequent encounter	59	Major Depressive, Bipolar, and Paranoid Disorders	60	0.309	0.164	0.299	0.127	0.306	0.109	0.187
X82.8XXS	Other intentional self-harm by crashing of motor vehicle, sequela	59	Major Depressive, Bipolar, and Paranoid Disorders	60	0.309	0.164	0.299	0.127	0.306	0.109	0.187
X83.0XXA	Intentional self-harm by crashing of aircraft, initial encounter	59	Major Depressive, Bipolar, and Paranoid Disorders	60	0.309	0.164	0.299	0.127	0.306	0.109	0.187
X83.0XXD	Intentional self-harm by crashing of aircraft, subsequent encounter	59	Major Depressive, Bipolar, and Paranoid Disorders	60	0.309	0.164	0.299	0.127	0.306	0.109	0.187
X83.0XXS	Intentional self-harm by crashing of aircraft, sequela	59	Major Depressive, Bipolar, and Paranoid Disorders	60	0.309	0.164	0.299	0.127	0.306	0.109	0.187
X83.1XXA	Intentional self-harm by electrocution, initial encounter	59	Major Depressive, Bipolar, and Paranoid Disorders	60	0.309	0.164	0.299	0.127	0.306	0.109	0.187

ICD-10-CM Code	ICD-10-CM Code Description	V24 CMS-HCC	V24 CMS-HCC Disease Group	V24 CMS-HCC Hierarchies	Community, NonDual, Aged	Community, NonDual, Disabled	Community, FBDual, Aged	Community, FBDual, Disabled	Community, PBDual, Aged	Community, PBDual, Disabled	Institutional
X83.1XXD	Intentional self-harm by electrocution, subsequent encounter	59	Major Depressive, Bipolar, and Paranoid Disorders	60	0.309	0.164	0.299	0.127	0.306	0.109	0.187
X83.1XXS	Intentional self-harm by electrocution, sequela	59	Major Depressive, Bipolar, and Paranoid Disorders	60	0.309	0.164	0.299	0.127	0.306	0.109	0.187
X83.2XXA	Intentional self-harm by exposure to extremes of cold, initial encounter	59	Major Depressive, Bipolar, and Paranoid Disorders	60	0.309	0.164	0.299	0.127	0.306	0.109	0.187
X83.2XXD	Intentional self-harm by exposure to extremes of cold, subsequent encounter	59	Major Depressive, Bipolar, and Paranoid Disorders	60	0.309	0.164	0.299	0.127	0.306	0.109	0.187
X83.2XXS	Intentional self-harm by exposure to extremes of cold, sequela	59	Major Depressive, Bipolar, and Paranoid Disorders	60	0.309	0.164	0.299	0.127	0.306	0.109	0.187
X83.8XXA	Intentional self-harm by other specified means, initial encounter	59	Major Depressive, Bipolar, and Paranoid Disorders	60	0.309	0.164	0.299	0.127	0.306	0.109	0.187
X83.8XXD	Intentional self-harm by other specified means, subsequent encounter	59	Major Depressive, Bipolar, and Paranoid Disorders	60	0.309	0.164	0.299	0.127	0.306	0.109	0.187
X83.8XXS	Intentional self-harm by other specified means, sequela	59	Major Depressive, Bipolar, and Paranoid Disorders	60	0.309	0.164	0.299	0.127	0.306	0.109	0.187
Y62.2	Failure of sterile precautions during kidney dialysis and other perfusion	134	Dialysis Status	135,136, 137,138	0.435	0.406	0.683	0.594	0.446	0.480	0.468
Z21	Asymptomatic human immunodeficiency virus [HIV] infection status	1	HIV/AIDS		0.335	0.287	0.595	0.396	0.482	0.200	1.722
Z43.0	Encounter for attention to tracheostomy	82	Respirator Dependence/Tracheostomy Status	83,84	1.000	0.781	2.183	1.465	0.836	0.769	1.622
Z43.1	Encounter for attention to gastrostomy	188	Artificial Openings for Feeding or Elimination		0.534	0.755	0.742	0.770	0.520	0.732	0.514
Z43.2	Encounter for attention to ileostomy	188	Artificial Openings for Feeding or Elimination		0.534	0.755	0.742	0.770	0.520	0.732	0.514
Z43.3	Encounter for attention to colostomy	188	Artificial Openings for Feeding or Elimination		0.534	0.755	0.742	0.770	0.520	0.732	0.514
Z43.4	Encounter for attention to other artificial openings of digestive tract	188	Artificial Openings for Feeding or Elimination		0.534	0.755	0.742	0.770	0.520	0.732	0.514
Z43.5	Encounter for attention to cystostomy	188	Artificial Openings for Feeding or Elimination		0.534	0.755	0.742	0.770	0.520	0.732	0.514
Z43.6	Encounter for attention to other artificial openings of urinary tract	188	Artificial Openings for Feeding or Elimination		0.534	0.755	0.742	0.770	0.520	0.732	0.514
Z43.8	Encounter for attention to other artificial openings	188	Artificial Openings for Feeding or Elimination		0.534	0.755	0.742	0.770	0.520	0.732	0.514
Z43.9	Encounter for attention to unspecified artificial opening	188	Artificial Openings for Feeding or Elimination		0.534	0.755	0.742	0.770	0.520	0.732	0.514
Z44.101	Encounter for fitting and adjustment of unspecified right artificial leg	189	Amputation Status, Lower Limb/Amputation Complications		0.519	0.437	0.795	0.934	0.697	0.626	0.357
Z44.102	Encounter for fitting and adjustment of unspecified left artificial leg	189	Amputation Status, Lower Limb/Amputation Complications		0.519	0.437	0.795	0.934	0.697	0.626	0.357
Z44.109	Encounter for fitting and adjustment of unspecified artificial leg, unspecified leg	189	Amputation Status, Lower Limb/Amputation Complications		0.519	0.437	0.795	0.934	0.697	0.626	0.357
Z44.111	Encounter for fitting and adjustment of complete right artificial leg	189	Amputation Status, Lower Limb/Amputation Complications		0.519	0.437	0.795	0.934	0.697	0.626	0.357
Z44.112	Encounter for fitting and adjustment of complete left artificial leg	189	Amputation Status, Lower Limb/Amputation Complications		0.519	0.437	0.795	0.934	0.697	0.626	0.357
Z44.119	Encounter for fitting and adjustment of complete artificial leg, unspecified leg	189	Amputation Status, Lower Limb/Amputation Complications		0.519	0.437	0.795	0.934	0.697	0.626	0.357
Z44.121	Encounter for fitting and adjustment of partial artificial right leg	189	Amputation Status, Lower Limb/Amputation Complications		0.519	0.437	0.795	0.934	0.697	0.626	0.357
Z44.122	Encounter for fitting and adjustment of partial artificial left leg	189	Amputation Status, Lower Limb/Amputation Complications		0.519	0.437	0.795	0.934	0.697	0.626	0.357

ICD-10-CM Code	ICD-10-CM Code Description	V24 CMS-HCC	V24 CMS-HCC Disease Group	V24 CMS-HCC Hierarchies	Community, NonDual, Aged	Community, NonDual, Disabled	Community, FBDual, Aged	Community, FBDual, Disabled	Community, PBDual, Aged	Community, PBDual, Disabled	Institutional
Z44.129	Encounter for fitting and adjustment of partial artificial leg, unspecified leg	189	Amputation Status, Lower Limb/ Amputation Complications		0.519	0.437	0.795	0.934	0.697	0.626	0.357
Z48.21	Encounter for aftercare following heart transplant	186	Major Organ Transplant or Replacement Status		0.832	0.445	0.728	0.865	0.438	0.613	1.046
Z48.23	Encounter for aftercare following liver transplant	186	Major Organ Transplant or Replacement Status		0.832	0.445	0.728	0.865	0.438	0.613	1.046
Z48.24	Encounter for aftercare following lung transplant	186	Major Organ Transplant or Replacement Status		0.832	0.445	0.728	0.865	0.438	0.613	1.046
Z48.28Ø	Encounter for aftercare following heart-lung transplant	186	Major Organ Transplant or Replacement Status		0.832	0.445	0.728	0.865	0.438	0.613	1.046
Z48.29Ø	Encounter for aftercare following bone marrow transplant	186	Major Organ Transplant or Replacement Status		0.832	0.445	0.728	0.865	0.438	0.613	1.046
Z49.Ø1	Encounter for fitting and adjustment of extracorporeal dialysis catheter	134	Dialysis Status	135,136, 137,138	0.435	0.406	0.683	0.594	0.446	0.480	0.468
Z49.Ø2	Encounter for fitting and adjustment of peritoneal dialysis catheter	134	Dialysis Status	135,136, 137,138	0.435	0.406	0.683	0.594	0.446	0.480	0.468
Z49.31	Encounter for adequacy testing for hemodialysis	134	Dialysis Status	135,136, 137,138	0.435	0.406	0.683	0.594	0.446	0.480	0.468
Z49.32	Encounter for adequacy testing for peritoneal dialysis	134	Dialysis Status	135,136, 137,138	0.435	0.406	0.683	0.594	0.446	0.480	0.468
Z68.41	Body mass index [BMI] 40.0-44.9, adult	22	Morbid Obesity		0.250	0.183	0.383	0.297	0.233	0.204	0.455
Z68.42	Body mass index [BMI] 45.0-49.9, adult	22	Morbid Obesity		0.250	0.183	0.383	0.297	0.233	0.204	0.455
Z68.43	Body mass index [BMI] 50.0-59.9, adult	22	Morbid Obesity		0.250	0.183	0.383	0.297	0.233	0.204	0.455
Z68.44	Body mass index [BMI] 60.0-69.9, adult	22	Morbid Obesity		0.250	0.183	0.383	0.297	0.233	0.204	0.455
Z68.45	Body mass index [BMI] 70 or greater, adult	22	Morbid Obesity		0.250	0.183	0.383	0.297	0.233	0.204	0.455
Z79.4	Long term (current) use of insulin	19	Diabetes without Complication		0.105	0.124	0.107	0.145	0.087	0.122	0.178
Z89.411	Acquired absence of right great toe	189	Amputation Status, Lower Limb/ Amputation Complications		0.519	0.437	0.795	0.934	0.697	0.626	0.357
Z89.412	Acquired absence of left great toe	189	Amputation Status, Lower Limb/ Amputation Complications		0.519	0.437	0.795	0.934	0.697	0.626	0.357
Z89.419	Acquired absence of unspecified great toe	189	Amputation Status, Lower Limb/ Amputation Complications		0.519	0.437	0.795	0.934	0.697	0.626	0.357
Z89.421	Acquired absence of other right toe(s)	189	Amputation Status, Lower Limb/ Amputation Complications		0.519	0.437	0.795	0.934	0.697	0.626	0.357
Z89.422	Acquired absence of other left toe(s)	189	Amputation Status, Lower Limb/ Amputation Complications		0.519	0.437	0.795	0.934	0.697	0.626	0.357
Z89.429	Acquired absence of other toe(s), unspecified side	189	Amputation Status, Lower Limb/ Amputation Complications		0.519	0.437	0.795	0.934	0.697	0.626	0.357
Z89.431	Acquired absence of right foot	189	Amputation Status, Lower Limb/ Amputation Complications		0.519	0.437	0.795	0.934	0.697	0.626	0.357
Z89.432	Acquired absence of left foot	189	Amputation Status, Lower Limb/ Amputation Complications		0.519	0.437	0.795	0.934	0.697	0.626	0.357
Z89.439	Acquired absence of unspecified foot	189	Amputation Status, Lower Limb/ Amputation Complications		0.519	0.437	0.795	0.934	0.697	0.626	0.357
Z89.441	Acquired absence of right ankle	189	Amputation Status, Lower Limb/ Amputation Complications		0.519	0.437	0.795	0.934	0.697	0.626	0.357
Z89.442	Acquired absence of left ankle	189	Amputation Status, Lower Limb/ Amputation Complications		0.519	0.437	0.795	0.934	0.697	0.626	0.357
Z89.449	Acquired absence of unspecified ankle	189	Amputation Status, Lower Limb/ Amputation Complications		0.519	0.437	0.795	0.934	0.697	0.626	0.357
Z89.511	Acquired absence of right leg below knee	189	Amputation Status, Lower Limb/ Amputation Complications		0.519	0.437	0.795	0.934	0.697	0.626	0.357

ICD-10-CM Code	ICD-10-CM Code Description	V24 CMS-HCC	V24 CMS-HCC Disease Group	V24 CMS-HCC Hierarchies	Community, NonDual, Aged	Community, NonDual, Disabled	Community, FBDual, Aged	Community, FBDual, Disabled	Community, PBDual, Aged	Community, PBDual, Disabled	Institutional
Z89.512	Acquired absence of left leg below knee	189	Amputation Status, Lower Limb/ Amputation Complications		0.519	0.437	0.795	0.934	0.697	0.626	0.357
Z89.519	Acquired absence of unspecified leg below knee	189	Amputation Status, Lower Limb/ Amputation Complications		0.519	0.437	0.795	0.934	0.697	0.626	0.357
Z89.611	Acquired absence of right leg above knee	189	Amputation Status, Lower Limb/ Amputation Complications		0.519	0.437	0.795	0.934	0.697	0.626	0.357
Z89.612	Acquired absence of left leg above knee	189	Amputation Status, Lower Limb/ Amputation Complications		0.519	0.437	0.795	0.934	0.697	0.626	0.357
Z89.619	Acquired absence of unspecified leg above knee	189	Amputation Status, Lower Limb/ Amputation Complications		0.519	0.437	0.795	0.934	0.697	0.626	0.357
Z91.15	Patient's noncompliance with renal dialysis	134	Dialysis Status	135,136, 137,138	0.435	0.406	0.683	0.594	0.446	0.480	0.468
Z93.0	Tracheostomy status	82	Respirator Dependence/Tracheostomy Status	83,84	1.000	0.781	2.183	1.465	0.836	0.769	1.622
Z93.1	Gastrostomy status	188	Artificial Openings for Feeding or Elimination		0.534	0.755	0.742	0.770	0.520	0.732	0.514
Z93.2	Ileostomy status	188	Artificial Openings for Feeding or Elimination		0.534	0.755	0.742	0.770	0.520	0.732	0.514
Z93.3	Colostomy status	188	Artificial Openings for Feeding or Elimination		0.534	0.755	0.742	0.770	0.520	0.732	0.514
Z93.4	Other artificial openings of gastrointestinal tract status	188	Artificial Openings for Feeding or Elimination		0.534	0.755	0.742	0.770	0.520	0.732	0.514
Z93.50	Unspecified cystostomy status	188	Artificial Openings for Feeding or Elimination		0.534	0.755	0.742	0.770	0.520	0.732	0.514
Z93.51	Cutaneous-vesicostomy status	188	Artificial Openings for Feeding or Elimination		0.534	0.755	0.742	0.770	0.520	0.732	0.514
Z93.52	Appendico-vesicostomy status	188	Artificial Openings for Feeding or Elimination		0.534	0.755	0.742	0.770	0.520	0.732	0.514
Z93.59	Other cystostomy status	188	Artificial Openings for Feeding or Elimination		0.534	0.755	0.742	0.770	0.520	0.732	0.514
Z93.6	Other artificial openings of urinary tract status	188	Artificial Openings for Feeding or Elimination		0.534	0.755	0.742	0.770	0.520	0.732	0.514
Z93.8	Other artificial opening status	188	Artificial Openings for Feeding or Elimination		0.534	0.755	0.742	0.770	0.520	0.732	0.514
Z93.9	Artificial opening status, unspecified	188	Artificial Openings for Feeding or Elimination		0.534	0.755	0.742	0.770	0.520	0.732	0.514
Z94.1	Heart transplant status	186	Major Organ Transplant or Replacement Status		0.832	0.445	0.728	0.865	0.438	0.613	1.046
Z94.2	Lung transplant status	186	Major Organ Transplant or Replacement Status		0.832	0.445	0.728	0.865	0.438	0.613	1.046
Z94.3	Heart and lungs transplant status	186	Major Organ Transplant or Replacement Status		0.832	0.445	0.728	0.865	0.438	0.613	1.046
Z94.4	Liver transplant status	186	Major Organ Transplant or Replacement Status		0.832	0.445	0.728	0.865	0.438	0.613	1.046
Z94.81	Bone marrow transplant status	186	Major Organ Transplant or Replacement Status		0.832	0.445	0.728	0.865	0.438	0.613	1.046
Z94.82	Intestine transplant status	186	Major Organ Transplant or Replacement Status		0.832	0.445	0.728	0.865	0.438	0.613	1.046
Z94.83	Pancreas transplant status	186	Major Organ Transplant or Replacement Status		0.832	0.445	0.728	0.865	0.438	0.613	1.046
Z94.84	Stem cells transplant status	186	Major Organ Transplant or Replacement Status		0.832	0.445	0.728	0.865	0.438	0.613	1.046
Z95.811	Presence of heart assist device	186	Major Organ Transplant or Replacement Status		0.832	0.445	0.728	0.865	0.438	0.613	1.046
Z95.812	Presence of fully implantable artificial heart	186	Major Organ Transplant or Replacement Status		0.832	0.445	0.728	0.865	0.438	0.613	1.046

ICD-10-CM Code	ICD-10-CM Code Description	V24 CMS-HCC	V24 CMS-HCC Disease Group	V24 CMS-HCC Hierarchies	Community, NonDual, Aged	Community, NonDual, Disabled	Community, FBDual, Aged	Community, FBDual, Disabled	Community, PBDual, Aged	Community, PBDual, Disabled	Institutional
Z99.11	Dependence on respirator [ventilator] status	82	Respirator Dependence/Tracheostomy Status	83,84	1.000	0.781	2.183	1.465	0.836	0.769	1.622
Z99.12	Encounter for respirator [ventilator] dependence during power failure	82	Respirator Dependence/Tracheostomy Status	83,84	1.000	0.781	2.183	1.465	0.836	0.769	1.622
Z99.2	Dependence on renal dialysis	134	Dialysis Status	135,136, 137,138	0.435	0.406	0.683	0.594	0.446	0.480	0.468

2020/2021/2022 CMS-HCC V24 Model Relative Factors for Continuing Enrollees

Variable	Community, NonDual, Aged	Community, NonDual, Disabled	Community, FBDual, Aged	Community, FBDual, Disabled	Community, PBDual, Aged	Community, PBDual, Disabled	Institutional
Female							
0-34 Years	—	0.241	—	0.349	—	0.383	0.902
35-44 Years	—	0.315	—	0.349	—	0.414	1.105
45-54 Years	—	0.348	—	0.374	—	0.418	1.043
55-59 Years	—	0.379	—	0.434	—	0.414	1.065
60-64 Years	—	0.428	—	0.490	—	0.412	1.067
65-69 Years	0.323	—	0.441	—	0.359	—	1.245
70-74 Years	0.386	—	0.519	—	0.406	—	1.150
75-79 Years	0.451	—	0.593	—	0.476	—	1.014
80-84 Years	0.528	—	0.716	—	0.550	—	0.882
85-89 Years	0.641	—	0.865	—	0.653	—	0.798
90-94 Years	0.783	—	0.987	—	0.783	—	0.668
95 Years or Over	0.787	—	1.041	—	0.873	—	0.501
Male							
0-34 Years	—	0.156	—	0.240	—	0.389	1.101
35-44 Years	—	0.199	—	0.235	—	0.282	1.002
45-54 Years	—	0.241	—	0.307	—	0.313	0.965
55-59 Years	—	0.287	—	0.402	—	0.340	1.017
60-64 Years	—	0.330	—	0.526	—	0.373	1.061
65-69 Years	0.308	—	0.494	—	0.370	—	1.288
70-74 Years	0.394	—	0.600	—	0.427	—	1.329
75-79 Years	0.473	—	0.710	—	0.500	—	1.317
80-84 Years	0.556	—	0.803	—	0.544	—	1.207
85-89 Years	0.686	—	1.000	—	0.659	—	1.122
90-94 Years	0.841	—	1.142	—	0.834	—	0.989
95 Years or Over	0.986	—	1.267	—	1.047	—	0.821

Medicaid and Originally Disabled Interactions

Variable	Community, NonDual, Aged	Community, NonDual, Disabled	Community, FBDual, Aged	Community, FBDual, Disabled	Community, PBDual, Aged	Community, PBDual, Disabled	Institutional
Medicaid	—	—	—	—	—	—	0.061
Originally Disabled, Female	0.250	—	0.173	—	0.136	—	—
Originally Disabled, Male	0.147	—	0.182	—	0.083	—	—

Disease Interactions

Variable	Description Label	Community, NonDual, Aged	Community, NonDual, Disabled	Community, FBDual, Aged	Community, FBDual, Disabled	Community, PBDual, Aged	Community, PBDual, Disabled	Institutional
HCC47_gCancer	Immune Disorders*Cancer	0.838	0.460	0.853	0.679	0.656	0.601	—
Diabetes_CHF	Congestive Heart Failure* Diabetes	0.121	0.024	0.192	0.043	0.113	—	0.169
CHF_gCopdCF	Congestive Heart Failure* Chronic Obstructive Pulmonary Disease	0.155	0.121	0.230	0.154	0.158	0.141	0.191
HCC85_gRenal_v24	Congestive Heart Failure* Renal	0.156	0.411	0.187	0.461	0.186	0.382	—
gCopdCF_CARD_RESP _FAIL	Cardiorespiratory Failure* Chronic Obstructive Pulmonary Disease	0.363	0.379	0.528	0.455	0.392	0.479	0.414
HCC85_HCC96	Congestive Heart Failure* Specified Heart Arrhythmias	0.085	0.282	0.138	0.361	0.101	0.303	—
gSubstanceUseDisord er_gPsych	Substance Use Disorder* Psychiatric	—	0.138	—	0.191	—	0.201	—
SEPSIS_PRESSURE_UL CER	Sepsis*Pressure Ulcer	—	—	—	—	—	—	0.155
SEPSIS_ARTIF_OPENIN GS	Sepsis*Artificial Openings for Feeding or Elimination	—	—	—	—	—	—	0.474
ART_OPENINGS_PRES SURE_ULCER	Artificial Openings for Feeding or Elimination* Pressure Ulcer	—	—	—	—	—	—	0.359
gCopdCF_ASP_SPEC_ BACT_PNEUM	Chronic Obstructive Pulmonary Disease* Aspiration and Specified Bacterial Pneumonias	—	—	—	—	—	—	0.216
ASP_SPEC_BACT_PNE UM_PRES_ULC	Aspiration and Specified Bacterial Pneumonias* Pressure Ulcer	—	—	—	—	—	—	0.472
SEPSIS_ASP_SPEC_BA CT_PNEUM	Sepsis*Aspiration and Specified Bacterial Pneumonias	—	—	—	—	—	—	0.346
SCHIZOPHRENIA_gCo pdCF	Schizophrenia*Chronic Obstructive Pulmonary Disease	—	—	—	—	—	—	0.417
SCHIZOPHRENIA_CHF	Schizophrenia*Congestive Heart Failure	—	—	—	—	—	—	0.127
SCHIZOPHRENIA_SEIZ URES	Schizophrenia*Seizure Disorders and Convulsions	—	—	—	—	—	—	0.573

Disabled/Disease Interactions

Variable	Description Label	Community, NonDual, Aged	Community, NonDual, Disabled	Community, FBDual, Aged	Community, FBDual, Disabled	Community, PBDual, Aged	Community, PBDual, Disabled	Institutional
DISABLED_HCC85	Disabled, Congestive Heart Failure	—	—	—	—	—	—	0.279
DISABLED_PRESSURE _ULCER	Disabled, Pressure Ulcer	—	—	—	—	—	—	0.544
DISABLED_HCC161	Disabled, Chronic Ulcer of the Skin, Except Pressure Ulcer	—	—	—	—	—	—	0.473
DISABLED_HCC39	Disabled, Bone/Joint Muscle Infections/Necrosis	—	—	—	—	—	—	0.456
DISABLED_HCC77	Disabled, Multiple Sclerosis	—	—	—	—	—	—	0.496
DISABLED_HCC6	Disabled, Opportunistic Infections	—	—	—	—	—	—	0.405

Payment HCC Counts

Variable	Description Label	Community, NonDual, Aged	Community, NonDual, Disabled	Community, FBDual, Aged	Community, FBDual, Disabled	Community, PBDual, Aged	Community, PBDual, Disabled	Institutional
D1	1 payment HCC	—	—	—	—	—	—	—
D2	2 payment HCCs	—	—	—	—	—	—	—
D3	3 payment HCCs	—	—	—	—	—	—	—
D4	4 payment HCCs	0.006	—	—	—	—	—	—
D5	5 payment HCCs	0.042	0.043	—	0.055	0.037	0.083	—
D6	6 payment HCCs	0.077	0.131	0.040	0.167	0.071	0.117	—
D7	7 payment HCCs	0.126	0.201	0.057	0.269	0.080	0.291	—
D8	8 payment HCCs	0.214	0.441	0.095	0.424	0.125	0.452	—
D9	9 payment HCCs	0.258	0.441	0.156	0.549	0.402	0.499	—
D10P	10 or more payment HCCs	0.505	0.897	0.373	1.056	0.548	0.893	—

2020/2021/2022 CMS-HCC V24 Model Relative Factors for Aged and Disabled New Enrollees

Variable	Non-Medicaid & Non-Originally Disabled	Medicaid & Non-Originally Disabled	Non-Medicaid & Originally Disabled	Medicaid & Originally Disabled
Female				
0-34 Years	0.804	0.969	—	—
35-44 Years	0.947	1.202	—	—
45-54 Years	1.016	1.306	—	—
55-59 Years	1.017	1.307	—	—
60-64 Years	1.122	1.408	—	—
65 Years	0.520	0.993	1.122	1.462
66 Years	0.515	0.897	1.174	1.887
67 Years	0.544	0.920	1.174	1.887
68 Years	0.598	0.951	1.174	1.887
69 Years	0.600	0.951	1.174	1.887
70-74 Years	0.690	0.985	1.174	1.887
75-79 Years	0.860	1.134	1.174	1.887
80-84 Years	1.014	1.353	1.174	1.887
85-89 Years	1.293	1.536	1.293	1.887
90-94 Years	1.293	1.701	1.293	1.887
95 Years or Over	1.293	1.701	1.293	1.887
Male				
0-34 Years	0.442	0.734	—	—
35-44 Years	0.657	1.059	—	—
45-54 Years	0.864	1.353	—	—
55-59 Years	0.904	1.418	—	—
60-64 Years	0.921	1.551	—	—
65 Years	0.518	1.144	0.921	1.811
66 Years	0.533	1.094	1.071	2.199
67 Years	0.582	1.151	1.123	2.199
68 Years	0.626	1.202	1.123	2.199
69 Years	0.690	1.202	1.320	2.199
70-74 Years	0.786	1.298	1.408	2.199
75-79 Years	1.060	1.407	1.408	2.199
80-84 Years	1.247	1.555	1.408	2.199
85-89 Years	1.498	1.777	1.498	2.199
90-94 Years	1.498	1.777	1.498	2.199
95 Years or Over	1.498	1.777	1.498	2.199

2020/2021/2022 CMS-HCC V24 Model Relative Factors for New Enrollees in Chronic Condition Special Needs Plans (C-SNPs)

	Non-Medicaid & Non-Originally Disabled	Medicaid & Non-Originally Disabled	Non-Medicaid & Originally Disabled	Medicaid & Originally Disabled
Female				
0-34 Years	1.513	1.776	—	—
35-44 Years	1.513	1.776	—	—
45-54 Years	1.513	2.010	—	—
55-59 Years	1.619	2.095	—	—
60-64 Years	1.686	2.126	—	—
65 Years	0.999	1.375	1.810	2.183
66 Years	0.999	1.375	1.810	2.209
67 Years	1.070	1.483	1.834	2.213
68 Years	1.108	1.559	1.834	2.248
69 Years	1.164	1.576	1.834	2.336
70-74 Years	1.310	1.789	2.006	2.424
75-79 Years	1.516	1.980	2.112	2.562
80-84 Years	1.746	2.194	2.476	2.772
85-89 Years	1.971	2.490	2.476	2.772
90-94 Years	2.161	2.680	2.476	2.772
95 Years or Over	2.161	2.680	2.476	2.772
Male				
0-34 Years	1.276	1.533	—	—
35-44 Years	1.276	1.533	—	—
45-54 Years	1.498	1.854	—	—
55-59 Years	1.630	2.041	—	—
60-64 Years	1.673	2.167	—	—
65 Years	0.980	1.525	1.664	2.173
66 Years	0.980	1.525	1.667	2.173
67 Years	1.020	1.646	1.725	2.179
68 Years	1.082	1.646	1.740	2.179
69 Years	1.140	1.646	1.797	2.179
70-74 Years	1.345	1.967	1.935	2.419
75-79 Years	1.581	2.140	2.073	2.509
80-84 Years	1.832	2.272	2.349	2.805
85-89 Years	2.095	2.630	2.349	2.805
90-94 Years	2.351	2.630	2.349	2.805
95 Years or Over	2.351	2.630	2.349	2.805